Group	Brand name	%	Generic name	Tube size (gm; unless noted)
IV	Halog cream	0.025	Halcinonide	15, 60, 240
	Halog ointment	0.025		15, 60, 240
	Kenalog ointment	0.1	Triamcinolone acetonide	15, 60, 80, 240, 2520
	Synalar ointment	0.025	Fluocinolone acetonide	15, 30, 60, 120, 425
	Synalar-HP cream	0.2		12
	Trymex ointment	0.1	Triamcinolone acetonide	15, 80
	Westcort ointment	0.2	Hydrocortisone	15, 45, 60
V	Aristocort cream	0.1	Triamcinolone acetonide	15, 60, 240, 2520
	Benisone cream	0.025	Betamethasone benzoate	15, 60
	Beta-Val cream	0.1	Betamethasone valerate	15, 45
	Betatrex cream	0.1	Betamethasone valerate	15, 45
	Betatrex lotion	0.1		15, 60 ml
	Cloderm cream	0.1	Clocortolone pivalate	15, 45
	Cordran cream	0.05	Flurandrenolide	15, 30, 60
	Cordran lotion	0.5		15, 60 ml
	Cordran ointment	0.025		30, 60
	Cutivate cream	0.05	Fluticasone propionate	15, 30, 60
	Dermatop cream	0.1	Prednicarbate	15, 60
	DesOwen ointment	0.05	Desonide	15, 60
	Fluonide cream	0.025	Fluocinolone acetonide	15, 60
	Kenalog cream	0.1	Triamcinolone acetonide	15, 60, 80, 240, 2520
	Kenalog lotion	0.1		15, 60 ml
	Kenalog ointment	0.025		15, 60, 80, 240
	Locoid cream	0.1	Hydrocortisone butyrate	15, 45
	Locoid ointment	0.1		15, 45
	Locoid solution			20, 60 cc
	Synalar cream	0.025	Fluocinolone acetonide	15, 30, 60, 425
	Synemol cream	0.025	Fluocinolone acetonide	15, 30, 60
	Tridesilon ointment	0.05	Desonide	15, 60
	Trymex cream	0.1	Triamcinolone acetonide	15, 80, 480
	Trymex ointment	0.025		15, 80
	Uticort cream	0.025	Betamethasone benzoate	15, 60
	Uticort lotion	0.025		15, 60 ml
	Valisone cream	0.1	Betamethasone valerate	15, 45, 110, 430
	Valisone lotion	0.1		20, 60 ml
	Westcort cream	0.2	Hydrocortisone	15, 45, 60
VI	Aclovate cream	0.05	Prednicarbate	15, 60
	Aclovate ointment	0.05	Prednicarbate	15, 60
	Aristocort cream	0.025	Triamcinolone acetonide	15, 60, 240, 2520
	DesOwen cream	0.05	Desonide	15, 60, 90
	DesOwen ointment			15, 60
	DesOwen lotion			2, 4 oz
	Fluonid cream	0.01	Fluocinolone acetonide	15, 60
	Fluonid solution	0.01		20, 60 ml
	Kenalog cream	0.025	Triamcinolone acetonide	15, 60, 80, 240, 2520
	Kenalog lotion	0.025		60 ml
	Locorten cream	0.03	Flumethasone pivalate	15, 60
	Synalar cream	0.01	Fluocinolone acetonide	15, 45, 60, 425
	Synalar solution	0.01		20, 60 ml
	Tridesilon cream	0.05	Desonide	15, 60
	Trymex cream	0.025	Triamcinolone acetonide	15, 80, 480
	Valisone cream	0.01	Betamethasone valerate	15, 60
VII	Celestone cream	0.2	Betamethasone valerate	15
	Decaderm gel	0.1	Dexamethasone	15, 30
	Epifoam	1.0	Hydrocortisone acetate	10
	Hytone cream	1.0	Hydrocortisone	1
		2.5		1, 2 oz
	Hytone lotion	1.0		4 oz
		2.5		2 oz
	Hytone ointment	1.0		1
		2.5		1 oz
	Lacticare HC lotion	1.0	Hydrocortisone	4 oz
		2.5		2 oz
	Medrol cream	0.25	Methylprednisolone	7.5, 30, 45
	Oxylone cream	0.025	Fluoromethalone	15, 60, 120
	Synacort cream	1.0	Hydrocortisone	15, 30, 60
		2.5		30

CLINICAL DERMATOLOGY

A Color Guide to Diagnosis and Therapy

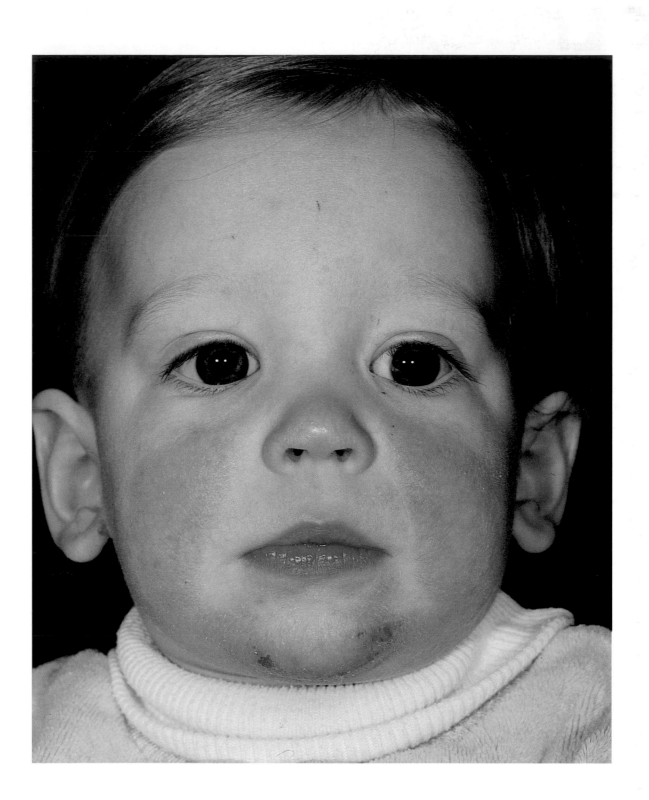

CLINICAL DERMATOLOGY

A Color Guide to Diagnosis and Therapy

THOMAS P. HABIF, M.D.

Adjunct Professor of Medicine (Dermatology),
Dartmouth Medical School,
Hanover, New Hampshire

Publisher: Anne S. Patterson
Editor: Susie Baxter
Developmental Editor: Anne Gunter
Project Manager: John Rogers
Production Editor: Lavon Wirch Peters
Manuscript Editor: Patricia Clewell
Design Coordinator: Renée Duenow
Manufacturing Manager: Theresa Fuchs
Electronic Production Coordinators: Peggy Hill, Chris Robinson
Layout Design: Jeanne Genz
Proofreaders: Jean Babrick, Katherine Aiken
Illustrator: Jeanne Robertson

Project Organization: Laura A. McCann
Technical Advice: David V. Habif, Jr., M.D.
Librarian: Darryl Hamson, Portsmouth Regional Hospital
Digital Color Scanning: Aurora Graphics, Portsmouth, NH
  Project Coordination: Norman E. O'Neil and William P. James
  Color Manager: Christopher R. Donovan
Photographs: Barry M. Austin, M.D., Richard D. Baughman, M.D., Alan N. Binnick, M.D.,
  William E. Clendenning, M.D., Daniel W. Collison, M.D., Robert L. Dimond, M.D., Thomas Hokanson, P.A.,
  Warren M. Pringle, M.D., Cameron L. Smith, M.D., and Steven K. Spencer, M.D.
Moral Support: Dorothy, Tommy, and David

THIRD EDITION
with over 1000 *illustrations*

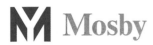

A *Harcourt Health Sciences Company*
Dedicated to Publishing Excellence

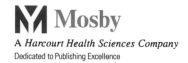

A *Harcourt Health Sciences Company*
Dedicated to Publishing Excellence

Printed in the United States of America

Mosby, Inc.
11830 Westline Industrial Drive
St. Louis, Missouri 63146

Library of Congress Cataloging-in-Publication Data

Habif, Thomas P.
    Clinical dermatology: a color guide to diagnosis and therapy /
Thomas P. Habif. — 3rd ed.
        p.   cm.
    Includes bibliographical references and index.
    ISBN 0-8151-4242-0 (hardcover)
    1. Dermatology—Atlases.   I. Title
    [DNLM: 1. Skin Diseases—atlases.   WR 17 H116c 1995]
RL81.H3   1995
616.5' 0022'2—dc20
DNLM/DLC   95-35912

00 01 / 9 8 7 6 5

Preface

This book is written for the practicing physician. I have attempted to combine illustrations with current and comprehensive therapeutic information to create the kind of practical resource a busy practicing physician needs. Bold headings are used extensively to facilitate rapid access to information.

The classic method of organizing skin diseases is used. A discussion of the most up-to-date therapeutic practice follows the description of each disease. Common diseases are covered in depth. Care was taken to include illustrations of classic examples of these disorders and to incorporate photographs of variations seen at different stages. Basic dermatologic surgical techniques are covered in detail. Highly specialized techniques such as Mohs' micrographic surgery and liposuction are described so that the physician can be better prepared to suggest referral.

How to Use This Book

MEDICAL STUDENTS

Medical students should first study the basics of dermatology, which involves learning the primary and secondary lesions and the distribution of diseases in Chapter One and studying the differential diagnosis of each lesion. Select a few familiar diseases from each list and read about them. Study the close-up pictures carefully. Obtain an overview of the text. Turn the pages, look at the pictures, and read the captions.

You examine or are shown patients every day in clinical rotations. Almost every patient has some skin abnormality. Try to identify these diseases, or ask for assistance. Make a habit of studying all diseases, especially tumors, with a magnifying glass or ocular lens. Make a list of what you see and what you read about those entities each night. You will rapidly gain a broad fund of knowledge.

INTERNS AND RESIDENTS

Interns and residents can follow the same system as medical students to build a fund of knowledge. Study thoroughly Chapters Twenty (Benign Skin Tumors), Twenty-one (Premalignant and Malignant Nonmelanoma Skin Tumors), and Twenty-two (Nevi and Malignant Melanoma). Skin growths are common, and it is important to recognize their features.

House officers are responsible for patient management. Read Chapter Two carefully, and study all aspects of the use of topical steroids. These valuable agents are used to treat a great variety of inflammatory skin conditions. It is tempting to use these agents as a therapeutic trial and ask for a consultation only if therapy fails. Topical steroids mask some diseases, make some diseases worse, and create other diseases. Do not develop bad habits; if you do not know what a disease is, do not treat it.

The diagnosis of skin disease is deceptively easy. Do not make hasty diagnoses. Take a history, study primary lesions and the distribution, and be deliberate and methodical. Ask for help. With time and experience you will feel comfortable managing many common skin diseases.

THE PRACTICING PHYSICIAN

Most skin diseases in the United States are treated by physicians other than dermatologists. The training that practicing physicians have varies with the medical school that they attended. With this in mind, read the above guidelines for using this book and plan an appropriate course. Learn a few topical steroids in each potency group. There are a great number of agents in the Formulary. Many in each table contain similar ingredients and have the same therapeutic effect. Develop an armamentarium of agents and gain experience in their use.

Inflammatory conditions are often confusing, and sometimes biopsies are of limited value in their diagnosis. The clinical diagnosis of pigmented lesions is complicated. Punch biopsies make scars. A dermatologist can often make a specific diagnosis without the need for a biopsy.

THE DERMATOLOGIST

The dermatologist's experience and fund of knowledge is great enough so that an illustrated text is not as critical. The pictures can be useful as an aid to reassure patients. Examine the patient, make a diagnosis, and then show them an illustration of their disease. Many patients see the similarity and are reassured.

This is not meant to be a textbook but rather a practical manual. All of the most current descriptive and therapeutic information that is practical and relevant for the clinician has been included. All topics are researched on MEDLINE. Details about basic science and complex mechanisms of disease can be found elsewhere.

Photography

The photographs were taken specifically for this project with large-format cameras and 35-mm macrocameras. Large negatives require little enlargement and thus preserve maximum detail and full color saturation. The "point source" lighting technique was used to minimize glare and enhance detail. The macrocamera takes pictures that simulate the view through a hand lens. Therefore the distribution of the disease and the primary lesion can be accurately illustrated.

Illustrations

The illustrations were all digitized for this edition. Digital photographic files are dynamic. They can be color-balanced and infinitely manipulated in size to produce clear, accurate images. The pictures were scanned and printed at a very high resolution (175 line screen).

Thomas P. Habif

Contents

CLINICAL DERMATOLOGY

A Color Guide to Diagnosis and Therapy

CHAPTER ONE

Principles of Diagnosis and Anatomy

Diagnosis of Skin Disease

What could be easier than the diagnosis of skin disease? The pathology is before your eyes! Why then do nondermatologists have such difficulty interpreting what they see?

There are three reasons. First, there are literally hundreds of cutaneous diseases. Second, a single entity can vary in its appearance. A common seborrheic keratosis, for example, may have a smooth, rough, or eroded surface and a border that is either uniform or as irregular as a melanoma. Third, skin diseases are dynamic and change in morphology. Many diseases undergo an evolutionary process: herpes simplex may begin as a red papule, evolve into a blister, and then become an erosion that heals with scarring. If hundreds of entities can individually vary in appearance and evolve through several stages, then it is necessary to recognize thousands of permutations to diagnose cutaneous entities confidently. What at first glance appeared to be simple to diagnose may later appear to be simply impossible.

Dermatology is a morphologically oriented specialty. As in other specialties the medical history is important; however, the ability to interpret what is observed is even more important. The diagnosis of skin disease must be approached in an orderly and logical manner. The temptation to make rapid judgments after hasty observation must be controlled.

A METHODICAL APPROACH

The recommended approach to the patient with skin disease is as follows:

History. Obtain a brief history, noting duration, rate of onset, location, symptoms, family history, allergies, occupation, and previous treatment.

Distribution. Determine the extent of the eruption by having the patient disrobe completely.

Primary lesion. Determine the primary lesion. Examine the lesions carefully; a hand lens is a valuable aid for studying skin lesions. Determine the nature of any secondary or special lesions.

Differential diagnosis. Formulate a differential diagnosis.

Tests. Obtain a biopsy and perform laboratory tests, such as skin biopsy, potassium hydroxide examination for fungi, skin scrapings for scabies, Gram stain, fungal and bacterial cultures, cytology (Tzanck test), Wood's light examination, patch tests, dark field examination, and blood tests.

EXAMINATION TECHNIQUE

Distribution. The skin should be examined methodically. An eye scan over wide areas is inefficient. It is most productive to mentally divide the skin surface into several sections and carefully study each section. For example, when studying the face, examine the area around each eye, the nose, the mouth, the cheeks, and the temples.

During an examination, patients may show small areas of their skin, tell the doctor that the rest of the eruption looks the same, and expect an immediate diagnosis. The rest of the eruption may or may not look the same. Patients with rashes should receive a complete skin examination to determine the distribution and confirm the diagnosis. Decisions about quantities of medication to dispense require visualization of the big picture. Many dermatologists now advocate a complete skin examination for all their patients. Because of an awareness that some patients are uncomfortable undressing completely when they have a specific request such as treatment of a plantar wart, other dermatologists advocate a case-by-case approach.

Primary lesions and surface characteristics. Lesions should be examined carefully. Standing back and viewing a disease process provides valuable information about the distribution. Close examination with a magnifying device provides much more information. Often the primary lesion is identified and the diagnosis is confirmed at this step. The physician should learn the surface characteristics of all the common entities and gain experience by examining known entities. A flesh-colored papule might be a wart, sebaceous hyperplasia, or a basal cell carcinoma. The surface characteristics of many lesions are illustrated throughout this book.

APPROACH TO TREATMENT

Most skin diseases can be managed successfully with the numerous agents and techniques available. If a diagnosis has not been established, medications should not be prescribed; this applies particularly to prescription of topical steroids. Some physicians are tempted to experiment with various medications and, if the treatment fails, to refer the patient to a specialist. This is not a logical or efficient way to practice medicine.

PRIMARY LESIONS

Most skin diseases begin with a basic lesion that is referred to as a *primary lesion*. Identification of the primary lesion is the key to accurate interpretation and description of cutaneous disease. Its presence provides the initial orientation and allows the formulation of a differential diagnosis. Definitions of the primary lesions and their differential diagnoses are listed and illustrated on pp. 3 to 11.

SECONDARY LESIONS

Secondary lesions develop during the evolutionary process of skin disease or are created by scratching or infection. They may be the only type of lesion present, in which case the primary disease process must be inferred. The differential diagnoses of secondary lesions are listed and illustrated on pp. 12 to 16.

SPECIAL LESIONS

A certain number of unique structures and changes called *special lesions* occur (p. 17).

Regional Differential Diagnoses

Most skin diseases have preferential areas of involvement. Regional differential diagnosis locations are illustrated on p. 18 and listed on pp. 19 to 22.

PRIMARY SKIN LESIONS—MACULES

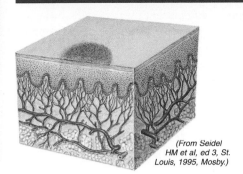

(From Seidel HM et al, ed 3, St. Louis, 1995, Mosby.)

MACULE

A circumscribed, flat discoloration that may be brown, blue, red, or hypopigmented

Brown
Becker's nevus (p. 694)
Café-au-lait spot (p. 793)
Erythrasma (p. 373)
Fixed drug eruption (p. 439)
Freckle (p. 622)
Junction nevus (p. 690)
Lentigo (p. 622)
Lentigo maligna (p. 707)
Melasma (p. 622)
Photoallergic drug eruption (p. 614)
Phototoxic drug eruption (p. 614)
Stasis dermatitis (p. 74)
Tinea nigra palmaris

Blue
Ink (tatoo)
Maculae ceruleae (lice) (p. 455)
Mongolian spot
Ochronosis

Red
Drug eruptions (p. 435)
Juvenile rheumatoid arthritis
   (Still's disease)
Rheumatic fever
Secondary syphilis (p. 283)
Viral exanthems (p. 424)

Hypopigmented
Idiopathic guttate hypomelanosis (p. 620)
Nevus anemicus (p. 621)
Piebaldism
Postinflammatory psoriasis (p. 202)
Radiation dermatitis
Tinea versicolor (p. 402)
Tuberous sclerosis (p. 797)
Vitiligo (p. 616)

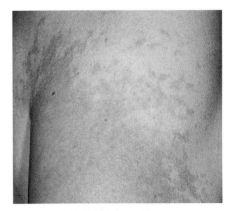

Becker's nevus

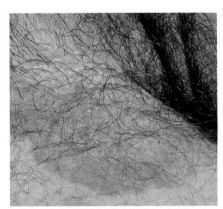

Erythrasma

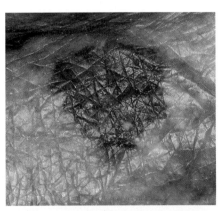

Lentigo

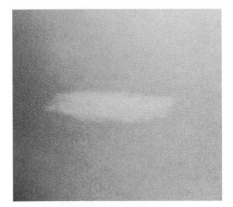

Tuberous sclerosis

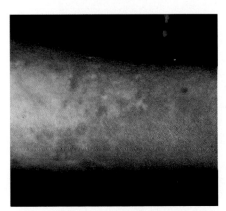

Phototoxic drug eruption

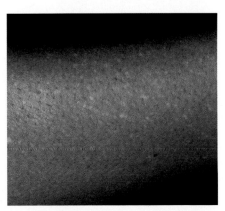

Idiopathic guttate hypomelanosis

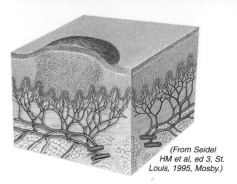

(From Seidel HM et al, ed 3, St. Louis, 1995, Mosby.)

PAPULE

An elevated solid lesion up to 0.5 cm in diameter; color varies; papules may become confluent and form plaques

Flesh colored, yellow, or white
Achrochordon (skin tag) (p. 635)
Adenoma sebaceum (p. 798)
Basal cell epithelioma (p. 649)
Closed comedone (acne) (p. 170)
Flat warts (p. 328)
Granuloma annulare (p. 786)
Lichen nitidus
Lichen sclerosis et atrophicus (p. 228)
Milium (p. 179)
Molluscum contagiosum (p. 30)
Nevi (dermal) (p. 690)
Neurofibroma (p. 794)
Pearly penile papules (p. 297)
Pseudoxanthoma elasticum (p. 803)
Sebaceous hyperplasia (p. 646)
Skin tags (p. 635)
Syringoma (p. 647)

Brown
Dermatofibroma (p. 636)
Keratosis follicularis
Melanoma (p. 699)
Nevi (p. 688)
Seborrheic keratosis (p. 627)
Urticaria pigmentosa (p. 144)
Warts (p. 325)

Red
Acne (p. 148)
Atopic dermatitis (p. 100)
Cat-scratch disease (p. 476)
Cherry angioma (p. 730)
Cholinergic urticaria (p. 135)
Chondrodermatitis helicis (p. 643)
Eczema (p. 45)
Folliculitis (p. 248)
Insect bites (p. 480)
Keratosis pilaris (p. 112)
Leukocytoclastic vasculitis (p. 579)
Miliaria (p. 186)
Polymorphic light eruption (p. 605)
Psoriasis (p. 190)
Pyogenic granuloma (p. 732)
Scabies (p. 445)
Urticaria (p. 122)

Blue or violaceous
Angiokeratoma (p. 730)
Blue nevus (p. 696)
Lichen planus (p. 221)
Lymphoma (p. 674)
Kaposi's sarcoma (pp. 322, 733)
Melanoma (p. 699)
Mycosis fungoides (p. 674)
Venous lake (p. 731)

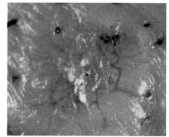

Basal cell epithelioma

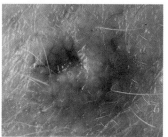

Sebaceous hyperplasia

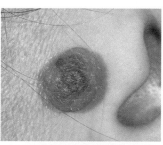

Nevi (dermal)

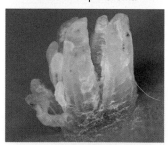

Wart (filiform)

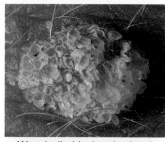

Wart (cylindrical projections)

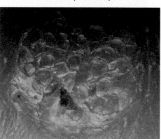

Wart (mosaic surface)

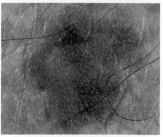

Seborrheic keratosis

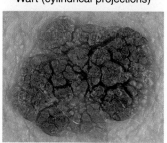

Seborrheic keratosis

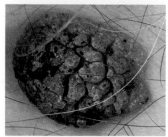

Seborrheic keratosis

PRIMARY SKIN LESIONS—PAPULES

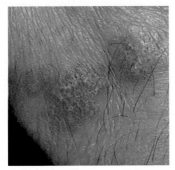

Lichen planus

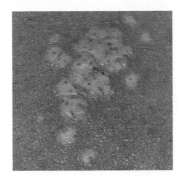

Lichen sclerosis et atrophicus

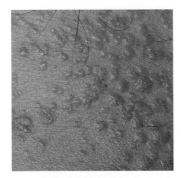

Melanoma

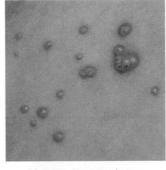

Granuloma annulare

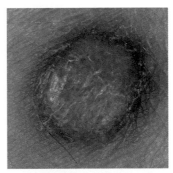

Dermatofibroma

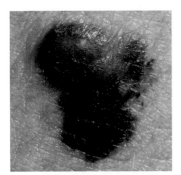

Flat warts

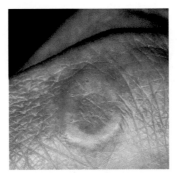

Molluscum contagiosum

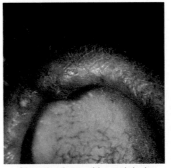

Chondrodermatitis nodularis
chronica helicis

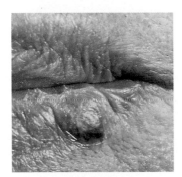

Venous lake

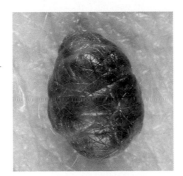

Cherry angioma

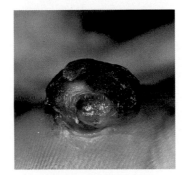

Pyogenic granuloma

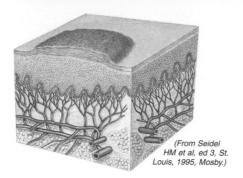

(From Seidel HM et al, ed 3, St. Louis, 1995, Mosby.)

PLAQUE

A circumscribed, elevated, superficial, solid lesion more than 0.5 cm in diameter, often formed by the confluence of papules

Eczema (p. 45)
Cutaneous T-cell lymphoma (p. 674)
Paget's disease (p. 679)
Sweet's syndrome (p. 589)
Papulosquamous (papular and scaling) lesions (p. 190)
Discoid lupus erythematosus (p. 540)
Lichen planus (p. 221)
Pityriasis rosea (p. 218)
Psoriasis (p. 190)
Seborrheic dermatitis (p. 214)
Syphilis (secondary) (p. 283)
Tinea corporis (p. 374)
Tinea versicolor (p. 402)

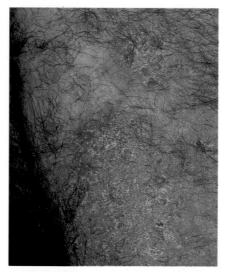

Eczema

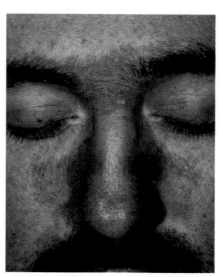

Seborrheic dermatitis

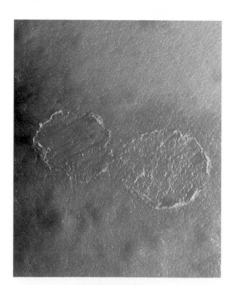

Pityriasis rosea

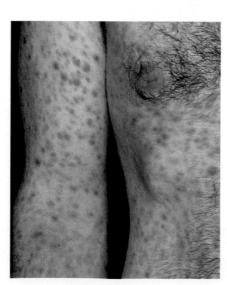

Syphilis (secondary)

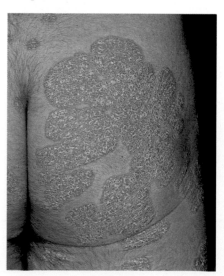

Psoriasis

PRIMARY SKIN LESIONS—PLAQUES

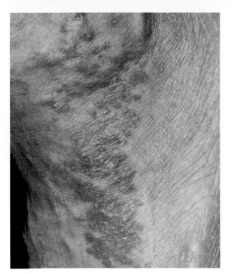

Lichen planus

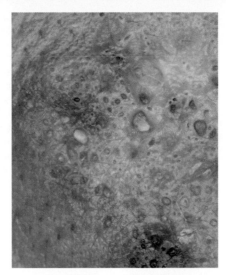

Discoid lupus erythematosus

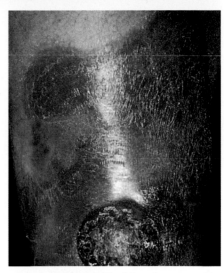

Cutaneous T-cell lymphoma

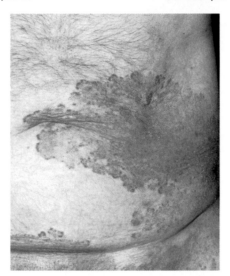

Tinea corporis

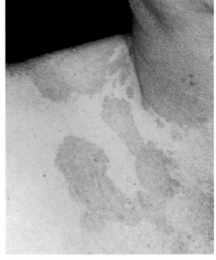

Tinea versicolor

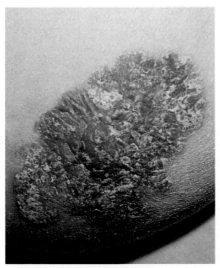

Paget's disease

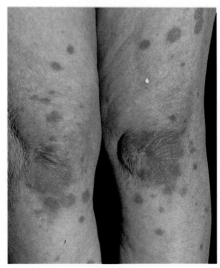

Sweet's syndrome

PRIMARY SKIN LESIONS—NODULES

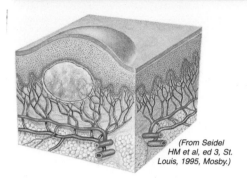

(From Seidel HM et al, ed 3, St. Louis, 1995, Mosby.)

NODULE

A circumscribed, elevated, solid lesion more than 0.5 cm in diameter; a large nodule is referred to as a *tumor*

Basal cell carcinoma (p. 649)
Erythema nodosum (p. 575)
Furuncle (p. 252)
Hemangioma (p. 722)
Kaposi's sarcoma (pp. 322, 733)
Keratoacanthoma (p. 638)
Lipoma
Lymphoma (p. 674)
Melanoma (p. 699)

Metastatic carcinoma (p. 681)
Cutaneous T-cell lymphoma (p. 674)
Neurofibromatosis (p. 793)
Prurigo nodularis (p. 72)
Sporotrichosis
Squamous cell carcinoma (p. 666)
Warts (p. 325)
Xanthoma (p. 790)

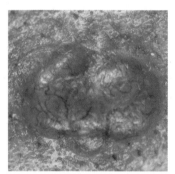

Basal cell carcinoma

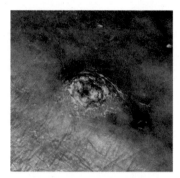

Squamous cell carcinoma

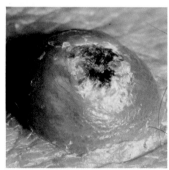

Keratoacanthoma

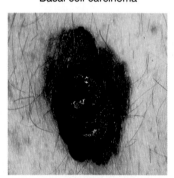

Melanoma

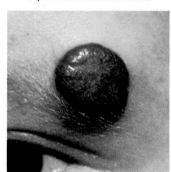

Hemangioma

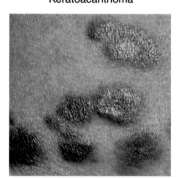

Kaposi's sarcoma

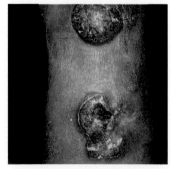

Cutaneous T-cell lymphoma

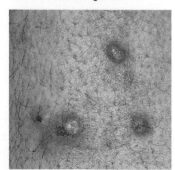

Prurigo nodularis

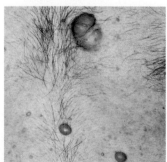

Neurofibromatosis

PRIMARY SKIN LESIONS—PUSTULES

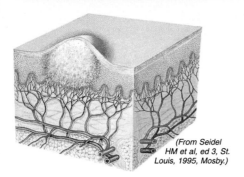

(From Seidel HM et al, ed 3, St. Louis, 1995, Mosby.)

PUSTULE
A circumscribed collection of leukocytes and free fluid that varies in size

Acne (p. 148)
Candidiasis (p. 391)
Chicken pox (p. 345)
Dermatophyte infection (p. 362)
Dyshidrosis (p. 63)
Folliculitis (p. 248)
Gonococcemia (p. 277)
Hidradenitis suppurativa (p. 184)
Herpes simplex (p. 337)
Herpes zoster (p. 351)
Impetigo (p. 236)
Keratosis pilaris (p. 112)
Pseudomonas folliculitis (p. 258)
Psoriasis (p. 190)
Pyoderma gangrenosum (p. 591)
Rosacea (p. 182)
Scabies (p. 445)
Varicella (p. 345)

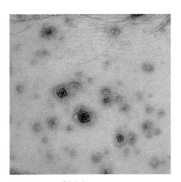

Chicken pox

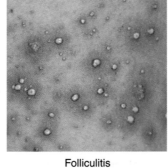

Folliculitis

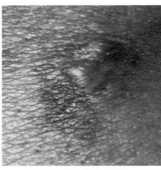

Gonococcemia

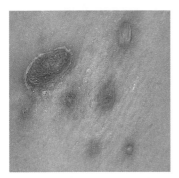

Impetigo

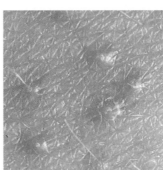

Keratosis pilaris

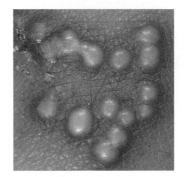

Herpes simplex

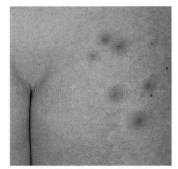

Pseudomonas folliculitis

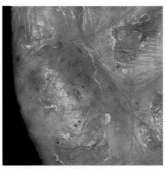

Dyshidrosis

PRIMARY SKIN LESIONS—VESICLES AND BULLAE

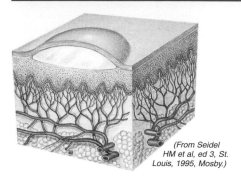

(From Seidel HM et al, ed 3, St. Louis, 1995, Mosby.)

VESICLE
A circumscribed collection of free fluid up to 0.5 cm in diameter

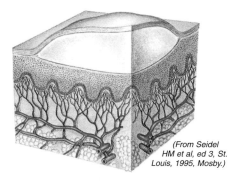

(From Seidel HM et al, ed 3, St. Louis, 1995, Mosby.)

BULLA
A circumscribed collection of free fluid more than 0.5 cm in diameter

Vesicles
Benign familial chronic pemphigus (p. 521)
Cat-scratch disease (p. 476)
Chicken pox (p. 345)
Dermatitis herpetiformis (p. 506)
Eczema (acute) (p. 45)
Erythema multiforme (p. 566)
Herpes simplex (p. 337)
Herpes zoster (p. 351)
Impetigo (p. 236)
Lichen planus (p. 222)
Pemphigus foliaceus (p. 510)
Porphyria cutania tarda (p. 609)
Scabies (p. 445)

Bullae
Bullae in diabetics (p. 508)
Bullous pemphigoid (p. 514)
Cicatricial pemphigoid (p. 516)
Epidermolysis bullosa acquisita (p. 519)
Fixed drug eruption (p. 439)
Herpes gestationis (p. 518)
Lupus erythematosus
Pemphigus (p. 508)

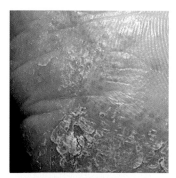

Eczema (acute)

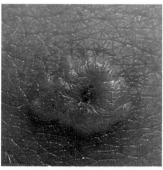

Chicken pox

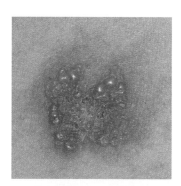

Dermatitis herpetiformis

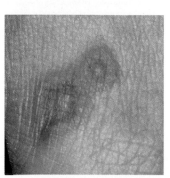

Erythema multiforme

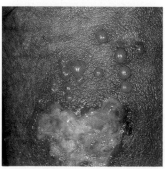

Herpes simplex

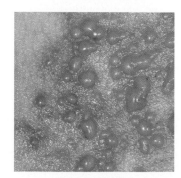

Herpes zoster

PRIMARY SKIN LESIONS—WHEALS (HIVES)

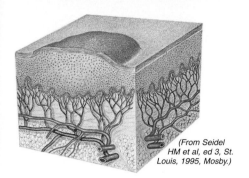

(From Seidel HM et al, ed 3, St. Louis, 1995, Mosby.)

WHEAL (HIVE)
A firm edematous plaque resulting from infiltration of the dermis with fluid; wheals are transient and may last only a few hours

Angioedema (p. 138)
Dermographism (p. 134)
Hives (p. 122)
Cholinergic urticaria (p. 135)
Urticaria pigmentosa (mastocytosis) (p. 144)

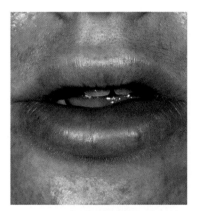

Angioedema

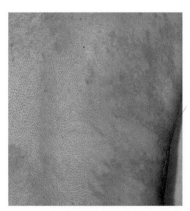

Angioedema

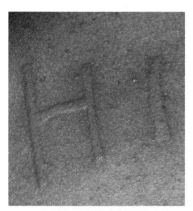

Dermographism

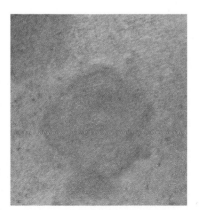

Hives

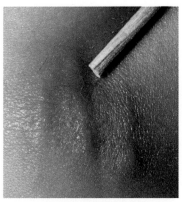

Urticaria pigmentosa

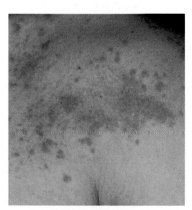

Cholinergic urticaria

SECONDARY SKIN LESIONS—SCALES

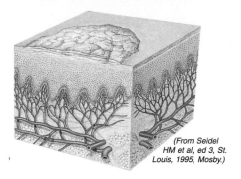

(From Seidel HM et al, ed 3, St. Louis, 1995, Mosby.)

SCALES
Excess dead epidermal cells that are produced by abnormal keratinization and shedding

Fine to stratified
Erythema craquele (p. 64)
Ichthyosis—dominant (quadrangular) (p. 111)
Ichthyosis—sex-linked (quadrangular) (p. 111)
Lupus erythematosus (carpet tack) (p. 540)
Pityriasis rosea (collarette) (p. 218)
Psoriasis (silvery) (p. 191)
Scarlet fever (fine, on trunk) (p. 414)
Seborrheic dermatitis (p. 214)
Syphilis (secondary) (p. 283)
Tinea (dermatophytes) (p. 366)
Tinea versicolor (p. 402)
Xerosis (dry skin) (p. 25)

Scaling in sheets (desquamation)
Kawasaki syndrome (p. 425)
Scarlet fever (hands and feet) (p. 414)
Staphylococcal scalded skin syndrome (p. 256)
Toxic shock syndrome (p. 431)

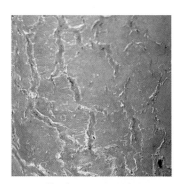

Erythema craquele
(dense scale)

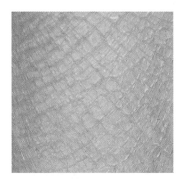

Ichthyosis—dominant
(quadrangular)

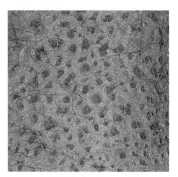

Ichthyosis—sex-linked
(quadrangular)

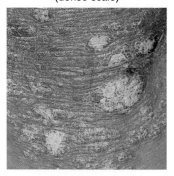

Psoriasis (silvery)

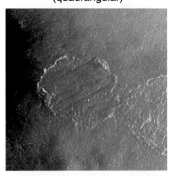

Pityriasis rosea (collarette)

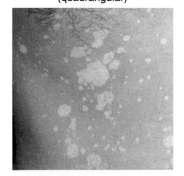

Tinea versicolor (fine)

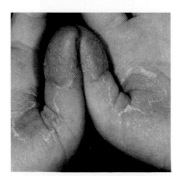

Scarlet fever (desquamation)

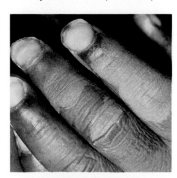

Kawasaki syndrome
(desquamation)

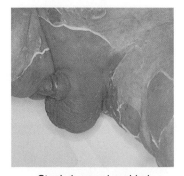

Staphylococcal scalded
skin syndrome (desquamation)

SECONDARY SKIN LESIONS—CRUSTS

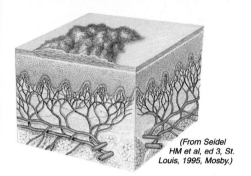

(From Seidel HM et al, ed 3, St. Louis, 1995, Mosby.)

CRUST
A collection of dried serum and cellular debris; a scab

Acute eczematous inflammation (p. 46)
Atopic (face) (p. 105)
Impetigo (honey colored) (p. 240)
Pemphigus foliaceus (p. 510)
Tinea capitis (p. 383)

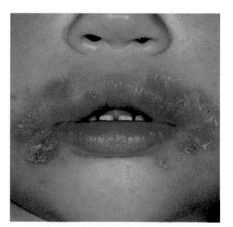

Atopic (lips)

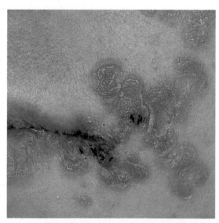

Impetigo (honey colored)

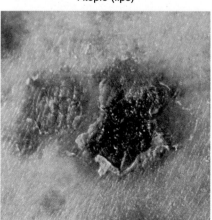

Pemphigus foliaceus

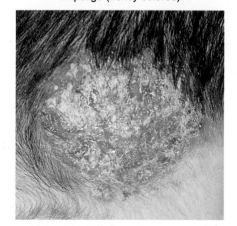

Tinea capitis

SECONDARY SKIN LESIONS—EROSIONS AND ULCERS

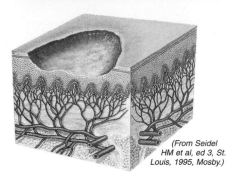

(From Seidel HM et al, ed 3, St. Louis, 1995, Mosby.)

EROSION

A focal loss of epidermis; erosions do not penetrate below the dermo-epidermal junction and therefore heal without scarring

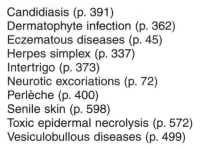

Candidiasis (p. 391)
Dermatophyte infection (p. 362)
Eczematous diseases (p. 45)
Herpes simplex (p. 337)
Intertrigo (p. 373)
Neurotic excoriations (p. 72)
Perlèche (p. 400)
Senile skin (p. 598)
Toxic epidermal necrolysis (p. 572)
Vesiculobullous diseases (p. 499)

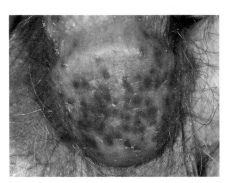

Candidiasis

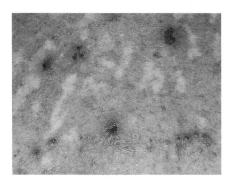

Neurotic excoriations

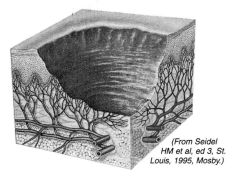

(From Seidel HM et al, ed 3, St. Louis, 1995, Mosby.)

ULCER

A focal loss of epidermis and dermis; ulcers heal with scarring

Aphthae
Chancroid (p. 292)
Decubitus
Factitial (p. 68)
Ischemic
Necrobiosis lipoidica (p. 784)
Neoplasms (p. 649)
Pyoderma gangrenosum (p. 591)
Radiodermatitis
Syphilis (chancre) (p. 280)
Stasis ulcers (p. 75)

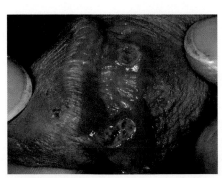

Chancroid

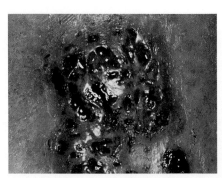

Pyoderma gangrenosum

SECONDARY SKIN LESIONS—FISSURES AND ATROPHY

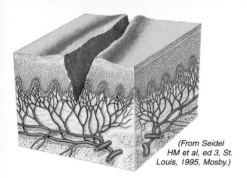

(From Seidel HM et al, ed 3, St. Louis, 1995, Mosby.)

Chapping (hands, feet) (p. 66)
Eczema (fingertip) (p. 61)
Intertrigo (p. 373)
Perlèche (p. 400)

FISSURE
A linear loss of epidermis and dermis with sharply defined, nearly vertical walls

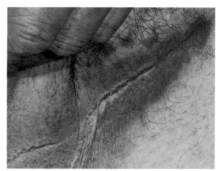

Intertrigo

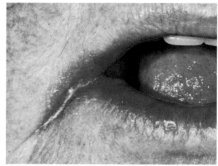

Perlèche

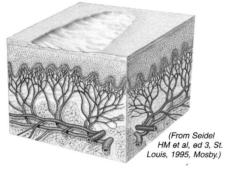

(From Seidel HM et al, ed 3, St. Louis, 1995, Mosby.)

Aging (p. 598)
Dermatomyositis (p. 549)
Discoid lupus erythematosus (p. 540)
Lichen sclerosis et atrophicus (p. 228)
Morphea (p. 560)
Necrobiosis lipoidica diabeticorum (p. 784)
Radiodermatitis
Striae (p. 40)
Topical and intralesional steroids (p. 40)

ATROPHY
A depression in the skin resulting from thinning of the epidermis or dermis

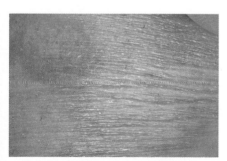

Lichen sclerosis et atrophicus

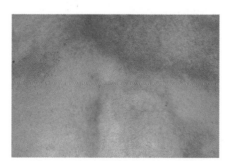

Morphea

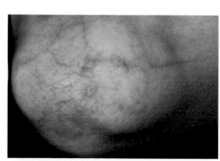

Topical and intralesional steroids

SECONDARY SKIN LESIONS—SCARS

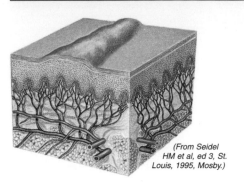

(From Seidel HM et al, ed 3, St. Louis, 1995, Mosby.)

SCAR
An abnormal formation of connective tissue implying dermal damage; after injury or surgery scars are initially thick and pink but with time become white and atrophic

Acne (p. 148)
Burns
Herpes zoster (p. 351)
Hidradenitis suppurativa (p. 184)
Keloid (p. 637)
Porphyria (p. 608)
Varicella (p. 345)

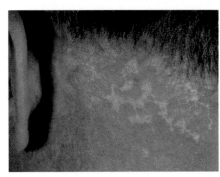

Herpes zoster

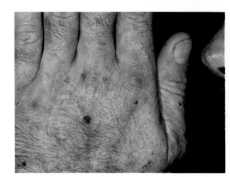

Porphyria

SPECIAL SKIN LESIONS	
Description	**Differential diagnosis**

EXCORIATION

An erosion caused by scratching; excoriations are often linear — —

COMEDONE

A plug of sebaceous and keratinous material lodged in the opening of a hair follicle; the follicular orifice may be dilated (blackhead) or narrowed (whitehead or closed comedone) — —

MILIA

A small, superficial keratin cyst with no visible opening — —

CYST

A circumscribed lesion with a wall and a lumen; the lumen may contain fluid or solid matter — —

BURROW

A narrow, elevated, tortuous channel produced by a parasite — —

LICHENIFICATION

An area of thickened epidermis induced by scratching; the skin lines are accentuated so that the surface looks like a washboard — —

TELANGIECTASIA

Dilated superficial blood vessels

Actinically damaged skin (p. 598)
Adenoma sebaceum (p. 799)
Ataxia-telangiectasia
Basal cell carcinoma (p. 649)
Bloom's syndrome
CREST syndrome (p. 557)
Hereditary hemorrhagic telangiectasia (p. 736)
Keloid (p. 637)
Lupus erythematosus (p. 536)
Necrobiosis lipoidica diabeticorum (p. 784)
Of the proximal nailfold
    Dermatomyositis (p. 549)
    Lupus erythematosus (p. 536)
    Scleroderma (p. 553)
Poikiloderma (p. 674)
Radiodermatitis
Rosacea (p. 182)
Scleroderma (p. 553)
Vascular spiders (p. 735)
    Pregnancy
    Cirrhosis
Xeroderma pigmentosum

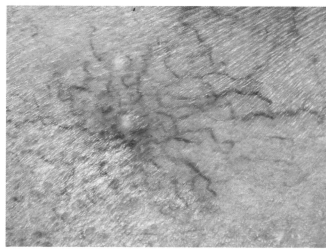

Vascular spider

PETECHIAE

A circumscribed deposit of blood less than 0.5 cm in diameter

Gonococcemia (p. 277)
Leukocytoclastic vasculitis (p. 579)
Meningococcemia (p. 265)

PURPURA

A circumscribed deposit of blood greater than 0.5 cm in diameter

Platelet abnormalities
Progressive pigmentary purpura (p. 585)
Rocky Mountain spotted fever (p. 472)
Scurvy
Senile (traumatic) purpura (p. 601)

REGIONAL DIFFERENTIAL DIAGNOSES

Most skin diseases have preferential areas of involvement. Disease locations are illustrated below; diseases are listed alphabetically by location on pp. 19 to 22. Common diseases that are obvious to most practitioners are not included. Diseases such as contact dermatitis and herpes zoster that can be found on any skin surface have also been left out of most of the lists.

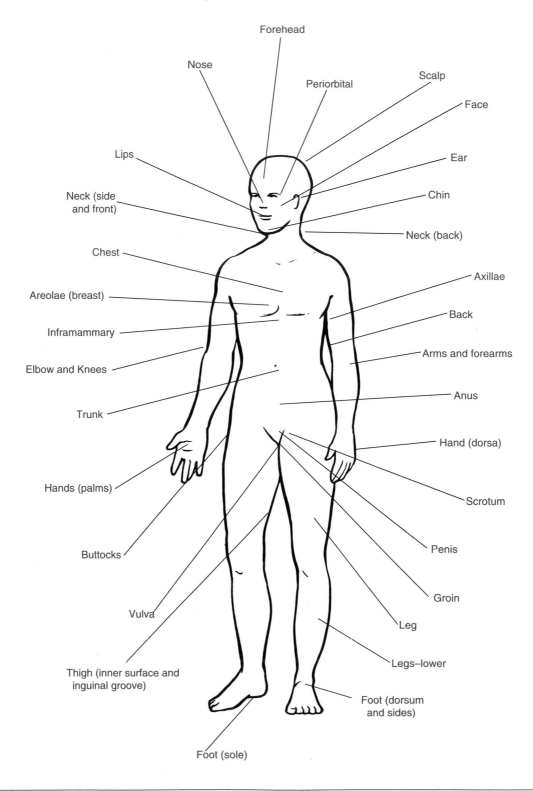

Forehead

Nose

Periorbital

Scalp

Face

Lips

Ear

Neck (side and front)

Chin

Neck (back)

Chest

Axillae

Areolae (breast)

Back

Inframammary

Arms and forearms

Elbow and Knees

Anus

Trunk

Hand (dorsa)

Hands (palms)

Scrotum

Buttocks

Penis

Groin

Vulva

Leg

Legs–lower

Thigh (inner surface and inguinal groove)

Foot (dorsum and sides)

Foot (sole)

REGIONAL DIFFERENTIAL DIAGNOSES

Anus

Candidiasis
Condyloma lata (secondary syphilis)
Extramammary Paget's disease
Gonorrhea
Herpes simplex/zoster
Hidradenitis suppurativa
Lichen sclerosis et atrophicus
Lichen simplex chronicus
Psoriasis (gluteal pinking)
Streptococcal cellulitis
Syphilis (primary—chancre)
Vitiligo
Warts

Areolae (breast)

Eczema
Fox-Fordyce spots
Paget's disease
Seborrheic keratosis

Arms and forearms

Acne
Atopic dermatitis
Cat-scratch disease
Dermatitis herpetiformis (elbows)
Dermatomyositis
Eruptive xanthoma
Erythema multiforme
Granuloma annulare
Herpes zoster
Insect bite
Keratoacanthoma
Keratosis pilaris
Leukocytoclastic vasculitis
Lichen planus
Lupus erythematosus
Neurotic excoriations
Nummular eczema
Pigmentary demarcation lines
Pityriasis alba (white spots)
Polymorphic light eruption
Prurigo nodularis
Purpura (in sun damaged skin)
Scabies
Scleroderma
Seborrheic keratosis (flat)
Sporotrichoid spread
Squamous cell carcinoma
Stellate pseudo scars
Sweet's syndrome
Swimming pool granuloma (mycobacteria)
Tinea

Axillae

Acanthosis nigricans
Acrochordons
Candidiasis
Contact dermatitis
Erythrasma
Fox-Fordyce spots
Freckling-Crowe's Sign (von Recklinghausen's disease)
Furunculosis
Hailey-Hailey disease
Hidradenitis suppurativa
Impetigo
Lice
Pseudoxanthoma elasticum
Scabies
Striae distensae
Tinea
Trichomycosis axillaris

Back

Acne
Amyloidosis
Atrophoderma
Becker's nevus
Cutaneous T cell lymphoma
Dermatographism
Erythema ab igne
Keloids—acne scars
Lichen spinulosis
Melanoma
Nevus anemicus
Notalgia paresthetica
Pityriasis lichenoides et varioliformis acuta (PLEVA)
Seborrheic keratosis
Striae distensae
Tinea versicolor
Transient acantholytic dermatosis (Grover's disease)

Buttocks

Cutaneous T cell lymphoma
Erythema ab igne
Furunculosis
Herpes simplex (females)
Hidradenitis suppurativa
Psoriasis
Scabies
Striae distensae
Tinea

Chest

Acne
Actinic keratosis
Darier's disease
Eruptive syringoma
Eruptive vellus hair cyst
Keloids
Nevus anemicus
Seborrheic dermatitis
Steatocystoma multiplex
Tinea versicolor
Transient acantholytic dermatitis (Grover's disease)

Chin

Acne
Atopic dermatitis
Basal cell carcinoma
Dental sinus
Epidermal cyst
Impetigo
Perioral dermatitis
Warts (flat)

Ear

Actinic keratosis
Atypical fibroxanthoma
Basal cell carcinoma
Bowen's disease
Cellulitis
Chondrodermatitis nodularis chronica helicis
Eczema (infected)
Epidermal cyst
Hydroa vacciniforme
Keloid (lobe)
Lupus erythematosus (discoid)
Lymphangitis
Melanoma
Ochronosis
Pseudocyst
Psoriasis
Ramsey-Hunt syndrome (herpes zoster)
Relapsing polychondritis
Seborrheic dermatitis
Squamous cell carcinoma
Tophi (gout)
Venous lake

Elbows and knees

Calcinosis cutis/CREST
Dermatitis herpetiformis
Erythema multiforme
Gout

Granuloma annulare
Lichen simplex chronicus
Psoriasis
Rheumatoid nodule
Scabies
Xanthoma

Face

Actinic keratosis
Adenoma sebaceum
Alopecia mucinosa
Angioedema
Atopic dermatitis
Basal cell carcinoma
Cowden's disease
CREST
Dermatosis papulosa nigra
Eczema
Erysipelas
Favre Racouchot (senile comedones)
Granuloma faciale
Herpes simplex
Herpes zoster
Impetigo
Keratoacanthoma
Lentigo maligna
Lupus erythematosus (discoid)
Lupus erythematosus (systemic)
Lymphocytoma cutis
Melasma
Molluscum contagiosum
Nevus sebaceous
Pemphigus erythematosus
Perioral dermatitis
Pilomatrixoma
Pityriasis alba (white spots)
Psoriasis
Rosacea
Scleroderma
Sebaceous hyperplasia
Seborrheic dermatitis
Seborrheic keratosis
Secondary syphilis
Spitz's nevus
Squamous cell carcinoma
Steroid rosacea
Sweet's syndrome
Sycosis barbae (folliculitis-beard)
Tinea
Trichoepitheliomas
Warts (flat)
Wegener's granulomatosis

REGIONAL DIFFERENTIAL DIAGNOSES

Foot (dorsum and sides)

Calcaneal petechiae
  (black heel)
Contact dermatitis
Cutaneus larva migrans
Erythema multiforme
Granuloma annulare
Hand, foot, and mouth disease
Keratoderma blennorrhagica
  (Reiter's disease)
Lichen planus
Lichen simplex chronicus
Painful fat herniation (piezo-
  genic papules)
Pernio
Pyogenic granuloma
Scabies
Stucco keratosis
Tinea

Foot (sole)

Arsenical keratosis
Corn (clavus)
Cutaneus larva migrans
Dyshidrotic eczema
Epidermolysis bullosum
Erythema multiforme
Hand, foot, and mouth disease
Hyperkeratosis
Immersion foot
Juvenile plantar dermatosis
Keratoderma
Keratoderma blennorrhagica
  (Reiter's disease)
Lichen planus
Melanoma
Nevi
Pitted keratolysis
Pityriasis rubra pilaris
Psoriasis (pustular)
Pyogenic granuloma
Rocky Mountain spotted fever
Scabies (infants)
Syphilis (secondary)
Tinea
Tinea (bullous)
Verrucous carcinoma
Wart

Forehead

Actinic keratosis
Basal cell carcinoma
Flat warts
Herpes zoster
Psoriasis
Scleroderma (en coup de
  sabre)

Sebaceous hyperplasia
Seborrheic dermatitis
Seborrheic keratosis
Sweet's syndrome

Groin

Acrochordons (skin tags)
Candidiasis
Condyloma
Erythrasma
Extramammary Paget's dis-
  ease
Hailey-Hailey disease
Hidradenitis suppurativa
Histiocytosis X
Intertrigo
Lichen simplex chronicus
Molluscum contagiosum
Pemphigus vegetans
Psoriasis (without scale)
Seborrheic keratosis
Striae (topical steroids)
Tinea

Hand (Dorsa)

Acquired digital fibrokeratoma
Acrosclerosis
Actinic keratosis
Atopic dermatitis
Atypical mycobacteria
Blue nevus
Calcinosis cutis/CREST
Cat-scratch disease
Contact dermatitis
Cowden's disease
Dermatomyositis
Erysipeloid
Erythema multiforme
Gonorrhea
Granuloma annulare
Herpes simplex/zoster
Impetigo
Keratoacanthoma
Lentigo
Lichen planus
Lupus erythematosus
  (systemic)
Mucous cyst (finger)
Orf (finger)
Paronychia (acute, chronic)
Pityriasis rubra pilaris
Polymorphic light eruption
Porphyria cutanea tarda
Pseudo PCT (porphyria
  cutanea tarda)
Psoriasis
Pyogenic granuloma

Scabies
Scleroderma
Seborrheic keratosis
Sporotrichosis
Squamous cell carcinoma
Stucco keratosis
Sweet's syndrome
Swimming pool granuloma
Tinea
Tularemia (ulcer)
Vesicular "id reaction"
Xanthoma

Hands (palms)

Basal-cell nevus syndrome
  (pits)
Calluses/corns
Contact dermatitis
Cowden's disease
Dyshidrotic eczema
Eczema
Erythema multiforme
Hand, foot, and mouth disease
Keratoderma
Keratolysis exfoliativa
Lichen planus (vesicles)
Lupus erythematosus
Melanoma
Pityriasis rubra pilaris
Pompholyx
Psoriasis
Pyogenic granuloma
Rocky Mountain spotted fever
Scabies (infants)
Syphilis (secondary)
Tinea
Vesicular "id reaction"
Wart

Inframammary

Acrochordon (skin tags)
Candidiasis
Contact dermatitis
Intertrigo
Psoriasis (without scale)
Seborrheic keratoses
Tinea versicolor

Leg

Basal cell carcinoma
Bites
Bowen's disease
Dermatofibroma
Disseminated superficial
  actinic porokeratosis
Ecthyma
Ecthyma gangrenosum

Eruptive xanthomas
Kaposi's sarcoma
Livedo reticularis
Lupus panniculus
Majocchi's granuloma (tinea)
Melanoma
Nummular eczema
Panniculitis
Pityriasis lichenoides et vario-
  liformis acuta (PLEVA)
Porokeratosis of Mibelli
Prurigo nodularis
Pyoderma gangrenosum
Squamous cell carcinoma
Urticarial vasculitis
Vasculitis (nodular lesions)
  Wegener's granulomatosis
  Churg-Strauss syndrome
  Polyarteritis nodosa
Weber-Christian disease

Legs—lower

Bites
Cellulitis
Dermatofibroma
Diabetic bullae
Diabetic dermopathy (shin
  spots)
Erysipelas
Erythema induratum
Erythema nodosum
Flat Warts
Folliculitis
Granuloma annulare
Henoch-Schönlein purpura
Ichthyosis vulgaris
Idiopathic guttate hypome-
  lanosis
Leukocytoclastic vasculitis
Lichen planus
Lichen simplex chronicus
Majocchi's granuloma (tinea)
Myxedema (pretibial)
Necrobiosis lipoidica
Purpura
Schamberg's purpura
Stasis dermatitis
Subcutaneous fat necrosis
  (associated with
  pancreatitis)
Sweet's syndrome
Vasculitis (nodular lesions)
Weber-Christian disease
Xerosis

REGIONAL DIFFERENTIAL DIAGNOSES

Lips

Actinic cheilitis
Allergic contact dermatitis
Angioedema
Aphthous ulcer
Fordyce spots (upper lips)
Herpes simplex
Labial melanotic macule
Leukoplakia
Mucous cyst
Perleche
Pyogenic granuloma
Squamous cell carcinoma
Venous lake
Wart

Neck (side and front)

Acanthosis nigricans
Acne
Acrochordon (skin tags)
Atopic dermatitis
Berloque dermatitis
Contact dermatitis
Dental sinus
Elastosis perforans
  serpiginosa
Epidermal cyst
Folliculitis
Impetigo
Pityriasis rosea
Poikiloderma of Civatte
Pseudofolliculitis
Pseudoxanthoma elasticum
Sycosis barbae (fungal,
  bacterial)
Tinea
Wart

Neck (back)

Acne
Acne keloidalis
Actinic keratosis
Cutis rhomboidalis nuchae
Epidermal cyst
Folliculitis
Furunculosis
Herpes zoster
Lichen simplex chronicus
Neurotic excoriations
Salmon patch
Tinea

Nose

Acne
Actinic keratosis
Adenoma sebaceum

Basal cell carcinoma
Discoid lupus erythematosus
Fissure (nostril)
Granulosa rubra nasi
Herpes simplex
Herpes zoster
Impetigo
Lupus erythematosus
Nasal crease
Nevus
Rhinophyma
Rosacea
Seborrheic dermatitis
Squamous cell carcinoma
Telangiectasias
Trichofolliculoma
Wegener's granulomatosis

Penis

Aphthae (Behcet's syndrome)
Balanitis circinata (Reiter's
  syndrome)
Bite (human)
Bowenoid papulosis
Candidiasis (under foreskin)
Chancroid
Condyloma (warts)
Contact dermatitis (condoms)
Erythroplasia of Queyrat
  (Bowen's disease)
Factitious
Fixed drug eruption
Giant condyloma (Buschke-
  Lowenstein)
Granuloma inguinale
Herpes simplex/zoster
Lichen nitidus
Lichen planus
Lichen sclerosis et atrophicus
  (balanitis xerotica obliterans)
Lymphogranuloma venereum
Molluscum contagiosum
Nevus
Pearly penile papules
Pediculosis (lice)
Penile melanosis
Psoriasis
Scabies
Sclerosing lymphangitis (non
  venereal)
Seborrheic keratosis
Squamous cell carcinoma
Syphilis (chancre)
Zoon's (plasma cell) balanitis

Periorbital

Acrochordons (skin tags)
Angioedema
Atopic dermatitis
Cat-scratch disease
Colloid degeneration (milium)
Contact dermatitis
Dermatomyositis
Milia
Molluscum contagiosum
Nevus of Ota
Seborrheic dermatitis
Senile comedones
Syringoma
Xanthelasma

Scalp

Acne necrotica
Actinic keratosis
Alopecia neoplastica
  (metastases)
Atypical fibroxanthoma
Basal cell carcinoma
Contact dermatitis
Cylindroma
Dermatitis occipital
  (excoriation)
Eczema
Folliculitis
Herpes zoster
Kerion (inflammatory tinea)
Lichen planopilaris
Lupus erythematosus (discoid)
Melanoma
Neurotic excoriations
Nevi
Nevus sebaceous
Pediculosis capitis
Pilar cyst (wen)
Prurigo nodularis
Psoriasis
Seborrheic dermatitis
Seborrheic dermatitis
  (Histiocytosis X)
Seborrheic keratosis
Tinea

Scrotum

Angiokeratoma (Fordyce)
Condyloma
Epidermal cyst
Extramammary Paget's
  disease
Henoch-Schönlein syndrome
Lichen simplex chronicus
Nevus

Scabies
Seborrheic keratosis

Thigh (inner surface and inguinal groove)

Acrochordons (skin tags)
Candidiasis
Eczema
Erythrasma
Extramammary Paget's
  disease
Fissures
Granuloma inguinale
Hidradenitis suppurativa
Intertrigo
Keratosis pilaris (anterior)
Lichen sclerosis et atrophicus
Striae distensae
Tinea

Trunk

Accessory nipple
Anetoderma
Ash leaf spot
Atopic dermatitis
Capillary hemangiomas
Chickenpox
CTCL (mycosis fungoides)
Drug eruption (maculopapular)
Epidermal cyst
Erythema annulare
  centrifugum
Familial atypical mole
  syndrome
Fixed drug eruption
Folliculitis (classical and
  hot tub)
Granuloma annulare
  (generalized)
Hailey-Hailey disease
Halo nevus
Herpes zoster
Keloids
Lichen planus (generalized)
Lichen sclerosis et atrophicus
Lupus erythematosus (sub-
  acute cutaneous)
Measles
Miliaria
Nevus anemicus
Nevus spilus
Parapsoriasis
Pediculosis (lice)
Pemphigus foliaceous
Pityriasis rosea
Pityriasis rubra pilaris

REGIONAL DIFFERENTIAL DIAGNOSES

Pityrosporum folliculitis
Poikiloderma vasculare
    atrophicans
Psoriasis (guttate)
Sarcoid
Scabies
Scleroderma (localized,
    morphea)
Seborrheic dermatitis
Steatocystoma multiplex
Syphilis (secondary)
Tinea
Tinea versicolor
Transient acantholytic der-
    matosis (Grover's disease)
Unilateral nevoid telangiectasia
Urticaria pigmentosa
Viral exanthem
von Recklinghausen's
    neurofibromatosis

Vulva
Allergic contact dermatitis
Angiokeratoma (of Fordyce)
Behcet's syndrome
Bowen's disease
Candidiasis
Chancroid
Cicatricial pemphigoid
Epidermal cyst
Erythrasma
Extramammary Paget's
    disease
Fibroepithelial polyp
Folliculitis
Fox-Fordyce spots
Furunculosis
Granuloma inguinale
Herpes simplex/zoster
Hidradenitis suppurativa
Intertrigo

Leukoplakia
Lichen planus
Lichen sclerosis et atrophicus
Lichen simplex chronicus
Melanoma
Molluscum contagiosum
Nevus
Pediculosis
Psoriasis
Squamous cell carcinoma
Steven-Johnson syndrome
Verrucous carcinoma
Warts

Skin Anatomy

The skin (Figure 1-1) is divided into three layers: the epidermis, the dermis, and the subcutaneous tissue. The skin is thicker on the dorsal and extensor surfaces than on the ventral and flexor surfaces.

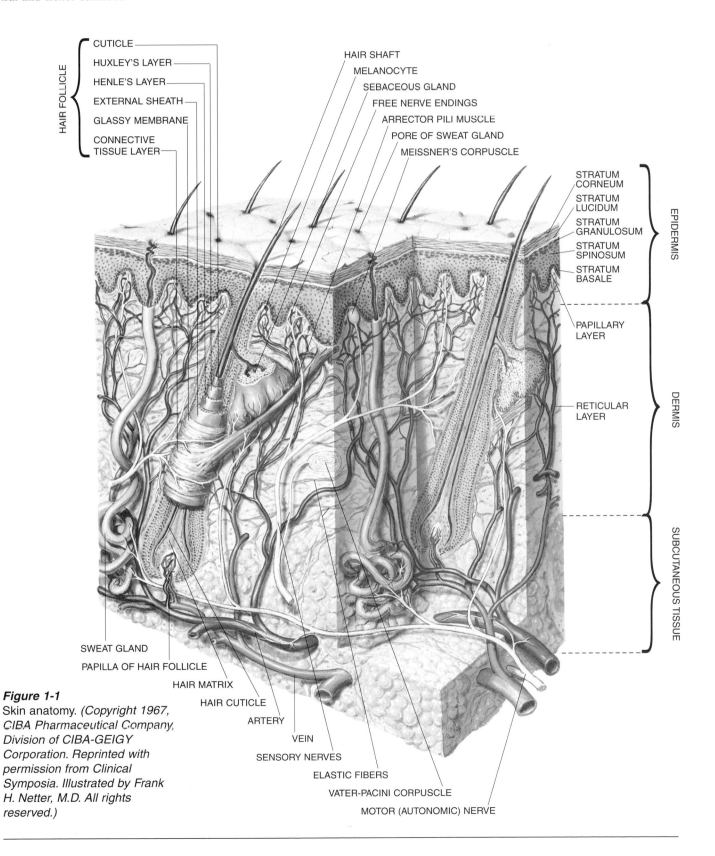

Figure 1-1

Skin anatomy. *(Copyright 1967, CIBA Pharmaceutical Company, Division of CIBA-GEIGY Corporation. Reprinted with permission from Clinical Symposia. Illustrated by Frank H. Netter, M.D. All rights reserved.)*

EPIDERMIS

The epidermis is the outermost part of the skin; it is stratified squamous epithelium. The thickness of the epidermis ranges from 0.05 mm on the eyelids to 1.5 mm on the palms and soles. The microscopic anatomy of the epidermal-dermal junction is complex; it is discussed in detail in Chapter Sixteen. The innermost layer of the epidermis consists of a single row of columnar cells called *basal cells*. Basal cells divide to form keratinocytes (prickle cells), which comprise the spinous layer. The cells of the spinous layer are connected to each other by intercellular bridges or spines, which appear histologically as lines between cells. The keratinocytes synthesize insoluble protein, which remains in the cell and eventually becomes a major component of the outer layer (the stratum corneum). The cells continue to flatten, and their cytoplasm appears granular (stratum granulosum); they finally die as they reach the surface to form the stratum corneum. There are three types of branched cells in the epidermis: the melanocyte, which synthesizes pigment (melanin); Langerhans' cell, which serves as a frontline element in immune reactions of the skin; and Merkel's cell, the function of which is not clearly defined.

DERMIS

The dermis varies in thickness from 0.3 mm on the eyelid to 3.0 mm on the back; it is composed of three types of connective tissue: collagen, elastic tissue, and reticular fibers. The dermis is divided into two layers: the thin upper layer, called the *papillary layer*, is composed of thin, haphazardly arranged collagen fibers; the thicker lower layer, called the *reticular layer*, extends from the base of the papillary layer to the subcutaneous tissue and is composed of thick collagen fibers that are arranged parallel to the surface of the skin. Histiocytes are wandering macrophages that accumulate hemosiderin, melanin, and debris created by inflammation. Mast cells, located primarily about blood vessels, manufacture and release histamine and heparin.

DERMAL NERVES AND VASCULATURE

The sensations of touch and pressure are received by Meissner's and the Vater-Pacini corpuscles. The sensations of pain, itch, and temperature are received by unmyelinated nerve endings in the papillary dermis. A low intensity of stimulation created by inflammation causes itching, whereas a high intensity of stimulation created by inflammation causes pain. Therefore, scratching converts the intolerable sensation of itching to the more tolerable sensation of pain and eliminates pruritis.

The autonomic system supplies the motor innervation of the skin. Adrenergic fibers innervate the blood vessels (vasoconstriction), hair erector muscles, and apocrine glands. Autonomic fibers to eccrine sweat glands are cholinergic. The sebaceous gland is regulated by the endocrine system and is not innervated by autonomic fibers. The anatomy of the hair follicle is described in Chapter Twenty-four.

CHAPTER TWO

Topical Therapy and Topical Corticosteroids

Topical Therapy

A wide variety of topical medications are available for treating cutaneous disease (see the Dermatologic Formulary, pp. 833 to 859). Specific medications are covered in detail in the appropriate chapters. Basic principles of topical treatment are discussed here.

The skin is an important barrier that must be maintained to function properly. Any insult that removes water, lipids, or protein from the epidermis alters the integrity of this barrier and compromises its function. Restoration of the normal epidermal barrier is accomplished with the use of mild soaps and emollient creams and lotions. There is an old and often-repeated rule: "If it is dry, wet it; if it is wet, dry it."

Dry diseases. Dry skin or dry cutaneous lesions have lost water and, in many instances, the epidermal lipids and proteins that help contain epidermal moisture. These substances are replaced with emollient creams and lotions.

Wet diseases. Exudative inflammatory diseases pour out serum that leaches the complex lipids and proteins from the epidermis. A wet lesion is managed with wet compresses that suppress inflammation and debride crust and serum. Repeated cycles of wetting and drying eventually make the lesion dry. Excessive use of wet dressings causes severe drying and chapping. Once the wet phase of the disease has been controlled, the lipids and proteins must be restored with the use of emollient creams and lotions.

EMOLLIENT CREAMS AND LOTIONS

Emollient creams and lotions restore water and lipids to the epidermis (see the Formulary, pp. 849 and 850). Preparations that contain urea or lactic acid have special lubricating properties and may be the most effective. Creams are thicker and more lubricating than lotions. Petroleum jelly and mineral oil contain no water; water should be applied to the skin prior to application. Greasy lubricants should not be applied to wet skin. Emollients should be applied as frequently as necessary to keep the skin soft. Chemicals such as menthol and phenol are added to lubricating lotions to control pruritis (see the Formulary, p. 842).

SEVERE DRY SKIN (XEROSIS)

Dry skin is more severe in the winter months when the humidity is low. ``Winter itch'' most commonly affects the hands and lower legs. Initially the skin is rough and covered with fine white scales. Thicker tan or brown scales may appear. The most severely affected skin may be crisscrossed with shallow red fissures. Dry skin may itch or burn. Preparations listed in the Formulary on p. 850 should be used for mild cases; severe dry skin responds to 12% lactate lotion (Lac-Hydrin).[1]

WET DRESSINGS

Wet dressings, or compresses, are a valuable aid in the treatment of exudative (wet) skin diseases (see the box at right). Their importance in topical therapy cannot be overstated. The technique for wet compress preparation and application is described in the list below.

1. Obtain a clean, soft cloth such as bedsheeting or shirt material. The cloth need not be new or sterilized. Compress material must be washed at least once daily if it is to be used repeatedly.
2. Fold the cloth so there are at least four to eight layers and cut to fit an area slightly larger than the area to be treated.
3. Wet the folded dressings by immersing them in the solution, and wring them out to the point of sopping wet (neither running nor just damp).
4. Place the wet compresses on the affected area. Do not pour solution on a wet dressing to keep it wet because this practice increases the concentration of the solution and may cause irritation. Remove the compress and replace it with a new one.
5. Dressings are left in place for 30 minutes to 1 hour. Dressings may be used two to four times a day or continuously. Discontinue the use of wet compresses when the skin becomes dry. Excessive drying causes cracking and fissures.

Wet compresses provide the following benefits:

- Antibacterial action: Different chemicals may be added to the water to provide an antibacterial effect (Table 2-1).
- Wound debridement: A wet compress macerates vesicles and crust, helping to debride these materials when the compress is removed.
- Inflammation suppression: Compresses have a strong antiinflammatory effect. The evaporative cooling causes constriction of superficial cutaneous vessels, thereby decreasing erythema and the production of serum. Wet compresses control acute inflammatory processes, such as acute poison ivy, faster than either topical or orally administered corticosteroids.
- Drying: Wet dressings cause the skin to be dry. Wetting something to make it dry seems paradoxical, but the effects of repeated cycles of wetting and drying are observed in lip chapping, caused by lip licking; irritant hand dermatitis, caused by repeated washing; and the soggy sock syndrome in children, caused by perspiration.

The temperature of the compress solution should be cool when an antiinflammatory effect is desired and tepid when the purpose is to debride an infected, crusted lesion. Covering a wet compress with a towel or plastic inhibits evaporation, promotes maceration, and increases skin temperature, which facilitates bacterial growth.

DISEASES TREATED WITH WET COMPRESSES

Acute eczematous inflammation (poison ivy)
Eczematous inflammation with secondary infection (pustules)
Bullous impetigo
Herpes simplex and herpes zoster (vesicular lesions)
Infected exudative lesions of any type
Insect bites
Intertrigo (groin or under breasts)
Nummular eczema (exudative lesions)
Stasis dermatitis (exudative lesions)
Stasis ulcers
Sunburn (blistering stage)
Tinea pedis (vesicular stage or macerated web infections)

TABLE 2-1 Wet Dressing Solutions

Solution	Preparation	Indications
Burow's solution (aluminum sulfate and calcium acetate) Bulboro powder Domeboro powder and tablets	One packet or tablet in a pint of water produces a modified 1:40 Burow's solution	Mildly antiseptic; for acute inflammation
Silver nitrate, 0.1%-0.5%	Supplied as a 50% aqueous solution. Stains skin dark brown and metal black.	Bactericidal; for exudative infected lesions (e.g., stasis ulcers and stasis dermatitis)
Acetic acid, 1%-2.5%	Vinegar is 5% acetic acid. Make 1% solution (approximate) by adding ½ cup of vinegar (white or brown) to 1 pint of water.	Bactericidal; for certain gram-negative bacteria (e.g., *Pseudomonas aeruginosa*), otitis externa, *Pseudomonas* intertrigo
Water	Tap water does not have to be sterilized.	Poison ivy, sunburn, any noninfected exudated or inflamed process

---

SUGGESTED STRENGTH OF TOPICAL STEROIDS TO INITIATE TREATMENT*

GROUPS I-II

Psoriasis
Lichen planus
Discoid lupus†
Severe hand eczema
Poison ivy (severe)
Lichen simplex chronicus
Hyperkeratotic eczema
Chapped feet
Lichen sclerosis et atrophicus (skin)
Alopecia areata
Nummular eczema (severe)
Atopic dermatitis (resistant adult cases)

GROUPS III-V

Atopic dermatitis
Nummular eczema
Asteatotic eczema
Stasis dermatitis
Seborrheic dermatitis
Lichen sclerosis et atrophicus (vulva)
Intertrigo (brief course)
Tinea (brief course to control inflammation)
Scabies (after scabicide)
Intertrigo (severe cases)
Anal inflammation (severe cases)
Severe dermatitis (face)

GROUPS VI-VII

Dermatitis (eyelids)
Dermatitis (diaper area)
Mild dermatitis (face)
Mild anal inflammation
Mild intertrigo

*Stop treatment, change to less potent agent, or use intermittent treatment once inflammation is controlled.
†Use on the face may be justified.

Topical Corticosteroids

Topical corticosteroids are a powerful tool for treating skin disease. Understanding the correct use of these agents will result in the successful management of a variety of skin problems. There are many products available, and new ones appear almost monthly. Pharmaceutical companies have responded to the great demand for these agents with an increasing number of products, but all of these preparations have basically the same antiinflammatory properties. They differ only in strength, base, and price.

STRENGTH

Potency: groups I through VII. The antiinflammatory properties of topical corticosteroids result in part from their ability to induce vasoconstriction of the small blood vessels in the upper dermis. This property is used in an assay procedure to determine the strength of each new product. These products are subsequently tabulated in seven groups, with group I the strongest and group VII the weakest (see the Formulary and the inside front cover of this book).[2] The treatment sections of this book recommend topical steroids by group number rather than by generic or brand name because the agents in each group are essentially equivalent in strength. When a new topical corticosteroid appears on the market, ask to which group it belongs and add it to the list in the Formulary.

Lower concentrations of some brands may have the same effect in vasoconstrictor assays as much higher concentrations of the same product. One study showed that there was no difference in vasoconstriction between Kenalog 0.025%, 0.1%, or 0.5% creams.[3]

Choosing the appropriate strength. Guidelines for choosing the appropriate strength of topical steroid are presented in the box above. The best results are obtained when preparations of adequate strength are used for a specified length of time. Weaker, "safer" strengths often fail to provide adequate control. Patients who do not respond after 1 to 4 weeks of treatment should be reevaluated.

Megapotent topical steroids (group I). Temovate (clobetasol propionate), Ultravate (halobetasol propionate), Diprolene (betamethasone dipropionate), and Psorcon (diflorasone diacetate) are the most potent topical steroids available. Temovate and Ultravate are the most potent,[4] and Psorcon and Diprolene are equipotent.

In general no more than 45 to 60 gm of cream or ointment should be used each week (Table 2-2). Side effects are minimized and efficacy increased when medication is applied once or twice daily for 2 weeks followed by 1 week of rest. This cyclic schedule (pulse dosing) is continued until resolution occurs.[5] Intermittent dosing (e.g., one or two times per week) can lead to a prolonged remission of psoriasis if used after initial clearing.[6] Alternatively, intermittent use of a weaker topical steroid can be used for maintenance. Psorcon can be used with plastic dressing occlusion. Temovate, Ultravate, and Diprolene should not be used with occlusive dressings.

TABLE 2-2	Restrictions on the Use of Group I Topical Steroids*		
	Length of therapy	**Grams per week**	**Use under occlusion**
Temovate	14 days	60	No
Ultravate	14 days	60	No
Diprolene	Unrestricted	45	No
Psorcon	Unrestricted	Unrestricted	Unrestricted

*Restrictions are listed in the package inserts.

Patients must be monitored carefully. Side effects such as atrophy and adrenal suppression[7] (see Table 2-3) are a real possibility, especially with unsupervised use of Temovate. Refills should be strictly limited.

Concentration. The concentration of steroid listed on the tube cannot be used to compare its strength with other steroids. Some steroids are much more powerful than others and need be present only in small concentrations to produce the maximum effect. Nevertheless, it is difficult to convince some patients that Lidex cream 0.05% (group II) is more potent than hydrocortisone 1.0% (group VII).

It is unnecessary to learn many steroid brand names. Familiarity with one preparation from groups II, V, and VII gives one the ability to safely and effectively treat any steroid-responsive skin disease. Most of the topical steroids are fluorinated (i.e., a fluorine atom has been added to the hydrocortisone molecule). Fluorination increases potency and the possibility of side effects. Products such as Westcort Cream increase potency without fluorination. However, side effects are possible with this midpotency steroid.

Compounding. Avoid having the pharmacist prepare or dilute topical steroid creams. The active ingredient may not be dispersed uniformly, resulting in a cream of variable strength. The cost of pharmacist preparation is generally higher because of the additional labor required. High-quality steroid creams, such as triamcinolone acetonide (Kenalog, Aristocort), are available in large quantities at a low cost.

Generic vs. brand names. Many generic topical steroid formulations are available (e.g., betamethasone valerate, betamethasone dipropionate, fluocinolone acetonide, fluocinonide, hydrocortisone, and triamcinolone acetonide). In many states, generic substitutions by the pharmacist are allowed unless the physician writes "no substitution." Vasoconstrictor assays have shown large differences in the activity of generic formulations compared with brand-name equivalents: many are inferior,[8] a few are equivalent,[9] and a few are more potent than brand-name equivalents. Many generic topical steroids have vehicles with different ingredients (e.g., preservatives) than brand-name equivalents.[10]

VEHICLE

The vehicle, or base, is the substance in which the active ingredient is dispersed. The base determines the rate at which the active ingredient is absorbed through the skin.[11,12] Components of some bases may cause irritation or allergy.

Creams. The cream base is a mixture of several different organic chemicals (oils) and water, and it usually contains a preservative. Creams have the following characteristics:

- White color and somewhat greasy texture
- Components that may cause irritation, stinging, and allergy
- High versatility (i.e., may be used in nearly any area), therefore creams are the base most often prescribed
- Cosmetically most acceptable, particularly emollient bases (e.g., Lidex-E, Topicort, and Cyclocort)
- Possible drying effect with continued use, therefore best for acute exudative inflammation
- Most useful for intertriginous areas (e.g., groin, rectal area, and axilla)

Ointments. The ointment base contains a limited number of organic compounds consisting primarily of greases such as petroleum jelly, with little or no water. Many ointments are preservative-free. Ointments have the following characteristics:

- Translucent (look like petroleum jelly)
- Greasy feeling persists on skin surface
- More lubrication, thus desirable for drier lesions
- Greater penetration of medicine than creams and therefore enhanced potency (see inside front cover; Synalar Cream in group V and Synalar Ointment in group IV)
- Too occlusive for acute (exudative) eczematous inflammation or intertriginous areas, such as the groin

Gels. Gels are greaseless mixtures of propylene glycol and water; some also contain alcohol. Gels have the following characteristics:

- A clear base, sometimes with a jellylike consistency
- Useful for acute exudative inflammation, such as poison ivy, and in scalp areas where other vehicles mat the hair

Solutions and lotions. Solutions may contain water and alcohol as well as other chemicals. Solutions have the following characteristics:

- Clear or milky appearance
- Most useful for scalp because they penetrate easily through hair, leaving no residue
- May result in stinging and drying when applied to intertriginous areas, such as the groin

Aerosols. Aerosols are composed of steroids suspended in a base and delivered under pressure. Aerosols have the following characteristics:

- Useful for applying medication to the scalp (long probe attached to the can may be inserted through the hair to deliver medication more easily to the scalp)
- Useful for moist lesions such as poison ivy
- Convenient for patients who lack mobility and have difficulty reaching their lower legs

STEROID-ANTIBIOTIC MIXTURES

Lotrisone cream. Lotrisone cream contains a combination of the antifungal agent clotrimazole and the corticosteroid betamethasone dipropionate. It is indicated for the topical treatment of tinea pedis, tinea cruris, and tinea corporis. This product is used by many physicians as their topical antiinflammatory agent of first choice. Most inflammatory skin disease is not infected or contaminated by fungus. Lotrisone is a marginal drug for cutaneous fungal infections. Lotrisone cream costs approximately $25.00 for 15 gm and $45.00 for 45 gm. Generic betamethasone dipropionate cream costs approximately $12.00 for 15 gm and $18.00 for 45 gm. Generic clotrimazole costs approximately $10.00 for 30 gm.

Some products contain a combination of antibiotics and corticosteroids. Generic neomycin-steroid products and Neo-synalar are available. Mycolog II does not contain neomycin. Dermatologists disagree about the desirability of these combination products.[13,14] The majority of steroid-responsive skin diseases can be managed successfully without topical antibiotics. Oral antibiotics have demonstrated more effectiveness than topical antibiotics. Neomycin is a sensitizer and may complicate an already prolonged and difficult-to-control problem such as stasis dermatitis. Present governmental guidelines for welfare recipients prohibit compensation for steroid-antibiotic mixtures.

AMOUNT OF CREAM TO DISPENSE

The amount of cream dispensed is very important. Patients do not appreciate being prescribed a $60.00, 60-gm tube of cream to treat a small area of hand dermatitis. Unrestricted and unsupervised use of potent steroid creams can lead to side effects. Patients rely on the judgment of the physician to determine the correct amount of topical medicine. If too small a quantity is prescribed, patients may conclude that the treatment did not work. It is advisable to allow for a sufficient amount of cream, and then to set limits on duration and frequency of application. Many steroids (e.g., triamcinolone, hydrocortisone) are available in generic form. They are purchased in bulk by the pharmacist and can be dispensed in large quantities at considerable savings.

The amount of cream required to cover a certain area can be calculated by remembering that 1 gm of cream covers 10 cm × 10 cm, or 100 square cm, of skin.[15] The entire skin surface of the average-size adult is covered by 20 to 30 gm of cream.

The fingertip unit and the rule of hand provide the means to assess how much cream to dispense and apply.

Fingertip unit. A fingertip unit (FTU) is the amount of ointment expressed from a tube with a 5-mm diameter nozzle, applied from the distal skin crease to the tip of the index finger. One FTU weighs approximately 0.5 gm. The number of FTUs required to cover specific body areas is illustrated on the inside of the back cover.[16]

The rule of hand. The hand area can be used to estimate the total area of involvement of a skin disease and to assess the amount of ointment required. The area of one side of the hand is defined as one hand area. One hand area of involved skin requires 0.5 FTU or 0.25 gm of ointment, or four hand areas equal 2 FTUs equal 1 gm. The area of one side of the hand represents approximately 1.0% of body surface area; therefore, it requires 1 FTU (2 hand units) to cover 2.0% of the body surface. Approximately 282 gm is required for twice-daily applications to the total body surface (except the scalp) for 1 week.[17]

APPLICATION

Frequency

Tachyphylaxis. *Tachyphylaxis* refers to the decrease in responsiveness to a drug as a result of enzyme induction. The term is used in dermatology in reference to acute tolerance to the vasoconstrictive action of topically applied corticosteroids. Experiments revealed that vasoconstriction decreased progressively when a potent topical steroid was applied to the skin three times a day for 4 days.[18] The vasoconstrictive response returned 4 days after termination of therapy. These experiments support years of complaints by patients about initially dramatic responses to new topical steroids that diminish with constant use. It would, therefore, seem reasonable to instruct patients to apply creams on an interrupted schedule.

Intermittent dosing

Group I topical steroids. Optimum dosing schedules for the use of potent topical steroids have not been determined. Studies show that steroid-resistant diseases, such as plaque psoriasis and hand eczema, respond most effectively when clobetasol (Temovate) is applied twice a day for 2 to 3 weeks.[19,20] Treatment is resumed after 1 week of rest. The schedule of 2 weeks of treatment followed by 1 week of rest is repeated until the lesions have cleared.

Intermittent treatment of healed lesions can lead to prolonged remission. Psoriatic patients with lingering erythema remained clear with applications three times a day on 1 day a week.[6] Twice weekly applications of clobetasol kept 75% of psoriatic patients[10] and 70% of hand eczema patients[20] in remission.

Groups II through VII topical steroids. The optimum frequency of application and duration of treatment for topical steroids has not been determined. Adequate results and acceptable patient compliance occur when the following steps are taken:

1. Apply groups II through VI topical steroids twice each day.
2. Limit the duration of application to 2 to 6 weeks.
3. If adequate control is not achieved, stop treatment for 4 to 7 days and begin another course of treatment.

These are general guidelines; specific instructions and limitations must be established for each individual case.

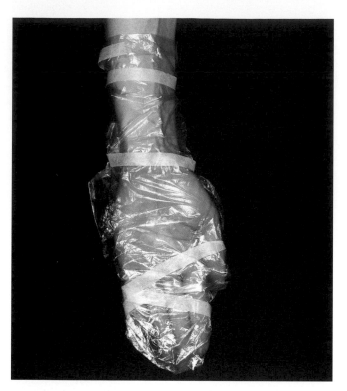

Figure 2-1
Occlusion of the hand. A plastic bag is pulled on and pressed against the skin to expel air. Tape is wound snugly around the bag.

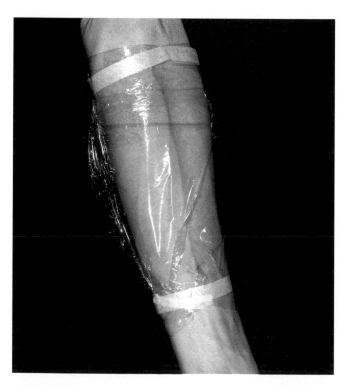

Figure 2-2
Occlusion of the arm. A plastic sheet (e.g., Saran Wrap) is wound about the extremity and secured at both ends with tape. A plastic bag with the bottom cut out may be used as a sleeve and held in place with tape or an Ace bandage.

Methods

Simple application. Creams and ointments should be applied in thin layers and slowly massaged into the site one to four times a day. Patients should be informed that it is unnecessary to wash before each application. Patients must be encouraged to continue treatment until the lesion is clear. Many patients decrease the frequency of applications or stop entirely when lesions appear to improve quickly. Other patients are so impressed with the efficacy of these agents that they continue treatment after the disease has resolved in order to prevent recurrence. Adverse reactions may follow this practice.

Different skin surfaces vary in the ability to absorb topical medicine. The thin eyelid skin heals quickly with group VI or VII steroids, whereas thicker skin on palms and soles offers a greater barrier to the penetration of topical medicine and requires more potent therapy. Intertriginous (skin touches skin) areas (e.g., axilla, groin, rectal area, and underneath the breasts) respond more quickly with weaker strength creams. The apposition of two skin surfaces performs the same function as an occlusive dressing, which greatly enhances penetration. The skin of infants and young children is more receptive to topical medicine and responds

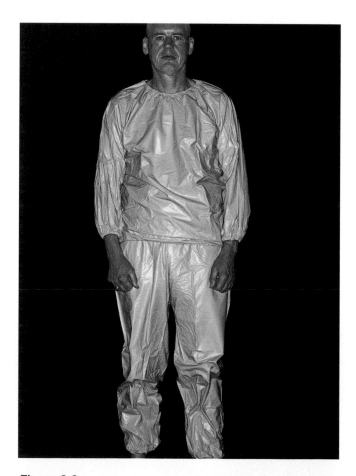

Figure 2-3
Occlusion of the entire body. A vinyl exercise suit is a convenient way to occlude the entire body.

quickly to weaker creams. A baby's diaper has the same occlusive effect as covering with a plastic dressing. Penetration of steroid creams is greatly enhanced; therefore, only group V, VI, or VII preparations should be used under a diaper. Inflamed skin absorbs topical medicines much more efficiently. This explains why red inflamed areas generally have such a rapid initial response when treated with weaker topical steroids.

Occlusion. Occlusion with a plastic dressing (e.g., Saran Wrap) is an effective method for enhancing absorption of topical steroids. The plastic dressing holds perspiration against the skin surface, which hydrates the top layer of the epidermis (stratum corneum). Topical medication penetrates a moist stratum corneum from 10 to 100 times more effectively than it penetrates dry skin.[21] Eruptions that are resistant to simple application may heal quickly with the introduction of a plastic dressing. Nearly any area can be occluded; the entire body may be occluded with a vinyl exercise suit, available at most sporting goods stores.

Discretion should be used with occlusion. Occlusion of moist areas may encourage the rapid development of infection.[21] Occlusive dressings are used more often with creams than with ointments, but ointments may be covered if the lesions are particularly dry. Weaker, less expensive products (e.g., triamcinolone cream, 0.1%) provide excellent results. Large quantities of this medicine may be purchased at a substantial savings.

Method of occlusion. The area should be cleaned with mild soap and water. Antibacterial soaps are unnecessary. The medicine is gently rubbed into the lesions, and the entire area is covered with plastic (e.g., Saran Wrap, Handi-Wrap, plastic bags, or gloves) (Figures 2-1 to 2-3). The plastic dressing should be secured with tape so that it is close to the skin and the ends are sealed. An airtight dressing is unnecessary. The plastic may be held in place with an Ace bandage or a sock. The best results are obtained if the dressing remains in place for at least 2 hours. Many patients find that bedtime is the most convenient time to wear a plastic dressing and therefore wear it for 8 hours. More medicine is applied shortly after the dressing is removed and while the skin is still moist.

Dressings should not remain on the area continuously because infection or follicular occlusion may result. If an occluded area suddenly becomes worse or pustules develop, infection, usually with staphylococci, should be suspected (Figure 2-4). Oral antistaphylococcal antibiotics should be given (e.g., cephalexin [Keflex] 500 mg twice a day).

A reasonable occlusion schedule is twice daily for a 2-hour period or 8 hours at bedtime, with simple application once or twice during the day.

Occluded areas often become dry, and the use of lubricating cream or lotion should be encouraged. Cream or lotion may be applied shortly after medicine is applied, when the plastic dressing is removed, or at other convenient times.

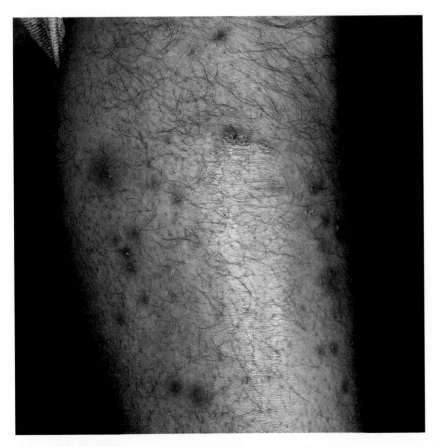

Figure 2-4
Infection following occlusion. Pustules have appeared at the periphery of an eczematous lesion. Plastic dressing had been left in place for 24 hours.

Systemic absorption

The possibility of producing systemic side effects from absorption of topical steroids concerns all physicians who use these agents. Several case reports in the past 20 years have documented systemic effects after topical application of glucocorticoids for prolonged periods. Cataracts, retardation of growth,[22] failure to thrive, and Cushing's syndrome[23] have all been reported.

Avoid weaker, "safe" preparations. In an attempt to avoid complications, physicians often choose a weaker steroid preparation than that indicated; the weaker preparations all too frequently fall short of expectations and fail to give the desired antiinflammatory effect. The disease does not improve, but rather becomes worse because of the time wasted using the ineffective cream. Pruritis continues, infection may set in, and the patient becomes frustrated. Treatment of intense inflammation with hydrocortisone cream 0.5% is a waste of time and money. Generally, a topical steroid of adequate strength (see the box on p. 27) should be used 2 to 4 times daily for a specific length of time, such as 7 to 21 days, in order to obtain rapid control. Even during this short interval, adrenal suppression may result when groups I through III steroids are used to treat wide areas of inflamed skin. This suppression of the hypothalamic-pituitary-adrenal axis is generally reversible in 24 hours and is very unlikely to produce side effects characteristic of long-term systemic use.[24]

Children. Many physicians worry about systemic absorption and will not use any topical steroids stronger than 1% hydrocortisone on infants. One study revealed that stronger creams can be used safely.[25] Children (7 months to 8 years old) with severe atopic dermatitis were treated with triamcinolone acetonide ointment 0.1% (Kenalog), applied four times each day for 6 weeks. The total quantities of ointment used during the 6-week period were large, varying from 414 to 1191 gm. No patient showed suppression of the hypothalamic-pituitary-adrenal axis. The author concluded that the use of placebo concentrations of hydrocortisone and the tendency to abandon the use of fluorinated steroids, such as triamcinolone acetonide 0.1%, in infants and children are not justified.[26]

The relative safety of moderately strong topical steroids and their relative freedom from serious systemic toxicity despite widespread use in the very young has been clearly demonstrated. Patients should be treated for a specific length of time with a medication of appropriate strength. Steroid creams should not be used continually for many weeks, and patients who do not respond in a predictable fashion should be reevaluated.

Group I topical steroids should be avoided in prepubertal children. Use only group VI or VII in the diaper area for only 3 to 10 days. Monitor growth parameters in children on chronic topical glucocorticoid therapy.

Adults. Tables 2-3 and 2-4 list the degree of adrenal suppression that can be expected with topical steroids.[24] Suppression may occur during short intervals of treatment with group I or II topical steroids, but recovery is rapid when treatment is discontinued. Physicians may prescribe strong agents when appropriate, but the patient must be cautioned that the agent should be used only for the length of time dictated.

TABLE 2-3 Percentage of Patients Experiencing Adrenal Suppression with Use of Topical Steroids*

	Daily dosage (amount per week)	Percentage of body surface treated	Duration of administration	Use with occlusion	Percentage of patients experiencing suppression
Temovate (ointment or cream)	3.5 gm twice daily (49 gm/wk)	30	7 days	No	75
	1.75 gm twice daily (25 gm/wk)	<30	7 days	No	22
	1 gm twice daily (14 gm/wk)	<30	7 days	No	10
Diprolene	>7 gm once daily (>49 gm/wk)	30	7 days	No	Significant depression
Psorcon	15 gm twice daily (210 gm/wk)	>30	7 days	No	0

Modified from Stoughton RB, Cornell RC: *Semin Dermatol* 6:72-76, 1987.
*The potential for topically applied corticosteroids to produce adrenal suppression depends on the condition of the skin, the method and extent of application, the potency, and, possibly, the amount of topical steroid used.

TABLE 2-4 Presence of Adrenal Suppression with Various Topical Steroids

Steroid group	Frequency	Body surface treated (%)	Duration	Occlusion	Suppression*
II†	Twice daily	50	5 days	No	None
II†	Twice daily	50	5 days	Yes	Yes
II	Twice daily	30	5 days	No	Immediate, but decreases during treatment
II	Twice daily	30	5 days	Yes	Marked; persists throughout treatment period
V	Twice daily	30	5 days	No	Mild decrease
V	Twice daily	30	5 days	Yes	Moderate decrease
II	Three times daily	5-50	4 to 6 weeks	No	Little or none
V	Three times daily	5-50	4 to 6 weeks	No	None

Modified from Gomez EC, Kaminester L, Frost P: *Arch Dermatol* 113:1196, 1977.
*Adrenal suppression was rapidly reversible in all cases.
†Normal skin.

ADVERSE REACTIONS

Because information concerning the potential dangers of potent topical steroids has been so widely disseminated, some physicians have abandoned their use. Topical steroids have been used for approximately 30 years with an excellent safety record. They do, however, have the potential to produce a number of adverse reactions. Once these are understood, the most appropriate strength can be prescribed confidently. The reported adverse reactions to topical steroids are listed below.

Rosacea, perioral dermatitis, acne

Skin atrophy with telangiectasia, stellate pseudoscars (arms), purpura, stria (from anatomic occlusion, e.g., groin)

Tinea incognito, impetigo incognito, scabies incognito

Ocular hypertension, glaucoma, cataracts

Allergic contact dermatitis

Systemic absorption

Burning, itching, irritation, dryness caused by vehicle (e.g., propylene glycol)

Miliaria and folliculitus following occlusion with plastic

Skin blanching from acute vasoconstriction

Rebound phenomenon (i.e., psoriasis becomes worse after treatment is stopped)

Nonhealing leg ulcers; steroids applied to any leg ulcer retard healing process

Hypopigmentation

Hypertrichosis of face

A brief description of some of the more important adverse reactions is presented in the following pages.

Steroid rosacea and perioral dermatitis

Steroid rosacea[27] is a side effect frequently observed in fair-skinned females who initially complain of erythema with or without pustules, the "flusher blusher complexion." In a typical example, the physician prescribes a mild topical steroid, which initially gives pleasing results. Tolerance (tachyphylaxis) occurs, and a new, more potent topical steroid is prescribed to suppress the erythema and pustules that have reappeared following the use of the weaker preparation. This progression to more potent creams may continue until group II steroids are applied several times each day. Figure 2-5, *A*, shows a middle-aged woman who has applied a group V steroid cream once each day for 5 years. Intense erythema and pustulation occurs each time attempts are made to discontinue topical treatment (Figure 2-5, *B*).

Perioral dermatitis (see Chapter Seven) is sometimes caused by the chronic application of topical steroids to the lower face. Pustules, erythema, and scaling occur about the nose, mouth, and chin.

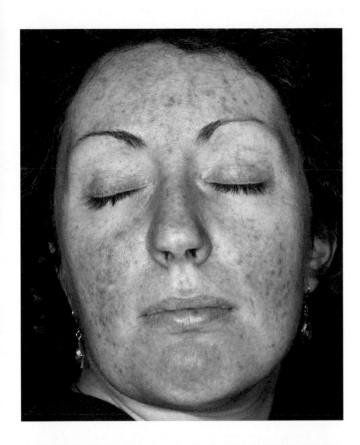

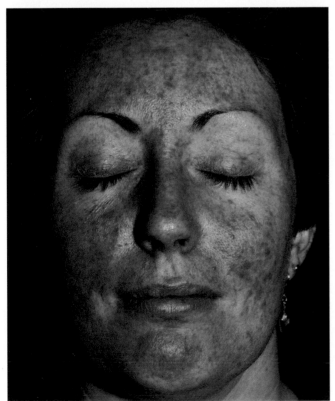

B, Ten days after discontinuing use of group V topical steroid.

Figure 2-5
Steroid rosacea.

A, Numerous red papules formed on the cheeks and forehead with constant daily use of a group V topical steroid for more than 5 years.

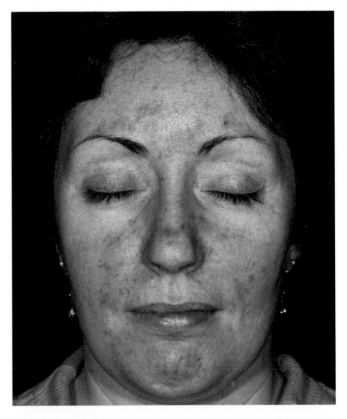

C, Two months after use of topical steroids was discontinued. Telangiectasia has persisted; rosacea has improved with oral antibiotics.

Management. Strong topical steroids must be discontinued. Tetracycline (250 mg four times a day) or erythromycin (250 mg four times a day) may reduce the intensity of the rebound erythema and pustulation that predictably occur during the first 10 days (Figures 2-6, 2-7, 2-8, and 2-9). Occasionally, cool, wet compresses, with or without 1% hydrocortisone cream, are necessary if the rebound is intense. Thereafter, mild noncomedogenic lubricants (those that do not induce acne, such as Nutraderm lotion) may be used for the dryness and desquamation that occur. Erythema and pustules are generally present at a low-grade level for months. Low dosages of tetracycline or erythromycin (250 mg two or three times a day) may be continued until the eruption clears. The pustules and erythema eventually subside, but some telangiectasia and atrophy may be permanent.

Figure 2-6
Steroid rosacea.

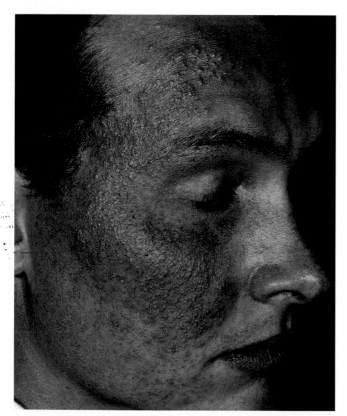

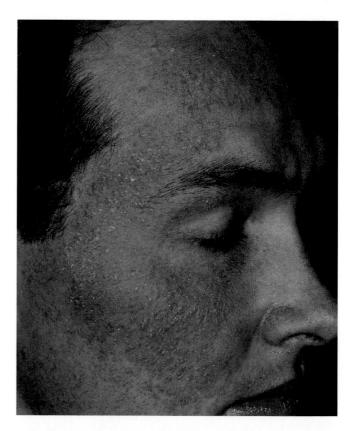

A, Intense erythema and pustulation appeared 10 days after discontinuing use of a group V topical steroid. The cream had been applied every day for 1 year.

B, Patient shown in *A* 24 days after discontinuing the group V topical steroid. Pustules have cleared without any treatment. Gradual improvement followed over the next several months.

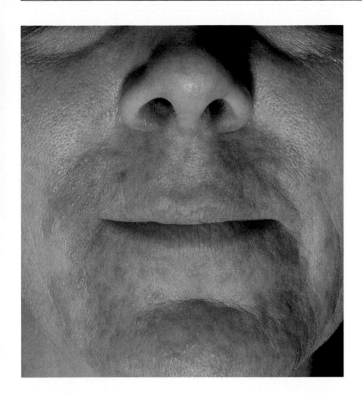

Figure 2-7
Perioral dermatitis. Pustules and erythema have appeared in a perioral distribution following several courses of a group III topical steroid to the lower face. The inflammation flares shortly after the topical steroid is discontinued.

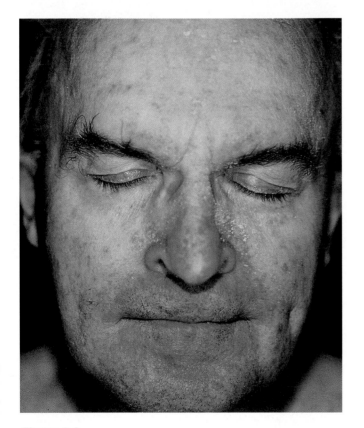

Figure 2-8
Steroid rosacea. A painful, diffuse pustular eruption occurred following daily application for 12 weeks of the group II topical steroid fluocinonide.

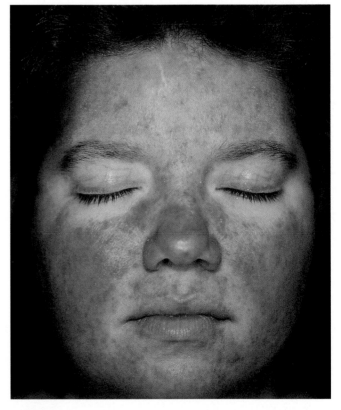

Figure 2-9
Steroid acne. Repeated application to the entire face of a group V topical steroid resulted in this diffuse pustular eruption. The inflammation improved each time the topical steroid was used but flared with increasing intensity each time the medication was stopped.

Atrophy

Long-term use of strong topical steroids in the same area may result in thinning of the epidermis and regressive changes in the connective tissue in the dermis. The affected areas are often depressed slightly below normal skin and usually reveal telangiectasia, prominence of underlying veins, and hypopigmentation. Purpura and ecchymosis result from minor trauma. The face (Figures 2-10, 2-11, 2-12, and 2-13), dorsa of the hands (Figure 2-14), extensor surfaces of the forearms and legs, and intertriginous areas are particularly susceptible. In most cases atrophy is reversible and may be expected to disappear in the course of several months.[28] Diseases (such as psoriasis) that respond slowly to strong topical steroids require weeks of therapy. Some atrophy may subsequently be anticipated (Figure 2-15).

Occlusion. Occlusion enhances penetration of medicine and accelerates the occurrence of this adverse reaction. Many patients are familiar with this side effect and must be assured that the use of strong topical steroids is perfectly safe when used as directed for 2 to 3 weeks. They must also be assured that if some atrophy does appear, it resolves in most cases when therapy is discontinued.

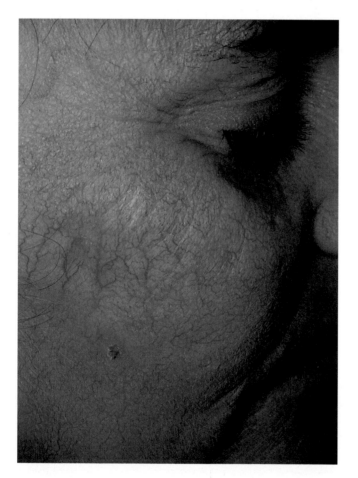

Figure 2-10
Atrophy and telangiectasia after continual use of a group IV topical steroid for 6 months. Atrophy may improve after the topical steroid is discontinued, but telangiectasia often persists.

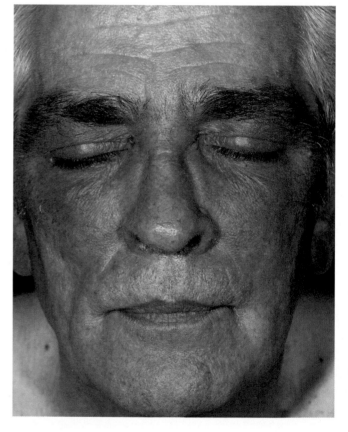

Figure 2-11
Steroid-induced erythema. This patient used the group II topical steroid fluocinonide almost constantly for 12 years. Erythema rather than pustules occurred each time the medication was stopped.

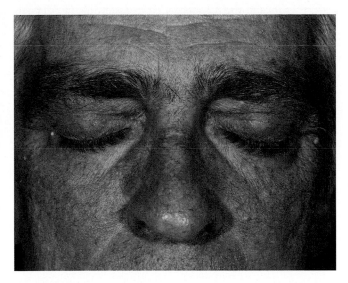

Figure 2-12
Steroid-induced telangiectasia. The patient in Figure 2-11 stopped all topical steroids. One year later he has permanent telangiectasia on the cheeks. His intraocular pressure was elevated but returned to near normal levels 3 months after stopping the fluocinonide.

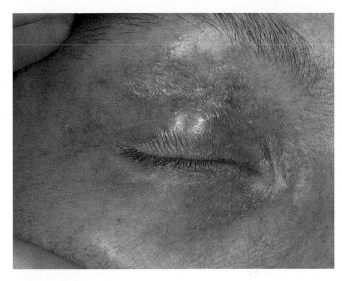

Figure 2-13
Steroid atrophy. Daily application of the group II topical steroid desoximetasone to the lids resulted in almost complete atrophy of the dermis. The lids bleed spontaneously when touched. The intraocular pressure was elevated. There was marked improvement in the atrophy and intraocular tension 8 weeks after stopping the topical steroid.

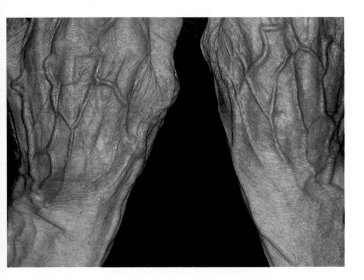

Figure 2-14
Severe steroid atrophy after continual occlusive therapy over several months. Significant improvement in the atrophy occurs after topical steroids are discontinued.

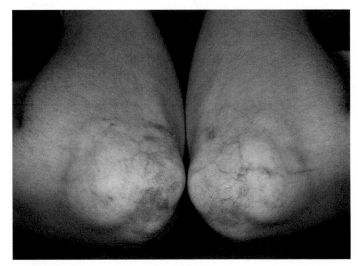

Figure 2-15
Steroid atrophy. Atrophy with prominence of underlying veins and hypopigmentation following use of Cordran Tape applied daily for 3 months to treat psoriasis. Note that small plaques of psoriasis persist. Atrophy improves after topical steroids are discontinued, but some hypopigmentation may persist.

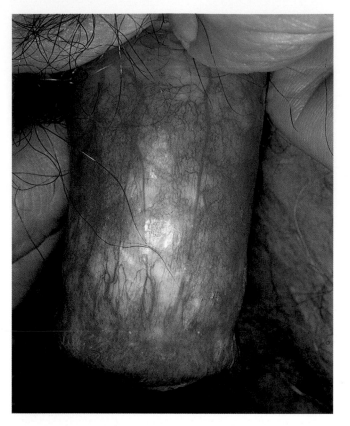

Figure 2-16
Steroid atrophy under the foreskin. Application of the group V topical steroid triamcinolone acetonide under the foreskin each day for 8 weeks produced severe atrophy and prominent telangiectasia of the shaft of the penis. The foreskin acted like an occlusive dressing to greatly enhance penetration of the steroid. Bleeding occurred with the slightest trauma. There was marked improvement 3 weeks after the medication was stopped.

Mucosal areas. Atrophy under the foreskin (Figure 2-16) and in the rectal and vaginal areas may appear much more quickly than in other areas.[29] The thinner epidermis offers less resistance to the passage of corticosteroids into the dermis. These are intertriginous areas where the apposition of skin surfaces acts in the same manner as a plastic dressing, retaining moisture and greatly facilitating absorption. These delicate tissues become thin and painful, sometimes exhibiting a susceptibility to tear or bleed with scratching or intercourse. The atrophy seems to be more enduring in these areas. Therefore, careful instruction about the duration of therapy must be given (e.g., twice a day for 10 days). If the disease does not resolve quickly with topical therapy, reevaluation is necessary.

Steroid injection sites. Atrophy may appear very rapidly after intralesional injection of corticosteroids (e.g., for treatment of acne cysts or in attempting to promote hair growth in alopecia areata). The side effect of atrophy is utilized to reduce the size of hypertrophic scars and keloids. When injected into the dermis, 5 mg/ml of triamcinolone acetonide (Kenalog) may produce atrophy; 10 mg/ml of triamcinolone acetonide almost always produces atrophy. For direct injection into the skin, stronger concentrations should probably be avoided.

Long-term use. Long-term use (over months) of even weak topical steroids on the upper inner thighs or in the axillae results in striae similar to those on the abdomens of pregnant women (Figure 2-17). These changes are irreversible. Pruritis in the groin area is common and patients are considerably relieved by the less potent steroids. Symptoms often recur after treatment is terminated. It is a great temptation to continue topical treatment on an ``as needed'' basis. Every attempt must be made to determine the underlying process and discourage long-term use.

Figure 2-17
Striae of the groin after long-term use of group V topical steroids for pruritus. These changes are irreversible.

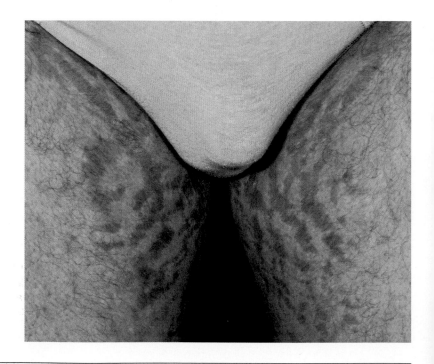

Alteration of infection

Cortisone creams applied to cutaneous infections may alter the usual clinical presentation of those diseases and produce unusual atypical eruptions.[30,31] Cortisone cream suppresses the inflammation that is attempting to contain the infection and allows unrestricted growth.

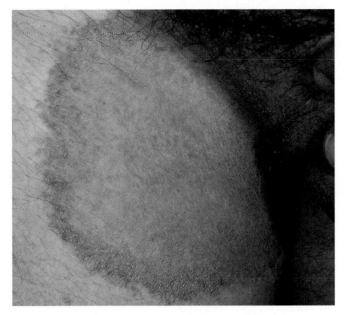

Figure 2-18
Typical presentation of tinea of the groin before treatment. Fungal infections of this type typically have a sharp, scaly border and show little tendency to spread.

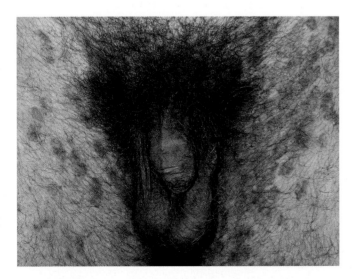

Figure 2-19
Tinea incognito. A bizarre pattern of widespread inflammation created by applying a group II topical steroid twice daily for 3 weeks to an eruption similar to that seen in Figure 2-18. A potassium hydroxide preparation showed numerous fungi.

Tinea incognito. Tinea of the groin is characteristically seen as a localized superficial plaque with a well-defined scaly border (Figure 2-18). A group II corticosteroid applied for 3 weeks to this common eruption produced the rash seen in Figure 2-19. The fungus rapidly spreads to involve a much wider area, and the typical sharply defined border is gone. Untreated tinea rarely produces such a florid eruption in temperate climates. This altered clinical picture has been called *tinea incognito.*

Figure 2-20 shows a young girl who applied a group II cream daily for 6 months to treat "eczema." The large plaques retain some of the characteristics of certain fungal infections by having well-defined edges. The red papules and nodules are atypical and are usually observed exclusively with an unusual form of follicular fungal infection seen on the lower legs.

Boils, folliculitis, rosacea-like eruptions, and diffuse fine scaling resulting from treatment of tinea with topical steroids have been reported. If a rash does not respond after a reasonable length of time or if the appearance changes, the presence of tinea, bacterial infection, or allergic contact dermatitis from some component of the steroid cream should be considered.

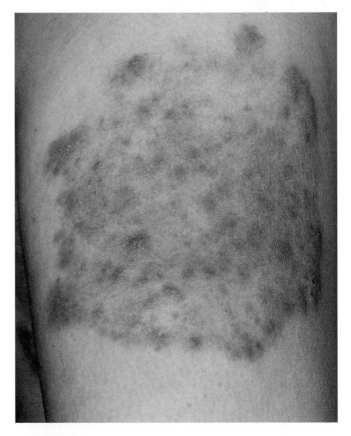

Figure 2-20
Tinea incognito. A plaque of tinea initially diagnosed as eczema was treated for 6 months with a group II topical steroid. Red papules have appeared where only erythema was once present.

Infestations and bacterial infections. Scabies and impetigo may initially improve as topical steroids suppress inflammation. Consequently, both diseases become worse when the creams are discontinued (or, possibly, continued). Figure 2-21 shows numerous pustules on a leg; this appearance is characteristic of staphylococcal infection after treatment of an exudative, infected plaque of eczema with a group V topical steroid.

Figure 2-21
Impetiginized eczema with satellite pustules after treatment of exudative, infected eczema with a group V topical steroid.

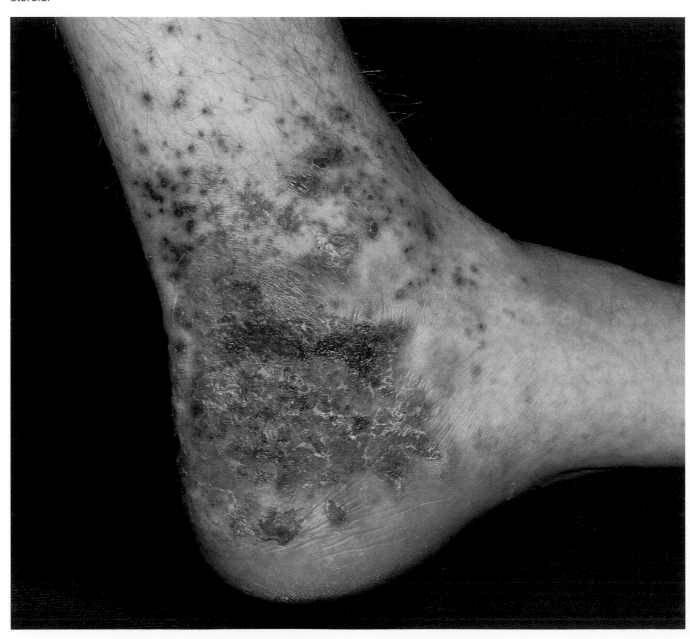

Contact dermatitis

Topical steroids are the drug of choice for allergic and irritant contact dermatitis, but occasionally topical steroids cause such dermatitis.[32] Allergic reactions to various components of steroid creams (e.g., preservatives [parabens], vehicle [lanolin], antibacterials [neomycin], and perfumes [Mycolog cream]) have all been documented. Figure 2-22 shows allergic contact dermatitis to a preservative in a group II steroid gel. The cream was prescribed to treat seborrheic dermatitis. Allergic reactions may not be intense. Inflammation created by a cream component (e.g., a preservative) may be suppressed by the steroid component of the same cream and the eruption simply smolders, neither improving nor worsening, presenting a very confusing picture.

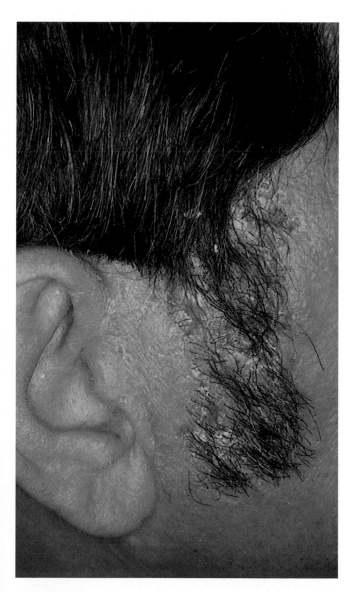

Figure 2-22
Acute contact allergy to a preservative in a group II steroid gel.

Hydrocortisone Sensitivity

Allergic hypersensitivity to topical steroids is becoming increasingly recognized. Patients with any condition that does not improve or that deteriorates after administration of hydrocortisone may be allergic to a component of the base or to the medication itself.[33] Patients with stasis dermatitis and leg ulceration who are apt to use several topical medications for extended periods are more likely to be allergic to hydrocortisone.[34] The over-the-counter availability of hydrocortisone makes long-term, unsupervised use possible. Allergy to hydrocortisone is demonstrated by patch or intradermal testing.

If inflammation improves and then suddenly worsens during treatment with a topical steroid, allergic contact dermatitis to some component of that cream should be considered.

Glaucoma

There are isolated case reports of glaucoma occurring after the long-term use of topical steroids about the eyes.[35] Glaucoma induced by the chronic use of steroid-containing eyedrops instilled directly into the conjunctival sac is encountered more frequently by ophthalmologists. The mechanism by which glaucoma develops from topical application is not understood, but presumably, cream applied to the lids seeps over the lid margin and into the conjunctival sac. It also seems possible that enough steroid could be absorbed directly through the lid skin into the conjunctival sac to produce the same results.

Inflammation about the eye is a common problem. Offending agents that cause inflammation may be directly transferred to the eyelids by rubbing with the hand, or they may be applied directly, as with cosmetics. Women who are sensitive to a favorite eye makeup often continue using that makeup on an interrupted basis, not suspecting the obvious source of allergy. Patients have been known to alternate topical steroids with a sensitizing makeup. Unsupervised use of over-the-counter hydrocortisone cream might also induce glaucoma.

No studies have yet determined what quantity or strength of steroid cream is required to produce glaucoma. The patient shown in Figure 2-13 used a group II topical steroid on the eyelids daily for 3 years. Severe atrophy and bleeding with the slightest trauma occurred, and ocular pressure was elevated.

It is good practice to restrict the use of topical steroids on the eyelids to a 2- to 3-week period and use only groups VI and VII preparations.

REFERENCES

1. Dahl MV, Dahl AC: 12% lactate lotion for the treatment of xerosis, *Arch Dermatol* 119:27-30, 1983.
2. Stoughton RB: A perspective of topical corticosteroid therapy. In Farber E, Cox A, editors: *Psoriasis: proceedings of the second international symposium*, New York, 1976, Yorke Medical Books.
3. Stoughton RB: Are generic formulations equivalent to brand name topical glucocorticosteroids? *Arch Dermatol* 121:1312-1314, 1987.
4. Olsen EA, Cornell RC: Topical clobetasol-17-propionate: review of its clinical efficacy and safety, *J Am Acad Dermatol* 15:246-255, 1986.
5. Gammon WR, Krueger GG, Van Scott EJ, et al: Intermittent short courses of clobetasol propionate ointment 0.05% in the treatment of psoriasis, *Curr Ther Res* 42:419-427, 1987.
6. Hardil E, Lindstrom C, Moller H: Intermittent treatment of psoriasis with clobetasol propionate, *Act Derm Venereol* (Stockh) 58:375-377, 1978.
7. Katz HI, Hien NT, Prawer SE, et al: Superpotent topical steroid treatment of psoriasis vulgaris: clinical efficacy and adrenal function, *J Am Acad Dermatol* 16:804-811, 1987.
8. Olsen EA: A double-blind controlled comparison of generic and trade-name topical steroids using the vasoconstriction assay, *Arch Dermatol* 127:197-201, 1991.
9. Stoughton RB: Are topical glucocorticosteroids equivalent to the brand name? *J Am Acad Dermatol* 18:138-139, 1988 (editorial).
10. Fisher AA: Problems associated with "generic" topical medications, *Cutis* 41:313-314, 1988.
11. Stoughton RB: Bioassay systems for formulations of topically applied glucocorticoids, *Arch Dermatol* 106:825, 1972.
12. McKenzie AW: Percutaneous absorption of steroids, *Arch Dermatol* 86:911, 1972.
13. Leyden JJ, Kligman AM: The case for topical antibiotics, *Prog Dermatol* 10(4) 1976.
14. Rasmussen JE: The case against topical antibiotics, *Prog Dermatol* 11(1) 1977.
15. Schlagel CA, Sanborn ED: The weights of topical preparations required for total and partial body inunction, *J Invest Dermatol* 42:252, 1964.
16. Long CC, Finlay AY: The finger-tip unit—a new practical measure, *Clin Exp Dermatol* 16:444-447, 1991.
17. Long CC, Averill RW: The rule of hand: 4 hand areas—2 FTU=1 g, *Arch Dermatol* 128:1129-1130, 1992.
18. duVivier A: Tachyphylaxis to topically applied steroids, *Arch Dermatol* 112:1245-1248, 1976.
19. Svartholm H, Larsson L, Frederiksen B: Intermittent topical treatment of psoriasis with clobetasol propionate ('Dermovate'), *Curr Med Res Opin* 8:154-157, 1982.
20. Moller H, Svartholm H, Dahl G: Intermittent maintenance therapy in chronic hand eczema with clobetasol propionate and fluprednidan acetate, *Curr Med Res Opin* 8:640-644, 1983.
21. Sulzberger MD, Witten VH: Thin pliable plastic films in topical dermatologic therapy, *Arch Dermatol* 84:1027, 1961.
22. Munto DD: *Percutaneous absorption in humans with particular reference to topical steroids and their systemic influence*, doctoral thesis, 1975, University of London.
23. May P, Stein EJ, Ryter RJ, et al: Cushing's syndrome from percutaneous absorption of triamcinolone cream, *Arch Intern Med* 136:612, 1976.
24. Gomez EC, Kaminester L, Frost P: Topical halcinonide cream and betamethasone valerate: effects on plasma cortisol, *Arch Dermatol* 113:1196, 1977.
25. Rasmussen JE: Percutaneous absorption of topically applied triamcinolone acetonide in children, *Arch Dermatol* 114:1165, 1978.
26. Rasmussen JE: Percutaneous absorption in children. In Dobson RL, editor: *1979 Year Book of Dermatology*, Chicago, Year Book Medical Publishers.
27. Leyden JJ, Thew M, Kligman AM: Steroid rosacea, *Arch Dermatol* 110:619, 1974.
28. Sneddon IB: The treatment of steroid-induced rosacea and perioral dermatitis, *Dermatologica* 152(suppl 1):231, 1976.
29. Goldman L, Kitzmiller KW: Perianal atrophoderma from topical corticosteroids, *Arch Dermatol* 107:611, 1973.
30. Ive FA, Mark SR: Tinea incognito, *Br Med J* 3:149-152, 1968.
31. Burry J: Topical drug addiction: adverse effects of fluorinated corticosteroid creams and ointments, *Med J Aust* 1:393, 1973.
32. Fisher AA, Pascher F, Kanof N: Allergic contact dermatitis due to ingredients of vehicles, *Arch Dermatol* 104:286, 1971.
33. Wilkinson SM, Cartwright PH, et al: Hydrocortisone: an important cutaneous allergen, *Lancet* 337:761-762, 1991.
34. Wilkinson SM, English JSC: Hydrocortisone sensitivity: clinical features of fifty-nine cases, *J Am Acad Dermatol* 27:683-687, 1992.
35. Brubaker RF, Halpin JA: Open angle glaucoma associated with topical administration of flurandrenolide to the eye, *Mayo Clin Proc* 50:320, 1975.

CHAPTER THREE

Eczema and Hand Dermatitis

Eczema (eczematous inflammation) is the most common inflammatory skin disease. Although the term *dermatitis* is often used to refer to an eczematous eruption, the word means inflammation of the skin and is not synonymous with *eczematous processes*. Recognizing a rash as eczematous rather than psoriasiform or lichenoid, for example, is of fundamental importance if one is to effectively diagnose skin disease. Here, as with other skin diseases, it is important to look carefully at the rash and to determine the primary lesion.

It is essential to recognize the quality and characteristics of the components of eczematous inflammation (erythema, scale, and vesicles) and to determine how these differ from other rashes with similar features. Once familiar with these features, the experienced clinician can recognize a process as being eczematous even in the presence of secondary changes produced by scratching, infection, or irritation. With the diagnosis of eczematous inflammation established, a major part of the diagnostic puzzle has been solved.

Three stages of eczema. There are three stages of eczema: acute, subacute, and chronic. Each represents a stage in the evolution of a dynamic inflammatory process (Table 3-1). Clinically, an eczematous disease may start at any stage and evolve into another. Most eczematous diseases, if left alone (i.e., neither irritated, scratched, nor medicated), resolve in time without complication. This ideal situation is almost never realized; scratching, irritation, or attempts at topical treatment are almost inevitable. Some degree of itching is a cardinal feature of eczematous inflammation.

TABLE 3-1 Eczematous Inflammation

Stage	Primary and secondary lesions	Symptoms	Etiology and clinical presentation	Treatment
Acute	Vesicles, blisters, intense red	Intense itch	Contact allergy (poison ivy), severe irritation, id reaction, acute nummular eczema, stasis dermatitis, pompholyx (dyshidrosis), fungal infections	Cold wet compresses, oral or intramuscular steroids, topical steroids, antihistamines, antibiotics
Subacute	Red, scale, fissuring, parched appearance, scalded appearance	Slight to moderate itch, pain, stinging, burning	Contact allergy, irritation, atopic dermatitis, stasis dermatitis, nummular eczema, asteatotic eczema, fingertip eczema, fungal infections	Topical steroids with or without occlusion, lubrication, antihistamines, antibiotics, tar
Chronic	Thickened skin, skin lines accentuated (lichenified skin), excoriations, fissuring	Moderate to intense itch	Atopic dermatitis, habitual scratching, lichen simplex chronicus, chapped fissured feet, nummular eczema, asteatotic eczema, fingertip eczema, hyperkeratotic eczema	Topical steroids (with occlusion for best results), intralesional steroids, antihistamines, antibiotics, lubrication

Stages of Eczematous Inflammation

ACUTE ECZEMATOUS INFLAMMATION

Etiology. Inflammation is caused by contact with specific allergens such as *Rhus* (poison ivy, oak, or sumac) and chemicals. In the id reaction, vesicular reactions occur at a distant site during or after a fungal infection, stasis dermatitis, or other acute inflammatory processes.

Physical findings. The degree of inflammation varies from moderate to intense. A bright red, swollen plaque with a pebbly surface evolves in hours. Close examination of the surface reveals tiny, clear, serum-filled vesicles (Figures 3-1 and 3-2). The eruption may not progress or it may go on to develop blisters. The vesicles and blisters may be confluent and are often linear. Linear lesions result from dragging the offending agent across the skin with the finger during scratching. The degree of inflammation in cases caused by allergy is directly proportional to the quantity of antigen deposited on the skin. Excoriation predisposes to infection and causes serum, crust, and purulent material to accumulate.

Symptoms. Acute eczema itches intensely. Patients scratch the eruption even while sleeping. A hot shower temporarily relieves itching because the pain produced by hot water is better tolerated than the sensation of itching; however, heat aggravates acute eczema.

Course. Lesions may begin to appear from hours to 2 to 3 days after exposure and may continue to appear for a week or more. These later-occurring, less inflammatory lesions are confusing to the patient, who cannot recall additional exposure. Lesions produced by small amounts of allergen are slower to evolve. They are not produced, as is generally felt, by contact with the serum of ruptured blisters, because the blister fluid does not contain the offending chemical. Acute eczematous inflammation evolves into a subacute stage before resolving.

Treatment

Cool wet dressings. The evaporative cooling produced by wet compresses causes vasoconstriction and rapidly suppresses inflammation and itching. Burow's powder, available in a 12-packet box, may be added to the solution to suppress bacterial growth, but water alone is usually sufficient. A clean cotton cloth is soaked in cool water, folded several times, and placed directly over the affected areas (see p. 26). Evaporative cooling produces vasoconstriction and decreases serum production. Wet compresses should not be held in place and covered with towels or plastic wrap because this prevents evaporation. The wet cloth macerates vesicles and, when removed, mechanically debrides the area and prevents serum and crust from accumulating. Wet compresses should be removed after 30 minutes and replaced with a freshly soaked cloth. It is tempting to leave the drying compress in place and rewet it by pouring solution onto the cloth. Although evaporative cooling will continue, irritation may occur from the accumulation of scale, crust, serum, and the increased concentration of aluminum sulfate and calcium acetate, the active ingredients in Burow's powder.

Oral corticosteroids. Oral corticosteroids such as prednisone are useful for controlling intense or widespread inflammation and may be used in addition to wet dressings. Prednisone controls most cases of poison ivy when it is taken in 20-mg doses twice a day for 7 to 14 days (for adults); however, to treat intense or generalized inflammation, prednisone may be started at 30 mg or more twice a day and maintained at that level for 3 to 5 days. Sometimes 21 days of treatment are required for adequate control. The dosage should not be tapered for these relatively short courses because lower dosages may not give the desired antiinflammatory effect. Inflammation may reappear as diffuse erythema and may even be more extensive if the dosage is too low or is tapered too rapidly. Commercially available steroid dose packs taper the dosage and treat for too short a time, therefore they should not be used. Topical corticosteroids are of little use in the acute stage because the cream does not penetrate through the vesicles.

Antihistamines. Antihistamines, such as diphenhydramine (Benadryl) and hydroxyzine (Atarax), do not alter the course of the disease, but they relieve itching and provide enough sedation so patients can sleep. They are given every 4 hours as needed.

Antibiotics. The use of oral antibiotics may greatly hasten resolution of the disease if signs of superficial secondary infection, such as pustules, purulent material, and crusts, are present. *Staphylococcus* is the usual pathogen, and cultures are not routinely necessary. Deep infection (cellulitis) is rare with acute eczema. Erythromycin, cephalexin, and dicloxacillin are effective. Topical antibiotics are much less effective.

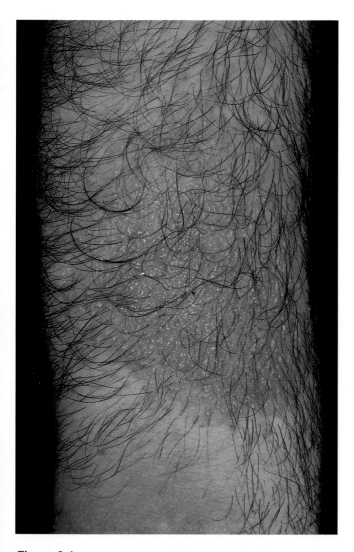

Figure 3-1
Acute eczematous inflammation. Numerous vesicles on an erythematous base. The vesicles may become confluent with time.

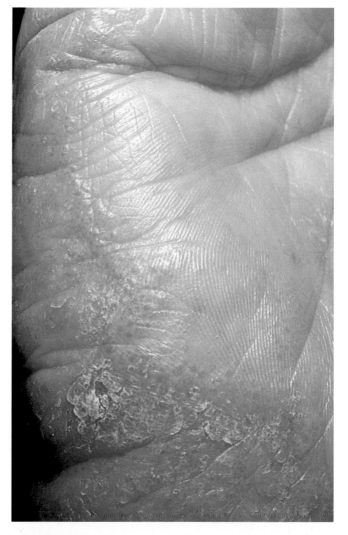

Figure 3-2
Acute eczematous inflammation. Vesicle appeared during a 24-hour period in this patient with chronic hand eczema. Episodes of acute inflammation had occurred several times in the past.

SUBACUTE ECZEMATOUS INFLAMMATION

Physical findings. Erythema and scale are present in various patterns, usually with indistinct borders (Figures 3-3 and 3-4). The redness may be faint or intense (Figures 3-5, 3-6, 3-7, and 3-8). Psoriasis, superficial fungal infections, and eczematous inflammation may have a similar appearance (Figures 3-9, 3-10, and 3-11). The borders of the plaques of psoriasis and superficial fungal infections are well defined. Psoriatic plaques have a deep, rich red color and silvery white scales.

Symptoms. These vary from no itching to intense itching.

Course. Subacute eczematous inflammation may be the initial stage or it may follow acute inflammation. Irritation, allergy, or infection can convert a subacute process into an acute one. Subacute inflammation resolves spontaneously without scarring if all sources of irritation and allergy are withdrawn. Excess drying created from washing or continued use of wet dressings causes cracking and fissures. If excoriation is not controlled, the subacute process can be converted to a chronic one. Diseases that have subacute eczematous inflammation as a characteristic are listed in the box at right.

SUBACUTE ECZEMATOUS INFLAMMATION AS A CHARACTERISTIC

Allergic contact dermatitis	Intertrigo
Asteatotic eczema	Irritant contact dermatitis
Atopic dermatitis	Irritant hand eczema
Chapped fissured feet	Nipple eczema
(sweaty sock dermatitis)	(nursing mothers)
Circumileostomy eczema	Nummular eczema
Diaper dermatitis	Perioral lick eczema
Exposure to chemicals	Statis dermatitis

Treatment. It is important to discontinue wet dressings when acute inflammation evolves into subacute inflammation. Excess drying creates cracking and fissures, which predispose to infection.

Topical corticosteroids. These agents are the treatment of choice (see Chapter Two). Creams may be applied 2 to 4 times a day or with occlusion. Ointments may be applied 2

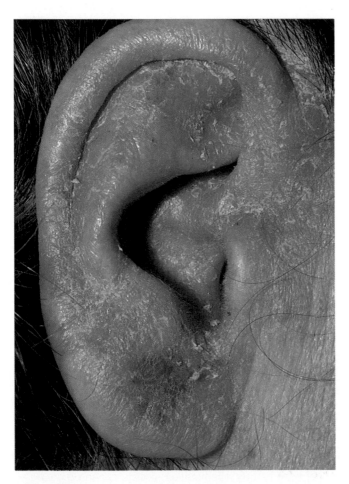

Figure 3-3
Subacute and chronic eczematous inflammation. The skin is dry, red, scaling, and thickened.

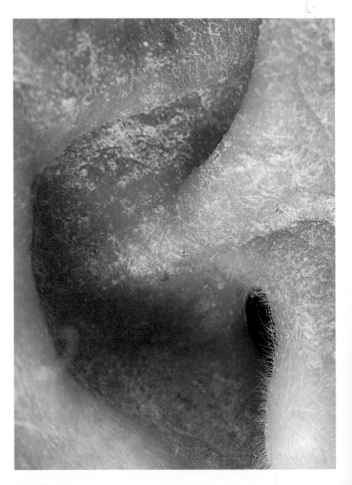

Figure 3-4
Subacute and chronic eczematous inflammation. The ear canal is red, scaling, and thickened from chronic excoriation.

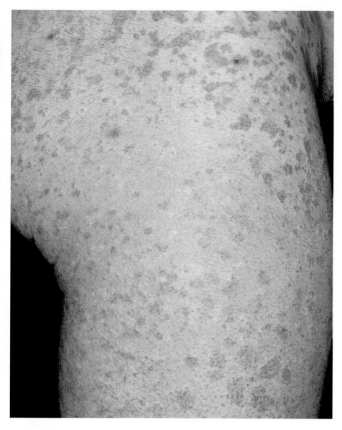

Figure 3-5
Subacute eczematous inflammation. Red, scaling, nummular (round) superficial plaques occurred during the winter months from excessive washing.

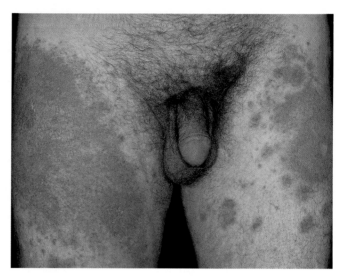

Figure 3-6
Subacute eczematous inflammation. Erythema and scaling are present, the surface is dry, and the borders are indistinct.

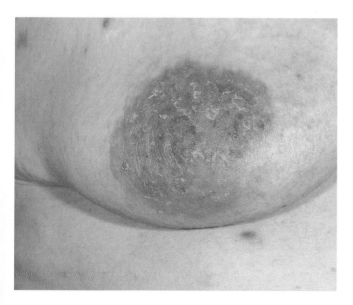

Figure 3-7
Subacute eczematous inflammation. The areolae of both breasts are red and scaly. Inflammation of one areola is characteristic of Paget's disease.

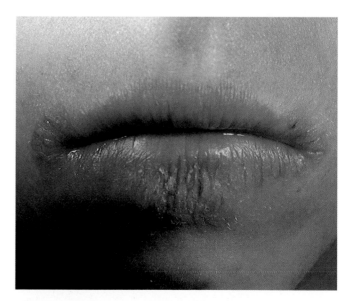

Figure 3-8
Subacute eczematous inflammation. Wetting the lip by licking will eventually cause chapping and then eczema.

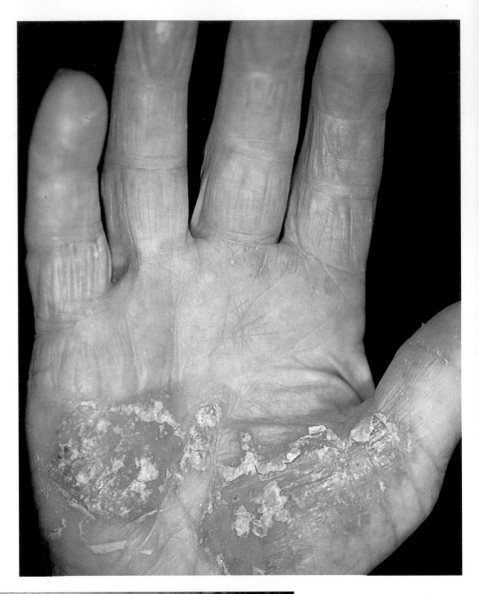

Figure 3-9
Subacute eczematous inflammation.
Acute vesicular eczema has evolved
into subacute eczema with redness and
scaling.

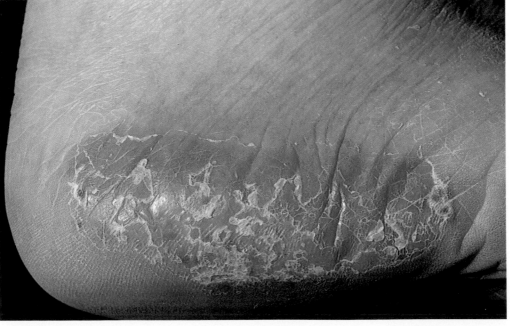

Figure 3-10
Acute and subacute
eczematous inflammation.
Acute vesicular eczema
is evolving into subacute
eczema. Vesicles, redness,
and scaling are all present
in this lesion undergoing
transition.

to 4 times a day for drier lesions. Subacute inflammation requires groups III through V corticosteroids for rapid control. Occlusion with creams hastens resolution, and less expensive, weaker products such as triamcinolone cream 0.1% (Kenalog) give excellent results. *Staphylococcus aureus* colonizes eczematous lesions, but studies show their numbers are significantly reduced following treatment with topical steroids.[1]

Lubrication. This is a simple but essential part of therapy. Inflamed skin becomes dry and is more susceptible to further irritation and inflammation. Resolved dry areas may easily relapse into subacute eczema if proper lubrication is neglected. Lubricants are best applied a few hours after topical steroids and should be continued for days or weeks after the inflammation has cleared. Frequent application (3 to 4 times a day) should be encouraged. Applying lubricants directly after the skin has been patted dry following a shower seals in moisture (the skin should be dried before the lubricants are applied). Lotions or creams with or without the hydrating chemicals urea and lactic acid may be used. Bath oils are very useful if used in amounts sufficient to make the skin feel oily when the patient leaves the tub.

Lotions. Keri, Lacticare (lactic acid), Nutraderm, Nutraplus (10% urea), or any of the other lotions listed in the Formulary, are useful.

Creams. Nutraderm, Nutraplus (10% urea), Keri, Neutrogena, Nivea, Purpose, Eucerin, and Shepard's creams, or any of the other creams listed in the Formulary, are useful.

Mild soaps. Frequent washing with a drying soap, such as Ivory, delays healing. Infrequent washing with mild or superfatted soaps (e.g., Dove, Cetaphil, Keri, Purpose, or Basis [see the Formulary]) should be encouraged. It is usually not necessary to use hypoallergenic soaps or to avoid perfumed soaps. Although allergy to perfumes occurs, the incidence is low.

Antibiotics. Eczematous plaques that remain bright red during treatment with topical steroids may be infected. Infected subacute eczema should be treated with appropriate systemic antibiotics, which are usually those active against staphylococci. Systemic antibiotics are more effective than topical antibiotics or antibiotic-steroid combination creams.

Tar. Tar ointments, baths, and soaps were among the few effective therapeutic agents available for the treatment of eczema before the introduction of topical steroids. Topical steroids provide rapid and lasting control of eczema in most cases. Some forms of eczema, such as atopic dermatitis and irritant eczema, tend to recur. Topical steroids become less effective with long-term use. Tar is an effective alternative in this setting. Tar ointments or creams may be used for long-term control or between short courses of topical steroids.

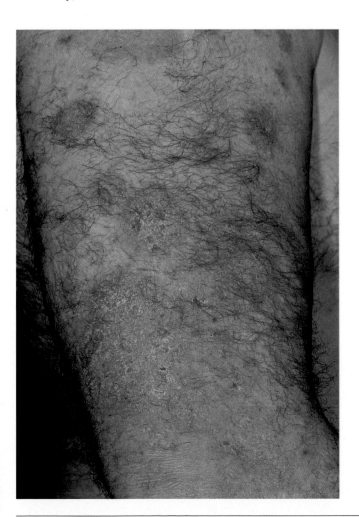

Figure 3-11
Subacute eczematous inflammation. Erythema and scaling in a round or nummular pattern.

CHRONIC ECZEMATOUS INFLAMMATION

Etiology. Chronic eczematous inflammation may be caused by irritation of subacute inflammation, or it may appear as lichen simplex chronicus.

Physical findings. Chronic eczematous inflammation is a clinical-pathologic entity and does not indicate simply any long-lasting stage of eczema. If scratching is not controlled, subacute eczematous inflammation can be modified and converted to chronic eczematous inflammation (Figure 3-12). The inflamed area thickens, and surface skin markings may become more prominent. Thick plaques with deep parallel skin marking ("washboard lesion") are said to be lichenified (Figure 3-13). The border is well defined but not as sharply defined as it is in psoriasis (Figure 3-14). The sites most commonly involved are those areas that are easily reached and associated with habitual scratching (e.g., dorsal feet, lateral forearms, anus, and occipital scalp), areas where eczema tends to be long lasting (e.g., the lower legs, as in stasis dermatitis), and the crease areas (antecubital and popliteal fossa, wrists, and ankles) in atopic dermatitis (Figures 3-15, 3-16, and 3-17).

Symptoms. There is moderate to intense itching. Scratching sometimes becomes violent, leading to excoriation and digging, and ceases only when pain has replaced the itch. Patients with chronic inflammation scratch while asleep.

Course. Scratching and rubbing become habitual and are often done unconsciously. The disease then becomes self-perpetuating. Scratching leads to thickening of the skin, which itches more than before. It is this habitual manipulation that causes the difficulty in eradicating this disease. Some patients enjoy the feeling of relief that comes from scratching and may actually desire the reappearance of their disease after treatment.

Treatment. Chronic eczematous inflammation is resistant to treatment and requires potent steroid therapy.

Topical steroids. Groups II through V topical steroids are used with occlusion each night until the inflammation clears—usually in 1 to 3 weeks. Group I topical steroids are used without occlusion.

Intralesional injection. Intralesional injection (Kenalog, 10 mg/ml) is a very effective mode of therapy. Lesions that have been present for years may completely resolve after one injection or a short series of injections. The medicine is delivered with a 27- or 30-gauge needle, and the entire plaque is infiltrated until it blanches white. Resistant plaques require additional injections given at 3- to 4-week intervals.

Excision. Excision is rarely necessary, but should be considered if multiple intralesional injections fail and if the lesion is very hypertrophic.

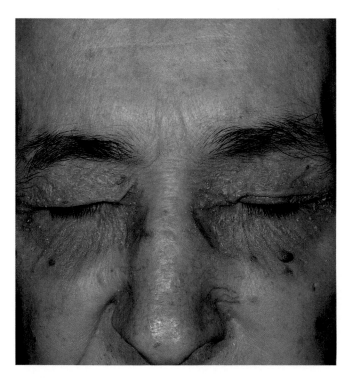

Figure 3-12
Subacute and chronic eczema. Dermatitis of the lids may be allergic, irritant, or atopic in origin. This atopic patient rubs the lids with the back of the hands.

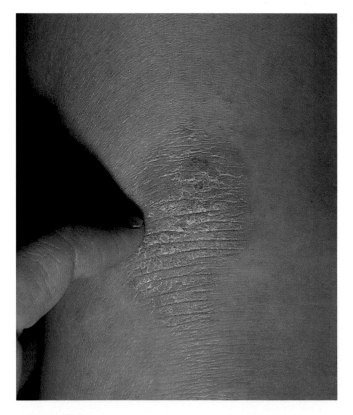

Figure 3-13
Chronic eczematous inflammation. Chronic excoriations thicken the epidermis, which results in accentuated skin lines. Chronic eczema created by picking is called lichen simplex chronicus.

CHRONIC ECZEMATOUS INFLAMMATION

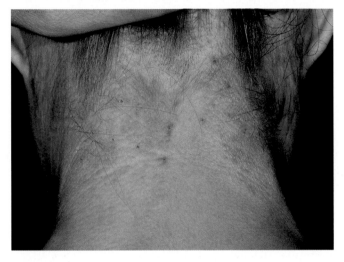

Figure 3-14
Erythema and scaling are present, and the skin lines are accentuated, creating a lichenified or "washboard" lesion.

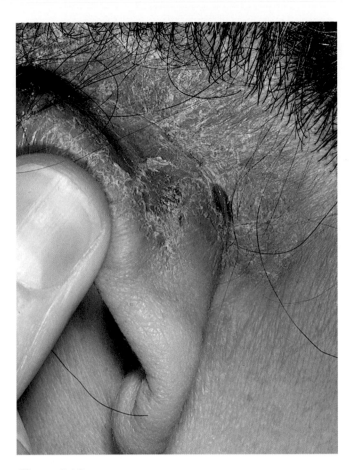

Figure 3-15
Picking and rubbing thickened the skin behind the ear.

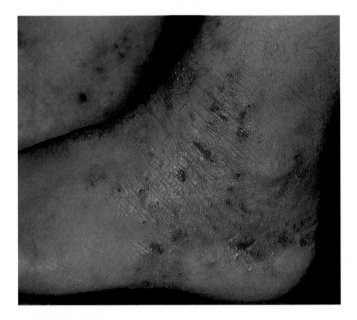

Figure 3-16
Atopic dermatitis. Atopic dermatitis is common in the crease areas. Atopic patients scratch, lichenify the skin, and often create a chronic process.

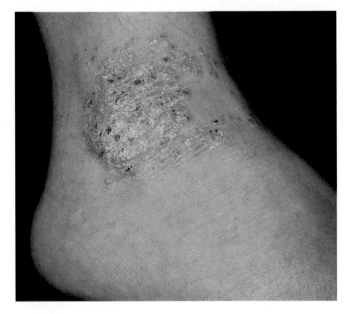

Figure 3-17
A plaque of lichen simplex chronicus created by excoriation is present. Accentuated skin lines and eczematous papules beyond the border help to differentiate this process from psoriasis.

From Meding B, Swanbeck G: Predictive factors for hand eczema, *Contact Dermatitis* 23:154-161, 1990.

Hand Eczema

Inflammation of the hands is one of the most common problems encountered by the dermatologist. Hand dermatitis causes discomfort and embarrassment and, because of its location, interferes significantly with normal daily activities. Hand dermatitis is common in industrial occupations:[2] it can threaten job security if inflammation cannot be controlled.[3] The box at left lists instructions for patients with irritant hand dermatitis.

Epidemiology. A large study provided the following statistics: the prevalence of hand eczema was approximately 5.4%. It was twice as common in females as in males. The most common type of hand eczema was irritant contact dermatitis (35%), followed by atopic hand eczema (22%), and allergic contact dermatitis (19%). The most common contact allergies were to nickel, cobalt, fragrance mix, balsam of Peru, and colophony. Of all the occupations studied, cleaners had the highest prevalence, at 21.3%. Hand eczema was more common among people reporting occupational exposure. The most harmful exposure was to chemicals, water and detergents, dust, and dry dirt. A change of occupation was reported by 8% and was most common in service workers. Hairdressers had the highest frequency of change. Hand eczema was shown to be a long-lasting disease with a relapsing course. Sixty-nine percent of the patients had consulted a physician, and 21% had been on sick leave at least once because of hand eczema. The mean total sick-leave time was 18.9 weeks, the median was 8 weeks.[4]

The most important predictive factors for hand eczema are listed in the box at left.

Diagnosis. The diagnosis and management of hand eczema is a challenge. There is almost no association between clinical pattern and etiology. No distribution of eczema is typically allergic, irritant, or endogenous.[5] Not only are there many patterns of eczematous inflammation (Table 3-2), but there are other diseases, such as psoriasis, that may appear eczematous. The original primary lesions and their distribution become modified with time by irritants, excoriation, infection, and treatment. All stages of eczematous inflammation may be encountered in hand eczema.

Various types of hand eczema

Irritant	Keratolysis exfoliativa
Atopic	Fingertip
Allergic	Hyperkeratotic
Nummular	Pompholyx (dyshidrosis)
Lichen simplex chronicus	Id reaction

TABLE 3-2 Hand Dermatitis: Differential Diagnosis and Distribution

Location	Redness and scaling	Vesicles	Pustules
Back of hand	Atopic dermatitis Irritant contact dermatitis Lichen simplex chronicus Nummular eczema Psoriasis Tinea	Id reaction Scabies (web spaces)	Bacterial infection Psoriasis Scabies (web spaces) Tinea
Palmar surface	Fingertip eczema Hyperkeratotic eczema Keratolysis exfoliativa Psoriasis Tinea	Allergic contact dermatitis Pompholyx (dyshidrosis)	Bacterial infection Pompholyx (dyshidrosis) Psoriasis

IRRITANT CONTACT DERMATITIS

Irritant hand dermatitis (housewives' eczema, dishpan hands, detergent hands) is the most common type of hand inflammation. Some people can withstand long periods of repeated exposure to various chemicals and maintain normal skin. At the other end of the spectrum, there are those who develop chapping and eczema from simple hand washing. Patients whose hands are easily irritated may have an atopic diathesis.

Pathophysiology. The stratum corneum is the protective envelope that prevents exogenous material from entering the skin and prevents body water from escaping. The stratum corneum is composed of dead cells, lipids (from sebum and cellular debris), and water-binding organic chemicals. The stratum corneum of the palms is thicker than that of the dorsa and is more resistant to irritation. The pH of this surface layer is slightly acidic. Environmental factors or elements that change any component of the stratum corneum interfere with its protective function and expose the skin to irritants. Factors such as cold winter air and low humidity promote water loss. Substances such as organic solvents and alkaline soaps extract water-binding chemicals and lipids. Once enough of these protective elements have been extracted, the skin decompensates and becomes eczematous.

Clinical presentation. The degree of inflammation depends on factors such as strength and concentration of the chemical, individual susceptibility, site of contact, and time of year. Allergy, infection, scratching, and stress modify the picture.

Stages of inflammation. Dryness and chapping are the initial changes (Figure 3-18). Very painful cracks and fissures occur, particularly in joint crease areas and around the fingertips. The backs of the hands become red, swollen, and tender. The palmar surface, especially that of the fingers, becomes red and continues to be dry and cracked. A red, smooth, shiny, delicate surface that splits easily with the slightest trauma may develop. These are subacute eczematous changes (Figures 3-19 and 3-20).

Acute eczematous inflammation occurs with further irritation creating vesicles that ooze and crust. Itching intensifies, and excoriation leads to infection (Figure 3-21).

Necrosis and ulceration followed by scarring occur if the irritating chemical is too caustic.

Patients at risk. Individuals at risk include mothers with young children (changing diapers), individuals whose jobs require repeated wetting and drying (e.g., surgeons, dentists, dishwashers, bartenders, fishermen), industrial workers whose jobs require contact with chemicals (e.g., cutting oils), and patients with the atopic diathesis.

Prevention. One study revealed that hospital staff members who used an emulsion cleanser (e.g., Cetaphil lotion, Aquanil lotion, Duosoft [in Europe]) had significantly less dryness and eczema than those who used a liquid soap.[6] Regular use of emollients prevented irritant dermatitis caused by a detergent.[7]

Treatment. The inflammation is treated as outlined in the section on stages of eczematous inflammation. Lubrication and avoidance of further irritation helps to prevent recurrence. A program of irritant avoidance should be carefully outlined for each patient (see the box on p. 54). Photochemotherapy (PUVA) may be considered for chronic dermatitis that does not respond to any other form of therapy.[8]

IRRITANT HAND DERMATITIS

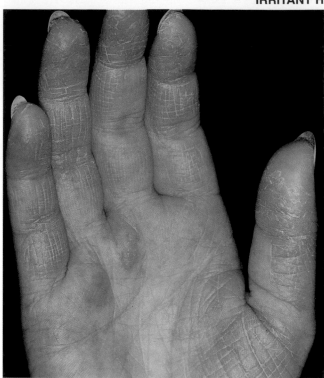

Figure 3-18
Early irritant hand dermatitis with dryness and chapping.

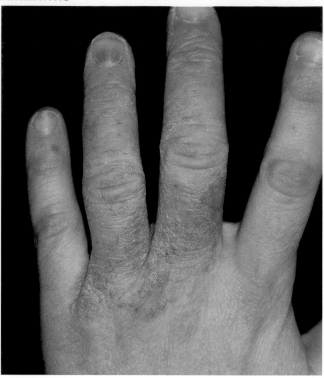

Figure 3-19
Subacute eczematous inflammation appeared on the dry, chapped third and fourth fingers.

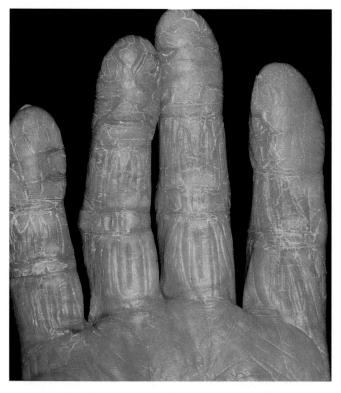

Figure 3-20
Subacute and chronic eczematous inflammation with severe drying and splitting of the fingertips.

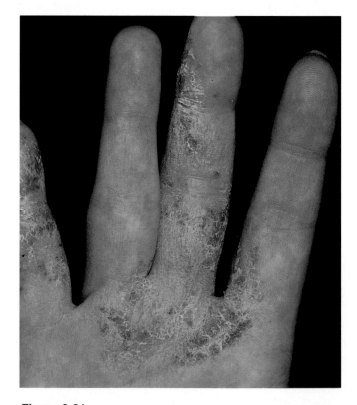

Figure 3-21
Numerous tiny vesicles suddenly appeared on these chronically inflamed fingers.

ATOPIC HAND DERMATITIS

Hand dermatitis may be the most common form of adult atopic dermatitis (see Chapter Five). Hand eczema is significantly more common in people with a history of atopic dermatitis than in others.[9] The following factors predict the occurrence of hand eczema in adults with a history of atopic dermatitis:[10]

- Hand dermatitis before age 15
- Persistent eczema on the body
- Dry or itchy skin in adult life
- Widespread atopic dermatitis in childhood

Many people with atopic dermatitis develop hand eczema independently of exposure to irritants, but such exposure causes additional irritant contact dermatitis.

The backs of the hands, particularly the fingers, are affected (Figure 3-22). The dermatitis begins as a typical irritant reaction with chapping and erythema. Several forms of eczematous dermatitis evolve. Erythema, edema, vesiculation, crusting, excoriation, scaling, and lichenification appear and are intensified by scratching.[11] Management for atopic hand eczema is the same as that for irritant hand eczema.

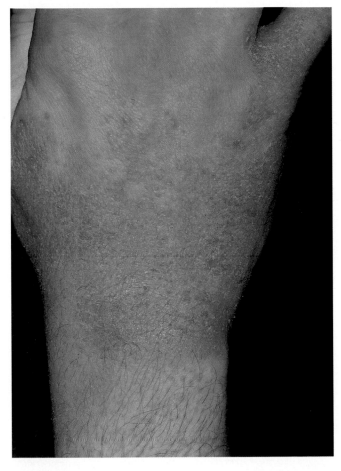

Figure 3-22
Irritant hand dermatitis in a patient with the atopic diathesis. Irritant eczema of the backs of the hands is a common form of adult atopic dermatitis.

ALLERGIC CONTACT DERMATITIS

Allergic contact dermatitis of the hands is not as common as irritant dermatitis. However, allergy as a possible cause of hand eczema, no matter what the pattern, should always be considered in the differential diagnosis; it may be investigated by patch testing in appropriate cases. The incidence of allergy in hand eczema was demonstrated by patch testing in a study of 220 patients with hand eczema.[12] In 12% of the 220 patients, the diagnosis was established with the aid of a standard screening series now available in a modified form from the Glaxo Pharmaceutical Company (T.R.U.E. TEST).[13] Another 5% of the cases were diagnosed as a result of testing with additional allergens. The hand eczema in these two groups (17%) changed dramatically after identification and avoidance of the allergens found by patch testing. Table 3-3 lists some possible causes of allergic hand dermatitis.

Physical findings. The diagnosis of allergic contact dermatitis is obvious when the area of inflammation corresponds exactly to the area covered by the allergen (e.g., a round patch of eczema under a watch or inflammation in the shape of a sandal strap on the foot). Similar clues may be present with hand eczema, but in many cases allergic and irritant hand eczemas cannot be distinguished by their clinical presentation. Hand inflammation, whatever the source, is increased by further exposure to irritating chemicals, washing, scratching, medication, and infection. Inflammation of the dorsum of the hand is more often irritant or atopic than allergic.

Treatment. Allergy may initially appear as acute, subacute, or chronic eczematous inflammation and is managed accordingly.

TABLE 3-3 Allergic Hand Dermatitis: Some Possible Causes	
Allergens	**Sources**
Nickel	Door knobs, handles on kitchen utensils, scissors, knitting needles, industrial equipment, hairdressing equipment
Potassium dichromate	Cement, leather articles (gloves), industrial machines, oils
Rubber	Gloves, industrial equipment (hoses, belts, cables)
Fragrances	Cosmetics, soaps, lubricants, topical medications
Formaldehyde	Wash and wear fabrics, paper, cosmetics, embalming fluid
Lanolin	Topical lubricants and medications, cosmetics

NUMMULAR ECZEMA

Eczema that appears as one or several coin-shaped plaques is called *nummular eczema*. This pattern often occurs on the extremities, but may present as hand eczema. The plaques are usually confined to the backs of the hands (Figure 3-23). The number of lesions may increase, but once the lesions are established they tend to remain the same size. The inflammation is either subacute or chronic. Itching is moderate to intense. The cause is unknown. Thick, chronic, scaling plaques of nummular eczema look like psoriasis. Treatment for nummular eczema is the same as that for subacute or chronic eczema.

LICHEN SIMPLEX CHRONICUS

A localized plaque of chronic eczematous inflammation that is created by habitual scratching is called *lichen simplex chronicus* or *localized neurodermatitis*. The back of the wrist is a typical site. The plaque is thick with prominent skin lines (lichenification) and the margins are fairly sharp. Once established, the plaque does not usually increase in area. Lichen simplex chronicus is treated in the same manner as chronic eczematous inflammation.

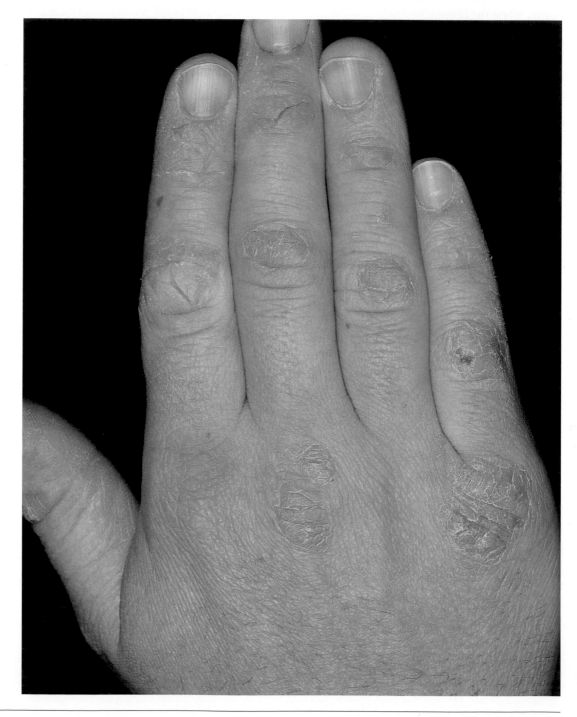

Figure 3-23
Nummular eczema. Eczematous plaques are round (coin-shaped).

KERATOLYSIS EXFOLIATIVA

Keratolysis exfoliativa is a common, chronic, asymptomatic, noninflammatory, bilateral peeling of the palms of the hands and the soles of the feet; its cause is unknown (Figure 3-24). The eruption is most common during the summer months and is often associated with sweaty palms and soles.[14] Some people experience this phenomenon only once, whereas others have repeated episodes. Scaling starts simultaneously from several points on the palms or soles with 2 or 3 mm of round scale that appears to have originated from a ruptured vesicle; however, these vesicles are never seen. The scale continues to peel and extend peripherally, forming larger, roughly circular areas that resemble ringworm, while the central area becomes slightly red and tender. The scaling borders may coalesce. The condition resolves in 1 to 3 weeks and requires no therapy other than lubrication.

HYPERKERATOTIC ECZEMA

A very thick, chronic form of eczema that occurs on the palms and occasionally the soles is seen almost exclusively in men. One or several plaques of yellow-brown, dense scale increase in thickness and form deep interconnecting cracks over the surface, similar to mud drying in a river bed (Figure 3-25). The dense scale, unlike callus, is moist below the surface and is not easily pared with a blade. Patients discover that the scale is firmly adherent to the epidermis when they attempt to peel off the thick scale and this exposes tender bleeding areas of dermis. Hyperkeratotic eczema may result from allergy or excoriation and irritation, but in most cases the cause is not apparent. The disease is chronic and may last for years. Psoriasis and lichen simplex chronicus must be considered in the differential diagnosis. The disease is treated like chronic eczema; although the plaques respond to group II steroid cream and occlusion, recurrences are frequent. Patch testing is indicated for recurrent disease.

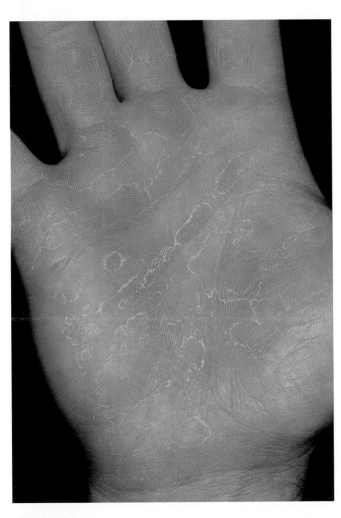

Figure 3-24
Keratolysis exfoliativa. Noninflammatory peeling of the palms that is often associated with sweating. The eruption must be differentiated from tinea of the palms.

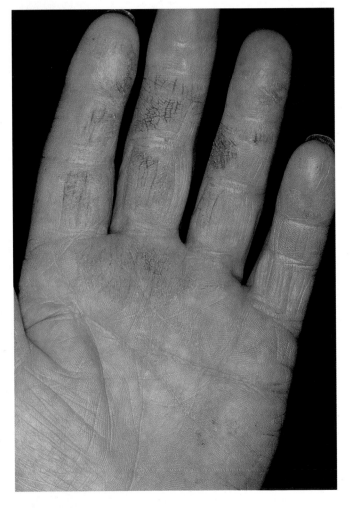

Figure 3-25
Hyperkeratotic eczema. Patches of dense yellow-brown scale occur on the palms. This patient was allergic to a steering wheel.

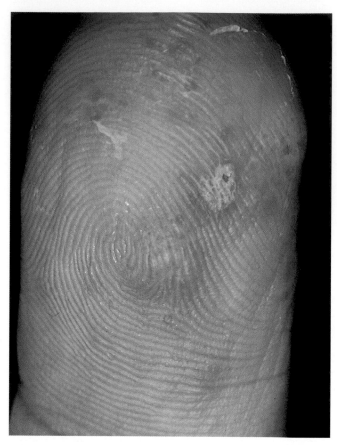

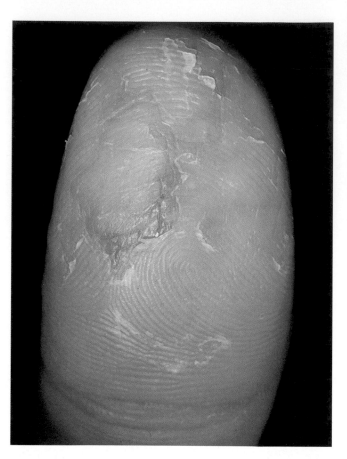

Figure 3-26
Fingertip eczema. An early stage. The skin is moist.
A vesicle is present. Redness and cracking have occurred
in the central area.

Figure 3-27
Fingertip eczema. A more advanced stage. Peeling occurs
constantly. The skin lines are lost.

Figure 3-28
Fingertip eczema may have a variety
of causes. The skin is extremely dry
and peels continuously, revealing a
red, cracked, smooth surface.

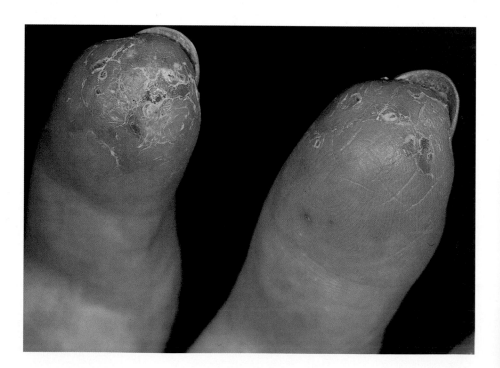

FINGERTIP ECZEMA

A very dry, chronic form of eczema of the palmar surface of the fingertips may be the result of an allergic reaction (e.g., to plant bulbs or resins) or may occur in children and adults as an isolated phenomenon of unknown cause. One finger or several fingers may be involved. Initially the skin may be moist. Moist skin becomes dry, cracked, and scaly (Figure 3-26). The skin peels from the fingertips distally, exposing a very dry, red, cracked, fissured, tender, or painful surface without skin lines (Figures 3-27, 3-28, and 3-29). The process usually stops shortly before the distal interphalangeal joint is reached (Figures 3-30 and 3-31). Fingertip eczema may last for months or years and is resistant to treatment. Topical steroids with or without occlusion give only temporary relief. Once allergy and psoriasis have been ruled out, fingertip eczema should be managed the same way as subacute and chronic eczema, by avoiding irritants and lubricating frequently. Tar creams such as Fototar applied twice each day have, at times, provided relief.

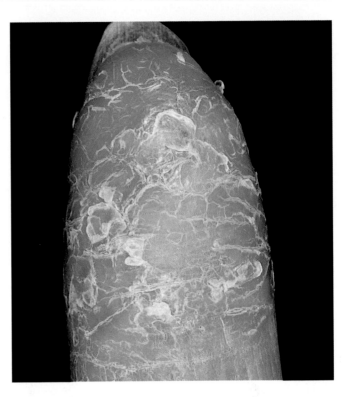

Figure 3-29
Fingertip eczema. Severe chronic inflammation. The skin lines are lost. The dry skin is fragile and cracks easily. Patients are tempted to peel away the dry loose scale.

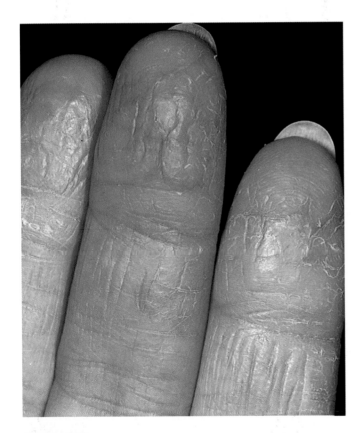

Figure 3-30
Fingertip eczema. The fingers are dry and wrinkled, and the skin is fragile. The skin peels but does not form the thick scale shown in Figures 3-26 through 3-29.

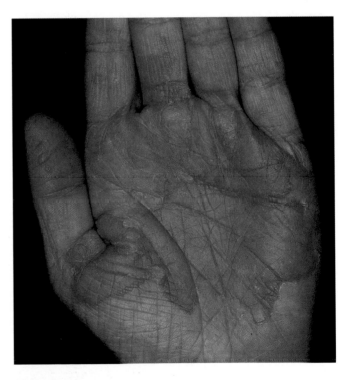

Figure 3-31
Eczema of the palm. The palms are red, but there is no scale. It appears as if a layer of skin has been peeled away. This pattern of inflammation is seen in patients with the pattern of fingertip eczema shown in Figure 3-30.

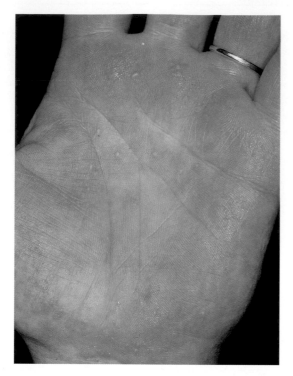

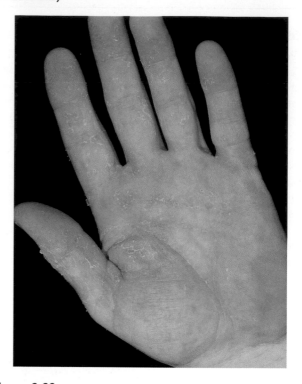

Figure 3-32
The palms are red and wet with perspiration, and numerous vesicles are present.

Figure 3-33
The vesicles have evolved, and the skin peels over the entire surface of the palm.

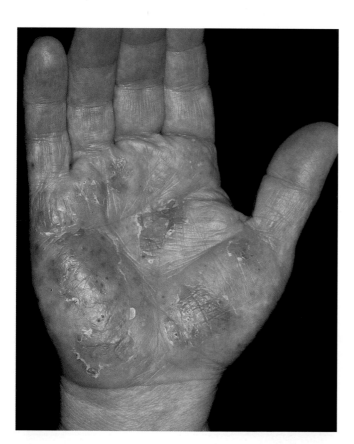

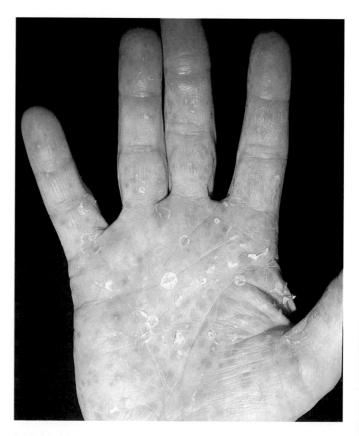

Figure 3-34
The acute process ends as the skin peels, revealing a red, cracked base with brown spots. The brown spots are sites of previous vesiculation.

Figure 3-35
A severe form (with large, deep vesicles and blisters) that is indistinguishable from pustular psoriasis of the palms and soles.

POMPHOLYX

Pompholyx (dyshidrosis) is a distinctive reaction pattern of unknown etiology presenting as symmetric, vesicular hand and foot dermatitis. Moderate to severe itching precedes the appearance of vesicles on the palms and sides of the fingers. The palms may be red and wet with perspiration; therefore the name dyshidrosis (Figure 3-32). The vesicles slowly resolve in 3 to 4 weeks and are replaced by 1- to 3-mm rings of scale. Chronic eczematous changes with erythema, scaling, and lichenification may follow. Waves of vesiculation may appear indefinitely (Figures 3-33 and 3-34). Pustular psoriasis of the palms and soles may resemble pompholyx, but the vesicles of psoriasis rapidly become cloudy with purulent fluid, and pain, rather than itching, is the chief complaint (Figure 3-35). Pustular psoriasis is chronic and the pustules do not evolve and disappear as rapidly as those of pompholyx. Patients with atopic dermatitis are affected as frequently as others.

The cause of pompholyx is unknown, but there seems to be some relationship to stress. Pompholyx is a disease that disrupts the skin and allows sensitization to contact allergens to occur, but direct contact with the allergen does not seem to be the cause of the disease. Ingestion of allergens such as chromate, neomycin, quinoline, or nickel may cause some cases.[15] Ingestion of nickel, cobalt, and chromium can elicit pompholyx in patients who are patch test negative to these metals.[16,17] The perspiration volume of pompholyx patients was found to be 2.5 times higher than that of age-matched normal controls. Twenty percent of patients showed sensitivity to chromate, 16% to cobalt, and 28% to nickel on patch testing. Some patients with positive results who are challenged orally with nickel, cobalt, or chromium show vesicular reactions on their hands. Sensitivity to orally ingested metal compounds in combination with local hyperhidrosis may contribute to the development of vesicular lesions in pompholyx.[18]

Treatment. Topical steroids, cold wet compresses, and oral erythromycin are always used as the initial treatment, but the response is often disappointing. Short courses of oral steroids are sometimes needed to control acute flares. Resistant cases might respond to PUVA.[19] Patients (64%) who flared after oral challenge to metal salt cleared or markedly improved on diets low in the incriminated metal salt, and 78% of those patients remained clear when the diet was rigorously followed (a suggested diet for nickel-sensitive patients with pompholyx appears on p. 91).[20] Attempts to control pompholyx with elimination diets may be worth a trial in difficult cases. Oral disodium cromoglycate helped selected cases of pompholyx.[21]

Administration of disulfiram (Antabuse, 200 mg/day for 8 weeks) improved the conditions of 8 of 11 women and healed 2 others with nickel sensitivity and pompholyx hand dermatitis.[22] Controlling stress and changing to a less competitive life-style is often the most effective treatment.

ID REACTION

Intense inflammatory processes, such as active stasis dermatitis or acute fungal infections of the feet, can be accompanied by an itchy, dyshidrotic-like vesicular eruption ("id reaction") (Figure 3-36). These eruptions are most common on the sides of the fingers but may be generalized. The eruptions resolve as the inflammation that initiated them resolves. The id reaction may be an allergic reaction to fungi or to some antigen created during the inflammatory process. Almost all dyshidrotic eruptions are incorrectly called *id reactions*. The diagnosis of an id reaction should not be made unless there is an acute inflammatory process at a distant site and the id reaction disappears shortly after the acute inflammation is controlled.

Figure 3-36
Id reaction. An acute vesicular eruption most often seen on the lateral aspects of the fingers.

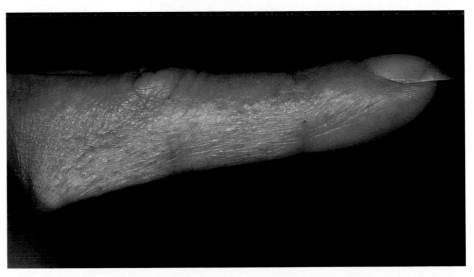

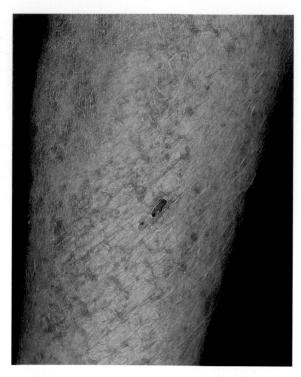

Figure 3-37
Asteatotic eczema (xerosis). The skin is extremely dry, cracked, and scaly. This pattern appears in the winter months when the air is dry.

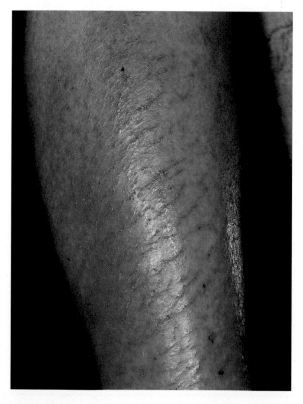

Figure 3-38
Asteatotic eczema (xerosis). Excessive washing of the dry skin shown in Figure 3-37 may result in horizontal, parallel cracks.

Eczema: Various Presentations
ASTEATOTIC ECZEMA

Asteatotic eczema (eczema craquele) occurs after excess drying, especially during the winter months and among the elderly. Patients with an atopic diathesis are more likely to develop this distinctive pattern. The eruption can occur on any skin area, but it is most commonly seen on the anterolateral aspects of the lower legs. The lower legs become dry and scaly and show accentuation of the skin lines (xerosis) (Figure 3-37). Red plaques with thin, long, horizontal superficial fissures appear with further drying and scratching (Figure 3-38). Similar patterns of inflammation may appear on the trunk and upper extremities as the winter progresses. A cracked porcelain or "crazy paving" pattern of fissuring develops when short vertical fissures connect with the horizontal fissures. The term *eczema craquele* is appropriately used to describe this pattern. The severest form of this type of eczema shows an accentuation of the above pattern with deep, wide, horizontal fissures that ooze and are often purulent (Figure 3-39). Pain, rather than itching, is the chief complaint with this condition. Scratching or treatment with drying lotions such as calamine aggravates the eczematous inflammation and leads to infection with accumulation of crusts and purulent material.

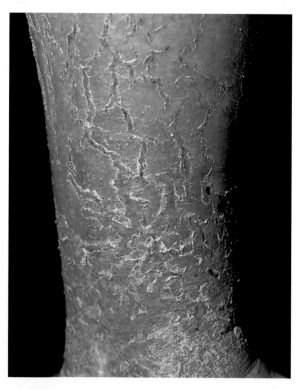

Figure 3-39
Asteatotic eczema (eczema craquele). Excessive drying on the lower legs may eventually become so severe that long, horizontal, superficial fissures appear. The fissures eventually develop a cracked porcelain or "crazy paving" pattern when short vertical fissures connect with the horizontal fissures.

Treatment. The initial stages are treated as subacute eczematous inflammation. The severest form may have to be treated as acute eczema. The treatment involves wet compresses and antibiotics to remove crust and suppress infection before group V topical steroids and lubricants are applied. Wet compresses should be used only for a short time. Prolonged use of wet compresses results in excessive drying. Lubricating the dry skin during and after topical steroid use is essential. The use of oral steroids should be avoided; the disease flares within 1 or 2 days once they are discontinued.

NUMMULAR ECZEMA

Nummular eczema is a common disease of unknown cause that occurs primarily in the middle-aged and elderly. The typical lesion is a coin-shaped, red plaque that averages 1 to 5 cm in diameter (Figure 3-40). The lesions itch, and scratching often becomes habitual. In these cases, the term *nummular neurodermatitis* has been used (Figure 3-41). With infection, the plaque becomes thicker and vesicles appear on the surface; vesicles in ringworm, if present, are at the border. Unlike the thick, silvery scale of psoriasis, this scale is thin and sparse. The erythema in psoriasis is darker. Once the disease is established, lesions may become more numerous, but individual lesions tend to remain in the same area and do not increase in size. The disease is worse in the winter. The back of the hand is the most commonly involved site; usually only one lesion or a few lesions are present (see Figure 3-23). Other frequently involved areas are the extensor aspects of the forearms and lower legs, the flanks, and the hips. Lesions in these other sites tend to be more numerous. An extensive form of the disease can occur suddenly in patients with dry skin that is exposed to an irritating medicine or chemical, or in patients who have an active eczematous process at another site, such as stasis dermatitis on the lower legs. The lesions in these cases are round, faintly erythematous, dry, cracked, superficial, and usually confluent.

The course is variable, but it is usually chronic, with some cases resisting all attempts at treatment. Many cases become inactive after several months. Lesions may reappear at previously involved sites in recurrent cases.

Treatment. Treatment depends on the stage of activity; all stages of eczematous inflammation may be present simultaneously. The red vesicular lesions are treated as acute, the red scaling plaques as subacute, and the habitually scratched thick plaques as chronic eczematous inflammation.

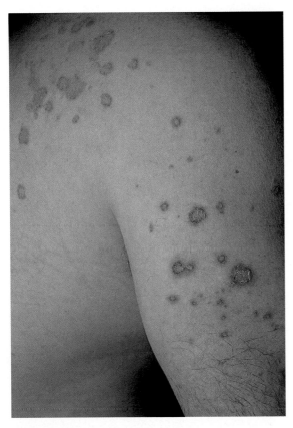

Figure 3-40
Nummular eczema. This form of eczema is of undetermined origin and is not necessarily associated with dry skin or atopy. The round, coin-shaped, eczematous plaques tend to be chronic and resistant to treatment.

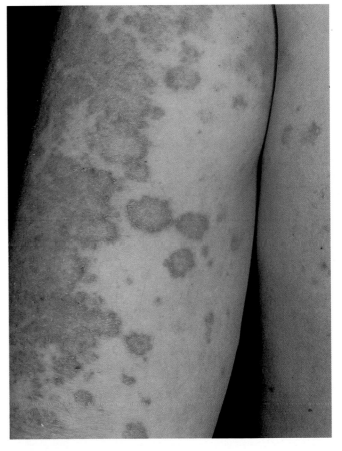

Figure 3-41
Nummular eczema. Round, eczematous plaques formed on the trunk and arms become confluent.

Chapped Fissured Feet

Clinical presentation. Chapped fissured feet (sweaty sock dermatitis, peridigital dermatitis, juvenile plantar dermatosis) are seen initially with scaling, erythema, fissuring, and loss of the epidermal ridge pattern. The tendency to severe chapping declines with age and is gone around the age of puberty. The mean age of onset is 7.3 years; the mean age of remission is 14.3 years.[23] Onset is in early fall when the weather becomes cold and heavy socks and impermeable shoes or boots are worn. An artificial intertrigo is created when moist socks are kept in contact with the soles. The skin in pressure areas, toes, and metatarsal regions becomes dry, brittle, and scaly and then fissured (Figure 3-42, *A*). The chapping extends onto the sides of the toes. Eventually, the entire sole may be involved; sometimes the hands are also affected (Figure 3-42, *B*).

The eruption lasts throughout the winter, clears without treatment in the late spring, and predictably recurs the next fall. Earlier descriptions referred to this entity as atopic winter feet in children, but the name has been changed to include patients who do not have atopic dermatitis. Atopic dermatitis of the feet in children occurs on the dorsal toes and usually not on the plantar surface, and it is itchy. The role of atopy is not yet defined.[24] Children with chapped fissured feet complain of soreness and pain. Affected individuals must be predisposed to chapping because their wearing of moist socks and impermeable boots does not differ from that of unaffected children.

Figure 3-42
Chapped fissured feet.

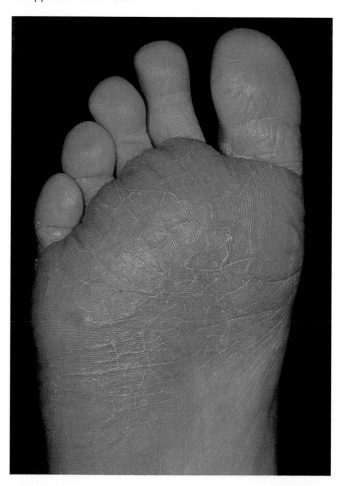

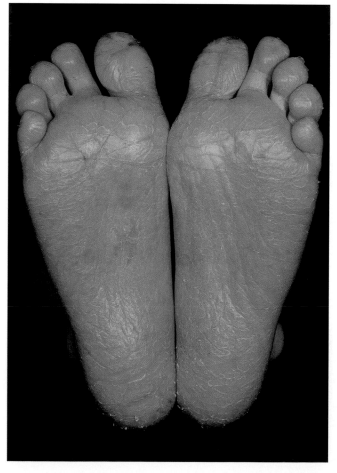

A, An early stage with erythema and cracking on pressure areas.

B, An advanced case in which the entire plantar surface is severely dried and fissured.

Differential diagnosis. The differential diagnosis includes psoriasis, tinea pedis, and allergic contact dermatitis. The erythema in psoriasis is darker and the scales shed; the scales in chapped fissured feet are adherent, and removal of the scales causes bleeding. Tinea of the feet in children is rare. Feet with the rare case of familial *Trichophyton rubrum* are pale brown and have a fine scale. Fissuring is minimal, and there is little seasonal variation. Allergic contact dermatitis to shoes usually affects the dorsal aspect and spares the soles, webs, and sides of the feet. The eruption is bright red and scaly rather than pale red and chapped.

Treatment. Treatment is less than satisfactory. Topical steroids and lubrication provide some relief. Group II or III topical steroids are applied twice each day or, preferably, with plastic wrap occlusion at bedtime. Lubricating creams are applied several times each day, especially directly after removing moist socks to seal in moisture. The feet should not be allowed to remain moist inside shoes. Preventative measures include changing into light leather shoes after removing boots at school and changing cotton socks 1 or 2 times each day.

Self-Inflicted Dermatoses

A number of skin disorders are created or perpetuated by manipulation of the skin surface (Table 3-4; Figures 3-43 and 3-44).[25-35] Patients may benefit from both dermatologic and psychiatric care. The most common self-inflicted dermatoses are discussed here.

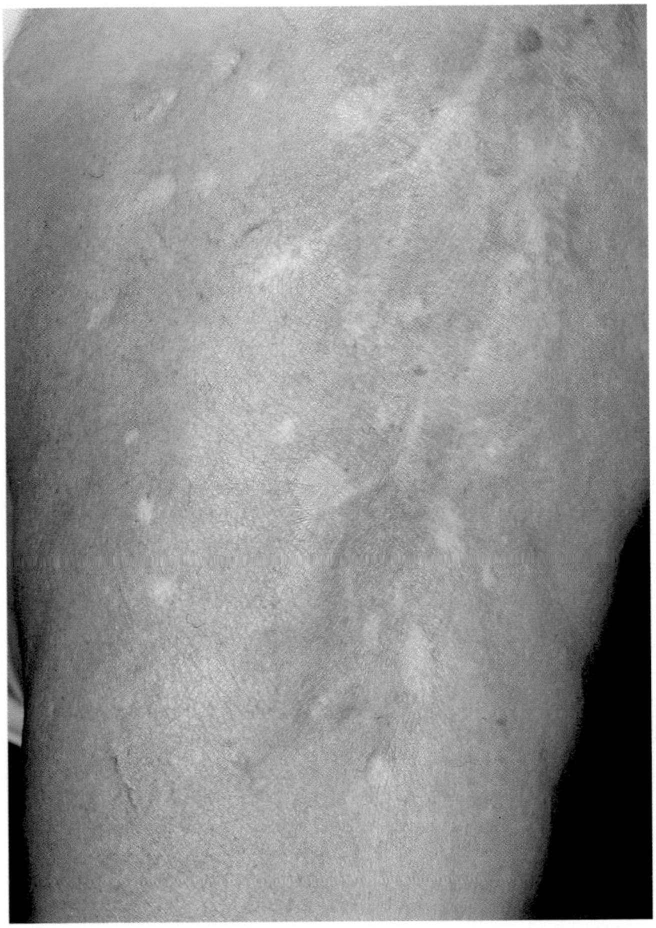

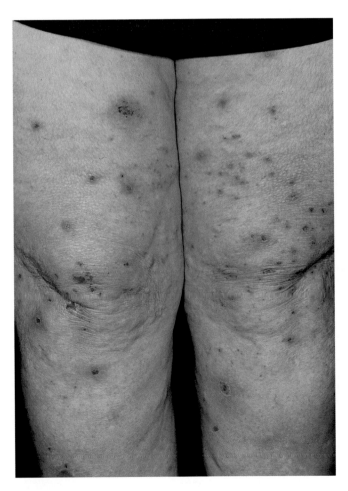

Figure 3-43
Factitial dermatitis. Self-inflicted injury in the past caused this unusual pattern of scars on the thigh.

Figure 3-44
Delusions of parasitosis. Attempts to pick "bugs" out of the skin produce focal erosions on easily accessed areas such as the arms and legs.

TABLE 3-4 Self-Inflicted and Self-Perpetuated Dermatoses

Type of dermatosis	Dermatologic features	Psychiatric features	Diagnosis	Treatment
Neurotic excoriation	Possibly initiated by itchy skin disease Linear excoriations in easily reached areas Groups of round or linear scars suggest diagnosis	Repetitive self-excoriation Patients admit self-inflicted nature Scratching "derived" from frustration and stress Perfectionistic and compulsive traits and depression Suicide possible	Exclude systemic causes of itching Patient admits self-inflicted nature	Empathic, supportive approach Amitriptyline Benzodiazepines
Factitial dermatitis	Wide range of lesions, blisters, ulcers, burns Bizarre patterns not characteristic of any disease	Immature personality Lesions are "an appeal for help" Suicide uncommon	Ratio of female to male patients is 4 to 1 Sudden appearance of lesions "Hollow history": patient cannot describe how lesions evolved	Supportive, empathic approach Avoid direct discussion of self-inflicted nature Occlusive dressings or casts
Delusions of parasitosis	Focal erosions and scars	Patients are convinced they are infested and angry with all doctors because "no one believes them" A monosymptomatic hypochondriacal psychosis	Most patients are women over 50 years old	Pimozide (Orap) 2-12 mg in morning Psychotherapy Patients who deny self-mutilation have poor prognosis
Lichen simplex chronicus	Created and perpetuated by constant scratching and rubbing Very thick oval plaques Usually just one lesion Severe itching Lasts indefinitely Recurs frequently	No known psychopathology Triggered by stress	Biopsy shows eczematous inflammation or resembles psoriasis	Steroids and plastic occlusion Cordran tape Intralesional steroids
Prurigo nodularis	Exaggerated form of lichen simplex chronicus 0.5-1.0 cm itchy nodules on arms and legs Lasts for years	Severe pruritis interferes with life activities and sleep	Biopsy shows very thick epidermis and hyperplasia of nerve fibers	Intralesional steroids Cryotherapy Excision Tranquilizers
Trichotillomania	Compulsive extraction of hair Hairs of various lengths Area not completely devoid of hair	"Neurotic children" Disturbed parent-child relationship Precipitated by stress	Most patients are girls between 5 and 12 years old Patients may deny hair pulling KOH exam rules out tinea Biopsy shows no hairs in follicles Hair pluck shows 100% of hairs in anagen	Psychotherapy and family therapy if persistent

LICHEN SIMPLEX CHRONICUS

Lichen simplex chronicus (Figures 3-45 through 3-50), or circumscribed neurodermatitis, is an eczematous eruption that is created by habitual scratching of a single localized area. The disease is more common in adults, but may be seen in children. The areas most commonly affected are those that are conveniently reached. These are listed in the box at right in approximate order of frequency. Patients derive great pleasure in the relief that comes with frantically scratching the inflamed site. Loss of this pleasurable sensation or continued subconscious habitual scratching may explain why this eruption frequently recurs.

A typical plaque stays localized and shows little tendency to enlarge with time. Red papules coalesce to form a red, scaly, thick plaque with accentuation of skin lines (lichenification). Lichen simplex chronicus is a chronic eczematous disease, but acute changes may result from sensitization with topical medication. Moist scale, serum, crust, and pustules are signs of infection.

Lichen simplex nuchae occurs almost exclusively in women who reach for the back of the neck during stressful situations (see Figure 3-46). The disease may spread beyond the initial well-defined plaque. Diffuse dry or moist scale, crust, and erosions extend into the posterior scalp beyond the neck. Secondary infection is common. Nodules, usually less than 1 cm and scattered randomly in the scalp, occur in patients who frequently pick at the scalp. There may be few nodules or many.

Treatment. The patient must first understand that the rash will not clear until even minor scratching and rubbing is stopped. Scratching frequently takes place during sleep, and the affected area may have to be covered. Lichen simplex chronicus is chronic eczema and is treated as outlined in the section on eczematous inflammation. Treatment of the anal area or the fold behind the ear does not require potent topical steroids as do other forms of lichen simplex; rather, these intertriginous areas respond to group V or VI topical steroids. Lichen simplex nuchae, because of its location, is difficult to treat. Dry inflammation that extends into the scalp may be treated with a group II steroid gel such as fluocinonide (Lidex) applied twice each day. Moist, secondarily infected areas respond to oral antibiotics and topical steroid lotions. A 2- to 3-week course of prednisone (20 mg twice daily) should be considered when an extensively inflamed scalp does not respond rapidly to topical treatment. Nodules caused by picking at the scalp may be very resistant to treatment, requiring monthly intralesional injections with triamcinolone acetonide (Kenalog 10 mg/ml).

LICHEN SIMPLEX CHRONICUS: AREAS MOST COMMONLY AFFECTED LISTED IN APPROXIMATE ORDER OF FREQUENCY	
Outer lower portion of lower leg	Scrotum, vulva, anal area, pubis
Wrists and ankles	Upper eyelids
Back (lichen simplex nuchae) and side of neck	Orifice of the ear
Extensor forearms near elbow	Fold behind the ear
Scalp-picker's nodules	

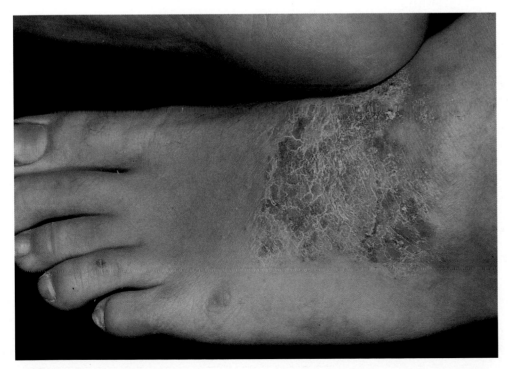

Figure 3-45
Lichen simplex chronicus. This localized plaque of chronic eczematous inflammation was created by rubbing with the opposite heel.

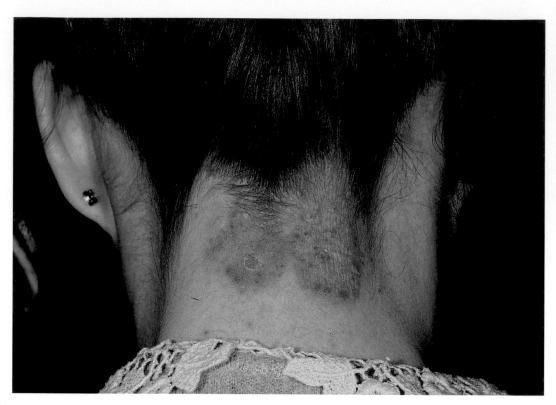

Figure 3-46
Lichen simplex nuchae occurs almost exclusively in women who scratch the back of their neck in stressful situations.

Figure 3-47
Lichen simplex chronicus of the scrotum. The skin is thickened and skin lines are accentuated, unlike the adjacent scrotal skin.

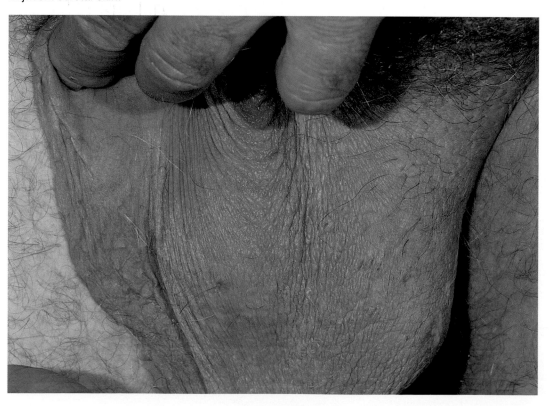

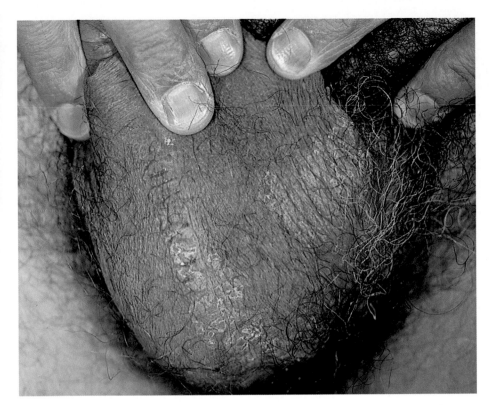

Figure 3-48
Lichen simplex chronicus of the scrotum. Two linear areas are picked and scratched, causing the skin to become very thick. The patient scratches during the day and while asleep.

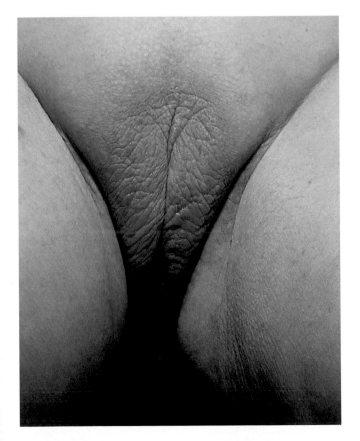

Figure 3-49
Lichen simplex chronicus of the vulva. The skin lines are markedly accentuated from years of rubbing and scratching.

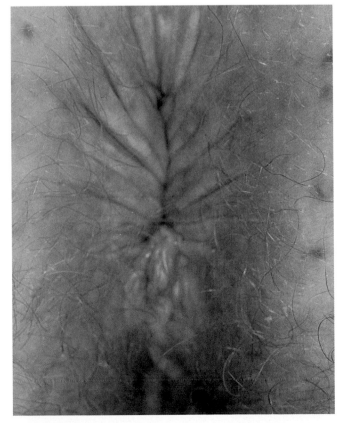

Figure 3-50
Anal excoriations. Scratching has produced focal erosions and thickening of the skin about the anus.

PRURIGO NODULARIS

Prurigo nodularis is a rare disease of unknown cause that may be considered a nodular form of lichen simplex chronicus. It resembles picker's nodules of the scalp except that the few to 20 or more nodules are randomly distributed on the extensor aspects of the arms and legs (Figure 3-51). They are created by repeated scratching. The nodules are red or brown, hard, and dome-shaped with a smooth, crusted, or warty surface; they measure 1 to 2 cm in diameter. Hypertrophy of cutaneous papillary dermal nerves is a relatively constant feature.[36] Complaints of pruritis vary. Some patients claim there is no itching and that scratching is only habitual, whereas others complain pruritus is intense.

Treatment. Prurigo nodularis is resistant to treatment and lasts for years. As with picker's nodules of the scalp, repeated intralesional steroid injections may be necessary for control. Excision of individual nodules is sometimes helpful. Cryotherapy is sometimes successful.

In one study, thalidomide, 50 to 300 mg daily, produced an immediate pronounced effect on the tormenting itching. Patients had a significant decrease in size and numbers of skin lesions after 1 to 2 months of treatment. Therapy had to be discontinued in 59% due to side effects. The most important side effect was neuropathy. This treatment might be offered to patients with the most severe symptoms.[37]

NEUROTIC EXCORIATIONS

Neurotic excoriations are patient-induced linear excoriations. Patients dig at their skin to relieve itching or to extract imaginary pieces of material that they feel is imbedded or extruding from the skin. Itching and digging become compulsive rituals. Most patients are aware that they create the lesions. The most consistent psychiatric disorders reported are perfectionistic and compulsive traits. Patients manifest repressed aggression and self-destructive behavior.[38]

Clinical appearance. Repetitive scratching and digging produces few to several hundred excoriations. All lesions are of similar size and shape. They tend to be grouped in areas that are easily reached, such as the arms, legs, and upper back (Figures 3-52 and 3-53). Recurrent picking at crusts delays healing. Groups of white scars surrounded by brown hyperpigmentation are typical; their presence alone can indicate past difficulty.

Treatment. The use of group I topical steroids applied twice a day or group V topical steroids under plastic wrap occlusion combined with systemic antibiotics produces gratifying results. Frequent lubrication and infrequent washing only with mild soaps should be encouraged once areas are healed. Patients should try to substitute a ritual of applying lubricants for the ritual of digging. An empathic, supportive approach has been reported to be significantly more effective than insight-oriented psychotherapy, which often exacerbates the symptoms.

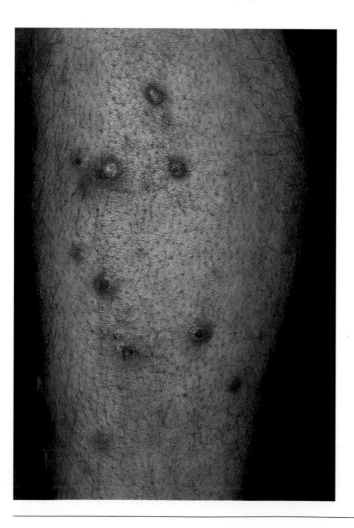

Figure 3-51
Prurigo nodularis. Thick, hard nodules usually present on the extensor surfaces of the forearms and legs from chronic picking.

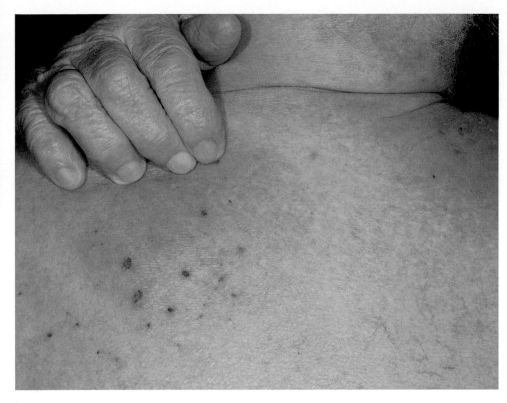

Figure 3-52
Neurotic excoriations. The upper back is one of the most common sites attacked by chronic pickers. Several white, round scars are evidence of past activity.

Figure 3-53
Neurotic excoriations. Severe involvement of the upper back. Picking causes shallow erosions and small, round scars. Long, linear scars occur from deep gouging.

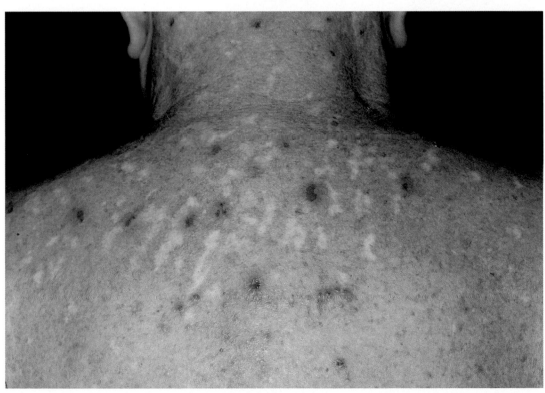

Stasis Dermatitis and Venous Ulceration: The Postphlebitic Syndromes

STASIS DERMATITIS

Etiology. Stasis dermatitis is an eczematous eruption that occurs on the lower legs in some patients with venous insufficiency. The dermatitis may be acute, subacute, or chronic and recurrent, and it may be accompanied by ulceration. Most patients with venous insufficiency do not develop dermatitis; this suggests that genetic or environmental factors may play a role. The reason for its occurrence is unknown. Some have speculated that it represents an allergic response to an epidermal protein antigen created through increased hydrostatic pressure, whereas others feel that the skin has been compromised and is more susceptible to irritation and trauma.

Allergy to topical agents. Patients with stasis dermatitis have significantly more positive reactions when patch tested with components of previously used topical agents. Topical medications that contain potential sensitizers such as lanolin, benzocaine, parabens, and neomycin should be avoided by patients with stasis disease.

TYPES OF ECZEMATOUS INFLAMMATION

Subacute inflammation

Subacute inflammation usually begins in the winter months when the legs become dry and scaly. Brown staining of the skin (hemosiderin) may have appeared slowly for months (Figure 3-54). The pigment is iron left after disintegration of red blood cells that leaked out of veins because of increased hydrostatic pressure. Scratching induces first subacute and then chronic eczematous inflammation (Figure 3-55). Attempts at self-treatment with drying lotions (calamine) or potential sensitizers (e.g., neomycin-containing topical medicines) exacerbate and prolong the inflammation.

Acute inflammation

A red, superficial, itchy plaque may suddenly appear on the lower leg. This acute process may be eczematous inflammation, cellulitis, or both. Weeping and crusts appear (Figure 3-56). A vesicular eruption (id reaction) on the palms, trunk, and/or extremities sometimes accompanies this acute inflammation. The inflammation responds to systemic antibiotics, wet compresses, and group V topical steroids. Wet compresses should be discontinued before excessive drying occurs. The id reaction resolves spontaneously as the primary site improves.

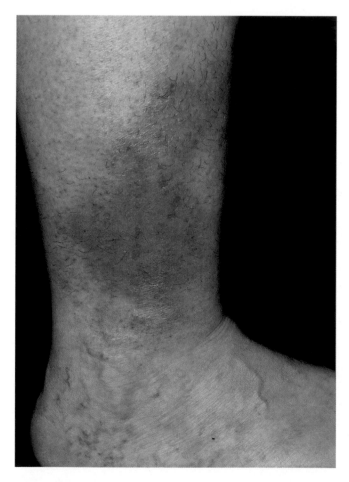

Figure 3-54
Stasis dermatitis in an early stage. Erythema and erosions produced by excoriations are shown.

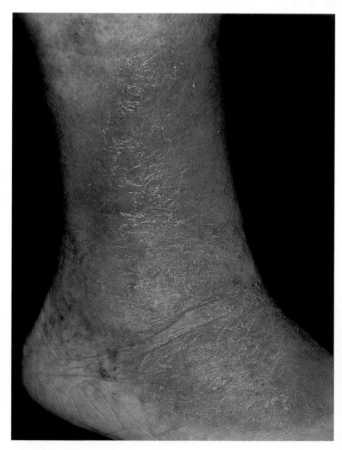

Figure 3-55
Stasis dermatitis (subacute and chronic inflammation). A broad area of redness and scaling has been present for months.

Chronic inflammation

Recurrent attacks of inflammation eventually compromise the poorly vascularized area, and the disease becomes chronic and recurrent. The typical presentation is a cyanotic red plaque over the medial malleolus. Fibrosis following chronic inflammation leads to permanent skin thickening. The skin surface in these irreversibly changed areas may have a bumpy, cobblestone appearance that results from fibrosis and venous and lymph stasis. The skin remains thickened and diffusely dark brown (postinflammatory hyperpigmentation) during quiescent periods.

Treatment of stasis dermatitis

Topical steroids and wet dressings. The early, dry, superficial stage is managed as subacute eczematous inflammation. Oral antibiotics (usually those active against staphylococci) hasten resolution if cellulitis is present. Moist exudative inflammation and moist ulcers respond to tepid wet compresses of Burow's solution or silver nitrate (0.25%) applied for 30 to 60 minutes several times a day. Wet dressings suppress bacteria and inflammation while debriding the ulcer. Adherent crust may be carefully freed with blunt-tipped scissors. Group V topical steroids are applied to eczematous skin at the periphery of the ulcer. Patients must be warned that steroid creams placed on the ulcer stop the healing process. Elevation of the legs encourages healing.

VENOUS LEG ULCERS

Etiology. Venous insufficiency followed by edema is the fundamental change that predisposes to dermatitis and ulceration. Venous insufficiency occurs when venous return in the deep, perforating, or superficial veins is impaired by vein dilation and valve dysfunction.[39] Deep vein thrombophlebitis, which may have been asymptomatic earlier, is the most frequent precursor of lower leg venous insufficiency. Blood pools in the deep venous system and causes deep venous hypertension and dilation of the perforators that connect the superficial and deep venous systems. Venous hypertension is then transmitted to the superficial venous system. The largest perforators are posterior and superior to the lateral and medial malleoli. These are the same areas where dermatitis and ulceration are most prevalent. Superficial varicosities alone are unlikely to produce venous insufficiency.

Clinical features. Ulceration is almost inevitable once the skin has been thickened and circulation is compromised. Ulceration may occur spontaneously or after the slightest trauma (Figure 3-57). The ulcer may remain small or may enlarge rapidly without any further trauma. A dull, constant pain that improves with leg elevation is present. Pain from ischemic ulcers is more intense and does not improve with elevation.

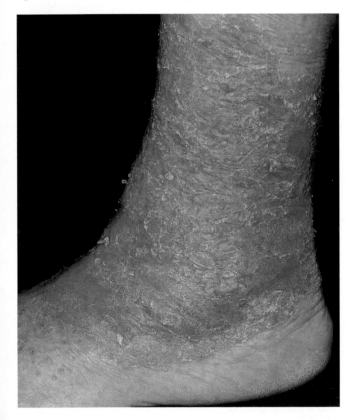

Figure 3-56
Stasis dermatitis (severe inflammation). A red, itchy plaque may suddenly develop acute inflammation and/or cellulitis. Weeping, crusts, and fissuring may be extensive.

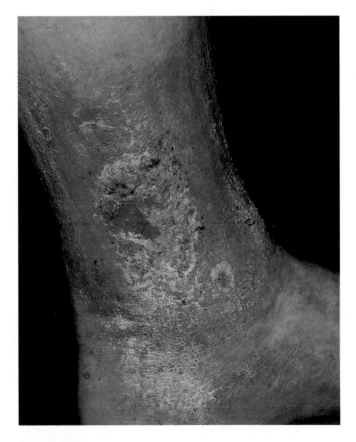

Figure 3-57
The skin is diffusely red, thickened, and bound down by fibrosis. Ulceration occurs with the slightest trauma.

Ulcers have a sharp or sloping border and are deep or superficial. Removal of crust and debris reveals a moist base with granulation tissue. The base and surrounding skin is often infected. Healing is slow, taking several weeks or months. After healing, it is not uncommon to see ulcers rapidly recur. The ulcers are replaced with ivory-white sclerotic scars. Despite the pain and the inconvenience of treatment, most patients tolerate this disease well and remain ambulatory.

Changes in surrounding skin. Edema is a common finding; it is usually pitting and disappears at night with elevation. Chronic edema, trauma, infection, and inflammation lead to subcutaneous tissue fibrosis, giving the skin a firm, nonpitting, "woody" quality. Fat necrosis may follow thrombosis of small veins, and this may be the most important underlying change that predisposes to ulceration. Recurrent ulceration and fat necrosis is associated with loss of subcutaneous tissue and a decrease in lower leg circumference (lipodermatosclerosis). Advanced disease is represented by an "inverted bottle leg," in which the proximal leg swells from chronic venous obstruction and the lower leg shrinks from chronic ulceration and fat necrosis.

Stasis papillomatosis. Stasis papillomatosis is a condition usually found in chronically congested limbs. Lesions vary from small to large plaques that consist of aggregated brownish or pinkish papules with a smooth or hyperkeratotic surface. The lesions most frequently affect the dorsum of the foot, the toes, the extensor aspect of the lower leg, or the area surrounding a venous ulcer. It occurs in patients with local lymphatic disturbances. Patients with primary lymphedema, chronic venous insufficiency, trauma, and recurrent erysipelas are at greatest risk.[40]

Postphlebitic syndromes (clinical variants). Impairment of venous return leads to increased hydrostatic pressure and interstitial fluid accumulation. Six clinical variants (Table 3-5) occur with venous hypertension.

TABLE 3-5 Venous Ulceration Syndromes (the Postphlebitic Syndromes)

Syndrome	Clinical features	Pathophysiology	Management
Dependent edema and ulceration	Pitting edema reversed by elevation Hyperpigmentation	Increased capillary hydrostatic pressure	Compression bandages Unna's boot Bed rest (short periods) Elevation
Lipodermatosclerosis and ulceration	Induration of skin and subcutaneous tissue Extensive hyperpigmentation Pitting edema Erythema secondary to capillary proliferation	Prolonged high pressure in veins Biopsy shows fibrin deposits around capillaries Fibrin prevents O_2 diffusion to epidermis	Fibrinolytic therapy; stanozol 5 gm twice daily Hyperbaric O_2
Atrophie blanche	White, smooth, flat scars with focal dilated capillaries May be preceded by small painful ulcers	Statis and platelet sludging causes platelet thrombi Dermal capillary occlusion causes infarction of overlying dermis; heals with white scars	Antiplatelet therapy; aspirin Compression therapy makes ulcers worse Elevation promotes venous return
Ankle blow-out syndrome	Multiple small, tortuous veins below and behind the malleoli Ulcers usually above and behind medial malleolus in midst of veins Trauma, eczema, bursting of vein causes ulcer	Localized venous valvular incompetence of lower third of leg Exercise makes condition worse	Surgical ligation of localized incompetent veins
Secondary venous varicosity with ulceration	Tortuous saphenous systems	Transmission of hypertension to saphenous system	Compression bandages Hyperbaric O_2
Secondary lymphedema with ulceration	Nonpitting edema	Lymphedema may complicate the lipodermatosclerosis syndrome because of involvement of lymphatic channels by the fibrotic process	Hyperbaric O_2

Modified from Heng MCY: *Int J Dermatol* 26:14-21, 1987.

Management of venous ulcers

Initial evaluation and treatment. Refer to the boxes at right and below. Once other causes of lower leg ulcers have been excluded, the area around the ulcer must be prepared for definitive treatment. Ulcers do not heal if edema, infection, and eczematous inflammation are present.[41] The venous system should be investigated. Surgery or sclerotherapy may be needed to control venous reflux.

Varicose veins. Varicose veins are superficial vessels that are caused by defective venous valves. Perforator vein incompetence may lead to ulceration. Varicose veins cause venous hypertension that leads to edema, cutaneous pigmentation, stasis dermatitis, and ulceration. The goal of therapy is to normalize venous physiology. Deep venous hypertension is managed with compression therapy. Sclerotherapy is used to treat isolated perforator incompetence, even through an ulcer if necessary. Saphenous vein insufficiency is usually managed by surgery.

Noninvasive diagnostic techniques

Ultrasound studies. Ultrasound is used to identify the presence and source of significant venous reflux. The venous Doppler ultrasound attempts to detect sites of valvu-

---

LOWER EXTREMITY ULCER: INITIAL EVALUATION AND TREATMENT

CONDITIONS TO EXCLUDE	DIAGNOSTIC TESTS OR TREATMENTS
Arterial disease, venous thrombosis	Arteriography, Doppler flow studies, venography, Doppler plethysmography
Squamous cell cancer, basal cell cancer, vasculitis	Biopsy
Infectious disease	Biopsy and culture
Diabetes, neuropathy, nutritional deficiencies	Appropriate laboratory studies, physical examination
Cellulitis	Systemic antibiotics
Eczema (skin around ulcer)	Patch test to topical agents (to rule out allergy); topical steroids, systemic antibiotics, wet compresses

---

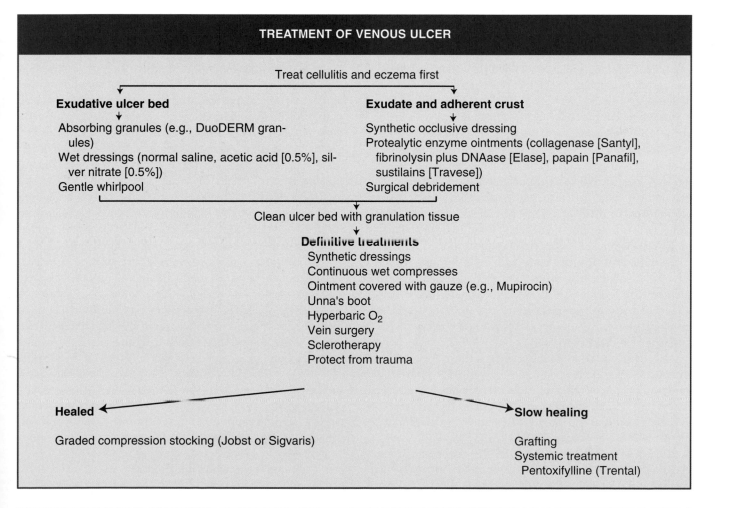

TREATMENT OF VENOUS ULCER

Treat cellulitis and eczema first

Exudative ulcer bed

Absorbing granules (e.g., DuoDERM granules)
Wet dressings (normal saline, acetic acid [0.5%], silver nitrate [0.5%])
Gentle whirlpool

Exudate and adherent crust

Synthetic occlusive dressing
Protealytic enzyme ointments (collagenase [Santyl], fibrinolysin plus DNAase [Elase], papain [Panafil], sustilains [Travese])
Surgical debridement

Clean ulcer bed with granulation tissue

Definitive treatments
Synthetic dressings
Continuous wet compresses
Ointment covered with gauze (e.g., Mupirocin)
Unna's boot
Hyperbaric O_2
Vein surgery
Sclerotherapy
Protect from trauma

Healed

Graded compression stocking (Jobst or Sigvaris)

Slow healing

Grafting
Systemic treatment
Pentoxifylline (Trental)

lar incompetence. It assesses both the presence of venous thrombosis and the sites of incompetent perforators. When bulging varicosities are present in the mid or distal thigh, or extend into the groin, the anteromedial calf, or distally from the popliteal fossa, a continuous-wave Doppler ultrasound examination is advisable. Varicosities in a saphenous system distribution or anatomic region suggest major axial venous incompetence. Duplex ultrasound allows direct visualization of the veins and identification of flow through venous valves. The scan maps superficial and deep veins with precise identification of the sources of venous reflux. Duplex scanning combines echo-pulsing with Doppler velocity recording. These units are found in fully equipped vascular laboratories.

Controlling edema. Contributing systemic disease, local infection, and inflammation should be treated. Pneumatic compression devices are especially effective.[42] Unna's boots or graded elastic stockings help to maintain the leg free of edema.

Inflammation surrounding the ulcer. Tepid saline or silver nitrate (0.5%) wet compresses rapidly control inflammation. Silver nitrate is preferred when infection is present. Fresh compresses (replaced hourly) should be kept in place almost continuously for 24 to 72 hours. Fluids should not be added to dressings that are in place. Group V topical steroids are applied 2 to 4 times each day and may be covered with the compress. Patients with venous ulcers are prone to develop allergic reactions to topical medications in the surrounding compromised skin. Neomycin, paraben preservatives, and lanolin should be avoided. If inflammation persists after appropriate treatment, patch testing should be undertaken.

Infection. Ulcers are typically contaminated with different aerobic and anaerobic bacteria,[43] but routine administration of systemic antibiotics does not increase healing rates.[44] Topical and/or systemic antibiotics may enhance wound healing when heavy bacterial contamination is present. In one study,[45] quantitative measurements showed that ulcers with greater than 10^6 organisms per square centimeter (collected by swab culture) did not heal. Cellulitis must be treated with systemic antibiotics (see Chapter Nine).

Debridement of ulcer bed. Once cellulitis and eczematous inflammation have been controlled, the ulcer must be prepared for definitive treatment. Exudate and crust must be removed to expose granulation tissue, the foundation for new epithelium.

Exudative ulcer bed

WET COMPRESSES. Exudate that turns into a yellow slough can be softened and removed with wet-to-dry saline compresses. As the dressing dries, solubilized exudate is drawn into the absorbent gauze. If the dressings become too dry, they should be resoaked before removal to prevent tearing the delicate new epithelium.

ABSORBING GRANULES AND PASTE. Debrisan wound cleaning paste and DuoDERM hydroactive granules and paste absorb low-molecular weight substances. The ability of unsaturated beads and paste to remove exudates rapidly and continuously from the ulcer results in a reduction of inflammation and edema. The beads and paste are not effective for cleaning dry ulcers and should be discontinued once healthy granulation tissue appears. Patients can be ambulatory during treatment, and healing time is significantly decreased.

Adherent exudate and crust

SYNTHETIC OCCLUSIVE DRESSINGS. Synthetic occlusive dressings (see the Formulary, p. 857) hydrate crust, which facilitates surgical debridement.

PROTEOLYTIC ENZYME OINTMENTS. Necrotic tissue, slough, and exudate consist largely of nucleoproteins and fibrinous materials. Enzymatic debridement with proteolytic enzyme ointments is effective for debridement and stimulation of granulation tissue.[46]

SURGICAL REMOVAL. Mechanical removal of crust and exudate is best performed on soft material. Curved, blunt-tipped dissecting scissors are used to cut adhesions that anchor crust and exudate to the ulcer bed. Great care must be exercised so that new epithelium is not disturbed.

Definitive treatment

1. Measure the ulcer at each visit.
2. Encourage elevation and periods of exercise and ambulation.
3. Minimize bacteria and necrotic debris.
4. Promote granulation tissue formation.
5. Induce reepithelialization.
6. Reduce edema.
7. Protect from trauma.

Occlusive dressings. An occlusive film promotes rapid healing of leg ulcers.[47] Crust formation is suppressed, and epidermis migrates rapidly over the moist granulation tissue. Patients remain ambulatory, and relief of pain is significant. Patients should be warned that an unpleasant odor occurs with fluid buildup. A bewildering variety of synthetic dressings[48] are available (see the Formulary, p. 857). Clinical judgment is necessary to decide which type of the many occlusive dressings should be used. In general, hydrocolloid dressings (e.g., DuoDERM CGF) are effective and easy to use. The surface of the dressing that faces the wound "melts" onto the wound bed. This minimizes disruption of the healing tissues when the dressing is removed. Hydrocolloids allow accumulation of wound fluid that may frighten patients into thinking that an infection is present. A DuoDERM adhesive compression bandage may be applied over the dressing to provide sustained compression. These are 2 yards longer than standard elastic bandages, which ensures thorough coverage of the leg from the toes to the knee. Ulcers treated with hydrocolloid dressings may granulate well but sometimes fail to epithelialize. If this occurs, change to a nonadherent hydrogel dressing such as Vigilon. Hydrogels are semitransparent, comfortable, and absorbent.

APPLICATION TECHNIQUES. Good preparation of surrounding skin assures secure adhesion:

1. Cleanse the wound with hydrogen peroxide and dry it with gauze.

2. Apply alcohol to the area surrounding the wound to remove excess skin oil.
3. Irrigate the ulcer with 2% hydrogen peroxide for 1 minute, then rinse with normal saline solution for 1 minute.
4. When applying the dressing, allow at least 2.5 cm of margin around the wound to prevent leakage.

There is no set amount of time that occlusive dressings should stay on a wound. Dressings should be left in place until fluid begins to leak from around their edges. Early removal of dressings can lead to stripping of delicate new epithelium. Initially, dressings usually need to be changed every other day. Thereafter they may be left in place for many days if excess fluid does not accumulate. Dressings applied over fresh wounds accumulate large amounts of fluid. This can be removed by needle aspiration. Patients who disrupt new epithelium by careless removal of adherent dressings should use a nonadherent dressing such as Vigilon.[49] Dressings should not be applied to inflamed eczematous skin at the borders of stasis ulcers because this increases bacterial flora. Treatment should be interrupted only if clinical signs of infection appear.

Wet compressing. Continuous wet compressing during the waking hours with solutions such as silver nitrate (0.5%) or normal saline is effective. Because of the inconvenience, this technique is usually reserved for hospitalized patients.

Antibacterial compounds covered with gauze. Silver sulfadiazine, mupirocin (Bactroban) ointment, or benzoyl peroxide (10% water based acne lotions [e.g., Panoxy AQ 10]) are applied to the ulcer bed and covered with a nonstick gauze. Wounds are cleaned and redressed every 24 to 48 hours. This treatment can be considered for patients who object to synthetic dressings.

Hyperbaric oxygen. Topical hyperbaric oxygen may be beneficial for venous ulcers. A simplified technique using disposable polyethylene bags has been described[50] and modified to treat venous ulcers. The pressure of oxygen is reduced to 18 mm Hg to minimize obstruction of venous return. Patients receive 4 to 6 hours of topical oxygen administration on 4 consecutive days each week, interspersed by rest periods of 3 consecutive days.[51]

External compression. Elimination of edema is essential during treatment and after resolution. This is accomplished by applying external compression bandages such as DuoDERM adhesive compression bandage, graded compression stockings, or Unna's boots.

GRADED COMPRESSION STOCKINGS (HIGH PRESSURE AT THE ANKLE, DECREASING TO THE THIGH). Once ulcers have healed, pressure-graded lower leg compression can be maintained by a custom-fitted (Jobst or Sigvaris) or premade compression stocking (Sigvaris or Venes) (the so-called support stockings available in department stores do not provide sufficient compression and are not useful). Measurements of the circumference at several points on the leg are made and preserved on paper tape in a measuring kit provided by the company. The measurements are taken after the leg has been elevated and edema has drained. The amount of compression can be specified by the physician. Patients with chronic venous insufficiency who have had stasis dermatitis or ulceration require a compression of between 35 and 40 mm Hg. Various lengths can be purchased, but an above-the-knee length stocking may give the best results. The stockings are difficult to apply and must be replaced periodically because of stretching. Firmly applied Ace bandages are a less effective but convenient alternative.

UNNA'S BOOT (HARD CAST). A commercially available Unna's paste boot (Dome-paste bandage, Gelocast bandage) impregnated with zinc oxide paste may be applied soon after acute inflammation has subsided. In one study, seven of 10 stasis leg ulcers healed in an average of 7.3 weeks.[52] Unna's boots are not applied over synthetic dressings.

Because the boot does not eliminate existing edema fluid, it should be applied in the morning after edema has drained. At home on the morning of the day when the boot is to be applied, the patient places gauze over the ulcer and firmly wraps a rubberized Ace bandage in a pressure gradient fashion with the greatest pressure at the ankle and the least at the knee. The patient then comes directly to the physician's office. The Ace bandage is removed, the skin is cleansed, and the ulcer, if present, is debrided. A group V topical steroid is applied to the surrounding skin if chronic inflammation is present, and lubricating creams are applied to normal skin.

An Unna's boot is applied, as the instructions in each box indicate, in layers starting behind the first metatarsal and ending just below the knee. Care must be taken to avoid folding or creasing the bandage during application. In approximately 1 hour, the moist bandage dries to form a firm cast. The cast may be left exposed. Many patients prefer to have the cast covered with an Ace bandage or long stocking to protect the other leg from abrasion from the hard cast. The boot is changed every 7 to 10 days, or more frequently if drainage from the ulcer penetrates through it. After healing, elastic Ace bandages or pressure gradient stockings are applied each morning, indefinitely, to prevent dependent edema.

Systemic therapy. Systemic therapy should be considered for treatment-resistant disease.

Pentoxifylline. Pentoxifylline (Trental) increases fibrinolytic activity. Presumably, improvements are obtained because the drug has a specific blood-flow–promoting effect in ischemic areas. A double-blind trial demonstrated that pentoxifylline (Trental, 400 mg, three times per day) improved therapy-resistant venous leg ulcers.[53] Systemic therapy was used in conjunction with topical treatment for a minimum of 6 to 8 weeks. Its effectiveness is still controversial.

Vitamins. Patients with signs of malnutrition, such as low serum albumin or transferrin concentrations, may benefit from dietary supplementation. Ascorbic acid (1 to 2 gm/day), zinc sulfate (220 mg, three times per day), and vitamin E (200 mg/day) may be used for supplementation.

These vitamins are essential for wound healing but should not be prescribed in excessively high dosages.

Grafting. Skin grafting should be considered if response to medical treatment is inadequate. Split-thickness grafts, meshed grafts, and partial-thickness pinch grafts have all been successful. Grafts are most successful when applied to granulation tissue that is free of exudate and when edema has been controlled.

REFERENCES

1. Nilsson E, Henning C, Hjorleifsson M-L: Density of the microflora in hand eczema before and after topical treatment with a potent corticosteroid, *J Am Acad Dermatol* 15:192-197, 1986.
2. Meding B, Swanbeck G: Occupational hand eczema in an industrial city, *Contact Dermatitis* 22:13-23, 1990.
3. Meding B, Swanbeck G: Consequences of having hand eczema, *Contact Dermatitis* 23:6-14, 1990.
4. Meding B: Epidemiology of hand eczema in an industrial city, *Acta Derm Venereol* 153-161 (Suppl):1-43, 1990.
5. Cronin E: Clinical patterns of hand eczema in women, *Contact Dermatitis* 13:153-161, 1985.
6. Lauharanta J, Ojajarvi J, et al: Prevention of dryness and eczema of the hands of hospital staff by emulsion cleansing instead of washing with soap, *J Hosp Infect* 17:207-215, 1991.
7. Hannuksela A, Kinnunen T: Moisturizers prevent irritant dermatitis, *Acta Derm Venereol* 72:42-44, 1992.
8. Rosen K, Mobacken H, Swanbeck G: Chronic eczematous dermatitis of the hands: a comparison of PUVA and UVB treatment, *Acta Derm Venereol* (Stockh) 67:48-54, 1987.
9. Rystedt I: Atopy, hand eczema, and contact dermatitis: summary of recent large scale studies, *Semin Dermatol* 5:290-300, 1986.
10. Rystedt I: Factors influencing the occurrence of hand eczema in adults with a history of atopic dermatitis in childhood, *Contact Dermatitis* 12:185-191, 1985.
11. Rystedt I: Hand eczema in patients with history of atopic manifestations in childhood, *Acta Derm Venereol* (Stockh) 65:305-312, 1985.
12. Jordan WP Jr: Allergic contact dermatitis in hand eczema, *Arch Dermatol* 110:567, 1974.
13. Adams RM: Patch testing: a recapitulation, *J Am Acad Derm* 5: 629-643, 1981.
14. MacKee GM, Lewis GM: Keratolysis exfoliative, *Arch Derm Syph* 23:445, 1931.
15. Thelin I, Agrup G: Pompholyx; a one year series, *Acta Derm Venereol* (Stockh) 65:214-217, 1985.
16. Veien NK et al: Oral challenge with metal salts: vesicular patch-test negative reaction, *Contact Dermatitis* 9:402, 1983.
17. Lodi A, Betti R, et al: Epidemiological, clinical and allergological observations on pompholyx, *Contact Dermatitis* 26:17-21, 1992.
18. Yokozeki H, Katayama I, et al: The role of metal allergy and local hyperhidrosis in the pathogenesis of pompholyx, *J Dermatol* 19:964-967, 1992.
19. LeVine MJ, Parrish JA, Fitzpatrick TB: Oral methoxsalen photochemotherapy (PUVA) of dyshidrotic eczema, *Acta Derm Venereol* (Stockh) 61:570-571, 1981.
20. Gawkrodger DJ et al: Nickel dermatitis: the reaction to oral nickel challenge, *Br J Dermatol* 115:33, 1986.
21. Pigatto PD, Gibelli E, et al: Disodium cromoglycate versus diet in the treatment and prevention of nickel-positive pompholyx, *Contact Dermatitis* 22:27-31, 1990.
22. Christensen OB, Kristensen M: Treatment with disulfiram in chronic nickel hand dermatitis, *Contact Dermatitis* 8:59-63, 1982.
23. Jones SK, English JSC, Forsyth A, et al: Juvenile plantar dermatosis: an 8-year follow-up of 102 patients, *Clin Exp Dermatol* 12:5-7, 1987.
24. Ashton RE, Griffiths WAD: Juvenile plantar dermatosis: atopy or footwear? *Clin Exp Dermatol* 11:529-534, 1986.
25. Lyell A: Cutaneous artifactual disease, *J Am Acad Dermatol* 1:391-407, 1979.
26. Doran AR, Roy A, Wolkowitz OW: Self-destructive dermatoses, *Psychiatr Clin North Am* 8:291-298, 1985.
27. Gupta MA, Gupta AK, Haberman HF: The self-inflicted dermatoses: a critical review, *Gen Hosp Psychiatry* 9:45-52, 1987.
28. Medansky RS, Handler RM: Dermatopsychosomatics: classification, physiology, and therapeutic approaches, *J Am Acad Dermatol* 5:125-136, 1981.
29. Munro A: Delusional parasitosis: a form of monosymptomatic hypochondriacal psychosis, *Semin Dermatol* 2:197-202, 1983.
30. Koo JY, Pham CT: Psychodermatology: practical guidelines on pharmacotherapy, *Arch Dermatol* 128:381-388, 1992.
31. Van Moffaert M: Psychodermatology: an overview, *Psychother Psychosom* 58:125-126, 1992.
32. Koblenzer CS: Cutaneous manifestations of psychiatric disease that commonly present to the dermatologist—diagnosis and treatment, *Int J Psychiatry Med* 22:47-63, 1992.
33. Folks DG, Kinney FC: The role of psychological factors in dermatologic conditions, *Psychosomatics* 33:45-54, 1992.
34. Moffaert MV: Localization of self-inflicted dermatological lesions: What do they tell the dermatologist? *Act Derm Venereol* (Stockh)156 (Suppl):23-27, 1991.
35. Hatch ML, Paradis C, et al: Obsessive-compulsive disorder in patients with chronic pruritic conditions: case studies and discussion, *J Am Acad Dermatol* 26:549-551, 1992.
36. Harris B, Harris K, et al: Demonstration by S-100 protein staining of increased numbers of nerves in the papillary dermis of patients with prurigo nodularis, *J Am Acad Dermatol* 26:56-58, 1992.
37. Johnke H, Zachariae H: Thalidomide treatment of prurigo nodularis, *Ugeskr Laeger* 155:3028-3030, 1993.
38. Fruensgaard K et al: Neurotic excoriations, *Int J Dermatol* 17:761-767, 1978.
39. Goldman MP, Weiss RA, Bergan JJ: Diagnosis and treatment of varicose veins: a review, *J Am Acad Dermatol* 31:393-413, 1994.
40. Schultz-Ehrenburg U, Niederauer HH, et al: Stasis papillomatosis. Clinical features, etiopathogenesis and radiological findings, *J Dermatol Surg Oncol* 19:440-446, 1993.
41. Ryan TJ: Current management of leg ulcers, *Drugs* 30:461-468, 1985.
42. Kolari PJ, Pekanmaki P: Intermittent pneumatic compression in healing of venous ulcers, *Lancet* 2:1108, 1986 (letter).
43. Eriksson G, Eklund A-E, Kallings LO: The clinical significance of bacterial growth in venous leg ulcers, *Scand J Infect Dis* 16:175-180, 1984.
44. Alinovi A, Bassissi P, Pini M: Systemic administration of antibiotics in the management of venous ulcers, *J Am Acad Dermatol* 15:186-191, 1986.
45. Lookingbill DP, Miller SH, Knowles RC: Bacteriology of chronic leg ulcers, *Arch Dermatol* 114:1765-1768, 1978.
46. Westerhof W, Jansen FC, de Wit FS, et al: Controlled double-blind trial of fibrinolysin-desoxyribonuclease (Elase) solution in patients with chronic leg ulcers who are treated before autologous skin grafting, *J Am Acad Dermatol* 17:32-39, 1987.
47. Friedman SJ, Daniel Su WP: Management of leg ulcers with hydrocolloid occlusive dressing, *Arch Dermatol* 120:1329-1336, 1984.
48. Witkowski JA, Parish LC: Cutaneous ulcer therapy, *Int J Dermatol* 25:420-426, 1986 (review).
49. Falanga V: Occlusive wound dressings: why, when, which? *Arch Dermatol* 124:872-877, 1988.
50. Heng MCY, Pilgrim JP, Beck FWJ: A simplified hyperbaric oxygen technique for leg ulcers, *Arch Dermatol* 120:640-645, 1984.
51. Heng MCY: Venous leg ulcers, *Int J Dermatol* 26:14-21, 1987.
52. Hendricks WM, Swallow RT: Management of stasis leg ulcers with Unna's boots versus elastic support stockings, *J Am Acad Dermatol* 12:90-98, 1985.
53. Weitgasser H: The use of pentoxifylline (Trental 400) in the treatment of leg ulcers: results of a double-blind trial, *Pharmatherapeutica* 3(suppl):143-151, 1983.

CHAPTER FOUR

Contact Dermatitis and Patch Testing

Contact dermatitis is an eczematous dermatitis caused by exposure to substances in the environment. Those substances act as irritants or allergens and may cause acute, subacute, or chronic eczematous inflammation. To diagnose contact dermatitis, one must first recognize that an eruption is eczematous. Contact allergies often have characteristic distribution patterns indicating that the observed eczematous eruption is caused by external rather than internal stimuli. Elimination of the suspected offending agent and appropriate treatment for eczematous inflammation usually serve to manage patients with contact dermatitis effectively. However, there are many cases in which this direct approach fails; then patch testing is useful.

It is important to differentiate contact dermatitis resulting from irritation from that caused by allergy. An outline of these differences is listed in Table 4-1.

TABLE 4-1 Contact Dermatitis: Irritant vs. Allergic

	Irritant	Allergic
People at risk	Everyone	Genetically predisposed
Mechanism of response	Nonimmunologic; a physical and chemical alteration of epidermis	Delayed hypersensitivity reaction
Number of exposures	Few to many; depends on individual's ability to maintain an effective epidermal barrier	One or several to cause sensitization
Nature of substance	Organic solvent, soaps	Low-molecular weight hapten (e.g., metals, formalin, epoxy)
Concentration of substance required	Usually high	May be very low
Mode of onset	Usually gradual as epidermal barrier becomes compromised	Once sensitized, usually rapid; 12 to 48 hours after exposure
Distribution	Borders usually indistinct	May correspond exactly to contactant (e.g., watch band, elastic waistband)
Investigative procedure	Trial of avoidance	Trial of avoidance, patch testing, or both
Management	Protection and reduced incidence of exposure	Complete avoidance

Irritant Contact Dermatitis

Irritation of the skin is the most common cause of contact dermatitis. The epidermis is a thin cellular barrier with an outer layer composed of dead cells in a water-protein-lipid matrix. Any process that damages any component of the barrier compromises its function, and a nonimmunologic eczematous response may result. Repeated use of strong alkaline soap or industrial exposure to organic solvents extract lipid from the skin. Acids may combine with water in the skin and cause dehydration. When the skin is compromised, exposure to even a weak irritant sustains the inflammation. The intensity of the inflammation is related to the concentration of the irritant and the exposure time. Mild irritants cause dryness, fissuring, and erythema; a mild eczematous reaction may occur with continuous exposure. Continuous exposure to moisture in areas such as the hand, the diaper area, or the skin around a colostomy may eventually cause eczematous inflammation. Strong chemicals may produce an immediate reaction. Figures 4-1 through 4-4 show examples of irritant dermatitis.

Patients vary in their ability to withstand exposure to irritants. Some people cannot tolerate frequent hand washing, whereas others may work daily with harsh cleaning solutions without any difficulty.

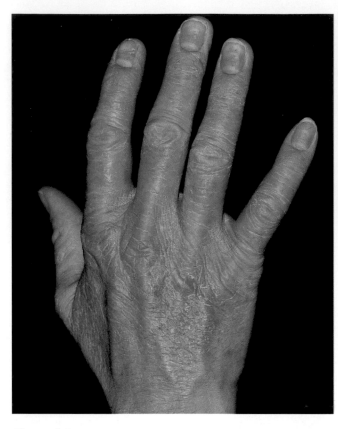

Figure 4-1
Irritant dermatitis. Chronic exposure to soap and water has caused subacute eczematous inflammation over the backs of the hands and fingers.

Figure 4-2
Irritant dermatitis. Long exposure to wet diapers followed by frequent washing has resulted in diffuse erythema and dry, cracked, fissured skin.

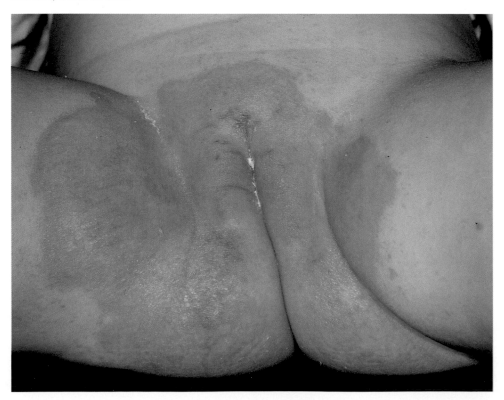

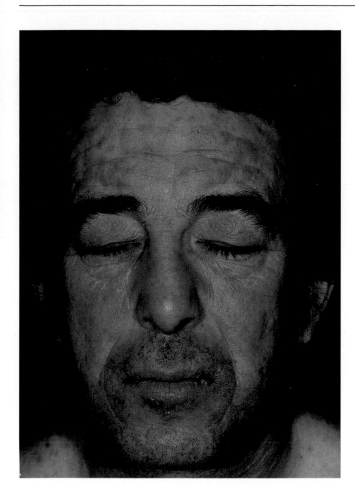

Figure 4-3
Irritant dermatitis. Exposure to industrial solvents has resulted in diffuse erythema with dryness and fissuring about the mouth.

Figure 4-4
Irritant dermatitis. Repeated cycles of wetting and drying by lip licking resulted in irritant dermatitis.

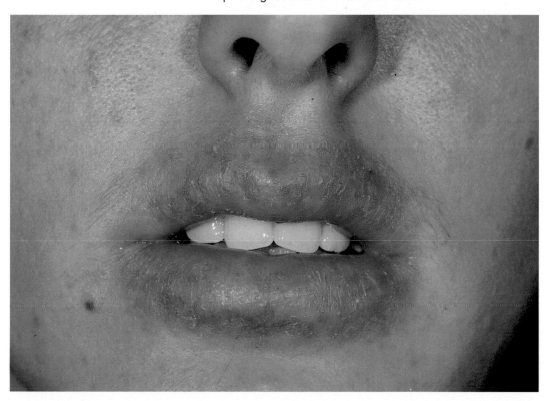

Allergic Contact Dermatitis

Allergic contact dermatitis is a delayed hypersensitivity reaction that affects a limited number of individuals after one or a few exposures to an antigenic substance.

Allergic contact dermatitis phases

Sensitization phase. A hapten, a low-molecular weight substance (e.g., nickel), penetrates into the epidermis and combines with epidermal protein to form an antigen. This hapten-protein binding takes place either on or in the vicinity of Langerhans' cells, which act as an epidermal reticuloendothelial trap for antigens. The Langerhans' cell is met by macrophages and T cells in the epidermis, and initial processing takes place. A message is directed to T cell precursors in the lymph nodes, and sensitized T cells are formed.

Elicitation phase. On reexposure to the antigen-protein complex, the sensitized T cells release lymphokines, which recruit inflammatory cells that cause eczematous inflammation. The time required for a previously sensitized individual to develop clinically apparent inflammation is generally 12 to 48 hours but may vary from 8 to 120 hours.

Cross-sensitization

A hapten, the chemical structure of which is similar to the original sensitizing hapten, may cause inflammation because the immune system is unable to differentiate between the original and the chemically related antigen. For example, the skin of patients who are allergic to balsam of Peru, which is present in numerous topical preparations, may become inflamed when exposed to the chemically related benzoin in tincture of benzoin.

SYSTEMICALLY INDUCED ALLERGIC CONTACT DERMATITIS

Patients who have been sensitized to topical medications may develop generalized eczematous inflammation if those medications or chemically related substances are ingested. Patients sensitized to ethylenediamine from contact with that chemical in topical medicines may develop generalized inflammation following treatment with aminophylline, which contains ethylenediamine. Patients allergic to poison ivy develop diffuse inflammation following the ingestion of raw cashew nuts (Figure 4-5). Cashew nut oil[1,2] is chemically related to the oleoresin of the poison ivy plant.

CLINICAL PRESENTATION

The intensity of inflammation depends on the degree of sensitivity and the concentration of the antigen. Strong sensitizers such as the oleoresin of poison ivy may produce intense inflammation in low concentrations, whereas weak sensitizers may cause only erythema.

The pattern of inflammation is an important consideration when attempting to differentiate allergic contact dermatitis from other causes of eczematous inflammation. The pattern of inflammation may correspond exactly to the shape of the offending substance. The diagnosis is obvious when inflammation is confined specifically to the area under a watch band, shoe, or elastic waistband.

The location of inflammation may provide a clue to the source of the antigen. Table 4-2 lists substances that are common causes of inflammation in specific body regions. Table 4-3 lists substances commonly encountered in specific professions.

Direct vs. airborne contact. Acute and chronic dermatitis of exposed parts of the body, especially the face, may be caused by chemicals suspended in the air. Sprays, perfumes, chemical dusts, and plant pollen (e.g., ragweed) are possible sources.[3] Inflammation from airborne sensitizers tends to be more diffuse. Photodermatitis can have the same distribution. Airborne material easily collects on the upper eyelids; this area is particularly susceptible. Volatile substances can collect in clothing.

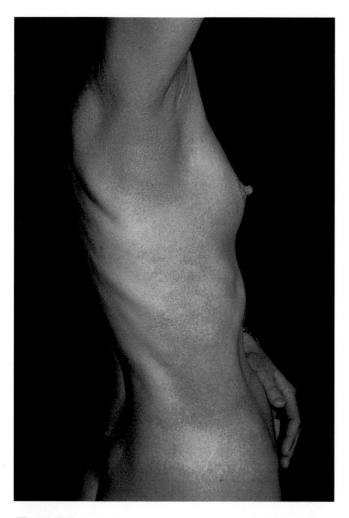

Figure 4-5
Diffuse allergic reaction occurring in a patient allergic to poison ivy who has ingested raw cashew nuts, the oil of which cross-reacts with the oleoresin of poison ivy.

TABLE 4-2 Contact Dermatitis: Distribution Diagnosis

Location	Material
Scalp and ears	Shampoo, hair dyes, topical medicines, metal earrings, eyeglasses
Eyelids	Nail polish (transferred by rubbing), cosmetics, contact lens solution, metal eyelash curlers
Face	Airborne allergens (poison ivy from burning leaves, ragweed), cosmetics, sunscreens, acne medications (e.g., benzoyl peroxide), after-shave lotion
Neck	Necklaces, airborne allergens (ragweed), perfumes, after-shave lotion
Trunk	Topical medication, sunscreens, poison ivy, plants (phototoxic reactions), clothing undergarments (e.g., spandex bra, elastic waistband), metal belt buckles
Axillae	Deodorant (axillary vault), clothing (axillary folds)
Hands	Soaps and detergents, foods, spices, poison ivy, industrial solvents and oils, cement, metal (pots, rings), topical medications, rubber gloves in surgeons
Arms	Same as hands; watch and watchband
Genitals	Poison ivy (transferred by hand), rubber condoms
Anal region	Hemorrhoid preparations (benzocaine, nupercaine)
Lower legs	Topical medication (benzocaine, lanolin, neomycin, parabens), dye in socks
Feet	Shoes (rubber or leather), cement spilling into boots

TABLE 4-3 Contact Dermatitis: Occupational Exposure

Occupation	Irritant	Allergens
Beauticians	Wet work (shampoos)	Hair tints, permanent solution, shampoos (formaldehyde)
Construction workers	Fuels, lubricants, cement	Cement (chromium, cobalt), epoxy, glues, paints, solvents, rubber, chrome-tanned leather gloves
Chefs, bartenders, bakers	Moist foods, juices, corn, pineapple juice	Orange and lemon peel (oil of limonene), mango, carrot, parsnips, parsley, celery; spices (e.g., capsicum, cinnamon, cloves, nutmeg, vanilla)
Farmers	Milker's eczema (detergents), tractor lubricants and fuels	Malathion, pyrethrum insecticides, fungicides, rubber, ragweed, marsh elder
Forest products industry	Wet work (wood processing)	Poison ivy and oak, plants growing on bark (e.g., lichens, liverworts)
Medical and surgical personnel	Surgical scrubbing	Rubber gloves, glutaraldehyde (germicides), acrylic monomer in cement (orthopedic surgeons), penicillin, chlorpromazine, benzalkonium chloride, neomycin
Printing industry	Alcohols, alkalis, grease	Polyfunctional acrylic monomers, epoxy acrylate oligomers, isocyanate compounds (all used in a new ink-drying method)

Allergic contact dermatitis in children

Allergic contact dermatitis may account for as many as 20% of all cases of dermatitis in children. Poison ivy, nickel (jewelry), rubber (shoe dermatitis), balsam of Peru (hand and face dermatitis), formaldehyde (cosmetics and shampoos), and neomycin (topical antibiotic ointments) are the most common allergens.[4]

RHUS DERMATITIS

In the United States, poison ivy, poison oak, and poison sumac produce more cases of allergic contact dermatitis than all other contactants combined. The allergens responsible for poison ivy and poison oak allergic contact dermatitis are contained within the resinous sap material termed *urushiol*. Urushiol is composed of a mixture of catechols. All parts of the plant contain the sap. These plants belong to the Anacardiaceae family and the genus *Rhus*. Other plants in that family, such as cashew trees, mango trees, Japanese laquer trees, and ginkgo contain allergens identical or related to those in poison ivy. Thousands of workers on cashew nut farms in India develop hand dermatitis from direct contact with the irritating resinous oil from cashew nut shells.[5]

Poison ivy and poison oak are neither ivy nor oak species.

Clinical presentation. *Rhus* dermatitis occurs from contact with the leaf or internal parts of the stem or root and can be acquired from roots or stems in the fall and winter. The clinical presentation varies with the quantity of oleoresin that contacts the skin, the pattern in which contact was made, individual susceptibility, and regional variations in cutaneous reactivity. Small quantities of oleoresin produce only erythema, whereas large quantities cause intense vesiculation (Figures 4-6 and 4-7).

The highly characteristic linear lesions are created when part of the plant is drawn across the skin or from streaking the oleoresin while scratching. Diffuse or unusual patterns of inflammation occur when the oleoresin is acquired from contaminated animal hair or clothing or from smoke while burning the plant. The eruption may appear as quickly as 8 hours after contact or may be delayed for a week or more. The appearance of new lesions a week after contact may be confusing to the patient, who may attribute new lesions to the spread of the disease by touching active lesions or to contamination with blister fluid. Blister fluid does not contain the oleoresin and, contrary to popular belief, cannot spread the inflammation.

Treatment of inflammation. Washing the skin with any type of soap inactivates and removes all surface oleoresin,

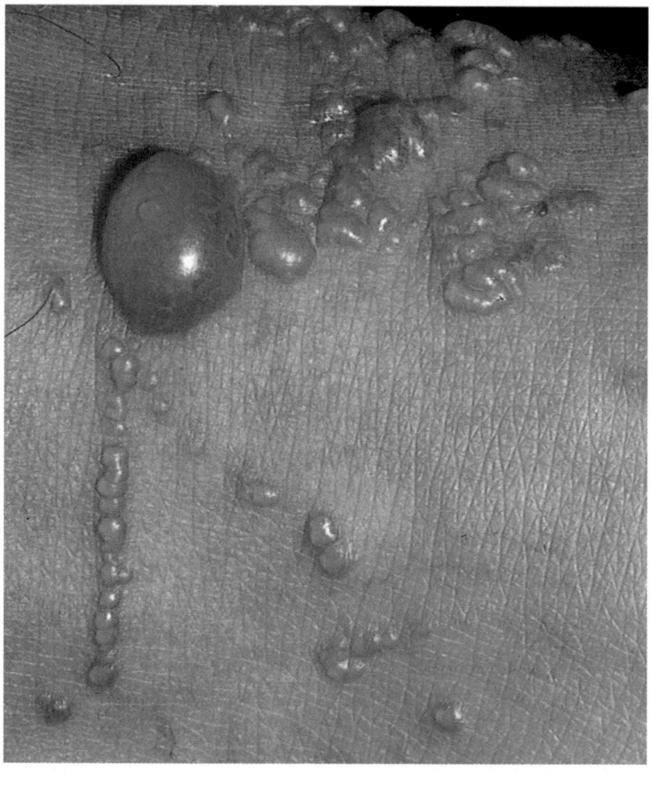

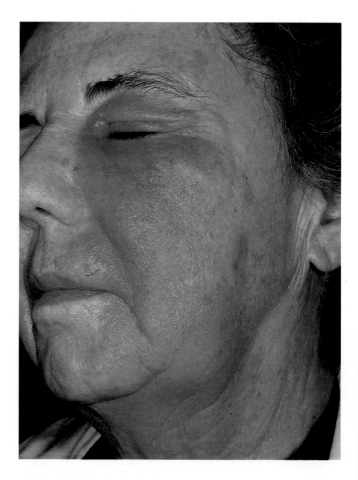

Figure 4-6
Poison ivy. A classic presentation with vesicles and blisters. A line of vesicles (linear lesions) caused by dragging the resin over the surface of the skin with the scratching finger is a highly characteristic sign of plant contact dermatitis.

Figure 4-7
Poison ivy dermatitis. Diffuse erythema with vesicles over the entire surface.

thereby preventing further contamination. Washing is most effective if done within 15 minutes of exposure.

Blisters and intense erythema. Cold wet compresses are highly effective during the acute blistering stage. They should be used for 15 to 30 minutes several times a day for 1 to 3 days until blistering and severe itching is controlled. Topical steroids do not penetrate through blisters.

Prednisone, administered in a dosage of 20 mg twice each day for at least 6 days, is used for severe, widespread inflammation. Patients who may have trouble adhering to a medication schedule may be treated with triamcinolone acetonide (Kenalog, Aristocort; 40 mg suspension) given intramuscularly. Commercially available steroid dose packs should be avoided; they provide an inadequate amount of medicine. Patients who do not initially seem to require medication may become much worse 1 or 2 days after an office visit; they should be advised that prednisone is available if their conditions worsen.

Short, cool tub baths with or without colloidal oatmeal (Aveeno) are very soothing and help to control widespread acute inflammation. Calamine lotion controls itching but prolonged use causes excessive drying. Hydroxyzine and diphenhydramine control itching and encourage sleep.

Mild to moderate erythema. Topical steroid gels or creams (groups III through V) applied 2 to 4 times a day rapidly suppress erythema and itching.

Prophylactic treatment. Complete desensitization cannot be accomplished. Poison ivy oleoresin in capsules and injectable syringes for hyposensitization has been removed from the market by the FDA.

SHOE DERMATITIS, GLOVE DERMATITIS, AND RUBBER ALLERGY

Shoe allergy. Fungal infections, psoriasis, and atopic dermatitis are common causes of inflammation of the feet. Shoe allergy, although less common, should always be considered in the differential diagnosis of inflammation of the feet, particularly in children.

Shoe allergy typically appears as subacute eczematous inflammation with redness and scaling over the dorsa of the feet, particularly the toes (Figures 4-8 and 4-9). The interdigital spaces are spared, in contrast to tinea pedis. Inflammation is usually bilateral, but unilateral involvement does not preclude the diagnosis of allergy. The thick skin of the soles is more resistant to allergens.

Sweaty sock dermatitis, an irritant reaction in children caused by excessive perspiration, presents as diffuse dryness with fissuring on the toes, webs, and soles (see Figure 3-42). These irritated areas may become eczematous and appear as shoe contact dermatitis.

Mercaptobenzothiazole, a rubber component of adhesives used to cement shoe uppers, and potassium bichromate, a leather tanning agent, are common causes of shoe allergy. These chemicals are leached out by sweat.

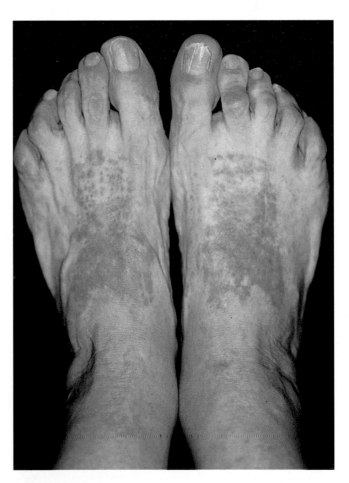

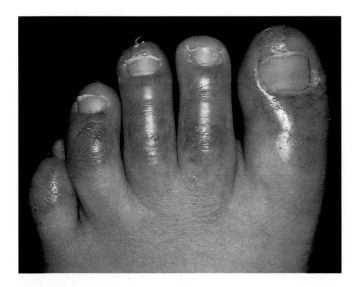

Figure 4-8
Shoe contact dermatitis. The toe webs are spared, in contrast to tinea pedis.

Figure 4-9
Shoe contact dermatitis. Sharply defined plaques formed under a shoe lining impregnated with rubber cement.

Diagnosis. Patch testing is required to confirm the diagnosis of allergy. Pieces of the shoe that cover the inflamed site should be used for the patch test (Figure 4-10).

1. Cut a 1-inch square piece of material from the shoe and round off the corners.
2. Separate glued surfaces and patch test with all layers.
3. Moisten each layer with water, apply the samples to the upper outer arm, cover with tape, and proceed as described in the section on patch testing.

In some cases, patch testing with the standard patch test series may be required to establish the diagnosis.

Management. Patients with shoe allergy must control perspiration. Socks should be changed at least once each day. An absorbent powder such as Z-Sorb applied to the feet may be helpful. Aluminum chloride hexahydrate in a 20% solution (Drysol) applied at bedtime is a highly effective antiperspirant. Most vinyl shoes are acceptable substitutes for rubber-sensitive and chrome-sensitive patients. Inflammation of the soles may be prevented by inserting a barrier such as Dr. Scholl's Air Foam Pads or Johnson's Odor-Eaters. Once perspiration is controlled, it may be possible for sensitized patients to wear both leather shoes and shoes that contain rubber cement.

Rubber and surgical glove allergy. Allergy to rubber compounds is also seen with adhesive bandages and surgical gloves. Spandex rubber in bras and underpants may cause allergic contact dermatitis (Figures 4-11 and 4-12). Of 100 cases of chronic hand dermatitis in surgeons, dentists, and surgical personnel, 11 patients were allergic to latex rubber surgical gloves.[6] Latex allergy occurs in up to 10% of operating room nurses.[7] Allergic patients are vulnerable in the hospital setting. Latex allergy can present as IgE-mediated anaphylaxis during surgery, barium enema, or dental work. Systemic effects have occurred intraoperatively as a result of mucosal latex absorption at the time of surgery or procedure, due to the surgeon's latex gloves.[8] Symptoms often occur immediately after exposure. Skin exposure causes contact urticaria. Exposure to latex in the air elicits allergic rhinitis, conjunctivitis, and asthma. Anaphylactic shock includes the above symptoms with tachycardia and hypotension.[9]

Antioxidants and accelerators added to rubber in the manufacturing process are the major allergens. Patients should be patch tested with a 2-cm square section of the rubber glove. Patients may test negative to the rubber allergens found in the standard patch test series.[10] Surgeons with rubber sensitivity may use Elastyren hypoallergenic surgical gloves.* Unlike latex rubber, Elastyren is not vulcanized and therefore contains no metal oxides, sulfur, accelerators, or mercaptobenzothiazole—sensitizers commonly found in rubber products. Other brands of hypoallergenic surgical gloves are Dermaprene and Neolon. Allerderm vinyl gloves, meant for household use, can be used with a cotton liner. Hypoallergenic vinyl examination gloves include TriFlex, TruTouch, and Surgikos.

---

*Available from Allerderm Laboratories; P.O. Box 931; Mill Valley, CA 94942-0931; (415) 381-0106.

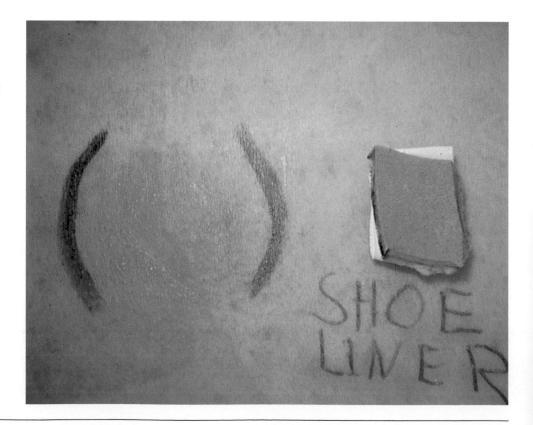

Figure 4-10
Patient in Figure 4-9 was patch tested with a piece of shoe lining. A 2+ positive allergic reaction occurred within 48 hours.

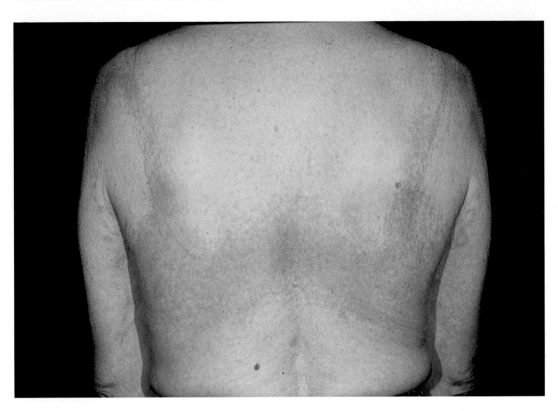

Figure 4-11
Allergic contact dermatitis to spandex rubber in a bra.

Figure 4-12
Allergic contact dermatitis to rubber band of underwear.
Washing clothes with bleach may make the rubber
allergenic.

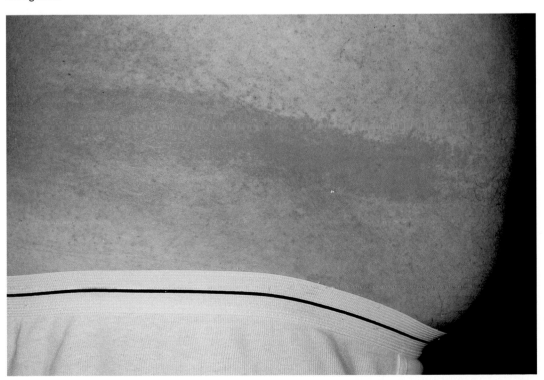

METAL DERMATITIS
Nickel

Nickel is the most common contact allergen affecting females in Europe and the United States. Women are affected much more frequently than men. Men are usually sensitized in an industrial setting. Ear piercing or wearing clip-on earrings brings metal into direct contact with skin, an ideal setting for sensitization to occur (Figure 4-13).[11, 12] Ears should be pierced with stainless steel instruments, and stainless steel or plastic studs should be worn until complete epithelialization takes place. So-called hypoallergenic earrings may sensitize a person to a metal. Some gold earrings contain nickel. A catalogue of earrings that have been clinically tested to be safe for nickel-sensitive patients[13] is available.* All-plastic earrings with fronts, posts, and backs made of hard nylon are now available.

---

*From Roman Research, Inc.; 45 Accore Park Dr.; Norwell, MA 02061.

Avoidance is the only way to prevent inflammation. Sources of contact are necklaces, scissors, door handles, watchbands, bracelets, belt buckles (Figure 4-14), and coined money (common in cashiers).[14] Nickel-sensitive persons are not at greater risk of developing discomfort in the oral cavity when wearing an intraoral orthodontic appliance.[15]

Modern plastic-to-metal joint replacements rarely cause sensitization to composite metals and are safe for nickel-sensitive patients.[16, 17] Acrylic bone cement has never been implicated in causing dermatitis, although orthopedic surgeons have become sensitized to the methyl methacrylate monomer used in the cement. Surgical skin clips should not be used in nickel-sensitive patients.[18]

The dimethylglyoxime spot test for nickel involves adding two solutions to a metal surface.* If the solution turns pink, the test is positive. All nickel-sensitive patients should be taught how to use the dimethylglyoxime test. This enables them to determine which metallic objects they should avoid.

---

*Test kits (Allertest-Ni) can be ordered from Allerderm Laboratories; P.O. Box 931; Mill Valley, CA 94942-0931; (415) 381-0106.

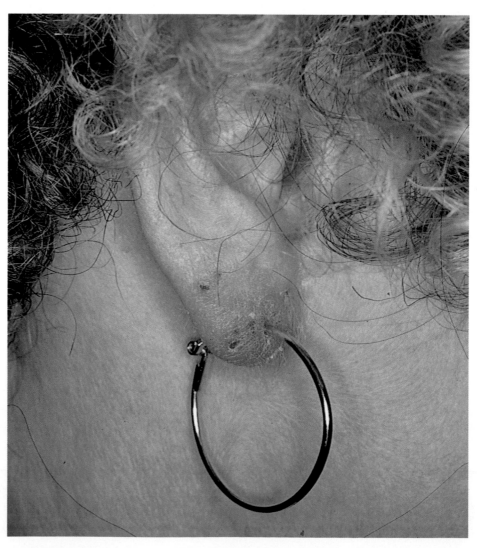

Figure 4-13
Nickel allergy. A classic presentation.

Some nickel-sensitive patients with periodic vesicular, palmar eczema (pompholyx) may benefit from a low-nickel diet (see the box at right).[19-22] Some cases of so-called endogenous pompholyx-like eruptions in nickel-sensitive persons may be due to exogenous contact with nickel-plated objects.

Mercury dental amalgam

The mercury amalgam that dentists use to fill decayed teeth does not contain nickel. Allergy to mercury is very rare. Patch testing to mercury is unreliable and rarely done.[23, 24] Gold alloyed with metal other than mercury is used for mercury-sensitive patients. Gold, however, is also a possible cause of allergic contact dermatitis.[25]

SUGGESTED DIET FOR NICKEL-SENSITIVE INDIVIDUALS WITH POMPHOLYX

Permitted foods: All meats, fish (except herring), poultry, eggs, milk, yogurt, butter, margarine, cheese, one medium-sized potato per day, small amounts of the following: cauliflower, cabbage, carrots, cucumber, lettuce, polished rice, flour (except whole grain), fresh fruits, except pears, marmalade/jam, coffee, wine, beer

Prohibited foods: Canned foods, foods cooked in nickel-plated utensils, herring, oysters, asparagus, beans, mushrooms, onions, corn (maize), spinach, tomatoes, peas, whole grain flour, fresh and cooked pears, rhubarb, tea, cocoa and chocolate, baking powder

Foods preferably should be cooked in aluminum or stainless steel utensils or in utensils that give a negative test for nickel with dimethylglyoxime.

Figure 4-14
Nickel allergy. Belt buckle rubbed against abdomen when the patient bent over.

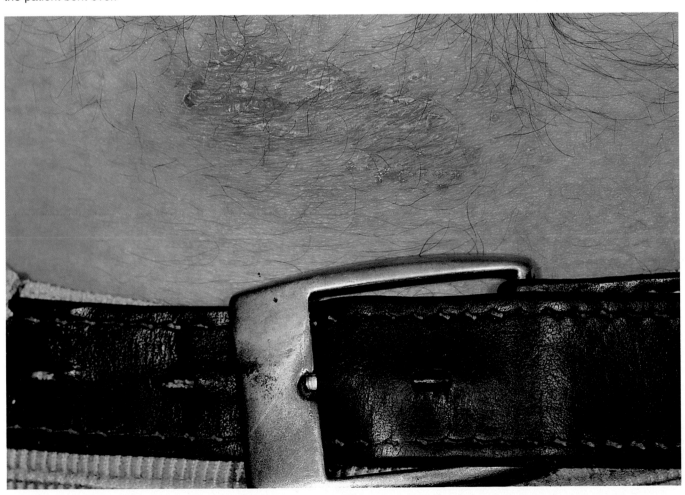

Chromates

Trivalent chromium (insoluble) and hexavalent chromium (soluble) compounds are sensitizers. Trivalent chromium is found in leather gloves and shoes. Hexavalent chromium is found in cement. Chromate is possibly the most common sensitizer for men in industrialized countries. Sources are cement, photographic processes, metal, and dyes. Cement is the most common cause of chromate allergy. Cement acts both as an irritant and a sensitizer.

CEMENT DERMATITIS AND BURNS

Most cement workers experience dryness of the skin when first exposed, but most seem to adapt. Severe deep cutaneous alkali (pH 12) burns may occur on the lower legs of men whose skin is in direct contact with wet cement. Initial symptoms are burning and erythema; ulceration develops after 12 hours.[26] The most severe burns occur when cement spills over the boot top and is held next to the skin[27] (Figure 4-15). Chronic pain and scarring may follow severe burns.[28] Industrial workers sensitized to chromates in cement develop eczematous inflammation on the backs of the hands and forearms. The source of contact frequently is not appreciated until these patients do not respond to both topical and systemic steroids. Once the patient is removed from contact with cement, response to treatment is rapid.

Hexavalent chromate in cement can be removed with iron sulfate. A proposal has been made that iron sulfate should be used in the construction industry to prevent cement dermatitis in construction workers.[29]

Further examples of allergic contact dermatitis are illustrated in Figures 4-16 through 4-19.

PATIENTS WITH LEG ULCERS

Patients with leg ulcers, venous insufficiency, and lower leg edema may have an altered sensitivity to chemicals and are particularly susceptible to contact dermatitis of the lower legs. Topical medicines containing wool alcohols, fragrance, parabens, and neomycin should be avoided.[30]

COSMETIC ALLERGY

Cosmetics are frequently suspected of causing allergic reactions. Preservatives, fragrances, and emulsifiers are frequently implicated.[31] Patch testing can be done with suspected products. A booklet entitled *C.T.F.A Cosmetic Industry On Call* is a directory of persons employed by individual cosmetic manufacturers who can provide useful information on product formulation and ingredient characteristics.*

---

*Contact The Cosmetic, Toiletry and Fragrance Association; 1110 Vermont Avenue, NW, Suite 800; Washington, DC 20005; (202) 331-1770.

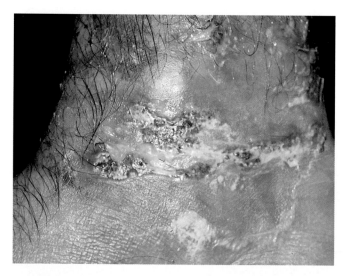

Figure 4-15
Severe irritant dermatitis from contact with wet cement.

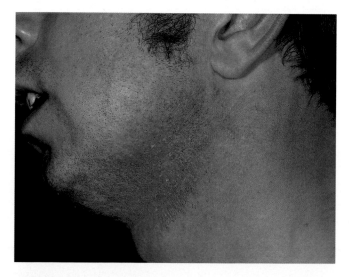

Figure 4-16
Allergic contact dermatitis to benzoyl peroxide in topical acne preparation.

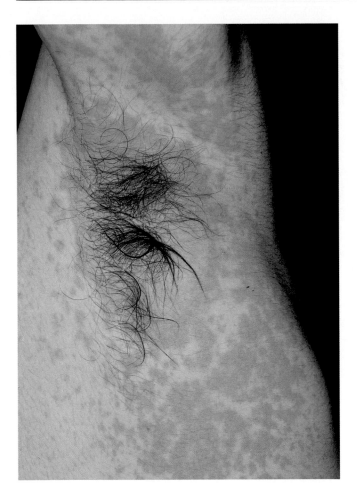

Figure 4-17
Allergic contact dermatitis to a spray deodorant.

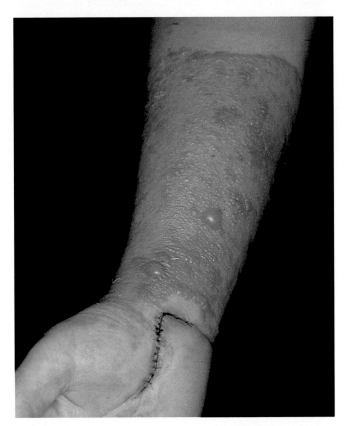

Figure 4-18
Allergic contact dermatitis to benzoin under a cast.

A

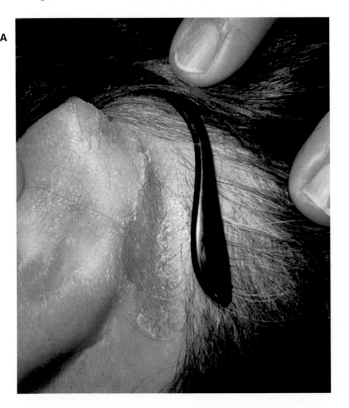

B

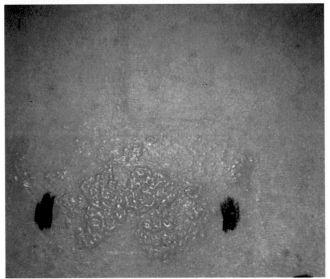

Figure 4-19
A, Allergic contact dermatitis to the plastic in a pair of glasses. **B**, Patch testing with the plastic handle applied to the skin under tape for 2 days shows a 3+ positive reaction.

Diagnosis of Contact Dermatitis

Determining the allergens responsible for allergic contact dermatitis requires a medical history, physical examination, and, in some instances, patch testing. Historical points of interest are date of onset, relationship to work (i.e., improves during weekends or vacations), and types of products used in skin care. The number of different creams, lotions, cosmetics, and topical medications that patients can accumulate is amazing. Persistent questioning may eventually uncover the responsible antigen.

Patch testing should not be attempted until the patient has had time to ponder the questions raised by the physician. In many cases all that is required is to avoid the suspected offending material. Patch testing is indicated for cases in which inflammation persists despite avoidance and appropriate topical therapy. Patch testing is not useful as a diagnostic test for irritant contact dermatitis, since irritant dermatitis is a nonimmunologically mediated inflammatory reaction.

PATCH TESTING

Open patch test. The suspected allergen is applied to the skin of the upper outer arm and left uncovered. Application is repeated twice daily for 2 days and read as described below.

Use test. The suspected cream or cosmetic is used on a site distant from the original eruption. Suitable areas for testing are the outer arm or the skin of the antecubital fossa. The material is applied twice daily for at least 7 days. The test is stopped if a reaction occurs.

Closed patch test. The material is applied to the skin and covered with an adhesive bandage. The adhesive bandage is removed in 48 hours for initial interpretation (Figures 4-20, 4-21, and 4-22).

Solid objects such as shoe leather, wood, or rubber materials, or nonirritating material such as skin moisturizers, topical medicines, or cosmetics are well suited to this technique.

Only bland material should be applied directly to the skin surface. Caustic industrial solvents must be diluted. Patch testing with a high concentration of caustic material may lead to skin necrosis. Petrolatum is generally the most suitable vehicle for dispersion of test materials. The concentration required to elicit a response varies with each chemical, and appropriate concentrations for testing can be found in standard textbooks dealing with contact dermatitis. If intense itching occurs, patches should be removed from test sites. A negative patch test with this direct technique does not rule out the diagnosis of allergy. The concentration of material tested may be too weak to elicit a response, or one component of a topical medication (e.g., topical steroids) may suppress the allergic reaction induced by another component of the same cream.

If this technique fails or if the clinical presentation is that of allergic contact dermatitis but a source cannot be uncovered by the history and physical examination, then patch testing with the standard patch test series should be considered.

Steroids and patch testing. Corticosteroids such as prednisone in dosages of 15 mg/day or the equivalent may inhibit patch test reactions.[32] The prior application of the group V topical steroid triamcinolone acetonide to skin does not strongly influence patch test reactions.[33] The presence of triamcinolone in the materials used for patch testing is capable of blocking both irritant and allergic reactions.[34] Allergic contact dermatitis to topical glucocorticosteroids is uncommon but possible.[35, 36]

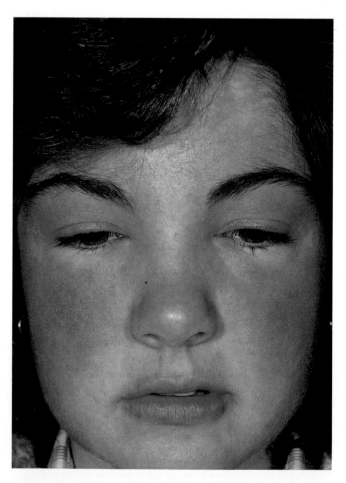

Figure 4-20
A beautician with diffuse erythema of the face.

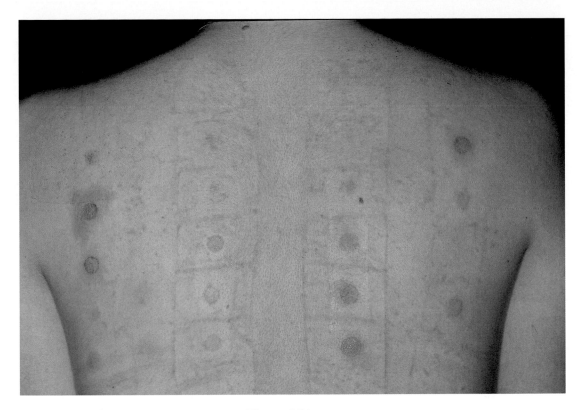

Figure 4-21
The patient in Figure 4-20 was patch tested with several of the preparations used at work. Many positive reactions of varying intensity appeared.

Figure 4-22
Patch testing. Individual allergens are tested on strips obtained from companies that sell individual allergens in syringes.

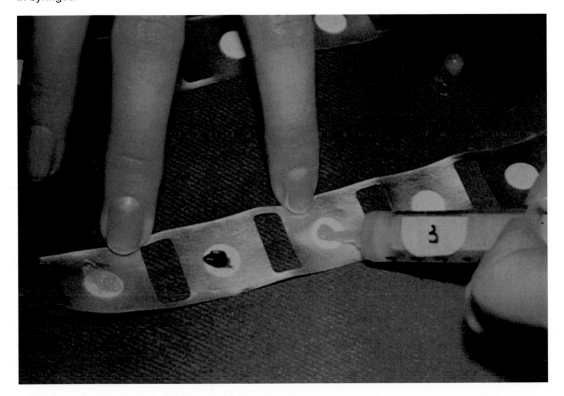

Standard patch test series

Testing with groups of allergens is generally performed by physicians who frequently see contact dermatitis and have experience with the problems involved in accurately determining the significance of test results. A group of chemicals that have proved to be frequent or important causes of allergic contact dermatitis have been assembled into standard patch test series. T.R.U.E. TEST (distributed by Glaxo Pharmaceutical Company) is a ready-to-use patch test for the diagnosis of allergic contact dermatitis. It contains 24 allergens and allergen mixes responsible for as much as 80% of allergic contact dermatitis (Table 4-4). Hermal Laboratories distributes an Allergen Patch Test Kit (1-800-HERMAL-1). The kit contains 20 allergens in syringe dispensers, instructions, and data collection forms. TROLAB patch test allergens from Europe are distributed by Omniderm Inc., Montreal, Quebec (1-514-340-1114). They have a very large number of different allergens available.[37]

These test kits are only a screening procedure and do not test for all possible environmental allergens.

Technique for T.R.U.E. TEST. Each of the two T.R.U.E. TEST panels employs 12 standardized allergens or allergen mixes fixed in thin, dehydrated gel layers attached to a waterproof backing. Moisture from the skin after application causes the gels to be rehydrated and to release small amounts of allergen onto the patient's skin. After 48 hours, T.R.U.E. TEST is removed; reactions are then interpreted at 72 to 96 hours after test application (Figure 4-23).

TABLE 4-4 T.R.U.E. TEST* Allergen Patch Test of 24 Allergens

Component	Occurrence	Reaction frequency (%)
1. Nickel sulfate	Jewelry, metal and metal-plated objects	24.2
2. Wool alcohols	Cosmetics and topical medications	0.8
3. Neomycin sulfate	Topical antibiotics	6.7
4. Potassium dichromate	Cement, chrome-tanned leather, welding fumes, cutting oils, antirust paints	2.4
5. Caine mix	Topical anesthetics	3.3
6. Fragrance mix	Fragrances, toiletries, scented household products, flavorings	8.3
7. Colophony	Cosmetics, adhesives, industrial products	1.6
8. Epoxy resin	Two-part adhesives, surface coatings, paints	0.5
9. Quinoline mix	Medicated creams and ointments, paste bandages, veterinary products	1.7
10. Balsam of Peru	Fragrances, flavorings, cosmetics	3.3
11. Ethylenediamine dihydrochloride	Topical medications, eyedrops, industrial solvents, anticorrosive agents	2.5
12. Cobalt dichloride	Metal-plated objects, paints, cement, metal	6.6
13. p-tert Butylphenol formaldehyde resin	Waterproof glues, leather, construction materials, paper, fabrics	1.6
14. Paraben mix	Preservative in topical formulations, industrial preparations	3.3
15. Carba mix	Rubber products, glues for leather, pesticides, vinyl	2.5
16. Black rubber mix	All black rubber products, some hair dye	1.7
17. Cl + Me- Isothiazolinone	Cosmetics and skin care products, topical medications, household cleaning products	2.5
18. Quaternium-15	Preservative in cosmetics and skin care products, household polishes and cleaners, industrial products	5.0
19. Mercaptobenzothiazole	Rubber products, adhesives, industrial products	0.8
20. p-Phenylenediamine (PPD)	Dyed textiles, cosmetics, hair dyes, printing ink, photodeveloper	4.2
21. Formaldehyde	Plastics, synthetic resins, glues, textiles, construction material	4.2
22. Mercapto mix	Rubber products, glues for leather and plastics, industrial products	1.6
23. Thimerosal	Preservative in contact lens solutions, cosmetics, nose and ear drops, injectable drugs	10.8
24. Thiuram mix	Rubber products, adhesives, pesticides, drugs	5.0

*Thin-layer Rapid Use Epicutaneous Test.

ALLERGEN PATCH TEST T.R.U.E. TEST
(Thin-layer Rapid Use Epicutaneous Test)

A, The two test panels are packaged in foil.

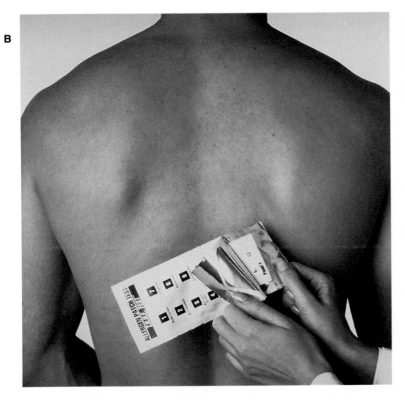

B, Each panel contains 12 allergens fixed to an adhesive tape.

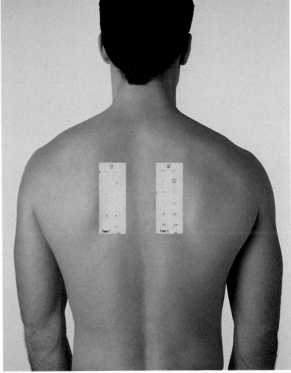

C, The tape is removed and applied to the back.

Figure 4-23

Patch test reading and interpretation. The test reactions are graded at each reading as follows:

+ = Weak (nonvesicular) positive reaction: erythema, infiltration, possibly papules

+ + = Strong (edematous or vesicular) positive reaction (Figure 4-24)

+ + + = Extreme (spreading, bullous, ulcerative) positive reaction (Figure 4-25)

− = Negative reaction

IR = Irritant reactions of different types

NT = Not tested ·

Doubtful reaction (macular erythema only)

Figure 4-24
A 2+ positive patch test reaction with erythema and vesicles.

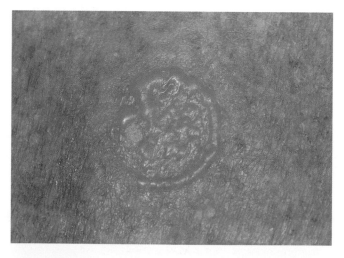

Figure 4-25
A 3+ positive patch test reaction with vesicles and bullae.

Allergic vs. irritant test reactions

It is important to determine whether the test response is caused by allergy or by a nonspecific irritant reaction. Strong allergic reactions are vesicular and may spread beyond the test site. Strong irritant reactions exhibit a deep erythema, resembling a burn. There is no morphologic method of distinguishing a weak irritant patch test from a weak allergic test. Commercially prepared antigens are formulated to minimize irritant reactions. Irritant test responses are caused by either hyperirritability of the skin or by the application of an irritating concentration of a test substance. Irritation is avoided by applying tests only on normal skin that has not been washed or cleaned with alcohol.

The excited skin syndrome (angry back). "Eczema creates eczema." The excited skin syndrome is a major cause of false-positive patch test reactions. Single or multiple concomitant positive patch test reactions may produce a state of skin hyperreactivity in which other patch test sites, particularly those with minimal irritation, may become reactive.[38] Patients who have multiple strong test reactions should be retested at a later date with one antigen at a time (Figure 4-26).[39] Retesting may show that some of the original tests were false positives. The excited skin syndrome may also be caused by even minimal dermatitis elsewhere.

Relevance of test results. A number of possible conclusions may be drawn from the test results:

- The allergen eliciting the positive test is directly responsible for the patient's dermatitis.
- A chemically related or cross-reacting material is responsible for the dermatitis.
- The patient has not recently been in contact with the indicated allergen and, although he or she is allergic to that specific chemical, it is not relevant to the present condition.
- The test is negative but would be positive if a sufficient concentration of the test chemical were used.
- The positive test is an irritant reaction and is irrelevant.

Contact allergen alternatives

A list of safe and practical alternatives to common allergens has been published in the *Journal of the American Academy of Dermatology*.[20]

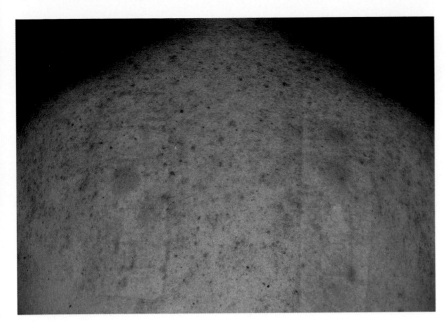

Figure 4-26
The excited skin syndrome. Several tests have become positive, and the severe reactions have stimulated inflammation over the entire back.

REFERENCES

1. Marks JG Jr et al: Dermatitis from cashew nuts, *J Am Acad Dermatol* 10:627-631, 1984.
2. Ratner JH, Spencer SK, Grainge JM: Cashew nut dermatitis, *Arch Dermatol* 110:921-923, 1974.
3. Dooms-Goossens An E et al: Contact dermatitis caused by airborne agents, *J Am Acad Dermatol* 15:1-10, 1986.
4. Weston WL, Weston JA: Allergic contact dermatitis in children, *Am J Dis Child* 138:932-936, 1984.
5. Behl PN: Dermatitis from cashew nuts, *J Am Acad Dermatol* 12:117, 1985.
6. Fisher AA: Contact dermatitis in surgeons, *J Dermatol Surg Oncol* 1:3, 63-67, 1975.
7. Lagier F, Vervloet D, et al: Prevalence of latex allergy in operating room nurses, *J Allergy Clin Immunol* 90:319-322, 1992.
8. Sussman GL: Latex allergy: its importance in clinical practice, *Allergy Proc* 13:67-69, 1992.
9. Sussman GL, Tarlo S, et al: The spectrum of IgE-mediated responses to latex , *JAMA* 265:2844-2847, 1991.
10. Rich P, Belozer ML, et al: Allergic contact dermatitis to two antioxidants in latex gloves: 4,4'-thiobis(6-tert-butyl-*meta*-cresol) and butylhydroxyanisole. Allergen alternatives for glove-allergic patients [published erratum appears in *J Am Acad Dermatol* 26(1):144], *J Am Acad Dermatol* 24.37-43, 1991.
11. Emmett EA et al: Allergic contact dermatitis to nickel: bioavailability from consumer products and provocation threshold, *J Am Acad Dermatol* 19:314-322, 1988.
12. Nielsen NH, Menne T: Nickel sensitization and ear piercing in an unselected Danish population. Glostrup Allergy Study, *Contact Dermatitis* 29:16-21, 1993.
13. Dobson RL: Earrings for nickel-sensitive women, *J Am Acad Dermatol* 16:631, 1987.
14. Gollhausen R, Ring J: Allergy to coined money: nickel contact dermatitis in cashiers, *J Am Acad Dermatol* 25:365-369, 1991.
15. Staerkjaer L, Menne T: Nickel allergy and orthodontic treatment, *Eur J Orthod* 12:284-289, 1990.
16. Fisher AA: The safety of artificial hip replacement in nickel-sensitive patients, *Cutis*, May, p 333, 1986.
17. Gawkrodger DJ: Nickel sensitivity and the implantation of orthopaedic prostheses, *Contact Dermatitis* 28:257-259, 1993.
18. Oakley AMM, Ive FA, Carr MM: Skin clips are contraindicated when there is nickel allergy, *J R Soc Med* 80:290, 1987.
19. Nielsen GD, Jepsen LV, et al: Nickel-sensitive patients with vesicular hand eczema: oral challenge with a diet naturally high in nickel, *Br J Dermatol* 122:299-308, 1990.
20. Adams RM, Fisher AA: Contact allergen alternatives: 1986, *J Am Acad Dermatol* 14:951-969, 1986.
21. Veien NK, Hattel T, et al: Low nickel diet: an open, prospective trial, *J Am Acad Dermatol* 29:1002-1007, 1993.
22. Moller H: Yes, systemic nickel is probably important, *J Am Acad Dermatol* 28:511-513, 1993.
23. Fisher AA: The misuse of the patch test to determine "hypersensitivity" to mercury amalgam dental fillings, *Cutis* 35:112-117, 1985.
24. Mackert JR Jr: Hypersensitivity to mercury from dental amalgams, *J Am Acad Dermatol* 12:877-880, 1985.
25. Laeijendecker R, van Joost T: Oral manifestations of gold allergy, *J Am Acad Dermatol* 30:205-209, 1994.
26. Robinson SM, Tachakra SS: Skin ulceration due to cement, *Arch Emerg Med* 9:326-329, 1992.
27. Peters WJ: Alkali burns from wet cement, *Can Med Assoc J* 130:902-903, 1984.
28. Lane PR, Hogan DJ: Chronic pain and scarring from cement burns, *Arch Dermatol* 121:368-369, 1985.
29. Goh CL, Kwok SF: Prevention of cement dermatitis in construction workers with iron sulphate, *Asia-Pac J Pub Health* 1:91-93, 1987.
30. Malten KE, Kuiper JP: Contact allergic reactions in 100 selected patients with ulcus cruris, *VASA* 14:340-345, 1985.
31. de Groot AC et al: The allergens in cosmetics, *Arch Dermatol* 124:1525-1529, 1988.
32. Feverman E, Levy A: A study of the effect of prednisone and antihistamines on patch test reactions, *Br J Dermatol* 86:68, 1972.
33. Dahl MV, Jordan WP Jr: Topical steroids and patch tests, *Arch Dermatol* 119:3-4, 1983.
34. Rietschel RL: Irritant and allergic responses as influenced by triamcinolone in patch test materials, *Arch Dermatol* 121:68-69, 1985.
35. Belsito DV: Allergic contact dermatitis to topical glucocorticosteroids, *Cutis* 52:291-294, 1993.
36. Lauerma AI, Reitamo S: Contact allergy to corticosteroids. *J Am Acad Dermatol* 28:618-622, 1993.
37. Adams RM: Patch testing: a recapitulation, *J Am Acad Dermatol* 5:629-643, 1981.
38. Bruynzeel DP et al: Angry back or the excited skin syndrome: a prospective study, *J Am Acad Dermatol* 8:392-397, 1983.
39. Bruynzeel DP, Maibach HI: Excited skin syndrome (angry back), *Arch Dermatol* 122:323-328, 1986.

Atopic Dermatitis

Definition. The term *atopy* was introduced years ago to designate a group of patients who had a personal or family history of one or more of the following diseases: hay fever, asthma, very dry skin, and eczema. Atopic dermatitis is an eczematous eruption that is itchy, recurrent, flexural, and symmetric. It generally begins early in life, follows periods of remission and exacerbation, and usually resolves by the age of 30. The disease characteristics vary with age. Infants have facial and patchy or generalized body eczema. Adolescents and adults have eczema in flexural areas and on the hands. The pattern of inheritance is unknown, but available data suggest that it is polygenic.

Diagnostic criteria. There are no specific cutaneous signs, no known distinctive histologic features, and no characteristic laboratory findings for atopic dermatitis. There are a variety of characteristics that indicate that the patient has atopic dermatitis (see the box on p. 101). The diagnosis is made when the patient has three or more of the major features and three or more of the minor features. Each patient is different, with a unique combination of major and minor features.

There may be two major subgroups of patients with atopic dermatitis: (1) those with atopic respiratory disease predisposition and an enhanced IgE-producing potential, and (2) those with neither respiratory disease predisposition nor an enhanced potential for IgE production.[1]

Incidence. Between 7 and 24 individuals per 1000 have atopic dermatitis. The highest incidence is among children. The lifetime prevalence of atopic eczema is 20% in children aged 3 to 11 years.[2]

Course and prognosis. Factors associated with a low frequency of healing and increased severity of persistent or recurring dermatitis are listed in order of relative importance in the box on p. 101.[3] More than 50% of young children with generalized atopic dermatitis develop asthma and allergic rhinitis by the age of 13. Dermatitis improves in most children.[4]

Seventy percent of atopic patients have a family history of one or more of the major atopic characteristics: asthma, hay fever, or eczematous dermatitis.

Misconceptions. There are two common misconceptions about atopic dermatitis. The first is that it is an emotional disorder. It is true that patients with inflammation that lasts for months or years seem to be irritable, but this is a normal response to a frustrating disease. The second misconception is that atopic skin disease is precipitated by an allergic reaction. Atopic individuals frequently have respiratory allergies and, when skin tested, are informed that they are allergic to "everything." Atopics may react with a wheal when challenged with a needle during skin testing, but this is a characteristic of atopic skin and is not necessarily a manifestation of allergy. All evidence to date shows that most cases of atopic dermatitis are precipitated by environmental stress on genetically compromised skin and not by interaction with allergens.

CRITERIA FOR DIAGNOSIS OF ATOPIC DERMATITIS

MAJOR FEATURES (MUST HAVE THREE OR MORE)

Pruritus
Typical morphology and distribution
    Flexural lichenification in adults
    Facial and extensor involvement in infants and
      children
    Dermatitis—chronically or chronically relapsing
    Personal or family history of atopy—asthma,
      allergic rhinitis, atopic dermatitis

MINOR FEATURES (MUST HAVE THREE OR MORE)

Cataracts (anterior-subcapsular)
Cheilitis
Conjunctivitis—recurrent
Eczema—perifollicular accentuation
Facial pallor/facial erythema
Food intolerance
Hand dermatitis—nonallergic, irritant
Ichthyosis
IgE—elevated
Immediate (type 1) skin test reactivity
Infections (cutaneous)—*Staphylococcus aureus*,
    herpes simplex
Infraorbital fold (Dennie-Morgan lines)
Itching when sweating
Keratoconus
Keratosis pilaris
Nipple dermatitis
Orbital darkening
Palmar hyperlinearity
Pityriasis alba
White dermographism
Wool intolerance
Xerosis

Data from Roth HL:*Int J Dermatol* 26:139-149, 1987; Hanifin JM, Rajka G: *Acta Derm Venereol* (Stockh) 92(suppl):44-47, 1980; and Hanifin JM, Lobitz WC Jr: *Arch Dermatol* 113:663-670, 1977.

ATOPIC DERMATITIS UNFAVORABLE PROGNOSTIC FACTORS*

Persistent dry or itchy skin in adult life
Widespread dermatitis in childhood
Associated allergic rhinitis
Family history of atopic dermatitis
Associated bronchial asthma
Early age at onset
Female sex

Data from Rystedt I: *Acta Derm Venereol* (Stockh) 65:206-213, 1985.
*In order of relative importance.

Pathogenesis and Immunology

Atopic dermatitis seems to result from a vicious circle of dermatitis associated with elevated T-lymphocyte activation, hyperstimulatory Langerhans' cells, defective cell-mediated immunity, and B-cell IgE overproduction.[5]

IgE-binding structures on Langerhans' cells in the epidermis capture and present IgE-targeted allergens to specific T cells, which elicit an IgE-inducing lymphokine interleukin-4. New therapies based on these facts are being tested. Cyclosporine, which targets T-cell activation and antigen presentation, is effective for severe atopic dermatitis. Interferon gamma normalizes immune responsiveness rather than directly suppressing the immune system.[6,7] Recent therapeutic trials have focused on the reduction of trigger factors, such as house-dust mite exposure, foods, and the abnormal epidermal lipid barrier to irritation.

Aeroallergens. Aeroallergens may play an important role in causing eczematous lesions. Patch testing patients caused reactions with house dust (70%), mites (70%), cockroaches (63%), mold mix (50%), and grass mix (43%). Only 10% of atopic children without atopic dermatitis had eczematous lesions.[8] Patients with atopic dermatitis frequently show positive scratch and intradermal reactions to a number of antigens. Avoidance of these antigens rarely improves the dermatitis.

Elevated IgE and the inflammatory response. Elevated IgE levels are the most consistent immune defect. Serum IgE levels are elevated above 200 IU/ml in 80% to 90% of patients with atopic dermatitis and are less than 200 IU/ml in 70% of normal adults. Patients with very active disease may have IgE levels greater than 1000 IU/ml. However, 20% of patients with atopic dermatitis have normal or below normal levels of IgE, suggesting that IgE elevations are a coincident feature of disordered cell regulation rather than a pathogenic factor. The levels of IgE do not necessarily correlate with the activity of the disease; therefore, elevated serum IgE levels can only be considered supporting evidence for the disease.[9] Total IgE is significantly higher in children with coexistent atopic respiratory disease in all age groups.

Because there are many false positives resulting from nonspecific IgE binding to the solid-phase radioimmunosorbent, radioallergosorbent tests (RASTs) are of little value for patients with atopic dermatitis who have high IgE levels. RAST findings correlated with positive findings from food-challenge tests in only one third of cases. Negative RAST findings are, however, predictive of negative results from food-challenge tests. The frequency of positive RAST for food allergens decreases with age; the frequency of positive RAST for inhalant allergens increases with age.[10]

Blood eosinophilia. Eosinophil levels roughly correlate with disease severity. Very high eosinophil counts are common with severe cases of atopic dermatitis in patients who have a personal or family history of respiratory atopy, whereas normal or moderately elevated eosinophil values are seen in severe cases of atopic dermatitis in patients who have neither a personal nor a family history of respiratory atopy.[11] There is no accumulation of tissue eosinophils; however, degranulation of eosinophils in the dermis with release of major basic protein may play a pathogenic role.[12] Major basic protein may induce histamine release from basophils and mast cells, which stimulates itching, irritation, and lichenification.

Reduced cell-mediated immunity. Patients with atopic dermatitis may have a primary T-cell defect. Several facts suggest that atopic patients have disordered cell-mediated immunity. Patients may develop severe diffuse cutaneous infection with the herpes simplex virus (eczema herpeticum) whether or not their dermatitis is active. Mothers with active herpes labialis should avoid direct contact of their active lesion with their children's skin, as in kissing, especially if the child has dermatitis.

Atopic patients have an increased susceptibility to cutaneous viral infections, such as molluscum contagiosum, and to cutaneous fungal infections.[13] The incidence of contact allergy may be lower than normal in atopic patients;[14] however, some studies show equal rates of sensitization.[15,16] Humoral immunity seems to be normal.

Altered T-cell regulation of IgE may be responsible for the overabundant IgE production. High levels of IgE sensitize mast cells to environmental antigens, resulting in excess histamine release.

Histamine. Histamine and other mediators of mast cells and basophils may be responsible for the acute inflammation. A basic disorder of cyclic AMP metabolism may alter the ability of mast cells toward hyperreleasability, leading to the high amounts of plasma and tissue histamine observed experimentally.[17,18] An IgE-mediated late-phase reaction initiated by food allergens, for example, may cause deposition of major basic protein and release of histamine.

Clinical Aspects

Major and minor diagnostic features. The box on p. 101 lists the major and minor diagnostic features for atopic dermatitis and atopy. Each patient has his or her own unique set of features.

Itching, the primary lesion. "It is not the eruption that is itchy but the itchiness that is eruptive." Atopic dermatitis starts with itching. Abnormally dry skin and a lowered threshold for itching are important features of atopic dermatitis. It is the scratching that creates most of the characteristic patterns of the disease. Most patients with atopic dermatitis make a determined effort to control their scratching, but during sleep conscious control is lost; under warm covers the patients scratch and a rash appears. The itch-scratch cycle is established, and conscious effort is no longer sufficient to control scratching. The act of scratching becomes habitual, and the disease progresses.

Patterns of inflammation. Atopic inflammation begins abruptly with erythema and severe pruritis. The skin surface is modified by scratching to produce lichenification, and the episode resolves slowly, leaving the skin in a dry, scaly, compromised condition called *xerosis*. There is no single primary lesion in atopic dermatitis. Rather, several patterns and types of lesions may be produced by exposure to external stimuli or may be precipitated by scratching. These types of lesions are papules (Figure 5-1), eczematous dermatitis with redness and scaling (Figure 5-2), and lichenification (Figure 5-3). Lichenification represents a thickening of the epidermis. It is a highly characteristic lesion, with the normal skin lines accentuated to resemble a washboard. These so-called primary responses are altered by excoriation and infection.

Although the cutaneous manifestations of the atopic diathesis are varied, they have characteristic age-determined patterns. Knowledge of these patterns is useful; many patients, however, have a nonclassic pattern. Atopic dermatitis may terminate after an indefinite period or may progress from infancy to adulthood with little or no relief. Fifty-eight percent of infants with atopic dermatitis were found to have persistent inflammation 15 to 17 years later.[19] Atopic dermatitis is arbitrarily divided into three phases.

ATOPIC DERMATITIS—PATTERNS OF INFLAMMATION

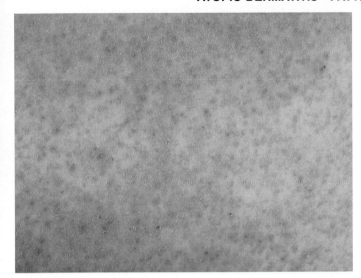

Figure 5-1
Papular lesions are common in the antecubital and popliteal fossae. Papules become confluent and form plaques.

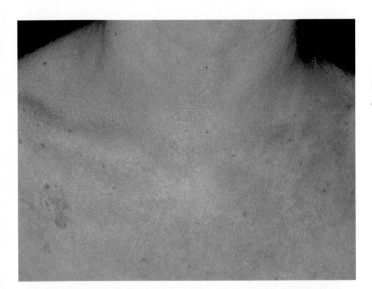

Figure 5-2
Eczematous dermatitis with diffuse erythema and scaling on the neck and chest.

Figure 5-3
Lichenification with accentuation of normal skin lines. This lichenified plaque is surrounded by papules.

INFANT PHASE (BIRTH TO 2 YEARS)

Infants are rarely born with atopic eczema, but they typically develop the first signs of inflammation during the third month. The most common occurrence is that of a baby who during the winter months develops dry, red, scaling areas confined to the cheeks, but sparing the perioral and paranasal areas (Figures 5-4 and 5-5). This is the same area that becomes flushed with exposure to cold. The chin is often involved and initially may be more inflamed than are the cheeks. This may result from the irritation of drooling and subsequent repeated washing. Inflammation may spread to involve the paranasal and perioral area as the winter progresses (Figure 5-6). Habitual lip licking by an atopic child results in oozing, crusting, and scaling on the lips and perioral skin (Figure 5-7). Many infants do not excoriate during these early stages, and the rash remains localized and chronic. Repeated scratching or washing creates red, scaling, oozing plaques on the cheeks, a classic presentation of infantile eczema. At this stage the infant is uncomfortable and becomes restless and agitated during sleep.

A small but significant number of infants have a generalized eruption consisting of papules, redness, scaling, and areas of lichenification. The diaper area is often spared (Figure 5-8). Lichenification may occur in the fossae and crease areas, or it may be confined to a favorite, easily reached spot, such as directly below the diaper, the back of the hand, or the extensor forearm (Figures 5-9 and 5-10). Prolonged atopic dermatitis with increasing discomfort disturbs sleep, and both the parents and the child are distraught.

For years, foods such as milk, wheat, eggs, juices, and beef have been suspected as etiologic factors.[20] Food testing and breast-feeding are discussed at the end of this chapter. The course of the disease may be influenced by events such as teething, respiratory infections, and adverse emotional stimuli. The disease is chronic, with periods of exacerbation and remission. Atopic dermatitis resolves in approximately 50% of infants by 18 months, but the others progress to the childhood phase, and a different pattern evolves.

Growth in atopic eczema. Height is significantly correlated with the surface area of skin affected by eczema. The growth of children with eczema affecting less than 50% of the skin surface area appears to be normal, and impaired growth is confined to those with more extensive disease. Treatment with topical steroids has only marginal additional effect on impaired growth.[21]

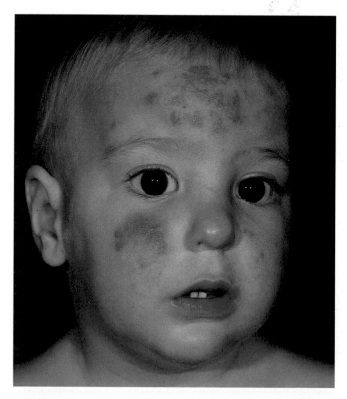

Figure 5-4
Red scaling plaques confined to the cheeks are one of the first signs of atopic dermatitis in an infant.

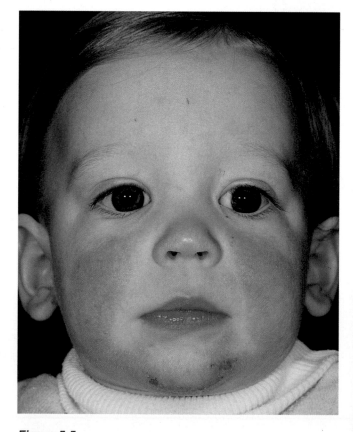

Figure 5-5
Atopic dermatitis. A common appearance in children with erythema and scaling confined to the cheeks and sparing the perioral and paranasal area.

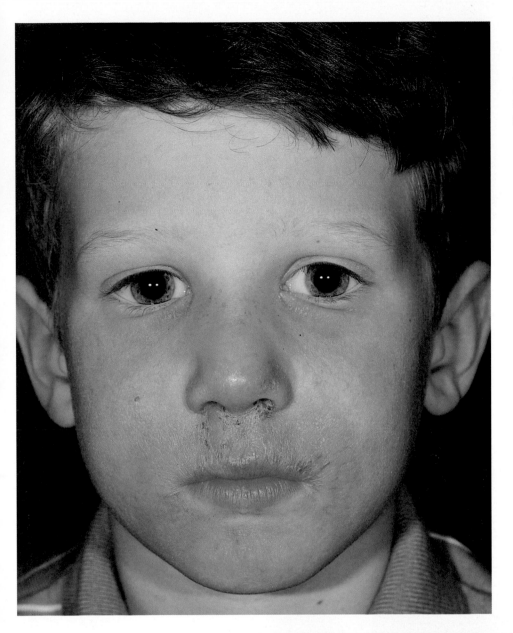

Figure 5-6
Atopic dermatitis. Progression of inflammation to involve the perioral and paranasal areas.

Figure 5-7
Habitual lip licking in an atopic child produces erythema and scaling that may eventually lead to secondary infection.

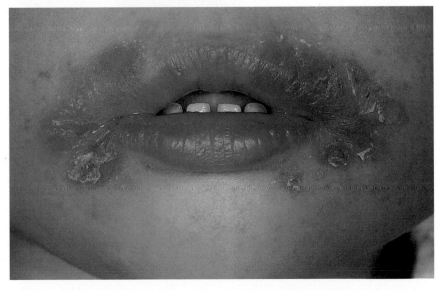

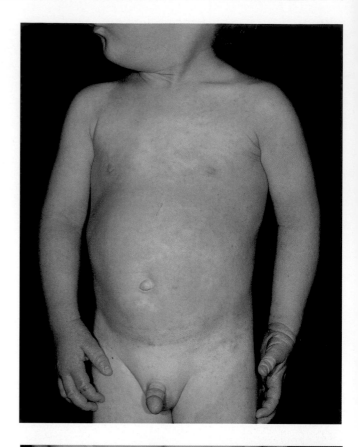

Figure 5-8
Generalized infantile atopic dermatitis sparing the diaper area, which is protected from scratching.

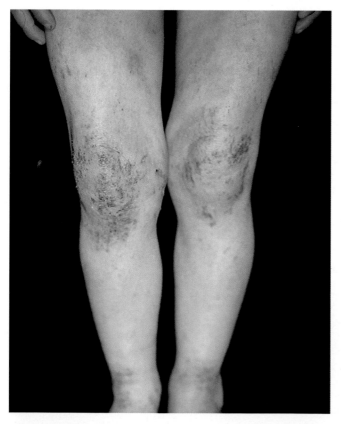

Figure 5-9
Inflammation in the flexural areas is the most common presentation of atopic dermatitis in children.

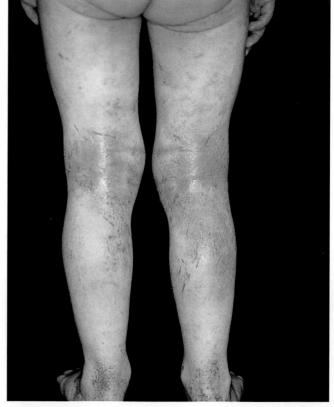

Figure 5-10
Rubbing and scratching the inflamed flexural areas causes thickened (lichenified) skin. These lesions form fissures and are infected with *Staphylococcus aureus*.

CHILDHOOD PHASE (2 TO 12 YEARS)

The most common and characteristic appearance of atopic dermatitis is inflammation in flexural areas (i.e., the antecubital fossae, neck, wrists, and ankles [Figures 5-11 through 5-14]). These areas of repeated flexion and extension perspire with exertion. The act of perspiring stimulates burning and intense itching and initiates the itch-scratch cycle. Tight clothing that traps heat about the neck or extremities further aggravates the problem. Inflammation typically begins in one of the fossae or about the neck. The rash may remain localized to one or two areas or progress to involve the neck, antecubital and popliteal fossae, wrists, and ankles. The eruption begins with papules that rapidly coalesce into plaques, which become lichenified when scratched. The plaques may be pale and mildly inflamed with little tendency to change (see Figure 5-13); if they have been vigorously scratched, they may be bright red and scaling with erosions. The border may be sharp and well defined, as it is in psoriasis (Figure 5-14), or poorly defined with papules extraneous to the lichenified areas. A few patients do not develop lichenification even with repeated scratching. The exudative lesions typical of the infant phase are not as common. Most patients with chronic lesions tolerate their disease and sleep well.

Figure 5-11
Atopic dermatitis. Classic appearance of confluent papules forming plaques in the antecubital fossa.

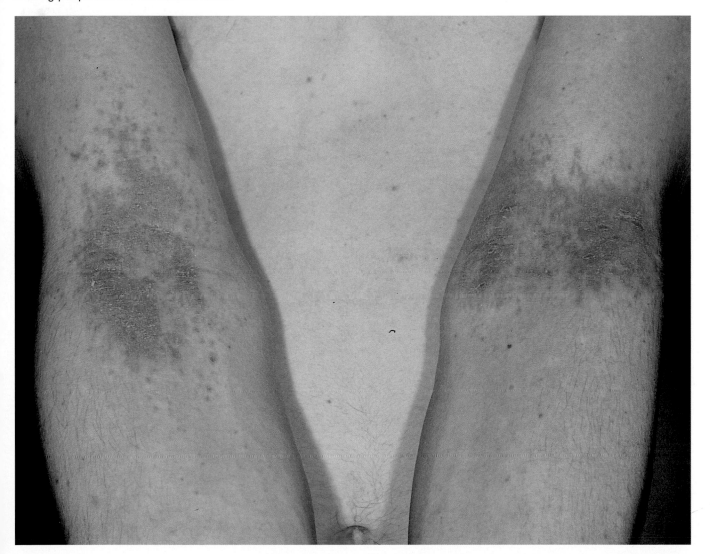

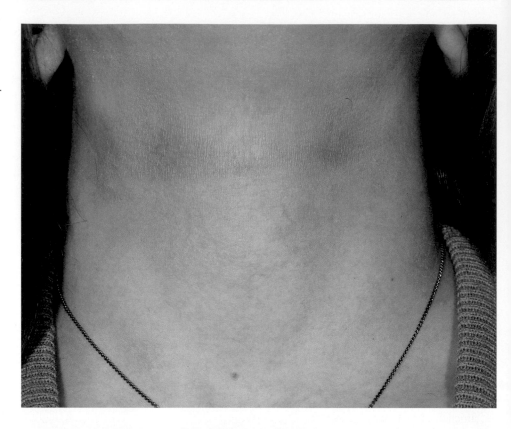

Figure 5-12
Atopic dermatitis. Classic appearance of erythema and diffuse scaling about the neck.

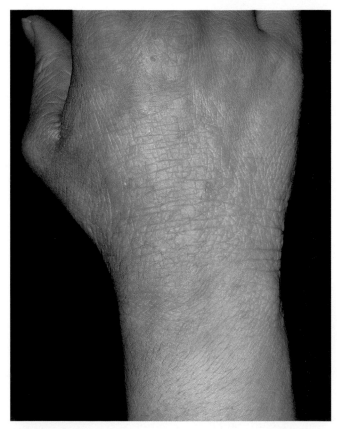

Figure 5-13
Atopic dermatitis. A chronically inflamed lichenified plaque on the wrist.

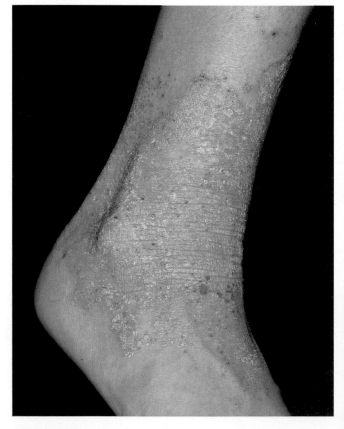

Figure 5-14
Sharply defined lichenified plaque with a silvery scale showing some of the features of psoriasis. Erosions are present.

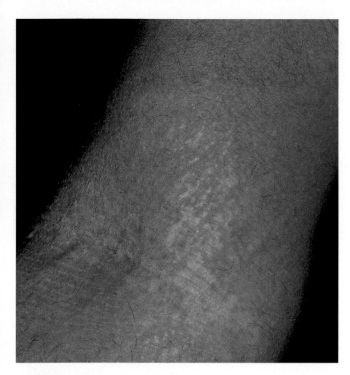

Constant scratching may lead to destruction of melanocytes, resulting in areas of hypopigmentation that become more obvious when the inflammation subsides. These hypopigmented areas fade with time (Figure 5-15). Additional exacerbating factors such as heat, cold, dry air, or emotional stress may lead to extension of inflammation beyond the confines of the crease areas (Figures 5-16 and 5-17). The inflammation becomes incapacitating. Normal duration of sleep cannot be maintained, and schoolwork or job performance deteriorates; these people are miserable. They discover that standing in a hot shower gives considerable temporary relief, but further progression is inevitable with the drying effect produced by repeated wetting and drying. In the more advanced cases, hospitalization is required. Most patients with this pattern of inflammation are in remission by age 30, but in a few patients the disease becomes chronic or improves only to relapse during a change of season or at some other period of transition. Then dermatitis becomes a lifelong ordeal.

Figure 5-15
Hypopigmentation in the antecubital fossa caused by destruction of melanocytes by chronic scratching.

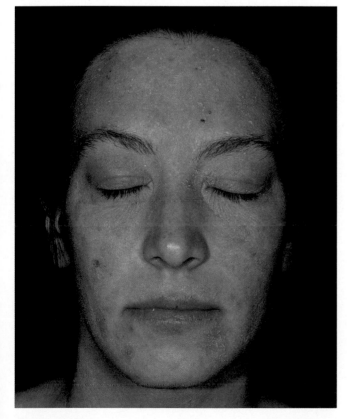

Figure 5-16
Generalized atopic dermatitis. Diffuse erythema and scaling are present.

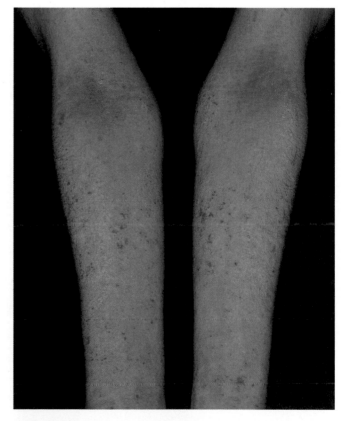

Figure 5-17
The dermatitis has generalized to involve the entire body. Secondary skin infection with *Staphylococcus aureus* is almost always present with this degree of inflammation.

ADULT PHASE (12 YEARS TO ADULT)

The adult phase of atopic dermatitis begins near the onset of puberty. The reason for the resurgence of inflammation at this time is not understood, but it may be related to hormonal changes or to the stress of early adolescence. Adults may have no history of dermatitis in earlier years, but this is unusual. As in the childhood phase, localized inflammation with lichenification is the most common pattern. One area or several areas may be involved. There are several characteristic patterns.

Inflammation in flexural areas. This pattern is commonly seen and is identical to childhood flexural inflammation.

Hand dermatitis. Hand dermatitis may be the most common expression of the atopic diathesis in the adult. (See the section on hand dermatitis in Chapter Three.) Adults are exposed to a variety of irritating chemicals in the home and at work, and they wash more frequently than do children. Irritation causes redness and scaling on the dorsal aspect of the hand or about the fingers. Itching develops, and the inevitable scratching results in lichenification or oozing and crusting. A few or all of the fingertip pads may be involved. They may be dry and chronically peeling or red and fissured. The eruption may be painful, chronic, and resistant to treatment. Psoriasis may have an identical presentation.

Inflammation around eyes. The lids are thin, frequently exposed to irritants, and easily traumatized by scratching. Many adults with atopic dermatitis have inflammation localized to the upper lids (Figure 5-18). They may claim to be allergic to something, but elimination of suspected allergens may not solve the problem. Habitual rubbing of the inflamed lids with the back of the hand is typical. If an attempt to control inflammation fails, then patch testing should be considered to eliminate allergic contact dermatitis.

Lichenification of the anogenital area. Lichenification of the anogenital area is probably more common in patients with atopic dermatitis than in others. Intertriginous areas that are warm and moist can become irritated and itch. Lichenification of the vulva (see Figure 3-49), scrotum (see Figure 3-48), and rectum (see Figure 3-50) may develop with habitual scratching. These areas are resistant to treatment, and inflammation may last for years. The patient may delay visiting a physician because of modesty, and the untreated lichenified plaques become very thick. Emotional factors should also be considered with this isolated phenomenon.

Figure 5-18
Atopic dermatitis of the upper eyelids, an area that is often rubbed with the back of the hand.

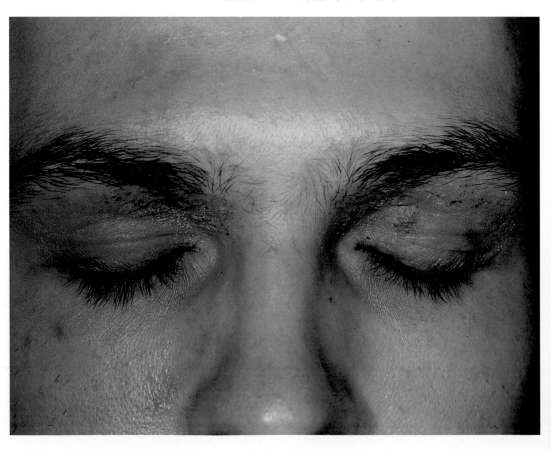

Associated Features

DRY SKIN AND XEROSIS

Dry skin is an important feature of the atopic state. It is commonly assumed that patients with atopic dermatitis have inherited dry skin. The dryness may, however, reflect mild eczematous changes, concomitant ichthyosis, or a complex of both of these changes.[22]

Dry skin may appear at any age, and it is not unusual for infants to have dry scaling skin on the lower legs. Dry skin is sensitive, easily irritated by external stimuli, and, more important, itchy. It is the itching that provides the basis for the development of the various patterns of atopic dermatitis. Scratched itchy skin develops eczema. In other words, it is the itch that rashes.

Dry skin is most often located on the extensor surfaces of the legs and arms, but in susceptible individuals it may involve the entire cutaneous surface. Dryness is worse in the winter when humidity is low. Water is lost from the outermost layer of the skin. The skin becomes drier as the winter continues, and scaling skin becomes cracked and fissured. Dry areas that are repeatedly washed reach a point at which the epidermal barrier can no longer maintain its integrity; erythema and eczema occur. Frequent washing and drying may produce redness with horizontal linear splits, particularly on the lower legs of the elderly, giving a cracked or crazed porcelain appearance (see Chapter Three, Figures 3-37, 3-38, and 3-39).

ICHTHYOSIS VULGARIS

Ichthyosis is a disorder of keratinization characterized by the development of dry, rectangular scales. There are many forms of ichthyosis. Dominant ichthyosis vulgaris may occur as a distinct entity, or it may be found in patients with atopic dermatitis. Atopic patients with ichthyosis vulgaris often have keratosis pilaris and hyperlinear, exaggerated palm creases. Infants may show only dry, scaling skin during the winter, but, with age, the changes become more extensive, and small, fine, white, translucent scales appear on the extensor aspects of the arms and legs (Figure 5-19). These scales are smaller and lighter in color than the large, brown polygonal scales of sex-linked ichthyosis vulgaris, which occurs exclusively in males (Figure 5-20). The scaling of the dominant form does not encroach on the axillae and fossae, as is seen in the sex-linked type. Scaling rarely involves the entire cutaneous surface. The condition tends to improve with age.

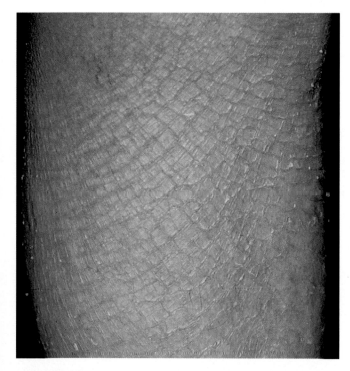

Figure 5-19
Dominant ichthyosis vulgaris. White, translucent, quadrangular scales on the extensor aspects of the arms and legs. This form is significantly associated with atopy.

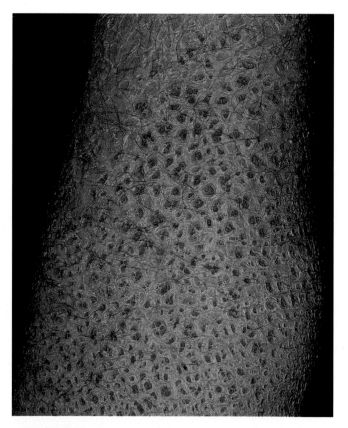

Figure 5-20
Sex-linked ichthyosis vulgaris. Large, brown, quadrangular scales that may encroach on the antecubital and popliteal fossae. Compare this presentation with Figure 5-19. There is no association with atopy.

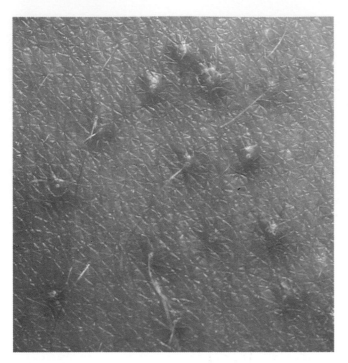

Figure 5-21
Keratosis pilaris. Small, rough, follicular papules or pustules occur most often on the posterolateral aspects of the upper arms and anterior thighs.

KERATOSIS PILARIS

Keratosis pilaris is so common that it is probably physiologic. It does, however, seem to be more common and more extensive in patients with atopic dermatitis. Small (1 to 2 mm), rough, follicular papules or pustules may appear at any age and are common in young children (Figure 5-21). The incidence peaks during adolescence, and the problem tends to improve thereafter.

The posterolateral aspects of the upper arms (Figure 5-22) and anterior thighs are frequently involved, but any area, with the exception of the palms and soles, may be involved. Lesions on the face may be confused with acne, but the uniform small size and association with dry skin and chapping differentiate keratosis pilaris from pustular acne (Figure 5-23). The eruption may be generalized, resembling heat rash or miliaria. Most cases are asymptomatic, but the lesions may be red, inflammatory, and pustular and resemble bacterial folliculitis, particularly on the thighs (Figure 5-24). In the adult generalized form, a red halo appears at the periphery of the keratotic papule. This unusual diffuse pattern in adults persists indefinitely (Figure 5-25). Systemic steroid therapy may greatly accentuate both the lesion and the distribution by creation of numerous follicular pustules.

Treatment with tretinoin (Retin-A) may induce temporary improvement, but the irritation is usually unacceptable. Short courses of group V topical steroids reduce the unsightly redness. Application of Lac-Hydrin cream is probably the most practical and effective way of reducing the roughness. Abrasive washing techniques cause further drying.

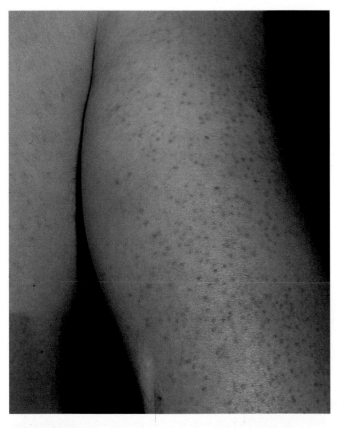

Figure 5-22
Keratosis pilaris. Small, follicular papules are most commonly found on the posterolateral aspects of the upper arms. Most lesions are not this red.

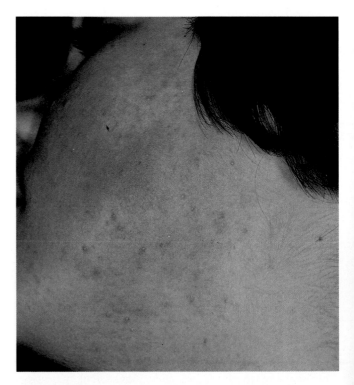

Figure 5-23
Keratosis pilaris. This is common on the face of children and is frequently confused with acne.

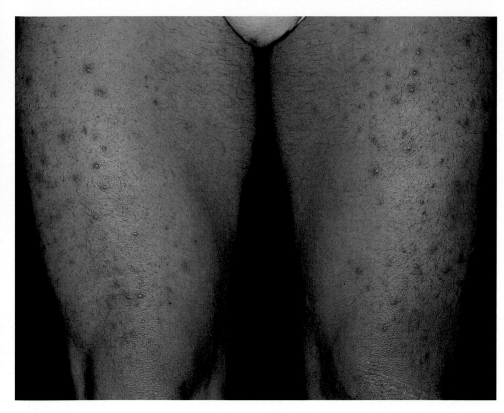

Figure 5-24
Keratosis pilaris. Infected lesions in a uniform distribution.
Typical bacterial folliculitis has a haphazard distribution.

Figure 5-25
Keratosis pilaris. Diffuse involvement of the buttock is
occasionally seen in adults. This type lasts indefinitely.

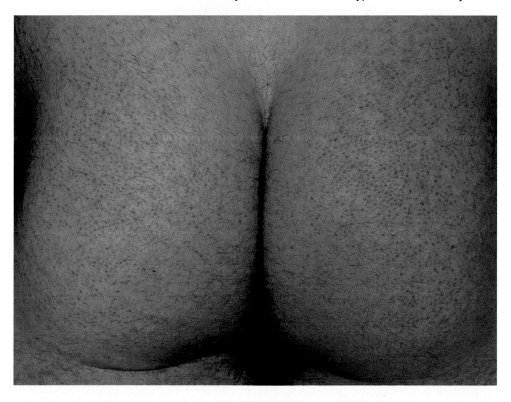

HYPERLINEAR PALMAR CREASES

Atopic patients frequently reveal an accentuation of the major skin creases of the palms (Figure 5-26). This accentuation may be present in infancy and become more prominent as age and severity of skin inflammation increase. The changes might be initiated by rubbing or scratching. Patients with accentuated skin creases seem to have more extensive inflammation on the body and experience a longer course of disease. Occasionally patients without atopic dermatitis have palm crease accentuation.

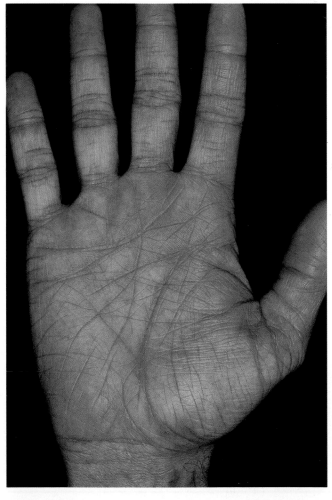

Figure 5-26
Hyperlinear palmar creases. Seen frequently in patients with severe atopic dermatitis.

PITYRIASIS ALBA

Pityriasis alba is a common disorder that is characterized by an asymptomatic, hypopigmented, slightly elevated, fine, scaling plaque with indistinct borders. The condition, which affects the face (Figures 5-27 and 5-28), lateral upper arms (Figure 5-29), and thighs (Figure 5-30), appears in young children and usually disappears by early adulthood. The white, round-to-oval areas vary in size, but generally average 2 to 4 cm in diameter (Figure 5-29). Lesions become obvious in the summer months when the areas do not tan.

Parents who are concerned about the appearance of pityriasis alba in their children should be assured that the loss of pigment is not permanent, as it is in vitiligo. Vitiligo and the fungal infection tinea versicolor both appear to be white, but the margin between normal and hypopigmented skin in vitiligo is distinct. Tinea versicolor is rarely located on the face, and the hypopigmented areas are more numerous and often confluent. A potassium hydroxide examination quickly settles the question. Patients should be assured that the hypopigmentation usually fades with time. No treatment other than lubrication should be attempted unless the patches become eczematous. Extensive pityriasis alba may respond to a short course of PUVA.[23]

ATOPIC PLEATS

The appearance of an extra line on the lower eyelid (Dennie-Morgan infraorbital fold) has been considered a distinguishing feature of patients with atopic dermatitis.[24] The line may simply be caused by constant rubbing of the eyes.[25] This extra line may also appear in people who do not have atopic dermatitis, and it is an unreliable sign of the atopic state.

CATARACTS AND KERATOCONUS

Analysis of a large group of atopic patients showed that the incidence of cataracts was approximately 10%.[26] The reason for their development is not understood. Most are asymptomatic and can only be detected by slit-lamp examination. Two types have been reported: the complicated type, which begins at the posterior pole in the immediate subcapsular region, and the anterior plaque or shieldlike opacity, which lies subcapsularly and in the pupillary zone. The anterior plaque type is the most frequently described. Posterior subcapsular cataracts are a well-established complication of systemic steroid therapy. Data suggest that there is no safe dosage of corticosteroids and that individual susceptibility may determine the threshold for development of cataracts.[27] It may be that atopic patients have a lower threshold or a greater tendency to develop cataracts, particularly when challenged with systemic steroids. This fact must be considered for the unusual atopic patient who requires systemic steroids for short-term control. Keratoconus (elongation and protrusion of the corneal surface) has been believed to be more common in the atopic state, but the incidence is low, and it does not appear to be associated with cataracts.

PITYRIASIS ALBA

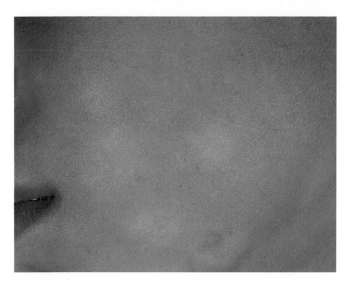

Figure 5-27
Hypopigmented round spots are a common occurrence on the faces of atopic children.

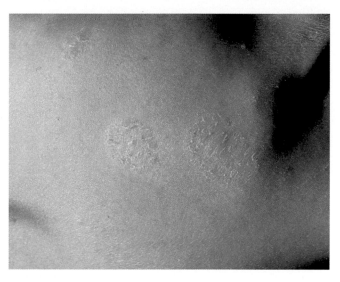

Figure 5-28
The superficial hypopigmented plaques become scaly and inflamed as the dry winter months progress.

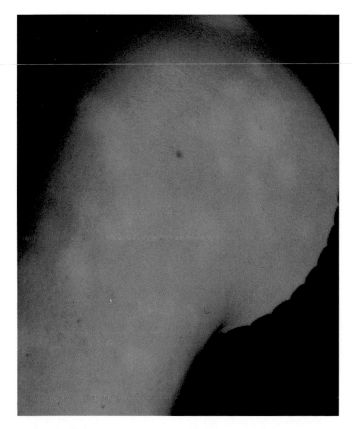

Figure 5-29
Irregular hypopigmented areas are frequently seen in atopic patients and are not to be confused with tinea versicolor or vitiligo.

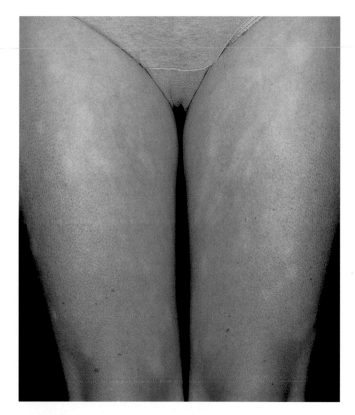

Figure 5-30
Lesions present here are more than are typically seen.

Triggering Factors

Factors that promote dryness or increase the desire to scratch worsen atopic dermatitis. Understanding and controlling these aggravating factors are essential to the successful management of atopic dermatitis.[28] A complete history is required since there is no standardized test scheme, like that for rhinitis or asthma, to identify specific triggering factors of atopic dermatitis.

TEMPERATURE CHANGE AND SWEATING

Atopic patients do not tolerate sudden changes in temperature. Sweating induces itching, particularly in the antecubital and popliteal fossae, to a greater extent in atopic patients than in other individuals. Lying under warm blankets, entering a warm room, and experiencing physical stress all intensify the desire to scratch. A sudden lowering of temperature, such as leaving a warm shower, promotes itching. Patients should be discouraged from wearing clothing that tends to trap heat.

DECREASED HUMIDITY

The beginning of fall heralds the onset of a difficult period for atopic patients. Cold air cannot support much humidity. The moisture-containing outer layer of the skin reaches equilibrium with the atmosphere and consequently holds less moisture. Dry skin is less supple, more fragile, and more easily irritated. Pruritis is established, the rash appears, and the long winter months in the northern states may be a difficult period to endure. Commercially available humidifiers can offer some relief by increasing the humidity in the house to above 50%.

EXCESSIVE WASHING

Repeated washing and drying removes water-binding lipids from the first layer of the skin. Daily baths may be tolerated in the summer months but lead to excessive dryness in the fall and winter.

CONTACT WITH IRRITATING SUBSTANCES

Wool, household and industrial chemicals, cosmetics, and some soaps and detergents promote irritation and inflammation in the atopic patient. Cigarette smoke may provoke eczematous lesions on the eyelids. The inflammation is frequently interpreted as an allergic reaction by patients, who claim that they are allergic to almost everything they touch. The complaints reflect an intolerance of irritation. Atopics do develop allergic contact dermatitis, but the incidence is lower than normal.

CONTACT ALLERGY

Contact allergic reactions to topical preparations, including corticosteroids, should be considered in patients who do not respond to therapy. Patch testing (see Chapter Four) may help to identify the offending agent.

AEROALLERGENS

The house-dust mite is the most important aeroallergen. Many patients with atopic dermatitis have anti-IgE antibodies to house-dust mite antigens, but the role of the house-dust mite in exacerbations of atopic dermatitis is controversial. Inhalation of house-dust antigen and allergen penetration through the skin may occur. Other aeroallergens such as pollens, allergens from pets, molds, or human dander may contribute to atopic dermatitis. Measures for allergen elimination should be undertaken. Hyposensitization may be effective, but there is little experience with this treatment.

MICROBIC AGENTS

Staphylococcus aureus. *S. aureus* is the predominant skin microorganism in atopic dermatitis lesions. It is significantly increased in nonaffected skin. Normally *S. aureus* represents less than 5% of the total skin microflora in persons without atopic dermatitis. Antibiotics given systemically or topically may dramatically improve atopic dermatitis.

Pityrosporum yeasts. *Pityrosporum* is part of the normal skin flora. Prick or patch tests to extracts of *Pityrosporum* may give positive results in patients with atopic dermatitis, and specific IgE antibodies have been demonstrated, but the data concerning the relevance of *Pityrosporum* as a provocative factor are inconclusive.

FOOD

Certain foods can provoke exacerbations of atopic dermatitis. Many patients who react to food are not aware of their hypersensitivity. Foods can provoke allergic and nonallergic reactions. The most common offenders are eggs, peanuts, milk, fish, soy, and wheat. Urticaria, an exacerbation of eczema, gastrointestinal or respiratory tract symptoms, or anaphylactic reactions may be signs of a food-induced reaction. Preservatives, colorants, and other low-molecular weight substances in foods may be offenders, but there are no tests for these substances.

EMOTIONAL STRESS

Stressful situations can have a profound effect on the course of atopic dermatitis. A stable course can quickly degenerate, and localized inflammation may become extensive almost overnight. Patients are well aware of this phenomenon and, regrettably, believe that they are responsible for their disease. This notion may be reinforced by relatives and friends who assure them that their disease "is caused by your nerves." Explaining that atopic dermatitis is an inherited disease that is made worse, rather than caused, by emotional stress is reassuring.

Treatment

Treatment goals consist of attempting to eliminate inflammation and infection (see the box below), preserving and restoring the stratum corneum barrier by using emollients, using antipruritics to reduce the self-inflicted damage to the involved skin, and controlling exacerbating factors (see the box at right). Most patients can be brought under adequate control in less than 3 weeks. The following are possible reasons for failure to respond: poor patient compliance, allergic contact dermatitis to a topical medicine, the simultaneous occurrence of asthma or hay fever, inadequate sedation, and continued emotional stress.

TREATING ATOPIC DERMATITIS

TOPICAL THERAPY

Topical steroids should be used to treat dermatitis until the skin clears, then steroid application should be discontinued
   Group V creams or ointments for red, scaling skin
   Group I or II creams or ointments for lichenified skin
Parenteral steroids may be used for extensive flares
   Prednisone
Tar
   Creams (e.g., FotoTar)
   Bath oil (e.g., Balnatar)
Moisturizers should be applied after showers and after hand washing
Lipid-free lotion cleansers (e.g., Cetaphil)

ANTIBIOTICS

Antibiotics may be prescribed to suppress *Staphylococcus aureus*; they may be administered on a short- or long-term basis.
   Erythromycin 250 mg four times daily
   Cephalexin (Keflex) 250 mg four times daily
   Cefadroxil (Duricef) 500 mg twice daily
   Dicloxacillin 250 mg four times daily

ANTIHISTAMINES

Antihistamines control pruritus and induce sedation and sleep
   Hydroxyzine
   Doxepin HCl cream 5% (Zonalon)

TREATING SEVERE CASES

Corticosteroids
   Oral prednisone
   Intramuscular triamcinolone
Hospitalization
   Home hospitalization (see the box on p. 119)
   Topical steroids and rest
   Goeckerman regimen (tar plus UVB)
PUVA

CONTROLLING ATOPIC DERMATITIS

PROTECT SKIN FROM THE FOLLOWING AGENTS

Moisture
   Avoid frequent hand washing
   Avoid frequent bathing
   Avoid lengthy bathing
   Use tepid water for baths
   Avoid abrasive washcloths
Foods
   Avoid prolonged contact (clean food around baby's mouth)
Rough clothing
   Avoid wool
   Use 100% cotton
Irritants and allergens
   Use soaps only in axilla, groin, feet
   Avoid perfumes or makeup that burns or itches
   Avoid fabric softeners
Scratching
   Do not scratch
   Pat, firmly press, or grasp the skin
   Apply soothing lubricants

CONTROL ENVIRONMENT

Temperature
   Maintain cool, stable temperatures
   Do not overdress
   Limit number of bed blankets
   Avoid sweating
Humidity
   Humidify the house in winter
Airborne allergens and dust
   Do not have rugs in bedrooms
   Vacuum drapes and blankets
   Use plastic mattress covers
   Wet-mop floors
   Avoid aerosols
   Ventilate cooking odors
   Avoid cigarettes
   Use artificial plants
   Avoid ragweed pollen contact
   Minimize animal dander—no cats, dogs, rodents, or birds
Change geographic location
   Sudden improvement may occur

CONTROL EMOTIONAL STRESS

Pleasant work environment
Learn relaxation techniques

CONTROL DIET

Diet control is a controversial treatment method (see text for treatment)

INFLAMMATION AND INFECTION

Topical steroids and antibiotics. Topical steroids and, occasionally, tar ointments are used to control inflammation. Oral antibiotics are more effective than topical antibiotics for controlling infection.

INFANTS

Localized inflammation. Infants with dry, red, scaling plaques on the cheeks respond to group V or VI topical steroids applied twice a day for 7 to 14 days. Parents are instructed to decrease the frequency of washing and start lubrication with a bland lubricant during the initial phase of the treatment period and to continue lubrication long after topical steroids have been discontinued. Antistaphylococcal antibiotics are required only if there is moderate serum and crusting. Cracking about the lips is controlled in a similar fashion, but heavy lubricants (such as petroleum jelly or Eucerin) are used after the inflammation is clear.

Generalized inflammation. Infants with more generalized inflammation require treatment with a group V topical steroid cream or ointment applied two to three times a day for 10 to 21 days. Secondary infection often accompanies generalized inflammation and a 3- to 7-day course of an appropriate antistaphylococcal antibiotic, such as cephalexin suspension (Keflex) used twice daily, is required. Start oral antibiotics 2 days before initiating topical steroid treatment. Sedation with hydroxyzine (10 mg/5 ml) is useful during the initial treatment period. The bedtime dose gives the child a good night's sleep and seems to suppress the unconscious scratching that occurs during disturbed sleep. The parents are grateful; at last they are not up all night with a scratching, crying child.

Potent topical or systemic steroids are potentially hazardous and may be associated with relapse after therapy has been discontinued. Cyclosporine and photochemotherapy (see below) may be considered for severe, refractory cases, but they are also associated with relapse after cessation of therapy and have potentially serious side effects. Avoidance of certain foods, pets, and house-dust mites is an option; the major drawbacks are the lack of tests to identify triggers or predict response.[29]

CHILDREN AND ADULTS

Lichenified plaques. Lichenified plaques in older children and adults respond to groups II through V topical steroids used with occlusive dressings (Figure 5-31). Occlusive therapy for 10 to 14 days is preferred if the plaques are resistant to treatment or are very thick. Occlusion may be used as soon as infection has been controlled.

Diffuse inflammation. Diffuse inflammation involving the face, trunk, and extremities is treated with group V topical steroids applied two to four times a day. A 3- to 7-day course of systemic antistaphylococcal antibiotics is almost invariably required. Start oral antibiotics 2 days before initiating topical steroid treatment. Exudative areas with serum and crust are treated with a Burow's solution compress for

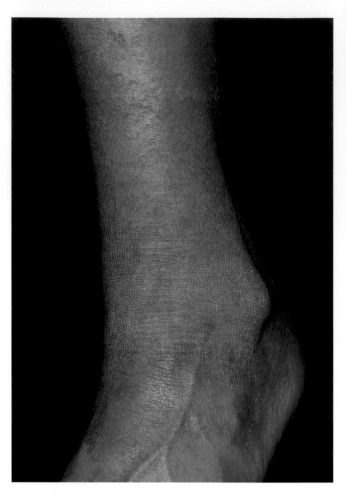

Figure 5-31
Response to treatment. Lichenified plaque shown in Figure 5-14 after 7 days of a group IV topical steroid under occlusive dressing.

20 minutes three times a day for 2 to 3 days. Dryness and cracking with fissures occur if compressing is prolonged. Resistant cases may be treated with group V topical steroids applied before and after vinyl suit occlusion. The suit may be worn to bed or worn for 2 hours twice a day. All signs of infection, such as serum and crust, should be clear before initiating occlusive therapy.

Systemic steroids. A 10-day course of 20 mg of prednisone twice daily is occasionally needed to control difficult cases in adults.

Oral and intramuscular steroid therapy has a number of disadvantages. The relapse rate is high, with inflammation returning shortly after the medication is discontinued. Enthusiasm for topical therapy diminishes once the patient has experienced the rapid clearing produced by systemic therapy, prompting some patients to request systemic therapy again. The answer should be no. Hospitalization with topical medication and sedation is indicated for the atopic patient with generalized inflammation who does not respond to routine measures. The association of atopic cataracts with systemic steroid therapy has been discussed.

HOSPITALIZATION FOR SEVERELY RESISTANT CASES

Some patients with severe, generalized inflammation do not respond to or flare soon after a reasonable trial of topical therapy. These patients are candidates for hospitalization. A short stay in the hospital can rapidly help to control a condition that has had a prolonged, unstable course. A program for "home hospitalization" is outlined in the box at right.

TAR

Tar ointments were the mainstay of therapy before topical steroids were introduced. They were effective and had few side effects but did not work quickly. Tar in a lubricating base such as T-Derm or Fototar applied twice daily is an effective alternative to topical steroids. Intensely inflamed areas should first be controlled with topical steroids. Tar ointments can then be used to complete therapy. Tar can be used as an initial therapy for chronic, superficial plaques.

LUBRICATION

Restoring moisture to the skin increases the rate of healing and establishes a durable barrier against further drying and irritation. A variety of lotions and creams is available, and most are adequate for rehydration. Petroleum jelly (Vaseline) is especially effective. Some products contain urea (e.g., Nutraplus); others contain lactic acid (e.g., Lac-Hydrin, Lacticare). Urea and lactic acid have special hydrating qualities and may be more effective than other moisturizers. Their use should be encouraged, particularly during the winter months. Patients should be cautioned that lotions may sting shortly after application. This may be a property of the base or of a specific ingredient such as lactic acid. If itching or stinging continue with each application, another product should be selected. If inflammation occurs after use of a lubricant, allergic contact dermatitis to a preservative or a perfume should be considered.

Lubricants are most effective when applied after a bath. The patient should gently pat the skin dry with a towel and immediately apply the lubricant to seal in the moisture. Bath oils are an effective method of lubrication, but they can make the tub slippery and dangerous for older patients. In order to be effective, a sufficient amount of oil must be used to create an oily feeling on the skin when leaving the tub. Septic systems may be adversely affected by prolonged use of bath oils. A mild bar soap should be used infrequently. Cetaphil, Dove, Keri, Purpose, Oilatum, and Basis are adequate. Ivory is very drying and should be avoided.

SEDATION AND ANTIHISTAMINES

Oral antihistamines. Antihistamines generally have offered only marginal therapeutic benefit. They do little to relieve itching,[30] but they do have a calming effect and aid more comfortable sleep. They should be considered for both infants and adults. Antihistamines may be prescribed on a continual basis or only before bedtime, depending on the needs of the individual. Continuing antihistamines for a

---

ATOPIC DERMATITIS—HOME HOSPITALIZATION (SHORT-TERM INTENSIVE TREATMENT)

Designate family member or friend as nurse.
All treatment is administered by nurse.
Write orders for home nurse.
Treatment starts Friday night and ends Monday morning.

ORDERS

1. Complete bed rest with bathroom privileges
2. Semidarkened room
3. No visitors other than nurse
4. Cotton bedclothes; dust-free and animal-free room
5. Temperature 68° to 70° F
6. Humidity 70%
7. Bland diet—no alcohol, spices, or caffeine

TOPICAL THERAPY

1. Tepid tub bath with bath oil, 20 minutes twice a day
2. Emollient bland cream applied to moist body immediately on emergence from tub
3. Body lesions covered with group V steroid cream or ointment twice daily
4. Face lesions covered with group V steroid cream or ointment twice daily
5. Scalp inflammation treated with daily shampoo followed by topical steroid lotion (e.g., Dermasmoothe F/S)

SYSTEMIC THERAPY

1. Antibiotics: erythromycin 250 mg four times daily; dicloxacillin 250 mg four times daily; or cefadroxil 500 mg twice daily
2. Sedating antihistamines: hydroxyzine 10 to 25 mg four times daily; doxepin 10 to 25 mg four times daily; or others
3. Phenothiazines for agitated patients: chlorpromazine 25 mg four times daily
4. May give a short-acting injectable steroid before hospitalization (such as dexamethasone 8 mg IM or betamethasone 6 mg IM)

Modified from Roth HL: *Int J Dermatol* 26:139-149, 1987.

---

short period after inflammation has subsided assists a smooth course of recovery. Hydroxyzine is well tolerated by most patients, and the dosage can be varied over a wide range with little chance of side effects. Newer, nonsedating H_1 antagonists, such as terfenadine, astemizole, loratadine, and cetirizine, have an antipruritic effect. Cetirizine exerts an additional inhibitory effect on eosinophils.[31]

Topical antihistamines. Doxepin HCl cream (Zonalon cream, 30-gm tube) is an antipruritic cream. The mechanism of action is unknown. Doxepin has potent H_1-receptor and

H_2-receptor blocking actions. Zonalon cream is indicated for the short-term (up to 8 days) management of moderate pruritus in adults with atopic dermatitis and lichen simplex chronicus. Drowsiness occurs in more than 20% of patients, especially patients receiving treatment to greater than 10% of their body surface area. The most common local adverse effect is burning and/or stinging. A thin film of cream is applied four times each day with intervals of at least 3 hours between applications.

PHOTOTHERAPY

Phototherapy is effective for mild or moderate atopic dermatitis. Combined UVA-UVB yields clearing or considerable improvement in 90% of patients, whereas UVA or UVB does so in approximately 70%. The effective dosage is considerably lower than that for UVB-treated psoriasis patients.[32]

PUVA (psoralen and ultraviolet light A) therapy is an effective treatment for older children and adolescents with refractory atopic dermatitis. A recent study showed that twice-weekly treatments resulted in clearance or near clearance of disease in 74% of patients after a mean of 9 weeks and that 82% of these children were able to achieve remission of disease following gradual withdrawal of treatment. The mean duration of treatment to remission was 37 weeks; the mean cumulative UVA dose was 1118 J/cm^2, and the mean number of treatments was 59.[33] The major benefit of this treatment is that it was associated with resumption of normal growth in children who were previously growing poorly.[34]

Cyclosporine. A few patients remain severely affected by atopic dermatitis into adult life despite treatment with systemic steroids and photochemotherapy. Cyclosporine (5 mg/kg per day) is effective short-term treatment for severe, refractory atopic dermatitis.[35,36] The disease may relapse despite continued treatment or may recur soon after stopping cyclosporine. After control is achieved, the dosage may be reduced until an increased activity of atopic dermatitis is noticed (the minimal effective dosage is approximately 4.0 mg/kg/day). Maintenance therapy may be hampered by side effects in the same way as therapy is hampered by side effects in the treatment of psoriasis.[37] Serum IgE levels and prick test responses are unchanged by cyclosporine.

Controlling aeroallergens. A regimen aimed at reducing the presence of house-dust mites can produce clinical improvement in patients with atopic dermatitis who show contact hypersensitivity to mite antigens on skin testing. Reduction of mites with a thorough housecleaning and by covering mattresses may result in dramatic improvement. These home-sanitation programs, which involve cleaning different surfaces, are often recommended by allergists to their rhinitis and asthma patients to control aeroallergens such as mites and molds.*

---

*Allergy Control Products, Inc.; 96 Danbury Road; Ridgefield, CT, 06877; (800) 422-DUST offers a guide and products for the control of aeroallergens.

DIET RESTRICTION AND BREAST-FEEDING

A small percentage of children and adults with atopic dermatitis have positive responses to food-challenge tests, resulting in eczematous flares. A child (especially younger than 7 years) with atopic dermatitis that is unresponsive to routine therapy may have a greater than 50% chance of having food hypersensitivity. Significant clinical improvement occurs within 1 or 2 months when an appropriately designed restricted diet is followed.

Food hypersensitivity is usually limited to one or two antigens and may be lost after several years. Six foods account for 90% of the positive oral challenges seen in children. In order of frequency, they are egg, peanut, milk, fish, soy, and wheat.

Evaluation. The most reliable and practical way of diagnosing food allergy has not been determined. The history is of marginal value in predicting which patients are likely to have food allergy. Skin tests and specific IgE antibodies (RAST) are ordered. Food challenges (provocation tests) are then performed.

Food testing

Radioallergosorbent test (RAST). The results of RAST are less reliable than skin and provocation tests. RAST results correlate with positive double-blind food challenges in only one third of cases, but negative tests are quite predictive of negative food challenges.

Skin tests. The prick skin test is an excellent preliminary test to exclude food antigens. A negative prick skin test excludes immediate food hypersensitivity. The test is useful for limiting the number of food antigens requiring evaluation with provocation tests. A positive reaction indicates the presence of antigen-specific IgE bound to cutaneous mast cells. Direct application of the native food to the skin or with a scratch test is probably more reliable than testing with commercial extracts.

Provocation tests. Food challenges may be positive in patients with negative skin tests or who show an absence of specific IgE by RAST, but patients with positive provocation tests almost always have positive skin tests to the food. Challenge tests must be performed to determine the clinical significance of the positive tests. Double-blind food challenges performed in the hospital are an accurate means of diagnosing immediate food hypersensitivity but are not practical in most cases. An open (single-blind) trial is less accurate but more practical. Patients are given a period of antigen avoidance. Foods that produce positive prick skin tests should be eliminated from the patient's diet for 1 to 2 weeks before the oral food challenge. The common food antigens are available in dried forms from supermarkets and camping stores.

Symptoms usually occur within 2 hours of ingesting the food antigen (early-phase reaction). They consist of pruritus, erythema, and edema. A recurrence of pruritus may occur 6 to 8 hours later. This late-phase reaction does not occur in the absence of early-phase reaction. Urticarial lesions are rarely seen. Many patients complain of nausea, abdominal pain, emesis, or diarrhea. Respiratory symptoms including stridor, wheezing, nasal congestion, and sneezing may develop. Anaphylactic reactions are uncommon but possible during food testing.

Prognosis. Food allergy does not last indefinitely. A gradual reintroduction of the offending foods should be carefully considered after the child is past the third birthday. Milk and soy allergies usually disappear with aging; egg and fish allergies tend to remain.

Elimination and restricted diets

Elimination tests. Some success has been reported with undirected elimination diets. One study showed that a standard elimination diet avoiding cow's milk, eggs, and tomatoes should help up to 75% of patients with moderate or severe atopic dermatitis. Patients who improved became worse on food challenges.[38] The response to food elimination could not be predicted by skin prick tests or by total or food-specific IgE. Most undirected elimination diets become confusing for the patient and the physician to interpret and manage. A complete evaluation should be performed before dietary restriction is started. Strict avoidance of the offending food is the only treatment. Consultation with a dietitian is helpful.

Breast-feeding. There is little evidence that prolonged breast-feeding or the delayed introduction of cow's milk or solid foods plays a role in modifying the prevalence, severity, or age of onset of the various atopic diseases. However, until more evidence is available, it is reasonable to breast-feed a child of atopic parents for at least 4 months. The mother should avoid ingestion of cow's milk and eggs. The infant should not be given cereals, eggs, peanuts, cow's milk, fish, soy, wheat, chocolate, fruits, nuts, peas, strawberries, or tomatoes during that time. The child should also not be fed distasteful foods.

Dietary histamine avoidance. After ingestion of foods that are rich in histamine (fish, cheese, hard-cured sausage, pickled cabbage, wine, beer), clear-cut recurrence of atopic eczema was seen in 50% of affected patients.

REFERENCES

1. Uehara M: Heterogeneity of serum IgE levels in atopic dermatitis, *Acta Derm Venereol* (Stockh) 66:404-408, 1986.
2. Kay J, Gawkrodger DJ, et al: The prevalence of childhood atopic eczema in a general population, *J Am Acad Dermatol* 30:35-39, 1994.
3. Rystedt I: Prognostic factors in atopic dermatitis, *Acta Derm Venereol* (Stockh) 65:206-213, 1985.
4. Linna O, Kokkonen J, et al: Ten-year prognosis for generalized infantile eczema, *Acta Paediatr Scand* 81:1013-1016, 1992.
5. Cooper KD: Atopic dermatitis: recent trends in pathogenesis and therapy, *J Invest Dermatol* 102:128-137, 1994.
6. Reinhold U, Kukel S, et al: Systemic interferon gamma treatment in severe atopic dermatitis, *J Am Acad Dermatol* 29:58-63, 1993.
7. Hanifin JM, Schneider LC, et al: Recombinant interferon gamma therapy for atopic dermatitis, *J Am Acad Dermatol* 28:189-197, 1993.
8. Wananukul S, Huiprasert P, et al: Eczematous skin reaction from patch testing with aeroallergens in atopic children with and without atopic dermatitis, *Pediatr Dermatol* 10:209-213, 1993.
9. Stone SP, Muller SA, Glech GJ: IgE levels in atopic dermatitis, *Arch Dermatol* 108:806-811, 1973.
10. Rudzki E, Litewska D: RAST and PRIST in children with atopic dermatitis, *Dermatologica* 180:82-85, 1990.
11. Uehara M, Izukura R, et al: Blood eosinophilia in atopic dermatitis, *Clin Exp Dermatol* 15:264-266, 1990.
12. Leiferman KM, Ackerman SJ, Sampson HA, et al: Dermal deposition of eosinophil-granule major basic protein in atopic dermatitis. Comparison with onchocerciasis, *N Engl J Med* 313:282-285, 1985.
13. Hanifin JM, Ray LF, Lobitz WC Jr: Immunologic reactivity in dermatophytosis, *Br J Dermatol* 90:1, 1974.
14. de Groot AC: The frequency of contact allergy in atopic patients with dermatitis, *Contact Dermatitis* 22:273-277, 1990.
15. Sutthipisal N, McFadden JP, et al: Sensitization in atopic and non-atopic hairdressers with hand eczema, *Contact Dermatitis* 29:206-209, 1993.
16. Cronin E, McFadden JP: Patients with atopic eczema do become sensitized to contact allergens, *Contact Dermatitis* 28:225-228, 1993.
17. Cooper KD: Immunologic aspects of atopic dermatitis, *Curr Concepts Skin Disorders* 7:19-23, 1986.
18. Ruzicka T, Gluck S: Cutaneous histamine levels and histamine releasability from the skin in atopic dermatitis and hyper IgE syndrome, *Arch Dermatol Res* 275:541-544, 1983.
19. Musgrove K, Morgan JK: Infantile eczema, *Br J Dermatol* 95:365-372, 1976.
20. Sampson HH, Jolie PL: Increased plasma histamine concentrations after food challenges in children with atopic dermatitis, *N Engl J Med* 311:372, 1984.
21. Massarano AA, Hollis S, et al: Growth in atopic eczema, *Arch Dis Child* 68:677-679, 1993.
22. Uehara M, Miyauchi H: The morphologic characteristics of dry skin in atopic dermatitis, *Arch Dermatol* 120:1186-1190, 1984.
23. Zaynoun S, Jaber LAA, Kurban AK: Oral methoxsalen photochemotherapy of extensive pityriasis alba, *J Am Acad Dermatol* 15:61-65, 1986.
24. Meenan FOC: The significance of Morgan's fold in children with atopic dermatitis, *Acta Derm Venereol* (Stockh) 92 (Suppl):42-44, 1980.
25. Uehara M: Infraorbital fold in atopic dermatitis, *Arch Dermatol* 117:627-630, 1981.
26. Roth HL, Kierland RR: The natural history of atopic dermatitis, *Arch Dermatol* 89:209, 1964.
27. Skalka HW, Prachal JT: Effects of corticosteroids on cataract formation, *Arch Opthalmol* 98:1773, 1980.
28. Morren M-A et al: Atopic dermatitis: triggering factors, *J Am Acad Dermatol* 31:467-473, 1994.
29. David TJ: Recent developments in the treatment of childhood atopic eczema, *J R Coll Physicians Lond* 25:95-101, 1991.
30. Wahlgren CF, Hagermark O, et al: The antipruritic effect of a sedative and a non-sedative antihistamine in atopic dermatitis, *Br J Dermatol* 122:545-551, 1990.
31. Behrendt H, Ring J: Histamine, antihistamines and atopic eczema, *Clin Exp Allergy* 20:25-30, 1990.
32. Jekler J: Phototherapy of atopic dermatitis with ultraviolet radiation, *Acta Derm Venereol* 171 (Suppl):1-37, 1992.
33. Sheehan MP, Atherton DJ, et al: Oral psoralen photochemotherapy in severe childhood atopic eczema: an update, *Br J Dermatol* 129:431-436, 1993.
34. Atherton DJ, Carabott F, Glover MT, et al: The role of psoralen photochemotherapy (PUVA) in the treatment of severe atopic eczema in adolescents, *Br J Dermatol* 118:791-795, 1988.
35. Sowden JM, Berth-Jones J, et al: Double-blind, controlled, crossover study of cyclosporin in adults with severe refractory atopic dermatitis, *Lancet* 338:137-140, 1991.
36. Salek MS, Finlay AY, et al: Cyclosporin greatly improves the quality of life of adults with severe atopic dermatitis. A randomized, double-blind, placebo-controlled trial, *Br J Dermatol* 129:422-430, 1993.
37. Korstanje MJ, van de Staak WJ: Cyclosporin maintenance therapy for severe atopic dermatitis, *Acta Derm Venereol* 71:356-357, 1991.
38. Sloper KS, Wadsworth J, et al: Children with atopic eczema. I: clinical response to food elimination and subsequent double-blind food challenge, *Q J Med* 80:677-693, 1991.

Urticaria

Urticaria, also referred to as *hives* or *wheals*, is a common and distinctive reaction pattern. Hives may occur at any age; up to 20% of the population will have at least one episode. Hives may be more common in atopic patients. Urticaria is classified as acute or chronic.[1] The majority of cases are acute, lasting from hours to a few weeks. Because most individuals can diagnose urticaria and realize that it is a self-limited condition, they do not seek medical attention.

The cause of acute urticaria is determined in many cases, but the cause of chronic urticaria (arbitrarily defined as hives lasting longer than 6 weeks) is determined in only 5% to 20% of cases. Patients with chronic urticaria present a major problem in diagnosis and management. These patients are often subjected to detailed and expensive medical evaluations that usually prove unrewarding. Recent studies have demonstrated the value of a complete history and physical examination followed by the judicious use of laboratory studies in evaluating the results of the history and physical examination.

Clinical Aspects

Definition. A hive or wheal is an erythematous or white, nonpitting, edematous plaque that changes in size and shape by peripheral extension or regression during the few hours or days that the individual lesion exists. The evolution of urticaria is a dynamic process. New lesions evolve as old ones resolve. Hives result from localized capillary vasodilation, followed by transudation of protein-rich fluid into the surrounding tissue; they resolve when the fluid is slowly reabsorbed.

Clinical presentation. Lesions vary in size from the 2 to 4 mm edematous papules of cholinergic urticaria to giant hives, a single lesion of which may cover an extremity. They may be round or oval; when confluent, they become polycyclic (Figures 6-1 and 6-2). A portion of the border either may not form or may be reabsorbed, giving the appearance of incomplete rings (Figure 6-2). Hives may be uniformly red or white, or the edematous border may be red and the remainder of the surface white. This variation in color is usually present in superficial hives. Thicker plaques have a uniform color (Figures 6-1, 6-2, 6-3, and 6-4).

Hives may be surrounded by a clear or red halo. Thicker plaques that result from massive transudation of fluid into the dermis and subcutaneous tissue are referred to as *angioedema*. These thick, firm plaques, like typical hives, may occur on any skin surface, but typically involve the lips, larynx (causing hoarseness or a sore throat), and mucosa of the gastrointestinal (GI) tract (causing abdominal pain) (Figures 6-5 and 6-6). Bullae or purpura may appear in areas of intense swelling. Purpura and scaling may result as the lesions of urticarial vasculitis clear. Hives usually have a haphazard distribution, but those elicited by physical stimuli have characteristic features and distribution.

Symptoms. Hives itch. The intensity varies, and some patients with a widespread eruption may experience little itching. Pruritus is milder in deep hives (angioedema) because the edema occurs in areas where there are fewer sensory nerve endings than there are near the surface of the skin.

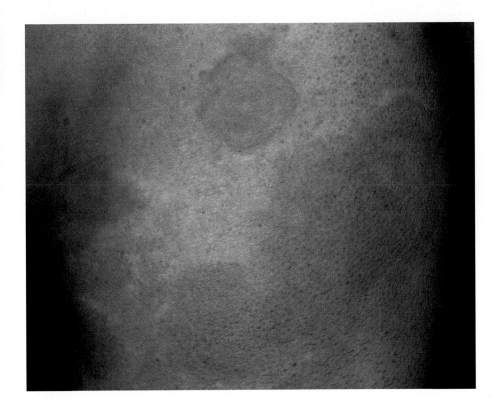

Figure 6-1
Hives. The most characteristic presentation is uniformly red edematous plaques surrounded by a faint white halo. These superficial lesions occur from transudation of fluid into the dermis.

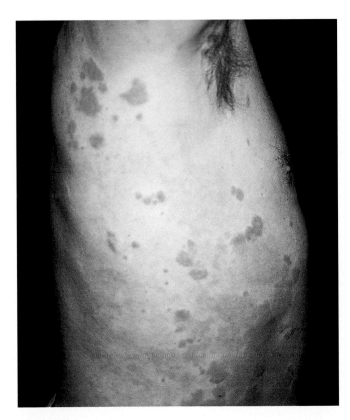

Figure 6-2
Hives. Urticarial plaques in different stages of formation.

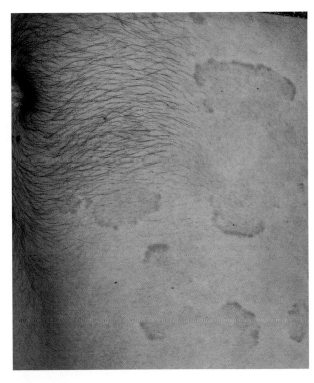

Figure 6-3
Hives. Polycyclic pattern.

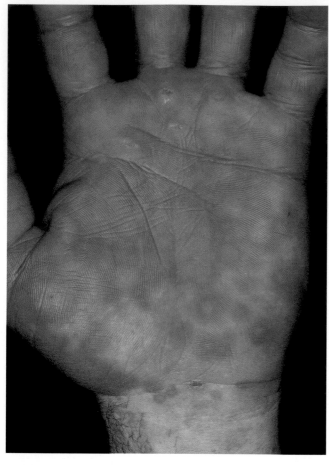

Figure 6-4
Hives. The entire palm is affected and is greatly swollen.
The lesions resemble those of erythema multiforme.

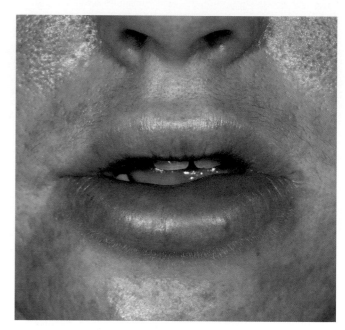

Figure 6-5
Angioedema is a deeper, larger hive than those shown in
Figures 6-1 through 6-3. It is caused by transudation of fluid
into the dermis and subcutaneous tissue. The lip is a common site.

Figure 6-6
Angioedema. Massive swelling of the entire central
area of the back.

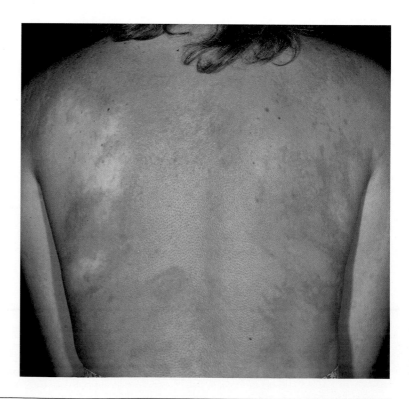

Pathophysiology

Histamine

Histamine mediates a variety of responses in different tissues and cells and is a mediator of inflammation in allergic disease. Histamine is the most important chemical mediator of urticaria. When injected into skin, histamine produces the triple response, the features of which are local erythema (vasodilation), the flare characterized by erythema beyond the border of the local erythema, and a wheal produced from leakage of fluid from the postcapillary venule.

Histamine causes endothelial cell contraction, which allows vascular fluid to leak between the cells through the vessel wall, contributing to tissue edema and wheal formation. Histamine is contained in the granules of mast cells. A variety of immunologic, nonimmunologic, physical, and chemical stimuli may be responsible for the degranulation of mast cell granules and the release of histamine into the surrounding tissue and circulation (Figure 6-7). All such stimuli appear to initiate the release of histamine by first reacting with different cell membrane receptors. Activation of one group of receptors stimulates the conversion of adenosine triphosphate (ATP) to cyclic adenosine monophosphate (cAMP), and activation of another group stimulates conversion of guanosine triphosphate (GTP) to cyclic guanosine monophosphate (cGMP). Increasing intracellular concentrations of cyclic GMP lead to histamine release, whereas increasing concentrations of cyclic AMP inhibit histamine release.

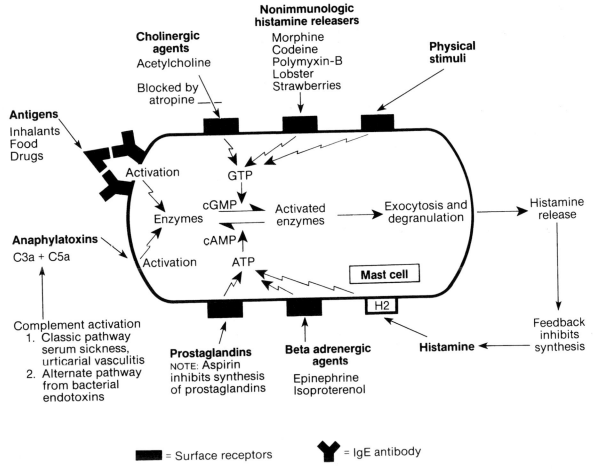

Figure 6-7
Mechanism of action of histamine on H_1 and H_2 cell receptors and endothelial cells.

Histamine receptors

Histamine induces vascular changes by a number of mechanisms (Figure 6-8). Blood vessels contain two (and possibly more) receptors for histamine. The two most studied are designated H_1 and H_2.

H_1 receptors. H_1 receptors, when stimulated by histamine, cause an axon reflex, vasodilation, and pruritus. Acting through H_1 receptors, histamine causes smooth-muscle contraction in the respiratory and gastrointestinal tracts and pruritis and sneezing by sensory-nerve stimulation. They are blocked by the vast majority of clinically available antihistamines called *H_1 antagonists* (e.g., chlorpheniramine), which occupy the receptor site and prevent attachment of histamine.

H_2 receptors. When H_2 receptors are stimulated, vasodilation occurs. H_2 receptors are also present on the mast cell membrane surface and, when stimulated, further inhibit the production of histamine. Activation of H_2 receptors alone increases gastric acid secretion. Cimetidine (Tagamet), ranitidine (Zantac), famotidine (Pepcid), and nizatidine (Axid) are clinically available H_2 blocking agents (antihistamines). H_2 receptors are present at other sites. Activation of both H_1 and H_2 receptors causes hypotension, tachycardia, flushing, and headache. The H_2 blocking agents are used most often to suppress gastric acid secretion. They are used only occasionally, usually in combination with an H_1 blocking agent, to treat urticaria.

HISTAMINE REGULATION
Factors increasing histamine release

Cell membrane–bound IgE plus antigen. Type I hypersensitivity reactions are probably responsible for most cases of acute urticaria. Circulating antigens such as foods, drugs, or inhalants interact with cell membrane–bound IgE to release histamine. Antigens produced in the skin by light (some cases of solar urticaria) may react with IgE. Some forms of cold urticaria are also IgE mediated.

Anaphylotoxins C3a and C5a. Type III hypersensitivity reactions (Arthus reactions) occur with deposition of insoluble immune complexes in vessel walls. The complexes are composed of IgG or IgM with an antigen such as a drug. Urticaria occurs when the trapped complexes activate complement to cleave the anaphylotoxins C5a and C3a from C5 and C3. C5a and C3a are potent releasers of histamine from mast cells. Serum sickness, hepatitis B prodromal reaction, urticarial vasculitis, and systemic lupus erythematosus are diseases in which hives may occur as a result of immune complex deposition.

Nonimmunologic release of histamine. Pharmacologic mediators such as acetylcholine, morphine, and strawberries react directly with cell membrane–bound mediators to release histamine. The physical urticarias may be induced by both direct stimulation of cell membrane receptors and immunologic mechanisms.

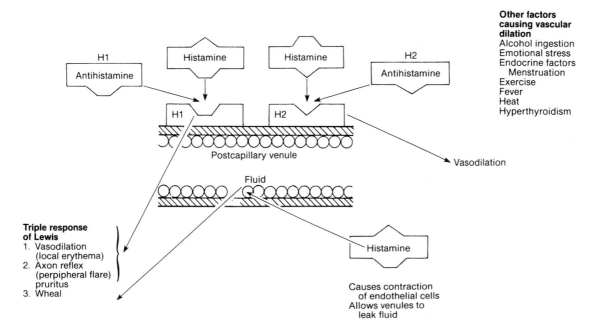

Figure 6-8
Physiology of histamine release.

Factors decreasing histamine release

Histamine. Histamine interacts with an H_2 mast cell surface receptor to inhibit further release of histamine. Therefore, in this case, histamine acts by feedback inhibition as an antihistamine.

Beta-adrenergic agents. Beta-adrenergic agents such as epinephrine are powerful suppressors of histamine release. Their function may be influenced by steroid hormones, which may help to explain why prednisone is sometimes useful for treating urticaria.

Prostaglandins. Prostaglandins may act as cell surface receptors to inhibit the release of histamine. Aspirin inhibits the synthesis of certain prostaglandins. This may explain why salicylates induce hives in a nonimmunologic way in many patients with chronic urticaria.

Evaluation

1. Determine by skin examination that the patient actually has urticaria and not bites.
2. Rule out the presence of physical urticaria to avoid an unnecessarily lengthy evaluation.
3. Determine whether hives are acute or chronic.
4. Review the known causes of urticaria listed in the box below. Knowledge of the etiologic factors helps to direct the history and physical examination.

ETIOLOGIC CLASSIFICATION OF URTICARIA

FOODS

Fish, shellfish, nuts, eggs, chocolate, strawberries, tomatoes, pork, cow's milk, cheese, wheat, yeast

FOOD ADDITIVES

Salicylates, dyes such as tartrazine, benzoates, penicillin. Aspartame (NutraSweet) probably does not cause hives.* Sulfites.

DRUGS

Penicillin, aspirin, sulfonamides, and drugs that cause a nonimmunologic release of histamine (e.g., morphine, codeine, polymyxin, dextran, curare, quinine)

INFECTIONS

Chronic bacterial infections (e.g., sinus, dental, chest, gallbladder, urinary tract), *Campylobacter enteritis*, fungal infections (dermatophytosis, candidiasis), viral infections (hepatitis B prodromal reaction, infectious mononucleosis, coxsackie), protozoal and helminth infections (intestinal worms, malaria)

INHALANTS

Pollens, mold spores, animal danders, house dust, aerosols, volatile chemicals

INTERNAL DISEASE

Serum sickness, systemic lupus erythematosus, hyperthyroidism, autoimmune thyroid disease, carcinomas, lymphomas, juvenile rheumatoid arthritis (Still's disease), leukocytoclastic vasculitis, polycythemia vera (acne urticaria—urticarial papule surmounted by a vesicle), rheumatic fever, some blood transfusion reactions

PHYSICAL STIMULI (THE PHYSICAL URTICARIAS)

Dermographism, pressure urticaria, cholinergic urticaria, exercise-induced anaphylactic syndrome, solar urticaria, cold urticaria, heat, vibratory, water (aquagenic)

NONIMMUNOLOGIC CONTACT URTICARIA

Plants (nettles), animals (caterpillars, jellyfish), medications (cinnamic aldehyde, compound 48/80, dimethyl sulfoxide)

IMMUNOLOGIC OR UNCERTAIN MECHANISM CONTACT URTICARIA

Ammonium persulfate used in hair bleaches, chemicals, foods, textiles, wood, saliva, cosmetics, perfumes, bacitracin

SKIN DISEASES

Urticaria pigmentosa (mastocytosis), dermatitis herpetiformis, pemphigoid, amyloidosis

HORMONES

Pregnancy, premenstrual flare-ups (progesterone)

GENETIC, AUTOSOMAL DOMINANT (ALL RARE)

Hereditary angioedema, cholinergic urticaria with progressive nerve deafness, amyloidosis of the kidney, familial cold urticaria, vibratory urticaria

*Geha R, Buckley CE, et al: *J Allergy Clin Immunol* 92:513-520, 1993.

Acute Urticaria

If the urticaria has been present for less than 6 weeks, it is considered acute. The evaluation and management of acute urticaria are outlined in the box below. A history and physical examination should be performed, and laboratory studies are selected to investigate abnormalities.[2] Histamine release that is induced by allergens (e.g., drugs, foods, or pollens) and mediated by IgE is a common cause of acute urticaria, and particular attention should be paid to these factors during the initial evaluation. There are no routine laboratory studies for the evaluation of acute urticaria. Once all possible causes are eliminated, the patient is treated with antihistamines to suppress the hives and stop the itching. Because urticaria clears spontaneously in most patients, an extensive workup is not advised during the early weeks of an urticarial eruption.[3,4]

Children with hives. Food origin is important in the etiology of infantile urticaria. In one series it accounted for 62% of patients, more often than drug etiology (22%), physical urticaria (8%), and contact urticaria (8%).[5]

Chronic Urticaria

Patients who have a history of hives lasting for 6 or more weeks are classified as having chronic urticaria. The etiology is often unclear.

Histamine-releasing IgG autoantibodies against a subunit of IgE receptors are present in the circulation of some patients with chronic urticaria. Autoantibody-induced cross-linking of IgE receptors may be an important mechanism in the pathogenesis of chronic urticaria.[6]

The patient must understand that the course of this disease is unpredictable; it may last for months or years. During the evaluation, the patient should be assured that antihistamines will decrease discomfort (see the box on p. 129). The patient should also be told that although the evaluation may be lengthy and is often unrewarding, in most cases the disease ends spontaneously. Patients who understand the nature of this disease do not become discouraged so easily, nor are they as apt to go from physician to physician seeking a cure.

There are many studies in the literature on chronic urticaria.[7,8] Most demonstrate that if the cause is not found after investigation of abnormalities elicited during the history and physical examination, there is little chance that it will be determined. It is tempting to order laboratory tests such as antinuclear antibody (ANA) levels and stool examinations for ova and parasites in an effort to be thorough, but results of studies do not support this approach. There are certain tests and procedures that might be considered when the initial evaluation has proved unrewarding.

Rule out physical urticarias. Unrecognized physical urticarias (see p. 133) may account for approximately 10% of all cases of chronic urticaria. In one large study, physical urticarias were present in 71% of patients with chronic urticaria: 22% had immediate dermographism, 37% had delayed pressure urticaria, 11% had cholinergic urticaria, and 2% had cold urticaria.[9]

The presence of physical urticaria should be ruled out by history and appropriate tests (see p. 133) before a lengthy evaluation and treatment program is undertaken. Dermographism is the most common type of physical urticaria; it begins suddenly following drug therapy or a viral illness, lasts for months or years, and clears spontaneously. Wheals that appear after the patient's arm is stroked prove the diagnosis.

ACUTE URTICARIA (LASTS A FEW DAYS TO A FEW WEEKS) EVALUATION AND MANAGEMENT

SKIN EXAMINATION FOR CHARACTERISTICS OF HIVES

Most cases present with typical urticarial plaques larger than 2 cm; stroke the patient's arm to rule out dermographism

Determine that lesions are not insect bites (an individual bite lesion lasts longer than 24 hours)

HISTORY

Exact time of onset
Food and drink
Medication (e.g., aspirin)
Change of environment, recent travel
Exposure to pollens, chemicals

PHYSICAL EXAMINATION

Signs of active infection
Recent viral infection

LABORATORY

No routine studies for acute urticaria
Studies to confirm findings of history and physical examination

MANAGEMENT

Stop aspirin and other suspected drugs
Stop suspected foods and drinks
Prescribe antihistamines (e.g., terfenadine [Seldane]—one or two tablets during the day to prevent sedation)
Hydroxyzine 10, 25, or 50 mg every 4 hours in the afternoon and evening
Prednisone in difficult-to-control cases
Epinephrine for extensive disease and intolerable itching

EVALUATION AND MANAGEMENT OF CHRONIC URTICARIA

SKIN EXAMINATION FOR THE CHARACTERISTICS OF HIVES

Size
    Papular—cholinergic urticaria, bites
    Plaque—most cases
Thickness
    Superficial—most cases
    Deep—angioedema
Distribution
    Generalized—ingestants, inhalants, internal disease
    Localized—physical urticarias, contact urticaria
Duration of individual lesion
    Less than 1 hour—physical urticarias, typical hives
    Less than 24 hours—typical hives
    More than 25 hours—urticarial vasculitis; scaling and purpura as lesions resolve

COMPLETE MEDICAL HISTORY

Medication
Food
Duration
    Acute—days to few weeks
    Chronic—more than 6 weeks
Time of appearance
    Time of day
    Time of year
        Constant—food, internal disease
        Seasonal—inhalant allergy
Environment
    Home—clear while at work or on vacation
    Work—contact or inhalation of chemicals
Appearance after physical stimuli (physical urticaria)
    Scratching, pressure, exercise, sun exposure, cold
Associated with arthralgia and fever
    Juvenile rheumatoid arthritis, rheumatic fever, serum sickness, systemic lupus erythematosus, urticarial vasculitis, viral hepatitis

COMPLETE PHYSICAL EXAMINATION

Sources of infection
    Sinus and gum infections
    Cystitis, vaginitis, prostatitis
Dental examination by dentist
    Fix carious teeth
    Treat periodontal disease
Internal disease, thyroid examination, gall bladder symptoms

LABORATORY EVALUATION

Studies to confirm findings of history and physical examination
Studies to consider if cause not found
Sinus and dental films
Thyroid microsomal antibodies
Skin biopsy of urticarial plaque (rule out urticarial vasculitis)

MANAGEMENT (POSSIBLE THERAPEUTIC STRATEGIES)

Antihistamines
Doxepin
Prednisone
Epinephrine
Stop aspirin and all other suspected drugs
Stop vitamins, laxatives, antacids, toothpaste, cigarettes, cosmetics and all toiletries, chewing gum, household cleaning solutions, aerosols
Salicylate- and additive-free diet
Highly restricted diet
Stop fruits, tomatoes, nuts, eggs, shellfish, chocolate, alcohol, milk, cheese, bread, diet drinks, junk food
Yeast elimination
    Yeast-free diet
    Treat with nystatin
Therapeutic trials of antibiotics
    Metronidazole (250 mg three times per day for 7 days)—*Trichomonas*
    Nizoral (200 mg two times per day for 14 days)—*Candida*, fungal infections
    Erythromycin (250 mg four times per day for 10 days)—*Campylobacter*, etc.
    Trimethoprim/sulfamethoxazole Four tablets, one dose (320/160 mg)—cystitis
    Thiabendazole (25 mg/kg twice a day for 5 days)—helminth infection
    Iodoquinol 650 mg three times per day for 20 days—*Entamoeba histolytica*
Change environment
    Take vacation
Admit to hospital
    Rule out internal disease
    No food for 48 hours
Scratch tests
    Molds, pollens, dust, animals

Sinus films. In one study,[2] sinus films were found to be abnormal in 17% of patients with chronic urticaria. The presence of sinus disease was not suspected in any of the patients prior to the radiologic studies. In all patients with sinus involvement who were also treated for acute sinusitis, the urticaria cleared and subsequent x-ray films showed no sinus disorder. Because the pathologic disorder was not evident on history or physical examination, the authors recommended that sinus films should be considered in all patients with chronic urticaria, especially of recent onset.

Thyroid autoimmune disease. There is a significant association between chronic urticaria and autoimmune thyroid disease (Hashimoto's thyroiditis, Grave's disease, toxic multinodular goiter).[10,11] Thyroid autoimmunity was found in 12% of 140 consecutively seen patients with chronic urticaria in one series; 88% were women.[12] Most patients with thyroid autoimmunity are asymptomatic and have thyroid function that is normal or only slightly abnormal. Thyroid autoimmunity is detected by measuring thyroid microsomal antibodies.

Change of environment. Because the environment consists of numerous antigens, patients should consider a trial period of 1 or 2 weeks of separation from home and work, preferably with a geographic change.

Salicylate-free diet. Salicylate-free diets[13] may be beneficial (see the Appendix, p. 831). Several studies revealed that a significant number of patients with chronic urticaria developed hives when challenged with food-coloring azo dyes (e.g., tartrazine), salicylates, or benzoic acid food preservatives.[14] These substances may not be the primary cause of the urticaria in such patients, but they may be an aggravating factor because they stimulate the release of histamine. The salicylate, azo dye, and benzoic acid free diet is not extremely restrictive and may be worth the effort for difficult cases.

Highly restricted diets. A highly restricted diet may be attempted. Patients are fed lamb, rice, sugar, salt, and water for 5 days. The occurrence of new hives after 3 days suggests that foods have no role. If hives disappear, a new food is reintroduced every other day until hives appear.

Elimination of yeast. *Candida albicans* sensitivity may be a factor in patients with chronic urticaria. Scratch tests can be performed to determine sensitivity to standard yeast allergens. Patients with a positive test, those who respond with hives when challenged with commercially available bakers' yeast, and those who have yeast antibodies are treated according to the protocol for elimination of yeast, which is outlined in the Appendix, p. 831.

Treatment of occult infections. Patients occasionally respond to antibiotics even in the absence of clinical infection.[15] See the box on p. 129.

Skin biopsy. Patients with hives that are characteristic of urticarial vasculitis should have a biopsy taken of the urticarial plaque. These hives burn rather than itch and last longer than 24 hours.

Treatment of Urticaria
ANTIHISTAMINES

For the majority of patients, acute and chronic urticaria may be controlled with antihistamines.

Mechanism of action. Antihistamines control urticaria by inhibiting vasodilation and vessel fluid loss. In a simplified form, Figure 6-8 shows that histamine and antihistamines have similar chemical structures and that both fit into and compete for the same receptor sites. Antihistamines do not block the release of histamine. If histamine has been released before an antihistamine is taken, the receptor sites will be occupied and the antihistamine will have no effect.

Side effects. Antihistamines are structurally similar to atropine, therefore they produce atropine-like peripheral and central anticholinergic effects such as dry mouth, blurred vision, constipation, and dizziness. First-generation antihistamines (H_1-receptor antagonists) such as chlorpheniramine, hydroxyzine, and diphenhydramine cross the blood-brain barrier and produce sedation. There is marked individual variation in response and side effects. Antihistamines may produce stimulation in children, especially in those ages 6 through 12. An increased sensitivity to antihistamines in patients known to undergo focal seizures may cause convulsions.

Long-term administration. Prolonged use of H_1 antagonists does not lead to autoinduction of hepatic metabolism. The efficacy of H_1-receptor blockade does not decrease with prolonged use. Tolerance of adverse central nervous system effects may or may not develop.

Different classes of antihistamines

Antihistamines are categorized according to the chemical group attached directly to the core ethylamine structure (see the Formulary, p. 841, and the box on p. 131). Drugs in each group have similar actions and side effects. If a patient does not respond to an agent in one group, it may be assumed that other drugs in that group will also be ineffective, and an agent from a different group should be selected.

H_1 and H_2 antihistamines. The majority of available antihistamines are H_1 antagonists (i.e., they compete for the H_1 receptor sites). Cimetidine, ranitidine, famotidine, and nizatidine are H_2 antagonists that are used primarily for the treatment of gastric hyperacidity. It would seem that the combination of H_1 and H_2 antihistamines would provide optimum effects. The results of studies are conflicting but generally show that the combination is no more effective than an H_1 blocking agent used alone, except for the treatment of dermographism, in which the combination of chlorpheniramine (H_1) and cimetidine (H_2) is more effective.[16]

Initiating treatment

First-generation (sedating) antihistamines. Acute and chronic urticaria should be treated with hydroxyzine, a drug with powerful antihistaminic, sedative, and antipruritic properties. The dosage may be regulated over a wide range to fit the needs of the individual patient. For adults, the ini-

FORMULATIONS AND DOSAGES OF REPRESENTATIVE H₁-RECEPTOR ANTAGONISTS*

H_1-RECEPTOR ANTAGONIST	FORMULATION	RECOMMENDED DOSE†
First generation		
Chlorpheniramine maleate (Chlor-Trimeton)	Tablets: 4 mg, 8 mg,‡ 12 mg‡ Syrup: 2.5 mg/5 ml Parenteral solution: 10 mg/ml	Adult: 8-12 mg bid§ Child: 0.35 mg/kg/q24h
Hydroxyzine hydrochloride (Atarax)	Capsules: 10 mg, 25 mg, 50 mg Syrup: 10 mg/5 ml	Adult: 25-50 mg bid (or qd, at bedtime) Child: 2 mg/kg/q24h
Diphenhydramine hydrochloride (Benadryl)	Capsules: 25 mg, 50 mg Elixir: 12.5 mg/5 ml Syrup: 6.25 mg/5 ml Parenteral solution: 50 mg/ml	Adult: 25-50 mg tid Child: 5 mg/kg/q24h
Second generation		
Terfenadine (Seldane)	Tablets: 60 mg, 120 mg‖ Suspension: 30 mg/5 ml‖	Adult: 60 mg bid or 120 mg/qd Child: 3-6 yr, 15 mg bid; 7-12 yr, 30 mg bid
Astemizole (Hismanal)	Tablets: 10 mg Suspension: 10 mg/5 ml‖	Adult: 10 mg/qd Child: 0.2 mg/kg/qd
Loratadine (Claritin)	Tablets: 10 mg Syrup: 1 mg/ml‖	Adult: 10 mg/qd Child: 2-12 yr, 5 mg/qd; >12 yr and >30 kg, 10 mg/qd
Cetirizine hydrochloride (Reactine)‖	Tablets: 10 mg	Adult: 5-10 mg/qd
Acrivastine (Semprex)	Tablets: 8 mg	Adult: 8 mg tid
Ketotifen fumarate (Zaditen)‖	Tablets: 1 mg, 2 mg‡ Syrup: 1 mg/5 ml	Adult with urticaria: 4 mg/qd Child >3 yr: 1 mg bid or 2 mg/qd§

*See the Formulary for the complete list of antihistamines.
†The dose for a child should be given if the patient weighs 40 kg (90 lb) or less.
‡A tablet of this size is a timed-release formulation.
§The timed-release formulation should be given.
‖Not approved for use in the United States at this time.

tial dosage should be 25 mg every 4 hours, and the dosage should be regulated as required to 10 to 100 mg every 4 hours. Some patients do not respond to hydroxyzine, and an antihistamine from another group, such as diphenhydramine, chlorpheniramine, clemastine, or azatadine, may be selected. Sometimes combinations of agents are more effective than a single agent. The combination of hydroxyzine and cyproheptadine is particularly useful. Some patients with chronic urticaria respond when an H_2 receptor antagonist such as cimetidine is added to conventional antihistamines. This may be worth trying in refractory cases.

Second-generation (nonsedating) antihistamines. Patients who do not tolerate sedation can take one of the nonsedating antihistamines during the day and hydroxyzine in the evening. Terfenadine (Seldane), astemizole (Hismanal),[17] and loratadine[18] (Claritin) are nonsedating antihistamines that, unlike other antihistamines, do not cross the blood-brain barrier.

Symptomatic, life-threatening ventricular arrhythmias have been reported with the concomitant use of terfenadine (Seldane) and ketoconazole (Nizoral). Similar effects have occurred with macrolide antibiotics. Concurrent use of macrolides (e.g., erythromycin, clarithromycin) should be approached with caution. Patients who are sensitive to salicylates or tartrazine must avoid antihistamines that contain tartrazine dyes. The tablet forms of Atarax and Periactin are examples of dye-free antihistamines.

The effects of second-generation antihistamines persist. A 7-day course of terfenadine or loratadine causes histamine blockade to persist another 7 days after the drug is stopped. Astemizole causes more prolonged histamine blockade.

Doxepin. Tricyclic antidepressants are potent blockers of histamine H_1 and H_2 receptors. The most potent is doxepin. It is approximately 775 times more potent as an H_1 blocker than diphenhydramine and approximately 56 times more potent than hydroxyzine. As an H_2 blocker, doxepin is approximately 6 times more potent than cimetidine. When taken in dosages between 10 and 25 mg three times a day, doxepin is effective for the treatment of chronic idiopathic urticaria. Few side effects occur at this low dosage. Higher dosages may be tolerated if taken in the evening. Doxepin is a good alternative for patients with chronic urticaria who are not controlled with conventional antihistamines.[19,20] Lethargy is commonly observed but diminishes with continued use. Dry mouth and constipation are also commonly observed.

EPINEPHRINE

Severe urticaria or angioedema requires epinephrine. Epinephrine solutions have a rapid onset of effect but a short duration of action. The dosage for adults is a 1:1000 solution (0.2 to 1.0 ml) given either subcutaneously or intramuscularly; the initial dose is usually 0.3 ml. The epinephrine suspensions provide both prompt and prolonged effect (up to 8 hours). For adults, 0.1 to 0.3 ml of the 1:200 suspension is given subcutaneously.

ORAL CORTICOSTEROIDS

Oral corticosteroids should be considered for refractory cases of urticaria. Prednisone 40 mg per day given in a single morning dose or 20 mg bid is effective in most cases.

Methotrexate in Corticosteroid-Resistant Urticaria

A single report describes the benefit of methotrexate in long-standing acute and chronically debilitating urticaria of unknown cause that had become unresponsive to corticosteroids over a 24-year period. All symptoms and signs resolved after two weekly cycles of methotrexate (2.5 mg orally twice a day for 3 days of the week). After two additional cycles of methotrexate the patient's therapy was halted. The patient remained in complete remission for 6 months when the full-blown syndrome recurred. Methotrexate alone was reinstituted and all symptoms and signs resolved after 3 days of therapy.[21]

Physical Urticarias

During the initial examination, the physician should determine whether the hives are elicited by physical stimuli (Table 6-1). Patients with these distinctive hives may be spared a detailed laboratory evaluation; they simply require an explanation of their condition and its treatment. Unrecognized physical urticarias may account for approximately 10% of all cases of chronic urticaria. A major distinguishing feature of the physical urticarias is that attacks are brief, lasting only 30 to 60 minutes.[22] In typical urticaria, individual lesions last from hours to a few days. The one exception among physical urticarias is pressure urticaria, in which swelling may last for several hours.

TABLE 6-1 Comparison of the Physical Urticarias

Urticaria	Relative frequency	Precipitant	Time of onset	Duration	Local symptoms	Systemic symptoms	Tests	Mechanism	Treatment
Symptomatic dermographism	Most frequent	Stroking skin	Minutes	2-3 hr	Irregular, pruritic wheals	None	Scratch skin	Passive transfer; IgE; histamine; possible role of adenosine triphosphate; substance P; possible direct pharmacologic mechannism	Continual hydroxyzine hydrochloride regimen; combined H_1 and H_2 blockers
Delayed dermographism	Rare	Stroking skin	30 min-8 hr	≤48 hr	Burning; deep swelling	None	Scratch skin; observe early and late	Unknown	Avoidance of precipitants
Pressure urticaria	Frequent	Pressure	3-12 hr	8-24 hr	Diffuse, tender swelling	Flulike symptoms	Apply weight	Unknown	Avoidance of precipitants; if severe, low dosages of corticosteroids given for systemic effect
Solar urticaria	Frequent	Various wavelengths of light	2-5 min	15 min-3 hr	Pruritic wheals	Wheezing; dizziness; syncope	Phototest	Passive transfer; reverse passive transfer; IgE; possible histamine	Avoidance of precipitants; antihistamines; sunscreens; chloroquine phosphate regimen for short time
Familial cold urticaria	Rare	Change in skin temperature from cold air	30 min-3 hr	≤48 hr	Burning wheals	Tremor; headache; arthralgia; fever	Expose skin to cold air	Unknown	Avoidance of precipitants
Essential acquired cold urticaria	Frequent	Cold contact	2-5 min	1-2 hr	Pruritic wheals	Wheezing; syncope; drowning	Apply ice-filled copper beaker to arm; immerse arm in cold water	Passive transfer; reverse passive transfer; IgE (IgM); histamine; vasculitis can be induced	Cyproheptadine hydrochloride regimen; other antihistamines; desensitization; avoidance of precipitants
Heat urticaria	Rare	Heat contact	2-5 min (rarely delayed)	1 hr	Pruritic wheals	None	Apply hot water–filled cylinder to arm	Possible histamine; possible complement	Antihistamines; desensitization; avoidance of precipitants
Cholinergic urticaria	Very frequent	General overheating of body	2-20 min	30 min-1 hr	Papular, pruritic wheals	Syncope; diarrhea; vomiting; salivation; headaches	Bathe in hot water; exercise until perspiring; inject methacholine chloride	Passive transfer; possible immunoglobulin; product of sweat gland stimulation; histamine; reduced protease inhibitor	Application of cold water or ice to skin; hydroxyzine regimen; refractory period; anticholinergics
Aquagenic urticaria	Rare	Water contact	Several min-30 min	30-45 min	Papular, pruritic wheals	None reported	Apply water compresses to skin	Unknown	Avoidance of precipitants; antihistamines; application of inert oil
Vibratory angioedema	Very rare	Vibrating against skin	2-5 min	1 hr	Angioedema	None reported	Apply body of vibrating mixer to forearm	Unknown	Avoidance of precipitants
Exercise-induced anaphylaxis	Rare	Exercise; some cases ingestion of certain foods	During or after exercise	Minutes to hours	Pruritic wheals	Respiratory distress; hypotension	Exercise testing; immersion tests	Unknown	Antihistamines; ketotifen

DERMOGRAPHISM

Also known as "skin writing," dermographism is the most common physical urticaria, occurring to some degree in approximately 5% of the population. Hives are produced by rubbing or stroking the skin. The onset is usually sudden; young patients are affected most commonly. The tendency to be dermographic lasts for weeks to months or years. It may be preceded by a viral infection, antibiotic therapy (especially penicillin), or emotional upset, but in most cases the cause is unknown.[23]

The degree of urticarial response varies. A patient will be highly reactive for months and then appear to be in remission, only to have symptoms recur (Figure 6-9). Patients complain of linear, itchy wheals from scratching or wheals at the site of friction from clothing. Delayed dermographism, in which the immediate urticarial response is followed in 1 to 6 hours by a wheal that persists for 24 to 48 hours, is rare.

Diagnosis. A tongue blade drawn firmly across the patient's arm or back produces whealing 2 mm or more in width in approximately 1 to 3 minutes, an exaggerated triple response (Figure 6-10).

1. A red line occurs in 3 to 15 seconds (capillary dilation).
2. Broadening erythema appears (axon reflex flare from arteriolar dilation).
3. A wheal with surrounding erythema replaces the red line (transudation of fluid through dilated capillaries).

As a control, the examining physician can perform this test on his or her own arm at the same time.

Treatment. Treatment is not necessary unless the patient is highly sensitive and reacts continually to the slightest trauma. Short courses of antihistamines (e.g., hydroxyzine) in relatively low dosages (10 to 25 mg every 4 hours) provide adequate relief. Some patients are severely affected and require continuous suppression with hydroxyzine for months. Ketotifen, a mast cell stabilizing agent, is as effective as antihistamines in controlling symptoms.[24] H_2 receptor antagonists have a small but therapeutically irrelevant additional effect compared with H_1 antagonists alone.[25]

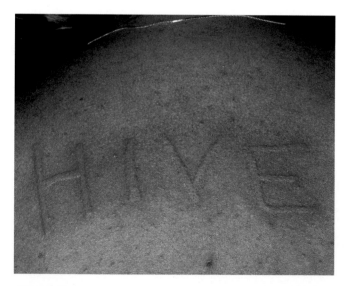

Figure 6-9
Dermographism. A highly sensitive patient. Swelling occurs 1 to 3 minutes after the skin is stroked.

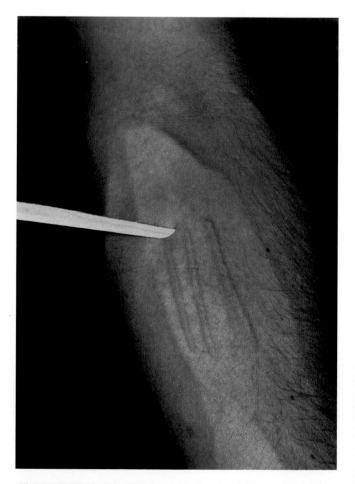

Figure 6-10
Dermographism. A tongue blade drawn firmly across the arm elicits urticaria in susceptible individuals. This simple test should be considered for any patient with acute or chronic urticaria.

PRESSURE URTICARIA

A deep, itchy, burning, or painful swelling occurring 4 to 6 hours after a pressure stimulus and lasting 8 to 72 hours is characteristic of this uncommon form of physical urticaria. The mean age of onset is the early 30s. The disease is chronic, and the mean duration is 9 years (range: 1 to 40 years). Malaise, fatigue, fever, chills, headache, or generalized arthralgia may occur. Many have moderate to severe disease that is disabling, especially for those who perform manual labor.[26] Pressure urticaria, chronic urticaria, and angioedema frequently occur in the same patient. In one study, delayed pressure urticaria was present in 37% of patients with chronic urticaria.[9] The hands, feet, trunk, buttock, lips, and face are commonly affected. Lesions are induced by standing, walking, wearing tight garments, or prolonged sitting on a hard surface.

Diagnosis. Because the swelling occurs hours after the application of pressure, the cause may not be immediately apparent. Repeated deep swelling in the same area is the clue to the diagnosis. Patients with dermographism may have whealing from pressure that occurs immediately, rather than hours later. Test for delayed pressure urticaria by placing a glass sphere (1.4 cm), such as a marble, on the back of the mid forearm. A strip of cloth is placed over the marble, allowed to hang down on either side, and tied below the arm. A 4-kg weight is suspended from the cloth loop for 5 minutes, and the pressure point under the marble is observed 4 to 8 hours later. A visible and palpable swelling at the site is evidence of pressure urticaria. After pressure stimulus, the mean onset of whealing occurs in 3½ hours, the mean peak swelling occurs after 10 hours, and the mean lesion duration is 36 hours. More accurate testing devices can be made.[27]

Treatment. Antihistamines are not helpful. Systemic steroids are the only effective treatment for severe, disabling delayed pressure urticaria. Dosages of prednisone greater than 30 mg/day may be required.[26]

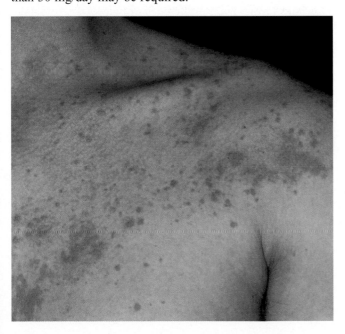

CHOLINERGIC URTICARIA

Round, papular wheals 2 to 4 mm in diameter that are surrounded by a slight to extensive red flare are diagnostic of this most distinctive type of hive[28] (Figure 6-11). Most cases begin in persons between the ages of 10 and 30 years and resolve spontaneously in only 14% of patients.[29] Typically, the hives occur during or shortly after exercise. However, their onset may be delayed for approximately an hour after stimulation. An attack begins with itching, tingling, burning, warmth, or irritation of the skin. Hives begin within 2 to 20 minutes after the patient experiences a general overheating of the body as a result of exercise, exposure to heat, or emotional stress, and they last for minutes to hours (median: 30 minutes). Cholinergic urticaria may become confluent and resemble typical hives. The incidence of systemic symptoms is very low; however, when they occur, systemic systems include angioedema, hypotension, wheezing, and GI tract complaints.[22,30]

Diagnosis. The diagnosis is suggested by the history and confirmed by experimentally reproducing the lesions. The most reliable and efficient testing method is to ask the patient to run in place or to use an exercise bicycle for 10 to 15 minutes, and then to observe the patient for 1 hour to detect the typical micropapular hives. Exercise testing should be done in a controlled environment; patients with exercise-induced anaphylaxis may need emergency treatment. Immersion of half the patient in a bath at 43° C can raise the patient's oral temperature by 1° C to 1.5° C and induce characteristic micropapular hives.[31] The immersion test does not induce hives in patients with exercise-induced anaphylaxis. An intradermal injection of 100 U of methacholine (Mecholyl) in saline solution elicits the characteristic lesions in only one third of affected patients and is not a reliable test.[29]

Treatment. Patients can avoid symptoms by limiting strenuous exercise. Showering with hot water may temporarily deplete histamine stores and induce a 24-hour refractory period. Hydroxyzine (10 to 50 mg) taken 1 hour before exercise attenuates the eruption, but the side effect of drowsiness is often unacceptable. Nonsedating antihistamines may be tried.

Figure 6-11
Cholinergic urticaria. Round, red, papular wheals that occur in response to exercise, heat, or emotional stress.

EXERCISE-INDUCED ANAPHYLAXIS

Exercise-induced anaphylaxis (EIA) was first described in 1980. Patients develop pruritis, urticaria, respiratory distress, and hypotension after exercise. Symptoms may progress to angioedema, laryngeal edema, bronchospasm, and hypotension, and there is a high frequency of progression to upper airway distress and shock .[32,33] It is associated with different kinds of exercise, although jogging is the most frequently reported. Exercise acts as a physical stimulus that, through an unknown mechanism, provokes mast cell degranulation and elevated serum histamine levels. In contrast to cholinergic urticaria, the lesions are large and are not produced by hot showers, pyrexia, or anxiety. It is differentiated from cholinergic urticaria by a hot-water immersion test (see cholinergic urticaria). Exercise-induced or exercise-accentuated anaphylaxis may occur only after ingestion of certain foods such as wheat or shellfish[34] (food-dependent EIA). Attacks occur when the patient exercises within 30 minutes after ingestion of the food; eating the food without exercising (and vice versa) causes no symptoms. Patients with wheat-associated EIA had positive skin tests to several wheat fractions.[35] Another precipitating factor includes drug intake; a familial tendency has been reported. The prognosis is not well defined, but a reduction of attacks occurs in 45% of patients by means of elimination diets and behavioral changes. The differential diagnosis includes exercise-induced asthma, idiopathic anaphylaxis, cardiac arrhythmias, and carcinoid syndrome.[36]

Treatment. Treatment includes the administration of epinephrine and antihistamines, airway maintenance, and cardiovascular support. H$_1$ antihistamines are recommended as pretreatment and acute therapy. Ketotifen, a mast cell–stabilizing agent, also controls symptoms.[24] Prophylactic treatment includes avoidance of exercise, abstention from coprecipitating foods and medications, pretreatment with antihistamines and cromolyn, or the induction of tolerance through regular exercise.

COLD URTICARIA

Cold urticaria occurs in both familial and acquired forms. The familial form is a rare, autosomal dominantly transmitted disorder.[37] The mean age of onset in acquired cold urticaria is 18 to 25 years; the mean duration of symptoms is 5 to 6 years (range: 3 weeks to 37 years).[38,39]

Nearly 25% of patients become asymptomatic in 1.6 years, but 20% have symptoms for more than 10 years. Dermographism and cholinergic urticaria are found relatively often in patients with cold urticaria. Hives occur with a sudden drop in air temperature or during exposure to cold water. Many patients have severe reactions with generalized urticaria, angioedema, or both.[38] Swimming in cold water is the most common cause of severe reactions and can result in massive transudation of fluid into the skin, leading to hypotension, fainting, shock, and possibly death. Like dermographism, cold urticaria often begins after infection, drug therapy, or emotional stress. The mast cell–derived mediators (histamine, eosinophil and neutrophil chemotactic factors, platelet activating factor, and prostaglandin D$_2$)[40] have been found in serum after cold challenge. There is no evidence of complement activation.

Diagnosis. The diagnosis is made by inducing a hive with an ice cube held against the skin for 1 to 5 minutes (Figure 6-12). A cold-water immersion test, in which the forearm is submerged for 5 to 15 minutes in water at 0° to 8° C, establishes the diagnosis when the results of the ice cube test are equivocal. The patient must be monitored closely because severe reactions are possible.

Treatment. Patients must learn to protect themselves from a sudden decrease in temperature. Cyproheptadine (Periactin) and doxepin are effective in suppressing cold urticaria despite the observation that they do not inhibit histamine release after cold challenges.[41] Cyproheptadine has a greater suppressive effect on cold urticaria than does chlorpheniramine. The dosage can be adjusted on an individual basis to as low as 2 mg orally once or twice a day to obtain optimum benefits with minimum side effects; side effects of cyproheptadine include sedation and increased appetite. Severe cold urticaria is associated with the release of platelet-activating factor into the circulation. Doxepin (10 mg two or three times a day) treatment is associated with a reduction of platelet-activating factor and improvement of symptoms.[40,42] Ketotifen, a mast cell stabilizing agent, is also effective.[24]

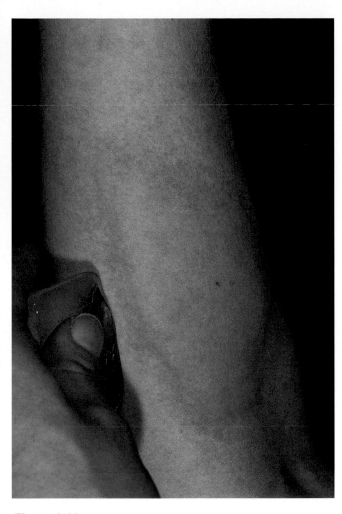

Figure 6-12
Cold urticaria. The hive occurred within minutes of holding an ice cube against the skin.

SOLAR URTICARIA

Hives that occur minutes after exposure to the sun and disappear in less than 1 hour are called *solar urticaria*. Previously exposed tanned skin may not react when exposed to ultraviolet light. Hives induced by exposure to ultraviolet light must be distinguished from the much more common sun-related condition of polymorphous light eruption. Lesions of polymorphous light eruption are rarely urticarial. They occur hours after exposure and persist for several days.

There are several different wavelengths that can cause solar urticaria.[43] The disease is classified into six types that correspond to six different wavelengths of light. An individual reacts to a specific wavelength or a narrow band of the light spectrum, usually within the range of 290 to 500 nm. In two types, type I (285 to 320 nm) and type IV (400 to 500 nm), the response can be transferred passively to the skin of a normal recipient. In at least some patients, the serum factor responsible for solar urticaria is present in the IgE fraction. The cause may be an allergic reaction to an antigen formed in the skin by light waves. Those reacting to light above 400 nm (visible light) develop hives even when exposed through glass. Solar urticaria has been described in patients with connective tissue diseases and porphyria. The wavelength responsible for solar urticaria is identified by phototesting. Antihistamines, sunscreens, and graded exposure to increasing amounts of light are effective treatments.

HEAT, WATER, AND VIBRATION URTICARIAS

Other physical stimuli such as heat, water of any temperature, or vibration are rare causes of urticaria. Aquagenic urticaria resembles the micropapular hives of cholinergic urticaria. One study[44] suggests that in aquagenic urticaria it is not the water but the epidermal substances dissolved in water that elicit hives; water acts only as a solvent to deliver these substances into the skin. This may explain why the palms, which have a thick epidermis, are resistant to aquagenic urticaria.

AQUAGENIC PRURITUS

Severe, prickling skin discomfort without skin lesions[45] occurs within 1 to 15 (or more) minutes after contact with water at any temperature and lasts for 10 to 120 minutes (average: 40 minutes). Histamine does not seem to play a key role in the pathogenesis of aquagenic pruritus. Capsaicin cream (Zostrix, Zostrix-HP) applied three times daily for 4 weeks resulted in complete relief of symptoms in the treated areas.[45a] Ultraviolet B phototherapy and antihistamines provide some relief.[46] One paper reported that sodium bicarbonate (25 to 200 gm) added to the bath or applied as a paste prevented the symptoms.[47] Polycythemia rubra vera should be ruled out.

Angioedema

Angioedema is a hivelike swelling caused by increased vascular permeability in the subcutaneous tissue of the skin and mucosa and the submucosal layers of the respiratory and GI tracts. A similar reaction occurs in the dermis with hives. Hives and angioedema commonly occur simultaneously. The deeper reaction produces a more diffuse swelling than is seen in hives. Itching is usually absent. Symptoms consist of burning and painful swelling. The lips, palms, soles, limbs, trunk, and genitalia are most commonly affected. Involvement of the GI and respiratory tracts produces dysphagia, dyspnea, colicky abdominal pain, and attacks of vomiting and diarrhea. GI symptoms are more common in the hereditary types of angioedema. Angioedema may occur as a result of trauma. Acquired and inherited types are identified below.

In one report of 17 patients admitted during a 5-year period, 94% had angioedema in the head and neck; three required urgent tracheotomy or intubation, 35% had recent initiation of angiotensin-converting enzyme inhibitor therapy for hypertension, and 6% demonstrated classic hereditary angioedema. The majority (59%) had unclear etiologies for their symptoms.[48]

Acquired angioedema
Acute angioedema
    Allergic IgE mediated (drugs, food, insect venom)
    Contrast dyes
    Serum sickness
    Cold urticaria
Chronic recurrent angioedema
    Idiopathic (most cases)
    Acquired C1 inhibitor deficiency (lymphoproliferative disease)
    Angioedema-eosinophilia syndrome
Hereditary angioedema
Type 1 (85%)—C1 inhibitor absent
Type 2 (15%)—C1 inhibitor not functional

ACQUIRED FORMS OF ANGIOEDEMA
Acute angioedema

Severe allergic type 1 immediate hypersensitivity IgE-mediated reactions can cause acute angioedema. IgE antibody unites with antigen (food, drug,[49] stinging insect venom, pollen) on the mast cell surface and precipitates an immediate and massive release of histamine and other mediators from mast cells. Angioedema occurs alone or with the other symptoms of systemic anaphylaxis (i.e., respiratory distress, hypotension). Some forms of cold urticaria are IgE mediated and occur initially as angioedema.

Contrast dyes used in radiology and drugs may also cause acute angioedema as a result of nonimmunologic mechanisms. Examples include nonsteroidal antiinflammatory drugs, such as aspirin and indomethacin, and angiotensin-converting enzyme–inhibiting drugs.

Angioedema occurs as part of serum sickness syndrome. Swelling, fever, arthralgias, and lymphadenopathy occur 7 to 10 days after exposure to heterologous serum or certain drugs.

Angiotensin-converting enzyme inhibitors. Angiotensin-converting enzyme inhibitors (ACEIs) are widely used for the treatment of mild forms of hypertension. Angioedema occurs in 0.1% to 0.2% of patients receiving an ACEI.[50,51] The onset usually occurs within hours to 1 week after starting therapy. Angioedema may occur suddenly even though the drug has been well tolerated for months or years; symptoms may regress spontaneously while the patient continues the medication, erroneously prompting an alternative diagnosis.

Most cases from the short-acting ACEI, captopril, present with mild angioedema that can be controlled with antihistamines and glucocorticosteroids. In contrast, the angioedema induced by the long-acting ACE inhibitors (lisinopril[52], enalapril) has been serious.[53] Angioedema that results from ACEIs is probably not IgE mediated and antihistamines and steroids may not alleviate the airway obstruction.

The pathology has a special predilection for the tongue, a circumstance that renders orotracheal and nasotracheal intubation difficult; symptoms may progress rapidly despite aggressive medical therapy, necessitating emergency airway procedures.[54] Individuals with a history of idiopathic angioedema probably should not be given ACE inhibitors.[55]

Treatment. Acute attacks are treated with epinephrine and high dosages of antihistamines. Prescribe Epi-pen or Epi-pen Jr for patients who experience severe reactions with insect stings. The epinephrine in Epi-pen is packaged in an auto-injector to avoid manual needle insertion.

Advise affected patients to wear a bracelet that identifies the diagnosis; their reactions could be misdiagnosed as symptoms related to alcoholism, stroke, myocardial infarction, or a foreign body in the airway.

Chronic recurrent angioedema

Idiopathic angioedema. Most cases of angioedema are idiopathic. Angioedema can occur at any age but is most common in the 40- to 50-year-old age group. Women are most frequently affected. The pattern of recurrence is unpredictable, and episodes can occur for 5 or more years. Involvement of the GI and respiratory tracts occurs, but asphyxiation is not a danger. Treat with antihistamines such as hydroxyzine. Long-term suppression may require corticosteroids. Alternate-day therapy is indicated with the lowest dosage of prednisone required to provide adequate control.

Acquired C1 inhibitor deficiency. Late-onset, recurrent angioedema may indicate an acquired deficiency of C1q esterase inhibitor. The characteristics are low levels or the absence of functional C1 inhibitor activity, CH_{50}, C1q, C1, C4, and C2; lack of evidence of inheritance; and the onset of symptoms in middle age.

The two types of acquired angioedema are described below. One form is associated with malignancy (B-cell lineage, breast cancer); the other is an autoimmune form.

Malignancy associated form. B-cell lymphoproliferative disorders (e.g., chronic lymphatic leukemia, non-Hodgkin's B-cell lymphoma)[56,57] may be characterized by circulating antiidiotypic antibodies to the monoclonal immunoglobulin synthesized by their B lymphocytes. The resulting activation of the early components of the complement pathway leads to increased consumption of C1 inhibitor; synthesis of C1 inhibitor is normal or increased.

Autoimmune form. IgGl autoantibodies are present in the absence of underlying lymphoproliferative disease. These anti–C1 inhibitor autoantibodies prevent the binding of Cl inhibitor to C1. Uncontrolled C1 degrades C1 inhibitor to an inactive degradation product.[58] As in other forms of C1 inhibitor deficiency, the unopposed activation of the complement system leads to angioedema.

Both types of acquired deficiency can be distinguished by low plasma levels of C1, an abnormality not seen in the hereditary form. Prophylaxis with attenuated androgens such as danazol is helpful in patients with lymphoproliferative disorders. Those with C1 inhibitor autoantibodies respond better to corticosteroid therapy.

Angioedema-eosinophilia syndrome. This rare, non–life-threatening syndrome consists of periodic attacks of angioedema, urticaria, myalgia, oliguria, and fever.[59] During attacks, body weights increase up to 18%, and leukocyte counts reach as high as 108,000/μl (88% eosinophils). Attacks resolve spontaneously or require corticosteroids to control symptoms and normalize the blood count.[60]

HEREDITARY ANGIOEDEMA

Hereditary angioedema is transmitted as an autosomal dominant trait. Attacks may be complicated by incapacitating cutaneous swelling, life-threatening upper airway impediment, and severe GI colic. There are episodes of acute subcutaneous or mucosal swelling, but hives do not occur. Obstruction of the upper respiratory tract is responsible for the 30% mortality rate.

In most cases the disease begins in late childhood or early adolescence. During an episode, the swelling increases slowly over 12 to 18 hours, then slowly subsides over the next 48 to 72 hours. Swelling involves the extremities (96%), face (85%), oropharynx (64%), and intestinal mucosa (88%). In one study, peripheral swelling accounted for 80% of all attacks, and abdominal pain, nausea, and vomiting for 20% of attacks.[61]

Women with hereditary angioedema frequently have cystic ovaries (polycystic or multifollicular) in the presence of high plasma beta-endorphin.[62]

Hereditary angioedema results from a lack of functional C1 esterase inhibitor. A lesion in the C1 inhibitor structural gene[63] can cause several different defects. There can be decreased production of the protein or the synthesis of a biologically inactive form. There are two types of hereditary angioedema. Type I is the most common and is characterized by an insufficient production of C1 inhibitor. This affects 85% of all patients with hereditary angioedema. Patients with type 2 have normal or elevated concentrations of C1 inhibitor but the protein is functionally deficient. A deficiency of active C1 inhibitor is the most commonly identified genetic defect of the complement system.

Diagnosis. The diagnosis is suggested by the family and personal history. Both types have low serum levels of CH_{50}, C4, and C2, and the absence of functional C1 inhibitor activity. The first step toward confirming the diagnosis is to order a serum C4 level test. Measurement of C4 should detect the abnormality in both types when the patient is in remission as well as during attacks. If the level is abnormal, two more tests should be ordered: (1) a C1 esterase inhibitor test and (2) a C1 esterase inhibitor, functional assay, and serum test. To distinguish the different forms of C1 inhibitor deficiencies, it is necessary to determine the amount of C1 inhibitor protein and the level of its functional activity. Family members of patients with hereditary angioedema may have markedly abnormal complement values despite being asymptomatic.

Treatment. Three main categories of substances have been proposed for the treatment of C1 deficiencies: the androgens, the antifibrinolytics, and fresh plasma or purified C1 inhibitor.

Acute attacks. Antihistamines, corticosteroids, and adrenergic drugs are not effective. In acute, life-threatening attacks, replacement therapy with purified C1 inhibitor concentrate[64] or fresh frozen plasma is required.

Prophylactic treatment. The best drugs for prophylaxis are the attenuated androgens danazol and stanozolol. Treatment is started for patients who have one or more severe attacks per month. Danazol (200 to 600 mg/day)[65] and stanozolol (2 mg/day) provide short- and long-term prophylaxis.[66] They correct the lowered C1 esterase inhibitor and C4 levels by inducing hepatic synthesis through the increase of serum levels of C1 esterase inhibitor, and they are effective in hereditary angioedema types I and II. Stanozolol and danazol are equally effective, but stanozolol costs less.

Menstrual abnormalities (79%), weight gain (60%), muscle cramps/myalgias (40%), and transaminase elevations (40%) are the most common adverse reactions.[67] To minimize these complications use the following schedule: daily for 1 month, then 5 days on, 5 days off. Adjust the dosage to prevent acute attacks.[68] This dosage may be less than that required to return C1 esterase inhibitor to normal levels. Spontaneous improvement occurs and the need for prophylactic treatment may diminish with time.

Contact Urticaria Syndrome

Clinical presentation. Contact urticaria is characterized by a wheal and flare that occur within 30 to 60 minutes after cutaneous exposure to certain agents. Direct contact of the skin with these agents may cause a wheal-and-flare response restricted to the area of contact, generalized urticaria, urticaria and asthma, or urticaria combined with an anaphylactoid reaction. Most patients give a history of relapsing dermatitis or generalized urticarial attacks rather than a localized hive; others complain only of localized sensations of itching, burning, and tingling. In addition, some patients experience rhinitis, laryngeal edema, and abdominal disturbances.

Precipitating factors. Urticaria occurs after the absorption of material through the skin and is elicited by nonimmunologic and immunologic mechanisms. Nonimmunologic, histamine-releasing substances are produced by certain plants (nettles), animals (caterpillars, jellyfish), and medications (dimethyl sulfoxide [DMSO]).[69,70] Anaphylaxis may occur after application of bacitracin ointment.[71] The mechanism by which wood, plants, foods, cosmetics, and animal hair and dander cause contact urticaria has not been defined. The term *protein contact dermatitis* is used when an immediate reaction occurs after eczematous skin is exposed to certain types of food (fish, garlic, onion, chives, cucumber, parsley, tomato), animal (cow hair and dander), or plant substances. Cooks who complain of burning or stinging when handling certain foods may have contact urticaria syndrome.

Diagnosis. Because there is no standard test battery for routine evaluation of contact urticaria, a careful history concerning the occurrence of immediate reactions, whether localized or generalized, is essential. An open patch test may be performed by applying a drop of the suspected substance to the ventral forearm and observing the site for a wheal 30 to 60 minutes later. Closed tests may be associated with more intense or generalized reactions.

Prick testing (using fresh samples of the food suspected from the patient's history) is an accurate method of investigation for selected cases of hand dermatitis in patients who spend considerable time handling foods (e.g., catering workers, cooks).[72] Seafood is a common allergen.

PRURITIC URTICARIAL PAPULES AND PLAQUES OF PREGNANCY

PUPPP,[73-79] or polymorphic eruption of pregnancy, is the most common gestational dermatosis with an incidence of approximately 1 in 160 pregnancies. It is seen most frequently in primigravidas and begins late in the third trimester of pregnancy or occasionally in the early postpartum period. The eruption appears suddenly, begins on the abdomen in 90% of patients (Figure 6-13, *A*), and in a few days may spread in a symmetric fashion to involve the buttock, proximal arms, and backs of the hands (Figure 6-13, *B*). The initial lesions may be confined to striae. The face is not involved. Itching is moderate to intense, but excoriations are rarely seen. The lesions begin as red papules that are often surrounded by a narrow, pale halo. They increase in number and may become confluent, forming edematous urticarial plaques or erythema multiforme-like target lesions that may look like the lesions of herpes gestationis. In other patients, the involved sites acquire broad areas of erythema, and the papules remain discrete. Papulovesicles have been reported. The mean duration is 6 weeks, but the rash is usually not severe for more than 1 week. Unlike urticaria, the eruption remains fixed and increases in intensity, clearing in most cases before or within 1 week after delivery. Recurrence with future pregnancies is unusual. There have been no fetal or maternal complications. Infants do not develop the eruption.

Significantly increased maternal weight gain, newborn birth weight, and twin birth rate have been reported in patients with PUPPP. It was postulated that abdominal distension or a reaction to it may play a role in the development of PUPPP.

The biopsy reveals a nonspecific perivascular lymphohistiocytic infiltrate. Eosinophils have also been noted in most biopsies. There are no laboratory abnormalities, and direct immunofluorescence of lesional and perilesional skin is negative.

Treatment is supportive. The expectant mother can be assured that pruritus will quickly terminate before or after delivery. Itching can be relieved with group V topical steroids; cool, wet compresses; oatmeal baths; and antihistamines. Prednisone (40 mg/day) may be required if pruritus becomes intolerable.

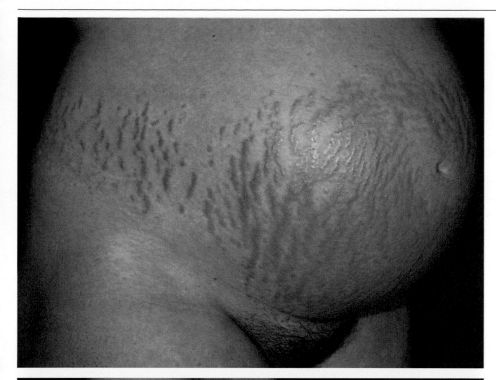

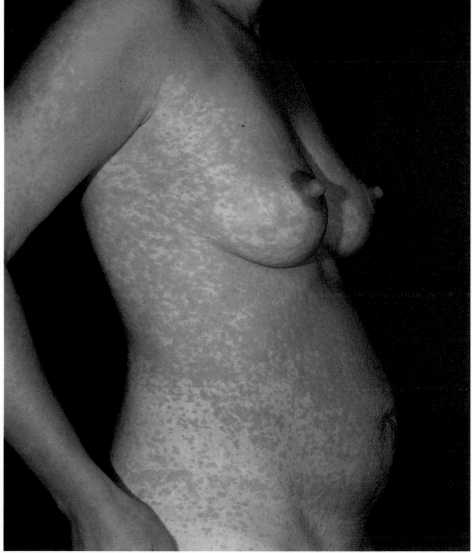

Figure 6-13
Pruritic urticarial papules and plaques of pregnancy.

A, The abdomen is often the initial site of involvement. Initial lesions may be confined to striae.

B, Fully evolved eruption.

Urticarial Vasculitis

Urticarial vasculitis is a subset of vasculitis characterized clinically by urticarial skin lesions and histologically by necrotizing vasculitis.[81-84] Immune complex deposition (a type II immune complex reaction) in the postcapillary venules is the probable cause. There is a spectrum of clinical and laboratory features.

Many patients have minimal signs or symptoms of systemic disease. Systemic symptoms include angioedema (42%), arthralgias (49%), pulmonary disease (21%), and abdominal pain (17%). Thirty-two percent have hypocomplementemia, 64% have lesions that last more than 24 hours, 32% have painful or burning lesions, and 35% have lesions that resolve with purpura.[85]

Patients with urticarial vasculitis have been categorized into two subgroups: those with hypocomplementemia and those with normal complement levels. Patients with hypocomplementemia are more likely to have systemic involvement than patients with normal complement levels. Overall, patients with urticarial vasculitis tend to have a benign course.

Urticarial plaques in most patients with typical chronic urticaria resolve completely in less than 24 hours and disappear while new plaques appear in other areas. Urticarial vasculitis plaques persist for 24 to 72 hours and may have residual changes of purpura, scaling, and hyperpigmentation (Figure 6-14). The lesions are burning and painful rather than itchy.

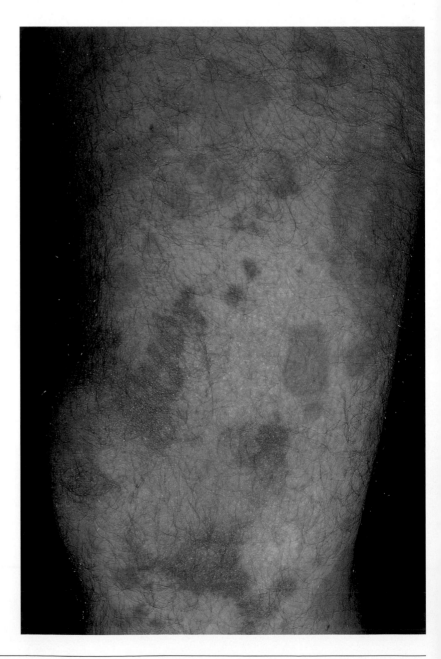

Figure 6-14
Urticarial vasculitis. Purpura occurs as the hive resolves.

Diagnosis. Biopsy shows a histologic picture that is indistinguishable from that seen in cutaneous necrotizing vasculitis (palpable purpura). Fragmentation of leukocytes and fibrinoid deposition occur in the walls of postcapillary venules, a pattern called *leukocytoclastic vasculitis*. There is an interstitial neutrophilic infiltrate of the dermis. Anti-C1q autoantibody develops in disorders characterized by immune complex–mediated injury and appears in most patients with hypocomplementemic urticarial vasculitis syndrome.[86]

Patients with hypocomplementemia may have an immunofluorescent pattern of immunoglobulins or C3 as determined by routine direct immunofluorescence. As with typical cutaneous vasculitis, most patients have an elevated erythrocyte sedimentation rate. Patients with more severe involvement have hypocomplementemia (hypocomplementemic urticarial vasculitis syndrome) with depressed CH_{50}, C1q, C4, or C2. Direct immunofluorescence in patients with hypocomplementemia shows deposition of Ig and C3; 87% have fluorescence of the blood vessels, and 70% have fluorescence of the basement membrane zone.[85] Rule out other diseases in which cutaneous vasculitis may present as an urticarial-like eruption (e.g., viral illness, systemic lupus erythematosus, Sjögren's syndrome, and serum sickness).

Treatment. Prednisone in dosages exceeding 40 mg/day is effective. Other medications reported to be effective are indomethacin (25 mg three times daily to 50 mg four times daily),[87] colchicine (0.6 mg two or three times daily),[88,89] dapsone (up to 200 mg/day), low-dose oral methotrexate,[89-91] and antimalarial drugs.

Serum Sickness

Serum sickness is a disease produced by exposure to drugs (e.g., cefaclor),[92,93] blood products, or animal-derived vaccines. After exposure to these antigens, a strong host-antibody response occurs. These circulating antibodies react with the newly introduced antigen to form precipitating antigen-antibody complexes. This is a type III (immune complex) reaction, or Arthus reaction—named after its discoverer. These circulating immune complexes are trapped in vessel walls of various organs, where they activate complement. A rise in the level of immune complexes is accompanied by a decrease in serum levels of C3 and C4 and an increase in C3a/C3a des-arginine, a split product of C3 whose presence indicates that the complement system has been activated by immune complexes. Inflammatory mediators are released. C3a/C3a des-arginine, a potent anaphylotoxin, induces mast cell degranulation to produce hives.

Clinical manifestations. Symptoms (Table 6-2) appear 8 to 13 days after exposure to the drug or antisera and last for 4 or more days. They include fever, malaise, skin eruptions, arthralgias, nausea, vomiting, occult blood in the stool, and lymphadenopathy. The disease resolves without sequelae in most cases. The skin eruption begins with the onset of other symptoms. A morbilliform rash or urticaria is limited to the trunk or may become generalized. The hands and feet may be involved.

Diagnosis. The white blood count may be as high as 25,000. Serum C3 and C4 are below normal. Proteinuria occurs in 40% of patients. Direct immunofluorescence of skin lesions less than 24-hours old shows Ig deposits (IgM, IgE, IgA, or C3) in the superficial small blood vessels.[94] Drugs are now the most common cause of serum sickness. Penicillin, sulfa drugs, thiouracils, cholecystographic dyes, hydantoins, aminosalicylic acid, and streptomycin are most often implicated.[95]

Treatment. The offending agent must be avoided. Antihistamines such as hydroxyzine control the hives. Prednisone 40 mg/day is used if symptoms are intense.

TABLE 6-2 Serum Sickness	
Symptom	**Incidence**
Fever	100%
Malaise	100%
Skin eruption	100%
Arthralgias	55%
Gastrointestinal symptoms	45%
Lymphadenopathy	18%
Proteinuria	40%
Circulating immune complexes (maximum level—12 days)	90%
Decreased C3, C4 (lowest level—10 days)	100%

Modified from Lawley TJ et al: *N Engl J Med* 311:1407-1413, 1984.

Mastocytosis

Mastocytosis is a disease in which there is an increased number of mast cells in various organs of the body.[96,97] In young children, the disease is usually confined to the skin; in adults, mastocytosis is usually systemic. Mast cells store histamine in granules. Histamine is released by scratching the lesions (Figure 6-15) or ingesting certain agents (see Figure 6-7). The cause is unknown, and familial occurrence is only rarely documented.[98] The skin is the most frequent site of involvement.

Mast cell disease of the skin is called *urticaria pigmentosa*. There are several types.

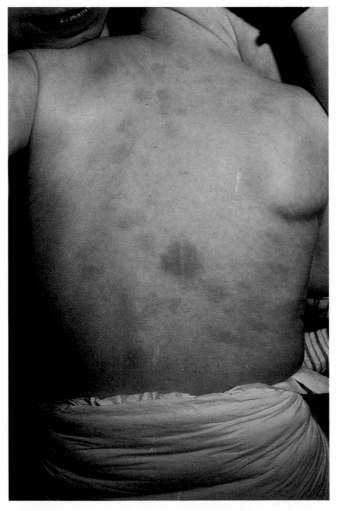

Figure 6-15
Cutaneous mastocytosis (urticaria pigmentosa). Red-brown, slightly elevated plaques averaging 0.5 to 3.5 cm in diameter typically occur in small groups on the trunk. One lesion turned red after being stroked.

Cutaneous mastocytosis (urticaria pigmentosa)

Infants and children. The onset of mastocytosis occurs between birth and 2 years of age in approximately 55% of all cases; an additional 10% develop the disease before the age of 15 years.[99] Internal organs, including the bone marrow and the GI tract, may be involved, but this is less common in children than in adults.

Clinical types

Localized cutaneous types. The typical presentation of pediatric-onset mastocytosis consists of red-brown, slightly elevated plaques averaging 0.5 to 1.5 cm in diameter. Typically they occur in small groups on the trunk and are often dismissed as variations of pigmentation. Large numbers can occur on any body surface. Erythema and blisters are seen during the first 2 years of life. A larger solitary collection of mast cells is called a *mastocytoma*.

Generalized cutaneous types. There are rare generalized forms of cutaneous disease. Telangiectasia macularis eruptiva perstans, seen in adults, consists of telangiectasias and sparse, widespread, mast cell infiltrates that resemble freckles. Diffuse generalized infiltration of the skin is called *pseudoxanthomatous mastocytosis*, or *xanthelasmoidea*. It begins in childhood and persists throughout life.

Symptoms. Symptoms are minimal with localized disease but troublesome when large numbers of lesions are present. Itching is the most common symptom. It is induced by scratching and usually remains confined to the lesion. Patients with a large number of lesions can experience widespread flushing, intense itching, headaches, bronchospasm, tachycardia, and abdominal pain. These symptoms are provoked by exercise, emotional stress, bathing in hot or cold water, rubbing lesions, or certain drugs, including aspirin and codeine.

Diagnosis. Stroking a lesion with the wooden end of a cotton-tipped applicator induces intense erythema of the entire plaque and a wheal that is usually confined to the stroked site (Darier's sign) (Figures 6-16 and 6-17). This test is highly characteristic and is as reliable as a biopsy for establishing the diagnosis. Metachromatic stains (Giemsa or toluidine blue) stain cytoplasmic mast cell granules in biopsy specimens deep blue. Injecting anesthetic directly into the biopsy site can degranulate mast cells.

The diagnosis of patients with systemic mast cell disease is accomplished by histologic examination of key tissues (bone, bone marrow, GI tract) with analysis of chemical markers of the mast cell.

Patients with proliferative systemic mast cell disease usually exhibit chronic overproduction of mast cell mediators. Mast cell secretory products that can be measured to obtain biochemical evidence of systemic mast cell activation include histamine, prostaglandin D_2, tryptase, and heparin.[100] Quantitation of urinary N-methylimidazoleacetic acid (MIAA), the major metabolite of histamine, is used as a measure of histamine release. Evaluation should include quantitation of urinary MIAA during periods of quiescence and for 4 to 6 hours after an episode. Patients should not consume histamine-rich foods (e.g., wine, yogurt, cheese, sauerkraut, spinach, tomatoes, eggplant, chicken livers, sirloin steak) for 24 hours prior to the start of or during the 24-hour urine collection. Plasma histamine levels may be elevated in pediatric-onset mastocytosis.

Prognosis. Most cases of urticaria pigmentosa occur before age 2. These cases gradually improve and usually clear spontaneously by puberty. Urticaria pigmentosa that begins after age 10 usually persists and may be associated with systemic disease. Systemic mastocytosis can occur at any age but is generally seen in adults. Systemic mast cell disease occurs in approximately 50% of adult patients with urticaria pigmentosa.[101] The GI tract and the skeletal system are most commonly involved. There is malignant transformation in 7% of patients with juvenile-onset systemic disease and in approximately 30% of patients with adult-onset systemic disease.[102]

Management. Systemic mastocytosis is managed in a stepwise manner: an H_1 antihistamine for flushing and pruritus, an H_2 blocker or proton-pump inhibitor for gastric and duodenal manifestations, oral cromolyn sodium for diarrhea and abdominal pain, and a nonsteroidal antiinflammatory agent to block mast cell biosynthesis of prostaglandin D_2 for severe flushing that is associated with vascular collapse and is unresponsive to H_1 and H_2 antihistamines.[103] Mast cell degranulation is prevented by cromolyn sodium (100 mg two to four times a day)[104,105] and ketotifen (2 mg daily).[106] Topical steroids are useful for treating limited areas. One study showed that the use of Diprolene ointment under occlusion[107] 8 hours a day for several weeks with intralesional triamcinolone acetonide (40 mg/ml) induced a prolonged remission. Marked cutaneous atrophy occurred at the injection sites.[107] Atrophy could be minimized by using lower concentrations of triamcinolone acetonide (e.g., 5 or 10 mg/ml). Photochemotherapy (PUVA) may be useful in extensive cases.[108] An average of 27 exposures was required to fade lesions and decrease pruritus. Relapse occurs weeks to months after therapy is discontinued.

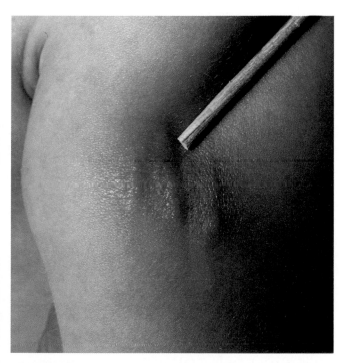

Figure 6-16
Cutaneous mastocytosis (urticaria pigmentosa): Darier's sign. Stroking a lesion with the wooden end of a cotton-tipped applicator produces a wheal that remains confined to the stroked site or enlarges.

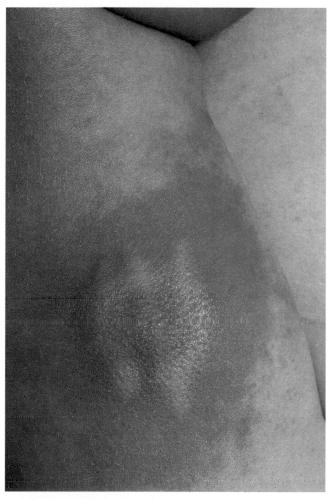

Figure 6-17
Cutaneous mastocytosis (urticaria pigmentosa): Darier's sign. Same plaque as in Figure 6-15. Minutes later the wheal has extended and intense erythema has appeared.

REFERENCES

1. Soter NA: Acute and chronic urticaria and angioedema, *J Am Acad Dermatol* 25:146-154, 1991.
2. Jacobson KW, Branch LB, Nelson HS: Laboratory tests in chronic urticaria, *JAMA* 243:1644, 1980.
3. Cooper KD: Urticaria and angioedema: diagnosis and evaluation, *J Am Acad Dermatol* 25:166-174, 1991.
4. Sorensen HT, Christensen B, Kjaerulff E: A two-year follow-up of children with urticaria in general practice, *Scand J Prim Health Care* 5:24-26, 1987.
5. Guillet MH, Guillet G: Food urticaria in children. Review of 51 cases, *Allerg Immunol* 25:333-338, 1993.
6. Hide M, Francis DM, et al: Autoantibodies against the high-affinity IgE receptor as a cause of histamine release in chronic urticaria, *N Engl J Med* 328:1599-1604, 1993.
7. Fisherman EW, Cohen GN: Recurring and chronic urticaria: identification of etiologies, *Ann Allergy* 36:401, 1976.
8. Juhlin L: Recurrent urticaria: clinical investigation of 330 patients, *Br J Dermatol* 104:369, 1981.
9. Barlow RJ, Warburton F, et al: Diagnosis and incidence of delayed pressure urticaria in patients with chronic urticaria, *J Am Acad Dermatol* 29:954-958, 1993.
10. Lanigan SW, Short P, Moult P: The association of chronic urticarial and thyroid autoimmunity, *Clin Exp Dermatol* 12:335-338, 1987.
11. Lanigan SW, Adams SJ, Robinson TWE, et al: Association of urticaria and hypothyroidism, *Lancet* 1:1476, 1984.
12. Leznoff A, Josse RG, Denburg J, et al: Association of chronic urticaria with thyroid autoimmunity, *Arch Dermatol* 119:636-640, 1983.
13. Noid HE, Schulze TW, Winkelmann RK: Diet plan for patients with salicylate-induced urticaria, *Arch Dermatol* 109:866, 1974.
14. Juhlin L: Additives and chronic urticaria, *Ann Allergy* 59:119-123, 1987.
15. Akers WA, Naversen DN: Diagnosis of chronic urticaria, *Int J Dermatol* 17:616-627, 1978.
16. Kaur S et al: Factitious urticaria (dermographism) treatment by cimetidine and chlorpheniramine in a randomized double-blind study, *Br J Dermatol* 104:185, 1981.
17. Kailasam V, Mathews KP: Controlled clinical assessment of astemizole in the treatment of chronic idiopathic urticaria and angioedema, *J Am Acad Dermatol* 16:797-804, 1987.
18. Monroe EW et al: Efficacy and safety of loratadine (10 mg once daily) in the management of idiopathic chronic urticaria, *J Am Acad Dermatol* 19:138-139, 1988.
19. Goldsobel AB et al: Efficacy of doxepin in the treatment of chronic idiopathic urticaria, *J Allergy Clin Immunol* 78:867-873, 1986.
20. Greene SL, Reed CE, Schroeter AL: Double-blind crossover study comparing doxepin with diphenhydramine for the treatment of chronic urticaria, *J Am Acad Dermatol* 12:669-675, 1985.
21. Weiner MJ: Methotrexate in corticosteroid-resistant urticaria, *Ann Intern Med* 110:848, 1989.
22. Jorizzo JL, Smith EB: The physical urticarias: an update and review, *Arch Dermatol* 118:194-201, 1982.
23. Wong RC, Fairley JA, Ellis CN: Dermographism: a review, *J Am Acad Dermatol* 11:643-652, 1984.
24. Huston DP et al: Prevention of mast-cell degranulation by ketotifen in patients with physical urticarias, *Ann Intern Med* 104:507-510, 1986.
25. Sharpe GR, Shuster S: In dermographic urticaria H_2 receptor antagonists have a small but therapeutically irrelevant additional effect compared with H_1 antagonists alone, *Br J Dermatol* 129:575-579, 1993.
26. Dover JS, Black AK, Ward AM, et al: Delayed pressure urticaria: clinical features, laboratory investigations, and response to therapy of 44 patients, *J Am Acad Dermatol* 18:1289-1298, 1988.
27. Estes SA, Yung CW: Delayed pressure urticaria: an investigation of some parameters of lesion induction, *J Am Acad Dermatol* 5:25-31, 1981.
28. Jorizzo JL: Cholinergic urticaria, *Arch Dermatol* 123:455-457, 1987.
29. Hirschmann JV et al: Cholinergic urticaria: a clinical and histologic study, *Arch Dermatol* 123:462-467, 1987.
30. Lawrence CM et al: Cholinergic urticaria with associated angioedema, *Br J Dermatol* 105:543-550, 1981.
31. Casale TB, Keahey TM, Kaliner M: Exercise-induced anaphylactic syndromes: insights into diagnostic and pathophysiologic features, *JAMA* 255:2049-2053, 1986.
32. Sheffer AL, Austen KF: Exercise-induced anaphylaxis, *J Allergy Clin Immunol* 60:106-111, 1980.
33. Sheffer AL et al: Exercise-induced anaphylaxis: a distinct form of physical allergy, *J Allergy Clin Immunol* 11:311-316, 1983.
34. Maulitz RM, Pratt DS, Schocket AL: Exercise-induced anaphylactic reaction to shellfish, *J Allergy Clin Immunol* 63:433-434, 1979.
35. Kushimoto H, Aoki T: Masked type I wheat allergy: relation to exercise-induced anaphylaxis, *Arch Dermatol* 121:355-360, 1985.
36. Nichols AW: Exercise-induced anaphylaxis and urticaria, *Clin Sports Med* 11:303-312, 1992.
37. Zip CM, Ross JB, et al: Familial cold urticaria, *Clin Exp Dermatol* 18:338-341, 1993.
38. Wanderer AA, Grandel KE, Wasserman SI, et al: Clinical characteristics of cold-induced systemic reactions in acquired cold urticaria syndromes: recommendations for prevention of this complication and a proposal for a diagnostic classification of cold urticaria, *J Allergy Clin Immunol* 78:417-423, 1986.
39. Neittaanmaki H: Cold urticaria: clinical findings in 220 patients, *J Am Acad Dermatol* 13:636-644, 1985.
40. Grandel KE et al: Association of platelet-activation factor with primary acquired cold urticaria, *N Engl J Med* 313:405-409, 1984.
41. Sigler RW et al: The role of cyproheptadine in the treatment of cold urticaria, *J Allergy Clin Immunol* 65:309-312, 1980.
42. Neittaanmaki H, Myohanen T, and Fraki JE: Comparison of cinnarizine, cyproheptadine, doxepin, and hydroxyzine in idiopathic cold urticaria: usefulness of doxepin, *J Am Acad Dermatol* 11:483-489, 1984.
43. Rauits M, Armstrong RB, Harber LC: Solar urticaria: clinical features and wavelength dependence, *Arch Dermatol* 118:228, 1982.
44. Czarnetzki BM, Traupe H: Evidence that water acts as a carrier for an epidermal antigen in aquagenic urticaria, *J Am Acad Dermatol* 15:623-627, 1986.
45. Greaves MW, Black AK, Eady RAJ, et al: Aquagenic pruritus, *Br Med J* 282:2008-2010, 1981.
45a. Lott T et al: Treatment of aquagenic pruritus with topical capsaicin cream, *J Am Acad Dermatol* 30:232-235, 1994.
46. Steinman HK, Greaves MW: Aquagenic pruritus, *J Am Acad Dermatol* 13:91-96, 1985.
47. Bayoumi A-HM, Highet AS: Baking soda baths for aquagenic pruritus, *Lancet* 23:464, 1986.
48. Megerian CA, Arnold JE, et al: Angioedema: 5 years' experience, with a review of the disorder's presentation and treatment, *Laryngoscope* 102:256-260, 1992.
49. Saxon A, Beall GN, Rohr AS, et al: Immediate hypersensitivity reactions to beta-lactam antibiotics, *Ann Intern Med* 107:204-215, 1987.
50. Thompson T, Frable MA: Drug-induced, life-threatening angioedema revisited, *Laryngoscope* 103:10-12, 1993.
51. Israili ZH, Hall WD: Cough and angioneurotic edema associated with angiotensin-converting enzyme inhibitor therapy. A review of the literature and pathophysiology, *Ann Intern Med* 117:234-242, 1992.
52. Rees RS, Bergman J, et al: Angioedema associated with lisinopril, *Am J Emerg Med* 10:321-322, 1992.
53. Bielory L, Lee SS, et al: Long-acting ACE inhibitor-induced angioedema, *Allergy Proc* 13:85-87, 1992.
54. Roberts JR, Wuerz RC: Clinical characteristics of angiotensin-converting enzyme inhibitor-induced angioedema, *Ann Emerg Med* 20:555-558, 1991.
55. Orfan N, Patterson R, et al: Severe angioedema related to ACE inhibitors in patients with a history of idiopathic angioedema, *JAMA* 264:1287-1289, 1990.

56. Sheffer AL, Austen KF, Rosen FS, et al: Acquired deficiency of the inhibitor of the first component of complement: report of five additional cases with commentary on the syndrome, *J Allergy Clin Immunol* 75:640-646, 1985.

57. Bain BJ, Catovsky D, et al: Acquired angioedema as the presenting feature of lymphoproliferative disorders of mature B-lymphocytes, *Cancer* 72:3318-3322, 1993.

58. Alsenz J, Bork K, Loos M: Autoantibody-mediated acquired deficiency of C1 inhibitor, *N Engl J Med* 316:1360-1366, 1987.

59. Putterman C, Barak V, et al: Episodic angioedema with eosinophilia: a case associated with T cell activation and cytokine production, *Ann Allergy* 70:243-248, 1993.

60. Gleich GJ et al: Episodic angioedema associated with eosinophilia, *N Engl J Med* 310:1621-1626, 1984.

61. Frank MM, Gelfand JA, Atkinson JP: Hereditary angioedema: the clinical syndrome and its management, *Ann Intern Med* 84:580-593, 1976.

62. Perricone R, Pasetto N, et al: Cystic ovaries in women affected with hereditary angioedema, *Clin Exp Immunol* 90:401-404, 1992.

63. Stoppa-Lyonnet D et al: Altered C1 inhibitor genes in type I hereditary angioedema, *N Engl J Med* 317:1-6, 1987.

64. Cicardi M et al: Hereditary angioedema: an appraisal of 104 cases, *Am J Med Sci* 284:2-9, 1982.

65. Gelfand JA, Sherins RJ, Alling DW, et al: Treatment of hereditary angioedema with danazol: reversal of clinical and biochemical abnormalities, *N Engl J Med* 295:1444-1448, 1976.

66. Cicardi M, Bergamaschini L, et al: Long-term treatment of hereditary angioedema with attenuated androgens: a survey of a 13-year experience, *J Allergy Clin Immunol* 87:768-773, 1991.

67. Zurlo JJ, Frank MM: The long-term safety of danazol in women with hereditary angioedema, *Fertil Steril* 54:64-72, 1990.

68. Greaves M, Lawlor F: Angioedema: manifestations and management, *J Am Acad Dermatol* 25:155-161, 1991.

69. Von Krogh, Maibach HI: The contact urticaria syndrome: an updated review, *J Am Acad Dermatol* 5:328, 1981.

70. Fisher AA: Contact urtiearia due to medicants, chemicals and foods, *Cutis* 30:168, 1982.

71. Schechter JF, Wilkinson RD, Del Carpio J: Anaphylaxis following the use of Bacitracin ointment, *Arch Dermatol* 120:909-911, 1984.

72. Freeman S, Rosen RH: Urticarial contact dermatitis in food handlers, *Med J Aust* 155:91-94, 1991.

73. Holmes RC, Black MM: The specific dermatoses of pregnancy, *J Am Acad Dermatol* 8:405-412, 1983.

74. Lawley TJ et al: Pruritic urticarial papules and plaques of pregnancy, *JAMA* 241:1696-1699, 1979.

75. Winton GB, Lewis CW: Dermatosis of pregnancy, *J Am Acad Dermatol* 6:977-998, 1982.

76. Yancey KB, Hall RP, Lawley TJ: Pruritic urticarial papules and plaques of pregnancy: clinical experience in twenty-five patients, *J Am Acad Dermatol* 10:473-480, 1984.

77. Callen JP, Hanno R: Pruritic urticarial papules and plaques of pregnancy (PUPPP): a clinical experience in twenty-five patients, *J Am Acad Dermatol* 5:401-405, 1981.

78. Holmes RC, Black MM: The specific dermatoses of pregnancy: a reappraisal with special emphasis on a proposed simplified clinical classification, *Clin Exp Dermatol* 7:65-73, 1982.

79. Weiss R, Hull P: Familial occurrence of pruritic urticarial papules and plaques of pregnancy, *J Am Acad Dermatol* 26:715-717, 1992.

80. Cohen LM, Capeless EL, et al: Pruritic urticarial papules and plaques of pregnancy and its relationship to maternal-fetal weight gain and twin pregnancy, *Arch Dermatol* 125:1534-1536, 1989.

81. Soter NA: Chronic urticaria as a manifestation of necrotizing venulitis, *N Engl J Med* 296:1440, 1977.

82. Monroe EF: Urticarial vasculitis: an updated review, *J Am Acad Dermatol* 5:88-95, 1981.

83. Sanchez NP, Winkelmann RK, Schroeter AL, et al: The clinical and histopathologic spectrums of urticarial vasculitis: study of forty cases, *J Am Acad Dermatol* 7:599-605, 1982.

84. Wanderer AA, Nuss DD, Tormey AD, et al: Urticarial leukocytoclastic vasculitis with cold urticaria: report of a case and review of the literature, *Arch Dermatol* 119:145-151, 1983.

85. Mehregan DR, Hall MJ, et al: Urticarial vasculitis: a histopathologic and clinical review of 72 cases, *J Am Acad Dermatol* 26:441-448, 1992.

86. Wisnieski JJ, Jones SM: IgG autoantibody to the collagen-like region of Clq in hypocomplementemic urticarial vasculitis syndrome, systemic lupus erythematosus, and 6 other musculoskeletal or rheumatic diseases, *J Rheumatol* 19:884-888, 1992.

87. Millns JL, Randle HW, Solley GO, et al: The therapeutic response of urticarial vasculitis to indomethacin, *J Am Acad Dermatol* 3:349-355, 1980.

88. Wiles JC, Hansen RC, Lynch PJ: Urticarial vasculitis treated with colchicine, *Arch Dermatol* 121:802-805, 1985.

89. Muramatsu C, Tanabe E: Urticarial vasculitis: response to dapsone and colchicine, *J Am Acad Dermatol* 13:1055, 1985.

90. Fortson JS, Zone JJ, Hammond E, et al: Hypocomplementemic urticarial vasculitis syndrome responsive to dapsone, *J Am Acad Dermatol* 15:1137-1142, 1986.

91. Stack PS: Methotrexate for urticarial vasculitis, *Ann Allergy* 72:36-38, 1994.

92. Hebert AA, Sigman ES, et al: Serum sickness-like reactions from cefaclor in children, *J Am Acad Dermatol* 25:805-808, 1991.

93. Heckbert SR, Stryker WS, et al: Serum sickness in children after antibiotic exposure: estimates of occurrence and morbidity in a health maintenance organization population, *Am J Epidemiol* 132:336-342, 1990.

94. Lawley TJ et al: A prospective clinical and immunologic analysis of patients with serum sickness, *N Engl J Med* 311:1407-1413, 1984.

95. Berman BA, Ross RN: Acute serum sickness, *Cutis* 32:420-422, 1983.

96. Stein DH: Mastocytosis: a review, *Pediatr Dermatol* 3:365-375, 1986.

97. DiBacco RS, DeLeo VA: Mastocytosis and the mast cell, *J Am Acad Dermatol* 7:709-722, 1982.

98. Fowler JF, Parsley WM, Gotter PG: Familial urticaria pigmentosa, *Arch Dermatol* 122:80-81, 1986.

99. Kettelhut BV, Metcalfe DD: Pediatric mastocytosis, *J Invest Dermatol* 96:15S-18S, 1991.

100. Roberts LW, Oates JA: Biochemical diagnosis of systemic mast cell disorders, *J Invest Dermatol* 96:24S-25S, 1991.

101. Czarnetzki BM et al: Bone marrow findings in adult patients with urticaria pigmentosa, *J Am Acad Dermatol* 18:45-51, 1988.

102. Webb TA, Li C-Y, Yam LT: Systemic mast cell disease: a clinical and hematopathologic study of 26 cases, *Cancer* 49:927-938, 1982.

103. Austen KF: Systemic mastocytosis, *N Eng J Med* 639-640, 1992.

104. Soter NA, Austen KF, Wasserman SI: Oral disodium cromoglycate in the treatment of systemic mastocytosis, *N Eng J Med* 301:465-469, 1979.

105. Welch EA, Alper JC, Bogaars H, et al: Treatment of bullous mastocytosis with disodium cromoglycate, *J Am Acad Dermatol* 9:349-353, 1983.

106. Czarnetzki BM: A double-blind crossover study of the effect of ketotifen in urticaria pigmentosa, *Dermatologica* 166:44-47, 1983.

107. Barton J et al: Treatment of urticaria pigmentosa with corticosteroids, *Arch Dermatol* 121:1516-1523, 1985.

108. Vella Briffa D et al: Photochemotherapy (PUVA) in the treatment of urticaria pigmentosa, *Br J Dermatol* 109:67-75, 1983.

CHAPTER SEVEN

Acne, Rosacea, and Related Disorders

Acne

Acne, a disease of the pilosebaceous unit, appears in males and females near puberty and in most cases becomes less active as adolescence ends. The intensity and duration of activity varies for each individual.

The disease may be minor, with only a few comedones or papules, or it may occur as the highly inflammatory and diffusely scarring acne conglobata. The severest forms of acne occur more frequently in males, but the disease tends to be more persistent in females, who may have periodic flares prior to menstrual periods, which continue until menopause.

Psychosocial effects of acne. Acne is too often dismissed as a minor affliction not worthy of treatment. Believing it is a phase of the growing process and that lesions will soon disappear, parents of children with acne postpone seeking medical advice. Permanent scarring of the skin and the psyche can result from such inaction. The disease has implications far beyond the few marks that may appear on the face. Lesions cannot be hidden under clothing; each is prominently displayed and detracts significantly from one's personal appearance and self-esteem. Taunting and ridicule from peers is demoralizing. Appearing in public creates embarrassment and frustration. Because acne is perceived by adolescents to have important negative personal and social consequences, improvement in these areas accompanies medical treatment. Facial appearance then becomes more acceptable to peers, embarrassment diminishes, and patients feel less socially inhibited.[1]

The physician-patient relationship. Many acne sufferers expect to be disappointed with the results of treatment.[2] They may be sensitive to actual or supposed lack of acceptance on the part of their physicians. Adolescence is usually characterized by the challenge of parental rules, and this transfers to the relationship with the physician. Noncompliance can be decreased by carefully explaining the goals and techniques of treatment and leaving the choice of implementation to the adolescent. Parents who offer to make sure the adolescent follows the treatment plan may encourage noncompliance by placing the treatment within the context of existing parent-child struggles.[3] Greater consideration of adolescents' psychologic situations improves the therapeutic outcome, increases compliance, and leads to a greater confidence in the physician.

Postadolescent acne in women. A low-grade, persistent acne is common in professional women. Closed comedones are the dominant lesions, with a few papulopustules. Premenstrual flares are typical. Many of these patients passed through adolescence without acne. One author postulated that chronic stress leads to enhanced secretion of adrenal androgens, resulting in sebaceous hyperplasia and subsequent induction of comedones.[4]

CLASSIFICATION

The Consensus Conference on Acne Classification (1990) proposed that acne grading be accomplished by the use of a pattern-diagnosis system, which includes a total evaluation of lesions and their complications such as drainage, hemorrhage, and pain. It takes into account the total impact of the disease, which is influenced by the disfigurement it causes. Degree of severity is also determined by occupational disability, psychosocial impact, and the failure of response to previous treatment.

Acne lesions. Acne lesions are divided into inflammatory and noninflammatory lesions. Noninflammatory lesions consist of open and closed comedones. Inflammatory acne lesions are characterized by the presence of one or more of the following types of lesions: papules, pustules, and nodules (cysts). Papules are less than 5 mm in diameter. Pustules have a visible central core of purulent material. Nodules are greater than 5 mm in diameter. Nodules may become suppurative or hemorrhagic. Suppurative nodular lesions have been referred to as cysts because of their resemblance to inflamed epidermal cysts. Recurring rupture and reepithelialization of cysts leads to epithelial-lined sinus tracks, often accompanied by disfiguring scars.

Classification. For inflammatory acne lesions, the Consensus Panel proposes that lesions be classified as papulopustular and/or nodular. A severity grade based on a lesion count approximation is assigned as mild, moderate, or severe. Illustrative examples of each category of severity are shown in Figure 7-2. Other factors in assessing severity include ongoing scarring, persistent purulent and/or serosanguineous drainage from lesions, and the presence of sinus tracks.

OVERVIEW OF DIAGNOSIS AND TREATMENT

An overview of diagnosis and treatment is presented in Figures 7-1 to 7-4.

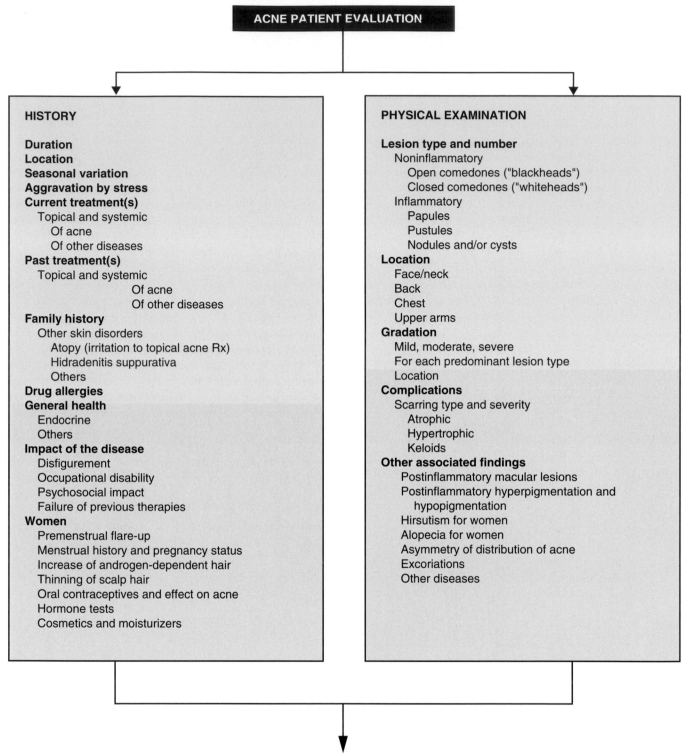

ACNE PATIENT EVALUATION

HISTORY

Duration
Location
Seasonal variation
Aggravation by stress
Current treatment(s)
  Topical and systemic
    Of acne
    Of other diseases
Past treatment(s)
  Topical and systemic
                Of acne
                Of other diseases
Family history
  Other skin disorders
    Atopy (irritation to topical acne Rx)
    Hidradenitis suppurativa
    Others
Drug allergies
General health
  Endocrine
  Others
Impact of the disease
  Disfigurement
  Occupational disability
  Psychosocial impact
  Failure of previous therapies
Women
  Premenstrual flare-up
  Menstrual history and pregnancy status
  Increase of androgen-dependent hair
  Thinning of scalp hair
  Oral contraceptives and effect on acne
  Hormone tests
  Cosmetics and moisturizers

PHYSICAL EXAMINATION

Lesion type and number
  Noninflammatory
    Open comedones ("blackheads")
    Closed comedones ("whiteheads")
  Inflammatory
    Papules
    Pustules
    Nodules and/or cysts
Location
  Face/neck
  Back
  Chest
  Upper arms
Gradation
  Mild, moderate, severe
  For each predominant lesion type
  Location
Complications
  Scarring type and severity
    Atrophic
    Hypertrophic
    Keloids
Other associated findings
  Postinflammatory macular lesions
  Postinflammatory hyperpigmentation and
    hypopigmentation
  Hirsutism for women
  Alopecia for women
  Asymmetry of distribution of acne
  Excoriations
  Other diseases

**IDENTIFY TYPES OF LESIONS AND SEVERITY;
FORMULATE TREATMENT PLAN**
Patients who appear similar differ in response to treatment.

Figure 7-1

TYPES OF LESIONS

Noninflammatory lesions

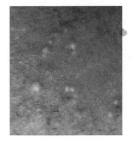 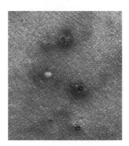

Closed comedones   Open comedones

Inflammatory lesions

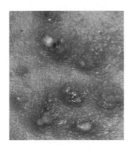 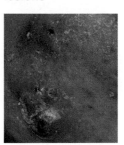

Papules/pustules   Nodules

ACNE CLASSIFICATION AND GRADING

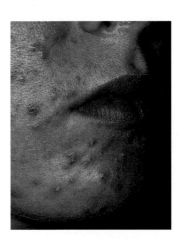 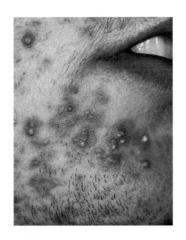 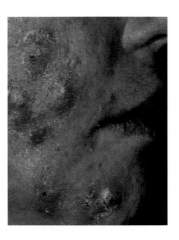

Mild
Papules/pustules +/++
Nodules 0

Moderate
Papules/pustules ++/+++
Nodules +/++

Severe
Papules/pustules +++/++++
Nodules +++

SEVERITY GRADING OF INFLAMMATORY LESIONS

Severity	Papules/pustules	Nodules	Additional factors that determine severity
Mild	Few to several	None	Psychosocial circumstances
Moderate	Several to many	Few to several	Occupational difficulties
Severe	Numerous and/or extensive	Many	Inadequate therapeutic responsiveness

Figure 7-2
Acne classification of lesions.

Figure 7-3

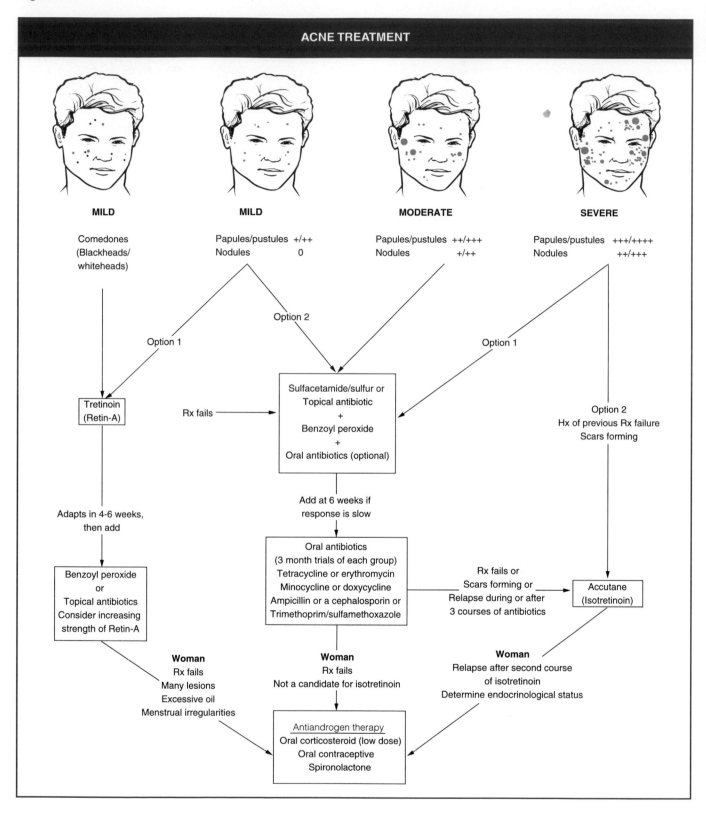

ACNE TREATMENT

MILD

MILD

MODERATE

SEVERE

Comedones
(Blackheads/
whiteheads)

Papules/pustules +/++
Nodules   0

Papules/pustules ++/+++
Nodules   +/++

Papules/pustules +++/++++
Nodules   ++/+++

Option 1

Option 2

Option 1

Tretinoin
(Retin-A)

Rx fails

Sulfacetamide/sulfur or
Topical antibiotic
+
Benzoyl peroxide
+
Oral antibiotics (optional)

Option 2
Hx of previous Rx failure
Scars forming

Adapts in 4-6 weeks,
then add

Add at 6 weeks if
response is slow

Benzoyl peroxide
or
Topical antibiotics
Consider increasing
strength of Retin-A

Oral antibiotics
(3 month trials of each group)
Tetracycline or erythromycin
Minocycline or doxycycline
Ampicillin or a cephalosporin or
Trimethoprim/sulfamethoxazole

Rx fails or
Scars forming or
Relapse during or after
3 courses of antibiotics

Accutane
(Isotretinoin)

Woman
Rx fails
Many lesions
Excessive oil
Menstrual irregularities

Woman
Rx fails
Not a candidate for isotretinoin

Woman
Relapse after second course
of isotretinoin
Determine endocrinological status

Antiandrogen therapy
Oral corticosteroid (low dose)
Oral contraceptive
Spironolactone

Figure 7-4

Acne Treatment (Overview)

Treatment	Mild Comedones (blackheads and whiteheads)	Mild Papules and pustules +/++ Nodules 0	Moderate Papules and pustules ++/+++ Nodules +/++	Severe Papules and pustules +++/++++ Nodules ++/+++	Very severe Acne conglobata, pyoderma faciale, acne fulminans
TRETINOIN (RETIN-A)					
Solution; gel 0.025%, 0.01%, cream 0.1%, 0.05%, 0.025%	Most effective agents; start with highest tolerable concentration	Effective as initial medication in many cases	Used after inflammation and number of lesions have been reduced	Possible use as maintenance medication after disease is controlled	Possible use as maintenance medication after disease is controlled
BENZOYL PEROXIDE (2.5%, 5%, AND 10%)					
Lotion—water- or alcohol-based; soaps—bar or liquid; masks	Start use after adapted to tretinoin—4-6 weeks or use alone as initial medication	Effective as initial medication and in combination with tretinoin or drying agent	Effective as initial medication and with tretinoin or drying agents	Aggressive use may control disease	Aggressive initial therapy if isotretinoin is not started
DRYING AGENTS					
Sulfacetamide/sulfur lotions; Sulfacet-R lotion or Novacet	Effective when combined with benzoyl peroxide or tretinoin	Effective, especially when used with benzoyl peroxide	Effective, especially when used with benzoyl peroxide	Aggressive use may control disease	Aggressive initial therapy combined with benzoyl peroxide if isotretinoin is not started
TOPICAL ANTIBIOTICS					
Lotions Erythromycin Clindamycin Tetracycline Pads Erythromycin Cleocin	Use if comedones become inflamed	Initial medication or used with benzoyl peroxide	Maintenance after control with oral antibiotics	Maintenance after disease is controlled	Maintenance after disease is controlled
ORAL ANTIBIOTICS					
Tetracycline Erythromycin Minocycline Ampicillin Trimethoprim with sulfamethoxazole Cephalosporins	In patients with excess sebum production who do not respond to above medications	Initial medication appropriate for many cases	Initial medication for most cases	Initial medication but not reliably effective	Use only when isotretinoin is not started as initial medication
INTRALESIONAL STEROIDS					
Triamcinolone acetonide 2.5-10 mg/ml	Used if comedones become inflamed	Produces rapid control; used for larger lesions	Produces rapid control; used for large lesions	Integral part of therapy	Integral part of therapy
ISOTRETINOIN (ACCUTANE)					
10, 20, and 40 mg	Consider for numerous lesions that fail above therapy especially if pitted scars form	Consider in patients who fail all forms of conventional therapy and who scar	Consider in patients who fail therapy especially if scarring is present	Initial medication or used after patients fail short vigorous course of drying agents and antibiotics	Intitial therapy especially if scarring is present
HORMONES					
Oral contraceptives with or without dexamethasone (0.25, 0.5 mg) or prednisone (5.0, 7.5 mg)	In women with excess sebum production who need contraception	For conventional therapy failures and women who need contraception	Conventional therapy failures and women who need contraception	For antibiotic therapy failures or relapse after taking isotretinoin	Oral contraceptives desirable for women who take isotretinoin
ACNE SURGERY					
#11 surgical blade Comedone extractor Schamberg	Expression of comedone hastens resolution	Gently unroof pustules and drain with Schamberg	Gently unroof pustules and drain with Schamberg	Incise thin-roofed cysts with #11 blade	Incise thin-roofed cysts with #11 blade

Figure 7-5
Pathogenesis of acne. (*Photographs courtesy Ortho Pharmaceutical Corporation.*)

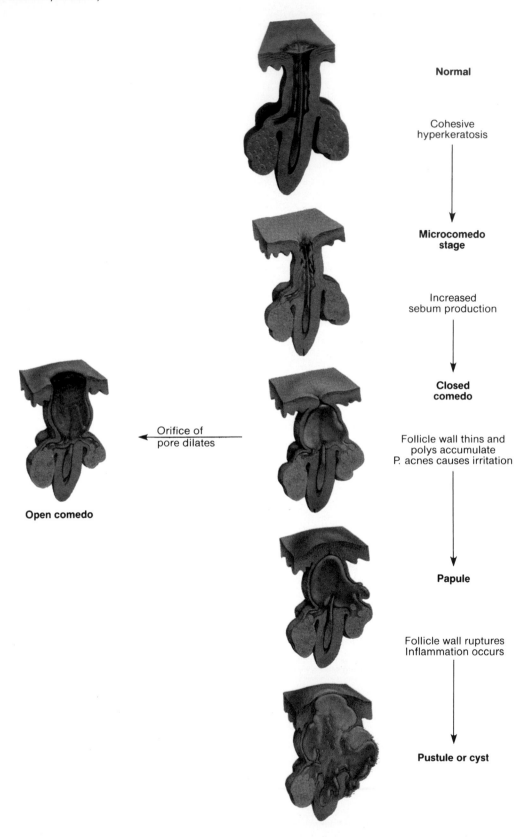

Normal

Cohesive
hyperkeratosis

**Microcomedo
stage**

Increased
sebum production

**Closed
comedo**

Orifice of
pore dilates

Open comedo

Follicle wall thins and
polys accumulate
P. acnes causes irritation

Papule

Follicle wall ruptures
Inflammation occurs

Pustule or cyst

Figure 7-6
Mode of action of therapeutic agents.

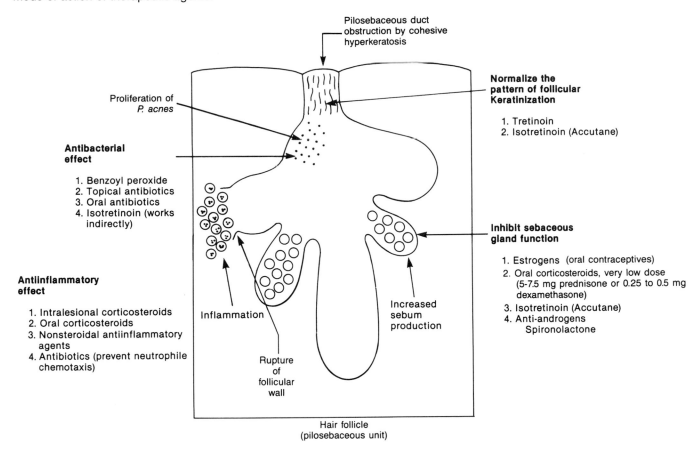

ETIOLOGY AND PATHOGENESIS

Much has been learned about the pathophysiology of acne. Figure 7-5 illustrates the evolution of the different acne lesions and Figure 7-6 illustrates the mechanism of action of therapeutic agents. Acne is a disease involving the pilosebaceous unit and is most frequent and intense in areas where sebaceous glands are largest and most numerous. Acne begins in predisposed individuals when sebum production increases. *Propionibacterium acnes* proliferates in sebum, and the follicular epithelial lining becomes altered and forms plugs called *comedones*. One study suggests that anxiety and anger are significant factors for severe acne patients.[5]

Sebaceous glands. Sebum is the pathogenic factor in acne; it is irritating and comedogenic, especially when the bacteria *P. acnes* proliferates and modifies its components. Most patients with acne have a higher-than-normal sebum level.

Sebaceous glands are located throughout the entire body except the palms, soles, dorsa of the feet, and lower lip. They are largest and most numerous on the face, chest, back, and upper outer arms. Clusters of glands appear as relatively large, visible, white globules on the buccal mucosa (Fordyce's spots), the vermilion border of the upper lip (Figure 7-7), the female areolae (Montgomery's tubercles), the labia minora, the prepuce, and around the anus.

Sebaceous glands are large in newborn infants, but regress shortly after birth. They remain relatively small in infancy and most of childhood, but enlarge and become more active in prepuberty. Hormones influence sebaceous gland secretion. Testosterone is converted to dihydrotestosterone in the skin and acts directly on the sebaceous gland to increase its size and metabolic rate. Estrogens, through a less well-defined mechanism, decrease sebaceous gland secretion. Sebaceous gland cells produce a complex mixture of oily material. Sebaceous cells mature, die, fragment, and then extrude into the sebaceous duct, where they combine with the desquamating cells of the lower hair follicle and finally arrive at the skin surface as sebum.

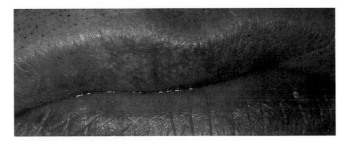

Figure 7-7
Clusters of sebaceous glands (tiny, white-yellow spots) are normally present on the vermilion border of the upper lip.

Pilosebaceous duct obstruction. The early acne lesion results from blockage in the follicular canal. Increased amounts of keratin result from hormonal changes and sebum modified by the resident bacterial flora *P. acnes*. The increased number of cornified cells remain adherent to the follicular canal (retention keratosis) directly above the opening of the sebaceous gland duct to form a plug (microcomedo). Factors causing increased sebaceous secretion (puberty, hormonal imbalances) influence the eventual size of the follicular plug. The plug enlarges behind a very small follicular orifice at the skin surface and becomes visible as a closed comedone (firm, white papule). An open comedone (blackhead) occurs if the follicular orifice dilates. Further increase in the size of a blackhead continues to dilate the pore, but usually does not result in inflammation. The small-pore, closed comedone is the precursor of inflammatory acne papules, pustules, and cysts.

Bacterial colonization and inflammation. *P. acnes*, an anaerobic diphtheroid, is a normal skin resident and the principal component of the microbic flora of the pilosebaceous follicle. The bacteria are thought to play a significant role in acne. *P. acnes* generates components that create inflammation, such as lipases, proteases, hyaluronidase, and chemotactic factors. Lipases hydrolyze sebum triglycerides to form free fatty acids, which are comedogenic and primary irritants. Chemotactic factors attract neutrophils to the follicular wall. Neutrophils elaborate hydrolases that weaken the wall. The wall thins, becomes inflamed (red papule), and ruptures, releasing part of the comedone into the dermis. An intense, foreign-body, inflammatory reaction results in the formation of the acne pustule or cyst. Other bacteria substances possibly mediate inflammation by stimulation of immune mechanisms.

P. acnes is sensitive to several antibiotics, such as tetracycline. Tetracycline also depresses neutrophil chemotaxis.

THERAPEUTIC AGENTS FOR TREATMENT OF ACNE

Topical and oral agents act at various stages (see Figure 7-6) in the evolution of an acne lesion and may be used alone or in combination to enhance efficacy. Most cases are controlled with combinations of vitamin A acid, benzoyl peroxide, drying and peeling agents, and antibiotics. Topical agents should be applied to the entire affected area to treat existing lesions and to prevent the development of new ones. Potent topical steroid creams produce no short-term improvement in patients with moderate acne.[6]

Tretinoin

Tretinoin (Retin-A), also known as *retinoic acid* or *Vitamin A acid* (VAA), is the agent of choice for noninflammatory acne consisting of open and closed comedones. It is available in various preparations: Retin-A solution (0.05%) is the strongest and most irritating. Retin-A gel (0.025% and 0.01%) is drying and is for oily skin. Retin-A cream (0.1%, 0.05%, and 0.025%) is lubricating and is for dry skin.

Mechanism of action. Vitamin A acid, an oxidation product of vitamin A, initiates increased cell turnover in both normal follicles and comedones and reduces the cohesion between keratinized cells. It acts specifically on microcomedones (the precursor lesion of all forms of acne), causing fragmentation and expulsion of the microplug, expulsion of comedones, and conversion of closed comedones to open comedones.[7] New comedone formation is prevented by continued use. Inflammation may occur during this process, temporarily making acne worse. Continual topical application leads to thinning of the stratum corneum, making the skin more susceptible to sunburn; sun damage; and irritation from wind, cold, or dryness. Irritants such as astringents, alcohol, and acne soaps will not be tolerated as they were previously. The incidence of contact allergy is very low. Because of the direct action of tretinoin on the microcomedone, many clinicians believe tretinoin is appropriate for all forms of acne.

Combination therapy—synergism. Vitamin A acid enhances the penetration of other topical agents such as topical antibiotics and benzoyl peroxide. The enhanced penetration results in a synergistic effect with greater overall drug efficacy and a faster response to treatment.

Figure 7-8
Response to treatment with vitamin A acid (Retin-A).

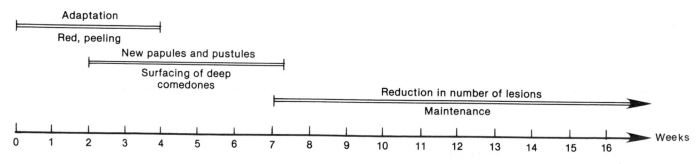

Application techniques. The skin should be washed gently with a mild soap (e.g., Purpose, Basis) no more than two to three times each day, using the hands rather than a washcloth. Special acne or abrasive soaps should be avoided. To minimize possible irritation, the skin should be allowed to dry completely by waiting 20 to 30 minutes before applying tretinoin. Tretinoin is applied in a thin layer once daily. Medication is applied to the entire area, not just to individual lesions. An amount the size of a pea is enough for a full facial application. Patients with sensitive skin or those living in cold, dry climates may start with an application every other or every third day. The frequency of application can be gradually increased to as often as twice each day if tolerated. The corners of the nose, the mouth, and the eyes should be avoided; these areas are the most sensitive and the most easily irritated. Tretinoin is applied to the chin less frequently during the initial stages of therapy; the chin is sensitive and is usually the first area to become red and scaly. Sunscreens should be worn during the summer months if exposure is anticipated.

Response to treatment (Figure 7-8)

One to four weeks. During the first few weeks, patients may experience redness, burning, or peeling. Those with excessive irritation should use less frequent applications (i.e., every other or every third day.) Most patients adapt to treatment within 4 weeks and return to daily applications. Those tolerating daily applications may be advanced to a higher dosage or to the more potent solution.

Three to six weeks. New papules and pustules may appear because comedones become irritated during the process of being dislodged. Patients unaware of this phenomenon may discontinue treatment. Some patients never get worse and sometimes begin to improve dramatically by the fifth or sixth week.

After six weeks. Most patients improve by the ninth to twelfth week and exhibit continuous improvement thereafter. Some patients never adapt to tretinoin and experience continuous irritation or continue to worsen. An alternate treatment should be selected if adaptation has not occurred by 6 to 8 weeks. Some patients adapt but never improve. Tretinoin may be continued for months to prevent appearance of new lesions.

Benzoyl peroxide

The primary effect of benzoyl peroxide is antibacterial, therefore it is most effective for inflammatory acne consisting of papules, pustules, and cysts, although many patients with comedone acne respond to it. Benzoyl peroxide is less effective than vitamin A acid at disrupting the microcomedo. Benzoyl peroxide and isotretinoin significantly reduce noninflamed lesions in 4 weeks. In one study, benzoyl peroxide had a more rapid effect on inflamed lesions with significant reductions at 4 weeks, whereas the use of isotretinoin showed a significant improvement at 12 weeks.[8]

Benzoyl peroxide is available over the counter and by prescription. Some examples of benzoyl peroxide preparations are water-based gel (Benzac AC 2.5%, 5%, and 10%), alcohol-based gel (Benzagel 5% and 10%), and acetone-based gel (Persa-gel 5% and 10%) (see the Formulary). Water-based gels are less irritating, but alcohol-based gels, if tolerated, might be more effective. Benzoyl peroxide is also available in a soap base in strengths from 2.5% to 10%.

Benzoyl peroxide produces a drying effect that varies from mild desquamation to scaliness, peeling, and cracking. Patients should be reassured that drying does not cause wrinkles. It causes a significant reduction in the concentration of free fatty acids via its antibacterial effect on *P. acnes*. This activity is presumably caused by the release of free radical oxygen, which is capable of oxidizing bacterial proteins. Benzoyl peroxide seems to reduce the size of the sebaceous gland, but whether sebum secretion is suppressed is still unknown. Patients should be warned that benzoyl peroxide is a bleaching agent that can ruin clothing.

Principles of treatment. Benzoyl peroxide should be applied in a thin layer to the entire affected area. Most patients experience mild erythema and scaling during the first few days of treatment, even with the lowest concentrations, but adapt in a week or two. It was previously held that vigorous peeling was necessary for maximum therapeutic effect; although many patients improved with this technique, others became worse. Recent studies show that an adequate therapeutic result can be obtained by starting with daily applications of the 2.5% or 5% gel and gradually increasing or decreasing the frequency of applications and strength until mild dryness and peeling occur.[9]

Allergic reaction. Approximately 2% of patients develop allergic contact dermatitis to benzoyl peroxide and must discontinue its use. The sudden appearance of diffuse erythema and vesiculation suggests contact allergy to benzoyl peroxide.

Drying and peeling agents

The oldest technique for treating acne is to use agents that induce a continuous mild drying and peeling of the skin. In selected patients, especially those with pustular acne, this technique may provide fast and effective results. Prescription and over-the-counter products used for this purpose contain sulfur, salicylic acid, resorcinol, and benzoyl peroxide. Before the use of tretinoin and antibiotics, this approach secured very acceptable results for many patients.

The goal is to establish a mild continuous peel by varying the frequency of application and strength of the agent. Treatment is stopped temporarily if dryness becomes severe. The drying and peeling technique can be recommended to patients who are reluctant to visit the physician or to parents inquiring about children who are beginning to develop acne. If improvement is negligible after an 8-week trial, the patient should consider evaluation by a physician. Two very effective agents are benzoyl peroxide 10% and sulfur 2% (Sulfoxyl-Strong) and sulfacetamide 10%, sulfur 5% lotion (Sulfacet-R, Novacet). One is used in the morning and the other in the evening or as often as tolerated.

Topical antibiotics

Topical antibiotics are useful for mild pustular and comedone acne. They can be prescribed initially or as adjunctive therapy after the patient has adapted to tretinoin or benzoyl peroxide. Clinical trials have demonstrated that application twice a day is as effective as oral tetracycline[10,11] 250 mg taken twice daily or minocycline 50 mg taken twice daily.[12] Most lotions are alcohol based and may produce some degree of irritation. Cleocin T lotion and Eryderm do not contain propylene glycol and for some patients may be less irritating. Commercially available topical antibiotics include erythromycin (A/T/S, Eryderm, Erygel, Erycette pads, Staticin, and T-Stat lotions), clindamycin (Cleocin-T pads, solution, and lotion), and Benzamycin (3% erythromycin, 5% benzoyl peroxide) (see the Formulary).

Oral antibiotics

Antibiotics have been used for approximately three decades for the treatment of papular, pustular, and cystic acne (Table 7-1).

Mechanism of action and dosage. The major effect of antibiotics is believed to ensue from their ability to decrease follicular populations of *P. acnes*. The role of *P. acnes* in the pathogenesis of acne is not completely understood. Neutrophil chemotactic factors are secreted during bacterial growth, and these may play an important role in initiating the inflammatory process. Because several antibiotics used to treat acne can inhibit neutrophil chemotaxis in vitro, they are thought to act as an antiinflammatory agent. Subminimal inhibitory concentrations of minocycline were shown to have an antiinflammatory effect by inhibiting the production of neutrophil chemotactic factors in comedonal bacteria.[13] Antibiotic-resistant strains of *P. acnes* have recently been discovered.

Antibiotic resistant propionibacteria. Antibiotic-resistant propionibacteria are being isolated with increasing frequency in patients treated with oral or topical antibiotics.[14] Emergence of resistant strains is associated with therapeutic failure. Tetracycline-resistant propionibacteria from acne patients were found to be cross-resistant to doxycycline but sensitive to minocycline. The recommended minocycline dosage to obtain adequate blood levels in male patients was 100 mg twice daily.[15]

TABLE 7-1 Antibiotics Used to Treat Acne

Antibiotic	Dosage available	Starting dosage	Adverse effects	Comments
Tetracycline	250, 500 mg	500 mg bid	GI intolerance Photosensitivity *Candida* vaginitis Reduce oral contraceptive efficacy Pseudotumor cerebri	Most widely prescribed antibiotic for acne Take on empty stomach
Erythromycin	250, 333, 400, 500 mg	500 mg bid	GI intolerance *Candida* vaginitis	Many forms absorbed with food Safe during pregnancy
Minocycline	50, 100 mg	50 or 100 mg bid	Vertigo	Expensive More effective than tetracycline Adequate absorption with food
Doxycycline	50, 100 mg	50 or 100 mg bid	Photosensitivity	As effective as minocycline Less expensive than minocycline
Clindamycin	75, 150, 300 mg	75 or 150 mg bid	Pseudomembranous colitis	Highly effective
Ampicillin	250, 500 mg	500 mg bid	Maculopapular rash	Alternative to tetracycline Gram-negative acne Safe during pregnancy
Cephalosporins (e.g. Cephalexin)	500 mg	500 mg bid	Urticaria Pseudomembranous colitis	Consider for resistant pustular acne
Trimethoprim/ sulfamethoxazole	Double strength (DS) tablets	One DS tablet bid	Rash, hives Photosensitivity	Consider for resistant pustular acne Gram-negative acne

Long-term treatment. Patients may express concern about long-term use of oral antibiotics but experience has shown that this is a safe practice.[16,17] Routine laboratory monitoring of patients who receive long-term oral antibiotics for acne rarely detects an adverse drug reaction and does not justify the cost of such testing. Laboratory monitoring should be limited to patients who may be at higher risk for an adverse drug reaction.[18]

Strategy of therapy with long-term antibiotics. A large study analyzed patients treated initially with erythromycin 1 gm/day and topical 5% benzoyl peroxide.[19] The median improvement at 6 months was 78%; 82% showed more than a 50% improvement, and 88% treated for a subsequent 6 months with benzoyl peroxide alone continued to do well. No significant benefit was gained by maintaining successfully treated patients on a further 6 months of systemic antibiotics. Some patients who did less well were given oral contraceptives or isotretinoin. Another group referred to as slow responders continued to take erythromycin or changed to another antibiotic; all continued benzoyl peroxide. Those prescribed minocycline for the second 6 months appeared to have greater benefit (64%) than those receiving erythromycin (57%). This level of improvement was still lower than that seen in those who responded well within 6 months (78%). Of the risk factors analyzed, the poorest response occurred in males with truncal acne. Age at presentation, duration, and severity did not adversely affect therapeutic outcome. Side effects were minimal.

Dosage and duration. Better clinical results and a lower rate of relapse after stopping antibiotics are achieved by starting at higher dosages and tapering only after control is achieved.[20] Typical starting dosages are tetracycline 1 gm/day, erythromycin 1 gm/day, minocycline 200 mg/day, and ampicillin 1 gm/day. Antibiotics are prescribed in divided doses; there is better compliance with twice-a-day dosing. Antibiotics must be taken for weeks to be effective and are used for many weeks or months to achieve maximum benefit. Attempts to control acne with short courses of antibiotics, as is often tried to prevent premenstrual flare-ups of acne, are usually not effective.[21]

Tetracycline. Tetracycline is the most widely prescribed oral antibiotic for acne.[22] One major disadvantage is the requirement that tetracycline not be taken with food (particularly dairy products), certain antacids, and iron, all of which interfere with the intestinal absorption of the drug. Failure to adhere to these restrictions accounts for many of the reported therapeutic failures of tetracycline.

DOSING. Efficacy and compliance are obtained by starting tetracycline administration at 500 mg twice each day and continuing this dosage until a significant decrease in the number of inflamed lesions occurs,[23] usually in 3 to 6 weeks. Thereafter the dosage may be decreased to 250 mg twice each day or oral therapy may be discontinued in favor of topical antibiotics. Patients with severe pustular and cystic acne or those who do not respond to 1 gm/day might respond to a higher dosage of tetracycline (1.5 to 3.0

gm/day).[24] These higher dosages may not be tolerated by some patients. Patients who do not respond after 6 weeks of adequate dosages of oral tetracycline should be introduced to an alternative treatment. For unknown reasons a significant number of patients who take tetracycline exactly as directed do not respond to high dosages, whereas others respond very favorably to 250 mg once a day or once every other day and flare when attempts are made to discontinue treatment.

ADVERSE EFFECTS. The incidence of photosensitivity to tetracycline is low, but it increases when higher dosages are used. All females should be warned about the increased incidence of *Candida albicans* vaginitis that occurs while taking antibiotics. The package labeling of oral contraceptives warns that reduced efficacy and increased incidence of breakthrough bleeding may occur with tetracycline and other antibiotics. Although this association has not been proven, it is prudent to inform patients of this potential risk. Pseudotumor cerebri, a self-limited disorder in which the regulation of intracranial pressure is impaired, is a rare complication of tetracycline treatment.[25] Increased intracranial pressure causes papilledema and severe headaches. Increased intraocular pressure can lead to progressive visual impairment and eventually blindness.

Erythromycin. Erythromycin (e.g., E-Mycin 250 mg or 333 mg; ERYC 250 mg; EES 400 mg) is as effective as tetracycline at the same dosage levels[26] but is more expensive. The advantages include better patient compliance with the newer enteric-coated forms, which are absorbed adequately when taken with food, and a lower incidence of *C. albicans* vaginitis than occurs with equivalent dosages of tetracycline. The dosage should be decreased only after control is achieved.

Minocycline. Minocycline (50-mg and 100-mg capsules and scored tablets) is a tetracycline derivative that has proved valuable in cases of pustular acne that have not responded to conventional oral antibiotic therapy. Minocycline is very expensive; generic forms are now available. One study comparing minocycline (50 mg three times a day) with tetracycline (250 mg four times a day) revealed that minocycline resulted in significant improvement in patients who did not respond to tetracycline. Patients who responded to tetracycline had significantly advanced improvement when switched to minocycline.[27] The inhibitory effect on gastrointestinal absorption with food and milk is significantly greater for tetracycline than for minocycline. Food causes a 13% inhibition of absorption with minocycline and a 46% inhibition with tetracycline, milk a 27% inhibition with minocycline and a 65% inhibition with tetracycline.[28] The simpler regime and early onset of clinical improvement are likely to result in better patient compliance. There is therefore justification for the use of minocycline as first-line oral therapy.

DOSING. The usual initial dosage is 50 to 100 mg twice each day. The dosage is tapered when a significant decrease in the number of lesions is observed, usually in 3 to 6 weeks.

ADVERSE EFFECTS. Minocycline is highly lipid-soluble and readily penetrates the cerebrospinal fluid, causing dose-related ataxia, vertigo, nausea, and vomiting in some patients. In susceptible individuals, central nervous system (CNS) side effects occur with the first few doses of medication. If CNS adverse reactions persist after the dosage is decreased or after the capsules are taken with food, alternative therapy is indicated. A blue-gray pigmentation of the skin, oral mucosa, nails, and thyroid gland has been found in some patients, usually those taking high dosages of minocycline for extended periods. Skin pigmentation has been reported in depressed acne scars, at sites of cutaneous inflammation, as macules resembling bruises on the lower legs, and as a generalized discoloration suggesting an off-color suntan.[29] Pigmentation may persist for long periods after minocycline has been discontinued.[30] The consequences of these deposits are unknown. Tooth staining (lasting for years) located on the incisal one half to three fourths of the crown has been reported in adults, usually after years of minocycline therapy.[31] In contrast, tooth staining produced by tetracycline occurs on the gingival third of the teeth in children treated before age 7.

Doxycycline. Studies of doxycycline (50 mg and 100 mg) showed no significant difference between its clinical efficacy and that of minocycline in treating acne.[32] Doxycycline is less expensive than minocyline.

Clindamycin. Clindamycin (75 mg and 150 mg capsules) is a highly effective oral antibiotic for the control of acne.[33]

Its use has been curtailed in recent years because of its association with severe pseudomembranous colitis caused by *Clostridium difficile*, which fortunately responds in most cases to oral or intravenous vancomycin hydrochloride. Clindamycin is effective in dosages ranging from 75 to 300 mg twice daily.

Ampicillin. Long-term use of oral antibiotics for treatment of acne may result in the appearance of cysts and pustules that yield gram-negative organisms when cultured.[34] Ampicillin (250 mg and 500 mg capsules) is effective for this so-called gram-negative acne. Ampicillin is often effective for the treatment of conventional mild to moderately inflammatory acne and is a safe alternative for patients who do not respond to tetracycline.[35] Ampicillin may be prescribed for acne during pregnancy or during lactation. A dosage of 500 mg twice each day is maintained until satisfactory control is achieved. The dosage is then decreased. Some patients experience a flare of activity at lower dosages and must resume taking 500 mg twice each day.

Cephalosporins. There are several anecdotal reports extolling the efficacy of cephalosporins.[36] These drugs may be considered for antibiotic-resistant pustular acne.

Trimethoprim and sulfamethoxazole. Trimethoprim and sulfamethoxazole (Bactrim, Septra) are useful for treating gram-negative acne and acne that is resistant to tetracycline.[37] The adult dosage is 160 mg of trimethoprim combined with 800 mg of sulfamethoxazole once or twice daily.

TABLE 7-2 Antiandrogen Therapy

Serum androgen levels	Androgen origin	Dexamethasone	Prednisone	Oral contraceptive (OC)
fT* (E)* DHEAS* (N)*	Ovarian			Treat with OC Improvement may not occur for 3 to 4 months Treat at least 1 year
fT (N) DHEAS (E)	Adrenal	0.125 to 0.5 mg qhs for 6 to 12 months	2.5 mg qAM 2.5 to 7.5 mg qhs for 6 to 12 months	
fT (E) DHEAS (E)	Adrenal (combined origin possible)	0.125 to 0.5 mg qhs for 6 to 12 months	2.5 mg qAM 2.5 to 7.5 mg qhs for 6 to 12 months	Add OC if no response to dexamethasone or prednisone after 4 to 5 months
fT (N) DHEAS (N)	Normal hormone levels but fails Rx with antibiotics and/or isotretinoin	Combine with OC 0.125 to 0.5 mg qhs	2.5 mg qAM 2.5 to 7.5 mg qhs	Start OC; add dexamethasone or prednisone after 4 to 5 months if response is poor

*Free testosterone (fT), dehydroepiandrosterone sulfate (DHEAS), (E) elevated, (N) normal.
NOTE: Spironolactone may be used alone or in combination with oral contraceptives in the above patients.

Antiandrogen therapy

The majority of patients with acne do not have serum androgen abnormalities. The profound sebum suppression produced by isotretinoin has to a large extent eliminated the need for antiandrogenic therapy. Antiandrogenic therapy is reserved for patients with acne who have clinical signs of androgen excess and for those in whom other treatments have failed.

Patient population. There is a group of women with treatment-resistant, late-onset, or persistent acne. Some of these women have signs suggesting hyperandrogenism, such as hirsutism, irregular menses, or menstrual dysfunction, but others are normal. Serum androgens may or may not be elevated.

Ovulation abnormalities. Ovulation disturbances have been found in 58.3% of women acne patients, with a prevalence of anovulation in juvenile acne and of luteal insufficiency in late-onset/persistent acne.[38] Women affected by late-onset or persistent acne have a high incidence of polycystic ovary disease.[39] Polycystic ovaries are not necessarily associated with menstrual disorders, obesity, or hirsutism. The presence of polycystic ovaries in acne patients does not correlate with acne severity, infertility, menstrual disturbance, hirsutes, or biochemical endocrinologic abnormalities.

Androgens. A combination of the effects of circulating androgens and the effects of their metabolism at the hair follicle modulates sebum production and acne severity. Androgens (free testosterone [fT], dehydroepiandrosterone sulfate [DHEAS]) are the most important hormones in the pathogenesis of acne. Plasma-free testosterone is the active fraction of testosterone and determines plasma androgenicity.

Diagnosis—serum androgen levels. fT and DHEAS are the most practical ways of evaluating hormonal influences in the female. DHEAS is the best index of adrenal androgen activity.

Treatment

Three options. There are three options for treating acne systemically with hormone manipulation. Estrogen suppresses ovarian androgen, glucocorticoids suppress adrenal androgen, and antiandrogens (spironolactone) act at the peripheral level (hair follicle, sebaceous gland). The recommended treatment is shown in Table 7-2.

Oral contraceptives. Ovarian hypersecretion of androgens can be suppressed with oral contraceptives. Most oral contraceptives contain combinations of estrogens and progestational agents. Oral contraceptives with estrogen (ethynyl estradiol or mestranol) and progestins of low androgenic activity are the most useful. Higher dose estrogen pills are more effective but not as safe.

Most synthetic progesterones have some degree of androgenic activity, which is undesirable in patients who already have signs of androgen excess. Oral contraceptives that appear to be useful in androgenic disorders and acne include Demulen, Ovcon 35, Modicon, Brevicon, and Ortho-Novum 7/7/7. The progesterone ethynodiol diacetate in Demulen is a relatively low androgenic progesterone. Norethindrone is more androgenic, but the low doses contained in Ovcon-35, Modicon, and Brevicon make these pills relatively nonandrogenic. Triphasil, containing levonorgestrel, and Diane (available outside the United States), containing cyproterone acetate, produced a 72% reduction in acne.[42]

The estrogenic and androgenic activity of various oral contraceptives are listed in the Formulary (p. 843). In many instances acne flares after the use of oral contraceptives is discontinued. Selection of an appropriate agent may provide the benefit of effective acne therapy for women who have chosen an oral contraceptive for birth control. Women in their thirties and forties without risk factors such as smoking or a family history of premature cardiovascular disease can safely use low-dose oral contraceptives to reduce ovarian androgen secretion.

Drugs that may reduce the effectiveness of oral contraceptives[43,43a]

Antibiotics: ampicillin, amoxicillin, isoniazid, metronidazole, penicillin, rifampin, tetracycline

Anticonvulsant drugs: barbiturates, carbamazepine, ethosuximide, phenytoin, primidone

Sedatives and hypnotics: barbiturates, benzodiazepines, chloral hydrate

Others: antacids, antimigraine preparations, clofibrate

Antiandrogens

Spironolactone. Spironolactone (SPL) has antiandrogenic properties and is used to treat acne, hirsutism, and androgenic alopecia. Men do not tolerate the high incidence of endocrine side effects, therefore it is only used in women. SPL decreases steroid production in adrenal and gonadal tissue. In women, total serum testosterone decreases and dehydroepiandrosterone sulfate is either decreased or remains unchanged. Free testosterone levels are unchanged or decreased. SPL acts as an antiandrogen peripherally by competitively blocking cytosol receptors for dihydrotestosterone in the sebaceous glands.

Indications. Spironolactone can be used with antibiotics or oral contraceptives or as a single drug therapy. Therefore it can be used when the source of androgen is either adrenal or ovarian or when screening for serum androgens is normal. Cyproterone acetate has similar effects (available outside the United States). A formulation of cyproterone acetate, in combination with 50 or 35 μg of estradiol, is available outside the United States. These drugs (Diane and Dianette) serve as an oral contraceptive and as an inhibitor of androgen receptors.

Acne. Spironolactone causes a significant reduction in sebum secretion and a decrease in the lesion counts of patients. Studies show that SPL at a dosage of 200 mg/day suppresses sebum production by 75% and can reduce lesion counts by up to 75% over a 4-month period.[44,45] Indications for its use are listed in the box on p. 163.

Adverse reactions. Side effects are dose related. The incidence is high, but the severity is generally mild and most women tolerate treatment. Menstrual irregularities (80%) such as amenorrhea, increased or decreased flow, midcycle bleeding, and shortened length of cycle occur. Oral contraceptives reduce the incidence and severity of menstrual irregularities. Breast tenderness or enlargement and decreased libido are infrequent. Other effects include mild hyperkalemia, headache, dizziness, drowsiness, confusion, nausea, vomiting, anorexia, and diarrhea. There are no documented cases of spironolactone-related tumors in human beings. The safety of spironolactone use during pregnancy is unknown.

Cyproterone. The antiandrogen cyproterone acetate (CPA) is available outside the United States. CPA (2 mg) in combination with either 0.035 mg ethynyl estradiol (Dianette) or 0.050 mg ethynyl estradiol (Diane) are oral contraceptives that are highly effective in improving acne. Its clinical benefit can be enhanced by giving 50 mg or 100 mg CPA from the fifth to fourteenth day of the cycle. Dianette is given for 24 months; thereafter a conventional contraceptive pill is used. There is no loss of clinical effectiveness with Dianette, and it provides the advantage of a 30% decrease in the amount of estrogen.[46] Diane formulations are available outside the United States.

Corticosteroids. Corticosteroids can be considered in recalcitrant cases of acne not responsive to oral contraceptives or spironolactone and for patients with elevated DHEAS. Corticosteroids can be used alone or in combination with oral contraceptives and antiandrogens. Elevated DHEAS indicates adrenal androgen overproduction. Either dexamethasone[40] (0.125 to 0.5 mg at bedtime) or prednisone (2.5 to 7.5 mg at bedtime and 2.5 mg on waking) is prescribed. Low-dose steroids administered at bedtime prevent the pituitary from producing extra ACTH and thereby reduce the production of adrenal androgens. Dexamethasone may be the more rational choice for adrenal suppression with its longer duration of action. The drug is given at bedtime so that effective levels will be present during the early morning hours when ACTH secretion is most active. Initial dosage should be dexamethasone 0.25 mg or prednisone 2.5 mg, and the dosage should be increased to dexamethasone 0.5 mg or prednisone 5.0 to 7.5 mg[41] if the DHEAS level has not been lowered after 3 to 4 weeks of treatment. Therapy is continued for 6 to 12 months, but the benefits may persist beyond that. This low dosage produces a clinical improvement and suppresses DHEAS levels. At these dosages, few patients experience shutdown of the adrenal-pituitary axis or other adverse effects of the drug. ACTH stimulation tests or early morning cortisol levels may be performed every few months to make sure that there is no adrenal suppression. Not all patients respond.

GUIDELINES FOR TREATMENT OF ACNE WITH SPIRONOLACTONE (ALDACTONE 25-, 50-, 100-MG TABLETS)

A. INDICATIONS

1. Adult women with inflammatory facial acne
2. Hormonal influence suggested by
   a. Premenstrual flares
   b. Onset after age 25 years
   c. Distribution on the lower face, including the mandibular line and chin
   d. Increase in oiliness on the face
   e. Coexistent facial hirsutism
3. Inadequate response or intolerance to standard treatment with topical therapies, systemic antibiotics, or isotretinoin
4. Presence of coexisting symptoms such as irregular menses, premenstrual weight gain, or other symptoms of premenstrual syndrome

B. PRETREATMENT EVALUATION

1. Evaluation of serum androgens generally is not required because most women with acne have normal serum levels. In the clinical setting of new onset of acne with other signs of virilization, evaluation by an endocrinologist may be required.
2. Determination of adequate birth control measures
3. Discussion of potential side effects with oral spironolactone
4. Obtaining baseline blood pressure

C. GUIDELINES FOR STARTING TREATMENT

1. Begin with 1 or 2 mg/kg/day (50 to 100 mg/day) as a single daily dose to minimize side effects. It is not known whether twice-daily dosing has an advantage over a single daily dose.
2. Check serum potassium levels and blood pressure in 1 month. Obtaining a CBC is optional because hematologic abnormalities occur only rarely.
3. Topical therapies and systemic antibiotics may be continued while spironolactone treatment is initiated. Tapering of the standard therapies may then be possible as a beneficial response to spironolactone is noted.
4. Oral contraceptives, if not contraindicated, may be given concomitantly at the start of treatment with spironolactone, or they can be considered if menstrual irregularities develop.
5. If no clinical response is seen in 1 to 3 months, consider increasing the dosage to 150 or 200 mg/day as tolerated. Good clinical responses can be followed by a reduction of the dosage to the lowest effective daily dose.
6. If adverse effects develop, consider lowering the dose; consider adding an oral contraceptive for menstrual irregularities.
7. Effective treatment of hirsutism usually requires longer treatment periods and higher dosages to obtain clinical benefit than is seen in the treatment of acne.

From Shaw JC: Spironolactone in dermatologic therapy, *J Am Acad Dermatol* 24:236-243, 1991.

Isotretinoin (Accutane 10-, 20-, 40-mg capsules)

Isotretinoin (13-cis retinoic acid), an oral retinoid related to vitamin A, is a very effective agent for control of acne and in the induction of long-term remissions, but it is not suitable for all types of acne. Isotretinoin affects all major etiologic factors implicated in acne. It dramatically reduces sebum excretion, follicular keratinization, and ductal and surface *Propionibacterium acnes* counts. These effects are maintained during treatment and persist at variable levels after therapy. A full list of indications and guidelines for treatment are found in Table 7-3 and the box below. A number of side effects occur during treatment. Isotretinoin is a potent teratogen; pregnancy must be avoided during treatment. Isotretinoin is not mutagenic; female patients should be assured that they may safely get pregnant but should wait for at least 1 month after stopping isotretinoin. Age is not a limiting factor in patient selection.

TABLE 7-3 Dosage of Isotretinoin by Body Weight

| Body weight | | Total mg/day | | |
Kilograms	Pounds	0.5 mg/kg	1 mg/kg	2 mg/kg
40	88	20	40	80
50	110	25	50	100
60	132	30	60	120
70	154	35	70	140
80	176	40	80	160
90	198	45	90	180
100	220	50	100	200

GUIDELINES FOR THE TREATMENT OF ACNE WITH ISOTRETINOIN (ACCUTANE 10-, 20-, 40-MG CAPSULES)

INDICATIONS

Severe recalcitrant cystic acne*
Severe recalcitrant nodular and inflammatory acne*
Moderate acne unresponsive to conventional therapy
Patients who scar
Excessive oiliness
Severely depressed or dysmorphic patients[47]
Unusual variants
Acne fulminans
Gram-negative folliculitis
Pyoderma faciale

DOSAGE

Total cumulative dose determines remission rate
Cumulative dose 120 to 150 mg/kg
88% of patients have a stable, complete remission when treated in this dosage range
No therapeutic benefit from doses >150 mg/kg
0.5 to 1.0 mg/kg/day for 4 months—typical course of Rx
Optimal long-term benefit: 1.0 mg/kg/day for initial course of Rx
1.0 mg/kg/day × 120 days = 120 mg/kg

Treat with 1 mg/kg/day especially in
Young patients
Males
Severe acne
Truncal acne
Treat with 0.5 mg/kg/day
Older patients, especially men
Double dosage at end of 2 months if no response

DURATION

Usually 85% clear in 4 months at 0.5 to 1.0 mg/kg/day; 15% require longer Rx
May treat at lower dosage for longer period to arrive at the optimum total cumulative dosage

RELAPSE

39% relapse (usually within 3 years, most within 18 months)
23% require antibiotics
16% require additional isotretinoin

ADDITIONAL COURSES OF ISOTRETINOIN

Appears to be safe
Response is predictable
Some patients require three to five courses
Cumulative dosage for each course should not exceed 150 mg/kg[48]

Adapted from Layton AM, Cunliffe WJ: *J Am Acad Dermatol* 27:S2-S7, 1992, and Lehucher-Ceyrac D, Weber-Buisset MJ: *Dermatology* 186:123-128, 1993.
*FDA-approved indication.

Indications

Severe, recalcitrant cystic or nodular and inflammatory acne. A few patients with severe disease respond to oral antibiotics and vigorous drying therapy with a combination of agents such as benzoyl peroxide and sulfacctamide/sulfur lotion. Those who do not respond after a short trial of this conventional therapy should be treated with isotretinoin to minimize scarring.

Moderate acne unresponsive to conventional therapy. Moderate acne usually responds to antibiotics (e.g., tetracycline or erythromycin 500 mg twice daily) plus topical agents. Change to a different antibiotic (e.g., minocycline 100 mg twice daily) if response is poor after 3 months. Change to a third antibiotic (e.g., ampicillin, a cephalosporin, or trimethoprim/sulfamethoxazole) if response is poor after 3 months on the second antibiotic. Change to isotretinoin if response is unsatisfactory after three consecutive 3-month courses of antibiotics. Patients who have a relapse during or after three courses of antibiotics are also candidates for isotretinoin.[49]

Patients who scar. Any patient who scars should be considered for isotretinoin therapy. Acne scars leave a permanent mark on the skin and psyche.

Excessive oiliness. Excessive oiliness is disturbing and can last for years. Antibiotics and topical therapy may provide some relief, but isotretinoin's effect is dramatic. Relief may last for months or years; some patients require a second or third course of treatment.

Severely depressed or dysmorphophobic patients. Some patients, even with minor acne, are depressed. Those who do not respond to conventional therapy are candidates for isotretinoin. They respond well to isotretinoin, although some may relapse quickly and require repeat courses.[47]

Dosage. The severity of the side effects of isotretinoin is proportional to the daily dose. Start with lower dosages and progressively increase the dosage in accordance with the tolerance.

The cumulative dose may be more important than the duration of therapy. A cumulative dose of greater than 120 mg/kg is associated with significantly better long-term remission.[50] This dosage level can be achieved by either 1 mg/kg/day for 4 months or a smaller dosage for a longer period. The therapeutic benefit from a total cumulative dose of more than 150 mg/kg is virtually nonexistent.[48] Analysis of 9 years of experience demonstrated that 1 mg/kg/day of isotretinoin for 4 months resulted in the longest remissions.[51] Relapse rates in patients receiving 0.5 mg/kg/day were approximately 40% and those receiving 1.0 mg/kg/day were approximately 20%. Younger patients, males, and patients with truncal acne derive maximum benefit from the higher dosages. In these patients, dosages less than 0.5 mg/kg/day for a standard 4-month course are associated with a high relapse rate. Treat older patients with facial acne with a dosage of 0.5 mg/kg/day. Double the dosage if there is no response at the end of 2 months. Side effects depend on the dosage and can be controlled through reduction.

Duration of therapy. A standard course of isotretinoin therapy is 16 to 20 weeks. Approximately 85% of patients are clear at the end of 16 weeks; 15% require longer treatment. Side effects are related to the dosage. Treat for a longer duration at a lower dosage if mucocutaneous side effects become troublesome. Patients with large, closed comedones may respond slowly and relapse early with inflammatory papules. Another ill-defined group responds slowly and requires up to 9 months until the condition begins to clear.

Relapse and repeat courses of isotretinoin. Approximately 39% of patients relapse and require oral antibiotics (23%) or additional isotretinoin (16%). Relapse usually occurs within the first 3 years after isotretinoin is stopped; most often during the first 18 months after therapy. Some patients require multiple courses of therapy. The response to repeat therapy is consistently successful, and side effects are similar to those of previous courses. Repeat courses of isotretinoin seem to be safe.

Isotretinoin therapy. Patients are seen frequently during the course of therapy (e.g., every 4 weeks). Isotretinoin is given in two divided doses daily, preferably with meals. Many patients experience a moderate to severe flare of acne during the initial weeks of treatment. This adverse reaction can be minimized by starting at 10 to 20 mg twice each day and gradually increasing the dosage during the first 4 to 6 weeks. Treatment is discontinued at the end of 16 to 20 weeks, and the patient is observed for 2 to 5 months. Those with persistently severe acne may receive a second course of treatment after the posttreatment observation period.

Response to therapy. At dosages of 1 mg/kg/day, sebum production decreases to approximately 10% of pretreatment values and the sebaceous glands decrease in size.[52] Maximum inhibition is reached by the third or fourth week. Within a week, patients normally notice drying and chapping of facial skin and skin oiliness disappears quickly. These effects persist for an indefinite period when therapy is discontinued.

During the first month, there is usually a reduction in superficial lesions such as papules and pustules. New cysts evolve and disappear quickly. A significant reduction in the number of cysts normally takes at least 8 weeks. Facial lesions respond faster than trunk lesions.

Resistant patients. Younger patients (14 to 19 years of age) and those who have severe acne relapse more often.[53] Truncal acne relapses more often than facial acne. A return of the reduced sebum excretion rate to within 10% of the pretreatment level is a poor prognostic factor.[54] Patients with microcystic acne (whiteheads) and women with gyneco-endocrinologic problems are resistant to treatment. Women who do not clear after a total cumulative dose of 150 mg/kg need laboratory and clinical evaluation of their endocrinologic status. They may benefit from antiandrogen therapy.

Psychosocial implications. Patients successfully treated with isotretinoin have significant posttreatment gains in social assertiveness and self-esteem.[55] There is also a significant reduction in anxiety and depression.[56]

TABLE 7-4 Laboratory Tests with Isotretinoin	
Test	**Comments**
Pregnancy	Performed prior to starting treatment
Triglyceride level*	Performed during pretreatment, after 2 to 3 weeks of treatment, and then at 4-week intervals. If levels exceeds 350 to 400 mg/dl, repeat blood lipids at 2 to 3-week intervals. Stop if the value exceeds 700 to 800 mg/dl to reduce the risk of pancreatitis
Complete blood count	Performed prior to treatment and after 4 to 6 weeks of treatment
Liver function*	Performed prior to treatment and after 4 to 6 weeks of treatment

*Liver and lipid abnormalities rarely necessitate dosage reduction, and the need for repeat laboratory tests after initial normal values has been questioned.[49]

TABLE 7-5 Adverse Events Among 404 Subjects who Discontinued Isotretinoin Therapy	
Event	**Frequency, No**
Mucous/skin effects	2.5
Elevated triglyceride levels	2.0
Musculoskeletal effects	1.3
Headaches	1.1
Elevated liver enzyme levels	0.6
Amenorrhea	0.4
Other	0.5

From McElwee NE, Schumacher MC, et al: *Arch Dermatol* 127:341-346, 1991.

TABLE 7-6 Frequency of Mucocutaneous and Musculoskeletal Events in 404 Subjects*	
Event	**Frequency, No**
Cheilitis	96
Dry skin	87
Pruritis	23
Dry mouth	29
Dry nose	40
Epistaxis	33
Conjunctivitis	40
Musculoskeletal symptoms	42
Rash	16
Hair thinning	6
Peeling	6

From McElwee NE, Schumacher MC, et al: *Arch Dermatol* 127:341-346, 1991.
*Mean initial isotretinoin dose was 1 mg/kg. Most commonly used initial dosage regimen for males is 80 or 120 mg/day, and 80 or 40 mg/day for females.

Patients with minimal facial acne but with symptoms of dysmorphophobia (inappropriate depression and/or anxiety response to mild acne) are often treated with long-term antibiotic therapy with no perceived improvement. These patients respond to isotretinoin in that they are satisfied with the cosmetic results achieved. The incidence of relapse is greater than that of other acne patients and often requires additional therapy in the form of antibiotics or further isotretinoin.[47]

Laboratory studies. Pregnancy tests, triglyceride tests, complete blood counts, and liver function tests are performed on patients taking isotretinoin (Table 7-4).

Side effects. Side effects occur frequently, are dose-dependent, and are reversible shortly after discontinuing treatment. Patients with side effects can be managed at a lower dosage for a period long enough to reach the 120 mg/kg cumulative dose level. Explain to patients that the long-term benefit is related to the cumulative dosage, not to the duration of therapy.

The incidence of side effects was documented in a large study. They are shown in Tables 7-5 and 7-6. Patients in that study stopped isotretinoin for the following reasons: mucous/skin effects (2.5), elevated triglyceride levels (2.0), musculoskeletal effects (1.3), headaches (1.1), elevated liver enzyme levels (0.6), amenorrhea (0.4), and other (0.5).

Teratogenicity—pregnancy prevention program. Isotretinoin is a potent teratogen primarily involving craniofacial, cardiac, thymic, and central nervous system structures.[57] A number of physicians inadvertently prescribed isotretinoin to pregnant women,[58] which resulted in birth defects. For this reason the FDA considered withdrawing isotretinoin in 1988. Roche Laboratories designed the pregnancy prevention program; as a result, isotretinoin is still available.

The pregnancy prevention program is available from Roche Laboratories in a box containing a qualification checklist for patients, information about treatment, contraception counseling and serum pregnancy testing information, an optional referral form for expert counseling on contraception and patient self-evaluation, consent forms, and a follow-up survey.

Women should be educated about the risks to the fetus and the need for adequate contraception. Sexually active women should have a pregnancy test and postpone therapy until their next normal menstrual period. Some physicians will not prescribe isotretinoin to women of child-bearing age unless they are taking oral contraceptives. Others withhold isotretinoin if abortion is not an option. Isotretinoin is not mutagenic, nor is it stored in tissue. It is recommended that contraception be continued for 1 month after stopping isotretinoin. Patients can be reassured that conception is safe after this 1-month period.[59] One study showed that from the fourth month of treatment onward, a statistically significant increase in the mean sperm density, sperm morphology, and motility were not affected. One year after treatment there was no evidence of any negative influence of 6 months of treatment with isotretinoin on spermatogenesis.[60]

Plasma lipid abnormalities. Accutane therapy induces an elevation of plasma triglycerides. In one study of patients (ages 14 to 40 years) treated for 20 weeks with 1 mg/kg/day, the maximum mean triglyceride levels rose 46.3 mg/dl in men and 52.3 mg/dl in women. In that study, 2 of 53 patients had a triglyceride elevation over 500 mg/dl, and 8 had elevations of 200 to 500 mg/dl. Triglyceride levels rise after 6 weeks of therapy and continue to rise while therapy continues.[61] Age, sex, and weighted dose do not appear to be risk factors for triglyceride elevations. Overweight subjects are 6 times more likely to develop significant elevations in serum triglyceride, and subjects with elevated baseline triglyceride levels are 4.3 times more likely to develop significant elevations.[62] Plasma lipid and lipoprotein levels return to baseline by 8 weeks after treatment.[63] Liver and lipid abnormalities rarely necessitate dosage reduction and the need for repeat laboratory tests after initial normal values has been questioned.[49]

Hyperostoses. Asymptomatic hyperostoses (spurs) of the spine and extremities can be documented radiographically[64] in some patients but do not seem to be of concern with a standard course of isotretinoin therapy.[65,66]

Cheilitis. Cheilitis is the most common side effect, occurring in virtually all patients. Application of emollients should be started with the initiation of therapy to minimize drying.

Approximately 40% of patients develop an elevated sedimentation rate during treatment. Isotretinoin does not specifically affect skeletal or myocardial muscles,[67] although 28% of patients complain of musculoskeletal symptoms. Accutane contains the preservative parabens; those patients with a proven allergy to parabens cannot receive Accutane. Exuberant granulation tissue may occur at the sites of healing acne lesions and is more likely to develop in patients who have preexisting crusted, draining, or ulcerated lesions. Granulation tissue can be controlled with intralesional steroid injections or silver nitrate sticks. Severe dry skin or eczema commonly occurs on the backs of the hands. Routine use of moisturizers and infrequent washing is recommended.

Prednisone

Prednisone has a limited but definite place in the management of acne. Nodulocystic acne can be resistant to all forms of conventional topical and antibiotic therapy. Nodulocystic acne can be destructive, producing widespread disfigurement through scarring. Intervention with powerful antiinflammatory agents should not be postponed in the case of rapidly advancing disease. Deep cysts improve only slowly with isotretinoin, and much permanent damage can be done while waiting for an effect.

Prednisone therapy. The dosage and duration of prednisone treatment is determined by the patient's response. The following program has been successful for treating extensive, rapidly advancing, painful cystic acne. Prednisone should be started at 40 to 60 mg per day given in divided doses twice daily. This dosage is maintained until the majority of lesions are significantly improved. Dosage is tapered. The dosage is lowered to 30 mg given as a single dose in the morning. The dosage can be tapered by 5 mg each week until 20 mg is reached, at which point prednisone can be further tapered to 30 mg every other day and withdrawn in 5-mg increments every 4 days. Patients with acne severe enough to require prednisone usually require isotretinoin for lasting control. Both drugs can be started simultaneously.

Intralesional corticosteroids

Individual nodulocystic and large pustular lesions can be effectively treated with a single injection of triamcinolone acetonide delivered with a 27- or 30-gauge needle. Commercial preparations include Kenalog (10 mg/ml) and Tac-3 (3 mg/ml). The 10 mg/ml suspension can be used at full strength or diluted with 1% Xylocaine or physiologic saline. Saline is preferred because injections of Xylocaine mixtures are painful. A 2.5 to 5.0 mg/ml concentration is usually an adequate injection for suppressing inflammation.

Intralesional corticosteroid therapy. The bottle of steroid solution needs to be shaken thoroughly in order to disperse the white suspension. The syringe should be shaken immediately prior to injection. The needle is inserted through the thinnest portion of the cyst roof and 0.1 to 0.3 ml of solution is deposited into the cyst cavity. This quantity momentarily blanches most cysts. Atrophy may occur if steroids are injected into the base of the cyst. Patients should be assured that if skin depression does occur, in most cases it is temporary and gradually resolves in 4 to 6 months. Multiple cysts can be injected in the course of one session. Intralesional injection is used specifically to supplement other programs.

It is comforting for patients to know that if a large, painful cyst appears, fast relief is available with this relatively painless procedure. Occasionally, intralesional steroid injections may be given for small papules and pustules when rapid resolution is desired. Prolonged, continual use of intralesional steroids has resulted in adrenal suppression.

ACNE SURGERY

Acne surgery is the manual removal of comedones and the drainage of pustules and cysts. When done correctly, acne surgery speeds resolution and rapidly enhances cosmetic appearance. Three instruments are used: the round loop comedone extractor; the oval loop acne extractor, or the Schamberg extractor; and the #11 pointed-tip scalpel blade.

Comedones. Removal of open comedones (blackheads) enhances the patient's appearance and discourages self-manipulation. By use of either type of extractor, most comedones can easily be expressed with uniform, smooth pressure. Lesions that offer resistance are loosened and sometimes disengaged by inserting the point of a #11 blade into the blackhead and elevating. The orifice of the closed comedone must be enlarged before pressure can be applied. Following the angle of the follicle, the scalpel point is inserted with the sharp edge up approximately 1 mm into the tiny orifice. The blade is drawn slightly forward and up, then pressure is applied with the extractor to remove the sometimes surprisingly large quantity of soft, white material. Macrocomedones (whiteheads, microcystic acne) can also be treated with light cautery.[68]

Pustules and cysts. After the head of the white pustule is nicked with the #11 blade, pustules are easily drained by pressing the material with the acne extractor. Cysts are preferably managed by intralesional injection because incision and drainage may cause scarring. Pustules and cysts that have a thin, effaced roof in which fluid contents are easily felt are drained through a small incision by manual pressure. To prevent scarring, a short incision (about 3 mm) should be made. After drainage, a #1 curette may be inserted through the incision on the cyst in order to dislodge chunks of necrotic tissue.

Scar revision

Many patients are very self-conscious about the pitted and craterlike scars that remain as a permanent record of previous inflammation. Some people will endure any procedure and spare no expense to rid themselves of the minutest scar. A variety of procedures is available to remove or revise scars. A dermatologic or plastic surgeon is best equipped to perform such procedures. Dermatologic surgeons are proficient at many innovative techniques to correct all types of acne scars.

Generally, it is advisable to wait until disease activity has been low or absent for several months. Scars improve with time as they become atrophied. The color contrast is often the most troublesome aspect of acne. Inflamed lesions may leave a flat or depressed red scar that is so obvious patients mistake the mark for an active lesion. The color will fade and approach skin tones in 4 to 12 months. The following techniques are those most commonly used for scar revision.

Dermabrasion. Dermabrasion (see also Chapter Twenty-seven) has been practiced for years and when performed correctly is a valuable technique for decreasing the depth of pitted scars (Figure 7-9). The epidermis and part of the dermis is planed away with a high-speed, motor-driven, finely abrasive brush or wheel. A major portion of the face may be treated during a single session. Reepithelialization takes 3 to 4 weeks. The procedure may have to be repeated one or two times to obtain optimum results. Adverse effects include the creation of additional scarring and permanent loss of pigment. The creation of hypopigmented areas is a common side effect, and for this reason many surgeons advise against using this technique for patients with dark skin.

Scar excision. Many pitted scars are too deep to be planed by dermabrasion. These deep or "ice pick" scars may be excised and closed carefully with gratifying results. Some dermatologic surgeons remove the scars with a punch biopsy. The plug is removed and the scar is separated from the subcutaneous tissue. The remaining round core of fat and dermis is replaced in the round hole and held at the surface with a Steri-strip. The autograft is rapidly fibrosed into place, and the epidermis subsequently regenerates. There are many modifications of this technique.

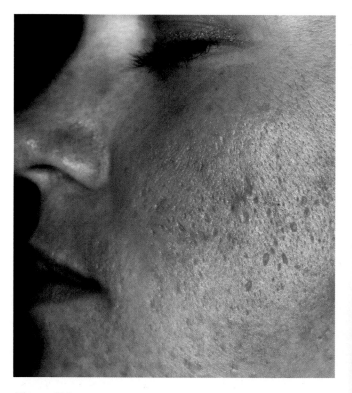

Figure 7-9
Pitted acne scars. An ideal candidate for dermabrasion.

Gelatin matrix collagen implant (Fibrel). Fibrel is a porcine collagen suspension that is injected intradermally to correct depressed cutaneous scars (see Chapter Twenty-seven). Fibrel is composed of absorbable gelatin powder (denatured collagen types I and III) and epsilon-aminocaproic acid (EAC) in a lyophilized form. Fibrel is reconstituted with equal amounts of the patient's plasma and 0.9% sodium chloride for injection. The reconstituted Fibrel suspension forms a fibrin network within a gelatin matrix, which initially restores the skin's contour. Over a period of months, the implant is colonized by the patient's own connective tissue cells.

Scars should be distensible by manual stretching of the scar borders. A custom needle is supplied with the Fibrel kit and is used for undermining fibrotic scars prior to injection. Improvement is maintained for up to 1 year in 85% of the treated scars. "Ice pick" or extremely fibrotic scars do not respond.

Bovine dermal collagen implants (Zyderm, Zyplast). Zyderm and Zyplast are bovine collagen suspensions indicated for the correction of scars and wrinkles. A processing technique renders collagen nonantigenic and suitable for augmenting scars in humans (see Chapter Twenty-seven). Collagen is supplied in preloaded syringes for intradermal injection. Soft, distensible lesions with smooth margins are the most amenable to correction, whereas "ice pick" acne and tiny, punched lesions do not respond as well. Zyplast, a newer cross-linked collagen product, can be placed deeper than Zyderm. The duration of correction is shorter than that of Fibrel.

APPROACH TO ACNE THERAPY
Initial visit

HISTORY. Many patients are embarrassed to ask for help. Any feeling of apathy or indifference on the part of the physician will be sensed, resulting in a loss of esteem and enthusiasm for the treatment. A careful history should be taken. Inquiring about many details reassures the patient that this is a disease to be taken seriously and managed carefully. Previous treatment should be documented—types of cleansers and lubricants, family history, and history of cyclic menstrual flares. The potential for irritation can be determined by past responses to drying therapy with over-the-counter benzoyl peroxide. This past experience helps to decide with which strength and base of benzoyl peroxide, tretinoin, or other topical agents to start.

PATHOGENESIS AND COURSE. Acne is an inherited disease. It is not possible to predict which members of a family will inherit it. The severity of acne in persons developing the disease is not necessarily related to the severity of acne in their parents. Acne does not end at age 19 but can persist into a person's forties. Many women have their first episode after age 25. Several myths should be discussed. Greasy foods cause obesity, not acne, but moderate dietary restriction is appropriate if the patient feels that certain foods are a problem. Acne is not caused by dirt. The pigment in black-heads is not dirt and may not be melanin as was once suspected.[69] Excessive washing is unnecessary and interferes with most treatment programs. Gentle manipulation of pustules is tolerated; aggressive pressure and excoriation produces permanent scarring. The erythema and pigmentation that follows resolution of acne lesions in some patients may take many months to fade.

Patients should not have inappropriate expectations. Acne can in most cases be controlled, but not cured.

COSMETICS AND CLEANSERS. Moderate use of nongreasy lubricants and water-based cosmetics is usually well tolerated, but a gradual decrease in the use of cosmetics is encouraged as acne improves. Cream-based cleansers should be avoided.

ORAL CONTRACEPTIVES. If women patients are taking oral contraceptives, a change in estrogen and progestin combinations may be all that is necessary.

Initial evaluation

Type of lesions. An overview of diagnosis and treatment is presented in the beginning of this chapter (see Figures 7-1 to 7-4). The types of lesions present are determined (i.e., comedones, papules, pustules, nodules, or cysts). The degree of severity (mild, moderate, severe) is also determined.

Degree of skin sensitivity. The degree of skin sensitivity can be determined by inquiring about past experiences with topical medicines and soaps. Degree of pigmentation and hair color are not the sole determinants of skin sensitivity. Atopic patients with dry skin and a history of eczema generally do not tolerate aggressive drying therapy.

Selection of therapy. Therapy appropriate to the type of acne is selected. (For initial orientation, refer to Figures 7-3 and 7-4 and to the previous section on therapeutic agents.) If antibiotics are selected for initial therapy, it is best to start with "therapeutic dosages" (see section on oral antibiotics, p. 158).

Course of treatment. A program can be established for most patients after three visits, but some difficult cases require continual supervision. For maximum effect treatment must be continual and prolonged. Patients who had only a few lesions that quickly cleared may be given a trial period without treatment 6 to 8 weeks after clearing. In an attempt to suppress further activity, those patients who have numerous lesions should remain on continual topical treatment for several months. The patient's propensity to scar must be ascertained. Patients vary in their tendency to develop scars. Some demonstrate little scarring even after significant inflammation, whereas others develop a scar from nearly every inflammatory papular or pustular lesion. This later group requires aggressive therapy in order to prevent further damage.

ACNE TREATMENT PROGRAMS

The following treatment programs are offered only as a guide. Modifications must be made for each individual (see Figures 7-3 and 7-4).

Comedone and closed comedone acne

Closed comedone acne (whiteheads) (Figures 7-10 and 7-11) responds slowly. A large mass of sebaceous material is impacted behind a very small follicular orifice. The orifice may enlarge during treatment, making extraction by acne surgery possible. Comedones may remain unchanged for months or evolve into a pustule or cyst.

First visit. Tretinoin is the most effective agent for this type of acne. The base and strength is selected according to skin sensitivity. Tretinoin is applied once each evening or less frequently if irritation develops. Large open comedones (blackheads) are expressed; many are difficult to remove. Several weeks of tretinoin treatment facilitates easier extraction.

Second visit (week 5). The strength and frequency of application of tretinoin are adjusted. If comedones become inflamed and form pustules during treatment, benzoyl peroxide gel, either 2.5% or 5%, or topical antibiotics may be added. The medication should be applied once each day or less frequently if irritation develops. Oral antibiotics should be considered for significant inflammation. Open comedones are expressed.

Third visit (week 10). The patient should have adapted to using combination treatment. The strength and frequency of the application of tretinoin and other topical agents should be adjusted as needed.

Pustular acne

Mild to moderate inflammation. Pustular acne with mild to moderate inflammation is defined here as fewer than 20 pustules (Figure 7-12).

First visit. Tretinoin and benzoyl peroxide gel are initially applied on alternate evenings. The lowest concentration of tretinoin gel or cream and 2.5% or 5% benzoyl peroxide gel are initially used. After the initial adjustment period, tretinoin is used each night and benzoyl peroxide each morning. A drying agent program can also be very effective. Sulfacetamide/sulfur lotion (Sulfacet-R, Novacet) is used in the morning and Sulfoxyl Regular in the evening. Patients using drying agents should adjust the frequency of application to induce a mild, continuous peel. Tetracycline or erythromycin is prescribed for patients with 10 to 20 pustules. Pustules and open comedones are expressed.

Second visit (week 5). The strength of tretinoin and/or benzoyl peroxide is increased. Patients using the drying treatment program may now tolerate Sulfoxyl Strong. Oral antibiotics (see Table 7-1) are introduced if the number of pustules has not decreased. Pustules and open comedones are expressed.

Third visit (week 10). By the tenth week a program of topical therapy that results in some dryness and mild erythema without irritation should have been established; there should be a significant decrease in the number of pustules. A few closed comedones will have disappeared, but they usually require much longer, continual therapy. If the number of pustules has not changed significantly, it should be established that tetracycline is being taken correctly. If directions have been followed, increasing the dosage of

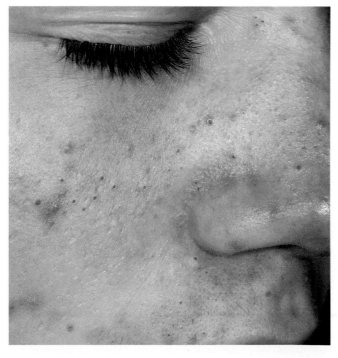

Figure 7-10
Comedones (blackheads) are occasionally inflamed.

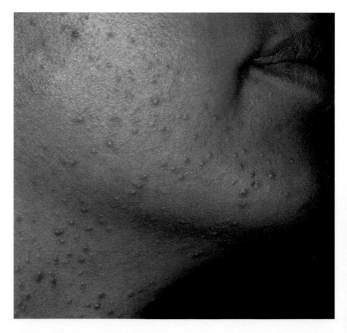

Figure 7-11
Closed comedones (whiteheads). Tiny, white, dome-shaped papules with a small follicular orifice. Stretching the skin accentuated these lesions.

tetracycline or starting minocycline at full dosage is necessary. If there are any signs of irritation, the frequency and strength of topical medicines should be decreased. Irritation, particularly about the mandibular areas and neck, worsens pustular acne. Resistant pustules are injected with triamcinolone acetonide (Kenalog).

Those who have responded well may begin to taper and eventually discontinue oral antibiotics. A topical antibiotic may be substituted for benzoyl peroxide. Topical therapy is continued for extended periods.

Moderate to severe inflammation. Patients who have moderate to severe acne (more than 20 pustules) are temporarily disfigured (Figure 7-13). Their disease may have been gradually worsening or may be virulent at the onset. The explosive onset of pustules can sometimes be precipitated by stress. There may be few to negligible visible comedones. Affected areas should not be irritated during the initial stages of therapy.

First visit. Begin tetracycline or erythromycin, 1 gm/day in divided doses. Patient compliance is highest with twice-a-day dosing. Consider using minocycline for the more extensive and acutely inflamed cases. Begin either 2.5% or 5% benzoyl peroxide and apply once or twice daily during the initial days of therapy; avoid irritation. A combination of agents may be very effective. Sulfacetamide/sulfur lotion (Sulfacet-R, Novacet) is used in the morning and Sulfoxyl Regular in the evening. The frequency of application is adjusted to induce a mild, continuous peel. Pustules are gently incised and expressed. Injecting each pustule with a very small amount of triamcinolone acetonide (Kenalog) can give immediate and very gratifying results.

Second visit (week 5). A significant response will have occurred in many patients. Antibiotic dosage at therapeutic levels is maintained to ensure control. Some patients have dramatic results and can slowly taper, but not discontinue, antibiotics. Those displaying little improvement should, if taking tetracycline or erythromycin, switch to minocycline or another antibiotic (see Table 7-1). Those on minocycline may have the dosage maintained or increased. Tretinoin can be introduced if the number of pustules and the degree of inflammation have decreased. Combination topical therapy is begun as tolerated (e.g., tretinoin gel 0.01%, benzoyl peroxide 2.5% or 5%). Frequency of use is increased until slight dryness and erythema occur.

Third visit (week 10). Many patients will have significantly improved; therefore plans should be made to taper and discontinue oral antibiotics. Some patients respond very well to lower dosages of oral antibiotics and require tetracycline, 250 mg/day or even every other day for control. Those patients may be safely maintained on low-dose oral antibiotics for extended periods. Patients who do not respond to conventional therapy may be colonized by gram-negative organisms. The pustules and cysts are cultured and an appropriate antibiotic such as ampicillin is started. The response may be dramatic.

Combinations of tretinoin, benzoyl peroxide, and topical antibiotics should be continued for months in an attempt to suppress recurrent activity. Consider isotretinoin or intralesional triamcinolone injections for antibiotic-resistant acne in patients who demonstrate a potential for scarring.

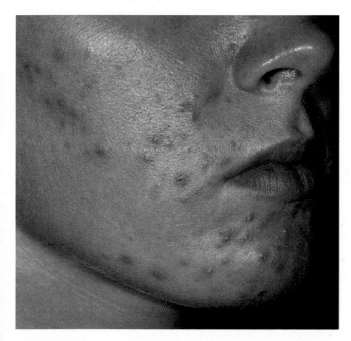

Figure 7-12
Papular and pustular acne (mild). Several papules are localized on the cheeks.

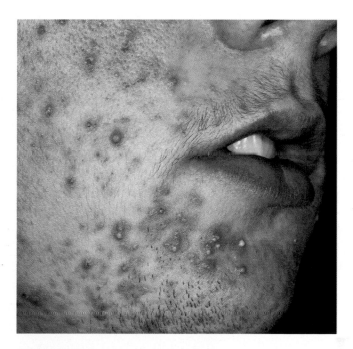

Figure 7-13
Papular and pustular acne (moderate). Many pustules are present, and several have become confluent on the chin area.

Nodulocystic acne

Nodulocystic acne includes localized cystic acne (few cysts on face, chest, or back) (Figure 7-14), diffuse cystic acne (wide areas of face, chest, and back) (Figures 7-15 through 7-22), pyoderma faciale (inflamed cysts localized on the face in females) (Figure 7-17), and acne conglobata (highly inflammatory, with cysts that communicate under the skin, abscesses, and burrowing sinus tracts) (Figures 7-18 and 7-23).

Cystic acne. Cystic acne is a serious and sometimes devastating disease that requires aggressive treatment. The face, chest, back, and upper arms may be permanently mutilated by numerous atrophic or hypertrophic scars. Patients sometimes delay seeking help, hoping that improvement will occur spontaneously; consequently, the disease may be quite advanced when first viewed by the physician.

Patients are often embarrassed by and preoccupied with their disease. They may experience anxiety, depression, insecurity, psychic suffering, and social isolation. The physical appearance may be so unattractive that teenagers refuse to attend school and adults fear going to work. Patients report difficulty securing employment when afflicted and problems being accepted in the working environment.

Patients with a few inflamed cysts can be managed with a program similar to that outlined for inflammatory acne. Oral antibiotics, conventional topical therapy, and periodic intralesional Kenalog injections may keep this problem under adequate control.

Extensive cystic acne requires a different approach. There are two less common variants of cystic acne.

Pyoderma faciale. Pyoderma faciale is a distinctive variant of cystic acne that remains confined to the face. It is a disease of adult women ranging in age from the teens to the forties. They experience the rapid onset of large, sore, erythematous-to-purple cysts, predominantly on the central portion of the cheeks. Erythema may be intense. Purulent drainage from cysts occurs spontaneously or with minor trauma. Comedones are absent and scarring occurs in most cases.[70] A traumatic emotional experience has been associated with some cases. Many patients do not have a history of acne.

Cultures help to differentiate this condition from gram-negative acne. Highly inflamed lesions can be managed by starting isotretinoin and oral corticosteroids. A study report-

Figure 7-14
Localized nodular and cystic acne. Cystic and nodular lesions appeared in this patient, who has chronic comedo and pustular acne.

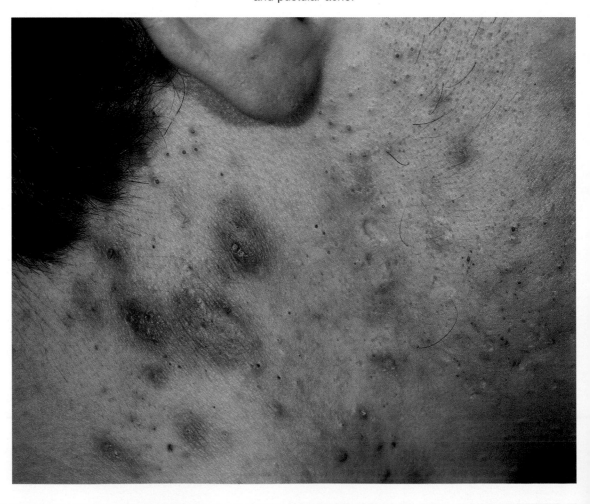

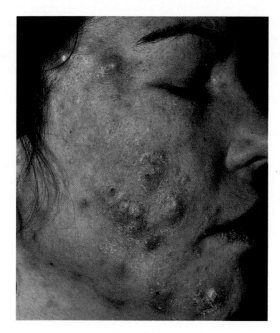

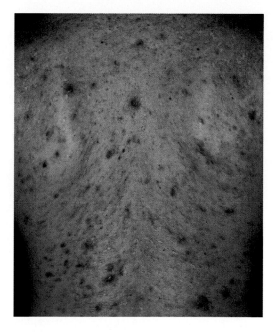

Figure 7-15
Cystic acne. The lesions in this patient are primarily cystic. Only a few pustules and comedones are present.

Figure 7-16
Nodular and cystic acne. Years of activity have left numerous scars over the entire back. Several active cysts are present.

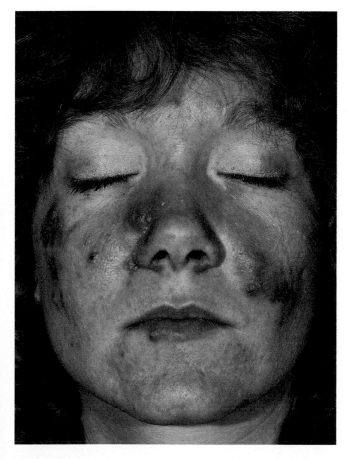

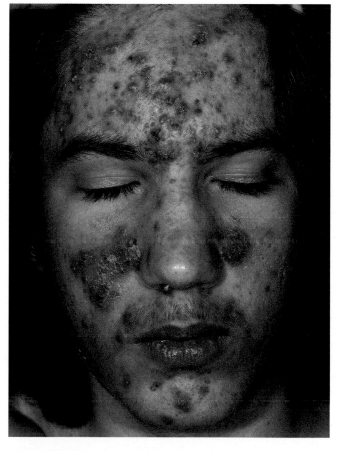

Figure 7-17
Pyoderma faciale. Confluent cysts remain localized to the face. This disease occurs almost exclusively in females.

Figure 7-18
Acne conglobata. Large communicating cysts are present on the cheeks; scarring is extensive.

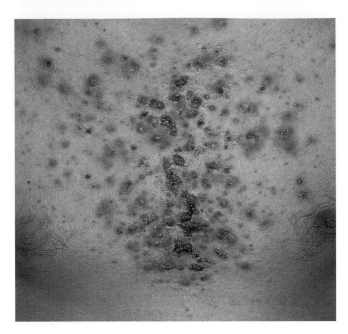

Figure 7-19
Nodular and cystic acne (severe). Many cysts have opened and drained.

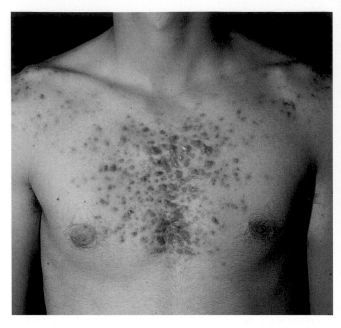

Figure 7-20
Nodular and cystic acne (severe). Patient in Figure 7-19 6 months after stopping isotretinoin. There are numerous atrophic and hypertrophic scars with postinflammatory pigmentation.

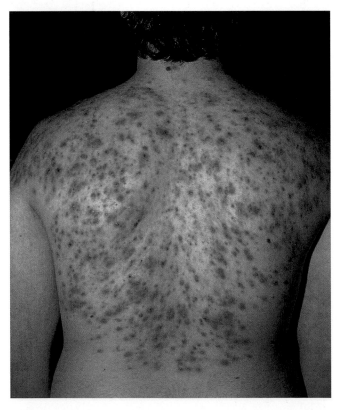

Figure 7-21
Nodular and cystic acne (severe). Active nodular and cystic acne covering the entire back.

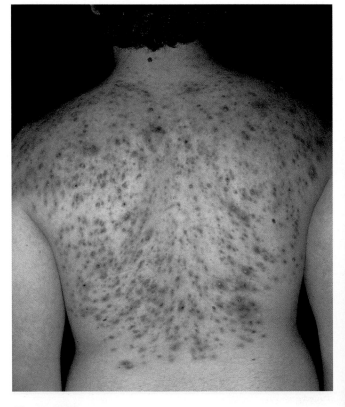

Figure 7-22
Nodular and cystic acne (severe). Patient in Figure 7-21 2 months after stopping isotretinoin. The disease is inactive, but there are numerous atrophic scars.

ed effective management with the following. Treatment was begun with prednisolone (1.0 mg/kg daily for 1 to 2 weeks). Isotretinoin was then added (0.2 to 0.5 mg/kg/day [rarely, 1.0 mg/kg in resistant cases]), with a slow tapering of the corticosteroid over the following 2 to 3 weeks. Isotretinoin was continued until all inflammatory lesions resolved. This required 3 to 4 months. None of the patients had a recurrence.[71] This group of patients were "flusher and blushers" and it was suggested that pyoderma faciale is a type of rosacea. The investigators proposed the term *rosacea fulminans*. Another review showed that the disease could be effectively managed by omitting prednisone and using Vlem Dome (sulfur solution compresses) and oral antibiotics.[72]

Acne fulminans. Acne fulminans (AF) is a rare ulcerative form of acne of unknown etiology with an acute onset and systemic symptoms. It most commonly affects adolescent white boys. A genetic predisposition is suspected.[73] Patients rapidly develop an ulcerative, necrotic acne with systemic symptoms. There are arthralgias or severe muscle pain, or both, that accompany the acne flare.[74] Episodes of arthritis, arthralgias, and myalgias may recur over many years.[75] Painful bone lesions occur in approximately 40% of patients. Weight loss, fever, leukocytosis, and elevated erythrocyte sedimentation rate (ESR) are common findings.

Antibiotic therapy is not effective. Oral corticosteroids (e.g., prednisolone, 0.5 to 1.0 mg/kg) are the primary therapy. They quickly control the skin lesions and systemic symptoms. Isotretinoin (0.5 to 1.0 mg/kg) is started simultaneously and, as in the therapy of severe cystic acne, is continued for 5 months.[76] The duration of steroid therapy is often at least 2 months. The bone lesions have a good prognosis; chronic sequelae are rare.

Acne conglobata. Acne conglobata is a chronic, highly inflammatory form of cystic acne in which involved areas contain a mixture of double comedones (two blackheads that communicate under the skin), papules, pustules, communicating cysts, abscesses, and draining sinus tracts. The disease may linger for years, ending with deep atrophic or keloidal scarring. Acne conglobata is part of the rare follicular occlusion triad syndrome of acne conglobata, hidradenitis suppurativa, and dissecting cellulitis of the scalp (Figure 7-24).[77] Musculoskeletal symptoms have been reported in some of these patients; 85% were black. There is no fever or weight loss as is seen in acne fulminans. The onset coincides with an acne flare. The pattern is that seen in seronegative spondyloarthropathies. Sacroiliitis occurs in a majority of cases. Peripheral joints may also be involved. X-ray studies show a variety of abnormalities. Recurrent episodes of axial and peripheral joint arthritis or arthralgias continue for weeks to years.[78]

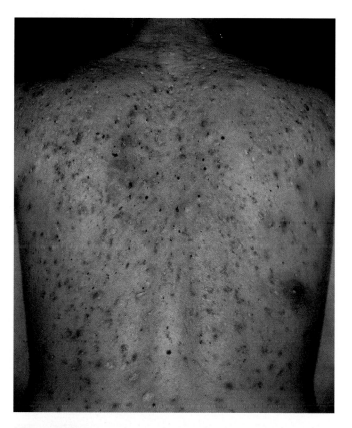

Figure 7-24
Follicular occlusion triad syndrome. Acne conglobata is part of the rare follicular occlusion triad syndrome of acne conglobata, hidradenitis suppurativa, and dissecting cellulitis of the scalp. Note the huge blackheads.

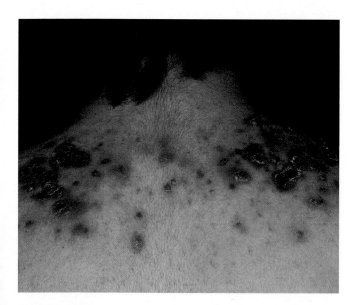

Figure 7-23
Acne conglobata. Abscesses and ulcerated cysts are found over most of the upper shoulder area.

Treatment of nodulocystic acne

First visit. The patient should be assured that effective treatment is available. Patients should be told that they will be followed closely and, if the disease becomes very active, they will be seen at least weekly until the condition is adequately controlled. Patients with numerous draining cysts may be better managed in the hospital. A primary therapeutic goal is to avoid scarring by terminating the intense inflammation quickly; prednisone is sometimes required. Cysts with thin roofs are incised and drained. Deeper cysts are injected with triamcinolone acetonide (Kenalog 2.5 to 10 mg/ml).

TOPICAL THERAPY. Begin either 5% or 10% benzoyl peroxide and apply once or twice daily during the initial days of therapy; avoid irritation. An alternate program with a combination of agents may be very effective. Sulfacetamide/sulfur lotion (Sulfacet-R, Novacet) is used in the morning and Sulfoxyl Regular or Sulfoxyl Strong in the evening. The frequency of application is adjusted to induce a mild, continuous peel.

SYSTEMIC THERAPY. Tetracycline, erythromycin, or minocycline are begun in full dosages. Initiating isotretinoin therapy for patients with extensive involvement or for patients who have a propensity to scar should be considered. The simultaneous use of tetracyclines (tetracycline or minocycline) and isotretinoin is avoided, because a higher incidence of pseudotumor cerebri may occur with this combination. For highly active cases, prednisone (adult dosage is 20 to 30 mg two times a day) is used. Prednisone should not be withheld in severe cases while waiting weeks or months for antibiotics to take effect.

Two to three weeks after initial visit. Intralesional triamcinolone acetonide injections and incision and drainage of cysts are important in the early weeks of management. Patients taking isotretinoin may taper other forms of therapy as improvement is noted. Drying agents should be continued as tolerated to produce a mild peel for many weeks.

Six weeks after initial visit. Patients who have not responded to aggressive conventional therapy may be started on isotretinoin. Patients who have responded may continue the same program outlined for the management of moderate to severe pustular acne.

OTHER TYPES OF ACNE

Several other types of papular, pustular, and nodular acne are described here.

Gram-negative acne

Patients with a long history of treatment with oral antibiotics for acne may have an increased carriage rate of gram-negative rods in the anterior nares. There are three presentations. The most common is the sudden development of superficial pustules around the nose and extending to the chin and cheeks. Others present with the sudden development of crops of pustules. Some patients develop deep nodular and cystic lesions. Cultures of these lesions and the anterior nares reveal *Escherichia aerogenes*, *Proteus mirabilis*, *Klebsiella pneumoniae*, *E. coli*, *Serratia marcescens*, and other gram-negative organisms.[79,80] Selection of the appropriate antibiotic is made after antibiotic culture and sensitivities.

Ampicillin or trimethoprim and sulfamethoxazole (Bactrim, Septra) are generally the appropriate drugs. Gram-negative acne responds quickly to the proper antibiotic, usually within 2 weeks. A quick relapse is common when antibiotics are stopped, even if given for 6 months. Elimination of the gram-negative organisms is difficult. Isotretinoin (1 mg/kg/day for 20 weeks) is successful for resistant cases of gram-negative acne.[79,81]

Steroid acne

In predisposed individuals, sudden onset of follicular pustules and papules may occur 2 to 5 weeks after starting oral corticosteroids.[82] The lesions of steroid acne (Figure 7-25) differ from acne vulgaris by being of uniform size and symmetric distribution, usually on the neck, chest, and back. They are 1- to 3-mm, flesh-colored or pink-to-red, dome-shaped papules and pustules.[83] Comedones may form later. There is no scarring. Steroid-induced acne is rare before puberty and in the elderly. There is no residual scarring. This drug eruption is not a contraindication to continued or future use of oral corticosteroids. Topical therapy with benzoyl peroxide and/or sulfacetamide/sulfur lotion (Sulfacet-R, Novacet) is effective. The eruption clears when steroids are stopped.

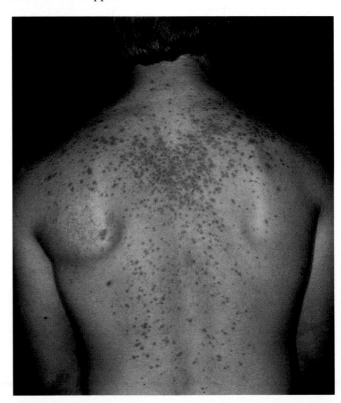

Figure 7-25
Steroid acne. Numerous papules and pustules are of uniform size and symmetrically distributed.

Neonatal acne

Acneiform lesions (Figure 7-26) confined to the nose and cheeks may be present at birth or may develop in early infancy. The lesions clear without treatment as the large sebaceous glands stimulated by maternal androgens become smaller and less active.

Occupational acne

An extensive, diffuse eruption of large comedones and pustules (Figure 7-27) may occur in some individuals who are exposed to certain industrial chemicals. These include chlorinated hydrocarbons[84] and other industrial solvents, coal tar derivatives, and oils. Lesions occur on the extremities and trunk where clothing saturated with chemicals has been in prolonged close contact with the skin. Patients predisposed to this form of acne must avoid exposure by wearing protective clothing or finding other work. Treatment is the same as for inflammatory acne.

Acne mechanica

Mechanical pressure may induce an acneiform eruption (Figure 7-28). Common causes include forehead guards and chin straps on sports helmets and orthopedic braces.

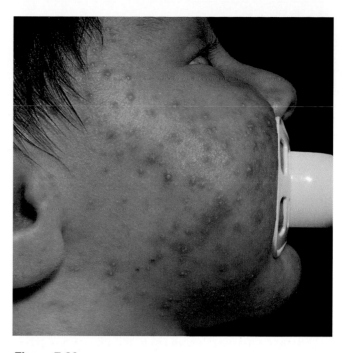

Figure 7-26
Neonatal acne. Small papules and pustules commonly occur on the cheeks and nose of infants.

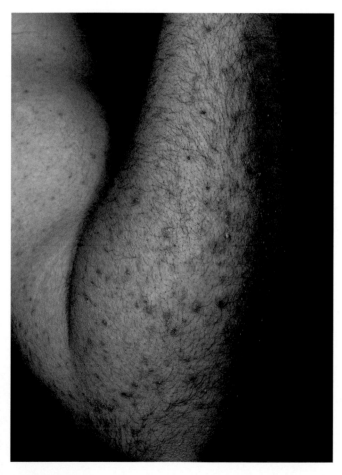

Figure 7-27
Occupational acne. Comedones, papules, and pustules occur in areas exposed to oils and industrial solvents.

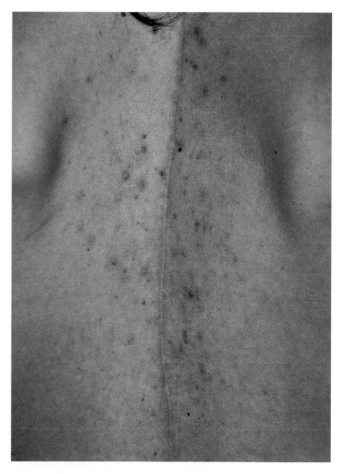

Figure 7-28
Acne mechanica. Comedones, papules, and pustules occurred after a few weeks of wearing a back brace.

Acne cosmetica

Postadolescent women who regularly apply layers of cosmetics may develop closed and open comedones, papules, and pustules. This may be the patient's first experience with acne. Traditionally, the comedogenicity of a given cosmetic formulation has been tested for its ability to produce comedones in the ear of a rabbit. More recently, trials with specific cosmetics on women have revealed that some formulations cause acne, some have no effect, and some may possibly result in decreasing the number of comedones. Until specific formulations are tested and their comedogenic potential is known, patients should be advised to use light, water-based cosmetics and to avoid cosmetic programs that advocate applying multiple layers of cream-based cleansers and coverups. Many patients are under the false impression that "facials" performed in beauty salons are therapeutic and clean pores. The various creams and cosmetics used during a facial are tolerated by most people, but acne can be precipitated by this practice.

One alternative to cosmetics is the use of tinted acne preparations (e.g., Sulfacet-R) (see the Formulary). These are generally very well received by patients.

Excoriated acne (acne excorieé des jeunes filles)

Most acne patients attempt to drain comedones and pustules with moderate finger pressure. Occasionally, a young woman with little or no acne develops several deep, linear erosions on the face (Figure 7-29). The skin has been picked vigorously with the fingernail and eventually forms a crust. These broad, red erosions with adherent crusts are obvious signs of manipulation and can easily be differentiated from resolving papules and pustules (Figure 7-30). This inappropriate attempt to eradicate lesions causes scarring and brown hyperpigmentation. Women may deny or be oblivious to their manipulation. It should be explained that such lesions can occur only with manipulation, and that the lesions may be unconsciously created during sleep. Once confronted, many women are capable of exercising adequate restraint. Those unable to refrain from excoriation may benefit from psychiatric care.

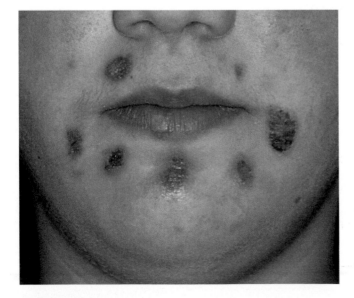

Figure 7-29
Acne excorieé des jeunes filles. Erosions and ulcers are created by inappropriate attempts to drain acne lesions.

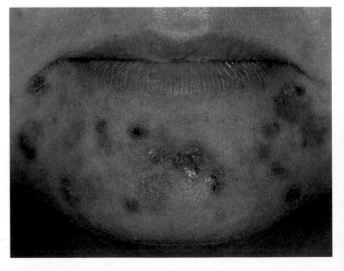

Figure 7-30
Excoriated acne. There are no primary lesions. Erosions have healed with postinflammatory hyperpigmentation.

Senile comedones

Excessive exposure to sunlight in predisposed individuals causes large open and closed comedones around the eyes and on the temples (Figure 7-31). Inflammation rarely occurs, and comedones can easily be expressed with acne surgery techniques. Tretinoin may be used to loosen impacted comedones and continued to discourage recurrence. Once cleared, the comedones may not return for months or years and tretinoin may be discontinued. Lesions that recur can be effectively treated with a 2-mm curette. The skin is held taut, and the comedone is lifted out with a quick flick of the wrist.[85] It is important to go deep enough to remove the entire lesion. Bleeding is controlled with Monsel's solution; electrocautery causes scars and should be avoided.

Milia

Milia are tiny, white, pea-shaped cysts that commonly occur on the face, especially around the eyes (Figure 7-32). They also occur during the healing process in lesions of porphyria cutanea tarda. Milia may occur spontaneously or after habitual rubbing of the eyelids. These tiny structures annoy patients, and drainage is frequently requested.

Milia have no opening on the surface and cannot be expressed like blackheads. A #11 pointed surgical blade tip is inserted with the sharp edge up and advanced laterally approximately 1 mm. Apply pressure with the Schamberg extractor to remove the soft, white material.

Solid facial edema

Solid, persistent, inflammatory edema of the face may occur in rare instances in patients with acne and last for years. The edema is often resistant to conventional treatment, including isotretinoin. The therapeutic combination of oral isotretinoin (0.5 mg/kg body weight daily) and ketotifen (2 mg daily) led to complete resolution of all facial lesions in one reported case.[86] The pathogenesis of persistent edema remains mysterious but may be related to chronic inflammation that results in obstruction of lymph vessels or fibrosis induced by mast cells.

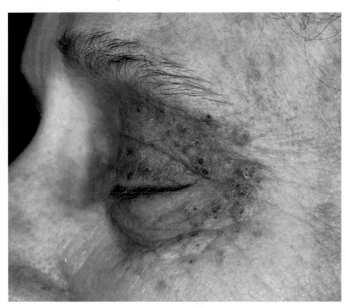

Figure 7-31
Senile comedones. Large comedones may appear around the eyes and temples in middle-aged and older individuals. Sunlight is a predisposing factor.

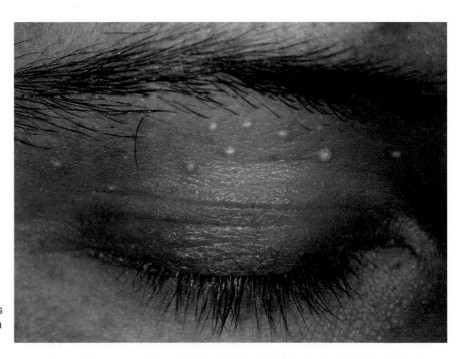

Figure 7-32
Milia. Tiny, white, dome-shaped cysts that occur about the eyes and cheeks. There is no obvious follicular opening like that seen in closed comedones.

Perioral dermatitis

Perioral dermatitis is a distinctive eruption. It occurs in young women and resembles acne. Papules and pustules on an erythematous and sometimes scaling base are confined to the chin and nasolabial folds while sparing a clear zone around the vermilion border (Figure 7-33). There are varying degrees of involvement. Patients may develop a few pustules on the chin and nasolabial folds. These cases resemble acne. Pustules on the cheeks adjacent to the nostrils are highly characteristic initially (Figure 7-34), and sometimes the disease remains confined to this area. Pustules and papules may also be seen lateral to the eyes (Figure 7-35).

Perioral dermatitis has been reported in children. Children often have periocular and perinasal lesions, as well as a higher relative incidence in boys. Topical steroids were used in several reported cases.[87] One group of children presented with flesh-colored "micronodules" in the typical perioral dermatitis distribution. Biopsy showed granulomatous inflammation. Lesions resolved in months to years without scars.[88]

Prolonged use of fluorinated steroid creams was thought to be the primary cause when this entity was described more than 25 years ago.[89] However, in recent years, most women have denied using of such creams. Perioral dermatitis occurs in an area where drying agents are poorly tolerated; topical preparations such as benzoyl peroxide, tretinoin, and alcohol-based antibiotic lotions aggravate the eruption.

The pathogenesis is unknown. A group of authors proposed that the dermatitis is a cutaneous intolerance reaction linked to constitutionally dry skin and often accompanied by a history of mild atopic dermatitis. It is precipitated by the habitual, regular, and abundant use of moisturizing creams. This results in persistent hydration of the horny layer, impairment of barrier function, and proliferation of the skin flora.[90]

Treatment. Perioral dermatitis uniformly responds in 2 to 3 weeks to 1 gm per day of tetracycline or erythromycin.[91] Once cleared, the dosage may be stopped or tapered and discontinued in 4 to 5 weeks. Patients with renewed activity should have an additional course of antibiotics. Long-term maintenance therapy with oral antibiotics is sometimes required. The twice-daily topical application of 1% metronidazole cream (Metrogel) reduces the number of papules, but oral antibiotics are more effective.[92] Short courses of group VII nonfluorinated steroids, such as hydrocortisone, may occasionally be required to suppress erythema and scaling. Stronger steroids should be avoided. Encourage patients to discontinue or limit the use of moisturizing creams.

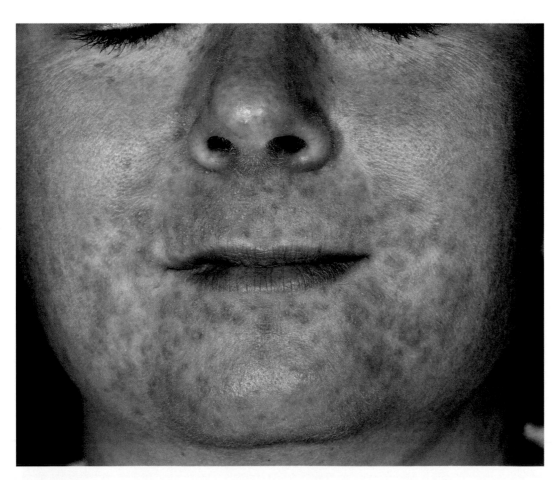

Figure 7-33
Perioral dermatitis. A florid case with numerous tiny papules and pustules located around the mouth.

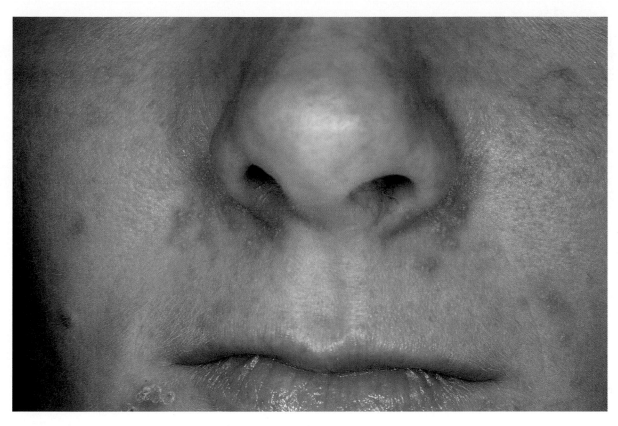

Figure 7-34
Perioral dermatitis. Pinpoint pustules next to the nostrils may be the first sign or the only manifestation of the disease.

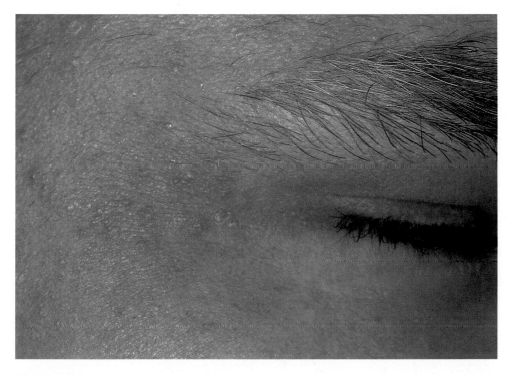

Figure 7-35
Perioral dermatitis. Pinpoint papules and pustules similar to those seen next to the nostrils are sometimes seen lateral to the eyes.

Rosacea (Acne Rosacea)

W.C. Fields drank excessively and had clusters of papules and pustules on red, swollen, telangiectatic skin of the cheeks and forehead. The red, bulbous nose completed the full-blown syndrome of active rosacea. Many patients with rosacea are defensive about their appearance and must explain to unbelieving friends that they do not imbibe. Rosacea with the same distribution and eye changes occurs in children but is rare.[93,94] The etiology is in fact unknown. Alcohol may accentuate erythema, but does not cause the disease. Sun exposure may precipitate acute episodes, but solar skin damage is not a necessary prerequisite for its development.[95] Coffee and other caffeine-containing products once topped the list of forbidden foods in the arbitrarily conceived elimination diets previously recommended as a major part of the management of rosacea. It is the heat of coffee, not its caffeine content, that leads to flushing.[96] Hot drinks of any type should be avoided. A significant increase in the hair follicle mites *Demodex folliculorum* is found in rosacea.[97,98]

One study showed that venous blood flow from the face via the emissary veins to the brain was suppressed in patients with rosacea. Therefore a functional impairment of venous flow resulting in facial vasodilation and an abnormal vascular response to heat and other stimuli may lead to a sequence of changes resulting in persistent erythema, telangiectasia, edema, and subsequent inflammatory events.[99]

Mite counts before and after a 1-month course of oral tetracycline showed no significant difference. Increased mites may play a part in the pathogenesis of rosacea by provoking inflammatory or allergic reactions, by mechanical blockage of follicles, or by acting as vectors for microorganisms.

Skin manifestations. Rosacea occurs after the age of 30 and is most common in people of Celtic origin. The resemblance to acne is at times striking. The cardinal features are erythema and edema, papules and pustules, and telangiectasia. One or all of these features may be present. The disease is chronic, lasting for years, with episodes of activity followed by quiescent periods of variable length. Eruptions appear on the forehead, cheeks, nose, and occasionally about the eyes (Figure 7-36). Most patients have some erythema, with less than 10 papules and pustules at any one time. At the other end of the spectrum are those with numerous pustules, telangiectasia, diffuse erythema, oily skin, and edema, particularly of the cheeks and nose. Granuloma formation occurs in some patients (granulomatous rosacea).[100,101] Chronic, deep inflammation of the nose leads to an irreversible hypertrophy called *rhinophyma* (Figure 7-37).[102]

Ocular rosacea. Manifestations of this disease range from minor to severe. Symptoms frequently go undiagnosed because they are too nonspecific. The prevalence in patients with rosacea is as high as 58%, with approximately 20% of those patients developing ocular symptoms before the skin lesions. A common presentation is a patient with mild conjunctivitis with soreness, grittiness, and lacrimation. Patients with ocular rosacea have been reported to have subnormal tear production (dry eyes),[103] and they frequently have complaints of burning that are out of proportion to the clinical signs of disease.[104] The reported signs are conjunctival hyperemia (86%), telangiectasia of the lid (63%), blepharitis (47%) (Figure 7-38), superficial punctate keratopathy (41%), chalazion (22%), corneal vascularization and infiltrate (16%), and corneal vascularization and thinning (10%).[105] Conjunctival epithelium is infiltrated by chronic inflammatory cells.[106]

Treatment

Oral antibiotics and isotretinoin. Both the skin and eye manifestations of rosacea respond to either tetracycline or erythromycin. One gm/day is used in divided doses. Resistant cases can be treated with 100 to 200 mg/day of minocycline or doxycycline[107] and with 200 mg of metronidazole twice daily.[108] Medication is stopped when the pustules have cleared. The response after treatment is unpredictable. Some patients clear in 2 to 4 weeks and stay in remission for weeks or months. Others flare and require long-term suppression with oral antibiotics. Treatment should be tapered to the minimum dosage that provides adequate control. Patients who remain clear should periodically be given a trial without medication. However, many patients promptly revert to the low-dose oral regimen. Isotretinoin, 0.5 mg/kg/day for 20 weeks, was effective in treating severe, refractory rosacea;[109] 85% had no relapse at the end of a year.[110]

Topical therapy. Topical metronidazole (Metrogel) is not as effective but may be used for initial treatment for mild cases or for maintenance after stopping oral antibiotics.[111] Metronidazole is not very effective in inhibiting anaerobic *P. acnes*, but it may exert its therapeutic effect by inhibiting oxidative tissue injury by neutrophils.[112] One study showed that clindamycin in a lotion base produced clinical results similar to those of oral tetracycline (250 mg four times a day for 3 weeks, then 250 mg twice a day for 9 weeks) and was superior in the eradication of pustules.[113]

Sulfacetamide/sulfur lotion (Sulfacet, Novacet) controls pustules. Sulfacet-R is flesh colored and hides redness. They are effective alone or when used with oral antibiotics.

Patients with rhinophyma may benefit from specialized procedures performed by plastic or dermatologic surgeons. These include electrosurgery,[114] carbon dioxide laser,[115] and surgery.[116] Unsightly telangiectatic vessels can be eliminated with careful electrocautery.

Patients who do not respond to antibiotics may have *Demodex folliculorum* mite infestation or tinea, in which the facial pustules and scales are usually localized to one cheek; a potassium hydroxide examination confirms the diagnosis (Figure 7-39). Crotamiton (Eurax) is reported to be effective.[117] Lindane lotion or Sulfur & Salicylic Acid soap should also be effective.

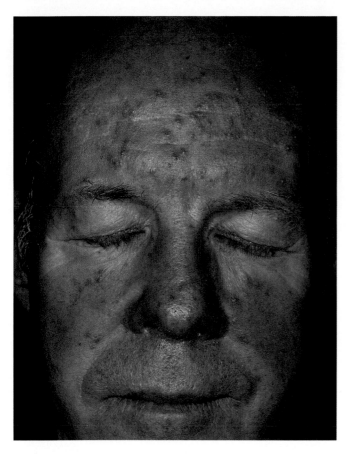

Figure 7-36
Rosacea. Pustules and erythema occur on the forehead, cheeks, and nose.

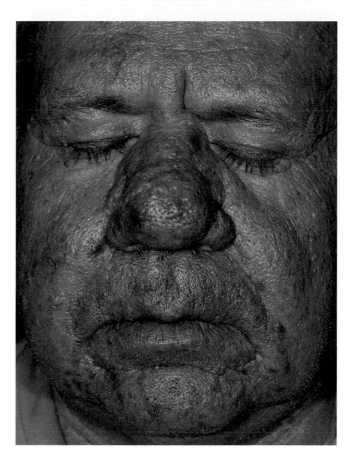

Figure 7-37
Rosacea and rhinophyma. Chronic rosacea of the nose has caused irreversible hypertrophy (rhinophyma).

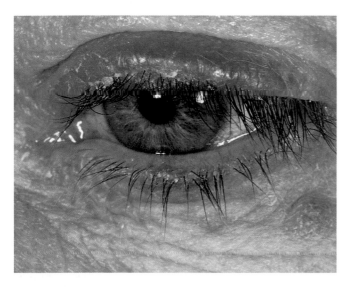

Figure 7-38
Ocular rosacea. The patient has conjunctivitis, soreness, and blepharitis.

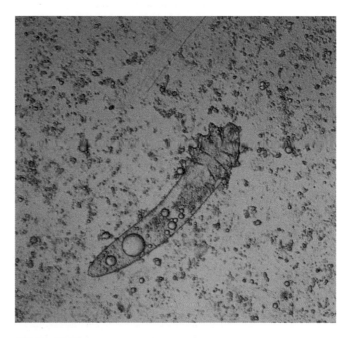

Figure 7-39
Demodex folliculorum. These mites are found as residents of human hair follicles and may be found in increased numbers in patients with rosacea.

Hidradenitis Suppurativa

Hidradenitis suppurativa is a chronic suppurative and scarring disease of the skin and subcutaneous tissue occurring in the axillae, the anogenital regions, and under the female breast (Figures 7-40 through 7-42). There is a great variation in clinical severity. Many cases, especially of the thighs and vulva, are mild and misdiagnosed as recurrent furunculosis. The disease is worse in the obese. One study reported inflammatory arthropathy in several patients with hidradenitis suppurativa and acne conglobata. Clinical and laboratory findings were similar to those seen in other seronegative spondyloarthropathies, except for the lack of association with HLA-B27.[118]

Clinical presentation. A hallmark of hidradenitis is the double comedone, a blackhead with two or sometimes several surface openings that communicate under the skin (Figure 7-42, *B*). This distinctive lesion may be present for years before other symptoms appear. Unlike acne, once the disease begins it becomes progressive and self-perpetuating. Extensive, deep, dermal inflammation results in large, painful abscesses. The healing process permanently alters the dermis. Cordlike bands of scar tissue criss-cross the axillae and groin. Reepithelialization leads to meandering, epithelial-lined sinus tracts in which foreign material and bacteria become trapped. A sinus tract may be small and misinterpreted as a cystic lesion. The course varies among individuals from an occasional cyst in the axillae to diffuse abscess formation in the inguinal region.

Pathogenesis. The pathogenesis is disputed. Some claim that, like acne, the initial event is the formation of a keratinous follicular plug, whereas others claim that apocrine duct occlusion is the primary event. Like acne, the plugged structure dilates, ruptures, becomes infected, and progresses to abscess formation, draining, and fistulous tracts. In the chronic state, secondary bacterial infection probably is a major cause of exacerbations.

The disease does not appear until after puberty, and most cases develop in the second and third decades of life. Studies show clustering in families, but inheritance patterns, if there are any, have not been established.[119] As with acne, there may be an excessive rate of conversion of androgens within the gland to a more active androgen metabolite or an exaggerated response of the gland to a given hormonal stimulus.[120]

Hidradenitis is part of the rare follicular occlusion triad syndrome of acne conglobata, hidradenitis suppurativa, and dissecting cellulitis of the scalp.[77]

Management

Antiperspirants, shaving, chemical depilatories, and talcum powder are probably not responsible for the initiation of the disease.[121] Tretinoin cream (0.05%) may prevent duct occlusion, but it is irritating and must be used only as tolerated. Large cysts should be incised and drained, whereas smaller cysts respond to intralesional injections of triamcinolone acetonide (Kenalog, 2.5 to 10 mg/ml). Weight loss helps to reduce activity.

Actively discharging lesions should be cultured. Repeated bacteriologic assessment is advisable in all cases. The laboratory should be instructed to look specifically for *Streptococcus milleri* and anaerobes and to assess sensitivity to erythromycin and tetracycline in particular.[122] Oral contraceptives do not seem to work nearly as well as they do with acne.

Antibiotics. Antibiotics are the mainstay of treatment, especially for the early stages of the disease. As with acne vulgaris, long-term oral antibiotics such as tetracycline (1 gm daily), erythromycin (1 gm daily), or minocycline (200 mg daily) may prevent disease activation. High dosages, such as 500 mg of erythromycin four times daily for an average-sized adult, are effective for active disease.

Isotretinoin. Isotretinoin (1 mg/kg/day for 20 weeks) may be effective in selected cases. The response is variable and unpredictable and complete suppression or prolonged remission is uncommon. Early cases with only inflammatory cystic lesions in which undermining sinus tracts have not developed have the best chance of being controlled,[123] but severe cases have also responded.[124,125]

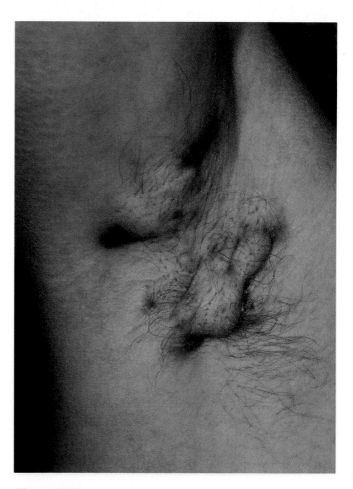

Figure 7-40
Hidradenitis suppurativa. A chronic suppurative and scarring disease occurs in the axillae, under the breast, in the groin, and on the buttocks.

Surgery. Surgical excision is at times the only solution. Residual lesions, particularly indolent sinus tracts, are a source of recurrent inflammation. Local excision is often followed by recurrence. Wide excision of affected skin, and healing by granulation[126] or applying split skin grafts or transposed or pedicle flaps, affords better control. Local recurrence after wide excision varies greatly with the disease site. The reported recurrence rates in one study were axillae (3%), inguinoperineal area (37%), and submammary area (50%). There were no recurrences in the perianal region. Treatment of the axillae by local excision and suture was found to result in a high rate (54%) of reoperation for recurrence at the same site when compared with groups treated by either wide excision and split skin grafting (13%) or excision and local flap cover (19%).[127]

HIDRADENITIS SUPPURATIVA

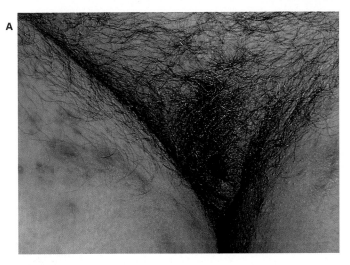

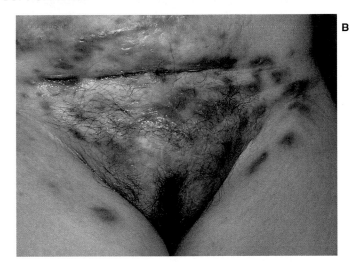

Figure 7-41

A, The buttock and anal area are inflamed with active cystic lesions.

B, Inflamed cysts have been present continuously for years.

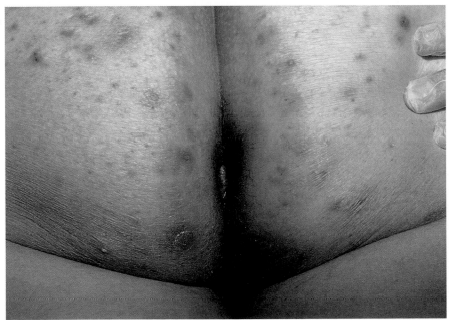

Figure 7-42

A, The disease may remain localized or involve large areas of the groin or anal area. The inflammation in this case is severe.

B, A hallmark of hidradenitis is the double and triple comedone, a blackhead with two or sometimes several surface openings that communicate under the skin.

Miliaria

Miliaria or heat rash is a common phenomenon occurring in predisposed individuals during periods of exertion or heat exposure. Eccrine sweat duct occlusion is the initial event. The duct ruptures, leaks sweat into the surrounding tissues, and induces an inflammatory response. Occlusion occurs at three different levels to produce three distinct forms of miliaria. The papular and vesicular lesions that resemble pustules of folliculitis have one major distinguishing feature: They are not follicular and therefore do not have a penetrating hair shaft. Follicular pustules are likely to be infectious, whereas nonfollicular papules, vesicles, and pustules, such as those seen in miliaria, are usually noninfectious.

MILIARIA CRYSTALLINA

In miliaria crystallina (Figure 7-43), occlusion of the eccrine duct at the skin surface results in accumulation of sweat under the stratum corneum. The sweat-filled vesicle is so near the skin surface that it appears as a clear dew drop. There is little or no erythema and the lesions are asymptomatic. The vesicles appear individually or in clusters and are most frequently seen in infants or bedridden, overheated patients. Rupture of a vesicle produces a drop of clear fluid. A cool water compress and proper ventilation are all that is necessary to treat this self-limited process.

Figure 7-43
Miliaria crystallina. Eccrine sweat duct occlusion at the skin surface results in a cluster of vesicles filled with clear fluid.

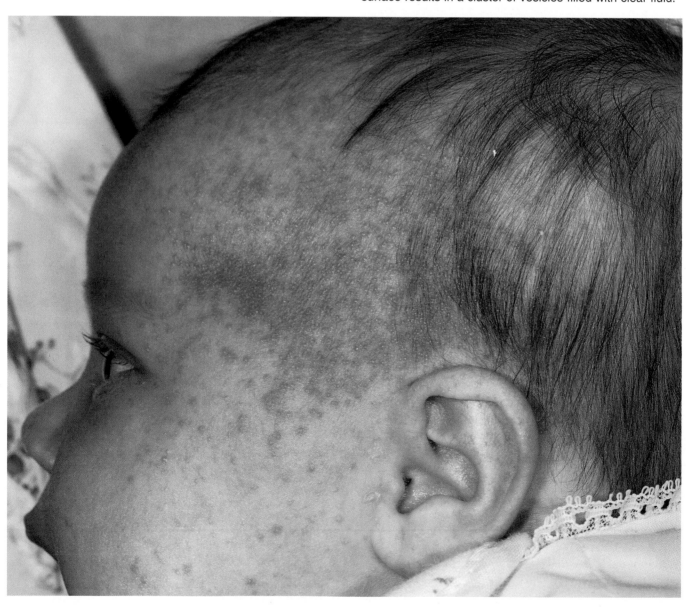

MILIARIA RUBRA

Miliaria rubra (prickly heat, heat rash) (Figure 7-44), the most common of the sweat-retention diseases, results from occlusion of the intraepidermal section of the eccrine sweat duct. Papules and vesicles surrounded by a red halo or diffuse erythema develop as the inflammatory response develops. Instead of itching, the eruption is accompanied by a stinging or "prickling" sensation. The eruption occurs underneath clothing or in areas prone to sweating after exertion or overheating; the palms and soles are spared. The disease is usually self-limited, but some patients never adapt to hot climates and must therefore make a geographic change to aid their condition.

Treatment consists of removing the patient to a cool, air-conditioned area. Frequent application of a mild antiinflammatory lotion relieves symptoms and shortens the duration of inflammation. The patient can prepare this lotion by adding the contents of a 15-gm tube of a group V steroid cream (e.g., betamethasone cream 0.1%) to 2 oz of water.

MILIARIA PROFUNDA

Miliaria profunda is observed in the tropics in patients who have had several bouts of miliaria rubra. Occlusion of the dermal section of the eccrine duct is followed by a white papular eruption.

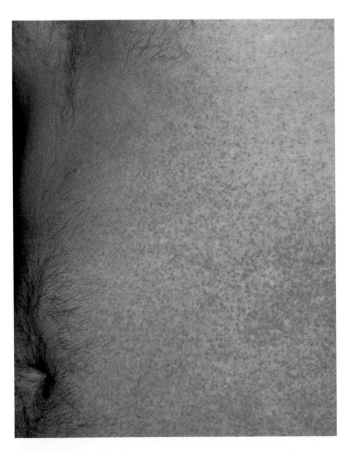

Figure 7-44
Miliaria (prickly heat). A diffuse eruption of tiny papules and vesicles occurs after exertion or overheating.

REFERENCES

1. Krowchuk DP, Stancin T, et al: The psychosocial effects of acne on adolescents, *Pediatr Dermatol* 8:332-338, 1991.
2. Korczak D: The psychological status of acne patients. Personality structure and physician-patient relations, *Fortschr Med* 107:309-313, 1989.
3. Rauch PK, Jellinek MS: Pediatric dermatology: developmental and psychological issues, *Adv Dermatol* 4:143-156, 1989.
4. Kligman AM: Postadolescent acne in women, *Cutis* 48:75-77, 1991.
5. Wu SF, Kinder BN, Trunnell TN, et al: Role of anxiety and anger in acne patients: a relationship with the severity of the disorder, *J Am Acad Dermatol* 18:325-333, 1988.
6. Hull SM, Cunliffe WJ: The use of a corticosteroid cream for immediate reduction in the clinical signs of acne vulgaris, *Acta Derm Venereol* 69:452-453, 1989.
7. Thomas JR, Doyle JA: The therapeutic uses of topical vitamin A acid, *J Am Acad Dermatol* 4:505-513, 1981.
8. Hughes BR, Norris JF, et al: A double-blind evaluation of topical isotretinoin 0.05%, benzoyl peroxide gel 5% and placebo in patients with acne, *Clin Exp Dermatol* 17:165-168, 1992.
9. Mills OH Jr, Kligman AM, Pochi P, et al: Comparing 2.5%, 5%, and 10% benzoyl peroxide on inflammatory acne vulgaris, *Int J Dermatol* 25:664-667, 1986.
10. Gratton D et al: Topical clindamycin versus systemic tetracycline in the treatment of acne: results of a multiclinic trial, *J Am Acad Dermatol* 7:50-53, 1982.
11. Norris JF, Hughes BR, et al: A comparison of the effectiveness of topical tetracycline, benzoyl-peroxide gel and oral oxytetracycline in the treatment of acne, *Clin Exp Dermatol* 16:31-33, 1991.
12. Sheehan-Dare RA, Papworth-Smith J, et al: A double-blind comparison of topical clindamycin and oral minocycline in the treatment of acne vulgaris, *Acta Derm Venereol* 70:534-537, 1990.
13. Akamatsu H, Niwa Y, et al: Effects of subminimal inhibitory concentrations of minocycline on neutrophil chemotactic factor production in comedonal bacteria, neutrophil phagocytosis and oxygen metabolism, *Arch Dermatol Res* 283:524-528, 1991.
14. Eady EA, Cove JH, et al: Erythromycin-resistant propionibacteria in antibiotic treated acne patients: association with therapeutic failure, *Br J Dermatol* 121:51-57, 1989.
15. Eady EA, Jones CE, et al: Tetracycline-resistant propionibacteria from acne patients are cross-resistant to doxycycline, but sensitive to minocycline, *Br J Dermatol* 128:556-560, 1993.
16. Ad Hoc Committee Report: Systemic antibiotics for treatment of acne vulgaris: efficacy and safety, *Arch Dermatol* 111:1630-1636, 1975.
17. Sauer GC: Safety of long-term tetracycline therapy for acne, *Arch Dermatol* 112:1603-1605, 1976.
18. Driscoll MS, Rothe MJ, et al: Long-term oral antibiotics for acne: is laboratory monitoring necessary? *J Am Acad Dermatol* 28:595, 1993.
19. Hughes BR, Murphy CE, et al: Strategy of acne therapy with long-term antibiotics, *Br J Dermatol* 121:623-628, 1989.
20. Greenwood R, Burke B, Cunliffe WJ: Evaluation of a therapeutic strategy for the treatment of acne vulgaris with conventional therapy, *Br J Dermatol* 114:353-358, 1986.
21. Rajka G: On therapeutic approaches to some special types of acne, *Acta Dermatovener* 120(suppl):39-42, 1986.
22. Humbert P, Treffel P, et al: The tetracyclines in dermatology, *J Am Acad Dermatol* 25:698-705, 1991.
23. Cunliffe WJ: Evolution of a strategy for the treatment of acne, *J Am Acad Dermatol* 16:591-599, 1987.
24. Baer RL, Leshaw SM, Shalita AR: High-dose tetracycline therapy in severe acne, *Arch Dermatol* 112:479-481, 1976.
25. Pierog SH, Al-Salihi FL, Cinotti D: Pseudotumor cerebri: a complication of tetracycline treatment of acne, *J Adolescent Health Care* 7:139-140, 1986.
26. Gammon WR et al: Comparative efficacy of oral erythromycin versus oral tetracycline in the treatment of acne vulgaris, *J Am Acad Dermatol* 14:183-186, 1986.

27. Rossman RE: Minocycline treatment of tetracycline-resistant and tetracycline-responsive acne vulgaris, *Cutis* 27:196-197, 1981.

28. Leyden JJ: Absorption of minocycline hydrochloride and tetracycline hydrochloride, *J Am Acad Dermatol* 12:308-312, 1985.

29. Basler RSW: Minocycline-related hyperpigmentation, *Arch Dermatol* 121:606-608, 1985.

30. Pepine M, Flowers FP, et al: Extensive cutaneous hyperpigmentation caused by minocycline, *J Am Acad Dermatol* 28:295-297, 1993.

31. Poliak SC et al: Minocycline-associated tooth discoloration in young adults, *JAMA* 254:2930-2932, 1985.

32. Laux B: Treatment of acne vulgaris. A comparison of doxycycline versus minocycline, *Hautarzt* 40:577-581, 1989.

33. Christian GL, Krueger GG: Clindamycin vs placebo as adjunctive therapy in moderately severe acne, *Arch Dermatol* 111:997-1000, 1975.

34. Leyden JJ et al: Gram-negative folliculitis: a complication of antibiotic therapy in acne vulgaris, *Br J Dermatol* 88:583, 1973.

35. Shore RN: Usefulness of ampicillin in treatment of acne vulgaris, *J Am Acad Dermatol* 9:604-605, 1983.

36. Sheeler RD: Cephalosporin for acne vulgaris, *J Am Acad Dermatol* 14:1091, 1986.

37. Nordin K, Hallander H, Fredriksson T, et al: A clinical and bacteriological evaluation of the effect of sulfamethoxazole trimethoprim in acne vulgaris, resistant to prior therapy with tetracyclines, *Dermatologica* 157:245-253, 1978.

38. Noto G, Arico M, et al: Ovulatory patterns in women with juvenile and late-onset/persistent acne vulgaris, *Acta Eur Fertil* 21:293-296, 1990.

39. Bunker CB, Newton JA, et al: Most women with acne have polycystic ovaries, *Br J Dermatol* 121:675-680, 1989.

40. Redmond GP, Bergfeld WF: Treatment of androgenic disorders in women: acne, hirsutism, and alopecia, *Cleve Clin J Med* 57:428-432, 1990.

41. Nader S, Rodriguez-Rigau LJ, Smith KD, et al: Acne and hyperandrogenism: impact of lowering androgen levels with glucocorticoid treatment, *J Am Acad Dermatol* 11:256-259, 1984.

42. An open study of Triphasil and Diane 50 in the treatment of acne, *Australas J Dermatol* 32(1):51-54, 1991.

43. Dickey RP: *Managing contraceptive pill patients,* ed 4, Creative Infomatics, Inc., PO Box 1607, Durant, OK 74702-1607.

43a. Miller DM et al: A practical approach to antibiotic treatment in women taking oral contraceptives, *J Am Acad Dermatol* 30:1008-1011, 1994.

44. Goodfellow A, Alaghband-Zadeh, et al: Oral spironolactone improves acne vulgaris and reduces sebum excretion, *Br J Dermatol* 111:209-214, 1984.

45. Burke BM, Cunliffe WJ: Oral spironolactone therapy for female patients with acne, hirsutism or androgenic alopecia, *Br J Dermatol* 112:124-125, 1985.

46. Fugere P, Percival-Smith RK, et al: Cyproterone acetate/ethinyl estradiol in the treatment of acne. A comparative dose-response study of the estrogen component, *Contraception* 42:225-234, 1990.

47. Hull SM, Cunliffe WJ, et al: Treatment of the depressed and dysmorphophobic acne patient, *Clin Exp Dermatol* 16:210-211, 1991.

48. Lehucher-Ceyrac D, Weber-Buisset MJ: Isotretinoin and acne in practice: a prospective analysis of 188 cases over 9 years, *Dermatology* 186:123-128, 1993.

49. Layton AM, Cunliffe WJ: Guidelines for optimal use of isotretinoin in acne, *J Am Acad Dermatol* 27:S2-S7, 1992.

50. Falk ES, Stenvold SE: Long-term effects of isotretinoin in the treatment of severe nodulocystic acne, *Riv Eur Sci Med Farmacol* 14:215-220, 1992.

51. Cunliffe WJ, Layton A, Knaggs HE, et al: Isotretinoin and acne: a long-term study. In Saurat J-H, editor: *Retinoids: 10 years on*, Basel, 1991, S Karger.

52. Strauss JS, Stranier AM: Changes in long-term sebum production from isotretinoin therapy, *J Am Acad Dermatol* 6:751-755, 1982.

53. Chivot M, Midoun H: Isotretinoin and acne—a study of relapses, *Dermatologica* 180:240-243, 1990.

54. Cunliffe WJ, Norris JFB: Isotretinoin: an explanation for its long-term benefit, *Dermatologica* 175(suppl 1):133-137, 1987.

55. Myhill JE, Leichtman SR, Burnett JW: Self-esteem and social assertiveness in patients receiving isotretinoin treatment for cystic acne, *Cutis* 41:171-173, 1988.

56. Rubinow DR, Peck GL, Squillace KM, et al: Reduced anxiety and depression in cystic acne patients after successful treatment with oral isotretinoin, *J Am Acad Dermatol* 17:25-32, 1987.

57. Lammer EJ et al: Retinoic acid embryopathy, *N Engl J Med* 313:837-841, 1985.

58. Dai WS, La Braico JM, et al: Epidemiology of isotretinoin exposure during pregnancy, *J Am Acad Dermatol* 26:599-606, 1992.

59. Dai WS, Hsu MA, et al: Safety of pregnancy after discontinuation of isotretinoin, *Arch Dermatol* 125:362-365, 1989.

60. Hoting VE, Schutte B, et al: Isotretinoin treatment of acne conglobata. Andrologic follow-up, *Fortschr Med* 110:427-430, 1992.

61. Walker BR, Mac Kie RM: Serum lipid elevation during isotretinoin therapy for acne in the west of Scotland, *Br J Dermatol* 122:531-537, 1990.

62. McElwee NE, Schumacher MC, et al: An observational study of isotretinoin recipients treated for acne in a health maintenance organization, *Arch Dermatol* 127:341-346, 1991.

63. Bershad S et al: Changes in plasma lipids and lipoproteins during isotretinoin therapy for acne, *N Engl J Med* 313:981-985, 1985.

64. Tangrea JA, Kilcoyne RF, et al: Skeletal hyperostosis in patients receiving chronic, very-low-dose isotretinoin, *Arch Dermatol* 128:921-925, 1992.

65. Ellis CN et al: Long-term radiographic follow-up after isotretinoin therapy, *J Am Acad Dermatol* 18:1252-1261, 1988.

66. Kilcoyne RF et al: Minimal spinal hyperostosis with low-dose isotretinoin therapy, *Invest Radiol* 21:41-44, 1986.

67. Oikarinen A, Vuori J, et al: Comparison of muscle-derived serum carbonic anhydrase III and myoglobin in dermatological patients: effects of isotretinoin treatment, *Acta Derm Venereol* 72:352-354, 1992.

68. Pepall LM, Cosgrove MP, Cunliffe WJ: Ablation of white-heads by cautery under topical anesthesia, *Br J Dermatol* 125:256-259, 1991.

69. Zelickson AS, Mottaz JH: Pigmentation of open comedones, *Arch Dermatol* 119:567-569, 1983.

70. Plewig G, Kligman AM: *Acne: morphogenesis and treatment*, Berlin, 1975, Springer-Verlag.

71. Plewig G, Jansen T, et al: Pyoderma faciale. A review and report of 20 additional cases: is it rosacea? *Arch Dermatol* 128:1611-1617, 1992.

72. Massa MC, Daniel WP: Pyoderma faciale: a clinical study of twenty-nine patients, *J Am Acad Dermatol* 6:85-91, 1982.

73. Wong SS, Pritchard MH, et al: Familial acne fulminans, *Clin Exp Dermatol* 17:351-353, 1992.

74. Reunala T, Pauli S-L, Rasasen L. Musculoskeletal symptoms and bone lesions in acne fulminans, *J Am Acad Dermatol* 22:144-146, 1990.

75. Jemec G BE, Rasmussen I: Bone lesions of acne fulminans, *J Am Acad Dermatol* 20:353-357, 1989.

76. Karvonen S-L: Acne fulminans: report of clinical findings and treatment of twenty-four patients, *J Am Acad Dermatol* 28:572, 1993.

77. Chicarilli ZN: Follicular occlusion triad: hidradenitis suppurativa, acne conglobata, and dissecting cellulitis of the scalp, *Ann Plast Surg* 18:230-237, 1987.

78. Knitzer RH, Neekleman BW: Musculoskeletal syndromes associated with acne, *Semin Arth Rheum* 20:247-255, 1991.

79. James WD, Leyden JJ: Treatment of gram-negative folliculitis with isotretinoin: positive clinical and microbiologic response, *J Am Acad Dermatol* 12:319-324, 1985.

80. Mostafa WZ: *Citrobacter freundii* in gram-negative folliculitis, *J Am Acad Dermatol* 20:504-505, 1989.

81. Plewig G, Nikolowski J, Wolff HH: Action of isotretinoin in acne rosacea and gram-negative folliculitis, *J Am Acad Dermatol* 6:766-785, 1982.

82. Hitch JM: Acneiform eruptions induced by drugs and chemicals, *JAMA* 200:879, 1967.

83. Hurwitz RM: Steroid acne, *J Am Acad Dermatol* 21:1179-1181, 1989.

84. Bond GG, McLaren EA, et al: Incidence of chloracne among chemical workers potentially exposed to chlorinated dioxins, *J Occup Med* 31:771-774, 1989.

85. Mohs FE, McCall MW, Greenway HT: Curettage for removal of the comedones and cysts of the Favre-Racouchot syndrome, *Arch Dermatol* 118:365-366, 1982.

86. Jungfer B, Jansen T, et al: Solid persistent facial edema of acne: successful treatment with isotretinoin and ketotifen, *Dermatology* 187:34-37, 1993.

87. Manders SM, Lucky AW: Perioral dermatitis in childhood, *J Am Acad Dermatol* 27:688-692, 1992.

88. Fricden IJ, Prose NS, et al: Granulomatous perioral dermatitis in children, *Arch Dermatol* 125:369-373, 1989.

89. Wells K, Brodell RT: Topical corticosteroid 'addiction.' A cause of perioral dermatitis, *Postgrad Med* 93:225-230, 1993.

90. Fritsch P, Pichler E, et al: Perioral dermatitis, *Hautarzt* 40:475, 1989.

91. Sneddon IB: Treatment of steroid-induced rosacea and perioral dermatitis, *Dermatologica* 152(suppl 1):231, 1976.

92. Veien NK, Munkvad JM, et al: Topical metronidazole in the treatment of perioral dermatitis, *J Am Acad Dermatol* 24:258-260, 1991.

93. Drolet B, Paller AS: Childhood rosacea, *Pediatr Dermatol* 9:22-26, 1992.

94. Erzurum SA, Feder RS, et al: Acne rosacea with keratitis in childhood, *Arch Ophthalmol* 111:228-230, 1993.

95. Dupont C: The role of sunshine in rosacea, *J Am Acad Dermatol* 15:713-714, 1986.

96. Wilkin JK: Oral thermal-induced flushing in erythematotelangiectatic rosacea, *J Invest Dermatol* 76:15-18, 1981.

97. Bonnar E, Eustace P, et al: The *Demodex* mite population in rosacea, *J Am Acad Dermatol* 28:443-448, 1993.

98. Sibenge S, Gawkrodger DJ: Rosacea: a study of clinical patterns, blood flow, and the role of *Demodex folliculorum*, *J Am Acad Dermatol* 26:590-593, 1992.

99. Brinnel H, Friedel J, et al: Rosacea: disturbed defense against brain overheating, *Arch Dermatol Res* 281:66-72, 1989.

100. Helm KF, Menz J, et al: A clinical and histopathologic study of granulomatous rosacea, *J Am Acad Dermatol* 25:1038-1043, 1991.

101. Patrinely JR, Font RL, et al: Granulomatous acne rosacea of the eyelids, *Arch Ophthalmol* 108:561-563, 1990.

102. Black AA, McCauliffe DP, et al: Prevalence of acne rosacea in a rheumatic skin disease subspecialty clinic, *Lupus* 1:229-237, 1992.

103. Gudmundsen KJ, O'Donnell BF, et al: Schirmer testing for dry eyes in patients with rosacea, *J Am Acad Dermatol* 26:211-214, 1992.

104. Browning DJ, Proia AD: Ocular rosacea, *Surv Ophthalmol* 31:145-158, 1986.

105. Jenkins MA, Brown SI, Lempert SL, et al: Ocular rosacea, *Am J Ophthalmol* 88:618-622, 1979.

106. Hoang-Xuan T, Rodriguez A, et al: Ocular rosacea. A histologic and immunopathologic study, *Ophthalmology* 97:1468-1475, 1990.

107. Frucht-Pery J, Sagi E, et al: Efficacy of doxycycline and tetracycline in ocular rosacea, *Am J Ophthalmol* 116:88-92, 1993.

108. Nielsen PG: Metronidazole treatment in rosacea, *Int J Dermatol* 27:1-5, 1988 (review).

109. Hoting E, Paul E, Plewig G: Treatment of rosacea with isotretinoin, *Int J Dermatol* 25:660-663, 1986.

110. Turjanmaa K, Reunala T: Isotretinoin treatment of rosacea, *Acta Derm Venereol* 67:89-91, 1987.

111. Bleicher PA, Charles JH, Sober AJ: Topical metronidazole therapy for rosacea, *Arch Dermatol* 123:609-614, 1987.

112. Akamatsu H, Oguchi M, et al: The inhibition of free radical generation by human neutrophils through the synergistic effects of metronidazole with palmitoleic acid: a possible mechanism of action of metronidazole in rosacea and acne, *Arch Dermatol Res* 282:449-454, 1990.

113. Wilkin JK, De Witt S: Treatment of rosacea: topical clindamycin versus oral tetracycline, *Int J Dermatol* 32:65-67, 1993.

114. Clark DP, Hanke CW: Electrosurgical treatment of rhinophyma, *J Am Acad Dermatol* 22:831-837, 1990.

115. Haas A, Wheeland RG: Treatment of massive rhinophyma with the carbon dioxide laser, *J Dermatol Surg Oncol* 16:645-649, 1990.

116. Lloyd KM: Surgical correction of rhinophyma, *Arch Dermatol* 126:721-723, 1990.

117. Shelley WB, Shelley ED, et al: Unilateral demodectic rosacea, *J Am Acad Dermatol* 20:915-917, 1989.

118. Rosner IA, Burg CG, et al: The clinical spectrum of the arthropathy associated with hidradenitis suppurativa and acne conglobata, *J Rheumatol* 20:684-687, 1993.

119. Fitzsimmons JS, Guilbert PR, Fitzsimmons EM: Evidence of genetic factors in hidradenitis suppurativa, *Br J Derm* 113:1-8, 1985.

120. Mortimer PS, Dawber RPR, Gales MA, et al: Mediation of hidradenitis suppurativa by androgens, *Br Med J* 292:245-248, 1986.

121. Morgan WP, Leicester G: The role of depilation and deodorants in hidradenitis suppurativa, *Arch Dermatol* 118:101-102, 1982.

122. Highet AS, Warren RE, Weekes AJ: Bacteriology and antibiotic treatment of perineal suppurative hidradenitis, *Arch Dermatol* 124:1047-1051, 1988.

123. Dicken CH, Powell ST, Spear KL: Evaluation of isotretinoin treatment of hidradenitis suppurativa, *J Am Acad Dermatol* 11:500-502, 1984.

124. Shalita AR et al: Isotretinoin treatment of acne and related disorders: an update, *J Am Acad Dermatol* 9:629-638, 1983.

125. Brown CF, Gallup DG, Brown VM: Hidradenitis suppurativa of the anogenital region: response to isotretinoin, *Am J Obstet Gynecol* 158:12-15, 1988.

126. Banerjee AK: Surgical treatment of hidradenitis suppurativa, *Br J Surg* 79:863-868, 1992.

127. Harrison BJ, Mudge M, Hughes LE: Recurrence after surgical treatment of hidradenitis suppurativa, *Br Med J* 294:487-489, 1987.

CHAPTER EIGHT

Psoriasis and Other Papulosquamous Diseases

Papulosquamous diseases are a group of disorders characterized by scaly papules and plaques. These entities have little in common except the clinical characteristics of their primary lesion. A complete list of diseases characterized by scaly plaques appears in the section on primary lesions in Chapter One. The major papulosquamous diseases are described here.

Psoriasis

Psoriasis occurs in 1% to 3% of the population worldwide. The disease is transmitted genetically, most likely with a dominant mode with variable penetrance; the origin is unknown. The disease is lifelong and characterized by chronic, recurrent exacerbations and remissions that are emotionally and physically debilitating. Men and women are equally affected.

There may be many millions of people with the potential to develop psoriasis, with only the correct combination of environmental factors needed to precipitate the disease. Stress, for example, may precipitate an episode.[1] Environmental influences may modify the course, severity, and age of the individual at the time of the onset of the disease. Extent and severity of the disease vary widely. Psoriasis frequently begins in childhood, when the first episode may be stimulated by streptococcal pharyngitis (as in guttate psoriasis).

"The heartbreak of psoriasis." Psoriasis for most patients is more emotionally than physically disabling. Psoriasis erodes the self-image and forces the victim into a life of concealment and self-conciousness. Patients may avoid activities, including sunbathing, the very activity that can clear the disease, for fear of being discovered.[2] Therefore, even when a patient has only a few asymptomatic, chronic plaques, the disease is more serious than it appears.

CLINICAL MANIFESTATIONS

The lesions of psoriasis are distinctive. They begin as red, scaling papules that coalesce to form round-to-oval plaques, which can easily be distinguished from the surrounding normal skin (Figure 8-1). The scale is adherent, silvery white, and reveals bleeding points when removed (Auspitz's sign). Scale may become extremely dense, especially on the scalp. Scale forms but is macerated and dispersed in intertriginous areas; therefore the psoriatic plaques of skin folds appear only as smooth, red plaques with a macerated surface. The most common site for an intertriginous plaque is the intergluteal fold; this is referred to as *gluteal pinking* (Figure 8-2). The deep rich red color is another characteristic feature and remains constant in all areas.

Psoriasis can develop at the site of physical trauma (scratching, sunburn, or surgery), the so-called isomorphic or Köebner's phenomenon (Figure 8-3; see also Figures 8-8 and 8-10). Pruritus is highly variable. Although psoriasis can affect any cutaneous surface, certain areas are favored and should be examined in all patients in whom the diagnosis of psoriasis is suspected. Those areas are the elbows, knees, scalp, gluteal cleft, fingernails, and toenails.

The disease affects the extensor more than the flexor surfaces and usually spares the palms, soles, and face. Most patients have chronic localized disease, but there are several other presentations. Localized plaques may be confused with eczema or seborrheic dermatitis, and the guttate form with many small lesions can resemble secondary syphilis or pityriasis rosea.

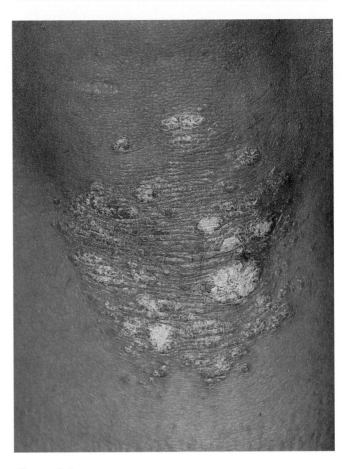

Figure 8-1
Psoriasis. Typical oval plaque with well-defined borders and silvery scale.

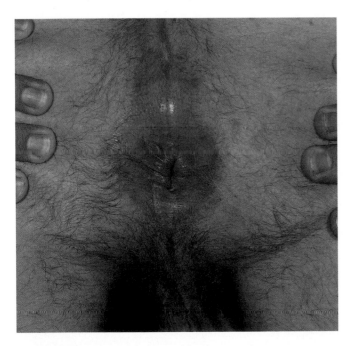

Figure 8-2
Psoriasis. Gluteal pinking, a common lesion in patients with psoriasis. Intertriginous psoriatic plaques retain the rich red color typical of skin lesions but do not retain scale.

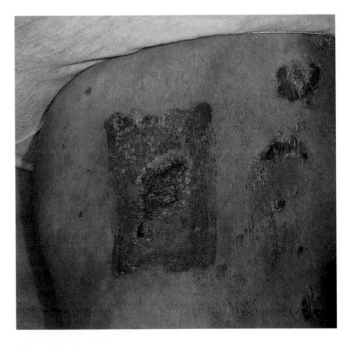

Figure 8-3
Psoriasis. Köebner's phenomenon. Psoriasis has appeared on the donor site of the skin graft.

Drugs that precipitate or exacerbate psoriasis

Lithium. Exacerbation of preexisting psoriasis during lithium treatment is well documented, but preexisting psoriasis is not a general contraindication to lithium treatment.[3] The disease does not worsen in many lithium-treated patients. Lithium dosage reduction or more intensive psoriasis treatment is indicated when lithium must be continued.

Beta-blocking agents. Beta-blockers may worsen psoriasis and should be carefully evaluated in the management of these patients.[4]

Antimalarials. Exfoliative dermatitis and exacerbation of psoriasis is reported in psoriatic patients treated with antimalarials,[5] but the incidence is low. Antimalarials are not contraindicated in psoriasis patients who need prophylactic treatment for malaria.[6]

Systemic steroids. Systemic steroids rapidly clear psoriasis; unfortunately, in many instances the disease worsens, occasionally evolving into pustular psoriasis, when corticosteroids are withdrawn.[7] For this reason systemic corticosteroids have been abandoned as a routine treatment for psoriasis.

HISTOLOGY

The psoriatic epidermis contains a large number of mitoses. There is epidermal hyperplasia and scale, the final product of the abnormally functioning epidermis. The dermis contains enlarged and tortuous capillaries that are very close to the skin surface and impart a characteristic erythematous hue to the lesions. Bleeding occurs (Auspitz's sign) when the capillaries are ruptured as scale is removed.

CLINICAL PRESENTATIONS

Variations in the morphology of psoriasis are listed here.

Chronic plaque psoriasis
Guttate psoriasis (acute eruptive psoriasis)
Pustular psoriasis
Erythrodermic psoriasis
Light-sensitive psoriasis
HIV-induced psoriasis
Keratoderma blenorrhagicum (Reiter's syndrome)

Variations in the location of psoriasis are listed here.

Scalp psoriasis
Psoriasis of the palms and soles
Pustular psoriasis of the palms and soles
Pustular psoriasis of the digits
Psoriasis inversus (psoriasis of flexural areas)
Psoriasis of the penis and Reiter's syndrome
Nail psoriasis
Psoriatic arthritis

Chronic plaque psoriasis. Chronic, noninflammatory, well-defined plaques are the most common presentation of psoriasis. Lesions can appear anywhere on the cutaneous surface. They enlarge to a certain size and then tend to remain stable for months or years (Figure 8-4). A temporary brown, white, or red macule remains when the plaque subsides.

Guttate psoriasis. More than 30% of psoriatic patients have their first episode before age 20; in many instances, an episode of guttate psoriasis is the first indication of the patient's propensity for the disease. Streptococcal pharyngitis or a viral upper respiratory infection may precede the eruption by 1 or 2 weeks.[8] Scaling papules suddenly appear on the trunk and extremities, not including the palms and soles (Figure 8-5, *A* and *B*). Their number ranges from a few to many, and their size may be that of a pinpoint up to 1 cm. Lesions increase in diameter with time. The scalp and face may also be involved. Pruritus is variable. Guttate psoriasis may resolve spontaneously in weeks or months; it responds more readily to treatment than does chronic plaque psoriasis. Throat cultures should be taken to rule out streptococcal infection. There is a high incidence of positive antistreptolysin O titers in this group.

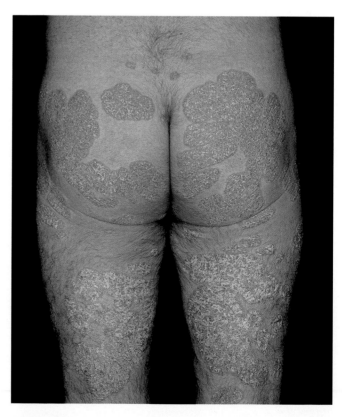

Figure 8-4
Chronic plaque psoriasis. Noninflamed plaques tend to remain fixed in position for months.

Figure 8-5 Guttate Psoriasis.

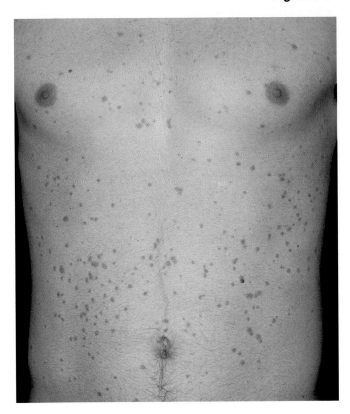

A, Numerous, uniformly small lesions may abruptly occur following streptococcal pharyngitis.

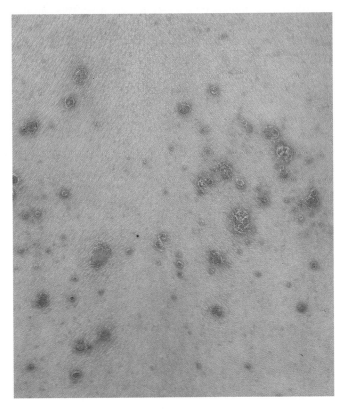

B, Numerous pinpoint to 1-cm lesions develop typical psoriatic scale soon after appearance.

Generalized pustular psoriasis. This rare form of psoriasis (also called *von Zumbusch psoriasis*) is a serious and sometimes fatal disease. Erythema suddenly appears in the flexural areas and migrates to other body surfaces. Numerous tiny, sterile pustules evolve from an erythematous base and coalesce into lakes of pus (Figure 8-6). The superficial, upper epidermal pustules are easily ruptured. The patient is toxic, febrile, and has leukocytosis. Topical medications such as tar and anthralin may precipitate episodes in patients with unstable or labile psoriasis. Withdrawal of both topical and systemic steroids has precipitated flares. Relapses are common. Wet dressings and group V topical steroids provide initial control. Systemic therapy may be necessary for severe cases. Etretinate yields rapid control. Methotrexate and cyclosporine are also effective.[9]

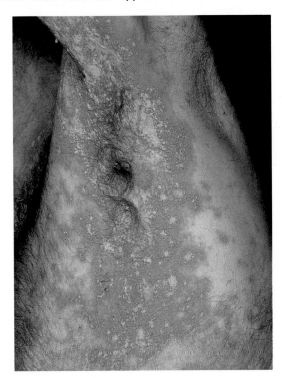

Figure 8-6
Generalized pustular psoriasis. An erythematous plaque has evolved into numerous sterile pustules, which have coalesced in many areas.

Erythrodermic psoriasis. Generalized erythrodermic psoriasis, like generalized pustular psoriasis, is a severe, unstable, highly labile disease that may appear as the initial manifestation of psoriasis but usually occurs in patients with previous chronic disease (Figure 8-7). Precipitating factors include the administration of systemic corticosteroids; the excessive use of topical steroids; overzealous, irritating topical therapy; phototherapy complications; severe emotional stress; and preceding illness, such as an infection. Treatment includes bed rest, initial avoidance of all UV light, Burow's solution compresses, colloidal oatmeal baths, the liberal use of emollients, increased protein and fluid intake, antihistamines for pruritus, avoidance of potent topical steroids, and, in severe cases, hospitalization.[10] Methotrexate or etretinate is used if rapid control is not obtained with conservative topical therapy. Tar and anthralin may exacerbate the disease and should be avoided.

Light-sensitive psoriasis. Psoriatic patients wait for sunny summer months when, in most cases, the disease responds predictably to ultraviolet light. However, too much of a good thing can be dangerous, especially for the patient who gets sunburned in an anxious attempt to clear the disease rapidly. As a result of Köebner's phenomenon, guttate lesions or a painful, diffusely inflamed plaque forms in the burned areas (Figure 8-8). Plaques subsequently converge onto the clear, previously protected sites. Some psoriatic patients do not tolerate ultraviolet light of any intensity.

Psoriasis of the scalp. The scalp is a favored site for psoriasis and may be the only site affected. Plaques are similar to those of the skin except that the scale is more readily retained; it is anchored by hair. Extension of the plaques onto the forehead is relatively common (Figure 8-9). A dense, tight-feeling scale can cover the entire scalp. Even in the most severe cases, the hair is not permanently lost. A distinct scaling eruption of the scalp observed in children is described in this chapter in the section concerning seborrheic dermatitis.

Psoriasis of the palms and soles. The palms and soles may be involved as part of a generalized eruption, or they may be the only locations involved in the manifestation of the disease. There are several presentations. Superficial red plaques with thick brown scale may be indistinguishable from chronic eczema (Figure 8-10). Smooth, deep red plaques are similar to those found in the flexural area (Figure 8-11).

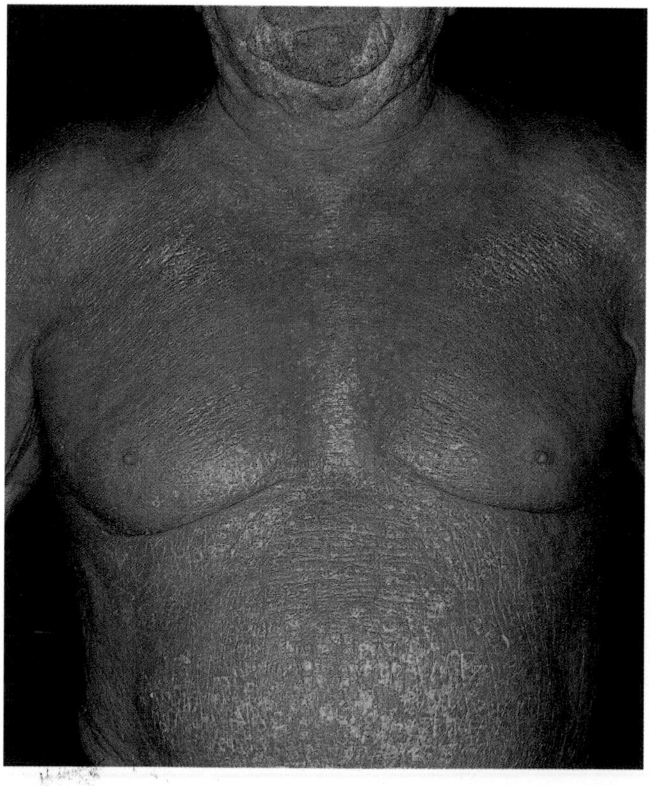

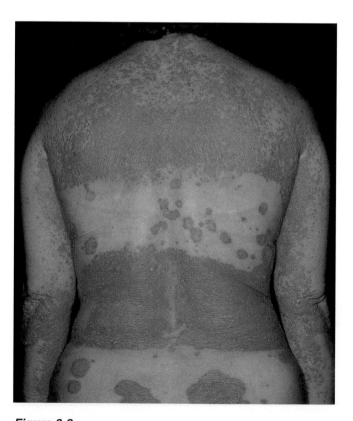

Figure 8-7
Psoriatic erythroderma. Generalized erythema occurred shortly after this patient discontinued use of methotrexate.

Figure 8-8
Light-induced psoriasis. Overexposure to sunlight precipitated this diffuse flare of psoriasis. The mid back was protected by a wide halter strap.

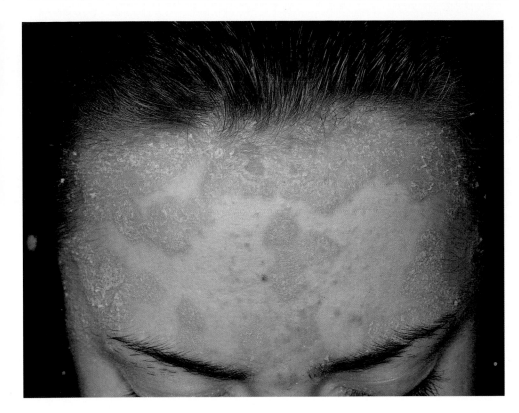

Figure 8-9
Psoriasis of the scalp. Plaques typically form in the scalp and along the hair margin. Occasionally plaques occur on the face.

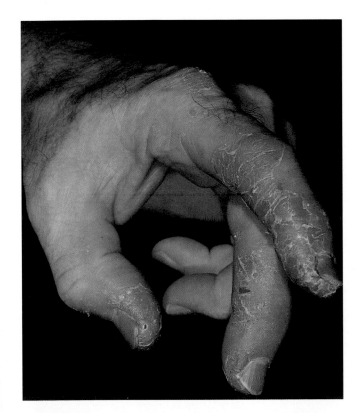

Figure 8-10
Psoriasis of the fingertips. The eruption appears eczematous, but the rich red hue is typical of psoriasis. This eruption occurred as a Köebner's phenomenon in a surgeon.

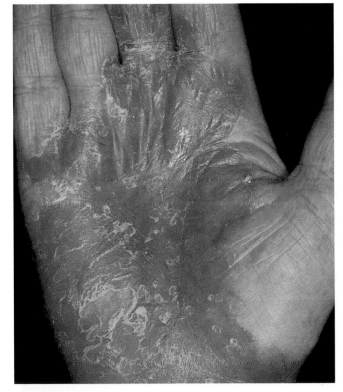

Figure 8-11
Psoriasis of the hand. Deep red, smooth plaque in a patient with typical lesions on the body.

Pustular psoriasis of the palms and soles. Deep pustules first appear on the middle portion of the palms and insteps of the soles; they may either remain localized or spread (Figure 8-12, *A* and *B*). The pustules do not rupture but turn dark brown and scaly as they reach the surface. The surrounding skin becomes pink, smooth, and tender. A thick crust may later cover the affected area. The course is chronic, lasting for years while the patient endures periods of partial remission followed by exacerbations so painful that mobility is affected. There is a considerably higher prevalence of smoking in these patients.[11] Etretinate, methotrexate, PUVA (psoralen ultraviolet light A), and intermittent courses of topical steroids under plastic occlusions are therapeutic alternatives.

Keratoderma blenorrhagicum (Reiter's syndrome). Reiter's syndrome appears to be a reactive immune response that is usually triggered in a genetically susceptible individual (60% to 90% of patients are HLA-B27 positive) by any of several different infections, especially those that cause dysentery or urethritis, such as *Yersinia enterocolitica* and *Y. pseudotuberculosis*. Patients with Reiter's syndrome (urethritis and/or cervicitis, peripheral arthritis of more than 1 month's duration) develop psoriasiform skin lesions usually 1 to 2 months after the onset of arthritis; 25% develop conjunctivitis. The distinctive lesions, keratoderma blenorrhagica, typically appear on the soles (Figure 8-13, *A*) and extend onto the toes (Figure 8-13, *B*) but also occur on the legs, scalp, and hands. Nail dystrophy, thickening, and destruction occur. The plaques are psoriasiform with a distinctive circular, scaly border. The scaly, scalloped-edged plaques develop from coalescence of expanding papulovesicular plaques with thickened yellow, heaped-up scale. Similar lesions occur on the penis. Skin and joint symptoms have responded to methotrexate, etretinate,[12] and ketoconazole.[13]

Psoriasis of the penis and Reiter's syndrome. Typical psoriatic scaling plaques with white scale can appear on the circumcised penis (Figure 8-14). Scale does not form when the penis is covered by a foreskin. A highly characteristic psoriasiform lesion, balanitis circinata, occurs in Reiter's syndrome when erosions covered by scale and crust on the corona and glans coalesce to form a distinctive winding pattern (Figure 8-15). A biopsy helps confirm the diagnosis. A KOH examination excludes *Candida*.

Figure 8-12 Pustular psoriasis of the soles.

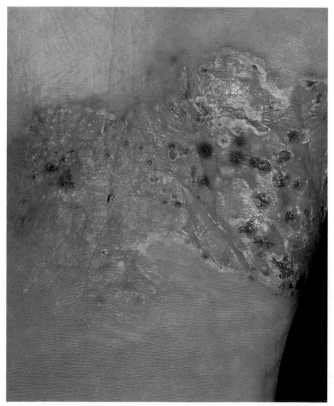

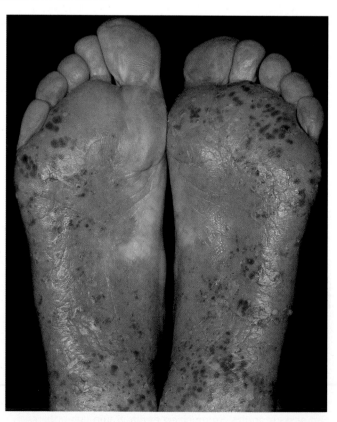

A, An early case in a typical location.

B, This is a chronic disease in which the soles may remain inflamed for years.

Figure 8-13 Keratoderma blenorrhagicum (Reiter's syndrome).

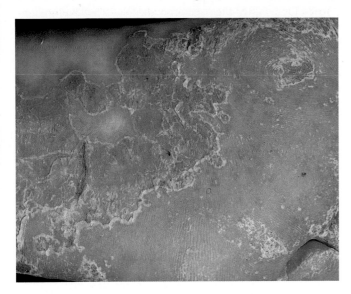

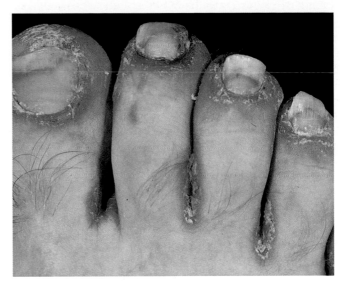

A, Patients with Reiter's syndrome develop psoriasiform skin lesions (keratoderma blenorrhagica) with a distinctive circular, scaly border. These distinctive lesions occur most frequently on the soles and toes.

B, Psoriasiform plaques develop from coalescence of expanding papulovesicular plaques and are typically found on the soles and toes.

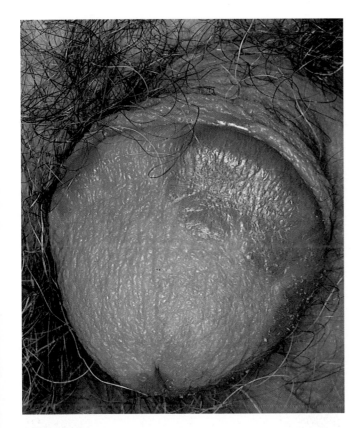

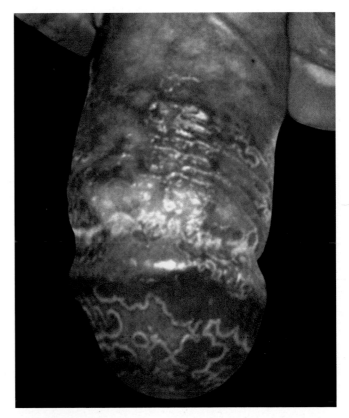

Figure 8-14
Psoriasis. Typical psoriatic scaling plaques with white scale can appear on the circumcised penis. Scale does not form when the penis is covered by a foreskin.

Figure 8-15
Reiter's syndrome. A highly characteristic psoriasiform lesion, balanitis circinata, occurs in Reiter's syndrome when erosions covered by scale and crust on the corona and glans coalesce to form a distinctive winding pattern.

Pustular psoriasis of the digits. This severe localized variant of psoriasis, also known as acrodermatitis continua, may remain localized to one finger for years. Vesicles rupture, resulting in a tender, diffusely eroded, and fissured surface that continually exudes serum. The loosely adherent, moist crust is easily shed, but recurs (Figure 8-16). Localized pustular psoriasis is very resistant to therapy.

Psoriasis inversus (psoriasis of the flexural or intertriginous areas). The gluteal fold, axillae, groin, submammary folds, retroauricular fold, and the glans of the uncircumcised penis may be affected. The deep red, smooth, glistening plaques may extend to and stop at the junction of the skin folds, as with intertrigo or candida infections. The surface is moist and contains macerated white debris. Infection, friction, and heat may induce flexural psoriasis, a Köebner's phenomenon. Cracking and fissures are common at the base of the crease, particularly in the groin, gluteal cleft, and superior and posterior auricular fold (Figure 8-17). As with typical psoriatic plaques, the margin is distinct. Pustules beyond the plaque border suggest secondary yeast infection. Infants and young children may develop flexural psoriasis of the groin that extends onto the diaper area.

HIV-induced psoriasis. Psoriasis may be the first or one of the first signs of acquired immunodeficiency syndrome (AIDS). Psoriasis in the setting of HIV disease may be mild, moderate, or severe.[14] It can be atypical and unusually severe with involvement of the groin, axilla, scalp, palms, and soles. An explosive onset with erythroderma or pustular lesions that rapidly become confluent should lead one to suspect AIDS. The disease is difficult to treat. PUVA, ultraviolet light B, and topical steroids are immunosuppressive and should be avoided. It is not clear that use of methotrexate adversely affects the natural course of HIV disease.[15] Etretinate is the drug of choice for severe disease. Zidovudine is effective and cleared an etretinate-resistant case.[16]

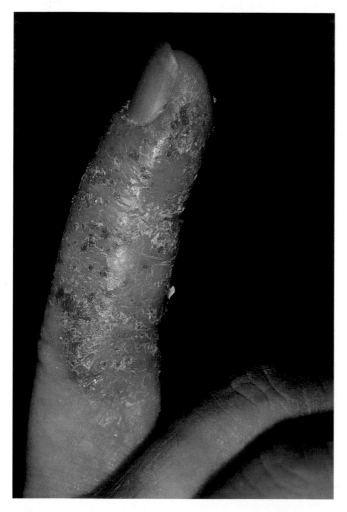

Figure 8-16
Pustular psoriasis of the digits. The eruption has remained localized in this one finger for years.

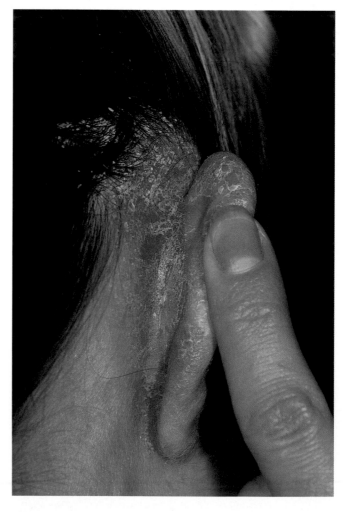

Figure 8-17
Psoriasis of the posterior auricular fold.

Psoriasis of the nails. Nail changes are characteristic of psoriasis and the nails of patients should be examined. (See Chapter Twenty-five.) These changes offer supporting evidence for the diagnosis of psoriasis when skin changes are equivocal or absent.

Pitting. Nail pitting is the best known and possibly the most frequent psoriatic nail abnormality (Figure 8-18). Nail plate cells are shed in much the same way as psoriatic scale is shed, leaving a variable number of tiny, punched-out depressions on the nail plate surface. They emerge from under the cuticle and grow out with the nail. Many other cutaneous diseases may cause pitting (e.g., eczema, fungal infections, and alopecia areata), or it may occur as an isolated finding as a normal variation.

Onycholysis. Psoriasis of the nail bed causes separation of the nail from the nail bed. Unlike the uniform separation caused by pressure on the tips of long nails, the nail detaches in an irregular manner. The nail plate turns yellow, simulating a fungal infection.

Subungual debris. This is analogous to fungal infection; the nail bed scale is retained, forcing the distal nail to separate from the nail bed.

Nail deformity. Extensive involvement of the nail matrix results in a nail losing its structural integrity, resulting in fragmentation and crumbling (Figure 8-19).

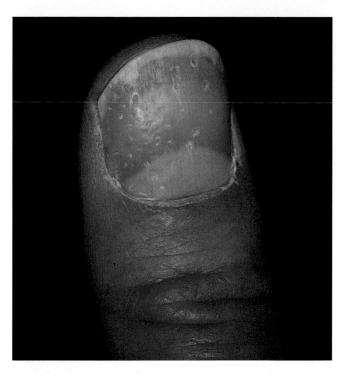

Figure 8-18
Psoriasis of the nails. Pitting is the best-known psoriatic nail abnormality.

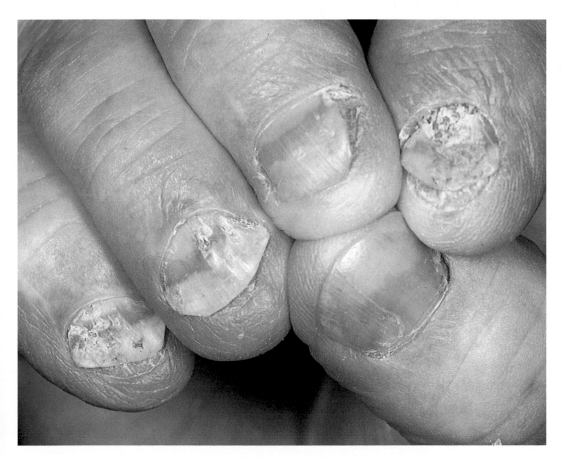

Figure 8-19
Psoriasis of the nails. Extensive involvement of each nail matrix has caused all nails to be poorly formed.

Psoriatic arthritis

Psoriatic arthritis is a distinct form of arthritis in which the rheumatoid factor is usually negative. It may precede, accompany, or, more often, follow the skin manifestations. Onset may occur at any age, but peak occurrence is between ages 20 and 40; women and men are equally affected. The incidence in the psoriatic population is approximately 5% to 8%, but up to 53% of psoriatic patients suffer from arthralgia.[17,18] The prevalence of psoriatic arthritis is higher among patients with more severe cutaneous disease. Nail involvement occurs in more than 80% of patients with psoriatic arthritis, compared with 30% of patients with uncomplicated psoriasis. The prevalence of nail psoriasis is highest among patients with psoriatic arthritis who have arthritic involvement of their fingers, but the presence of nail disease does not have predictive value in determining if a patient is at risk for psoriatic arthritis. Cases of arthritis have been reported to develop following trauma. Patients with psoriatic arthritis who become pregnant improve or even remit in 80% of cases.[19] Despite active treatment and a reduction in joint inflammation and the rate of damage, psoriatic arthritis may be a progressively deforming arthritis.[20]

Diagnosis. Laboratory tests are most useful to exclude other arthritic diseases. Although tests for antinuclear antibody (ANA) levels, erythrocyte sedimentation rate (ESR), white blood cell (WBC) counts, and uric acid sometimes identify elevated levels, they have little predictive value in diagnosing psoriatic arthritis. ESR is the best laboratory guide to disease activity. Rheumatoid factor levels are typically normal, but are elevated in a small percentage of patients.

Clinical features. There are five recognized presentations of psoriatic arthritis (Table 8-1).[21]

Asymmetric arthritis. The most common pattern is an asymmetric arthritis involving one or more joints of the fingers and toes (Figure 8-20). Usually one or more proximal interphalangeal (PIP), distal interphalangeal (DIP), metatarsophalangeal, or metacarpophalangeal joints are involved. During the acute phase, the joint is red, warm, and painful. Continued inflammation promotes soft-tissue swelling on either side of the joint ("sausage finger") and restricts mobility. HLA-DR7 is significantly increased in this group with peripheral arthritis.[22]

Symmetric arthritis. A symmetric polyarthritis resembling rheumatoid arthritis occurs, but the rheumatoid factor is negative. The small joints of the hands and feet, wrists, ankles, knees, and elbows may be involved.

Distal interphalangeal joint disease. Perhaps the most characteristic presentation of arthritis with psoriasis is the involvement of the DIP joints of the hands and feet with associated psoriatic nail disease. The disease is chronic but mild, is not disabling, and is responsible for approximately 5% of cases of psoriatic arthritis.

Arthritis mutilans. The most severe form of psoriatic arthritis involves osteolysis of any of the small bones of the hands and feet. Gross deformity and subluxation are attributed to this condition. Severe osteolysis leads to digital telescoping, producing the "opera glass" deformity. This deformity may be seen in rheumatoid arthritis.

Ankylosing spondylitis. This condition occurs as an isolated phenomenon or in association with peripheral joint disease. The association of HLA-B27 and spondylitis is well known. The strongest association is in males with sacroiliitis. Asymptomatic sacroiliitis occurs in as many as one third of cases of psoriasis. It is usually asymmetrical and may be associated with spondylitis.

TABLE 8-1 Psoriatic Arthritis

Type	Percentage of all psoriatic arthritis	Features
Asymmetric arthritis (one or more joints)	60%-70%	Joints of fingers and toes ("sausage finger")
Symmetric polyarthritis	15%	Clinically resembles rheumatoid arthritis, rheumatoid factor negative
Distal interphalangeal joint disease	5%	Mild, chronic, associated with nail disease
Destructive polyarthritis (arthritis mutilans)	5%	Osteolysis of small bones of hands and feet; gross deformity; joint subluxation
Ankylosing spondylitis	5%	With or without peripheral joint disease

Modified from Moll JMH: *Clin Orthop* 143:66, 1979.

Treatment of psoriatic arthritis. Management is similar to that of other chronic inflammatory joint diseases. Nonsteroidal antiinflammatory agents are the mainstay of therapy and usually provide adequate control, but they do not induce remissions. Parenteral gold salts, methotrexate, and azathioprine are effective for long-term treatment.

Methotrexate or etretinate controls advanced joint and skin diseases. Methotrexate is an effective second-line agent for psoriatic arthritis.[23] Pain and function improve dramatically 2 to 6 weeks after starting methotrexate therapy with 5 mg every 12 hours in three consecutive doses once a week. Lower dosages may not be effective.[24] Methotrexate may also be given as a single dose or divided into two doses taken 12 hours apart. The amount is increased to 25 to 30 mg/week, until control is obtained, and then tapered to a maintenance dose of around 5 to 15 mg/week.

The risk of liver toxicity in patients undergoing long-term, low-dose methotrexate therapy for psoriatic arthritis is substantial, and that risk increases with the total cumulative dose and with heavy consumption of alcohol. Liver biopsies should be done periodically to monitor for liver toxicity.[25]

Etretinate (1 mg/kg/day) has a beneficial effect on objective symptoms. The dosage is lowered after the initial response in an attempt to minimize side effects.[26] Sulfasalazine (2 gm/day) is also an effective second-line agent for psoriatic arthritis.[27]

Cyclosporine at daily doses ranging usually from 1.5 to 5.0 mg/kg provides impressive relief from arthralgias and improvement of joint function.[28] Although mild to moderate relapses occur, rebound phenomena is not observed after discontinuation of treatment.[29]

Antimalarials, particularly hydroxychloroquine, are usually avoided in psoriatic patients for fear of precipitating exfoliative dermatitis or exacerbating psoriasis. Two studies showed that these reactions did not occur in patients treated with hydroxychloroquine[30] or chloroquine.[31]

Systemic corticosteroids are usually avoided because of possible rebound of the skin disease on withdrawal.

Some psoriatic patients treated with photochemotherapy (PUVA) experience improvement in joint symptoms. Sulfasalazine (2 gm daily) was recently shown to be safe and effective.[32]

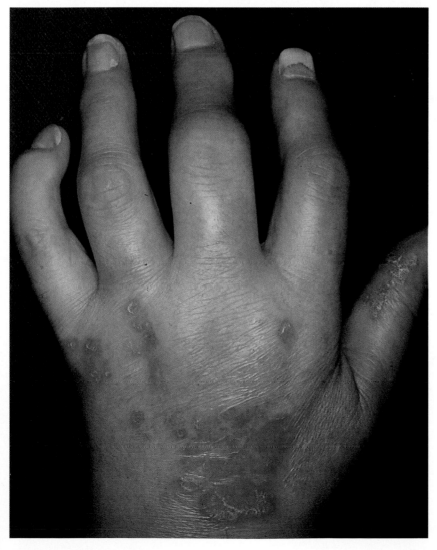

Figure 8-20
Psoriatic arthritis. Asymmetric arthritis pattern.

TREATMENT OF PSORIASIS

Overview. Many topical and systemic agents are available. All require lengthy treatment to give relief that is often only temporary. Patients with limited disease can be managed with topical therapy (Table 8-2). One intralesional steroid injection can heal a small plaque and keep it in remission for months. This is an ideal treatment for patients with a few, small plaques. Topical steroid creams and ointments, calcipotriol (Dovonex), anthralin, and tar are the mainstays of topical treatment. These agents are used with or without ultraviolet light exposure. Effective programs can be designed for patients who do not have access to a therapeutic light source and for patients who have limited disease. Without light, tar is moderately effective, but persistent use of anthralin or calcipotriol can clear the disease and offers the patient substantial remission periods. Topical steroids work quickly, but total eradication of the plaques is difficult to accomplish; remission times are short and the creams become less effective with continued use.

Patients with psoriasis covering more than 20% of the body need specialized treatment programs (Table 8-3).

Ultraviolet light B. The most effective topical programs use ultraviolet light in combination with topical steroids, tar, calcipotriol, or anthralin. Ultraviolet light in intensities high enough to be effective can be obtained from natural sunlight or commercially available light cabinets. Inexpensive single-bulb tanning lights and long-wave ultraviolet light (UVA) tanning salon lights are not effective. Most dermatologists have phototherapy units; many patients are best treated in that setting. There is a significant positive correlation between patients' responses to sunbathing and their responses to short-wave ultraviolet light (UVB) phototherapy. Sunlight nonresponders have a 70% chance of failure with UVB phototherapy; sunlight responders have an 80% chance that clearance treatment will succeed.[33]

Determining the degree of inflammation. The most common form of psoriasis is the localized chronic plaque disease involving the skin and scalp (see Figures 8-1 and 8-4). It must be determined whether the plaque is inflamed prior to instituting therapy (Figure 8-21). Red, sore plaques can be irritated by tar, calcipotriol, and anthralin. Irritation can induce further activity. Inflammation should be suppressed with topical steroids and/or antibiotics prior to initiating other treatments.

Determining the end of treatment. The plaque is effectively treated when induration has disappeared. Residual erythema, hypopigmentation, or brown hyperpigmentation is common when the plaque clears; patients frequently mistake the residual color for disease and continue treatment. If the plaque cannot be felt by drawing the finger over the skin surface, treatment may be stopped.

Control stress. A study demonstrated a positive correlation between the severity of psoriatic symptoms and psychologic distress.[34] Stress reduction techniques may be appropriate for certain patients.[35]

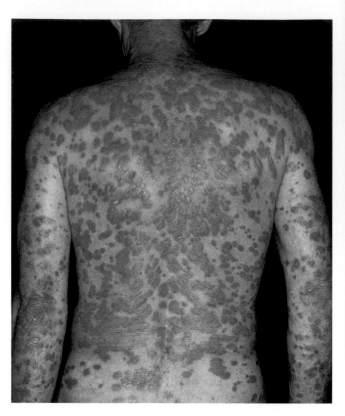

Figure 8-21
Inflammatory plaque psoriasis. A patient with such highly inflamed disease must not be treated initially with irritating medicines such as anthralin.

TOPICAL THERAPY
Calcipotriol (Dovonex)

Calcipotriol is a vitamin D_3 analogue that inhibits epidermal cell proliferation and enhances cell differentiation.

It is effective and safe for the short-and long-term treatment of psoriasis. Calcipotriol ointment should be applied twice daily in amounts up to 100 gm/week. Application for 6 to 8 weeks gives a 60% to 70% improvement in plaque-type psoriasis. No serious side effects have been reported when using up to 100 gm of the ointment weekly. Used according to these guidelines, calcipotriol treatment does not seem to affect calcium or bone metabolism.

Some patients experience mild and transient local irritation and erythema. Occlusion improves the response to calcipotriol by enhancing its penetration. Indices of calcium metabolism remained unchanged throughout a study of occlusive therapy.[36] Calcipotriol ointment applied twice daily was significantly more effective than betamethasone valerate and dithranol (anthralin).[37]

Topical steroids

Topical steroids (see Chapter Two) give fast but temporary relief. They are most useful for reducing inflammation and

TABLE 8-2 Therapeutic Options for Persons with Psoriasis on Less than 20% of the Body

Treatment	Advantages	Disadvantages	Comments
Topical steroids	Rapid response, controls inflammation and itching, best for intertriginous areas and face, convenient, not messy	Temporary relief (tolerance occurs), less effective with continued use, atrophy and telangiectasia occur with continued use, brief remissions, very expensive	Best results occur with pulse dosing (e.g., 2 weeks of medication and 1 week of lubrication only); plastic occlusion is very effective
Calcipotriol (Dovonex)	Well tolerated, long remissions possible	Burning, skin irritation, expensive	Best for moderate plaque psoriasis
Anthralin	Convenient short contact programs, long remissions, effective for scalp	Purple-brown staining, irritating, careful application (only to plaque) required	Used on chronic (not inflamed) plaques; best results occur when used with UVB light
Tar	New preparations are pleasant	Only moderately effective in a few patients	Most effective when combined with UVB (Goeckerman regimen)
UVB and lubricating agents or tar	Insurance may cover part or all of treatment, effective for 70% of patients, no need for topical steroids	Expensive, office-based therapy	Used only on plaque and guttate psoriasis, travel and time required
Tape or occlusive dressing	Convenient, no mess	Expensive; only for limited disease	May be used to occlude topical steroids
Intralesional steroids	Convenient, rapidly effective, long remissions	Only for limited areas, atrophy and telangiectasia occur at injection site	Ideal for chronic scalp and body plaques when small and few in number

TABLE 8-3 Therapeutic Options for Persons with Psoriasis on More than 20% of the Body

Treatment	Advantages	Disadvantages
UVB and tar administered in physician's office	More effective than UVB alone	More expensive and carcinogenic than UVB alone; requires many office visits
PUVA	Allows patient to be ambulatory; effective	Many treatments needed; many office visits required
SYSTEMIC TREATMENTS		
Methotrexate	"Gold standard" for efficacy; helps arthritis	Hepatotoxicity; liver biopsy periodically required
Hydrea	Effective in the few for whom it works at all	Hematopoietic toxicity; flulike syndrome
Etretinate	Effective for palmar-plantar-pustular, erythrodermic, and pustular types of psoriasis; fast, effective; helps arthritis	Teratogenic; usually ineffective as a single therapy for plaques
Cyclosporine	Fast, effective; helps arthritis	Experimental; hepatotoxic; nephrotoxic; immunosuppressive
Hospitalization or office day treatment for tar, anthralin, and combinations of all therapies above	Most effective for those who are unresponsive to topical agents or for whom systemic agents are inappropriate	Time-consuming; expensive

controlling itching. Initially, when the patient is introduced to topical steroids, the results are most gratifying. However, tachyphylaxis, or tolerance, occurs, and the medication becomes less effective with continued use. Patients remember the initial response and continue topical steroids in anticipation of continued effectiveness. Long-term use of topical steroids results in atrophy and telangiectasia. Topical steroids are useful for treating inflamed and intertriginous plaques.

A group I through V steroid applied one to four times a day in a cream or ointment base is required for best results. Plastic occlusion of topical steroids is much more effective than simple application. Diprolene and Temovate are extremely potent, and occlusion is not used with these drugs. Group V topical steroids applied once or twice a day should be used in the intertriginous areas and on the face. Some plaques resolve completely, but most remain only partially reduced with continued application. Continual application for more than 3 weeks should be discouraged. Remissions are usually brief and the plaques may return shortly after treatment is terminated. Topical steroid creams applied under an occlusive plastic dressing promote more rapid clearing, but remissions are not extended.

The rapid appearance of atrophy and telangiectasia occurs when the group I topical steroids Diprolene and Temovate are occluded. Topical steroid solutions are useful for scalp psoriasis. Intralesional injection of small plaques with triamcinolone acetonide (Kenalog, 5 to 10 mg/ml) almost invariably clears the lesion and accords long-term remission. Atrophy may occur with the 10 mg/ml concentration.

Intralesional steroids

Patients with a few, small, chronic psoriatic plaques of the scalp or body can be effectively treated with a single intralesional injection of triamcinolone acetonide (Kenalog, 5 to 10 mg/ml). The 10 mg/ml solution may be diluted with saline. Most injected plaques clear completely and remain in remission for months. Atrophy and telangiectasias may appear at the injection site. The face and intertriginous areas are avoided.

Anthralin

Anthralin is used only for chronic plaques. For years anthralin has been used effectively in the hospital to treat psoriasis. The principal objections were to the mess, long treatment times, and staining. Maximum patient compliance can be achieved with the new, short-treatment time schedules and commercially available preparations. There are several effective treatment programs. Psoriasis clears faster when UVB radiation is used in combination with anthralin.[38]

Preparations and use. Anthralin is commercially available in concentrations ranging from 0.1% to 1.0% (2.0% in some countries) (see the Formulary, p. 853). Higher concentrations must be compounded by the pharmacist (a formula is found in the Formulary, p. 854). Anthralin is expensive and some pharmacists are reluctant to compound it. Patients must be cautioned about irritation and staining. Hands

should be washed carefully after application, with care to avoid eye contact. Care must also be taken to protect normal skin, and anthralin should not be applied to intertriginous areas or to the face. Ointment-based anthralin is removed with petroleum jelly and followed by a shower with soap. Lubricants are applied to avoid dryness and to remove the last traces of anthralin. If irritation occurs, anthralin should be discontinued and the patient should be treated with group II through V topical steroids until improvement is noted. Skin stains fade in a matter of weeks, but purple clothing stains are permanent (Figure 8-22).

Short contact therapy. A prescription is written for several different strengths of anthralin so that adjustments in dosage can be made by the patient. The patient starts with 0.1% and washes it off in 20 minutes. The potency (0.1% to 4.0%) and contact time (10 to 60 minutes) can be adjusted according to tolerance. Potency is increased to the highest concentration that does not cause irritation. Contact time can be increased to an hour; longer times are probably no more effective and become inconvenient.[39] The goal is to maintain a daily schedule using the highest concentration of anthralin that can be tolerated without inducing inflammation.

Ingram regimen. The Ingram regimen of daily tar baths, UVB radiation, and anthralin applied at bedtime has been used for 30 years. Studies show that although this method produces a significantly faster rate of improvement than the short-contact regimen, the degree of relapse after 12 weeks is identical for both methods.[40]

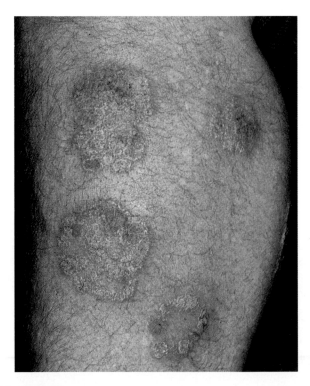

Figure 8-22
Psoriatic plaques under treatment with anthralin. As with all forms of treatment, plaques first clear in the center.

Ultraviolet light B and lubricating agents

Tar enhances the effectiveness of ultraviolet light,[41] but studies suggest that application of lubricants prior to UVB exposure provides results similar to those achieved with tar and UVB.[42] The ideal schedules for treatment frequency and increasing UVB dosages have not been established. Data suggest that aggressive treatment with UVB exposures intense enough to produce erythema (maximally erythemogenic UVB) at each treatment results in clearing with fewer treatments and less total UVB dosage.[43] Practically speaking, these aggressive techniques may be difficult to manage for routine office use; acceptable results have been achieved using suberythemogenic doses.[42] Optimal, long-term management may be achieved by continuing UVB phototherapy after initial clearing (average—six treatments per month).[44] Treatment with UVB and lubricating agents is just as effective as UVB and topical steroids, therefore costly topical steroids can be avoided during light therapy.[45] If not removed before phototherapy, preparations containing tar or thickly applied petrolatum or emollients can block UVB.[46] Tan Thru Swim Suits by Solar allow penetration of ultraviolet light.*

UVB and tar. Despite several studies that show lubricating agents are as effective as tar for treatment before UVB exposure, the final answer is not yet known. Tar and UVB phototherapy have been used for years with gratifying results, and this method continues to be used in both hospital and outpatient treatment programs. Tar preparations are applied 2 or more hours before ultraviolet light exposure. There are several commercially available tar preparations (see the Formulary, p. 854). Some of these preparations cause drying, whereas others, particularly those with a lubricating base (e.g., T-Derm and Fototar), are well tolerated.

Goeckerman regimen. This regimen combines the daily application of tar with UVB exposure; it is safe, highly effective, and possibly produces the longest remissions.[47] However, a major commitment of time and money is required. Many larger hospitals provide inpatient facilities for this program. Patients with diffuse or poorly responsive psoriasis may leave the hospital with gratifying results. The Goeckerman regimen can also be used on an outpatient basis. The addition of topical steroids to the Goeckerman regimen may interfere with treatment by shortening the duration of remission.[48] A tar concentrate such as Balnatar can be added to the bath water as a substitute for tar ointments and lotions. Tar-solution soaks are useful for psoriasis of the palms and soles. The feet can be soaked for 1 hour each day in a basin of warm water and Balnatar.

Tape or occlusive dressings

One study showed that adhesive occlusive dressings applied and changed every week were therapeutically supe-

rior to a group V topical steroid and comparable to UVB therapy.[49] Complete clearing occurred in 47% of the cases in an average of 5 weeks; another 41% improved. Waterproof tape with low-moisture vapor transmission applied continually for 1 week gave similar results. Two or more applications were required.[50] This treatment may be appropriate for treating localized chronic plaques. Actiderm, DuoDerm for Psoriasis, and Topiclude are self-adhesive patches marketed specifically for this treatment technique. They are applied alone or over topical steroids and changed every 1 to 7 days.

Treating the scalp

The scalp is difficult to treat because hair interferes with the application of medicine and shields the skin from ultraviolet light. Symptoms of tenderness and itching vary considerably. The goal is to provide symptomatic and cosmetic relief. It is unnecessary and impractical to attempt to keep the scalp constantly clear.

Removing scale. Scale must be removed first to facilitate penetration of medicine. Superficial scale can be removed with shampoos that contain tar and salicylic acid. Thicker scale is removed by applying Baker's P & S or 10% liquor carbonis detergens (LCD) in Nivea oil to the scalp and washing 6 to 8 hours later with shampoo or Dawn dishwashing liquid. Combing during the shampoo helps dislodge scale.

Baker's P & S liquid (phenol, sodium chloride, and liquid paraffin) applied to the scalp at bedtime and washed out in the morning is moderately effective in reducing scale. Baker's liquid is pleasant and well tolerated for extended periods.

LCD (10%), a tar extract of crude oil tar, is mixed with Nivea oil by the pharmacist. The unpleasant mixture is liberally massaged into the scalp at bedtime. Warming the mixture prior to application enhances scale penetration. A shower cap protects pillows and also encourages scale penetration. An impressive amount of scale is removed in the first few days. Nightly applications are continued until the scalp is acceptably clear.

Mild to moderate scalp involvement. When used at least every other day, tar shampoos (see the Formulary, p. 852) may be effective in controlling moderate scaling.

Corticosteroid solutions are very expensive, but a minute amount can cover a wide area. Steroid gels (e.g., Lidex gel, Temovate gel, Topicort gel), which have a keratolytic base and penetrate hair, are effective for localized plaques. Derma-smoothe FS lotion (peanut oil, mineral oil, fluocinolone acetonide 0.01%) is an effective topical steroid that can be applied to the entire scalp and occluded with a shower cap. The scalp is dampened before application. Treatment is repeated each night for 1 to 3 weeks until itching and erythema are controlled.

Small plaques are effectively treated with intralesional steroid injections of triamcinolone acetonide (Kenalog, 10 mg/ml). Remissions following use of intralesional steroids are much longer than those following topical steroids.

---

*Available from Solar Swim Wear; 1511-J East Fowler Avenue; Tampa, FL 33612; (813) 971-0090; FAX (813) 971-0509.

Ketoconazole cream is sometimes useful. Oral ketoconazole (400 mg daily) may be effective in some cases.[51] The possibility of drug toxicity limits its usefulness.

Treatment of diffuse and thick scalp psoriasis. Three different programs can be implemented, all of which use oil or ointment-based preparations for scale penetration. They are applied at bedtime and washed out each morning with strong detergents such as Dawn dishwashing liquid. Topical steroid solutions can be applied during the day.

TAR AND OIL. Ten percent LCD in Nivea oil applied to the scalp and washed out each morning removes scale and suppresses inflammation.

"20-10-5." A mixture of 20% cade oil, 10% sulfur precipitate, and 5% salicylic acid in unibase to make 3 oz is very effective for stubborn plaques. Warming the mixture prior to application enhances penetration. It is applied each night and washed out in the morning.

ANTHRALIN. Anthralin ointment applied each evening and removed in the morning is another method for treating resistant scalp psoriasis. A short-contact method similar to that previously described for anthralin is used. Apply 0.1% to 2% anthralin ointment and wash completely 10 to 20 minutes after application. Drithoscalp (0.25% and 0.5%) is packaged in a tube with a long nozzle for hair penetration.

SYSTEMIC THERAPY

Topical treatment has its limits. Many patients do not respond to the most vigorous topical programs, or the disease may be so extensive that topical treatment is not practical. A number of systemic drugs are available. All of them have potentially serious side effects. Photochemotherapy (PUVA) is the technique most commonly used for extensive, chronic, plaque psoriasis. It is highly effective and relatively safe. Etretinate is used to potentiate the effects of PUVA and as a monotherapy for the uncommon pustular and erythrodermic forms of psoriasis. Etretinate is less effective for chronic plaque psoriasis. Etretinate has many annoying side effects. Methotrexate is highly effective, relatively safe, and well tolerated, but the need for periodic liver biopsies discourages many patients and physicians. Hydrea is not hepatotoxic, but it is rarely used because it is effective in only a few patients. Cyclosporine is rapidly effective, but long-term use may be associated with loss of kidney function.

Rotational therapy. A rotational approach to therapy has been suggested (see the diagram below). Rotation of available therapies (UVB plus tar, PUVA, methotrexate, etretinate, and cyclosporine) for moderate to severe psoriasis may minimize long-term toxicity and allow effective treatments to be maintained for many years. Patients may receive each form of therapy for 1 to 2 years and then switch to the next form of treatment. By rotating each of the three or four treatments at these intervals, it may be 4 or 5 years before the patient needs to return to the first therapy, thereby minimizing the cumulative toxicity by long periods off each treatment.[52]

The physician and patient must make the final decision about which therapeutic modality is appropriate based on the unique features of each individual case.

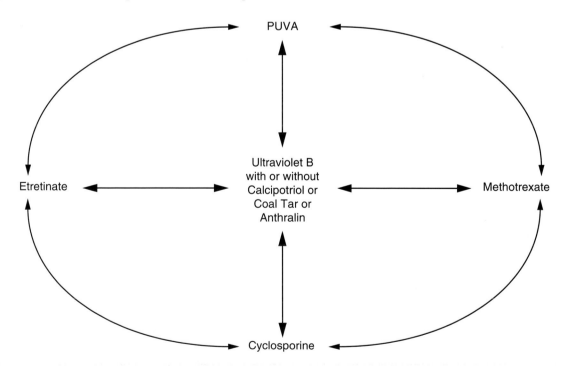

Rotational therapy. For moderate-to-severe psoriasis to minimize toxic effects from any one therapy. A reasonable sequence would start with phototherapy (PUVA or ultraviolet B), followed by methotrexate, then the other form of radiation, then another oral agent, and so on. Patients who do not tolerate radiation therapy rotate oral agents.

Photochemotherapy (PUVA)

Complete prescribing information can be found in the Formulary.

The FDA approved photochemotherapy treatment for psoriasis in 1982. The treatment, known as PUVA, is so designated because of the use of a class of drugs called *psoralens* (P), along with exposure to long-wave ultraviolet light (UVA). The specific psoralen drug approved for use in PUVA therapy is methoxsalen (8-methoxypsoralen). Oxsoralen-Ultra capsules are the newest encapsulated liquid formulation of methoxsalen (available in 10-mg capsules). Patients ingest a prescribed dose of methoxsalen approximately 2 hours before being exposed to a carefully measured amount of UVA in a uniquely designed enclosure. The drug apparently couples with and inhibits DNA synthesis after activation with ultraviolet light in the UVA region (320 to 400 nm), thereby decreasing cellular proliferation. A major advantage of PUVA is that it controls severe psoriasis with relatively few maintenance treatments, and it can be done on an outpatient basis. Light does not penetrate hair: scalp psoriasis must be treated with conventional therapy.

Indications. PUVA is an effective method of controlling but not curing psoriasis. Patients should be selected only by physicians who are experienced in the treatment of all forms of psoriasis. PUVA is indicated for the symptomatic control of severe, recalcitrant, disabling, plaque psoriasis that is not adequately responsive to other forms of therapy. Erythrodermic and pustular psoriasis are best treated with etretinate. Pustular psoriasis of the palms and soles responds best to PUVA-etretinate.[53,54] Because of the concerns about long-term toxicity, PUVA is most appropriate for severe psoriasis in patients over 50 years of age. The American Academy of Pediatrics has disapproved the use of PUVA therapy in children.

Psoriatic arthropathy of the nonspondylitic type may respond to PUVA with improvement in erythema, tenderness, and inflammation of the peripheral joints.[33]

Treatment regimen. The treatment regimen is divided into two phases: the clearance phase, in which continual treatment is given until clearing occurs, followed by the maintenance phase, in which treatments are given less frequently but in numbers sufficient to prevent a flare-up of the disease.

Clearance phase. Two treatment protocols are in use. In the United States protocols are as follows. Drug dosage is based on body weight (see the Formulary, p. 853) and the amount of initial energy delivered is based on the degree of skin pigmentation and ability to sunburn.[55,56] The UVA dosage is increased in increments of 0.5 to 1.5 J/cm^2, depending on erythema production and therapeutic response. Patients are treated two or three times each week during the clearing phase; this requires approximately 25 treatments in 13 weeks with a cumulative dosage of 245 J/cm^2. The European protocols are more aggressive. They are designed to clear the patient before tanning develops. The initial energy delivered is the patient's minimum photo-toxic dose. UVA is delivered on Monday, Tuesday, Thursday, and Friday and is increased in increments of 0.5 to 2 J/cm^2 only after the first four treatments if no more than a pink erythema has developed. This requires approximately 20 treatments in 6 weeks with a cumulative dosage of 96 J/cm^2.

Maintenance phase. The UVA dose that is administered at the time when the psoriasis has cleared is the most important single dose because it is used as a maintenance dose. Cumulative exposure to UVA radiation is usually greatest during the maintenance phase. Generally, the number of treatments needed for maintenance and during flare-ups is directly related to the total body surface area initially affected by psoriasis, but there is a wide variation among individuals.

Maintenance protocols. More than 80% of patients experience clearing of symptoms that is maintained with periodic treatments. The goal of maintenance is to keep the patient as symptom-free as possible with the least amount of UVA exposure. When patients have achieved 95% clearing, they are placed on a maintenance schedule. It is recommended that each maintenance schedule be adhered to for at least two treatments (unless erythema or a psoriatic flare occurs). At this time, if there is no clinical worsening, treatment can be discontinued. If a flare-up occurs at any time, then the frequency of treatments is either held at a number greater than the level at which worsening occurred or temporarily increased to the level of the clearing-phase protocol. The therapy is then gradually tapered according to the clinical response. Patients who relapse during the first 2 months of maintenance treatment continue on a maintenance regimen. In most instances, patients who experience a psoriasis flare after discontinuing therapy can be successfully re-treated.

Response to treatment. After the initial clearing phase, patients require a mean of 30 treatments per year during the first 1½ years.[57] Most patients who are clear after the initial 2- to 3-month maintenance period remain clear for at least 6 to 12 months. Disease control lasts longer after PUVA than after UVB therapy. Continued use of PUVA after initial clearing affords good disease control for prolonged periods. The recurrence rate is higher in patients who do not continue maintenance treatment; however, long-term maintenance results in high cumulative doses of energy.

During maintenance, flares occur in 35% of patients with guttate and plaque psoriasis, and in 58% of those with erythrodermic psoriasis.

The proportion of patients actively using PUVA decreases with time. It is burdensome for most patients with chronic disease to continue to rely on a suppressive, but not curative, therapy. Cost, frequency of treatments, time needed for treatment, distance to travel, short-term toxic effects, and concern about potential long-term side effects are reasons for stopping.[58]

PUVA combined with other modalities. Combining PUVA with other modalities reduces the number of PUVA treatments required to maintain remission, results in fewer adverse effects from treatment, increases efficacy, and reduces cost.

PUVA PLUS ETRETINATE. The combination of PUVA and etretinate is called *Re-PUVA*. A substantial reduction in PUVA burden may be accomplished when etretinate, in the 1 mg/kg/day range, is given for 1 to 3 weeks before starting PUVA. Some studies dispute this claim, citing the need for further studies.[59] The combination is claimed to accelerate the response to PUVA, reduce the number of exposures and treatment time required for clearing, clear PUVA-resistant cases, and at least halve the cumulative UVA dosage needed to clear the psoriasis when PUVA is used alone.[60] The same beneficial results were reported when isotretinoin (Accutane, 1.0 mg/kg/day) was used instead of etretinate.[61]

PUVA PLUS UVB. Simultaneous use of PUVA and UVB clears the disease more quickly and at a lower final dosage of light therapy than PUVA and UVB used separately.[62,63]

PUVA PLUS MTX. Combined methotrexate-PUVA therapy achieved a marked reduction in the total cumulative exposure to UVA radiation during the clearance phase of therapy and the early phase of maintenance PUVA therapy.[64] The combination of methotrexate and PUVA may be synergistic in the induction of cutaneous malignancy.[65]

PUVA PLUS CALCIPOTRIOL. Calcipotriol improved the response to PUVA in 82% of patients. The median UVA dose to clear plaques was reduced by 26.5%.[66]

ANTHRALIN. The use of anthralin with PUVA results in earlier clearing than does the use of PUVA alone.[67]

PUVA PLUS TAR OR TOPICAL STEROIDS. The combination of tar or topical steroids with PUVA does not produce any significant long-term benefits.[68]

Side effects

Long-term side effects. Most long-term side effects of PUVA are dose-dependent. Methods should be sought to control disease using the minimum amount of PUVA therapy. These include the use of appropriate dosage regimens, the avoidance of maintenance therapy as far as possible, and the use of combination therapies.

Short-term side effects. Short-term side effects include dark tanning, pruritus, nausea, and severe sunburn.

Cataracts. Concern has been expressed that PUVA therapy may cause cataracts, but the incidence seems to be very low in patients who use eye protection.[69] During the first day of PUVA treatment, patients should wear UVA-blocking, plastic, wraparound glasses when they are outdoors from the time they ingest the drug until bedtime. While indoors or in dim light, either wraparound glasses or clear UVA-blocking glasses should be worn. During the second day, either plastic wraparound or clear UVA-blocking glasses should be worn the entire day.

Skin tumors. PUVA promotes skin aging, actinic keratoses, and squamous cell carcinoma (SCC), especially in patients previously treated with arsenic or ionizing radiation and in patients with a history of skin cancer.[70,71,72] The risk of cutaneous SCC from PUVA is dose related. There is a strong, dose-dependent increase in the risk of genital tumors associated with exposure to PUVA and ultraviolet B radiation. Men should use genital protection when they are exposed to PUVA and to other forms of ultraviolet radiation for therapeutic, recreational, or cosmetic reasons.[73]

Methotrexate

Methotrexate (MTX) is the "gold standard" for the treatment of severe psoriasis and is particularly effective in controlling erythrodermic and generalized pustular psoriasis.[74] It induces remissions in the majority of treated patients and maintains remissions for long periods with continued therapy. MTX is also effective for psoriatic arthritis. It is relatively safe and well tolerated,[75] but the need for periodic liver biopsies discourages many patients and physicians from using it. Guidelines for the use of MTX are available.*[,76]

Mechanism of action. MTX is a folic acid antagonist that inhibits dihydrofolate reductase. DNA synthesis is inhibited as the concentrations of thymidine and purines fall after treatment with MTX.[77] There follows a marked suppressive effect on rapidly proliferating cells. Psoriatic skin has more cells in replication at any one time than normal skin. MTX, by its inhibitory effect on DNA synthesis, apparently functions as a direct suppressor of psoriatic epidermal cell reproduction.[78] MTX also has antiinflammatory and immunomodulatory effects.

Dosing. The oral triple-dose regimen is now the most common method of prescribing MTX for psoriasis. There is less toxicity, with effectiveness that equals other schedules. It is based on the psoriatic 36 hour cell cycle. A dose is taken at 12-hour intervals during a 36-hour period once each week. An initial test dose of 5 to 10 mg is given and complete blood counts and liver function tests are obtained 1 week later. If this dose was well tolerated, start the patient on one 2.5-mg tablet at 12-hour intervals for three doses. The next week the dosage is increased by one to two tablets (hour 0), one tablet (hour 12), and one tablet (hour 24). In the following weeks, titrate up or down by a 2.5-mg tablet to the most effective and best-tolerated dosage. Most patients are controlled and tolerate 15 mg/week (two-tablet, two-tablet, two-tablet dosage). Once the desired degree of clearing is obtained, the dosage is decreased by one tablet per week every few weeks to arrive at a maintenance regimen (i.e., 2.5 to 5.0 mg/week). The goal is not necessarily 100% clearance, but to reach 80% improvement. This is safer than pushing higher, more toxic dosages to obtain 100% clearance. Discontinue the drug for several months of rest; the summer months are a good time to attempt this, when sunlight may control the disease. Gradually tapering to withdraw MTX seems to present fewer problems of rebound than does a sudden discontinuance of the drug. Single oral and intramuscular weekly dosage schedules are described in the literature.[76] Mylan's MTX tablet (generic) is bioequivalent to Lederle's product.[79]

Side effects. Short-term side effects include nausea, anorexia, fatigue, oral ulcerations, mild leukopenia, and thrombocytopenia. These are dose-related and rapidly

---

*Available in *J Am Acad Dermatol* 19:145, 1988 (Methotrexate in psoriasis: revised guidelines).

reversible. Switching among triple dosing, weekly oral dosing, and intramuscular dosing may decrease these reactions. Gastrointestinal symptoms can be controlled with folic acid, 5 mg daily.[80] The therapeutic result may be better if folic acid is not given on the day MTX is taken.[81] An increase in the erythrocyte mean corpuscular volume may be a useful indicator of folate deficiency and impending toxicity.[82] Hepatic fibrosis or cirrhosis can develop with long-term treatment. Extensive alcohol intake, daily dosing, prior liver disease, and cumulative MTX intake predispose patients to fibrosis and cirrhosis. Male and female patients should discontinue MTX for 3 to 4 months before attempting conception.[83]

Drug Interactions. Salicylates, many nonsteroidal antiinflammatory agents, trimethoprim-sulfamethoxazole, ethanol, phenylbutazone, sulfonamides, probenecid, cephalothin, penicillins, colchicine, barbiturates, phenytoin, dipyridamole, and retinoids interact with MTX to increase toxicity. Concomitant therapy may result in neutropenia. Blood counts should be monitored after changes in therapy, especially in patients with impaired renal function, such as the elderly.[84,85]

Monitoring. Evaluate renal and liver functions prior to initiating therapy. MTX is excreted mainly via the kidney. Older individuals tend to have reduced renal function and require lower dosages of MTX.

Leukocyte and platelet counts are depressed maximally approximately 7 to 10 days after treatment. A drop in these counts below normal levels necessitates reducing or stopping therapy. Obtain CBCs every week during the first few weeks, then obtain monthly counts 1 week after the last dose. A patient whose CBC remains stable for 4 to 6 months may then obtain CBCs less frequently. LFTs are obtained at 3- to 4-month intervals, but at least 1 week after the last dose of the drug. MTX causes transient elevations in LFTs for 1 to 3 days after its administration, so a false-positive elevation might be seen if the patient is tested too soon.

Liver fibrosis, cirrhosis, and biopsy interval. Serum LFTs are not reliable indicators of liver disease. Data suggest that at 1.5 gm of cumulative drug usage, cirrhosis can occur in approximately 3% of patients.[76] Cumulative doses of 4 gm or more have led to an incidence as high as 25%.[86] MTX-induced cirrhosis may be of a "low aggressive" type.

If the patient has normal liver chemistry values, a normal history, a normal physical examination, and no risk factors, a liver biopsy is recommended after a cumulative MTX dose of approximately 1.5 gm. If the first postmethotrexate liver biopsy shows no significant abnormalities, repeat liver biopsies are recommended at 1.0 to 1.5 gm intervals of further cumulative doses. Patients taking 15 mg of MTX each week reach the 1.5-gm cumulative dose in 25 months.

Cyclosporine

Cyclosporine (CS) at dosages of 2.5 to 5.0 mg/kg/day administered to reliable, carefully selected patients who are closely monitored for both clinical and laboratory parameters currently produces the quickest and more consistently favorable results for severe plaque psoriasis. CS in doses of 3 to 5 mg/kg/day led to clinical remission in 77% of patients. Complete remission was observed in 70% of those patients within the first 5 months.[87] CS in dosages of 3 to 5 mg/kg/day has led to complete remission in 67% of patients with erythrodermic psoriasis in a median time of 2 to 4 months.[88] Palmoplantar pustulosis responds to 1.25 to 2.5 mg/kg/day.[89] Nephrotoxicity and hypertension are the major adverse reactions. Psoriasis returns in most cases when the drug is stopped.

Patients with malignancy, those on immunosuppressive therapy, those with abnormal renal function, and those who are pregnant should not be given CS. CS does not seem to be a definite contraindication to pregnancy, but the data are limited. CS can increase blood lipids.

Dosing. Start with a dosage of 2.5 or 5.0 mg/kg/day and follow up at 1-week intervals for the first month, every 2 weeks for the subsequent month, and monthly thereafter.[90,91] After remission (defined as a reduction of 75% of the body area involved), CS is slowly tapered (0.5 mg/kg/day every 2 weeks) until total discontinuation or the reappearance of signs of the disease. In one study, this allowed control over the disease (the absence of relapse) to be maintained for a median of 8 months in 59% of patients.[87] The dosage of CS is varied in case of any important change in renal function or blood pressure.

Nephrotoxicity. How CS produces nephrotoxicity is not understood. The risk of its development can be minimized by allowing a dosage no higher than 5 mg/kg/day and avoiding increases in serum creatinine of more than 30% above the patient's baseline value.[92] Short-term use (mean 2.4 months) of CS at a dosage of 5 mg/kg/day is associated with a significant increase in blood pressure, but only a transient, mild reduction in the glomerular filtration rate (GFR).[93] Monitor GFR 3, 6, and 12 months after initiating therapy, provided the serum creatinine level is stable. If the serum creatinine level increases by 30% over the baseline, the GFR should be monitored more frequently and the dosage of CS should be adjusted if there is a persistent decrease.

GFR is a more accurate assessment of renal function than is creatinine clearance or blood urea nitrogen. Both a fall in the GFR and a rise in the serum creatinine correlate with the severity of the features of CS nephrotoxicity seen on biopsy. The best predictor of abnormal biopsy findings is a failure of renal function to show significant improvement when CS is discontinued for a month.[94]

Hypertension occurred in 17% of patients in a 12-week study, 29% in a 2-year study and 44% in a 5-year study. Blood pressure returned to normal in all hypertensive patients when CS was discontinued for 1 month.[91]

Drug Interactions. Erythromycin, corticosteroids, oral contraceptives, verapamil, and nifedipine can increase the blood concentration of CS by inhibiting cytochrome P-450. Phenobarbital can decrease the blood concentration by inducing cytochrome P-450. Diuretics and nonsteroidal antiinflammatory drugs can potentiate nephrotoxicity.

Retinoids

Etretinate is the first retinoid to be approved for use in psoriasis. An analogue, acitretin, with a short half-life similar to that of isotretinoin, is available outside the United States. Etretinate is highly effective for generalized pustular and erythrodermic psoriasis, but is less effective for plaque-type psoriasis. Etretinate may be useful as a short-term adjunctive treatment in combination with PUVA and UVB phototherapy for treating chronic plaque psoriasis. The mechanism of action is unknown. Absorption is increased when the drug is taken with whole milk or a high-fat meal.

There are no known interactions of etretinate with other drugs, although vitamin A should be avoided (see the box below).

Patients should be monitored closely (Table 8-4). Many patients find the side effects intolerable and stop treatment. Etretinate is a teratogen. With continued therapy, the drug accumulates in high concentrations in adipose tissue and in the liver. After 6 months of therapy, it may be detectable in serum for at least 2 years after discontinuation. Because of its extended tissue half-life and its teratogenic capabilities, this drug should not be given to women capable of conceiving. Male patients should avoid fathering children during etretinate treatment until more knowledge is gained.

ETRETINATE SIDE EFFECTS

Hypervitaminosis A symptoms
  Dryness of lips and mucous membranes (cheilitis, epistaxis, conjunctivitis)
  Hair loss
  Bone and joint pain
  Peeling palms and soles (45%)
  Eye irritation
  Pseudotumor cerebri (papilledema, headache, nausea, vomiting, stiff neck)
Skin thinning and fragility (25%)
Thin, soft nails
Hair loss—reversible (75%)
Sticky smooth skin sensation
Retinoid rash (50%)
Granulation tissue (15%) (toe webs, nail sulcus, groin)
Extraspinal tendon and ligament calcification
Premature epiphysial closure
Multiple bone changes in children
Triglycerides and cholesterol increased
Teratogenic—effects last for years after stopping drug
Liver enzyme alteration (20%)
Hepatitis (1.5%)

TABLE 8-4 Etretinate Therapy: Patient Monitoring*

Type of evaluation	Comments
Clinical evaluation	Performed twice in first month monthly for 6 months, and every 3 months thereafter
Laboratory testing CBC, urinalysis, fasting glucose, kidney function tests, calcium	Performed at each visit during first year and twice yearly thereafter
Liver function tests	Performed at each visit
Fasting lipids	Performed at each visit in first 4 months and every 2 to 3 months thereafter; stop etretinate if serum triglycerides exceed 800 mg/ml to reduce the risk of pancreatitis
Pregnancy test	Performed prior to and monthly during and for at least 1 year after therapy
Radiographs	For adults—no routine radiographs if patient is over 40 years of age; children—radiographic monitoring for long-term (>0.5 years) treatment

Modified from Ellis CN, Voorhees JJ: *J Am Acad Dermatol* 16:267-291, 1987.
*Patients at risk for various side effects or who develop abnormalities may require more frequent evaluations.

Indications. Etretinate should be considered for initial treatment of patients with severe pustular[95] or erythrodermic psoriasis.[96] Patients with generalized pustular psoriasis showed complete or almost complete clearing after 1½ to 4½ months, with dramatic improvement occurring in 2 weeks. Etretinate is less effective for plaque-type psoriasis. Consider etretinate for moderate to severe plaque-type psoriasis and in the following cases: (1) for patients who have received extensive radiation with PUVA;[97] (2) as a 1- to 3-week pretreatment for PUVA to accelerate the response rate; (3) for patients who do not respond to UVB with anthralin or tar; or (4) for patients who are not candidates for methotrexate.

Liver biopsy is not a routine part of etretinate therapy. Most patients require maintenance or intermittent therapy to prevent relapses. Topical steroids reduce some of the cutaneous side effects of etretinate.

Dosage. Etretinate (Tegison) is available in 10-mg and 25-mg capsules and is prescribed in two daily doses. Etretinate can be effective in lower dosages with less toxicity when given concurrently with other types of antipsoriasis therapy, such as PUVA (Re-PUVA),[98] UVB, topical steroids, anthralin, methotrexate,[99] and cyclosporine.[100] Standard treatment consists of starting treatment in the 1 mg/kg/day range and reducing the dosage once control is achieved. In some patients the disease can initially worsen. This can be minimized by starting with a lower dosage and gradually increasing it during a 1- to 2-month period. The best results have been obtained when a drug "holiday" has been given after 9 months of therapy. Etretinate is not restarted for 3 months unless the disease flares.[101]

Generalized pustular psoriasis. Initial dosage is 1 mg/kg/day. The response is rapid. Pustules regress in days. Some patients clear after a short course of treatment,[102] and others require maintenance at a lower dosage.[95,102] Isotretinoin (1.5 to 2.0 mg/kg/day) may be as effective as etretinate for generalized pustular psoriasis.[103]

Pustular psoriasis of the palms and soles. Initial dosage is 1 mg/kg/day. In one study, complete remission occurred in 44% of patients. Pustule counts decreased by 71% within 3 weeks and by 94% within 10 weeks.[104] Adequate control can be maintained at a lower dosage (e.g., 30 mg/day),[105] but most patients require long-term treatment. The treatment of choice for severe recalcitrant disease is PUVA plus etretinate.[53,54]

Erythrodermic psoriasis. Initial dosage is 0.5 mg/kg/day. A prompt reduction in erythema occurs and may be completely resolved in 2 to 4 weeks.

Plaque-type psoriasis. Initial dosage is 0.5 to 0.75 mg/kg/day; this is increased gradually to 1.0 to 1.5 mg/kg/day if there is no response. Plaques increase in size in a few weeks in approximately 50% of patients and generally subside in 3 to 4 months.

Re-PUVA. Etretinate combined with PUVA, called *Re-PUVA*, accelerates the response to PUVA, reduces the number of exposures and treatment time required for clearing, clears PUVA-resistant cases, and at least halves the cumulative UVA dose needed to clear the psoriasis when PUVA is used alone. See the PUVA treatment section on p. 208.

The patient is pretreated with etretinate (1 mg/kg/day for 1 to 3 weeks), PUVA is combined with etretinate until the disease is controlled, and then PUVA is used for maintenance alone. The same beneficial results were reported when isotretinoin (Accutane, 1 mg/kg/day) was used instead of etretinate.[61]

Dubertret, who has treated more than 700 patients with etretinate, suggests a three-phase treatment schedule (described below) that clears psoriasis at a slower rate but with a lower incidence of side effects.[106]

1. Begin with low dosages of etretinate (i.e., 10 to 20 mg/day for an adult). Increase the daily dose by 10 mg every week until the appearance of bearable cheilitis.
2. When treatment is stabilized and if the skin lesions did not disappear, add another treatment (topical steroids, dithranol, PUVA, or UVB) until skin clearing occurs, while maintaining the same dosage of etretinate.
3. After the patient's condition has cleared, continue etretinate at the same dosage in order to prevent relapses. Others recommend tapering the etretinate dosage after the patient has been clear for 1 or 2 months and restarting only with recurrence.[100]

Figure 8-23
Pityriasis rubra pilaris. The entire surface of the palms and soles become thick (hyperkeratotic) and yellow.

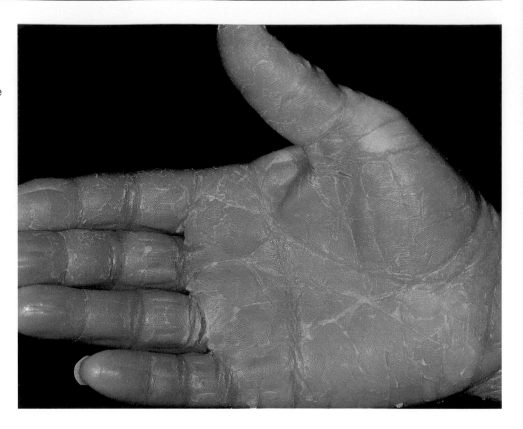

Figure 8-24
Pityriasis rubra pilaris. The classic presentation. Bright red follicular papules merge to form large, bright red-orange plaques.

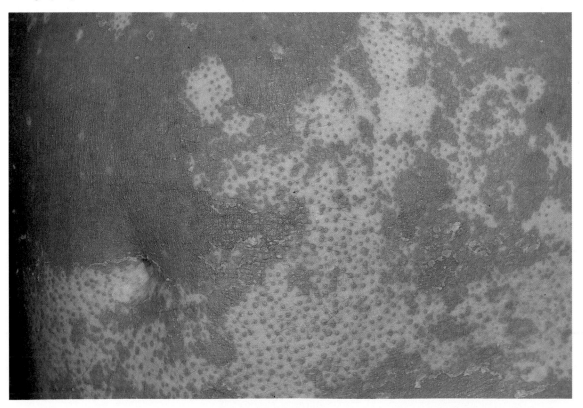

Pityriasis Rubra Pilaris

Pityriasis rubra pilaris (PRP) is a rare, chronic disease of unknown etiology with a unique combination of features. These are thick, smooth, yellow palms and soles, erythroderma, frequently with well-defined "skip spots" of normal skin surrounded by a background of erythema and red follicular papules on the dorsal aspects of the proximal phalanges, elbows, and knees. PRP may occur at any age, but most cases occur in the first and fifth or sixth decades of life. PRP has been divided into adult and childhood forms. Griffiths subclassified the disease into five groups, separating adult disease into classic and atypical types, and the juvenile form into classic, circumscribed, and atypical types.[107] Classic adult PRP (type I) and juvenile PRP are the most common.

A severe form of PRP may be unmasked, precipitated, or otherwise associated with HIV infection.[108,109]

Clinical manifestations. Classic adult PRP begins insidiously, usually in the fifth or sixth decade, with a small, indolent, red scaling plaque on the face or upper body. The plaque slowly enlarges over days and weeks, the palms and soles begin to thicken (Figure 8-23), and bright red-orange follicular papules appear on the dorsal aspects of the proximal phalanges, elbows, knees, and trunk as the disease evolves and progresses into a grotesque generalized eruption. The follicular keratotic papules coalesce on many areas of the trunk to produce a complex pattern of discrete papules and sharply bordered, red plaques with islands of normal skin (Figure 8-24). The eruption may spread to involve almost the entire cutaneous surface. Scaling is coarse on the lower half of the body and fine and powdery on the upper half. Ectropion is present with extensive facial involvement. The nails show distal yellow-brown discoloration, subungual hyperkeratosis, nail thickening, and splinter hemorrhages. Psoriatic nails show onycholysis (particularly marginal), salmon patches, small pits, and larger indentations of the nail plate.[110]

There is little or no itching. The patient is impaired by the thick, tight scales of the scalp, face, and palms and the painful fissures that develop on the soles. The diffuse, red, tight-scaling face destroys the self-image and these patients remain isolated. The eruption lasts for months and years; 80% are clear within 3 years.

Childhood pityriasis rubra pilaris. Childhood PRP begins on the scalp and face and simulates seborrheic dermatitis. The disease becomes more widespread and follicular keratotic papules develop. The childhood form tends to recur for years, which is not characteristic of the adult form. The circumscribed form is characterized by red-orange plaques, usually on the elbows and knees, consisting of sharply demarcated areas of follicular hyperkeratosis and erythema (Figure 8-25). The 3-year remission rate is 32%.[111]

Diagnosis. The distinctive clinical picture is the most valuable diagnostic feature. The disease looks like psoriasis when localized to the scalp, elbows, and knees. The biopsy shows thick scale and dense, keratotic, follicular plugs.

Treatment. Frequent use of lubricants such as Lac-Hydrin (12% lactic acid) and Eucerin or vaseline keeps the skin supple. Lac-Hydrin applied to the feet and covered with a plastic bag at bedtime is an effective approach for removing scale. Application of heavy moisturizers, such as equal parts Aquaphor and Unibase, followed by occlusion with a plastic suit for several hours makes the skin supple. Dovonex (calcipotriol, a vitamin D_3 analogue), the new topical agent approved for psoriasis (discussed earlier), may be effective for PRP.

Retinoids are the most effective systemic agents.[112] Isotretinoin provides symptomatic improvement of erythema, pruritus, scaling, ectropion, and keratoderma in 4 weeks, while significant improvement or clearing takes 16 to 24 weeks. Remission or maintained improvement persists after stopping therapy in many patients. Dosages in the range of 0.5 to 2.0 mg/kg/day are used for up to 6 months.[113]

A review suggested that etretinate may be superior to isotretinoin in the treatment of adult-onset pityriasis rubra pilaris. Of the patients treated with isotretinoin, 7 of 15 cleared. The duration of treatment ranged from 82 to 384 days; the total intake of isotretinoin ranged from 3.28 to 26.10 gm (average dose 1 mg/kg/day). Of the etretinate-treated patients, three of four cleared after 5 months of treatment at an average dosage of 0.5 mg/kg/day.[114]

The antimetabolites offer an alternative to retinoids[115] and methotrexate[116,117] and appear to be more effective than azathioprine.[118] Daily methotrexate (2.5 mg/day) is more effective than the standard weekly regimen used for psoriasis and may be more effective than retinoids. Improvement may be noted in the second or third week, and there may be marked improvement in 10 to 12 weeks, at which time the dose can be tapered. Megadose vitamin A (1 million IU/day) given for 5 to 14 days clears the skin in days in some reports but has been less effective in others.[119,120,121]

Penicillin, stanozolol,[122] and the Goeckerman regimen (UVB and crude coal tar) are probably not effective. PRP patients are photosensitive and the majority flare with either psoralens and ultraviolet A (PUVA) or ultraviolet B therapy.

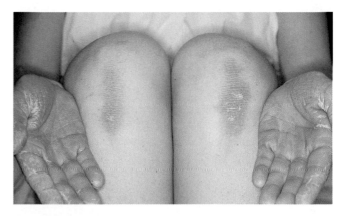

Figure 8-25
Childhood pityriasis rubra pilaris. Red-orange plaques usually remain confined to the elbows, knees, and palms.

Seborrheic Dermatitis

Seborrheic dermatitis is a common, chronic, inflammatory disease with a characteristic pattern for different age groups. The yeast *Pityrosporum ovale* probably is a causative factor, but both genetic and environmental factors seem to influence the onset and course of the disease. Many adult patients have an oily complexion, the so-called seborrheic diathesis. In adults, seborrheic dermatitis tends to persist, but it does undergo periods of remission and exacerbation. The extent of involvement among patients varies widely. Most cases can be adequately controlled.

INFANTS (CRADLE CAP)

Infants commonly develop a greasy adherent scale on the vertex of the scalp. Minor amounts of scale are easily removed by frequent shampooing with products containing sulfur and salicylic acid (e.g., Sebulex shampoo). Scale may accumulate and become thick and adherent over much of the scalp and may be accompanied by inflammation (Figure 8-26). Secondary infection can occur.

Treatment. Patients with serum and crust are treated with oral antistaphylococcal antibiotics. Once infection is controlled, erythema and scaling can be suppressed with group VI or VII topical steroid creams or lotions. Dense, thick, adherent scale is removed by applying warm mineral or olive oil to the scalp and washing several hours later with detergents such as Dawn dishwashing liquid. Remissions possibly can be prolonged with frequent use of salicylic acid or tar shampoos (see the Formulary, p. 852).

Figure 8-26
Seborrheic dermatitis (cradle cap). Diffuse inflammation with secondary infection. Much of the scale from this child's scalp was removed with shampoos.

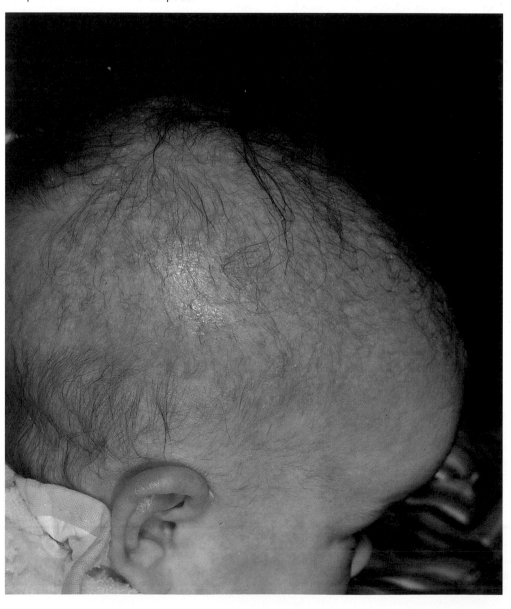

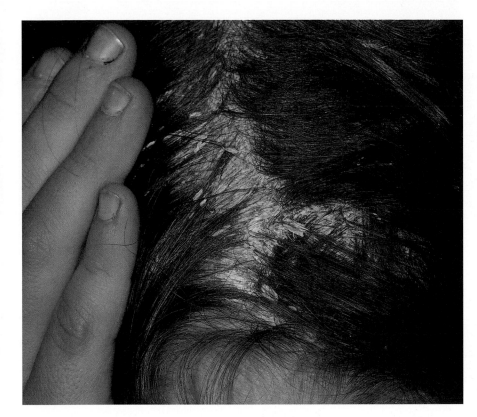

Figure 8-27
Seborrheic dermatitis (tinea amiantacea). The scalp contains dense patches of scale. Large plates of yellow-white scale firmly adhere to the hair shafts.

YOUNG CHILDREN (TINEA AMIANTACEA AND BLEPHARITIS)

Tinea amiantacea is a characteristic eruption of unknown etiology. Mothers of afflicted children often recall the child experiencing episodes of cradle cap during infancy. Some authors believe that tinea amiantacea is a form of eczema or psoriasis. One patch or several patches of dense scale appear anywhere on the scalp and may persist for months before the parent notices temporary hair loss or the distinctive large, oval, yellow-white plates of scale firmly adhered to the scalp and hair (Figure 8-27). Characteristically, the scale binds to the hair and is drawn up with the growing hair. Patches of dense scale range from 2 to 10 cm. The scale suggests fungal scalp disease, which explains the designation tinea. Amiantacea, meaning asbestos, refers to the platelike quality of the scale, which resembles genuine asbestos.

Treatment. Warm 10% liquor carbonis detergens (LCD) in Nivea oil (prescription is for 8 oz; it must be prepared by the pharmacist) is applied to the scalp at bedtime and removed by shampooing each morning with Dawn dishwashing liquid. Derma-smoothe FS lotion (peanut oil, mineral oil, fluocinolone acetonide 0.01%) is an effective topical steroid that can be applied to the entire scalp and occluded with a shower cap. The scalp is dampened before application. Treatments are repeated each night for 1 to 3 weeks until itching and erythema is controlled. The scale is completely removed in 1 to 3 weeks and tar shampoos such as T-gel are used for maintenance. Periodic recurrences are similarly treated.

White scale adherent to the eyelashes and lid margins with variable amounts of erythema is characteristic of seborrheic blepharitis (Figure 8-28). The disease produces some discomfort and is unbecoming. The disease persists for years and is resistant to treatment. Scale may be suppressed by frequent washing with zinc- or tar-containing antidandruff shampoos (see the Formulary, p. 851). Although topical steroid creams and lotions suppress this disease, prolonged use of such preparations around the eyes may cause glaucoma and must be avoided. Ketoconazole (Nizoral cream) applied once a day is worth a trial in resistant cases.

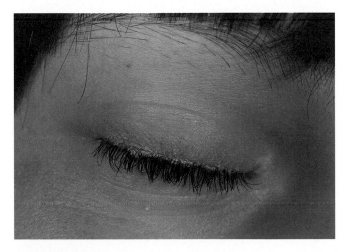

Figure 8-28
Seborrheic dermatitis (blepharitis). Dense adherent scale on the lids.

Figure 8-29
Seborrheic dermatitis in an adult with extensive involvement
in all of the characteristic sites.

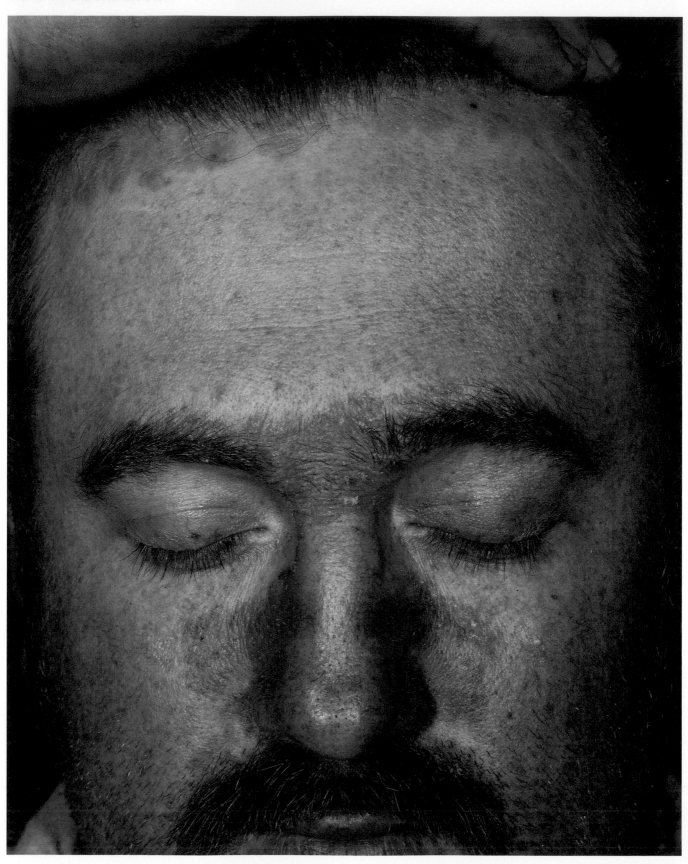

ADOLESCENTS AND ADULTS (CLASSIC SEBORRHEIC DERMATITIS)

Most individuals periodically experience fine, dry, white scalp scaling with minor itching; this is dandruff. They tend to attribute this condition to a dry scalp and consequently avoid hair washing. Avoidance of washing allows scale to accumulate and inflammation may occur. Patients with minor amounts of dandruff should be encouraged to wash every day or every other day with antidandruff shampoos (see the Formulary, p. 851). Fine, dry, white or yellow scale may occur on an inflamed base. The distribution of scaling and inflammation may be more diffuse and occur in the seborrheic areas: scalp and scalp margins, eyebrows, base of eyelashes, nasolabial folds, external ear canals, posterior auricular fold, and presternal area (Figure 8-29).

The axillae, inframammary folds, groin, and umbilicus are affected less frequently. Scaling of the ears may be misjudged as eczema or fungus infection. Its presence in association with characteristic scaling in other typical areas assists in supporting the diagnosis. Scaling may appear when a beard is grown and disappear when it is shaved (Figure 8-30). Once established, the disease tends to persist to a variable degree. Older patients, particularly those who are bedridden or those with neurologic problems such as Parkinson's disease, tend to have a more chronic and extensive form of the disease. Seborrheic dermatitis is seen in neuroleptic-induced parkinsonism.[123] Occasionally the scalp scale may be diffuse, thick, and adherent. Differentiation from psoriasis may be impossible.

Patients should be reassured that seborrheic dermatitis does not cause permanent hair loss. Tinea capitis caused by *Trichophyton tonsurans* has a dry, white, diffuse scale in the adult that does not fluoresce under Wood's light. Fungal culture and potassium hydroxide examination are indicated for atypical or resistant cases of scalp scaling.

AIDS

Seborrheic dermatitis is one of the most common cutaneous manifestations of AIDS. The onset usually occurs before the development of AIDS symptoms. The severity of the seborrheic dermatitis correlates with the degree of clinical deterioration.

Treatment of Seborrheic Dermatitis

Treatment consists of frequent washing of all affected areas, including the face and chest, with an antiseborrheic shampoo. Remaining inflamed areas respond quickly to group V topical steroid creams. Steroid lotions may be applied to the scalp twice daily. Patients must be cautioned that topical steroids should not be used as maintenance therapy.

Dense, diffuse scalp scaling is treated with 10% LCD in Nivea oil or Derma-smoothe FS lotion (peanut oil, mineral oil, fluocinolone acetonide 0.01%) as previously described for treating young children. Adults may apply oil preparations at bedtime and cover with a shower cap. Treatment is repeated each night until the scalp is clear, in approximately 1 to 3 weeks.

Ketoconazole (Nizoral cream) applied once a day is effective against even the most difficult and diffuse cases.[124] Patients with widespread disease involving the face, ears, chest, and upper back can now be treated effectively by using Nizoral to clear the scale and erythema. Frequent washing with zinc soaps (ZNP bar soap) or selenium lotions (Exsel, Selsun) suppresses activity and maintains the remission. Curiously, minor seborrheic dermatitis of the face may not respond as well and may require the addition of group V through VII topical steroids for control.

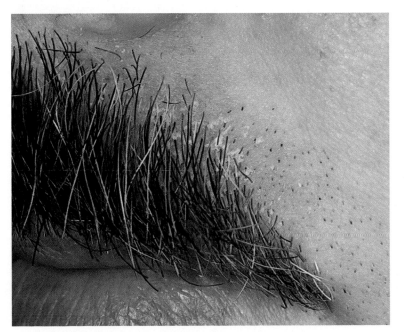

Figure 8-30
Seborrheic dermatitis. Redness and scaling can appear when a mustache or beard is grown. The scaling spontaneously clears when the hair is cut.

Pityriasis Rosea

Pityriasis rosea is a common, benign, usually asymptomatic, distinctive, self-limiting skin eruption of unknown etiology.[125] There is some evidence that it is viral in origin. Small epidemics have occurred in fraternity houses and military bases. It is predominant among women by a margin of 1.5 to 1. More than 75% of patients are between the ages of 10 and 35 years, with a mean age of 23 years and an age range of 4 months to 78 years. Two percent of patients have a recurrence.[126] The incidence of disease is higher during the colder months. Twenty percent of patients have a recent history of acute infection with fatigue, headache, sore throat, lymphadenitis, and fever; the disease may be more common in atopic patients. Pityriasis rosea has several unique features, but variant patterns do exist; these may create confusion between pityriasis rosea and secondary syphilis, guttate psoriasis, viral exanthems, tinea, nummular eczema, and drug eruptions.

Clinical manifestations. Typically, a single 2- to 10-cm round-to-oval lesion, the herald patch, abruptly appears. It may occur anywhere on the body, but is most frequently located on the trunk or proximal extremities. The herald patch retains the same features as the subsequent oval lesions. At this stage, many patients are convinced that they have ringworm.

Within a few days to several weeks (average 7 to 14 days) the disease enters the eruptive phase. Smaller lesions appear and reach their maximum number in 1 to 2 weeks (Figure 8-31). They are typically limited to the trunk and proximal extremities, but in extensive cases they develop on the arms, legs, and face (Figure 8-32). Lesions are typically benign and are concentrated in the lower abdominal area (Figure 8-33). Individual lesions are salmon pink in whites and hyperpigmented in blacks. Many of the earliest lesions are papular, but in most cases the typical 1- to 2-cm oval plaques appear (Figure 8-34). A fine, wrinkled, tissuelike scale remains attached within the border of the plaque giving the characteristic ring of scale, called *collarette scale* (Figure 8-35). The long axis of the oval plaques is oriented along skin lines. Numerous lesions on the back, oriented along skin lines, give the appearance of drooping pine-tree branches, which explains the designation Christmas-tree distribution. The number of lesions varies from a few to hundreds. In rare instances the lesions seem to cover the entire skin surface. A variety of oral lesions has been reported.[127,128]

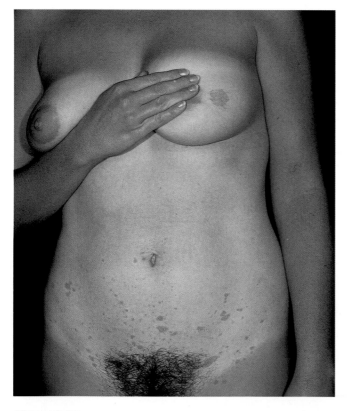

Figure 8-31
Pityriasis rosea. A herald patch is present on the breast. Subsequent lesions commonly begin in the lower abdominal region.

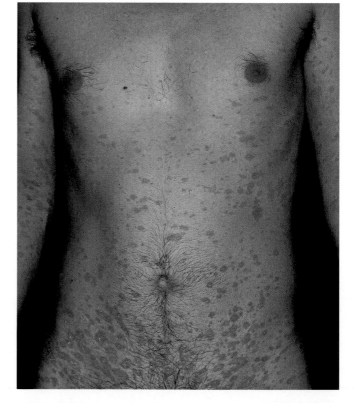

Figure 8-32
Pityriasis rosea. The fully evolved eruption 2 weeks after onset.

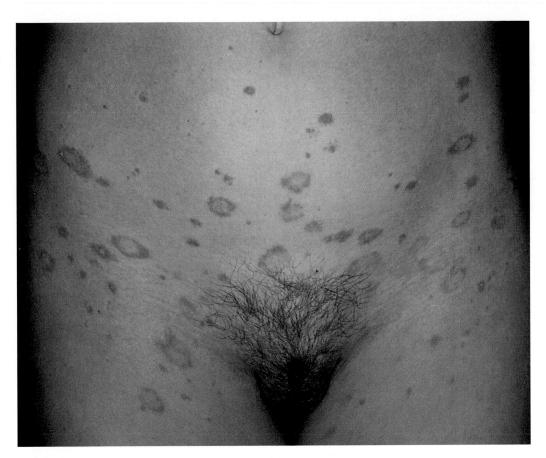

Figure 8-33
Pityriasis rosea. Lesions are typically concentrated in the lower abdominal area.

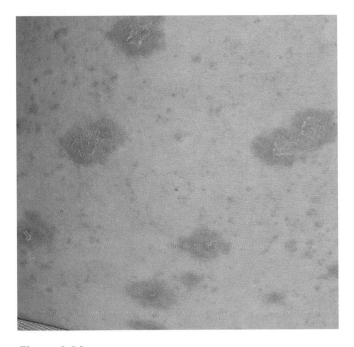

Figure 8-34
Pityriasis rosea. Both small, oval plaques and multiple, small papules are present. Occasionally the eruption consists only of small papules.

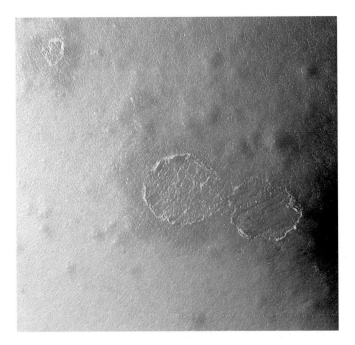

Figure 8-35
Pityriasis rosea. A ring of tissuelike scale (collarette scale) remains attached within the border of the plaque.

In some cases other types of lesions predominate. The papular variety is more common in young children, pregnant women, and blacks (Figures 8-36 and 8-37). Vesicular and, rarely, purpuric[129] lesions are seen in infants and children.

Most lesions are asymptomatic, but many patients complain of mild transient itching. Severe itching may accompany extensive inflammatory eruptions. The disease clears spontaneously in 1 to 3 months. There may be postinflammatory hyperpigmentation, especially in blacks.

Diagnosis. The experienced observer can rely on a clinical impression to make the diagnosis. Tinea can be ruled out with a potassium hydroxide examination. Secondary syphilis may be indistinguishable from pityriasis rosea, especially if the herald patch is absent. A serologic test for syphilis should be ordered if a clinical diagnosis cannot be made.[130] A biopsy is useful in atypical cases; it reveals extravasated erythrocytes within dermal papillae and dyskeratotic cells within the dermis. Pityriasis rosea may also be mimicked by psoriasis and nummular eczema.

Management. Whether or not PR is contagious is unknown. The disease is benign and self-limited and does not appear to affect the fetus; therefore, isolation is unnecessary. Group V topical steroids and oral antihistamines may be used as needed for itching. The rare extensive case with intense itching responds to a 1- to 2-week course of prednisone (20 mg twice a day). Direct sun exposure hastens the resolution of individual lesions, whereas those in protected areas, such as under bathing suits, remain (see Figure 8-31). Ultraviolet light B (UVB), administered in five consecutive daily erythemogenic exposures, results in decreased pruritus and hastens the involution of lesions. Therapy is most beneficial within the first week of the eruption.[131]

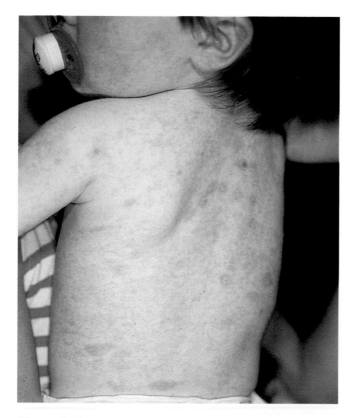

Figure 8-36
Pityriasis rosea. Papular lesions may be the predominant lesion in children.

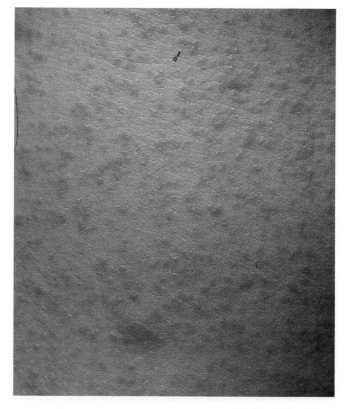

Figure 8-37
Pityriasis rosea. Papular lesions are seen in children, pregnant women, and blacks.

Lichen Planus

Lichen planus (LP) is a unique inflammatory cutaneous and mucous membrane reaction pattern of unknown etiology. The mean age of onset is 40.3 years in males compared with 46.4 years in females. The main eruption clears within 1 year in 68% of patients, but 49% recur.[132] Although the disease may occur at any age, it is rare in children younger than 5 years of age. Approximately 10% of patients have a positive family history. This supports the hypothesis that genetic factors are of etiologic importance in lichen planus.[133] Liver disease is a risk factor for LP although not a specific marker of it.[134] LP may be associated with hepatitis C virus–related, chronic, active hepatitis.[135]

There are several clinical forms, and the number of lesions varies from a few chronic papules to acute generalized disease (Table 8-5). Eruptions from drugs (e.g., gold, chloroquine, methyl-dopa, penicillamine), chemical exposure (film processing), bacterial infections (secondary syphilis), and post–bone marrow transplants (graft-vs.-host reaction) that have a similar appearance are referred to as lichenoid.

Primary lesions. The morphology and distribution of the lesions are characteristic (Figure 8-38). The clinical features of lichen planus can be remembered by learning the five P's of lichen planus: pruritic, planar (flat-topped), polyangular, purple papules. The primary lesion is a 2- to 10-mm flat-topped papule with an irregular angulated border (polygonal papules). Close inspection of the surface shows a lacy, reticular pattern of criss-crossed, whitish lines (Wickham's stria) that can be accentuated by a drop of immersion oil (Figure 8-39, *A* and *B*). (Histologically, Wickham's stria are areas of focal epidermal thickening.)

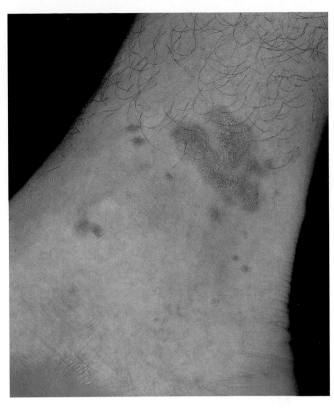

Figure 8-38
Lichen planus. A characteristic lesion of planar, polyangular, purple papules with lacy reticular, criss-crossed whitish lines (Wickham's striae) on the surface.

Figure 8-39 Lichen planus—primary lesions.

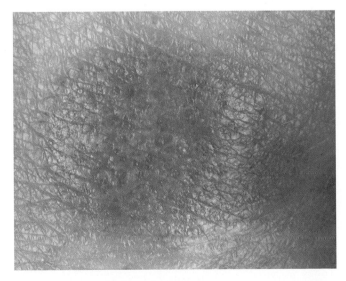

A, The primary lesion is a flat-topped papule with an irregular, angulated border (polygonal papules).

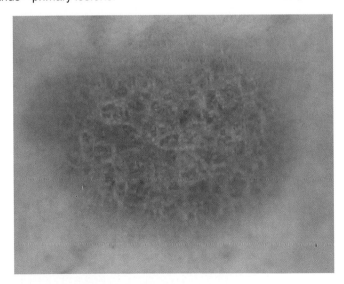

B, Close inspection of the surface shows a lacy, reticular pattern of criss-crossed whitish lines (Wickham's striae), accentuated here by a drop of immersion oil.

TABLE 8-5 Various Patterns of Lichen Planus

Various patterns of lichen planus	Most common site
Actinic	Sun-exposed areas
Annular	Trunk, external genitalia
Atrophic	Any area
Erosioulcerative	Soles of feet, mouth
Follicular (lichen plano pilaris)	Scalp
Guttate (numerous small papules)	Trunk
Hypertrophic	Lower limbs (especially ankles)
Linear	Zosteriform (leg), scratched area
Nail disease	Fingernails
Papular (localized)	Flexor surface (wrists and forearms)
Vesiculobullous	Lower limbs, mouth

Newly evolving lesions are pink-white, but over time they assume a distinctive violaceous, or purple, hue with a peculiar waxy luster. Lesions that persist for months may become thicker and dark red (hypertrophic lichen planus). Papules aggregate into different patterns. Patterns are usually haphazard clusters, but they may be annular, diffusely papular (guttate), or linear, appearing in response to a scratch (Köbner's phenomenon). Rarely, a line of papules may extend the length of an extremity. Vesicles or bullae may appear on preexisting lesions or on normal skin. Many patients have persistent brown staining many years after the rash has cleared.

LOCALIZED PAPULES

Papules are most commonly located on the flexor surfaces of the wrists and forearms (Figure 8-40), the legs immediately above the ankles (Figure 8-41), and the lumbar region (Figure 8-42). Itching is variable; 20% of patients with lichen planus do not itch. Some patients with generalized involvement have minimal symptoms, whereas others display intolerable pruritus. The course is unpredictable. Some patients experience spontaneous remission in a few months, but the most common localized papular form tends to be chronic and endures for an average of approximately 4 years.

HYPERTROPHIC LICHEN PLANUS

This second most common cutaneous pattern may occur on any body region, but it is typically found on the pretibial areas of the legs and ankles (Figure 8-43). After a long time, papules lose their characteristic features and become confluent as reddish-brown or purplish, thickened, round-to-elongated (bandlike) plaques with a rough or verrucose surface; itching may be severe. Lesions continue for months or years, averaging approximately 8 years, and may be perpetuated by scratching. After the lesions clear, a dark-brown pigmentation remains.

Figure 8-40
Localized lichen planus. Early lesions are present on the wrists **(A)** and ankles **(B)**, common sites for localized lichen planus.

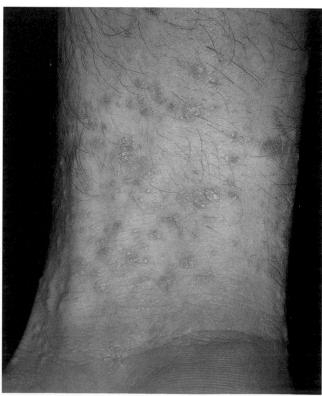

A

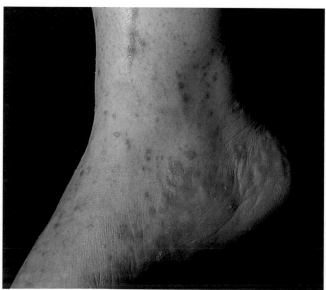

B

Figure 8-41 Localized lichen planus.

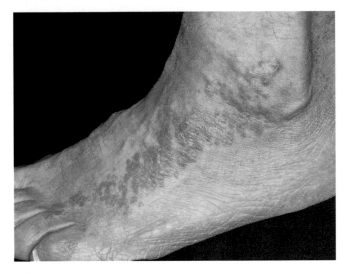

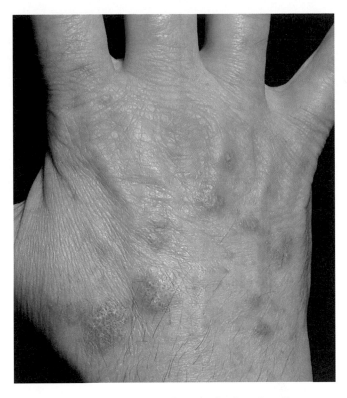

A, Papules become thicker and confluent with time.

B, Wickham's striae are prominently displayed on these lesions.

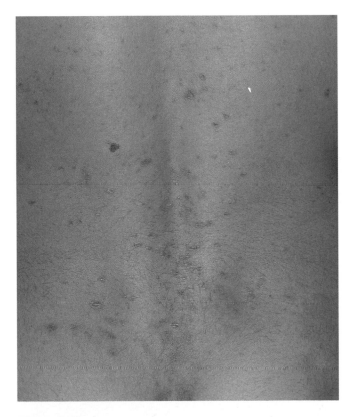

Figure 8-42
Lichen planus. Papules are larger and are confluent in the lower back region.

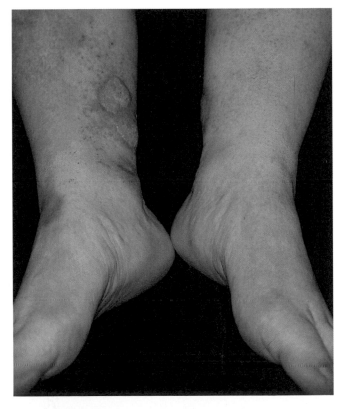

Figure 8-43
Hypertrophic lichen planus. Thick, reddish-brown plaques are most often present on the lower legs.

GENERALIZED LICHEN PLANUS AND LICHENOID DRUG ERUPTIONS

Lichen planus may occur abruptly as a generalized, intensely pruritic eruption (Figure 8-44). Initially, the papules are pinpoint, numerous, and isolated. The papules may remain discrete or become confluent as large, red, eczematous-like, thin plaques. A highly characteristic, diffuse, dark brown, postinflammatory pigmentation remains as the disease clears. Before resolving spontaneously, untreated generalized lichen planus continues for approximately 8 months. Lichenoid drug eruptions are frequently of this diffuse type.[136] Low-grade fever may be present in the first few days, and lesions appear on the trunk, extremities, and lower back (see Figure 8-42). The disease is seldom seen on the face or scalp and is rare on the palms and soles.

LICHEN PLANUS OF THE PALMS AND SOLES

Lichen planus of the palms and soles generally occurs as an isolated phenomenon, but may appear simultaneously with disease in other areas. The lesions differ from classic lesions of lichen planus in that the papules are larger and aggregate into semitranslucent plaques with a globular waxy surface (Figure 8-45). Itching may be intolerable. Ulceration may occur and lesions of the feet may be so resistant to treatment that surgical excision and grafting is required.[137] The disease may last indefinitely.

FOLLICULAR LICHEN PLANUS

Follicular lichen planus is also known as *lichen planopilaris*.[138] Lesions localized to the hair follicles may occur alone or with papular lichen planus. Follicular lichen planus,

manifested as pinpoint, hyperkeratotic, follicular projections, is the most common form of lichen planus found in the scalp, where papular lesions are rarely observed. Hair loss occurs and may be permanent if the disease is sufficiently active to cause scarring. Lichen planus of the scalp causes scarring alopecia. Patients with scarring alopecia should be evaluated histologically and with direct immunofluorescence. The immunofluorescence abnormalities differ from those associated with lichen planus, suggesting that lichen planopilaris and lichen planus are two different diseases.[139,140]

ORAL MUCOUS MEMBRANE LICHEN PLANUS

Oral lichen planus can occur without cutaneous disease. Onset before middle age is rare; the mean age of onset is in the sixth decade.[141] Women outnumber men by more than 2:1.[142] Mucous membrane involvement is observed in more than 50% of patients with cutaneous lichen planus. Lesions may be located on the tongue (Figure 8-46) and lips, but the most common site is the buccal mucosa (Figure 8-47). There are two stages of severity. The most common form is the nonerosive, generally asymptomatic, dendritic branching or lacy white network pattern seen on the buccal mucosa; papules and plaques may appear with time. The oral cavity should always be examined if the diagnosis of cutaneous lichen planus is suspected. The presence of this dendritic pattern is solid supporting evidence for the diagnosis of cutaneous lichen planus.

A more difficult form is erosive mucosal lichen planus (Figure 8-48). Localized or extensive ulcerations may involve any area of the oral cavity. Candidal infection was found in 17% to 25% of ulcerated and nonulcerated cases of lichen planus.[143] Malignant transformation occurs in 1.2% of patients.[144] Superficial and erosive lesions are less commonly found on the glans penis (Figure 8-49), vulvovaginal region, and anus.[145]

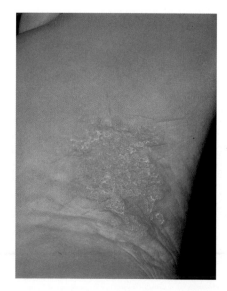

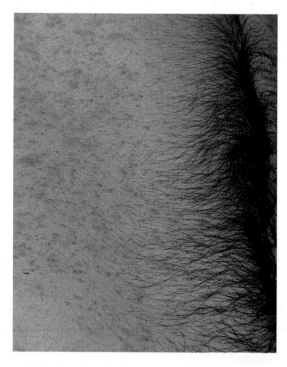

Figure 8-44
Generalized lichen planus.

Figure 8-45
Lichen planus of the soles. Thick, semitranslucent plaques.

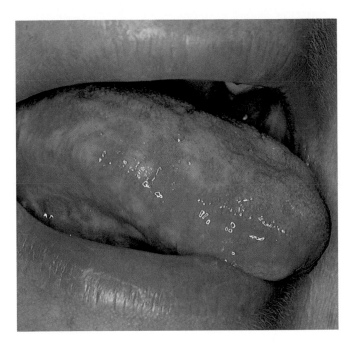

Figure 8-46
Mucous membrane lichen planus. The lacey white pattern is similar to that seen on the buccal mucosa.

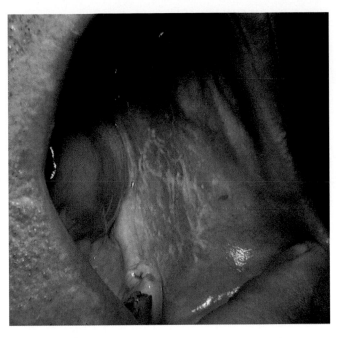

Figure 8-47
Mucous membrane lichen planus. A lacy, white pattern is present on the buccal mucosa. *(Courtesy Gerald Shklar, B.Sc., D.D.S., M.S., Harvard School of Dental Medicine.)*

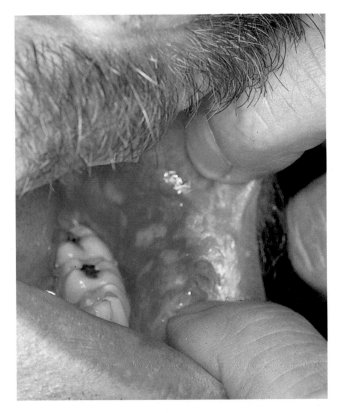

Figure 8-48
Erosive oral lichen planus. Localized or extensive ulcerations may involve any area of the oral cavity.

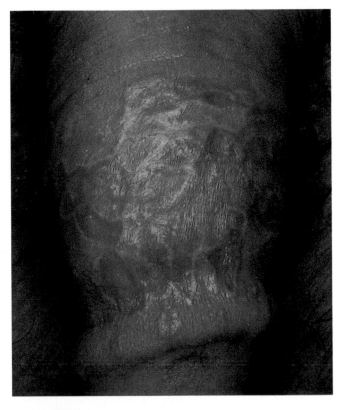

Figure 8-49
Lichen planus on the penis. A lacy, white pattern identical to that seen on the buccal mucosa.

EROSIVE VAGINAL LICHEN PLANUS

Lichen planus usually involves skin and oral cavity lesions, but erosive vaginal disease may be the first sign. Lichen planus may be the most common cause of desquamative vaginitis. There are flares and partial remissions but no tendency for complete remission. There is marked vaginal mucosal fragility and erythema (Figure 8-50). Agglutination of the labia minora may occur, and vaginal adhesions may render a patient unable to engage in sexual intercourse. Vaginal histology may be nonspecific, showing only a loss of epithelium. A biopsy taken from a white hyperkeratotic area on the labial skin may provide a specific histologic picture. Vaginal desquamation is not associated with lichen sclerosus. Topical and oral steroids are the most effective treatment. Some patients respond to dapsone. Many other systemic agents have been used.[146,147]

Estrogens are not effective.

NAILS

Nail changes frequently accompany generalized lichen planus, but may occur as the only manifestation of disease. Approximately 25% of patients with nail LP have LP in other sites before or after the onset of nail lesions. Nail LP usually appears during the fifth or sixth decade of life. The changes include proximal to distal linear depressions or grooves and partial or complete destruction of the nail plate. The development of severe and early destruction of the nail matrix characterizes a small subset of patients with nail LP.[148] Long-term observation indicates that permanent damage to the nail is rare even in patients with diffuse involvement of the matrix. (See Chapter Twenty-five.)

DIAGNOSIS

The diagnosis can be made clinically, but a skin biopsy eliminates any doubt. Direct immunofluorescence may help to establish the diagnosis.[149] The skin shows ovoid globular deposits of IgG, IgM, IgA, and complement. Basement membrane zone deposits of fibrin and fibrinogen are present in a linear pattern in both cutaneous and oral lesions in almost all patients. Circulating antibodies have not been found, therefore indirect immunofluorescence is negative.

TREATMENT

Therapy for cutaneous lichen planus

Topical steroids. Group I or II topical steroids (in a cream or ointment base applied three times daily) are used as initial treatment for localized disease. They relieve itching, but the lesions are slow to clear. Plastic occlusion enhances the effectiveness of topical steroids.

Intralesional steroids. Triamcinolone acetonide (Kenalog, 5 to 10 mg/ml) may reduce the hypertrophic lesions located on the wrists and lower legs. Injections may be repeated every 3 or 4 weeks.

Systemic steroids. Generalized, severely pruritic lichen planus responds to oral corticosteroids. For adults, a 2- to 4-week course of prednisone, 20 mg twice daily, is usually sufficient to clear the disease. To prevent recurrence, gradually decrease the dosage over a 3-week period.

Acitretin 30 mg/day is effective for severe LP. At the end of 8 weeks, 64% showed remission or marked improvement.[150]

Cyclosporine. Patients with severe, chronic lichen planus were successfully treated with oral CS (6 mg/kg/day). A response was noted within 4 weeks, and complete clearing was achieved after 8 weeks of treatment. No significant adverse effect was noted. The patients remained in remission up to 10 months after therapy.[151]

Antihistamines. Antihistamines such as hydroxyzine, 10 to 25 mg every 4 hours, may provide very satisfactory relief from itching.

PUVA. A bilateral comparison study demonstrated that PUVA is an effective therapy for generalized, symptomatic lichen planus and suggested that maintenance therapy might not be required once complete clearance is attained.[152]

Oral griseofulvin. Oral griseofulvin (250 mg twice daily for 3 to 6 months) has been reported to clear more than 80% of patients,[153] but another report claimed griseofulvin was ineffective.[154]

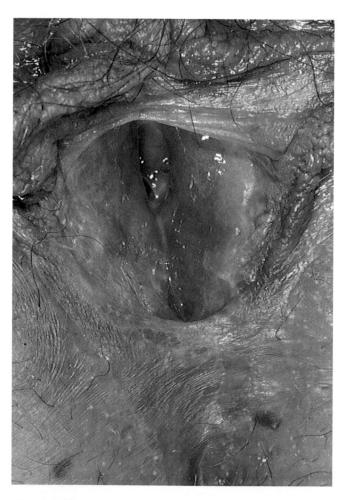

Figure 8-50
Erosive vaginal lichen planus. The entire vaginal tract is involved in this severe case.

Therapy for mucous membrane lichen planus

Topical application of corticosteroids (fluocinonide 0.025%,[155] fluocinolone acetonide, triamcinolone acetonide [Kenalog]) in an adhesive base (orabase) is safe and effective. These medicines are the initial treatment for oral lichen planus. The medication is placed on the lesions, but it is not rubbed in. Massaging the special cream base results in the loss of adhesiveness. Topical application of fluocinonide gel to the gingiva and buccal mucosa over a 3-week period in patients with erosive lichen planus produces no adrenal suppression.[156] Acute candidiasis may occur during treatment but responds to topical antifungal therapy.

Intralesional steroids in a single submucosal injection, 0.5 to 1.0 ml of methyl prednisolone acetate (Depo-Medrol 40 mg/ml) may be sufficient to heal erosive oral lichen planus within 1 week.[157]

Prednisone rapidly and effectively controls the disease, but recurrences may occur when the dosage is tapered.[141,158]

Dapsone (50 to 150 mg/day) is the treatment of choice if conservative medical treatment fails.[159,160]

Hydroxychloroquine sulfate (Plaquenil), 200 to 400 mg daily, is useful for oral LP. Pain relief and reduced erythema occur after 1 to 2 months; erosions required 3 to 6 months of treatment before they resolved.[161]

Azathioprine. Azathioprine is very effective for controlling oral lichen planus and may be considered for resistant, debilitating cases.[162]

Topical cyclosporine. In one study patients swished and expectorated 5 ml of solution (containing 100 mg of CS per ml) three times daily. There was marked improvement after 8 weeks. There were no systemic side effects. Blood CS levels were low or undetectable.[163]

Griseofulvin. Griseofulvin is not effective.[164]

Lichen Striatus

Lichen striatus is an uncommon, unilateral eruption of unknown etiology that has a linear distribution following the embryonic lines described in 1901 by Blaschko (see Figure 20-34). It is typically seen in girls; the mean age at diagnosis is 3 years (6 months to 14 years; median 2 years). Discrete, red or flesh-colored, flat-topped, lichenoid papules with adherent scale erupt suddenly, then coalesce in several areas to form a linear band that may extend the entire length of an extremity (Figure 8-51). Lesions extending to the proximal nailfold affect the nail.[165] Lesions are usually asymptomatic, but at times pruritus is intense. Spontaneous involution occurs. The mean duration was 9.5 months (4 weeks to 3 years; median 6 months) in one study.[166] Transient hyperpigmentation follows resolution in 50% of cases. A biopsy is useful when the diagnosis is in doubt. The differential diagnosis includes lichen planus, nevus unius lateris, and linear Darier's disease. Lesions are resistant to treatment.

Group I topical steroids or group II topical steroids under plastic occlusion may help, but intralesional steroids (triamcinolone acetonide, 2.5 to 10 mg/kg/ml) are more effective. Several courses of treatment may be necessary.

Figure 8-51
Lichen striatus. Discrete red or flesh-colored, flat-topped, lichenoid papules form a linear band that may extend the entire length of an extremity. Lesions extending to the proximal nailfold affect the nail.

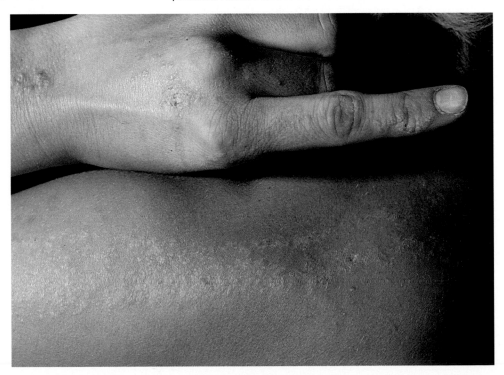

Lichen Sclerosus et Atrophicus

Lichen sclerosus et atrophicus (LSA) is an uncommon but distinctive chronic cutaneous disease of unknown origin. Cases in females outnumber those in males by 10:1. Although the trunk and extremities may be affected, the disease has a predilection for the vulva, perianal area, and groin. Most lesions appear spontaneously, but some may be induced by trauma or radiation (Köbner's phenomenon).[167]

At a glance, LSA may be confused with guttate morphea, lichen planus, or discoid lupus erythematosus. The difference becomes evident upon closer inspection of the surface features. Early lesions are small, smooth, pink or ivory, flat-topped, slightly raised papules. White-to-brown, horny follicular plugs appear on the surface; this feature is referred to as *delling* (Figures 8-52 and 8-53). Delling is not observed in lichen planus or morphea. In time, clusters of papules may coalesce to form small oval plaques with a dull or glistening, smooth, white, atrophic, wrinkled surface (Figure 8-53). Histologically, it appears that the interface area between the dermis and epidermis has dissolved. The overlying, unsupported, thin, atrophic epidermis contracts, giving the appearance of wrinkled tissue paper (Figure 8-54).

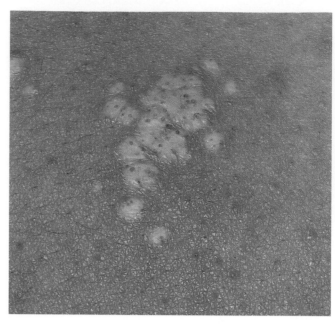

Figure 8-52
Lichen sclerosus et atrophicus. Early lesions are ivory-colored, flat-topped, slightly raised papules with follicular plugs.

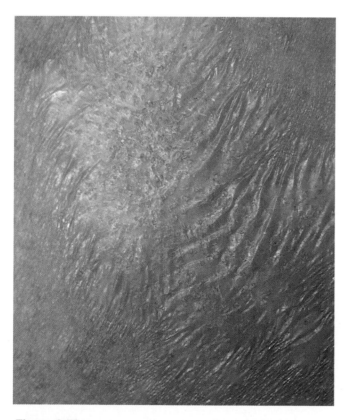

Figure 8-53
Papular lesions as illustrated in Figure 8-52 coalesce to form atrophic plaques with a wrinkled surface. White-to-brown, horny follicular plugs appear on the surface, a feature referred to as *delling*.

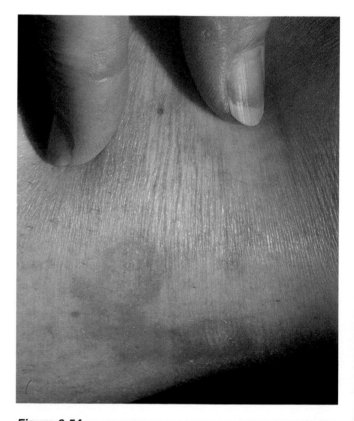

Figure 8-54
Lichen sclerosus et atrophicus. The epidermis is thin and atrophic and gives the appearance of wrinkled tissue paper when compressed.

ANOGENITAL LESIONS IN FEMALES

In most cases, anogenital lesions are distinctive. All of the following patterns may be present in the same individual. The first is a white atrophic plaque in the shape of an hourglass or inverted keyhole encircling the vagina and rectum (Figure 8 55). This most distinctive pattern is seen in prepubertal females, as well as in adults (Figure 8-56). Dysuria and pain on defecation is common.[168] Prepubertal LSA may occur in infants and resolves without sequelae in about two thirds of cases at or just before menarche, leaving a brown hyperpigmented area on skin that had been white and atrophic.[169] Purpura of the vulva is an occasional manifestation of pediatric LSA. It mimics sexual abuse and has led to false accusation and investigations.[170,171,172] The disease persists in approximately one third of patients.

Intertriginous (skin crease) lesions involve the groin and anal area and are subject to friction and maceration. The delicate, thin, white, wrinkled, compromised skin breaks down to become hemorrhagic and eroded, simulating irritant or candidal intertrigo. Bullae may precede erosions.

LSA of the vulva (kraurosis vulvae) is a very distressing problem. Typically, the adult form appears after menopause and has a lengthy duration. Lesions itch and may show evidence of excoriation. The disease is chronic, painful, and interferes with sexual activity. Fragile atrophic tissue erodes, becomes macerated, and heals slowly. Repeated cycles of erosion and healing induce contraction of the vaginal introitus and atrophy and shrinkage of the clitoris and labia minora (Figure 8-57). A watery discharge may be present. Squamous cell carcinoma, particularly of the clitoris or labia minora, has been reported in approximately 3% of patients with chronic LSA.[173] Therefore, biopsy should be considered in lesions that are white and raised (leukoplakia), fissured or ulcerated, and unresponsive to medical therapy.

One report showed that patients with untreated vulvar lichen sclerosus had significantly decreased serum levels of dihydrotestosterone and androstenedione and significantly higher serum levels of free testosterone. Estrogen and sex hormone–binding globulin levels were normal.[174]

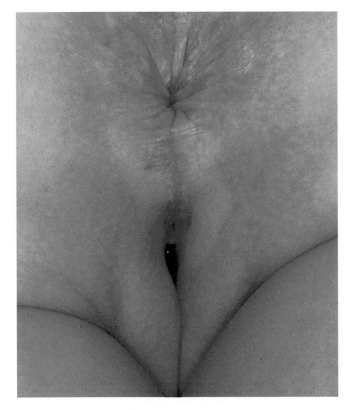

Figure 8-55
Lichen sclerosus et atrophicus. Prepubertal LSA typically involves the vulval and rectal areas. Spontaneous remission occurs in over two thirds of patients.

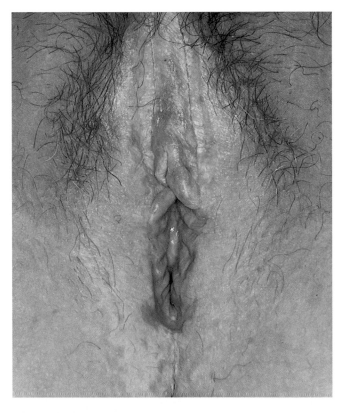

Figure 8-56
Lichen sclerosus et atrophicus. A white, atrophic plaque encircles the vagina and rectum (inverted keyhole pattern).

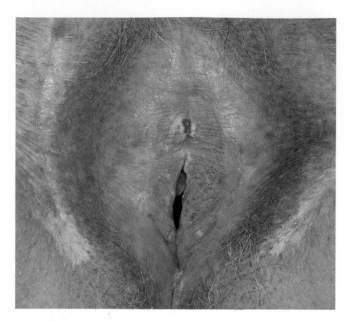

Figure 8-57
Lichen sclerosus et atrophicus of the vulva (kraurosis vulvae). The crease areas are atrophic and wrinkled, the labia is hyperpigmented, and the introitus is contracted and ulcerated.

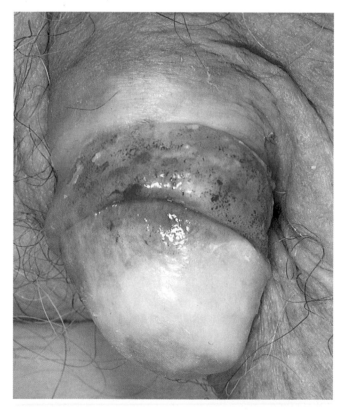

Figure 8-58
Lichen sclerosus et atrophicus of the penis (balanitis xerotica obliterans). The glans is smooth, white, and atrophic. Erosions are present on the prepuce.

LSA OF THE PENIS

In LSA of the penis in the adult (balanitis xerotica obliterans), the patient complains initially of recurrent balanitis, which may be intensified by intercourse; the shaft is rarely involved. The white atrophic plaques occur on the glans and prepuce and erode and heal with contraction (Figure 8-58). Most patients are uncircumcised. LSA may be caused by chronic occlusion.[175] Encroachment into the urinary meatus may lead to stricture. As with vaginal LSA, degeneration into squamous cell carcinoma is rare.[176]

LSA in boys was thought to be rare, but recent reports suggest that it has been overlooked in the past. Most boys are between 4 and 12 years of age at onset. Nearly all affected boys had severe phimosis in a previously retractable penis, with obvious scarring or sclerosis near the tip of the prepuce.[177] Purpura is an occasional manifestation of pediatric LSA. Genital purpura is also a sign of sexual abuse.[171]

MANAGEMENT

In general, the diagnosis of LSA can be made by clinical observation, but a biopsy may be necessary for confirmation. Chronically fissured, ulcerated, or hyperplastic lesions should be biopsied to rule out squamous cell carcinoma.

Topical steroids. Topical steroid creams should be the initial treatment for uncomplicated lesions. The creams suppress itching and may correct some of the pathologic changes. Group V topical steroid creams are applied twice daily for 2 weeks. Vaginal and vulvar candidiasis may occur. Atrophy of the vulva may result from continual application of topical steroids. Use should be discontinued when a favorable response is obtained (usually 2 weeks or less), and bland lubricants such as Nutraplus cream can be used daily to soothe dry tissues.

Treatment with topical testosterone propionate 2% was compared with a twice-daily application of a group I topical steroid (clobetasol dipropionate 0.05%) during a 24-week study. Testosterone suppressed symptoms, but clobetasol was highly effective in relation to symptoms (itching, burning, pain, dyspareunia), clinical aspects (atrophy, hyperkeratosis, sclerosis), and histologic alterations (atrophy of the epithelium, edema, inflammatory infiltrate, fibrosis).[178] Clobetasol is used even in children, and histologic regression of LSA, as well as remarkable relief of symptoms, may occur.[179]

Intralesional steroids such as triamcinolone acetonide (Kenalog, 2.5 to 5.0 mg/ml) may be useful for areas that do not respond to topical therapy.

Fissures and erosions are effectively treated with scarlet red gauze.

Testosterone. Testosterone propionate in a bland ointment has been reported to be partially effective for vulvar[174] and penile LSA. A 2% testosterone ointment is prescribed. The pharmacist is instructed to add 5 ml of testosterone propionate in oil (100 mg/ml) to 25 gm of white petrolatum. The ointment is applied at bedtime and in the morning each day until lesions improve. Two or three months may be required before improvement is noted. One report demonstrated that during the period of testosterone application both total testosterone and dihydrotestosterone levels increased significantly.[174] Side effects such as increased libido and clitoral hypertrophy may occur with chronic use.

Patients may benefit from a combined-treatment program. For example, testosterone ointment applied twice daily for 10 days, lubrication with Nutraplus cream for 7 days, Lotrisone cream applied twice daily for 7 days, lubrication again for 7 days, and the cycle is then repeated. This program can be modified to meet the needs of the individual.

Other treatments. Etretinate (1 mg/kg/day)[180] and Acitretin (20 to 30 mg/day for 16 weeks)[181] are effective in treating women with severe LSA of the vulva.

Carbon dioxide laser ablation to a depth of 1 to 2 mm is acceptable treatment for patients who have LSA of the penis or vulva that is refractory to other measures.[182] The procedure may be performed under general anesthesia. Healing is complete 6 weeks postoperatively, and patients were free of symptoms for up to 3 years.[183]

Cases refractory to medical treatment might benefit from surgical management. Symptoms are relieved by circumcision in men and boys. Skinning vulvectomy and split-thickness skin graft provide excellent cosmetic results and minimal adverse effects on sexual function.[184]

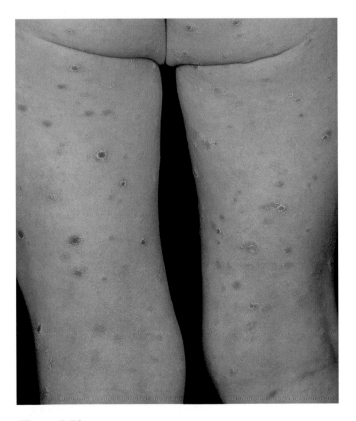

Figure 8-59
Pityriasis lichenoides et varioliformis acuta (PLEVA). Crops of red-to-brown papules that can become hemorrhagic, pustular, or necrotic appear on the trunk, thighs, and upper arms.

Pityriasis Lichenoides

Pityriasis lichenoides is a rare disease with two variants: acute (pityriasis lichenoides et varioliformis acuta [PLEVA] or Mucha-Habermann disease) and chronic (pityriasis lichenoides chronica). The terms *acute* and *chronic* refer to the characteristics of the individual lesions and not to the course of the disease. Most cases occur during the first three decades of the patient's life. The diseases are more common in males. Evidence suggests that PLEVA is a hypersensitivity reaction to an infectious agent. The prognosis for both forms is good.[185] Pityriasis lichenoides chronica, PLEVA, and lymphomatoid papulosis share several clinical and immunohistologic features, suggesting that these disorders are interrelated.[186] The histology of these entities is distinctive.

PLEVA. Mucha-Habermann disease, or PLEVA, is usually a benign, self-limited papulosquamous disorder. PLEVA has been documented in all age groups, with most cases occurring in the second and third decades. PLEVA begins insidiously, with few symptoms other than mild itching or a low-grade fever. Crops of round or oval, reddish-brown papules, usually 2 to 10 mm in diameter, appear, either singly or in clusters. They can occur anywhere, but they typically appear on the trunk, thighs, and upper arms (Figure 8-59). The face, scalp, palms, and soles are involved in approximately 10% of cases.

The papules may develop a violaceous center and a surrounding rim of erythema. There may be micaceous scale. Lesions can become vesicular or pustular and then undergo hemorrhagic necrosis, usually within 2 to 5 weeks, often leaving a postinflammatory hyperpigmentation and sometimes scars. Acute exacerbations are common and the disease may wax and wane for months or years. High fever is a rare complication, but it may be associated with an ulceronecrotic type of lesion.[187] Complications include a self-limited arthritis and superinfection of the skin lesions. Mucha-Habermann disease can mimic other common entities such as varicella and insect bites.

Pityriasis lichenoides chronica. Pityriasis lichenoides chronica (Juliusberg type) is a generalized eruption consisting of brownish papules with fine, micalike, adherent scale that becomes more evident when scratched. The disease may persist for years. Systemic symptoms are rare. The scale is less conspicuous than in psoriasis. Lesions clear without scarring and show only transient skin discolorations. The distribution is similar to PLEVA.

Treatment. Erythromycin produced a remission in 73% of the cases. It frequently took as long as 2 months before a significant therapeutic effect was noted. Clearing with oral erythromycin was reported in most cases at dosages of 30 to 50 mg/kg/day.[188] Erythromycin was tapered over several months, depending on the response. The disease usually recurred if erythromycin was tapered too rapidly. Psoralen ultraviolet light A (PUVA), ultraviolet light B (UVB) phototherapy,[189] tetracycline, gold, methotrexate, oral corticosteroids, and dapsone have all been used with some success.[190]

REFERENCES

1. Farber EM, Nickoloff BJ, Recht B, et al: Stress, symmetry, and psoriasis: possible role of neuropeptides, *J Am Acad Dermatol* 14:305-311, 1986.
2. Updike J: Personal history: at war with my skin, *The New Yorker*, Sept 2, 1985.
3. Skoven I, Thormann J: Lithium compound treatment and psoriasis, *Arch Dermatol* 115:1185-1187, 1979.
4. Gold MH, Holy AK, Roenigk HH: Beta-blocking drugs and psoriasis, *J Am Acad Dermatol* 19:837-841, 1988.
5. Slagel GA, James WD: Plaquenil-induced erythroderma, *J Am Acad Dermatol* 12:857-862, 1985.
6. Abel EA et al: Drugs in exacerbation of psoriasis, *J Am Acad Dermatol* 15:1007-1022, 1986.
7. Baker H, Ryan TJ: Generalized pustular psoriasis: a clinical and epidemiological study of 104 cases, *Br J Dermatol* 80:71-72, 1968.
8. Telfer NR, Chalmers RJ, et al: The role of streptococcal infection in the initiation of guttate psoriasis, *Arch Dermatol* 128:39-42, 1992.
9. Zelickson BD, Muller SA: Generalized pustular psoriasis. A review of 63 cases, *Arch Dermatol* 127:1339-1345, 1991.
10. Boyd AS, Menter A: Erythrodermic psoriasis. Precipitating factors, course, and prognosis in 50 patients, *J Am Acad Dermatol* 21:985-991, 1989.
11. O'Doherty CJ, Macintyre C: Palmoplantar pustulosis and smoking, *Br Med J* 291:861-864, 1985.
12. Benoldi D et al: Reiter's disease: successful treatment of the skin manifestations with oral etretinate, *Acta Derm Venereol* 64:352-354, 1984.
13. Lesher JL, Chalker DK: Response of the cutaneous lesions of Reiter's syndrome to ketoconazole, *J Am Acad Dermatol* 13:161-163, 1985.
14. Obuch ML, Maurer TA, et al: Psoriasis and human immunodeficiency virus infection, *J Am Acad Dermatol* 27:667-673, 1992.
15. Maurer TA et al: The use of methotrexate for psoriasis in patients with HIV infection, *J Am Acad Dermatol* 3:372-375, 1994.
16. Ruzicka T et al: Treatment of HIV-induced retinoid-resistant psoriasis with zidovudine, *Lancet* 2:1469, 1987.
17. Stern RS: The epidemiology of joint complaints in patients with psoriasis, *J Rheumatol* 12:315-320, 1985.
18. Zanolli MD, Wikle JS: Joint complaints in psoriasis patients, *Int J Dermatol* 31:488-491, 1992.
19. Ostensen M: The effect of pregnancy on ankylosing spondylitis, psoriatic arthritis, and juvenile rheumatoid arthritis, *Am J Reprod Immunol* 28:235-237, 1992.
20. Gladman DD, Stafford-Brady F, et al: Longitudinal study of clinical and radiological progression in psoriatic arthritis, *J Rheumatol* 17:809-812, 1990.
21. Moll JMH: The clinical spectrum of psoriatic arthritis, *Clinical Orthop* 143:66-79, 1979.
22. McHugh MJ et al: Psoriatic arthritis: clinical subgroups and histocompatibility antigens, *Ann Rheum Dis* 46:184-188, 1987.
23. Espinoza LR, Zakraoui L, et al: Psoriatic arthritis: clinical response and side effects to methotrexate therapy, *J Rheumatol* 19:872-877, 1992.
24. Willkens R et al: Randomized, double-blind, placebo controlled trial of low-dose pulse methotrexate in psoriatic arthritis, *Arthritis Rheum* 27:376-381, 1984.
25. Whiting-O'Keefe QE, Fye KH, et al: Methotrexate and histologic hepatic abnormalities: a meta-analysis, *Am J Med* 90:711-716, 1991.
26. Chieregato GC, Leoni A: Treatment of psoriatic arthropathy with etretinate: a two-year follow-up, *Acta Derm Verereol* 66:321-324, 1986.
27. Newman ED, Perruquet JL, et al: Sulfasalazine therapy in psoriatic arthritis: clinical and immunologic response, *J Rheumatol* 18:1379-1382, 1991.
28. Salvarani C, Macchioni P, et al: Low dose cyclosporine A in psoriatic arthritis: relation between soluble interleukin 2 receptors and response to therapy, *J Rheumatol* 19:74-79, 1992.
29. Wagner SA, Peter RU, et al: Therapeutic efficacy of oral low-dose cyclosporin A in severe psoriatic arthritis, *Dermatology* 186:62-67, 1993.
30. Kammer GM et al: Psoriatic arthritis: a clinical immunologic and HLA study of 100 patients, *Semin Arthritis Rheum* 9:75, 1979.
31. Gladman DD, Blake R, et al: Chloroquine therapy in psoriatic arthritis, *J Rheumatol* 19:1724-1726, 1992.
32. Farr M et al: Sulphasalazine in psoriatic arthritis. A double blind placebo-controlled study, *Br J Rheumatol* 26:46-49, 1990.
33. Boer J, Hermans J, Schothorst, et al: Comparison of phototherapy (UV-B) and photochemotherapy (PUVA) for clearing and maintenance therapy of psoriasis, *Arch Dermatol* 120:52-57, 1984.
34. Gaston L et al: Psoriasis and stress: a prospective study, *J Am Acad Dermatol* 17:82-86, 1987.
35. Gupta MA, Gupta AK, Haberman HF: Psoriasis and psychiatry: an update, *Gen Hosp Psychiatry* 9:157-166, 1987.
36. Bourke JF, Berth-Jones J, et al: Occlusion enhances the efficacy of topical calcipotriol in the treatment of psoriasis vulgaris, *Clin Exp Dermatol* 18:504-506, 1993.
37. Berth-Jones J, Chu AC, et al: A multicentre, parallel-group comparison of calcipotriol ointment and short-contact dithranol therapy in chronic plaque psoriasis, *Br J Dermatol* 127:266-271, 1992.
38. Farr PM, Diffey BL, Marks JM: Phototherapy and dithranol treatment of psoriasis: new lamps for old, *Br Med J* 294:205-207, 1987.
39. Jones SK, Campbell WC, Mackie RM: Out-patient treatment of psoriasis: short contact and overnight dithranol therapy compared, *Br J Dermatol* 113:331-337, 1985.
40. Statham BN, Ryatt KS, Rowell NR: Short-contact dithranol therapy—a comparison with the Ingram regime, *Br J Dermatol* 110:703-708, 1984.
41. Marsico AR, Eaglstein WH, Weinstein GD: Ultraviolet light and tar in the Goeckerman regimen for psoriasis, *Arch Dermatol* 112:1249-1250, 1976.
42. Stern RS et al: Contribution of topical tar oil to ultraviolet B phototherapy for psoriasis, *J Am Acad Dermatol* 14:742-747, 1986.
43. Adrain RM, Parrish JA, Momtaz TK, et al: Outpatient phototherapy of psoriasis, *Arch Dermatol* 117:623-626, 1981.
44. Stern RS et al: Effect of continued ultraviolet B phototherapy on the duration of remission of psoriasis: a randomized study, *J Am Acad Dermatol* 15:546-552, 1986.
45. Petrozzi JW: Topical steroids and UV radiation in psoriasis, *Arch Dermatol* 119:207-210, 1983.
46. Lebwohl M et al: Effects of topical preparations on the erythemogenicity of UVB: implications for phototherapy, *J Am Acad Dermatol* 32:469-471, 1995.
47. Perry HO et al: The Goeckerman treatment of psoriasis, *Arch Dermatol* 98:178, 1968.
48. Horwitz SN, Johnson RA, Sefton J, et al: Addition of a topically applied corticosteroid to a modified Goeckerman regimen for treatment of psoriasis: effect on duration of remission, *J Am Acad Dermatol* 13:784-791, 1985.
49. Friedman SJ: Management of psoriasis vulgaris with a hydrocolloid occlusive dressing, *Arch Dermatol* 123:1046-1052, 1987.
50. Shore RN: Treatment of psoriasis with prolonged application of tape, *J Am Acad Dermatol* 15:540-542, 1986.
51. Farr PM et al: Response of scalp psoriasis to oral ketoconazole, *Lancet* 2:921, 1985.
52. Weinstein GD, White GM: An approach to the treatment of moderate to severe psoriasis with rotational therapy, *J Am Acad Dermatol* 28:454-459, 1993.
53. Rosen K, Mobacken H, Swanbeck G: PUVA, etretinate, and PUVA-etretinate therapy for pustulosis palmoplantaris: a placebo-controlled comparative trial, *Arch Dermatol* 123:885-889, 1987.
54. Lawrence CM, Marks J, Parker S, et al: A comparison of PUVA-etretinate and PUVA-placebo for palmoplantar pustular psoriasis, *Br J Dermatol* 110:221-226, 1984.

55. Rampen FHJ, Fleuren BAM, de Boo TM, et al: Unreliability of self-reported burning tendency and tanning ability, *Arch Dermatol* 124:885-888, 1988.

56. Fitzpatrick TB: The validity and practicality of sun-reactive skin types I through VI, *Arch Dermatol* 124:869-871, 1988 (editorial).

57. Melski JW, Stern RS: Annual rate of psoralen and ultraviolet-A treatment of psoriasis after initial clearing, *Arch Dermatol* 118:404-408, 1982.

58. Stern RS et al: Long-term use of psoralens and ultraviolet A for psoriasis: evidence for efficacy and cost savings, *J Am Acad Dermatol* 14:520-526, 1986.

59. Morison WL: Etretinate and psoriasis, *Arch Dermatol* 123:879-881, 1987.

60. Lauharanta J, Juvakoski T, Lassus A: A clinical evaluation of the effects of an aromatic retinoid (Tigason), combination of retinoid and PUVA, and PUVA alone in severe psoriasis, *Br J Dermatol* 104:325-332, 1981.

61. Honigsmann H, Wolff K: Isotretinoin-PUVA for psoriasis, *Lancet* 1: 1983.

62. Momtaz TK, Parrish JA: Combination of psoralens and ultraviolet A and ultraviolet B in the treatment of psoriasis vulgaris: a bilateral comparison study, *J Am Acad Dermatol* 10:481-486, 1984.

63. Diette KM et al: Psoralens and UV-A and UV-B twice weekly for the treatment of psoriasis, *Arch Dermatol* 120:1169-1173, 1984.

64. Morison WL, Momtaz K, Parrish JA, et al: Combined methotrexate-PUVA therapy in the treatment of psoriasis, *J Am Acad Dermatol* 6:46-51, 1982.

65. MacKie RM, Fitzsimons CP: Risk of carcinogenicity in patients with psoriasis treated with methotrexate or PUVA singly or in combination, *J Am Acad Dermatol* 9:467-469, 1983.

66. Speight EL, Farr PM: Calcipotriol improves the response of psoriasis to PUVA, *Br J Dermatol* 130:79, 1994.

67. Cripps DJ, Lowe NJ: Photochemotherapy for psoriasis remission times: psoralens and UV-A and combined photochemotherapy with anthralin, *Clin Exp Dermatol* 4:477-483, 1979.

68. Meola T Jr, Soter NA, et al: Are topical corticosteroids useful adjunctive therapy for the treatment of psoriasis with ultraviolet radiation? A review of the literature, *Arch Dermatol* 127:1708-1713, 1991.

69. Stern RS et al: Ocular lens findings in patients treated with PUVA, *J Invest Dermatol* 103:534, 1994.

70. Studniberg HM, Weller P: PUVA, UVB, psoriasis, and nonmelanoma skin cancer, *J Am Acad Dermatol* 29:1013-1022, 1993.

71. Henseler T et al: Skin tumors in the European PUVA study: eight-year follow-up of 1,643 patients treated with PUVA for psoriasis, *J Am Acad Dermatol* 16:108-116, 1987.

72. Mali-Gerrits MG, Gaasbeek D, et al: Psoriasis therapy and the risk of skin cancers, *Clin Exp Dermatol* 16:85-89, 1991.

73. Stern RS: Genital tumors among men with psoriasis exposed to psoralens and ultraviolet A radiation (PUVA) and ultraviolet B radiation. The Photochemotherapy Follow-up Study, *N Engl J Med* 322:1093-1097, 1990.

74. Collins P, Rogers S: The efficacy of methotrexate in psoriasis—a review of 40 cases, *Clin Exp Dermatol* 17:257-260, 1992.

75. Van Dooren-Greebe RJ, Kuijpers AL, et al: Methotrexate revisited: effects of long-term treatment in psoriasis, *Br J Dermatol* 130:204-210, 1994.

76. Roenigk HH Jr et al: Methotrexate in psoriasis: revised guidelines, *J Am Acad Dermatol* 19:145-156, 1988.

77. Olsen EA: The pharmacology of methotrexate, *J Am Acad Dermatol* 25:306-318, 1991.

78. Bleyer WA: The clinical pharmacology of methotrexate, *Cancer* 41:36-51, 1978.

79. Teresi ME, Riggs CE, et al: Bioequivalence of two methotrexate formulations in psoriatic and cancer patients, *Ann Pharmacother* 27:1434-1438, 1993.

80. Duhra P: Treatment of gastrointestinal symptoms associated with methotrexate therapy for psoriasis, *J Am Acad Dermatol* 28:466-469, 1993.

81. Hills RJ, Ive FA: Folinic acid rescue used routinely in psoriatic patients with known methotrexate "sensitivity," *Acta Derm Venereol* 72:438-440, 1992.

82. Casserly CM, Stange KC, et al: Severe megaloblastic anemia in a patient receiving low-dose methotrexate for psoriasis, *J Am Acad Dermatol* 29:477-480, 1993.

83. Morris LF, Harrod MJ, et al: Methotrexate and reproduction in men: case report and recommendations, *J Am Acad Dermatol* 29:913-916, 1993.

84. Mayall B, Poggi G, et al: Neutropenia due to low-dose methotrexate therapy for psoriasis and rheumatoid arthritis may be fatal, *Med J Aust* 155:480-484, 1991.

85. King HW, MacFarlane AW, Graham RM, et al: Near fatal drug interactions with methotrexate given for psoriasis, *Lancet* 295:752-753, 1987.

86. Zachariae H, Kragballe K, Sogaard H. Methotrexate-induced liver cirrhosis, *Br J Dermatol* 102:407-412, 1980.

87. Short- and long-term considerations concerning the management of plaque psoriasis with low-dose cyclosporin. Studio Italiano Multicentrico nella Psoriasi (SIMPSO), *Dermatology* 1:19-29, 1993.

88. Cyclosporin versus etretinate: Italian multicenter comparative trial in severe plaque-form psoriasis. Italian Multicenter Study Group on Cyclosporin in Psoriasis, *Dermatology* 1:8-18, 1993.

89. Reitamo S, Erkko P, et al: Cyclosporine in the treatment of palmo-plantar pustulosis. A randomized, double-blind, placebo-controlled study, *Arch Dermatol* 129:1273-1279, 1993.

90. Christophers E, Mrowietz U, et al: Cyclosporine in psoriasis: a multicenter dose-finding study in severe plaque psoriasis. The German Multicenter Study, *J Am Acad Dermatol* 26:86-90, 1992.

91. Fry L: Psoriasis: immunopathology and long-term treatment with cyclosporin, *J Autoimmun* 5:277-283, 1992.

92. Feutren G, Mihatsch MJ: Risk factors for cyclosporine-induced nephropathy in patients with autoimmune diseases. International Kidney Biopsy Registry of Cyclosporine in Autoimmune Diseases, *N Engl J Med* 326:1654-1660, 1992.

93. Brown AL, Wilkinson R, et al: The effect of short-term low-dose cyclosporin on renal function and blood pressure in patients with psoriasis, *Br J Dermatol* 128:550-555, 1993.

94. Powles AV, Cook T, et al: Renal function and biopsy findings after 5 years' treatment with low-dose cyclosporin for psoriasis, *Br J Dermatol* 128:159-165, 1993.

95. Wolska H, Jablonska S, Bounameaux Y: Etretinate in severe psoriasis: results of a double-blind study and maintenance therapy in pustular psoriasis, *J Am Acad Dermatol* 9:883-889, 1983.

96. Kaplan RP, Russell DH, Lowe NJ: Etretinate therapy for psoriasis: clinical responses, remission times, epidermal DNA and polyamine responses, *J Am Acad Dermatol* 8:95-102, 1983.

97. Logan RA: Efficacy of etretinate for the PUVA-dependent psoriatic, *Clin Exp Dermatol* 12:98-102, 1987.

98. Rosen K, Mobacken H, Swanbeck G: PUVA, etretinate, and PUVA-etretinate therapy for pustulosis palmoplantaris, *Arch Dermatol* 123:885-889, 1987.

99. Tuyp E, MacKie RM: Combination therapy for psoriasis with methotrexate and etretinate, *J Am Acad Dermatol* 14:70-73, 1986.

100. Brechtel B et al: Combination of etretinate with cyclosporine in the treatment of severe recalcitrant psoriasis, *J Am Acad Dermatol* 30:1023-1024, 1994.

101. Ellis CN, Voorhees JJ: Etretinate therapy, *J Am Acad Dermatol* 16:267, 1987.

102. Rubin MG, Hanno R: Short-term etretinate for pustular psoriasis, *J Am Acad Dermatol* 12:896-897, 1985.

103. Moy RL, Kingston TP, Lowe NJ: Isotretinoin vs etretinate therapy in generalized pustular and chronic psoriasis, *Arch Dermatol* 121:1297-1301, 1985.

104. White SI, Marks JM, Shuster S: Etretinate in pustular psoriasis of palms and soles, *Br J Dermatol* 113:581-585, 1985.

105. White SI, Puttick L, Marks JM: Low-dose etretinate in the maintenance of remission of palmoplantar pustular psoriasis, *Br J Dermatol* 115:577-582, 1986.

106. Dubertret L: Etretinate (Tigason, Europe; Tegison, USA) in psoriasis: advantages of low doses progressively increased, *J Am Acad Dermatol* 13:830-831, 1985.

107. Griffiths WA: Pityriasis rubra pilaris: the problem of its classification, *J Am Acad Dermatol* 26:140-142, 1992.

108. Auffret N, Quint L, et al: Pityriasis rubra pilaris in a patient with human immunodeficiency virus infection, *J Am Acad Dermatol* 27:260-261, 1992.

109. Blauvelt A, Nahass GT, et al: Pityriasis rubra pilaris and HIV infection, *J Am Acad Dermatol* 24:703-705, 1991.

110. Sonnex TS et al: The nails in adult type 1 pityriasis rubra pilaris: a comparison with Sezary syndrome and psoriasis, *J Am Acad Dermatol* 15:956-960, 1986.

111. Griffiths WAD: Pityriasis rubra pilaris: an historical approach. II. Clinical features, *Clin Exp Dermatol* 1:37-50, 1976.

112. Dicken CH: Treatment of classic pityriasis rubra pilaris, *J Am Acad Dermatol* 31:997-999, 1994.

113. Dicken CH: Isotretinoin treatment of pityriasis rubra pilaris, *J Am Acad Dermatol* 16:297-301, 1987.

114. Borok M, Lowe NJ: Pityriasis rubra pilaris. Further observations of systemic retinoid therapy, *J Am Acad Dermatol* 22:792-795, 1990.

115. Griffiths W: Pityriasis rubra pilaris, *Clin Exp Dermatol* 5:105-112, 1980.

116. Hanke CW, Steck WD: Childhood-onset pityriasis rubra pilaris treated with methotrexate administered intravenously, *Cleve Clin Q* 50:201-203, 1983.

117. Knowles WR, Chernosky ME: Pityriasis rubra pilaris: prolonged treatment with methotrexate, *Arch Dermatol* 102:603-612, 1970.

118. Hunter GA, Forbes IJ: Treatment of pityriasis rubra pilaris with azathioprine, *Br J Dermatol* 87:42-45, 1972.

119. Randle HW, Diaz-Perez JL, Winkelmann RK: Toxic doses of vitamin A for pityriasis rubra pilaris, *Arch Dermatol* 116:888-892, 1980.

120. Griffiths WAD: Vitamin A and pityriasis rubra pilaris, *J Am Acad Dermatol* 7:555, 1982.

121. Murry JC, Gilgor RS, Lazarus GS: Serum triglyceride elevation following high-dose vitamin A treatment for pityriasis rubra pilaris, *Arch Dermatol* 119:675-676, 1983.

122. Brice SL, Spencer SK: Stanozolol in the treatment of pityriasis rubra pilaris, *Arch Dermatol* 121:1105-1106, 1985.

123. Binder RL, Jonelis FJ: Seborrheic dermatitis: a newly reported side effect of neuroleptics, *J Clin Psychiatry* 45:125-126, 1984.

124. Green CA, Farr PM, Shuster S: Treatment of seborrhoeic dermatitis with ketoconazole. II. Response of seborrhoeic dermatitis of the face, scalp and trunk to topical ketoconazole, *Br J Dermatol* 116:217-221, 1987.

125. Parsons JM: Pityriasis rosea update: 1986, *J Am Acad Dermatol* 15:159-167, 1986.

126. Chuang T-Y et al: Pityriasis rosea in Rochester, Minnesota, 1969 to 1978: a 10-year epidemiologic study, *J Am Acad Dermatol* 7:80-89, 1982.

127. Kay MH, Rapini RP, Fritz KA: Oral lesions in pityriasis rosea, *Arch Dermatol* 121:1449-1451, 1985.

128. Vidimos AT, Camisa C: Tongue and cheek: oral lesions in pityriasis rosea, *Cutis* 50:276-280, 1992.

129. Pierson JC, Dijkstra JW, et al: Purpuric pityriasis rosea, *J Am Acad Dermatol* 28:1021, 1993.

130. Horn T, Kazakis A: Pityriasis rosea and the need for a serologic test for syphilis, *Cutis* 39:81-82, 1987.

131. Arndt KA, Paul BS, Stern RS, et al: Treatment of pityriasis rosea with UV radiation, *Arch Dermatol* 119:381-382, 1983.

132. Irvine C, Irvine F, et al: Long-term follow-up of lichen planus, *Acta Derm Venereol* 71:242-244, 1991.

133. Kofoed ML, Wantzin GL: Familial lichen planus, *J Am Acad Dermatol* 13:50-54, 1985.

134. Lichen planus and liver diseases: a multicentre case-control study. Gruppo Italiano Studi Epidemiologici in Dermatologia (GISED), *Br Med J* 300:227-230, 1990.

135. Jubert C, Pawlotsky JM, et al: Lichen planus and hepatitis C virus—related chronic active hepatitis, *Arch Dermatol* 130:73-76, 1994.

136. Halevy S, Shai A: Lichenoid drug eruptions, *J Am Acad Dermatol* 29:249-255, 1993.

137. Grotty CP, Daniel SU WP, Winkelmann RK: Ulcerative lichen planus: follow-up of surgical excision and grafting, *Arch Dermatol* 116:1252-1256, 1980.

138. Matta M, Kibbi AG, et al: Lichen planopilaris: a clinicopathologic study, *J Am Acad Dermatol* 22:594-598, 1990.

139. Mehregan DA, Van Hale HM, et al: Lichen planopilaris: clinical and pathologic study of forty-five patients, *J Am Acad Dermatol* 27:935-942, 1992.

140. Ioannides D, Bystryn JC: Immunofluorescence abnormalities in lichen planopilaris, *Arch Dermatol* 128:214-216, 1992.

141. Silverman S Jr, Gorsky M, Lozada-Nur F: A prospective follow-up study of 570 patients with oral lichen planus: persistence, remission, and malignant association, *Oral Surg Oral Med Oral Pathol* 60:30-34, 1985.

142. Brown RS, Bottomley WK, et al: A retrospective evaluation of 193 patients with oral lichen planus, *J Oral Pathol Med* 22:69-72, 1993.

143. Vincent SD, Fotos PG, et al: Oral lichen planus: the clinical, historical, and therapeutic features of 100 cases, *Oral Surg Oral Med Oral Pathol* 70:165-171, 1990.

144. Barnard NA, Scully C, et al: Oral cancer development in patients with oral lichen planus, *J Oral Pathol Med* 22:421-424, 1993.

145. Eisen D: The vulvovaginal-gingival syndrome of lichen planus, *Arch Dermatol* 130:1379-1382, 1994.

146. Edwards L, Friedrich EG Jr: Desquamative vaginitis: lichen planus in disguise, *Obstet Gynecol* 71:832-836, 1988.

147. Ridley CM: Chronic erosive vulval disease, *Clin Exp Dermatol* 15:245-252, 1990.

148. Tosti A, Peluso AM, et al: Nail lichen planus: clinical and pathologic study of twenty-four patients, *J Am Acad Dermatol* 28:724-730, 1993.

149. Firth NA, Rich AM, et al: Assessment of the value of immunofluorescence microscopy in the diagnosis of oral mucosal lichen planus, *J Oral Pathol Med* 19:295-297, 1990.

150. Laurberg G, Geiger JM, et al: Treatment of lichen planus with acitretin. A double-blind, placebo-controlled study in 65 patients, *J Am Acad Dermatol* 24:434-437, 1991.

151. Ho VC, Gupta AK, et al: Treatment of severe lichen planus with cyclosporine, *J Am Acad Dermatol* 22:64-68, 1990.

152. Gonzalez E, Momtaz TK, Freedman S: Bilateral comparison of generalized lichen planus treated with psoralens and ultraviolet A, *J Am Acad Dermatol* 10: 958-961, 1984.

153. Levy A et al: Treatment of lichen planus with griseofulvin, *Int J Dermatol* 25:405-406, 1986.

154. Massa MC, Rogers RS III: Griseofulvin therapy of lichen planus, *Acta Derm Venereol* 61:547-550, 1981.

155. Voute AB, Schulten EA, et al: Fluocinonide in an adhesive base for treatment of oral lichen planus. A double-blind, placebo-controlled clinical study, *Oral Surg Oral Med Oral Pathol* 75:181-185, 1993.

156. Plemons JM, Rees TD, et al: Absorption of a topical steroid and evaluation of adrenal suppression in patients with erosive lichen planus, *Oral Surg Oral Med Oral Pathol* 69:688-693, 1990.

157. Ferguson MM: Treatment of erosive lichen planus of the oral mucosa with depot steroids, *Lancet* 2:771-772, 1977.

158. Silverman S, Lozada-Nur F, Magliorati C: Clinical efficacy of prednisone in the treatment of patients with oral inflammatory ulcerative diseases: a study of 55 patients, *Oral Surg* 59:360-363, 1985.

159. Beck H-I, Brandrup F: Treatment of erosive lichen planus with dapsone, *Acta Derm Venereol* (Stockh) 66:366-367, 1986.

160. Falk DK, Latour DL, King LE Jr: Dapsone in the treatment of erosive lichen planus, *J Am Acad Dermatol* 12:567-570, 1985.

161. Eisen D: Hydroxychloroquine sulfate (Plaquenil) improves oral lichen planus: an open trial, *J Am Acad Dermatol* 28:609-612, 1993.

162. Silverman S Jr, Gorsky M, et al: A prospective study of findings and management in 214 patients with oral lichen planus, *Oral Surg Oral Med Oral Pathol* 72:665-670, 1991.

163. Eisen D, Ellis CN, et al: Effect of topical cyclosporine rinse on oral lichen planus. A double-blind analysis, *N Engl J Med* 323.290-294, 1990.

164. Matthews RW, Scully C: Griseofulvin in the treatment of oral lichen planus: adverse drug reactions, but little beneficial effect, *Ann Dent* 51:10-11, 1992.

165. Karp DL, Cohen BA: Onychodystrophy in lichen striatus, *Pediatr Dermatol* 10:359-361, 1993.

166. Taieb A, el Youbi A, et al: Lichen striatus: a Blaschko linear acquired inflammatory skin eruption, *J Am Acad Dermatol* 25:637-642, 1991.

167. Yates VM, King CM, Dave VK: Lichen sclerosus et atrophicus following radiation therapy, *Arch Dermatol* 121:1044-1047, 1985.

168. Berth-Jones J, Graham-Brown RA, et al: Lichen sclerosus et atrophicus—a review of 15 cases in young girls, *Clin Exp Dermatol* 16:14-17, 1991.

169. Helm KF, Gibson LE, et al: Lichen sclerosus et atrophicus in children and young adults, *Pediatr Dermatol* 8:97-101, 1991.

170. Loening-Baucke V: Lichen sclerosus et atrophicus in children, *Am J Dis Child* 145:1058-1061, 1991.

171. Barton PG, Ford MJ, et al: Penile purpura as a manifestation of lichen sclerosus et atrophicus, *Pediatr Dermatol* 10:129-131, 1993.

172. Young SJ, Wells DL, et al: Lichen sclerosus, genital trauma and child sexual abuse, *Aust Fam Physician* 22:732-733, 1993.

173. Ridley CM: Lichen sclerosus et atrophicus, *Arch Dermatol* 123:457-460, 1987 (editorial).

174. Friedrich EG Jr, Kalra PS: Serum levels of sex hormones in vulvar lichen sclerosus and the effect of topical testosterone, *N Engl J Med* 310:488-491, 1984.

175. Weigand DA: Microscopic features of lichen sclerosus et atrophicus in acrochordons: a clue to the cause of lichen sclerosus et atrophicus? *J Am Acad Dermatol* 28:751-754, 1993.

176. Pride HB, Miller OF, Tyler QB: Penile squamous cell carcinoma arising from balanitis xerotica obliterans, *J Am Acad Dermatol* 29:469-473, 1993.

177. Chalmers RJG et al: Lichen sclerosus et atrophicus: a common and distinctive cause of phimosis in boys, *Arch Dermatol* 120:1025-1027, 1984.

178. Cattaneo A, De Marco A, et al: Clobetasol vs. testosterone in the treatment of lichen sclerosus of the vulvar region, *Minerva Ginecol* 44:567-571, 1992.

179. Meffert JJ, Davis DM, Grimwood RE: Lichen sclerosus, *J Am Acad Dermatol* 32:393-416, 1995.

180. Mork NJ, Jensen P, Hoel PS: Vulval lichen sclerosus et atrophicus treated with etretinate (Tigason), *Acta Derm Venereol* (Stockh) 66:363-365, 1986.

181. Bousema MT, Romppanen U, et al: Acitretin in the treatment of severe lichen sclerosus et atrophicus of the vulva: a double-blind, placebo-controlled study, *J Am Acad Dermatol* 30:225-231, 1994.

182. Windahl T, Hellsten S: Carbon dioxide laser treatment of lichen sclerosus et atrophicus, *J Urol* 150:868-870, 1993.

183. Stuart GC, Nation JG, et al: Laser therapy of vulvar lichen sclerosus et atrophicus, *Can J Surg* 34:469-470, 1991.

184. Rettenmaier MA et al: Treatment of cutaneous vulvar lesions with skinning vulvectomy, *J Reproductive Med* 30:478-480, 1985.

185. Gelmetti C, Rigoni C, et al: Pityriasis lichenoides in children: a long-term follow-up of eighty-nine cases, *J Am Acad Dermatol* 23:473-478, 1990.

186. Wood GS et al: Immunohistology of pityriasis lichenoides et varioliformis acuta and pityriasis lichenoides chronica: evidence for their interrelationship with lymphomatoid papulosis, *J Am Acad Dermatol* 16:559-570, 1987.

187. Luberti AA, Rabinowitz LG, et al: Severe febrile Mucha-Habermann's disease in children: case report and review of the literature, *Pediatr Dermatol* 8:51-57, 1991.

188. Truhan AP, Hebert AA, Esterly NB: Pityriasis lichenoides in children: therapeutic response to erythromycin, *J Am Acad Dermatol* 15:66-70, 1986.

189. LeVine MJ: Phototherapy of pityriasis lichenoides, *Arch Dermatol* 119:378-380, 1983.

190. Powell FC, Muller SA: Psoralens and ultraviolet A therapy of pityriasis lichenoides, *J Am Acad Dermatol* 10:59-64, 1984.

CHAPTER NINE

Bacterial Infections

Skin Infections

The two gram-positive cocci, *Staphylococcus aureus* and the group A beta-hemolytic streptococci, account for the majority of skin and soft tissue infections. The streptococci are secondary invaders of traumatic skin lesions and cause impetigo, erysipelas, cellulitis, and lymphangitis. *S. aureus* invades skin and causes impetigo, folliculitis, cellulitis, and furuncles. Elaboration of toxins by *S. aureus* causes the lesions of bullous impetigo and staphylococcal scalded skin syndrome.

IMPETIGO

Impetigo is a common, contagious, superficial skin infection that is produced by streptococci, staphylococci, or a combination of both bacteria. There are two different clinical presentations: bullous impetigo and nonbullous impetigo.

Both begin as vesicles with a very thin, fragile roof consisting only of stratum corneum. Bullous impetigo is primarily a staphylococcal disease. Nonbullous impetigo was once thought to be primarily a streptococcal disease, but staphylococci are isolated from the majority of lesions in both bullous and nonbullous impetigo. *S. aureus* is now known to be the primary pathogen in both bullous and nonbullous impetigo.[1]

Children in close physical contact with each other have a higher rate of infection than do adults. Symptoms of itching and soreness are mild; systemic symptoms are infrequent. Impetigo may occur after a minor skin injury such as an insect bite, but it most frequently develops on apparently unimpaired skin. The disease is self-limiting, but when untreated it may last for weeks or months. Poststreptococcal glomerulonephritis may follow impetigo. Rheumatic fever has not been reported as a complication of impetigo.

Bullous impetigo

Bullous impetigo (staphylococcal impetigo) is caused by an epidermolytic toxin produced at the site of infection, most commonly by staphylococci of phage Group II, and usually is not secondarily contaminated by streptococci. The toxin causes intraepidermal cleavage below or within the stratum granulosum.

Clinical manifestations. Bullous impetigo is most common in infants and children but may occur in adults. It typically occurs on the face, but it may infect any body surface. There may be a few lesions localized in one area, or the lesions may be so numerous and widely scattered that they resemble poison ivy. One or more vesicles enlarge rapidly to form bullae in which the contents turn from clear to cloudy. The center of the thin-roofed bulla collapses, but the peripheral area may retain fluid for many days in an inner tube–shaped rim. A thin, flat, honey-colored, "varnishlike" crust may appear in the center and, if removed, discloses a bright red, inflamed, moist base that oozes serum. The center may dry without forming a crust, leaving a red base with a rim of scale. In most cases, a tinea-like scaling border replaces the fluid-filled rim as the round lesions enlarge and become contiguous with the others (Figures 9-1 to 9-5). The border dries and forms a crust. The lesions have little or no surrounding erythema. In some untreated cases, lesions may extend radially and retain a narrow, bullous, inner tube rim. These individual lesions reach 2 to 8 cm and then cease to enlarge, but they may remain for months (Figures 9-6 and 9-7). Thick crust accumulates in these longer lasting lesions. Lesions heal with hyperpigmentation in black patients. Regional lymphadenitis is uncommon with pure staphylococcal impetigo. There is some evidence that the responsible staphylococci colonize in the nose and then spread to normal skin prior to infection.

Serious secondary infections (e.g., osteomyelitis, septic arthritis, and pneumonia) may follow seemingly innocuous superficial infections in infants.

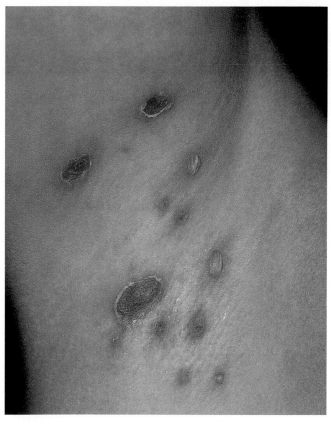

Figure 9-1
Bullous impetigo. Lesions are present in all stages of development. Bullae rupture, exposing a lesion with an eroded surface and a peripheral scale.

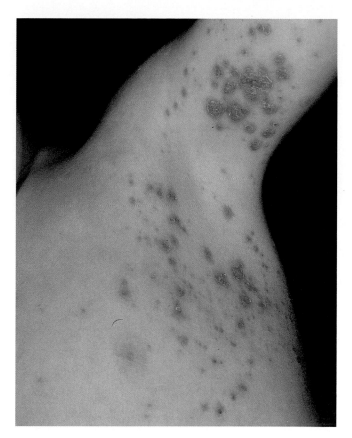

Figure 9-2
Bullous impetigo. The lesions initially were present on the arm and autoinoculated the chest.

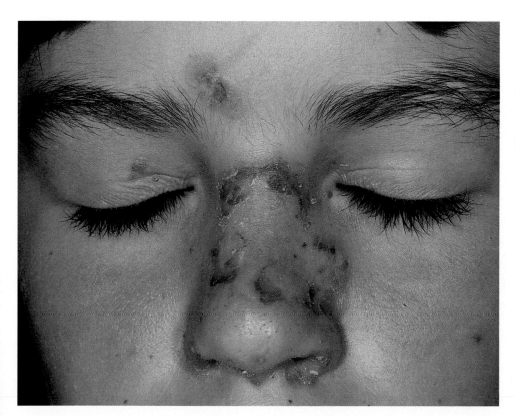

Figure 9-3
Bullous impetigo. Bullae have collapsed and disappeared. The lesion is in the process of peripheral extension. Note involvement of both nares.

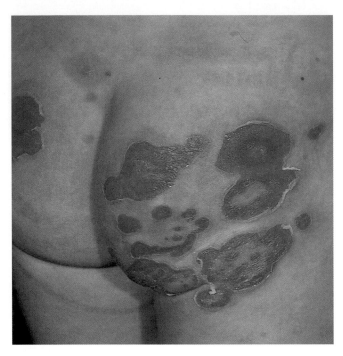

Figure 9-4
Bullous impetigo. Huge lesions with a glistening, eroded base and a collarette of moist scale.

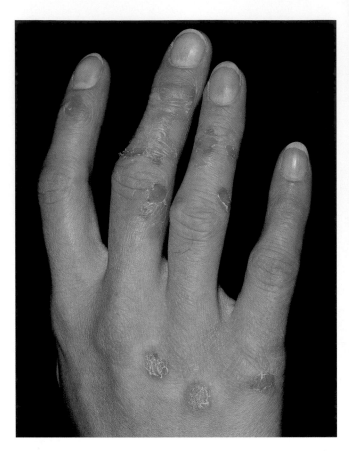

Figure 9-5
Bullous impetigo is occasionally seen on the hand and is often mistaken for eczema.

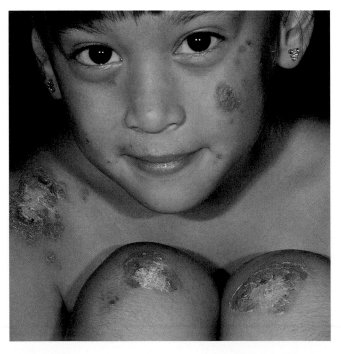

Figure 9-6
Impetigo. A bullous rim extended slowly for weeks. No topical or oral treatment had been attempted.

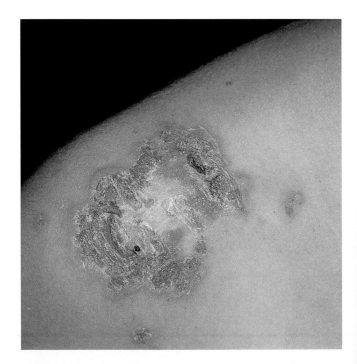

Figure 9-7
Impetigo. A bullous rim persists in this unusually large lesion.

Nonbullous impetigo

Nonbullous impetigo originates as a small vesicle or pustule that ruptures to expose a red, moist base. A honey-yellow to white-brown, firmly adherent crust accumulates as the lesion extends radially (Figures 9-8 to 9-11). There is little surrounding erythema. Satellite lesions appear beyond the periphery. The lesions are generally asymptomatic. The skin around the nose and mouth and the limbs are the sites most commonly affected. The palms and soles are not affected. Untreated cases last for weeks and may extend in a continuous manner to involve a wide area (Figure 9-12). Most cases heal without scarring. The sequence of events leading to nonbullous impetigo is exposure to the infectious agent, carriage on exposed normal skin, and finally skin infection after a minor trauma that is aggravated by scratching. The infecting strain has been found on normal skin surfaces 2 or more weeks prior to the appearance of lesions.

Intact skin is resistant to colonization or infection with group A beta-hemolytic streptococci, but skin injury by insect bites, abrasions, lacerations, and burns allows the streptococci to invade. A pure culture of group A beta-hemolytic streptococci may sometimes be isolated from early lesions, but most lesions promptly become contaminated with staphylococci.[2] Regional lymphadenopathy is common. The reservoirs for streptococcus infection include the unimpaired normal skin or the lesions of other individuals rather than the respiratory tract.[3] Children ages 2 to 5 years commonly have streptococcal impetigo. Warm, moist climates and poor hygiene are predisposing factors. The antistreptolysin O (ASO) titer does not rise to a significant level following impetigo. Anti-DNAase B rises to high levels and is a much more sensitive indicator of streptococcal impetigo.

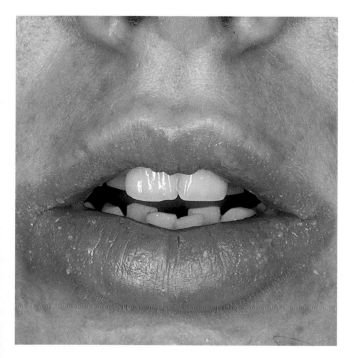

Figure 9-8
Impetigo. Serum and crust at the angle of the mouth is a common presentation for impetigo.

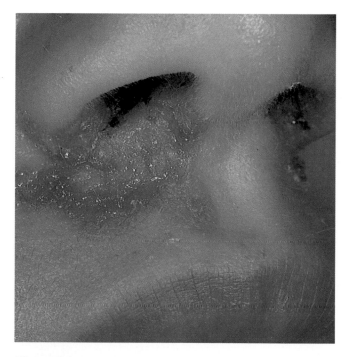

Figure 9-9
Impetigo. Serum and crust about the nostrils is a common presentation for impetigo.

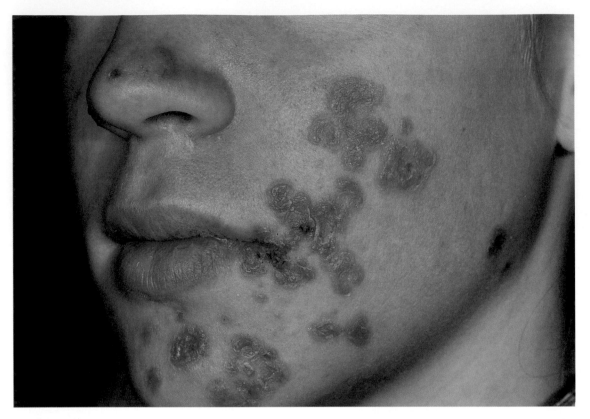

Figure 9-10
Impetigo. A thick, honey-yellow, adherent crust covers the
entire eroded surface.

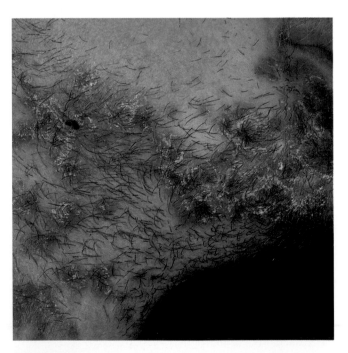

Figure 9-11
Impetigo. Shaving caused rapid dissemination of the
infection throughout the beard area.

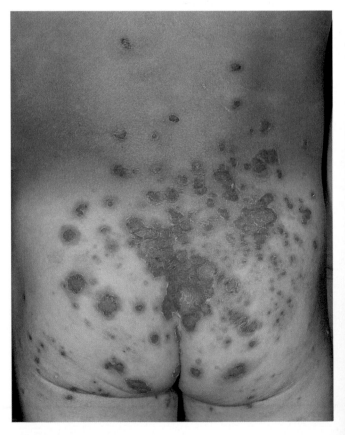

Figure 9-12
Impetigo. Widespread dissemination followed 3 weeks of
treatment with a group IV topical steroid.

Acute nephritis

Acute nephritis tends to occur when many individuals in a family have impetigo. Most cases occur in the southern part of the United States. Infants under $1\frac{1}{2}$ years of age are rarely affected by nephritis following impetigo. The highest incidence of nephritis following impetigo is in children between 2 and 4 years of age. After the appearance of the skin lesions, the anterior nares and, possibly later, the pharynx are colonized with streptococci responsible for the skin infection. The streptococci responsible for impetigo are of different strains than those causing pharyngeal infections. The latent period between the acquisition of a nephritogenic streptococcus in skin lesions and the onset of acute nephritis varies between 1 and 5 weeks and averages 10 days.[4] The overall incidence of acute nephritis with impetigo varies between 2% and 5%, but, in the presence of a nephritogenic strain of streptococcus, the rate varies between 10% and 15%. During the initial streptococcal infection, hematuria and proteinuria may be found in approximately one third of the patients. The urinary findings disappear for several days before development of poststreptococcal acute glomerulonephritis.

The overall incidence and clinical features of acute nephritis[4] are as follows. Hematuria occurs in 90% of patients. Gross hematuria occurs in 25% of patients, followed by microscopic hematuria with erythrocyte casts and proteinuria that last for a variable time. Edema occurs in the majority of patients; the degree varies with the amount of dietary sodium. In the early morning, there is periorbital edema and lower extremity swelling. Hypertension occurs in 60% of patients; adults have moderate elevation of 160/100 mm Hg; children are close to normal. The degree varies with dietary sodium. Cerebral symptoms (headache and disturbance of consciousness), congestive heart failure, and acute renal failure are less common.

Laboratory findings

After impetigo, ASO titer elevations are low or absent, but anti-DNAase B[5] and antihyaluronidase increase significantly. Total serum complement activity is low during the initial stages of acute nephritis. The C3 level parallels the total serum complement. The sedimentation rate parallels the activity of the disease. C-reactive protein is usually normal. Cultures of the pharynx and any skin lesion should be made and the serotype of the group A streptococcus that is responsible should be determined by typing with M-group and T-type antisera. M-T serotypes associated with acute nephritis are 2, 49, 55, 57, and 60.

Acute nephritis heals without therapeutic intervention. Symptoms and signs such as hypertension should be managed as they occur.

Prevention of impetigo

Mupirocin (Bactroban) or Triple antibiotic ointment, containing bacitracin, polysporin, and neomycin, applied three times daily to sites of minor skin trauma (e.g., mosquito bites and abrasions) can be efficacious as a preventative treatment.[6]

Recurrent impetigo

Patients with recurrent impetigo should be evaluated for carriage of *S. aureus*. The nares are the most common sites of carriage, but the perineum, axillae, and toe webs may also be colonized. Mupirocin ointment (Bactroban) applied to the nares twice each day for 5 days significantly reduces *S. aureus* carriage in the nose and hands at 3 days and in the nasal carriage for as long as 1 year.[7]

Treatment of impetigo

Impetigo may resolve spontaneously or become chronic and widespread. Studies show that 2% mupirocin ointment is as safe and effective as oral erythromycin in the treatment of patients with impetigo.[8] Local treatment does not treat lesions that evolve in other areas. Infected children should be briefly isolated until treatment is under way.

Oral antibiotics. Because some cases of impetigo have a mixed infection of staphylococci and streptococci, penicillin is inadequate for treatment.[9] A 5- to 10-day course of an oral antibiotic such as cloxacillin, dicloxacillin, or cephalexin induces rapid healing. Erythromycin may not be as effective because strains of resistant staphylococci are appearing in some areas. Azithromycin given over 5 days as a once-a-day regimen (500 mg on day 1, 250 mg on days 2 through 5) is as effective and better tolerated than either erythromycin or cloxacillin. Short-course therapy also may improve patient compliance.[10]

Mupirocin (Bactroban). Mupirocin ointment is the first topical antibiotic approved for the treatment of impetigo. It is active against staphylococci (including methicillin-resistant strains) and streptococci. The drug is not active against *Enterobacteriaceae*, *Pseudomonas aeruginosa*, or fungi. It is as effective as oral antibiotics and is associated with fewer adverse effects.[11] In superficial skin infections that are not widespread, mupirocin ointment offers several advantages. It is highly active against the most frequent skin pathogens, even those resistant to other antibiotics, and the topical route of administration allows delivery of high drug concentrations to the site of infection.[7] Mupirocin is applied three times a day until all lesions have cleared. If topical treatment is elected, then it might be worthwhile to wash the involved areas once or twice a day with an antibacterial soap such as Hibiclens or Betadine. Washing the entire body with these soaps may prevent recurrence at distant sites. Crusts should be removed because they block the penetration of antibacterial creams. To facilitate removal, crusts are softened by soaking with a wet cloth compress.

ECTHYMA

Ecthyma is characterized by ulcerations that are covered by adherent crusts. Poor hygiene is a predisposing factor. Ecthyma has many features similar to those of impetigo. The lesions begin as vesicles and bullae. They then rupture to form an adherent crust that covers an ulcer rather than the erosion of impetigo (see Figures 9-6 and 9-7). The lesion may remain fixed in size and resolve without treatment or may extend slowly, forming indolent ulcers with very thick, oyster shell–like crusts. This type of lesion occurs most commonly on the legs, where there are usually less than 10 lesions. Another more diffuse form occurs on the buttocks and legs of children who excoriate. Except for the thick crusts and underlying ulcers, the picture is approximately identical to diffuse streptococcal impetigo. Lesions heal with scarring. Ecthyma is initiated by group A beta-hemolytic streptococci, but quickly becomes contaminated with staphylococci. This should be treated with a 10-day course of an oral antibiotic such as dicloxacillin or a cephalosporin such as cephalexin.

CELLULITIS AND ERYSIPELAS

Cellulitis and erysipelas are skin infections characterized by erythema, edema, and pain.

Cellulitis is an infection of the dermis and subcutaneous tissue that is usually caused by a group A streptococcus and *S. aureus* in adults and *Haemophilus influenzae* type B in children less than 3 years of age. Cellulitis is sometimes caused by other organisms, such as non–group A streptococcus (seen most often in patients with underlying abnormalities of lymphatic and/or venous drainage),[12] *P. aeruginosa*, or *Campylobacter fetus*.[13] Cellulitis typically occurs near surgical wounds or a cutaneous ulcer or, like erysipelas, may develop in apparently normal skin. Recurrent episodes of cellulitis occur with local anatomic abnormalities that compromise the venous or lymphatic circulation. The lymphatic system can be compromised by a previous episode of cellulitis, surgery with lymph node resection, and radiation therapy.

Erysipelas is an acute, inflammatory form of cellulitis that differs from other types of cellulitis in that lymphatic involvement ("streaking") is prominent. Erysipelas is also more superficial and has margins that are more clearly demarcated from normal skin than does cellulitis. The lower legs, face, and ears are most frequently involved.

Diagnosis of cellulitis

Recognizing the distinctive clinical features (erythema, warmth, edema, and pain) is the most reliable way of making an early diagnosis of cellulitis. Isolation of the etiologic agent is difficult in most adult cases and is usually not attempted.[14] Fever, mild leukocytosis with a left shift, and a mildly elevated sedimentation rate may be present. Patients with cellulitis of the leg often have a preexisting lesion, such as an ulcer or erosion that acts as a portal of entry for the infecting organism.[15]

Adults. In adults with no underlying disease, yields of cultures of aspirates, biopsy specimens, and blood are low. In adults with underlying diseases (e.g., diabetes mellitus, hematologic malignancies, IV drug abuse, human immunodeficiency virus infection, chemotherapy) results of culture are more productive.[16] Cellulitis in these patients is often caused by organisms other than *S. aureus* or group A streptococcus, such as *Acinetobacter*, *Clostridium septicum*, *Enterobacter*, *Escherichia coli*, *H. influenzae*, *Pasteurella multocida*, *Proteus mirabilis*, *P. aeruginosa*, and group B streptococci. Cultures of entry sites, aspirates, biopsy specimens, and blood facilitate the selection of the appropriate antibiotic for these patients.

Children. Identification of the infectious agents causing cellulitis is more successful in children. *H. influenzae* is the most common etiologic agent. Buccal infection is the most common presentation. Blood cultures were positive in 6.4%[17] to 78%[18] of reported cases. Needle aspirate cultures are more productive in children than in adults but are usually not attempted. The organism responsible for facial cellulitis can be isolated from wounds, blood, and throat or ear cultures.

Culture. Optimal methods for etiologic diagnosis in adults have not been delineated. Culture of the lesion is a more predictable source of information than more invasive procedures. Leading-edge and midpoint aspirates after saline injection and blood cultures are of little value in normal hosts.[15,19,20] A higher concentration of bacteria may be found at the point of maximal inflammation. Needle aspiration from the point of maximal inflammation yielded a 45% positive culture rate, compared with a 5% rate from leading-edge cultures.[21] Needle aspiration is performed by piercing the skin with a 20-gauge needle mounted on a tuberculin syringe. A 22-gauge needle is used for facial lesions. The needle is introduced into subcutaneous tissue. Suction is applied as the needle is withdrawn.

Treatment of cellulitis

Adults. The low yield of needle aspiration and the predictability of the organisms recovered mean that empiric treatment with antibiotics aimed at staphylococcal and streptococcal organisms is appropriate in adults: a penicillinase-resistant penicillin (dicloxacillin 500 to 1000 mg orally every 6 hours) or a cephalosporin or erythromycin (250 to 500 mg orally every 6 hours). For more severe infections, an intravenous penicillinase-resistant penicillin such as nafcillin (500 to 1500 mg intravenously every 4 hours) or vancomycin should be used in persons allergic to penicillin. An aminoglycoside (gentamicin or tobramycin) should be considered in patients at risk for gram-negative infection. Some adults are infected with beta-lactamase–producing strains of *H. influenzae* type B (HIB) and require other appropriate antibiotics.[22] Pain can be relieved with cool Burow's compresses. Elevation of the leg hastens recovery for lower leg infections.

Children. *H. influenzae* cellulitis therapy must be prompt. Be sure that gas formation and/or purulent collections are not present, since these require aggressive surgical drainage and debridement. A decision must be made regarding the need for intubation or tracheotomy. Current resistance rates to ampicillin vary from 5% to 30%. Intravenous ampicillin with intravenous chloramphenicol is effective, but more institutions are using second-generation cephalosporins such as cefuroxime[23] or third-generation cephalosporins (e.g., ceftriaxone) with good cerebrospinal fluid (CSF) penetrance and coverage of HIB. Cephalosporins produce fewer drug-related side effects and provide good CSF penetrance.

H. influenzae type B can infect multiple members of a family and close contacts in day-care centers. Rifampin prophylaxis should be considered for the entire family of an index case where the household includes a child in the susceptible age group (less than 4 years old), in a day-care classroom where a case of systemic *H. influenzae* type B disease has occurred, and in circumstances where one or more children under 2 years old have been exposed.[24]

Prevention of recurrent infection. Prolonged antimicrobial prophylaxis is effective and safe in preventing recurrent episodes of soft tissue infections and may be continued for months or years. An antimicrobial agent with activity against both streptococci and staphylococci is used, such as erythromycin[25] (250 mg twice a day); however, patients with recurrent disease may also respond to phenoxymethyl penicillin 250 to 500 mg twice a day. Low-dose oral clindamycin has been advocated for the prevention of recurrent staphylococcal skin infections[26] and might also be useful for the prevention of recurrent cellulitis.

CELLULITIS OF SPECIFIC AREAS
Cellulitis and erysipelas of the extremities

Cellulitis of the extremities is most often caused by group A beta-hemolytic streptococci and is characterized by an expanding, red, swollen, tender-to-painful plaque with an indefinite border that may cover a small or wide area (Figures 9-13 and 9-14). Chills and fever occur as the red plaque spreads rapidly, becomes edematous, and sometimes develops bullae or suppurates. Less acute forms detected around a stasis leg ulcer spread slowly and may appear as an area of erythema with no swelling or fever. Erysipelas of the lower extremity is now more common than facial erysipelas. Group G streptococci may be a common pathogen, especially in patients older than 50 years.[27] Red, sometimes painful streaks of lymphangitis may extend toward regional lymph nodes. Repeated attacks can cause impairment of lymphatic drainage, which predisposes the patient to more infection and permanent swelling. This series of events takes place most commonly in the lower legs of patients with venous stasis and ulceration. The end stage, which includes dermal fibrosis, lymphedema, and epidermal thickening on the lower leg, is called *elephantiasis nostras*.

Treatment. Treatment with oral or intravenous antibiotics should be started immediately and, if appropriate, altered according to laboratory results. The mean time for healing after treatment is initiated is 12 days, with a range of 5 to 25 days.[19] See the section on the treatment of cellulitis for more details.

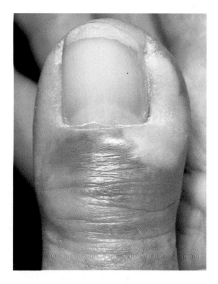

Figure 9-14
Cellulitis of the finger (acute paronychia). A painful, rapidly spreading form of localized cellulitis (see Chapter Twenty-five).

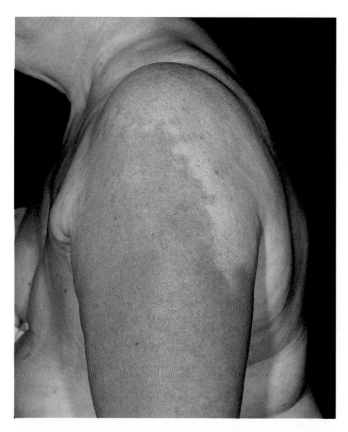

Figure 9-13
Cellulitis. Infected area is tender, deep red, and swollen.

Tinea pedis and recurrent cellulitis of the leg after saphenous venectomy

Tinea of the toe webs may predispose patients to cellulitis. Breaks in the dermal barrier caused by fungal infection may permit entry of bacteria through the skin. Recurrent cellulitis of the leg has been reported to occur following saphenous venectomy for coronary artery bypass grafting.[28] These patients have an acute onset of fever, erythema, and swelling of the leg arising months to years after coronary artery bypass surgery. Non–group A beta-hemolytic streptococci (groups C, G, and B) have been implicated.[12] Tinea pedis has been observed on the foot of the infected leg. The fungal infection may be an important factor in the pathogenesis of the cellulitis. The cellulitis responds to the treatment measures outlined and the fungal infection is treated topically or systemically as outlined in Chapter Thirteen.

Facial erysipelas and cellulitis in adults

Erysipelas. The archaic term *St. Anthony's Fire* accurately describes the intensity of this eruption. Erysipelas is a superficial cellulitis with lymphatic involvement. Isolated cases are the rule; epidemic forms are rare. Facial sites have become rare but erysipelas of the legs is common. It may originate in a traumatic or surgical wound, but no portal of entry can be found in most cases. In the preantibiotic era, erysipelas was a feared disease with a significant mortality rate, particularly in infants. Most contemporary cases are of moderate intensity and have a benign course. In the majority of cases, group A streptococci are the responsible organisms. The second most frequent causative organism is group G streptococci.[27]

After prodromal symptoms that last from 4 to 48 hours and consist of malaise, chills, fever (101° to 104° F), and occasionally anorexia and vomiting, there appears at the site of infection one or more red, tender, firm spots. These spots rapidly increase in size, forming a tense, red, hot, uniformly elevated, shining patch with an irregular outline and a sharply defined, raised border (Figure 9-15). As the process develops, the color becomes a dark, fiery red and vesicles appear at the advancing border and over the surface. Symptoms of itching, burning, tenderness, and pain may be moderate to severe. Without treatment, the rash reaches its height in approximately 1 week and subsides slowly over the next 1 or 2 weeks.

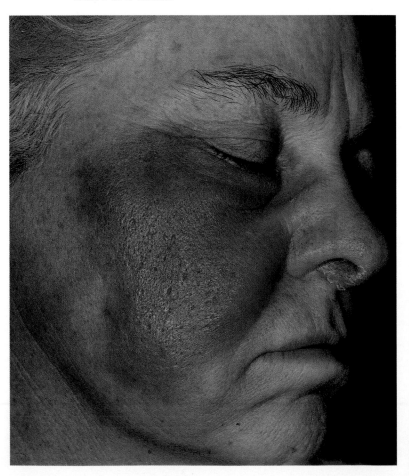

Figure 9-15
Erysipelas. Streptococcal cellulitis. The acute phase with intense erythema.

Recurrence. Recurrence after antibiotic treatment occurs in 18% to 30% of cases.[29] In particularly susceptible people, erysipelas may recur frequently for a long period and, by obstruction of the lymphatics, cause permanent thickening of the skin (lymphedema). Subsequent attacks may be initiated by the slightest trauma or may occur spontaneously to cause further irreversible skin thickening. The pinna and lower legs are particularly susceptible to this recurrent pattern (Figure 9-16).

Treatment. Treatment is the same as for streptococcal cellulitis. Recurrent cases may require long-term prophylactic treatment with low-dose penicillin or erythromycin.[30] If other organisms are found on culture, a different agent is needed. See the section on the treatment of cellulitis for more details.

Cellulitis (*Haemophilus influenzae* type B). *H. influenzae* type B is a rare but treatable event in adults. Suspect *H. influenzae* type B in any patient with cellulitis of the head or neck who appears toxic and/or in danger of airway compromise. The adult patient, who is usually older than 50 years of age, first develops pharyngitis, followed by high fever, rapidly progressive anterior neck swelling, tenderness, and erythema associated with dysphagia.[22] The erythema is usually not purple-red as is seen in children. Blood and respiratory tract cultures are positive.

Treatment. Cefuroxime (intravenously) or other appropriate cephalosporins such as cefotaxime or ceftriaxone are used. See the section on the treatment of cellulitis for more details.

Facial cellulitis in children

Facial cellulitis in children is potentially serious. Fever, irritability, and swelling and erythema of the cheek develop rapidly following a day or two of symptoms that are similar to those of an upper respiratory tract infection. Meningitis may occur.

The paramount factor in the evaluation of facial cellulitis is the presence or absence of a portal of entry. Patients over 3 years of age who have a laceration, insect bite, eczema, dental infections, or other obvious trauma that might allow a portal of entry can be treated for staphylococcal and streptococcal infection. Children without an obvious portal of entry may be infected with *H. influenzae*.

Haemophilus influenzae type B cellulitis. The cellulitis is thought to be caused either by local mouth trauma with subsequent soft tissue invasion or by lymphatic spread from ipsilateral otitis media. There is no obvious portal of entry. Infants are protected by maternal antibodies for the first few months of life. Children younger than 5 years of age are most susceptible. The child is typically between 6 months and 3 years of age. Symptoms usually develop after an upper respiratory infection with the rapid onset of a fever to 40° C. There is a unilateral, tender, warm, buccal discoloration, ranging from an intense erythema to a poorly demarcated violaceous hue ("bruised cheek syndrome") in approximately 50% of cases.[31] The color is not pathognomonic. Unilateral or bilateral otitis media is present in 68% of the patients. Meningitis is present in 8% of the infants, which in some cases is asymptomatic and requires lumbar puncture for demonstration. Therefore, a lumbar puncture should be considered for all patients. Blood cultures are positive in 75% of the cases. Blood cultures are the most sensitive test for identifying the organism. The organism may also be cultured from wounds (51%), middle ear fluid (96%), cerebrospinal fluid (CSF) (7.5%),[32] or the nasopharynx. Most cases of orbital cellulitis are associated with underlying ethmoid or maxillary sinusitis.[22] White blood counts are commonly more than 20,000 cells/mm³.

Treatment. See the section on the treatment of cellulitis on p. 243.

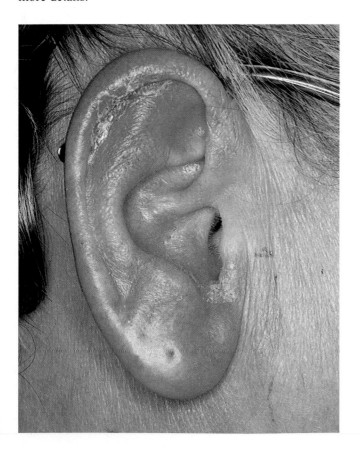

Figure 9-16
Erysipelas. Recurrent episodes of infection have resulted in lymphatic obstruction and caused permanent thickening of the skin.

Cellulitis around the eye

Cellulitis around the eye is a potentially dangerous disease. Preseptal or periorbital cellulitis (infection anterior to the orbital septum) must be differentiated from infection within the orbit, which is referred to as *postseptal* or *orbital cellulitis* (behind the orbital septum). The orbital septum or palpebral fascia in the upper and lower eyelids is continuous with the periosteum of the superior and inferior margins of the orbit and inserts into the anterior surfaces of the tarsal plates. The orbital septum is the primary barrier that prevents inflammatory processes of the eyelid (preseptal) from extending posteriorly into the orbit.

Periorbital cellulitis. Periorbital cellulitis is more common than orbital cellulitis and is limited to the eyelids in the preseptal region. It is more common in children. Sinusitis, upper respiratory infection, and eye trauma are the most frequently encountered predisposing diseases.[33] It is an acute inflammatory process associated with an elevated temperature, erythema and edema of the eyelid, conjunctivitis, and chemosis (Figure 9-17). As with orbital cellulitis, staphylo-

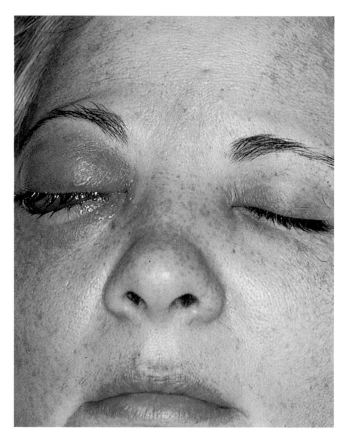

Figure 9-17
Periorbital cellulitis. An acute inflammatory process limited to the eyelids in the preseptal region. Patients are febrile. Erythema and edema of the eyelid, conjunctivitis, and chemosis occur. Sinusitis, upper respiratory infection, and eye trauma are common predisposing factors. *(Courtesy Shan R. Baker, M.D.)*

cocci and streptococci are common pathogens in adults and *H. influenzae* is prevalent in children. Periorbital cellulitis is rarely associated with central nervous system (CNS) involvement. Routine lumbar puncture is not warranted in children 6 months of age or older unless there are clinical signs and symptoms of CNS involvement.[34]

Treatment. Adults with nonfebrile, nontoxic periorbital cellulitis can be managed with warm soaks and oral antibiotics. Young children should be treated aggressively to prevent progression to orbital cellulitis. Patients should be treated with intravenous cefuroxime, ceftriaxone or other broad spectrum agents active against *H. influenzae* and various strains of *Streptococcus* and *Staphylococcus*. See the section on the treatment of cellulitis for more details.

Orbital cellulitis. Orbital cellulitis is an emergency. Proptosis, orbital pain, restricted movement of the eye, and chemosis occur in the majority of patients with this uncommon disease. The infection is most frequently attributed to acute sinusitis; in particular, involvement of the ethmoid and maxillary sinuses have been cited.[35] The infection spreads in two ways, direct extension and retrograde (thrombophlebitis/thromboembolism) along the valveless facial veins. Radiographic findings suggestive of sinusitis are present in 75% of patients. Visual disturbances occur in 56% of patients. *Staphylococcus* was isolated in a majority of cases in one series of adult patients.[36] *H. influenzae* is a common pathogen in children between the ages of 3 months and 4 years, and, when present, the blood cultures are positive in 10% to 60% of the cases.[37]

Complications included abscess formations, most of which are subperiosteal in location and well delineated by computed tomographic (CT) scanning, persistent blindness, limitation of movement of the globe, and diplopia. Cavernous sinus thrombosis and brain abscess are rare complications.[38,39] Meningitis occurred in 1% of 214 children with periorbital and orbital cellulitis. Therefore, lumbar puncture should not be a routine procedure in these patients.[40]

Treatment. Intravenous antibiotics are indicated for all patients. Cefuroxime is effective against all of the major etiologic agents and is especially effective against *H. influenzae*. Cefuroxime penetrates the CSF, thereby reducing the likelihood of secondary meningitis (see the section on the treatment of cellulitis for more details). CT should be used as an ancillary guide to the need for surgical exploration of the orbit in patients who do not rapidly respond to medical management.[41] CT is indicated when any degree of displacement of the globe is present or ophthalmoplegia or visual impairment is present. Serial assessment of the patient's visual acuity and ocular motility should be performed. Surgical intervention (exploration and decompression of the orbit) is indicated when there is CT evidence of intracranial involvement, a subperiosteal or orbital abscess, decreasing vision and worsening ocular motility, or the signs and symptoms do not rapidly improve over a 24- to 48-hour period in response to intravenous antibiotics.[42]

Perianal cellulitis

Cellulitis (group A beta-hemolytic *Streptococcus*) around the anal orifice is often misdiagnosed as candidiasis. It occurs more frequently in children than adults. Bright, perianal erythema extends from the anal verge approximately 2 to 3 cm onto the surrounding perianal skin (Figure 9-18). Boys are affected more than girls. Symptoms include painful defecation (52%), tenderness, soilage from oozing, and, sometimes, blood-streaked stool and perianal itching (78%).[43,44] These children are not systemically ill. Pharyngitis may precede the infection. The differential diagnosis includes *Candida* intertrigo, psoriasis, pinworm infection, inflammatory bowel disease, a behavioral problem, and child abuse. Culture confirms the diagnosis.

Initial treatment consists of a 10- to 14-day course of penicillin or erythromycin.[44] Relapses occurred in 39% of the patients.[45] After treatment, a new culture should be taken to check for recurrence. The topical antibiotic mupirocin (Bactroban) may also provide rapid relief of symptoms, but systemic therapy is also required.

Pseudomonas cellulitis

P. cellulitis is described in the section on *Pseudomonas* infection.

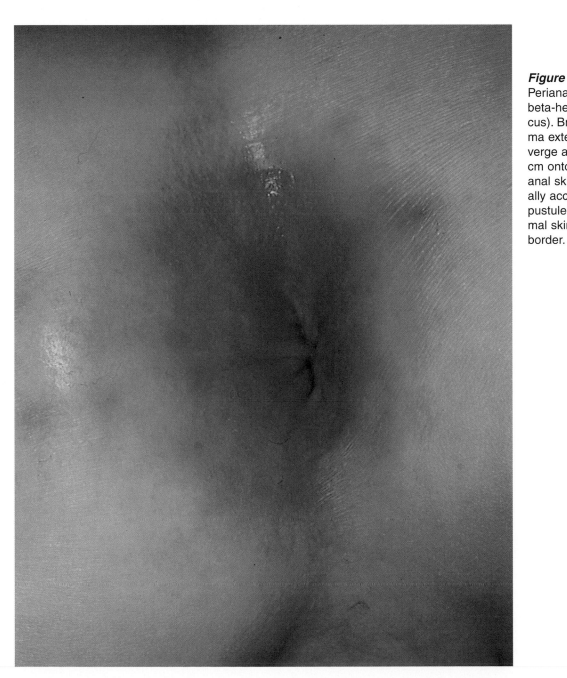

Figure 9-18
Perianal cellulitis (group A beta-hemolytic streptococcus). Bright perianal erythema extends from the anal verge approximately 2 to 3 cm onto the surrounding perianal skin. Candidiasis is usually accompanied by satellite pustules extending onto normal skin outside of the active border.

Folliculitis

Folliculitis is inflammation of the hair follicle caused by infection, chemical irritation, or physical injury. Inflammation may be superficial or deep in the hair follicle. Folliculitis is very common and is seen as a component of a variety of inflammatory skin diseases, which are listed in the box below.

In superficial folliculitis, the inflammation is confined to the upper part of the hair follicle. Clinically, it is manifested as a painless or tender pustule that eventually heals without scarring. In many instances, the hair shaft in the center of the pustule cannot be seen. Inflammation of the entire follicle or the deeper portion of the hair follicle initially appears as a swollen, red mass, which eventually may point toward the surface becoming a somewhat larger pustule than that seen in superficial folliculitis. Deeper lesions are painful and may heal with scarring.

STAPHYLOCOCCAL FOLLICULITIS

Staphylococcal folliculitis is the most common form of infectious folliculitis. One pustule or a group of pustules may appear, usually without fever or other systemic symptoms, on any body surface (Figure 9-19). Staphylococcal folliculitis may occur because of injury, abrasion, or nearby surgical wounds or draining abscesses. It may also be a complication of occlusive topical steroid therapy (Figure 9-20), particularly if moist lesions are occluded for many hours. Follicular pustules are cultured, not by touching the pustule with a cotton swab, but by scraping off the entire pustule with a #15 blade and depositing the material onto the cotton swab of a transport medium kit. Some cases can be treated with a tepid, wet Burow's compress, but oral antibiotics are used in most cases.

KERATOSIS PILARIS

Keratosis pilaris is a common finding on the posterolateral aspects of the upper arms and anterior thighs. The eruption is probably more common in atopics (see p. 112). Clinically, a group of small, pinpoint, follicular pustules remains in the same area for years. Histology shows that the inflammation actually occurs outside of the hair follicle. Scratching, wearing tight-fitting clothing, or undergoing treatment with abrasives may infect these sterile pustules and cause a diffuse eruption (see Figure 9-21). It is important to recognize this entity in order to avoid unnecessary and detrimental treatment. Many patients object to these small, sometimes unsightly bumps. Keratosis pilaris resists all types of treatment. Oral antibiotics active against *S. aureus* are used for folliculitis.

PSEUDOFOLLICULITIS BARBAE (RAZOR BUMPS)

Pseudofolliculitis is a foreign body reaction to hair. Clinically, there is less inflammation than with staphylococcal folliculitis. The condition occurs on the cheeks and neck in individuals who are genetically inclined to have tightly curled, spiral hair, which can become ingrown. This condition is found in 50% to 75% of blacks and 3% to 5% of whites who shave.[46] If cut below the surface by shaving, the sharp-tipped whisker may curve into the follicular wall or emerge and curve back to penetrate the skin. A tender, red papule or pustule occurs at the point of entry and remains until the hair is removed. Generally, the problem is more severe in the neck areas where hair follicles are more likely to be oriented at low angles to the skin surface, making repenetration of the skin more likely. Pseudofolliculitis can occur also in the axillae, pubic area, and legs. Normal bacterial flora may eventually be replaced by pathogenic organisms if the process becomes chronic. Pseudofolliculitis of the beard is a significant problem in the armed services (Figure 9-22) and in professions in which individuals are required to shave.

Treatment. This is a mechanical problem. Each imbedded hair shaft must be dislodged by inserting a firm, pointed instrument such as syringe needle under the hair loop and firmly elevating it. Shaving should be discontinued until all of the red papules have resolved. A short course of antistaphylococcal antibiotics may hasten resolution. Intra-

---

DISEASES INITIALLY MANIFESTING AS FOLLICULITIS

SUPERFICIAL FOLLICULITIS

Staphylococcal folliculitis
Pseudofolliculitis barbae (from shaving)
Superficial fungal infections (dermatophytes)
Cutaneous candidiasis (pustules also occur outside the hair follicle)
Acne vulgaris
Acne, mechanically or chemically induced
Steroid acne after withdrawal of topical steroids
Keratosis pilaris

DEEP FOLLICULITIS

Furuncle and carbuncle
Sycosis (inflammation of the entire depth of the follicle)
Sycosis (beard area): sycosis barbae, bacterial or fungal
Sycosis (scalp): bacterial
Acne vulgaris, cystic
Gram-negative acne
Pseudomonas folliculitis
Dermatophyte fungal infections

lesional triamcinolone acetonide (2.5 to 10 mg/ml) is useful for red papules that linger. Shaving may then be resumed using techniques that avoid close shaves and the production of sharply angled hair tips. Hydrating the beard prior to shaving by washing with soap and warm water softens the whiskers. The softened hairs are cut off directly, leaving a blunt hair and making ingrown hairs less likely. Use of a

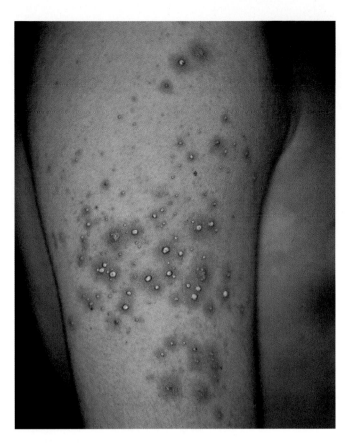

Figure 9-20
Staphylococcal folliculitis. Follicular pustules appeared after the patient's extremity had been occluded with a topical steroid and a plastic dressing for 24 hours. Gram-negative organisms may also flourish after long periods of plastic occlusion.

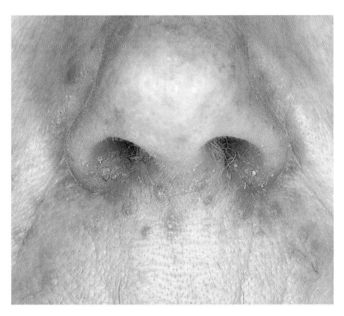

Figure 9-19
Staphylococcal folliculitis. The nares are a reservoir for *S. aureus*. Folliculitis may appear on the skin about the nose.

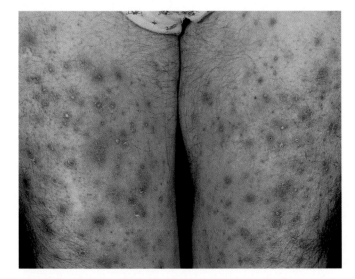

Figure 9-21
Keratosis pilaris and folliculitis. Keratosis pilaris is a common finding on the anterior thighs. A group of small, pinpoint, follicular pustules remains in the same area for years. Scratching, wearing tight-fitting clothing, or treating with abrasives may infect these sterile pustules and cause a diffuse eruption.

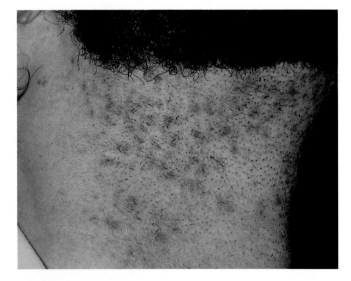

Figure 9-22
Pseudofolliculitis. Staphylococcal folliculitis is simulated when hair curves into and penetrates the skin, causing a foreign body–type reaction.

highly lubricating shaving gel (Edge Gel for Tough Beards) and a double-edged razor (e.g., Gillette Sensor) is recommended. Shaving closely with multiple razor strokes and shaving against the grain should be avoided. Electric clippers that cut hair as stubble can be an alternative to wet shaving. Specially designed electric razors (e.g., Remington's Black Man's Razor, Norelco Black Man's Razor) may also be used but they have not been very effective. Daily application of glycolic acid lotion (e.g., Aqua-Glycolic Lotion) facilitates a marked reduction in lesions, allowing some patients to shave daily with minimal irritation.[47] Depilatories with barium sulfide or calcium thioglycolate (available in all pharmacies) are the most practical and effective way of removing hair and preventing pseudofolliculitis. They are applied to the skin for 3 to 10 minutes and wiped off. The chemical reduces sulfide bonds in the cortex of the medulla of the hair shaft. The weakened hair fibers shear when the material is wiped off, leaving a soft, fluffy hair tip that is less likely to become ingrown. These products are irritating and can only be tolerated once or twice each week. If these measures fail, shaving must be discontinued indefinitely.

A surgical approach for removing hair follicles in patients with pseudofolliculitis has been described.[48] A flap of facial skin is undermined, turned inside out, and the hair roots are then cut using serrated scissors. Surgical depilation may be considered when conventional therapy has failed.

SYCOSIS BARBAE

Sycosis implies follicular inflammation of the entire depth of the hair follicle and may be caused by infection with *Staphylococcus aureus* or dermatophyte fungi. (See Chapter Thirteen on fungal infections for a discussion of fungal sycosis.) The disease occurs only in men who have commenced shaving. It begins with the appearance of small follicular papules or pustules and rapidly becomes more diffuse as shaving continues (Figure 9-23). Reaction to the disease varies greatly among individuals. Infiltration about the follicle may be slight or extensive. The more infiltrated cases heal with scarring. In chronic cases, the pustules may remain confined to one area, such as the upper lip or neck. The hairs are epilated with difficulty in staphylococcal sycosis and with relative ease in fungal sycosis. Hairs should be removed and examined for fungi and the purulent material should be cultured. Fungal infections tend to be more severe, producing deeper and wider areas of inflammation; bacterial follicular infections usually present with discrete pustules. Pseudofolliculitis (see previous section) has a similar appearance.

Localized inflammation is treated topically with mupirocin (Bactroban ointment). Extensive disease is treated with oral antibiotics (e.g., erythromycin, dicloxacillin, cephalexin) for at least 2 weeks or until all signs of inflammation have cleared. Recurrences are not uncommon and require an additional course of oral antibiotics. Shaving should be performed with a clean razor.

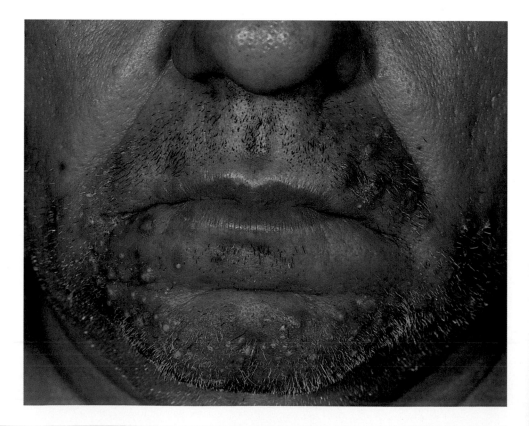

Figure 9-23
Sycosis barbae. Deep follicular pustules.

ACNE KELOIDALIS

Acne keloidalis is a chronic scarring folliculitis of unknown etiology located on the posterior neck that eventually results in the formation of a group of keloidal papules.[49] It occurs only in men and is more common in blacks. It may be initiated or aggravated by protective head devices.[50] Follicular papules or pustules (Figure 9-24) develop on the back of the neck. They coalesce into firm plaques and nodules. Histologic examination of early lesions shows that inflammation begins at the deep infundibular and isthmic levels of the hair follicle and is accompanied by absence of sebaceous glands. Scar forms at the isthmic levels, trapping hair fragments in the inferior portion of the follicle.[51] The inflammatory stage may be asymptomatic. The patient eventually discovers a group of hard papules (Figure 9-25). The inflammatory stage lasts for months or years. The degree of inflammation varies from a group of discrete pustules to abscess formation on the entire back of the neck.

Treatment

A bacterial etiology has never been proven but acne keloidalis usually responds to short- or long-term courses of oral antibiotics. Different classes of antibiotics may have to be tried before control is achieved. Erythromycin, cephalosporins, trimethoprim sulfamethoxazole (Bactrim, Septra), dicloxacillin, and amoxicillin-clavulanate potassium (Augmentin) have been successful in individual cases. Control with one antibiotic may diminish with time and the patient may have to be treated with a different antibiotic for continued long-term suppression. Intralesional injections of triamcinolone reduces the keloids, but this treatment should be delayed until infection has been controlled. Surgical excision may be necessary if persistent sinus tracts form. Successful surgical therapy of advanced cases can be carried out using a number of methods as long as subfollicular destruction of the process is achieved.[49]

SPONTANEOUS INFECTIOUS FOLLICULITIS

Infectious folliculitis may appear spontaneously. In this type, follicular pustules appear in crops on the face and limbs and resolve in 1 or 2 weeks.

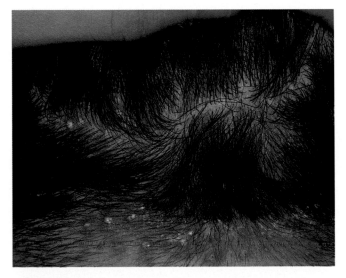

Figure 9-24
Deep folliculitis. Follicular pustules are surrounded by erythema and swelling. The entire follicular structure is inflamed. Staphylococci were isolated by culture.

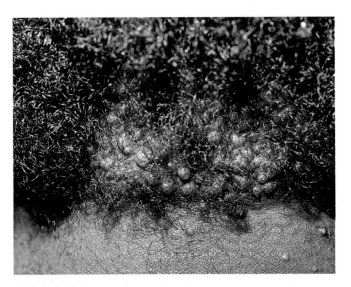

Figure 9-25
Acne keloidalis. Keloidal papules may eventually form on the back of the neck after chronic inflammation of the hair follicles.

Furuncles and Carbuncles

A furuncle (abscess or boil) is a walled-off collection of pus that is a painful, firm, or fluctuant mass. Cellulitis may precede or occur in conjunction with it. An abscess is not a hollow sphere, but a cavity formed by fingerlike loculations of granulation tissue and pus that extends outward along planes of least resistance. They may occur at any site, but they appear particularly in areas prone to friction or minor trauma, such as underneath a belt, the anterior thighs, buttocks, groin, axillae, and waist. Furuncles are uncommon in children, but increase in frequency after puberty. *S. aureus* is the most common pathogen. The infecting strain may be found during quiescent periods in the nares and perineum. There is evidence that the anterior nares is the primary site from which the staphylococcus is disseminated to the skin. Other organisms, either aerobic (*E. coli*, *P. aeruginosa*, *S. faecalis*) or anaerobic (*Bacteroides*, *Lactobacillus*, *Peptococcus*, *Peptostreptococcus*) may cause furuncles.[52] In general, the microbiology of abscesses reflects the microflora of the anatomic part of the body involved. Anaerobes are found in perineal and in some head and neck abscesses. Perirectal- and perianal-region abscesses often are reflective of fecal flora. Approximately 5% of abscesses are sterile.

Furunculosis occurs as a self-limited infection in which one or several lesions are present or as a chronic, recurrent disease that lasts for months or years, affecting one or several family members. Most patients with sporadic or recurrent furunculosis appear to be otherwise normal and have an intact immune system.

One disease in which an immune defect has been found to predispose a patient to recurrent furunculosis is the hyperimmunoglobulinemia E-staphylococcal abscess syndrome (Job's syndrome), in which large abscesses with little erythema or inflammation ("cold abscess") appear in young girls with an atopic-like dermatitis, eosinophilia, elevated IgE, and a profound defect in neutrophil granulocyte chemotaxis. Other immunodeficiency diseases with abscesses include chronic granulomatous disease, Chédiak-Higashi syndrome, C3 deficiency, C3 hypercatabolism, transient hypogammaglobulinemia of infancy, immunodeficiency with thymoma, and Wiskott-Aldrich syndrome. Diabetic patients probably do not have a predisposition to furunculosis or other cutaneous infections.

Predisposing conditions

A number of factors predispose the hair follicle to infection. Occlusion of the groin and buttocks by clothing, especially in patients with hyperhidrosis, encourages bacterial colonization. Follicular abnormalities, evident by the presence of comedones and acneiform papules and pustules are often found on the buttocks and axillae of patients with recurrent furunculosis of those areas; these findings suggest the diagnosis of hidradenitis suppurativa (see p. 184). Bacteria colonize the skin in patients with atopic dermatitis, eczema, and scabies.

Clinical manifestations

The lesion begins as a deep, tender, firm, red papule that enlarges rapidly into a tender, deep-seated nodule that remains stable and painful for days and then becomes fluctuant (Figure 9-26). The temperature is normal and there are no systemic symptoms. Pain becomes moderate to severe as purulent material accumulates. Pain is most intense in areas where expansion is restricted, such as the neck and external auditory canal. The abscess either remains deep and reabsorbs or points and ruptures through the surface. The abscess cavity contains a surprisingly large quantity of pus and white chunks of necrotic tissue. The point of rupture heals with scarring.

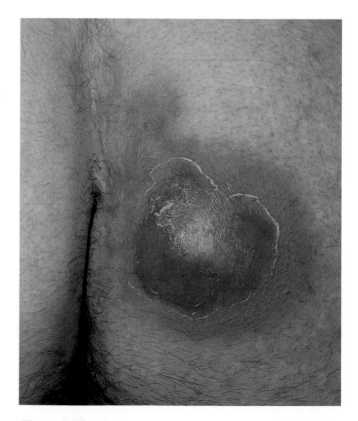

Figure 9-26
Furuncle (boil). Enlarged swollen mass with purulent material beginning to exude from several points on the surface.

Carbuncles are aggregates of infected follicles. The infection originates deep in the dermis and the subcutaneous tissue, forming a broad, red, swollen, slowly evolving, deep, painful mass that points and drains through multiple openings. Malaise, chills, and fever precede or occur during the active phase. Deep extension into the subcutaneous tissue may be followed by sloughing and extensive scarring. Areas with thick dermis (i.e., the back of the neck, the back of the trunk, and the lateral aspects of the thighs) are the preferred sites. In the preantibiotic era, there were some fatalities.

Differential diagnosis

A number of diseases can be manifested as a furuncle (Table 9-1). The most common structure that is misinterpreted as a furuncle is a ruptured epidermal cyst or pilar cyst of the scalp. The cyst wall ruptures spontaneously, leaking the white amorphous material into the dermis (Figure 9-27). An intense, foreign-body, inflammatory reaction occurs in hours, forming a sterile abscess.

Treatment of a ruptured cyst consists of making a linear incision over the surface and evacuating the white material with manual pressure and a curette. Sometimes the cyst wall can be forced through the incision and cut out. In many cases the wall cannot be removed because it is fused to the dermis during the inflammatory process. Antibiotics are unnecessary.

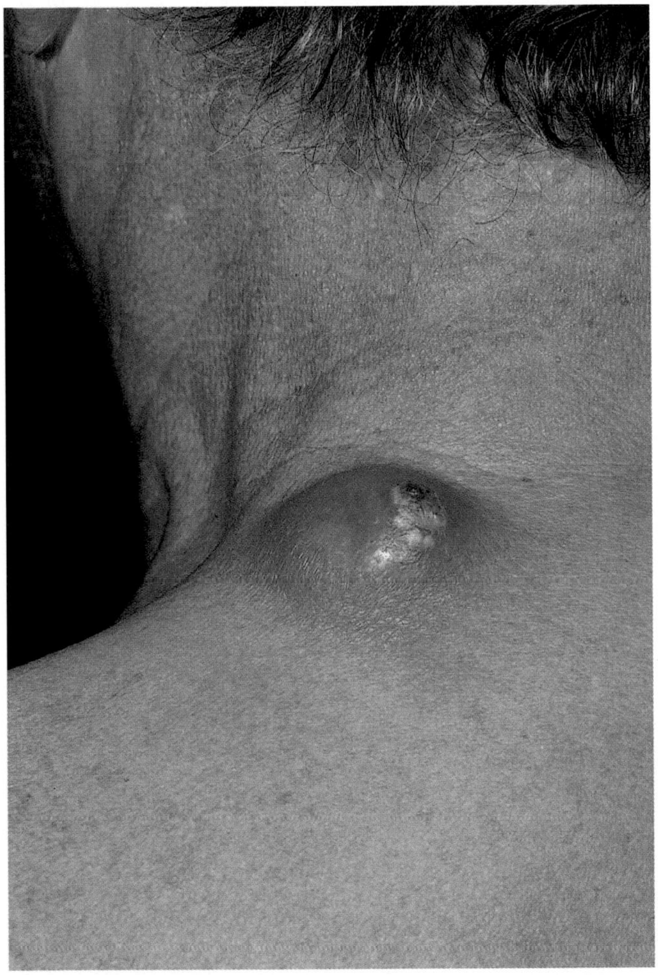

Figure 9-27
Ruptured epidermal cyst. This is commonly misinterpreted as a furuncle. A large mass of white, amorphous material and pus exudes after a linear incision is made over the surface.

TABLE 9-1 Disease Initially Manifesting as Furunculosis ("Boils")

Disease	Location
Bacterial furunculosis	Any body surface
Recurrent furunculosis in scarred tissue	Buttock or any location
Ruptured epidermal cyst	Preauricular and postauricular areas, face, chest, back
Hidradenitis suppurativa	Axilla, groin, buttock, under breasts
Cystic acne	Face, chest, back
Primary immunodeficiency diseases*	Any body surface
Secondary immunodeficiency†	Any body surface
Others: diabetes, alcoholism, malnutrition, severe anemia, debilitation	Any body surface

*Syndrome of hyperimmunoglobulinemia E associated with staphylococcal abscesses (Job's syndrome), chronic granulomatous disease, Chédiak-Higashi syndrome, C3 deficiency, C3 hypercatabolism, transient hypogammaglobulinemia of infancy, immunodeficiency with thymoma, Wiskott-Aldrich syndrome.
†Leukemia, leukopenia, neutropenia, therapeutic immunosuppression.

Treatment of furuncles

WARM COMPRESSES. Many furuncles are self-limited and respond well to frequent applications of a moist, warm compress, which provide comfort and probably encourage localization and pointing of the abscess.

INCISION, DRAINAGE, AND PACKING. The primary management of cutaneous abscesses should be incision and drainage. In general, routine culture and antibiotic therapy are not indicated for localized abscesses in patients with presumably normal host defenses.[53] The abscess is not ready for drainage until the skin has thinned and the underlying mass becomes soft and fluctuant. The skin around the central area is anesthetized with 1% lidocaine. A pointed, lance-shaped #11 surgical blade is inserted and drawn parallel to skin lines through the thin, effaced skin, creating an opening from which pus may be expressed easily with light pressure. Care must be taken to avoid extending the incision into firm, noneffaced skin. A curette is inserted through the opening and carefully drawn back and forth to break adhesions and dislodge fragments of necrotic tissue. Continuous drainage may be promoted in very large abscesses by packing the cavity with a long ribbon of iodoform gauze. The end of the ribbon is inserted through a curette loop. The curette is then turned to secure the gauze, inserted deep into the cavity, twisted in the reverse direction and removed concurrently, while the gauze is held in place with a thin-tipped forceps. Next, the gauze is worked into the cavity with the forceps until resistance is met. The gauze quickly becomes saturated and should be removed hours later and replaced with a fresh packing.

CULTURE AND GRAM STAIN. These studies are indicated when there are recurrent abscesses, a failure to respond to conventional therapy, systemic toxicity, involvement of the central face, abscesses that contain gas or involve muscle or fascia, or when the patient is immunocompromised. Material for culture and Gram stain is collected in a sterile syringe by inserting the needle through the unbroken effaced skin over the abscess. If anaerobic organisms are suspected, the material should be rapidly transported to the laboratory in the syringe or immediately inoculated into an anaerobic tube. Culturing of an abscess usually takes 48 hours or more to determine which bacteria are present. The Gram stain provides a rapid means of diagnosis.

ANTIBIOTICS. Patients with recurrent furunculosis learn that they can sometimes stop the progression of an abscess by starting antistaphylococcal antibiotics at the first sign of the typical localized swelling and erythema. They continue to use antibiotics for 5 to 10 days. Antibiotics should be started immediately in order to attenuate the evolving abscess. Antibiotics have little effect once the abscess has become fluctuant.

Recurrent furunculosis

Diseases manifesting as recurrent furunculosis are listed in Table 9-1.[54] Recurrent furunculosis in otherwise healthy patients with no predisposing factors is the most common manifestation.

Management. Although recurrent infection often ceases spontaneously after 2 years, a few patients have repeated episodes of furuncles that last for years. Several members of a family may be affected. Most of these patients are normal with an intact immune system. Most people do not carry *S. aureus* in the nose, but patients with recurrent furunculosis frequently carry the pathogenic strain of *S. aureus* in their nares and perineum.[55] Therapy goals are to decrease or eliminate the pathogenic strain. The treatment program for recurrent furunculosis is described in the box below.

TREATMENT PROGRAM FOR RECURRENT FURUNCULOSIS

ERADICATION OF *S. AUREUS* NASAL CARRIAGE

Program of first choice:
1. Instruct the patient to apply mupirocin (Bactroban) ointment to the anterior nares with a cotton swab applicator twice daily for 5 consecutive days. This treatment should be used for all verified familial carriers of the same strain (nasal carriage was 48% at 6 months and 53% at 1 year[7]).
2. Culture the anterior nares every 3 months to check for the effectiveness of the above measure. Retreat with mupirocin or consider oral antibiotics for treatment failures.

Program for topical treatment failures:
Prescribe an oral semisynthetic penicillin, 0.5 to 1 gm, to be taken twice daily for 10 to 14 days; treatment for 2 months offered no benefit in preventing recurrences.[127] (treatment with systemic antibiotics eradicates the pathogenic organisms from the nares, perineum, and furuncles*).

OTHER MEASURES TO ERADICATE *S. AUREUS*

Instruct the patient to:
1. Wash the entire body and the fingernails with a nail brush each day for 1 to 3 weeks with Betadine, Hibiclens, or pHisohex soap. The frequency of washing should be decreased if the skin becomes dry.
2. Change towels, washcloths, and sheets daily.
3. Change wound dressings frequently.
4. Clean shaving instruments thoroughly each day.
5. Avoid nose picking.

---

*The combination of 500 mg of cloxacillin every 6 hours for 7 to 10 days and 600 mg of rifampin once a day for 7 to 10 days may be more effective in eradicating coagulase-positive *staphylococci* from the anterior nares.[128] In one study, when culture of the anterior nares yielded *S. aureus*, rifampin alone (given at 3-month intervals) significantly reduced the incidence of infection.[129] In another study a 3-month course of oral clindamycin (150 mg daily) was effective in preventing infection.[29] Of nine patients who responded to clindamycin, six had no recurrences of their infection for at least 9 months after discontinuing therapy, and there were no side effects.

Erysipeloid

Erysipeloid is an acute skin infection caused by the gram-positive, rod-shaped, nonsporulating bacillus *Erysipelothrix rhusiopathiae* (or *insidiosa*). It has been found to cause infection in several dozen species of mammals and other animals.[56] Humans become infected through exposure to infected or contaminated animals or animal products.[57] By far the most common type of human infection is a localized, self-limited cutaneous lesion, erysipeloid. Diffuse cutaneous and systemic infections occur rarely. The disease is an occupational hazard for people who handle unprocessed meat and animal products, such as fishermen (fish poisoning, crab poisoning, seal finger, whale finger), meat handlers (swine erysipelas), butchers, farmers, and veterinarians. Patients who have repeated infections know that it responds to penicillin and treat themselves.

Approximately 1 to 7 days (an average of 3 days) after animal contact, a dull, red erythema appears at the inoculation site and extends centrifugally for 3 to 4 days to reach a fixed size of approximately 10 cm in diameter (Figure 9-28). Central clearing often occurs. Streptococcal cellulitis (erysipelas) is bright red, painful, and spreads rapidly. At times the lesions develop as dull-to-bright red, sharply demarcated "diamonds" with smooth, glistening surfaces. It often occurs on the hand, especially the finger webs, but spares the terminal phalanges. Infection also occurs on the face, neck, and sole of the foot. There is burning, itching, and discomfort; lymphangitis or constitutional symptoms develop in a few patients. The disease is self-limited and may subside spontaneously. Relapse may occur from 4 days to 2 weeks after the lesions are completely resolved. Diffuse and systemic forms with extensive, red, diamond-shaped

plaques, septic arthritis, and endocarditis[58] are rare. Systemic forms of the disease may occur at the time of skin inoculation or from 1 to 6 months after spontaneous resolution of skin lesions. Some patients with sepsis have no skin signs. The bacteria's apparent ability to revert to L forms (bacteria without cell walls)[59] may explain the phenomenon of recurrence and explain why *Erysipelothrix* is difficult to culture in wounds and blood or to demonstrate in stained smears or tissue sections. The obvious therapeutic implication is that other-than-cell-wall-active antibiotics may prove to be the drugs of choice for treatment. The organism may be isolated from biopsy or blood specimens on standard culture media. It is identified by morphology, lack of motility, and biochemical characteristics; identification may be confirmed by the mouse protection test.

Treatment. Although there are many instances of cutaneous forms of the disease running a self-limited course, all patients should receive antibiotics to prevent progression to systemic disease and the development of endocarditis.[60] The disease responds to penicillins, cephalosporins, erythromycin, and clindamycin, but it is often resistant to many other antibiotics, including vancomycin.

Blistering Distal Dactylitis

Blistering distal dactylitis is a superficial infection of the anterior fat pad of the fingertips. It is most commonly caused by group A beta-hemolytic streptococci (Figure 9-29).[61] *S. aureus* is the cause in a few reported patients.[62,63] A large blister filled with a watery, purulent fluid forms on the volar surface of the distal portion of the fingers. The age range of most of the reported patients is 2 to 16 years but adult cases are also reported.[64] A firm diagnosis can be made with a Gram stain and culture of the blister fluid. Treatment consists of incision, drainage, and a 10-day course of anti-streptococcal systemic antibiotics.

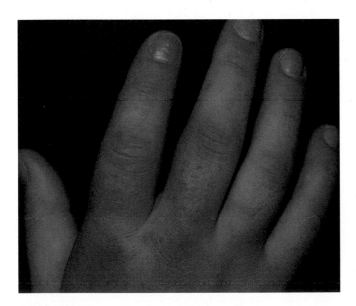

Figure 9-28
Erysipeloid. Approximately 3 days after animal or fish contact, a dull red erythema appears at the inoculation site and extends centrifugally.

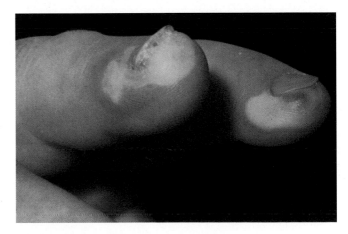

Figure 9-29
Blistering distal dactylitis. This superficial infection of the anterior fat pad of the distal portion of the fingers is caused most commonly by group A beta-hemolytic streptococci.
(Courtesy Lućia Martin-Moreno, M.D.)

Staphylococcal Scalded Skin Syndrome

Staphylococcal scalded skin syndrome (SSSS), also known as *Ritter's disease*, is a staphylococcal epidermolytic toxin syndrome.[65] This entity usually occurs in children under 5 years of age, and it is primarily explained by a lack of immunity to the toxins and to renal immaturity that leads to poor clearance of toxins.[66] Staphylococcal scarlatiniform eruption and bullous impetigo are also diseases that are caused by an epidermolytic toxin elaborated by *S. aureus*, phage group II, including types 55, 71, 3A, and 3B. The toxin is antigenic and when elaborated elicits an antibody response. Two antigenically distinct forms (ET A and ET B) have been identified.[67] Epidermolytic toxin antibody is present in 75% of normal people over the age of 10 years, a fact that explains the rarity of SSSS in adults. The epidermolytic toxins (A and B) directly cleave the epidermis beneath the granular cell layer by attacking the extracellular substance with subsequent rupture of desmosomes.[68]

The childhood form of SSSS is most often seen in otherwise healthy children. A review of the largest series of cases showed that 62% of children were younger than 2 years old, 98% were 6 years or younger, and only one child was older than 9 years old.[69] SSSS begins with a localized, often inapparent, *S. aureus* infection of the conjunctivae, throat, nares, or umbilicus. A diffuse, tender erythema appears; the skin has a sandpaper-like texture similar to that seen in scarlet fever. The erythema is often accentuated in flexural and periorificial areas. However, the rash of scarlet fever is not tender. The temperature rises and within 1 or 2 days the skin wrinkles, forms transient bullae, and peels off in large sheets, leaving a moist, red, glistening surface (Figure 9-30). Minor pressure induces skin separation (Nikolsky's sign). The area of involvement may be localized, but it is often generalized. Evaporative fluid loss from large areas is associated with increased fluid loss and dehydration. A yellow crust forms, and the denuded surface dries and cracks. Healing occurs in 7 to 10 days, accompanied by desquamation similar to that seen in scarlet fever. Reepithelialization is rapid because of the high level of the split in the epidermis. The distinction between the localized form of SSSS and bullous impetigo can be difficult. The criteria in favor of localized SSSS are (1) the absence of inflammatory cells in the dermis on biopsy, (2) erythematous skin with tenderness, (3) Nikolsky's phenomenon around lesions, and (4) a negative culture from intact bullae.[70]

Figure 9-30
Staphylococcal scalded skin syndrome. Exfoliative phase, during which the upper epidermis is shed.

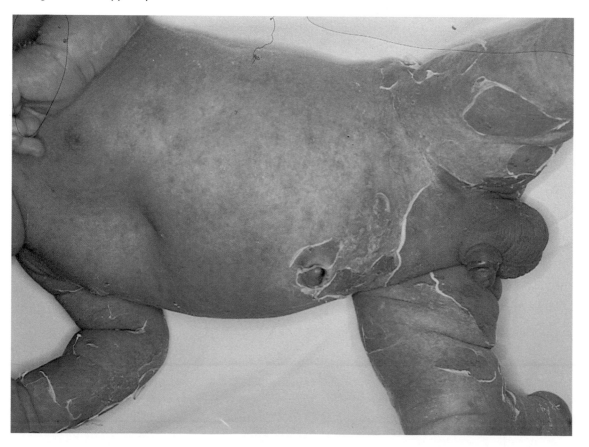

The rare, adult type of generalized SSSS is associated with underlying diseases related to immunosuppression, abnormal immunity,[71-73] and renal insufficiency. The epidermolytic toxin is filtered through the glomeruli and partially reabsorbed in the proximal tubule where it undergoes catabolism by the proximal tubule cells. The glomerular filtration rate of infants is less than 50% of the normal adult rate, which is reached in the second year of life. This may explain why infants, patients with chronic renal failure, and those on hemodialysis[69] may be predisposed to SSSS. Many of the reported adult cases had positive blood cultures; children younger than 5 years infrequently have sepsis. Cultures from bullae have also been reported to be positive, but this may have been the result of contamination. Several reported adult patients were on systemic steroids.

Staphylococcal scarlatiniform eruption is similar to SSSS, except that the skin does not blister or peel.

Diagnosis. In SSSS, a biopsy shows splitting of the epidermis in the stratum granulosum near the skin surface; there is scant inflammation. Thin-roofed bullae are flaccid and rupture easily. Cultures should be taken from the eye, nose, throat, bullae, and any obviously infected area. Skin and blood cultures are often negative in children and positive in adults. SSSS must be differentiated from toxic epidermal necrolysis, a rare, life-threatening disease in which full-thickness epidermal necrosis occurs. Histologically, toxic epidermal necrolysis shows dermal-epidermal separation, rather than the granular layer split in the epidermis seen in SSSS and an intense inflammatory infiltrate. A frozen section of peeled skin is a reliable way of rapidly establishing the diagnosis.

Treatment. Corticosteroids are contraindicated because they interfere with host defense mechanisms.[74] Hospitalization and intravenous antibiotic therapy are desirable for extensive cases. Most of the toxin-producing *S. aureus* produce penicillinase. Nafcillin 100 to 200 mg/kg daily is used in the hospital. Patients with limited disease may be managed at home with oral antibiotics. Dicloxacillin 25 mg/kg per day, or erythromycin 12.5 mg/kg every 6 hours is prescribed for a minimum of 1 week. Topical antibiotics are not necessary. The patient's skin should be lubricated with bland, light lotions and washed infrequently. Wet dressings may cause further drying and cracking and should be avoided.

Pseudomonas aeruginosa Infection

P. aeruginosa is a gram-negative aerobic bacillus found in less than 10% of nonhospitalized individuals. The incidence of fecal carriage increases with the length of the hospital stay. Antibiotic administration results in a much higher incidence. The bacteria may colonize warm, moist areas such as skin folds (toe webs), ear canals, burns, ulcers, and areas beneath nails. It is also found in the moist areas of sinks and drains and in poorly preserved topical creams and ointments. It produces diffusable fluorescent pigments including pyoverdin and a soluble phenazine pigment called pyocyanin. Pyocyanin appears blue or green at neutral or alkaline pH and is the source of the name *aeruginosa*. An organic metabolite may impart a fruity odor to some cutaneous lesions. That same odor in culture is a specific quality of *P. aeruginosa*. *Pseudomonas* survives poorly in an acid environment. There are many serotypes. Occasionally, other species such as *P. putrefaciens* are of clinical significance.

Pseudomonas infects warm, moist areas in healthy people. Hot tub folliculitis and toe-web intertrigo occur because of a temporary change in the skin moisture content and temperature that allows pseudomonal overgrowth. Correction of the altered environment results in resolution of the infection. Severe, life-threatening infections occur in patients with impaired immunity, such as those with serious burns or acute leukemia or those receiving immunosuppressive therapy.

Oral treatment of *Pseudomonas* infections is now possible with oral antibiotics such as the fluoroquinolone, ciprofloxacin hydrochloride (Cipro).

PSEUDOMONAS FOLLICULITIS

From 8 hours to 5 days or longer (mean incubation period is 48 hours) after using a contaminated whirlpool, home hot tub, waterslide, physiotherapy pool, or contaminated loofah sponge[75] 7% to 100% of those exposed develop *Pseudomonas* folliculitis. The attack rate is significantly higher in children than in adults, possibly because they tend to spend more time in the water. Showering after using the contaminated facility offers no protection. The typical patient has a few to more than 50 0.5- to 3-cm, pruritic, round, urticarial plaques with a central papule or pustule located on all skin surfaces except the head. The rash may be follicular, maculopapular, vesicular, pustular, or a polymorphous eruption that includes all of these types of lesions. Under normal conditions, *P. aeruginosa* infection cannot be induced by inoculation of the microorganism onto the intact skin surface of immune-competent persons. Occlusion and superhydration of the stratum corneum favors colonization of the skin with *P. aeruginosa*. This may explain why the rash is most severe in areas occluded by a snug bathing suit (Figures 9-31 and 9-32). Women who wear one-piece bathing suits are at an increased risk. The eruption, in most cases, clears in 7 to 10 days, leaving round spots of red-brown, postinflammatory hyperpigmentation, but patients have been reported to have recurrent crops of lesions for as long as 3 months. The spread of infection from person to person is not likely. Malaise and fatigue may occur during the initial few days of the eruption. Fever is uncommon and low grade when it appears.

P. aeruginosa serotype 0:9 and 0:11 are most commonly isolated from skin lesions, but other serotypes[76] have been reported.[77] Three conditions are associated with folliculitis: prolonged exposure to the water, an excessive number of bathers, and inadequate pool care. The organism gains entry via the hair follicles or breaks in the skin. The elevated water temperature promotes sweating, which enhances penetration of the skin by the bacteria. Also, with heavy use, there are desquamated skin cells in the water, providing a rich, organic nutrient source for the bacteria. The ubiquitous *P. aeruginosa* rapidly multiply in water at elevated temperatures. A heavy bather load, turbulent water, and aeration make it difficult to maintain satisfactory levels of chlorine. The risk of infection decreases when the water is changed frequently and the chlorine or bromine levels are kept well above the recommended concentration for the facility.

Figure 9-31
Pseudomonas folliculitis. Urticarial plaques surmounted by pustules located primarily in the areas covered by the bathing suit.

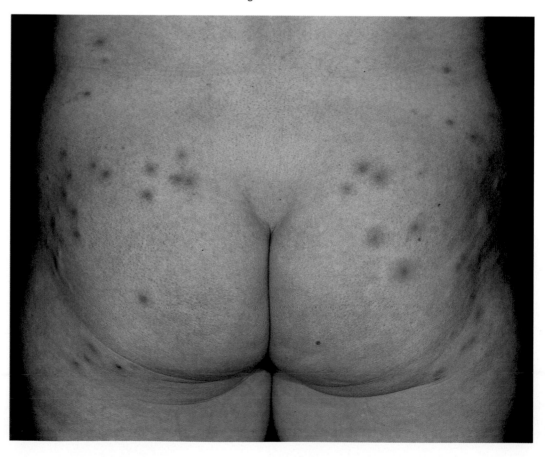

Management. The infection is self-limited, but a 5% acetic acid (white vinegar) wet compress applied for 20 minutes two to four times a day and/or silver sulfadiazine cream (Silvadene) might be of some help. Cases resistant to topical therapy can be treated orally with ciprofloxacin (Cipro) 500 or 750 mg twice each day.

The most effective preventative measures to be taken are continuous water filtration to eliminate desquamated skin, automatic chlorination to maintain a free residual chlorine level of at least 1 ppm, frequent monitoring of the disinfectant level, and frequent changing of the water, especially during heavy use.[78,79] The Centers for Disease Control's

Suggested Health and Safety Guidelines for Public Spas and Hot Tubs recommend a free chlorine concentration of 1 to 3 mg per liter and pH 7.2 to 7.8. Private hot tubs should be drained every 4 to 8 weeks depending on the amount of use. Public hot tubs and whirlpools with heavy use should be drained completely on a daily basis and the interior should be cleaned daily with an acidic solution. Bromine is an alternative to chlorine. Bromine is more effective in hot water than chlorine and it remains active for a longer period. Its effects are not inactivated so readily by ammonia compounds. Bromine is effective over a broader range and is more stable, but the odor is unpleasant.[80]

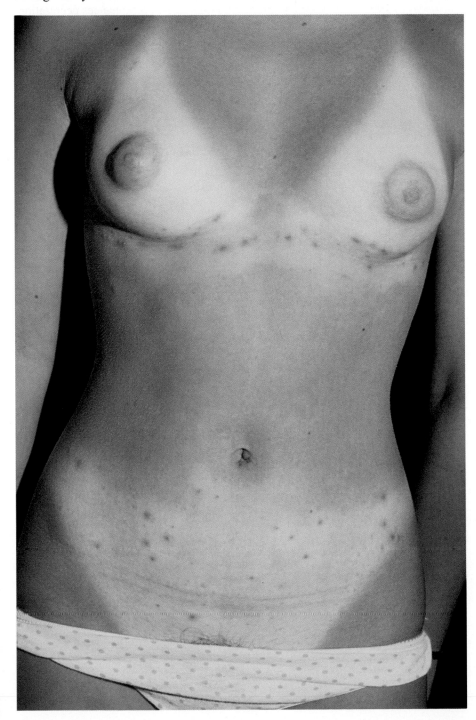

Figure 9-32
Pseudomonas folliculitis. Pustules form in occluded areas under the bathing suit.

PSEUDOMONAS CELLULITIS

Pseudomonas cellulitis may be localized or may occur during *Pseudomonas* septicemia. The localized form occurs as a secondary infection of tinea of the toe webs or groin (Figures 9-33 and 9-34), bed sores, stasis ulcers, burns, grafted areas, and under the foreskin of the penis[81,82] (Figures 9-35 and 9-36). Maceration or occlusion of these cutaneous lesions encourages secondary infection with *Pseudomonas*. Suppression of normal bacterial flora by broad-spectrum antibiotics encourages secondary infection. *Pseudomonas* infection is often unsuspected and appropriate therapy is therefore delayed. Deep erosions and tissue necrosis may occur before the correct diagnosis is made. Severe pain is highly characteristic of an evolving infection. The skin turns a dusky red (see Figure 9-34). Bluish green, purulent material with a fruity or "mousey" odor accumulates as the red, indurated area becomes macerated and then eroded. Vesicles and pustules may occur as satellite lesions. The eruption may spread to cover wide areas and be accompanied by systemic symptoms. *Pseudomonas* septicemia may produce a deep, indurated, necrotic cellulitis that resembles other forms of infectious cellulitis.

Treatment. Treatment consists of 5% acetic acid (white vinegar)[83] wet compresses applied 20 minutes four times a day. Localized infections respond to oral treatment with ciprofloxacin (Cipro) 500 or 750 mg twice each day. Application twice daily of mercurochrome to the infected penis can result in rapid control of infection.

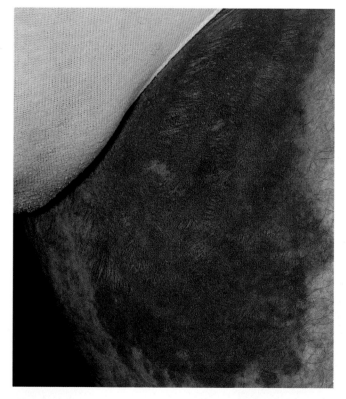

Figure 9-33
Pseudomonas cellulitis. Inflamed area has a "mousey" or grape juice–like odor.

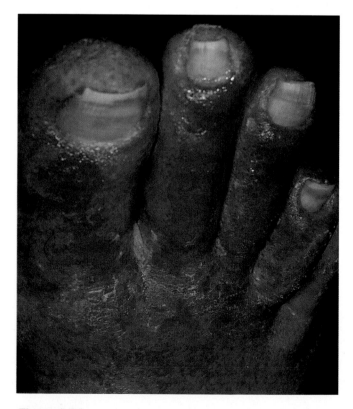

Figure 9-34
Pseudomonas cellulitis. The localized form occurs as a secondary infection of tinea of the toe webs. Maceration and occlusion in moist boots predisposes to secondary infection with *Pseudomonas*. The skin becomes painful and turns a dusky red.

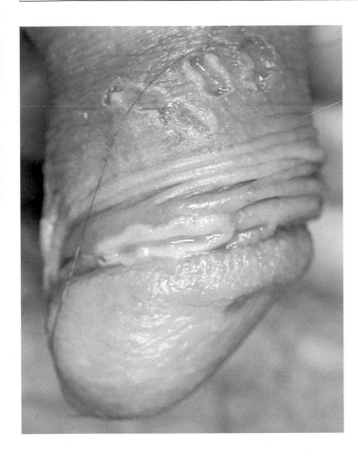

Figure 9-35
Erosions of the shaft of the penis exposed to the warmth and moisture under the foreskin may become infected with *Pseudomonas*.

Figure 9-36
Pseudomonas cellulitis. Maceration and abrasion under the foreskin can lead to secondary infection with *Pseudomonas*.

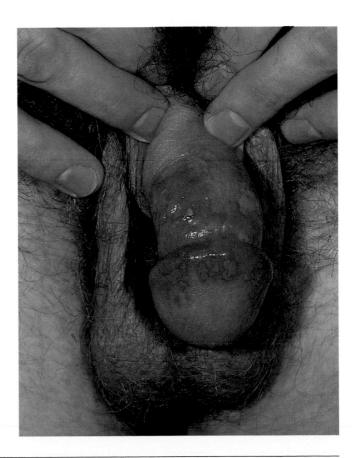

EXTERNAL OTITIS

External otitis is an inflammation of the external auditory canal. It occurs in a mild, self-limited form (swimmer's ear) or as an acute and chronic, recurrent, debilitating disease. The normally acidic cerumen inhibits gram-negative bacterial growth and forms a protective layer that discourages maceration. Swimming or excessive manipulation while cleaning the canal may disrupt this natural barrier. Inflammatory diseases such as psoriasis, seborrheic dermatitis, and eczematous dermatitis disrupt the normal barrier and encourage infection. *Pseudomonas* is the most common bacteria isolated from both mild and severe external otitis. Most cases, however, represent a mixed infection with other gram-negative (*Proteus mirabilis*, *Klebsiella pneumoniae*) and gram-positive (*Staphylococcus epidermidis*, beta-hemolytic streptococci) bacteria. Fungal infection with *Candida* or *Aspergillus niger* sometimes occurs, and these organisms may be the primary pathogens.

The early stages are characterized by erythema, edema, and an accumulation of moist, cellular debris in the canal.

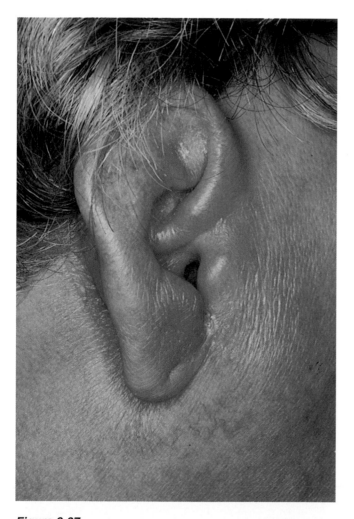

Figure 9-37
Pseudomonas cellulitis. The entire pinna and surrounding skin have become inflamed after an episode of external otitis.

Traction on the pinna or tragus may elicit pain. If the disease progresses, erythema radiates into the pinna and purulent material partly obstructs and exudes from the canal. Pain becomes constant and more intense. Cellulitis of the pinna and skin surrounding the ear accompanied by a dense mucopurulent exudate discharging from the canal may result from infection with *Pseudomonas* (Figure 9-37). However, in most cases, this indicates a secondary infection with staphylococci and streptococci.

The lymphatics of the external ear may be permanently damaged during an attack of cellulitis, predisposing the patient to recurrent episodes of streptococcal erysipelas of the pinna. Recurrent attacks are brought on by manipulation or even the slightest trauma.

Eczematous inflammation and infection of the external ear and surrounding skin may occur for a variety of reasons, such as irritation from purulent exudate, scratching and manipulation, or allergy to topical medications. Habitual manipulation may cause this disease to persist for years.

Treatment. The external auditory canal is cleansed. Squamous debris, cerumen, and pus are removed by suction or irrigation with an ear syringe.

Acidification is accomplished with 2% acetic acid (VōSol Otic Solution or Otic Domeboro) or 2% acetic acid with 1% hydrocortisone (VōSol Otic HC). Instill 5 drops in the canal four times each day. Acidification creates an environment that is inhospitable to gram-negative bacteria and fungi.

Topical antibiotics should be considered for infection localized to the canal. A culture of canal drainage is obtained. Antibiotic otic solutions such as Cortisporin Otic Suspension (a combination product made up of polymyxin B, neomycin, hydrocortisone, and bacitracin zinc) or Coly-Mycin S Otic (colistin sulfate, neomycin, and hydrocortisone) are instilled into the canal several times each day until the infection has resolved.

Ear wicks are made of strands of cotton or fine cloth and are inserted into the canal to act as a conduit for application of otic solutions. If properly saturated, they will keep medication in contact with all surfaces of the canal. Solution must be added almost hourly to maintain saturation. New wicks are inserted daily. The use of a wick is usually unnecessary for mild inflammation, but may be considered when the canal is partially obstructed by swelling and edema. The wick must be introduced before the canal swells and makes insertion painful or impossible.

Groups III to IV topical steroids, wet compresses, and oral antibiotics are used when eczematous inflammation and infection occur on the external ear and surrounding skin. These can be instilled deep in the canal by connecting a syringe filled with medication to a Zollinger or disposable metal sucker tip and the ear canal can be filled under direct microscopic vision.[84] (See the section on the treatment of eczematous inflammation.)

Infections that progress beyond the canal to the pinna and surrounding tissues are treated orally with ciprofloxacin (Cipro) 500 or 750 mg twice each day.

MALIGNANT EXTERNAL OTITIS

Patients with malignant external otitis present with a history of nonresolving otitis externa of many weeks or months duration (Figure 9-38). Most are diabetic. *Pseudomonas* infection penetrates the epithelium and invades underlying soft tissues. There is severe ear pain, which is worse at night, and purulent discharge. The external canal is edematous. Granulation tissue may be present, arising from the osseous cartilaginous junction at the floor of the canal or anteriorly. The infection then penetrates the floor of the canal at the bony cartilaginous junction and spreads to the base of the skull.[85] Malignant external otitis is an osteomyelitis of the skull base. More advanced cases demonstrate cranial nerve palsies, most frequently involving cranial nerve VII. The diagnosis is confirmed by nuclear scanning studies and CT scanning of the temporal bone and skull base. The criteria for diagnosis are listed in the box at right.

Treatment. The treatment of malignant external otitis has evolved from primarily surgical to one in which prolonged medical therapy of the underlying osteomyelitis with limited surgical debridement leads to a cure. Ciprofloxacin is the drug of choice. It is an orally administered, bactericidal, and antipseudomonal drug that is well absorbed from the GI tract and reaches high concentrations in tissue and bone. At least 6 weeks and up to 6 months of treatment in daily doses of 1.5 gm orally are required.[86]

CRITERIA FOR DIAGNOSIS OF MALIGNANT EXTERNAL OTITIS
Refractory otitis externa
Severe earache, worse at night
Purulent exudate
Granulation tissue
Recovery of *Pseudomonas aeruginosa*
Diabetes mellitus or other immune state compromise
Positive 99Tc bone scan of the temporal bone

From Levenson MJ, Parisier SC, et al: *Laryngoscope* 101:821-824, 1991.

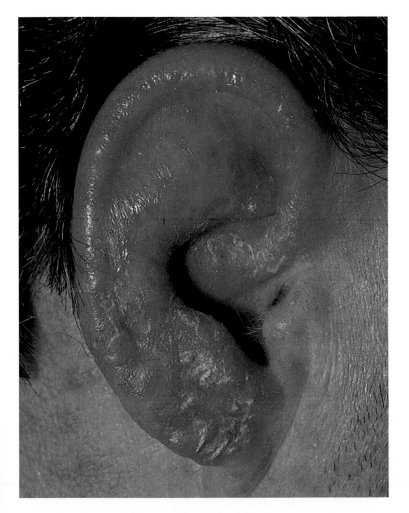

Figure 9-38
Malignant external otitis. Severe infection of the ear has occurred after months of chronic inflammation of the pinna.

TOE WEB INFECTION

Pseudomonas toe web infection is a distinctive clinical entity that is often misdiagnosed as tinea pedis.[87] A thick, white, macerated scale with a green discoloration may appear in the toe webs of people who wear heavy, wet boots. The most constant clinical feature is soggy wetness of the toe webs and immediately adjacent skin. In its mildest form, the affected tissue is damp, softened, boggy, and white. The second, third, and fourth toe webs are the most common sites of initial involvement. More severe forms may progress to denudation of affected skin and profuse, serous, or purulent discharge. In most cases, this sopping-wet denudation involves all toe webs and extends onto the plantar surface and the dorsal and plantar surfaces of the toes, and an area about 1 cm wide beyond the base of the toes on the plantar surface of the foot. All patients are males with broad feet, square toes, and tight interdigital spaces. Close skin-to-skin contact and friction between the toes is a constant feature. Wood's light examination may show a green-white fluorescence due to elaboration of pyoverdin and a green stain may be found on socks, bandages, toenails, and dried exudate. The green stain is due to elaboration of bacterial pyocyanin. *Pseudomonas* or a mixed flora of *Pseudomonas* organisms and fungi may be isolated from the soggy scale.

Treatment. First, the thickened, edematous, and devitalized layers of the epidermis are debrided.[88] Repeated applications of silver nitrate (0.5%) soaks or 5% acetic acid[83] (white vinegar) to the toe webs and the dorsal and plantar surfaces promote dryness and suppress bacteria. Gentamicin cream, silver sulfadiazine cream (Silvadene), or Castellani's paint (Derma-Cas gel) are then applied until the infection has resolved. Infections that do not respond to topical therapy are treated with ciprofloxacin (Cipro) 500 or 750 mg twice each day.

Measures to prevent reinfection include the use of gauze pledgets between toes to prevent occlusion, the use of sandals or open-weave shoes to enhance evaporation of sweat, and the use of astringents such as 20% aluminum chloride (Drysol) to promote dryness.

ECTHYMA GANGRENOSUM

Ecthyma gangrenosum (EG), not to be confused with pyoderma gangrenosum or streptococcal ecthyma, is a rare but highly characteristic entity that is pathognomonic of *Pseudomonas* infection. The lesions represent either a blood-borne, metastatic seeding of *P. aeruginosa* to the skin or a primary lesion with no bacteremia. The mortality rate is high for the septicemic form and approximately 15% without bacteremia.[89] The disease is rare, occurring in only 1.3% to 6.0% of patients with *Pseudomonas* sepsis.[90] There are usually less than 10 lesions.

All patients have predisposing factors that increase their risk for infection. EG occurs in immunocompromised patients (neoplasia, leukemia, immunosuppressive treatment, graft, malnutrition, diabetes), in burn patients, and in patients who have been treated with penicillin. Many patients have a disorder that leads to severe neutropenia or pancytopenia. Most cases arise during *P. aeruginosa* septicemia, but nonsepticemic forms are described in both infants and adults.[91-93] The nonsepticemic cases occur without overt immunosuppression or neutropenia and may occur following antibiotic therapy. Lesions consist of multiple noncontiguous ulcers or solitary ulcers. They begin as isolated, red, purpuric macules that become vesicular, indurated, and later, bullous or pustular. The pustules may be hemorrhagic. The lesions remain localized or, more typically, extend over several centimeters. The central area becomes hemorrhagic and necrotic (Figure 9-39). The lesion then sloughs to form a gangrenous ulcer with a gray-black eschar and a surrounding erythematous halo. Lesions occur mainly in the gluteal and perineal regions (57%), the extremities (30%), the trunk (6%), and the face (6%) but may occur anywhere.

Septicemic patients have high temperatures, chills, hypotension, and tachycardia or tachypnea or both. Neutropenia is a constant finding, and the absolute neutrophil count correlates closely with the clinical outcome. Most patients died when neutrophil counts were lower than 500/mm³ during or after appropriate therapy.[94] The skin lesions are slow to heal (an average of 4 weeks).

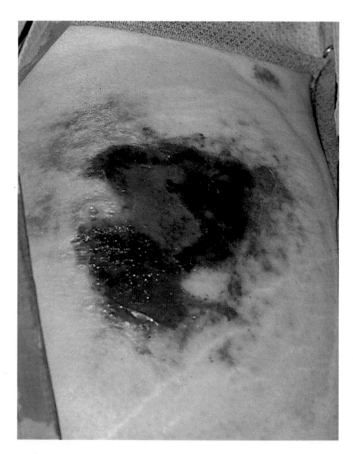

Figure 9-39
Ecthyma gangrenosum. A cutaneous manifestation of *Pseudomonas* septicemia. A large, vesicular, bullous, hemorrhagic mass is located on the thigh.

Management (septicemic form). Green et al.[94] recommend the following management program:

1. Take a deep skin biopsy (4 or 5 mm) for histopathology with special stains to identify bacteria in tissue.
2. Take a skin biopsy for culture.
3. Perform needle aspiration of lesions to perform Gram stain for rapid diagnosis.
4. Take blood cultures, especially during fever spikes.
5. Start appropriate systemic antibiotics after cultures have been taken. Effective therapy includes synergistic combination therapy with an aminoglycoside (tobramycin, gentamicin, amikacin) and an antipseudomonal penicillin (ticarcillin, piperacillin). Broad-spectrum antibiotics such as ceftazidime and imipenem are also effective.

Localized nonsepticemic disease may only require topical therapy such as silver nitrate (0.5%) or 5% acetic acid[83] (white vinegar) wet compresses or silver sulfadiazine cream.

Meningococcemia

Meningococcemia is a potentially fatal disease, with an overall case fatality rate of 6% to 10%. There are acute and chronic forms. The acute form is more common. Meningococci are present in the nasopharynx of approximately 10% to 20% of healthy persons. Most cases begin with acquisition of a new organism by nasopharyngeal colonization, followed by systemic invasion and development of bacteremia. CNS invasion then occurs. Protein and neutrophils move into the subarachnoid space causing cerebral edema and increased intracranial pressure.[95] Most cases of meningococcal infection occur in patients under 20 years of age, with half of the cases occurring in children under 5 years of age.[96] The highest rates of infection occur in the winter and spring. Epidemic outbreaks occur when crowded conditions prevail,[97] whereas sporadic cases appear throughout the year. Transmission is sometimes through airborne droplets from patients, but is more often transmitted by asymptomatic nasopharyngeal carriers. Most cases are asymptomatic, and susceptibility decreases with age.

Clinical manifestations. The incubation period varies from 2 to 10 days, but the disease typically begins 3 to 4 days after exposure. Clinical manifestations range from fever alone to fulminant septic shock with purpura fulminans. There is a sudden onset of fever, an intense headache, nausea, vomiting, a stiff neck, and a rash in more than 70% of cases.[98] Purpuric lesions (60%), erythematous papules (32%),[99] faint pink macules (28%), and conjunctival petechiae (10%) are the reported cutaneous signs.[100] Delirium and coma often appear. The skin lesions are caused by bacterial invasion, destruction of endothelial cells, and, possibly, endothelial damage by lipopolysaccharide meningococcal endotoxin. Decreased permeability and thrombosis lead to infarction, producing small areas of purpura with an irregular pattern.

With fulminating disease, accounting for approximately 3% of the cases, patients exhibit sudden prostration, ecchymoses, and shock at onset (purpura fulminans). This syndrome may lead to gangrene and autoamputation of distal extremities. It is particularly likely to complicate meningococcemia in children under 2 years of age. The rapidly fatal Waterhouse-Friderichsen syndrome or fulminating septicemia results in massive bleeding into the skin and hemorrhagic destruction in both adrenals.

Acquired deficiencies of proteins C and S may contribute to the pathogenesis of purpura fulminans. The immaturity of the protein C system in young children may explain the increased risk.[101]

Chronic meningococcemia. Chronic meningococcemia is rare. Clinical features are immunologically mediated and variable and include intermittent fever, rash, and arthritis that may mimic cutaneous vasculitis and reactive gonococcal arthritis. The skin lesions are similar to those seen in gonococcemia. A few macules, papules, tender nodules, or petechiae may occur. Patients deficient in certain complement components are prone to chronic disease.[102] Symptoms last a few weeks to 3 months. Meningitis may develop. Diagnosis is difficult to confirm because blood cultures commonly do not grow the organism, despite weeks of symptoms. Culture of the organism from the nasopharynx may provide supportive evidence for diagnosis. Chronic meningococcemia should be considered in the differential diagnosis of a cutaneous vasculitis. In the clinical setting of an undiagnosed fever with vasculitic rash and joint symptoms, an empiric trial of intravenously administered penicillin should be considered before steroid therapy because a rapid response may simplify the diagnostic dilemma.[103].

Diagnosis. Meningococci (*Neisseria meningitidis*) are gram-negative diplococci. They are separated into 13 groups on the basis of seroagglutination of capsular polysaccharides. Serogroups A, B, and C are identified in most recent cases, and groups W-135, X, Y and Z have also been implicated. Serogroups B and C are responsible for most cases throughout the world.[96,104] Petechiae are the clinical sign that best discriminates patients admitted with suspected meningococcal disease.[105] Ecchymoses are specific for meningococcal disease. Reduced general condition and reduced consciousness are other valuable diagnostic signs.[106] Evaluation of the CSF remains the gold standard for the diagnosis of bacterial meningitis.[107] Gram-negative diplococci are identified by Gram stain of the CSF, buffy coat, and smears taken from petechiae. A rapid diagnosis can be made with a biopsy of skin lesions. Bacteria are detected in specimens from hemorrhagic skin lesions by culture, Gram staining, or both in 63% of patients. In meningococcal sepsis, a Gram-stained skin lesion is significantly more sensitive (72%) than Gram-stained CSF (22%). The results for punch biopsy specimens are not affected by antibiotics because Gram staining gives positive results up to 45 hours after the start of treatment and culture gives positive results up to 13 hours.[108]

Histopathology of skin lesions shows that the primary damage is to the dermal vessels. Diplococci in Gram-stained sections are seen frequently in purpuric skin lesions compared with other skin lesions. They are located in degenerating neutrophils, endothelial cells, fibrin clots, or freely in the vascular lumen. Organisms are not present in the skin in chronic, recurrent disease. Cultures should be obtained from blood and CSF and held for 5 days before discarding them as negative because of their slow growth. The outcome of pediatric patients with meningococcal sepsis or the systemic inflammatory response syndrome with purpura can be predicted faster, more easily, and with better overall accuracy than that achieved with classic prognostication strategies by the simple presence or absence of coagulopathy (low serum fibrinogen, prolonged partial thromboplastin).[109,110] C-reactive protein (CRP) and thrombotest (TT) were the tests that most frequently were found to be abnormal in one large series.[105] Variables such as skin hemorrhages, body pain, CSF cell count, TT, CRP, and white blood cell count are the tests and signs that best support the diagnosis.

The differential diagnosis of acute petechial eruptions includes Rocky Mountain spotted fever, echovirus and cox-sackievirus infections, and toxic shock syndrome. Gonococcemia and allergic vasculitis (Henoch-Schönlein purpura, leukocytoclastic vasculitis) produce petechial and purpuric lesions that are usually elevated and palpable.

Management. Awareness of key symptoms and signs facilitates early diagnosis and reduces death and sequelae of meningococcal infections. Lowering the clinical admission threshold improves early antibiotic coverage of vaguely suspected cases.[111] Parenteral penicillin given before admission may contribute to a reduction in the case fatality rate from meningococcal disease. Such treatment should be given immediately on suspicion of the diagnosis before transferring the patient to hospital.[112] The presence of serious coagulopathy may be useful as an index of illness severity. There is a tetravalent (A, C, Y and W135) polysaccharide vaccine, which is immunogenic in children greater than 2 years.

ADULTS. Penicillin or ampicillin is the treatment of choice. Adults are treated with intravenous penicillin G, 2 million U every 2 hours, continued for 7 days after the fever has subsided. Cefotaxime and ceftriaxone can be used for patients who are allergic to penicillin, if bacteria resistance to penicillin is detected, or if *H. influenzae* is suspected.[113] Chloramphenicol and trimethoprim-sulfamethoxazole are alternatives for patients allergic to cephalosporins.

CHILDREN. Penicillin is the treatment of choice, but initial therapy must be directed at *H. influenzae* and *S. pneumoniae* until the organism is identified. Third-generation cephalosporins such as ceftriaxone[114] are effective and can be used pending culture reports. Chloramphenicol and trimethoprim-sulfamethoxazole are alternatives for patients who are allergic to cephalosporins. In many centers, when *H. influenzae* type B is suspected, dexamethasone is started before the first dose of antibiotic and is continued for 4 days to reduce neurologic and audiologic sequelae.[115]

Chemoprophylaxis is used for close contact during epidemics for prevention of secondary disease by eradication of nasopharyngeal carriage of the bacterial pathogen. The index case must also receive prophylaxis because penicillin G given for invasive disease does not necessarily eliminate nasopharyngeal carriage. Rifampin (10 mg per kg, not to exceed 600 mg) twice a day for 2 days or ciprofloxacin (500 or 750 mg) given as a single dose is effective. An appropriate drug must be given as soon as possible after the index case has been identified.[116]

Vaccines are used for epidemic control but are of no practical value for household contacts.

Heparin does not stop the progression of the purpuric lesions in meningococcemia. Repletion of proteins C and S with freshly frozen plasma may be important adjunctive therapy in patients with purpura fulminans complicating meningococcemia.[101]

Nontuberculous Mycobacteria

Mycobacteria are rods with a waxy coating that makes them resistant to stains and to many antibiotics. Once stained, they are not easily decolored and remain "acid-fast." The most common and important microbacteria are *M. tuberculosis* and *M. leprae*. Nontuberculous mycobacteria (previously referred to as *atypical mycobacteria*) usually cause systemic disease, but they may just infect the skin (Table 9-2).[117,118] They are widespread in nature and are found in soil, animal and human feces, and water in swimming pools and fish tanks. They differ in culture requirements, pigment production, disease manifestation, and drug susceptibility. The Runyon classification, which depends on colony pigment and growth-rate characteristics, is no longer used. The bacteria are simply referred to by genus and species. Most cutaneous disease is caused by *M. marinum*,[119] *M. ulcerans*,[120] *M. fortuitum*, *M. chelonei*,[121-123] and *M. avium–intracellulare*. *Mycobacterium–avium* complex causes disseminated disease in as many as 15% to 40% of patients with human immunodeficiency virus infection in the United States, causing fever, night sweats, weight loss, and anemia.[124,125] The bacteria are of low pathogenicity, and transmission between persons is rare. Predisposing conditions for infection are trauma, immunosuppression, HIV infection,[126] and chronic disease. Consider a nontuberculous mycobacterial infection when a lesion develops at the site of trauma and follows a chronic course.

Mycobacteria require different temperatures for culture. Instruct the laboratory to incubate the cultures at both 30° and 37° C. Isolation of these opportunistic, widespread organisms in culture does not prove that they cause the disease. DNA probes are now available to identify the species of mycobacteria; time for identification is within 3 to 4 weeks.

TABLE 9-2 Nontuberculous Mycobacteria Infection

	M. marinum	*M. ulcerans*	*M. fortuitum and M. chelonei*	*M. avium–intracellulare*	*M. kansasii*
Source of infection	Fresh and salt water (swimming pool, wells, contaminated fish, fish tanks); immunosuppressed patients	Water; swamp areas of Australia, Uganda, and Zaire.	Ocean and fresh water, dirt, dust, animal feed, sporadic postoperative infections; trauma; dialysis equipment; postinjection abscesses	Gulf coast; Pacific coast; north central U.S.; soil; house dust, water; dried plants	Unclear; has been isolated from tap water; opportunistic infection
Symptoms	Asymptomatic to painful swelling of skin	Asymptomatic to painful swelling of skin; decreased mobility of joint	Often develops in patients with preexisting lung disease. Disseminated disease associated with acquired immunodeficiency syndrome.	Asymptomatic fever, weight loss, bone pain	Pruritus, fever, plaques, swelling. The most common disease is a pulmonary infection in elderly men with chronic underlying pulmonary disease.
Skin lesion	Lesions occur at the inoculation site. Papules; nodules; verrucous plaques; ulcers/abscesses; sporotrichoid; disseminated	Large, solitary, deep, painless ulcer on the lower extremities. Secondary necrosis occurs. Primarily affects children and young adults.	Granulomatous nodules; draining abscesses; ulcers; sporotrichoid lesions; cellulitis; disseminated disease	Granulomatous synovitis; deep hand infection; panniculitis; subcutaneous nodule	Verrucous papules, sporotrichoid eruption, cellulitis, granulomatous plaques, ulcers, and necrotic papulopustules.
Treatment	Minocycline/doxycycline 100 mg twice daily; trimethoprim-sulfamethoxazole 160 to 800 mg twice daily; rifampin 600 mg daily and ethambutol 800 mg daily for resistant strains, sporotrichoid lesions, and disseminated infections. Treat for 1 month to 1 year	Wide excision with or without skin grafting is treatment of choice. Trimethoprim-sulfamethoxazole 80/400 mg twice daily followed by rifampin 600 mg daily, and minocyclin, 100 mg daily, or a combination of streptomycin, dapsone, and ethambutol. Heat area with occlusive wraps because *M. ulcerans* is heat sensitive.	Severe disease: surgical debridement; amikacin (15 mg/kg per day) plus cefoxitin (200 mg/kg per day) combined with oral administration of probenecid, followed by sulfonamide, erythromycin, or minocycline. Less severe disease: sulfonamide with erythromycin. Continue therapy for 4 to 6 weeks after wound healing.	Aggressive therapy with multiple drugs including INH, clofazimine, rifampin, streptomycin, ethambutol, ethionamide, cycloserine, or capreomycin	Rifampin in addition to ethambutol or isoniazid. Drug resistance has been reported with isoniazid. Treatment with higher dosages of isoniazid (900 mg) has been tried. Sulfonamides and amikacin have been added when rifampin-resistant strains occur.
Culture incubation temperature	30° to 33° C	30° to 33° C	Between 25° and 40° C	37° C	37° C

Adapted from Street ML, Umbert-Millet IJ, et al: *J Am Acad Dermatol* 24:208-215, 1991.

REFERENCES

1. Barton LL, Friedman AD: Impetigo: a reassessment of etiology and therapy, *Pediatr Dermatol* 4:185-188, 1987.
2. Dagan R, Bar-David Y: Comparison of amoxicillin and clavulanic acid (augmentin) for the treatment of nonbullous impetigo, *Am J Dis Child* 143:916-918, 1989.
3. Peter G, Smith AL: Group A streptococcal infections of the skin and pharynx, *N Engl J Med* 297:311-317, 1977.
4. Fine RN: Clinical manifestations and diagnosis of post-streptococcal acute glomerulonephritis. pp 79-82. In Nissen AR: Poststreptococcal acute glomerulonephritis: fact and controversy, *Ann Intern Med* 91:76-86, 1979.
5. Rajajee S: Post-streptococcal acute glomerulonephritis: a clinical, bacteriological and serological study, *Indian J Pediatr* 57:775-780, 1990.
6. Maddox JS, Ware JC, Dillon HC: The natural history of streptococcal skin infection: prevention with topical antibiotics, *J Am Acad Dermatol* 13:207-212, 1985.
7. Doebbeling BN et al: Long term efficacy of intranasal mupirocin ointment. A prospective cohort study of *Staphylococcus aureus* carriage, *Arch Intern Med* 154:1505-1508, 1994.
8. McLinn S: A bacteriologically controlled, randomized study comparing the efficacy of 2% mupirocin ointment (Bactroban) with oral erythromycin in the treatment of patients with impetigo, *J Am Acad Dermatol* 22:883-885, 1990.
9. Demidovich CW, Wittler RR, et al: Impetigo. Current etiology and comparison of penicillin, erythromycin, and cephalexin therapies, *Am J Dis Child* 144:1313-1315, 1990.
10. Daniel R: Azithromycin, erythromycin and cloxacillin in the treatment of infections of skin and associated soft tissues. European Azithromycin Study Group, *J Int Med Res* 19:433-445, 1991.
11. Mertz PM, Marshall DA, et al: Topical mupirocin treatment of impetigo is equal to oral erythromycin therapy, *Arch Dermatol* 125:1069-1073, 1989.
12. Baddour LM, Bisno AL: Non-group A beta-hemolytic streptococcal cellulitis: association with venous and lymphatic compromise, *Am J Med* 79:155-159, 1985.
13. Carbone KM, Heinrich MC, Quinn TC: Thrombophlebitis and cellulitis due to *Campylobacter fetus* ssp. *fetus*: report of four cases and a review of the literature, *Medicine* 64:244-250, 1985.
14. Sachs MK: Cutaneous cellulitis, *Arch Dermatol* 127:493-496, 1991.
15. Hook EW et al: Microbiologic evaluation of cutaneous cellulitis in adults, *Arch Intern Med* 146:295-297, 1986.
16. Kielhofner MA et al: Influence of underlying disease process on the utility of cellulitis needle aspirates, *Arch Intern Med* 148:451,1988.
17. Rudoy RC, Nakashima G: Diagnostic value of needle aspiration in *Haemophilus influenzae* type B cellulitis, *J Pediatr* 94:924, 1979.
18. Goetz JP et al: Needle aspiration in *Haemophilus influenzae* type B cellulitis, *Pediatrics* 54:504, 1974
19. Leppard BJ, Seal DV, Colman G, et al: The value of bacteriology and serology in the diagnosis of cellulitis and erysipelas, *Br J Dermatol* 112:559-567, 1985.
20. Epperly TD: The value of needle aspiration in the management of cellulitis, *J Fam Pract* 23:337-340, 1986.
21. Howe PM, Fajardo JE, Orcutt MA: Etiologic diagnosis of cellulitis: comparison of aspirates obtained from the leading edge and the point of maximal inflammation, *Pediatr Infect Dis J* 6:685-686, 1987.
22. McDonnell WM, Roth MS, Sheagren JN: *Hemophilus influenzae* type B cellulitis in adults, *Am J Med* 81:709-712, 1986.
23. Vallejo JG, Kaplan SL, et al: Treatment of meningitis and other infections due to ampicillin-resistant *Haemophilus influenzae* type B in children, *Rev Infect Dis* 13:197-200, 1991.
24. Broome CV et al: Special report: use of chemoprophylaxis to prevent the spread of *Hemophilus influenzae* B in day-care facilities, *N Engl J Med* 316:1226-1228, 1987.
25. Kremer M, Zuckerman R, et al: Long-term antimicrobial therapy in the prevention of recurrent soft-tissue infections, *J Infect* 22:37-40, 1991.
26. Klemper MS, Styrt B: Prevention of recurrent staphylococcal skin infections with low dose oral clindamycin therapy, *JAMA* 260:2682-2685, 1988.
27. Hugo-Persson M, Norlin K: Erysipelas and group G streptococci, *Infection* 15:36-39, 1987.
28. Baddour LM, Bisno AL: Recurrent cellulitis after saphenous venectomy for coronary bypass surgery, *Ann Intern Med* 97:493, 1982.
29. Jorup-Ronstrom C: Epidemiological, bacteriological and complicating features of erysipelas, *Scan J Infect Dis* 18:519-524, 1986.
30. Bitnun S: Prophylactic antibiotics in recurrent erysipelas, *Lancet* Feb 9, p 345, 1985 (letter).
31. Charnock DR, White T: Bruised cheek syndrome: *Haemophilus influenzae*, type B, cellulitis, *Otolaryngol Head Neck Surg* 103:829-830, 1990.
32. Ginsburg CM: *Hemophilus influenzae* type B buccal cellulitis, *J Am Acad Dermatol* 4:661, 1981.
33. Jackson K, Baker SR: Periorbital cellulitis, *Head Neck Surg* 9:227-234, 1987.
34. Antoine GA, Grundfast KM: Periorbital cellulitis, *Int J Pediatr Otorhinolaryngol* 13:273-278, 1987.
35. Mills RP, Kartush JM: Orbital wall thickness and the spread of infection from the paranasal sinuses, *Clin Otolaryngol* 10:209-216, 1985.
36. Jackson K, Baker SR: Clinical implications of orbital cellulitis, *Laryngoscope* 96:568-574, 1986.
37. Teele DW: Management of the child with a red and swollen eye, *Pediatr Infect Dis* 2:258-262, 1983.
38. Hodges E, Tabbara KF: Orbital cellulitis: review of 23 cases from Saudi Arabia, *Br J Ophthalmol* 73:205-208, 1989.
39. Spires JR, Smith RJH: Bacterial infection of the orbital and periorbital soft tissues in children, *Laryngoscope* 96:763-767, 1986.
40. Ciarallo LR, Rowe PC: Lumbar puncture in children with periorbital and orbital cellulitis, *J Pediatr* 122:355-359, 1993.
41. Noel LP, Clarke WN, et al: Clinical management of orbital cellulitis in children, *Can J Ophthalmol* 25:11-16, 1990.
42. Martin-Hirsch DP, Habashi S, et al: Orbital cellulitis, *Arch Emerg Med* 9:143-148, 1992.
43. Marks VJ, Maksimak M: Perianal streptococcal cellulitis, *J Am Acad Dermatol* 18:587-588, 1988.
44. Rehder PA, Eliezer ET, Lane AT: Perianal cellulitis: cutaneous group A streptococcal disease, *Arch Dermatol* 124:702-704, 1988.
45. Kokx NP, Comstock JA, Facklam RR: Streptococcal perianal disease in children, *Pediatrics* 80:659, 1987.
46. Brauner GJ, Flandermeyer KL: Pseudofolliculitis barbae, medical consequences of interracial friction in the Army, *Cutis* 23:61-66, 1979.
47. Perricone NV: Treatment of pseudofolliculitis barbae with topical glycolic acid: a report of two studies, *Cutis* 52:232-235, 1993.
48. Hage JJ, Bouman FG: Surgical depilation for the treatment of pseudofolliculitis or local hirsutism of the face: experience in the first 40 patients, *Plast Reconstr Surg* 88:446-451, 1991.
49. Dinehart SM, Herzberg AJ, Kerns BJ, et al: Acne keloidalis: a review, *J Dermatol Surg Oncol* 15:642-647,1989.
50. Harris H: Acne keloidalis aggravated by football helmets, *Cutis* 50:154, 1992.
51. Herzberg AJ, Dinehart SM, et al: Acne keloidalis. Transverse microscopy, immunohistochemistry, and electron microscopy, *Am J Dermatopathol* 12:109-121, 1990.
52. Meislin HW et al: Cutaneous abscesses: anaerobic and aerobic bacteriology and outpatient management, *Ann Intern Med* 87:145-149, 1977.
53. Llera JL, Levy RC: Treatment of cutaneous abscess: a double-blind clinical study, *Ann Emerg Med* 14:15-19, 1985.
54. Dahl MV: Strategies for the management of recurrent furunculosis, *South Med J* 80:352-356, 1987.
55. Hedstrom SA: Recurrent staphylococcal furunculosis: bacterial findings and epidemiology in 100 cases, *Scand J Infect Dis* 13:115-119, 1981.

56. Reboli AC, Farrar WE: *Erysipelothrix rhusiopathiae*: an occupational pathogen, *Clin Microbiol Rev* 2:354-359, 1989.

57. Molin G, Soderlind O, et al: Occurrence of *Erysipelothrix rhusiopathiae* on pork and in pig slurry, and the distribution of specific antibodies in abattoir workers, *J Appl Bacteriol* 67:347-352, 1989.

58. Gorby GL, Peacock JE: *Erysipelothrix rhusiopathiae* endocarditis; microbiologic, epidemiologic and clinical features of an occupational disease, *Rev Infect Dis* 10:317-325, 1988.

59. Pachas WN, Currid VR: L-form induction: morphology and development in two related strains of *Erysipelothrix rhusiopathiae*, *J Bacteriol* 119:576-582, 1974.

60. Barnett JH et al: Erysipeloid, *J Am Acad Dermatol* 9:116-123, 1983.

61. McCray MK, Esterly NB: Blistering distal dactylitis, *J Am Acad Dermatol* 5:592-594, 1981.

62. Norcross M Jr, Mitchell DF: Blistering distal dactylitis caused by *Staphylococcus aureus*, *Cutis* 51:353-354, 1993.

63. Zemtsov A, Veitschegger M: *Staphylococcus aureus*-induced blistering distal dactylitis in an adult immunosuppressed patient, *J Am Acad Dermatol* 26:784-785, 1992.

64. Benson PM, Solivan G: Group B streptococcal blistering distal dactylitis in an adult diabetic, *J Am Acad Dermatol* 17:310-311, 1987.

65. Lyell A: The staphylococcal scalded skin syndrome in historical perspective: emergence of dermopathic strains of *Staphylococcus aureus* and discovery of the epidermolytic toxin, *J Am Acad Dermatol* 9:285-294, 1983.

66. Resnick SD: Staphylococcal toxin-mediated syndromes in childhood, *Semin Dermatol* 11:11-18, 1992.

67. Elias PM, Fritsch P, Epstein EH: Staphylococcal scalded skin syndrome, *Arch Dermatol* 113:207-219, 1977.

68. Lillibridge CB, Melish ME, Glasgow LA: Site of action of exfoliative toxin in the staphylococcal scalded skin syndrome, *Pediatrics* 66:291-294, 1980.

69. Borchers SL, Gomez EC, Isseroff RR: Generalized staphylococcal scalded skin syndrome in an anephric boy undergoing hemodialysis, *Arch Dermatol* 120:912-918, 1984.

70. Elias PM, Levy SW: Bullous impetigo: occurrence of localized scalded skin syndrome in an adult, *Arch Dermatol* 112:856-858, 1976.

71. Goldberg NS, Ahmed T, et al: Staphylococcal scalded skin syndrome mimicking acute graft-vs-host disease in a bone marrow transplant recipient, *Arch Dermatol* 125:85-87, 1989.

72. Herzog JL, Sexton FM: Desquamative rash in an immunocompromised adult. Staphylococcal scalded skin syndrome (SSSS), *Arch Dermatol* 126:815-816, 1990.

73. Beers B, Wilson B: Adult staphylococcal scalded skin syndrome, *Int J Dermatol* 29:428-429, 1990.

74. Rudolph RI, Schwartz W, Leyden JJ: Treatment of staphylococcal toxic epidermal necrolysis, *Arch Dermatol* 110:559-562, 1974.

75. Bottone EJ, Perez A: *Pseudomonas aeruginosa* folliculitis acquired through use of a contaminated loofah sponge: an unrecognized potential public health problem, *J Clin Microbiol* 31:480-483, 1993.

76. Ratnam S, Hogan K, March SB, et al: Whirlpool-associated folliculitis caused by *Pseudomonas aeruginosa*: report of an outbreak and review, *J Clin Microbiol* 23:655-659, 1986.

77. Highsmith AK, Le PN, Khabbaz RF, et al: Characteristics of *Pseudomonas aeruginosa* isolated from whirlpools and bathers, *Infect Control Hosp Epidemiol* 6:407-412, 1985.

78. Chandrasekar PH et al: Hot tub-associated dermatitis due to *Pseudomonas aeruginosa*: case report and review of the literature, *Arch Dermatol* 120:1337-1340, 1984.

79. Breitenbach RA: *Pseudomonas* folliculitis from a health club whirlpool, *Postgrad Med* 90:169-170, 1991.

80. Penn C, Kain KC: *Pseudomonas* folliculitis: an outbreak associated with bromine-based disinfectants—British Columbia, *Can Dis Wkly Rep* 16:31-33, 1990.

81. Petrozzi JW, Alexander E: Pseudomonal balanitis, *Arch Dermatol* 113:952, 1977.

82. Manian FA, Alford RH: Nosocomial infectious balanoposthitis in neutropenic patients, *South Med J* 80(7):909-911, 1987.

83. Milner SM: Acetic acid to treat *Pseudomonas aeruginosa* in superficial wounds and burns, *Lancet* 340:61, 1992.

84. Dekker PJ: Alternative method of application of topical preparations in otitis externa, *J Laryngol Otol* 105:842-843, 1991.

85. Scherbenske JM, Winton GB, James WD: Acute pseudomonas infection of the external ear (malignant external otitis), *J Dermatol Surg Oncol* 14:165-169, 1988.

86. Levenson MJ, Parisier SC, et al: Ciprofloxacin: drug of choice in the treatment of malignant external otitis (MEO), *Laryngoscope* 101:821-824, 1991.

87. Westmoreland TA, Ross EV, Yeager JK: *Pseudomonas* toe web infections, *Cutis* 49:185-186, 1992.

88. King DF, King LAC: Importance of debridement in the treatment of gram-negative bacterial toe web infection, *J Am Acad Dermatol* 14:278-279, 1986.

89. Huminer D et al: Ecthyma gangrenosum without bacteremia: report of six cases and review of the literature, *Arch Intern Med* 147:299-301, 1987.

90. Bodey GP, Jadeja L, Elting L: *Pseudomonas* bacteremia: retrospective analysis of 410 episodes, *Arch Intern Med* 145:1621-1629, 1985.

91. Boisseau AM, Sarlangue J, et al: Perineal ecthyma gangrenosum in infancy and early childhood: septicemic and nonsepticemic forms, *J Am Acad Dermatol* 27:415-418, 1992.

92. Fergie JE, Patrick CC, et al: *Pseudomonas aeruginosa* cellulitis and ecthyma gangrenosum in immunocompromised children, *Pediatr Infect Dis* J 10:496-500, 1991.

93. el Baze P, Thyss A, et al: A study of nineteen immunocompromised patients with extensive skin lesions caused by *Pseudomonas aeruginosa* with and without bacteremia, *Acta Derm Venereol* 71:411-415, 1991.

94. Greene SL, Daniel Su WP, Muller SA: Ecthyma gangrenosum: report of clinical, histopathologic, and bacteriologic aspects of eight cases, *J Am Acad Dermatol* 11:781-787, 1984.

95. Tunkel AR, Scheld WM: Pathogenesis and pathophysiology of bacterial meningitis, *Clin Microbiol Rev* 6:118-136, 1993.

96. Berg S, Trollfors B, et al: Incidence, serogroups and case-fatality rate of invasive meningococcal infections in a Swedish region 1975-1989, *Scand J Infect Dis* 24:333-338, 1992.

97. Feigin RD et al: Epidemic meningococcal disease in an elementary-school classroom, *N Engl J Med* 307:1255-1257, 1982.

98. Wong VK, Hitchcock W, et al: Meningococcal infections in children: a review of 100 cases, *Pediatr Infect Dis J* 8:224-227, 1989.

99. Marzouk O, Thomson AP, et al: Features and outcome in meningococcal disease presenting with maculopapular rash, *Arch Dis Child* 66:485-487, 1991.

100. Ramesh V, Mukherjee A, et al: Clinical, histopathologic & immunologic features of cutaneous lesions in acute meningococcaemia, *Indian J Med Res* 91:27-32, 1990.

101. Powars DR et al: Purpura fulminans in meningococcemia: association with acquired deficiencies of proteins C and S, *N Engl J Med* 317:571-572, 1987.

102. Adams EM et al: Absence of the seventh component of complement in a patient with chronic meningococcemia presenting as vasculitis, *Ann Intern Med* 99:35, 1983.

103. Jennens ID, O'Reilley M, et al: Chronic meningococcal disease, *Med J Aust* 153:556-559, 1990.

104. Pinner RW, Gellin BG, et al: Meningococcal disease in the United States—1986. Meningococcal Disease Study Group, *J Infect Dis* 164:368-374, 1991.

105. Borchsenius F, Bruun JN, et al: Systemic meningococcal disease: the diagnosis on admission to hospital, *NIPH Ann* 14:11-22, 1991.

106. Tesoro LJ, Selbst SM: Factors affecting outcome in meningococcal infections, *Am J Dis Child* 145:218-220, 1991.

107. Pohl CA: Practical approach to bacterial meningitis in childhood, *Am Fam Physician* 47:1595-1603, 1993.

108. Van Deuren M, van Dijke BJ, et al: Rapid diagnosis of acute meningococcal infections by needle aspiration or biopsy of skin lesions, *Br Med J* 306:1229-1232, 1993.

109. McManus ML, Churchwell KB: Coagulopathy as a predictor of outcome in meningococcal sepsis and the systemic inflammatory response syndrome with purpura, *Crit Care Med* 21:706-711, 1993.

110. Giraud T, Dhainaut JF, et al: Adult overwhelming meningococcal purpura. A study of 35 cases, 1977-1989, *Arch Intern Med* 151:310-316, 1991.

111. Gedde-Dahl TW, Hoiby EA, et al: Some arguments on early hospital admission and treatment of suspected meningococcal disease cases, *NIPH Ann* 13:45-60, 1990.

112. Strang JR, Pugh EJ: Meningococcal infections: reducing the case fatality rate by giving penicillin before admission to hospital, *Br Med J* 305:141-143, 1992.

113. Wispelwey B, Tunkel AR, et al: Bacterial meningitis in adults, *Infect Dis Clin North Am* 4:645-659, 1990.

114. Schaad UB, Suter S, et al: A comparison of ceftriaxone and cefuroxime for the treatment of bacterial meningitis in children, *N Engl J Med* 322:141-147, 1990.

115. Kaplan SL: New aspects of prevention and therapy of meningitis, *Infect Dis Clin North Am* 6:197-214, 1992.

116. The Meningococcal Disease Surveillance Group, 1974: Meningococcal disease: secondary attack rate and chemoprophylaxis in the United States, 1974, *JAMA* 235:261-265, 1976.

117. Street ML, et al: Nontuberculous mycobacterial infections of the skin. Report of fourteen cases and review of the literature, *J Am Acad Dermatol* 24:208-215, 1991.

118. Wheeler AP, Graham BS: Atypical mycobacterial infections, *South Med J* 82:1250-1258, 1989.

119. Hoyt RE, Bryant JE, et al: *M. marinum* infections in a Chesapeake Bay community, *Va Med* 116:467-470, 1989.

120. Seevanayagam S, Hayman J: *Mycobacterium ulcerans* infection; is the "Bairnsdale ulcer" also a Ceylonese disease? *Ceylon Med J* 37:125-127, 1992.

121. Ingram CW, Tanner DC, et al: Disseminated infection with rapidly growing mycobacteria, *Clin Infect Dis* 16:463-471, 1993.

122. Drabick JJ, Duffy PE, et al: Disseminated *Mycobacterium chelonae* subspecies *chelonae* infection with cutaneous and osseous manifestations, Arch Dermatol 126:1064-1067, 1990.

123. Wallace R Jr.: The clinical presentation, diagnosis, and therapy of cutaneous and pulmonary infections due to the rapidly growing mycobacteria, *M. fortuitum* and *M. chelonae*, *Clin Chest Med* 10:419-429, 1989.

124. Masur H et al: Special report: recommendations on prophylaxis and therapy for disseminated *Mycobacterium avium* complex disease in patients infected with the human immunodeficiency virus, *N Engl J Med* 329:898-905, 1993.

125. Nightingale SD, et al: Two controlled trials of rifampin prophylaxis against mycobacterium complex infection in AIDS, *N Engl J Med* 329:828-833, 1993.

126. MacDonell KB, Glassroth J: *Mycobacterium avium* complex and other nontuberculous mycobacteria in patients with HIV infection, *Semin Respir Infect* 4:123-132, 1989.

127. Hedstrom SA: Treatment and prevention of recurrent staphylococcal furunculosis: clinical and bacteriological follow-up, *Scand J Infect Dis* 17:55-58, 1985.

128. Wheat LJ, Kohler RB, White A: Prevention of infections of skin and skin structures, *Am J Med* 76:187-190, 1984.

129. Yu VL et al: *Staphylococcus aureus* nasal carriage and infection in patients on hemodialysis: efficacy of antibiotic prophylaxis, *N Engl J Med* 315:91-96, 1986.

CHAPTER TEN

Sexually Transmitted Bacterial Infections

Gonorrhea

Gonorrhea is a common sexually transmitted disease. The responsible organism, *Neisseria gonorrhoeae*, can survive only in a moist environment approximating body temperature and is transmitted only by sexual contact (genital, genital-oral, or genital-rectal) with an infected person. It is not transmitted through toilet seats or the like. Purulent burning urethritis in males and asymptomatic endocervicitis in females are the most common forms of the disease, but gonorrhea is also found at other sites. All forms of the disease have the potential for evolving into a bacteremic phase, producing the arthritis-dermatitis syndrome. From an epidemiologic point of view the disease is becoming more difficult to control because of the increasing number of asymptomatic male carriers. All forms of the disease previously responded to penicillin, but resistant strains have emerged.

Neisseria gonorrhoeae

N. gonorrhoeae is a gram-negative coccus that is found in pairs (diplococci) within polymorphonuclear leukocytes in purulent material. The bacterium is an obligate aerobe that grows best at 35° to 37° C, in an atmosphere of 3% to 5% CO_2. A modified Thayer-Martin medium (chocolate agar) incubated in a candle jar to elevate CO_2 levels provides optimum conditions for isolation. *N. gonorrhoeae* is differentiated from nonpathogenic strains such as *N. meningitidis*, which may be normal flora in the pharynx, by colony morphology and sugar fermentation patterns. Specificity about the source of the culture is necessary so that the laboratory will perform all of the tests necessary for differentiation from normal flora.

N. gonorrhoeae is a fragile organism that survives only in humans and quickly dies if all of its environmental requirements are not met. The organism can survive only in blood and on mucosal surfaces including the urethra, endocervix, rectum, pharynx, conjunctiva, and prepubertal vaginal tract. It does not survive on the stratified epithelium of the skin and postpubertal vaginal tract. The bacteria must be kept moist with isotonic body fluids and will die if not maintained at body temperature. A slightly alkaline medium is required, such as that found in the endocervix and in the vagina during the immediate premenstrual and menstrual phases. The antibodies produced during the disease offer little protection from future attacks but can be measured with some newly developed tests. A fluorescent antibody test identifies the organism in tissue specimens such as in the skin in disseminated gonococcal infection (bacteremia-arthritis syndrome).

Virulent strains of gonococci contain surface structures called *pili* that are the primary mediators of adherence to epithelial cells. Other cell surface structures (e.g., proteins I, II, and III and lipopolysaccharide) give different strains of gonococci their unique characteristics and ability to infect different sites[1] and are utilized in serotyping. Presently serotyping is done only for epidemiologic purposes.

Nonculture gonococcal tests such as deoxyribonucleic acid (DNA) probes and enzyme immunoassay (EIA) tests are now available.

GENITAL INFECTION IN MALES

The risk of infection for a man after a single exposure to an infected woman is estimated to be 20% to 35%.[2] After a 3- to 5-day incubation period, most infected men have a sudden onset of burning, frequent urination, and a yellow, thick, purulent urethral discharge. In some men symptoms do not develop for 5 to 14 days. They then complain only of mild dysuria with a mucoid urethral discharge as observed in nongonococcal urethritis. Five to fifty percent of men who are infected never have symptoms and become chronic carriers for months, acting, as do women without symptoms, as major contributors to the ongoing gonorrhea epidemic.[3] Infection may spread to the prostate, seminal vesicles, and epididymis, but presently these complications are uncommon because most men with symptoms are treated.

Diagnosis. The diagnosis can be confirmed without culture in men with a typical history of acute urethritis by finding in urethral exudate gram-negative intracellular diplococci within polymorphonuclear leukocytes. Urethral culture is indicated when the result of Gram stain is negative, in tests of cure, or as a test for asymptomatic urethral infection. Material for culture is obtained by inserting a bacteriologic wire loop or a sterile narrow synthetic swab approximately 2 cm into the anterior urethra. No attempt should be made to insert the larger cotton-tipped swabs contained in standard culture kits.

GENITAL INFECTION IN FEMALES

The risk of infection for a woman after a single exposure to an infected man is estimated to be 60% to 90%.[4] Female genital gonorrhea has traditionally been described as an asymptomatic disease, but symptoms of urethritis and endocervicitis may be elicited from 40% to 60% of the women.[5] Urethritis begins with frequency and dysuria after a 3- to 5-day incubation period. These symptoms are of variable intensity. Pus may be seen exuding from the red external urinary meatus or after the urethra is "milked" with a finger in the vagina.

Endocervical infection may appear as a nonspecific, pale-yellow vaginal discharge, but in many cases this is not detected or is accepted as being a normal variation. The cervix may appear normal, or it may show marked inflammatory changes with cervical erosions and pus exuding from the os. Skene's glands, which lie on either side of the urinary meatus, exude pus if infected.

The Bartholin ducts, which open on the inner surfaces of the labia minora at the junction of their middle and posterior thirds near the vaginal opening, may, if infected, show a drop of pus at the gland orifice. After occlusion of the infected duct, the patient complains of swelling and discomfort while walking or sitting. A swollen, painful Bartholin gland may be palpated as a swollen mass deep in the posterior half of the labia majora.

Diagnosis

Gram stain. The diagnosis of acute urethritis can be made with a high degree of certainty if gram-negative intracellular diplococci are found in the purulent exudate from the urethra. Fifty percent of the cases of endocervical gonorrhea can be diagnosed by a carefully interpreted gram-stained smear of the endocervical canal. *Neisseria* species (e.g., *N. catarrhalis* and *N. sicca*) inhabit the female genital tract;

thus the diagnosis is considered only if gram-negative diplococci are present inside polymorphonuclear leukocytes.

Culture is the most reliable technique for establishing the presence of endocervical infection. However, the diagnosis will be missed in 10% of cases if reliance is exclusively on culture. An endocervical culture is taken by initially localizing the cervix with a water-moistened, nonlubricated speculum. Excess cervical mucus is most easily removed with a cotton ball held in a ring forceps. A sterile cotton-tipped swab is inserted into the endocervical canal, moved from side to side, and allowed to remain in place for 10 to 30 seconds before it is inoculated onto appropriate media. A culture of the anal canal need be performed only if there are anal symptoms, a history of rectal sexual exposure, or follow-up of treated gonorrhea in women.

Rapid laboratory tests are now available for diagnosis.

PELVIC INFLAMMATORY DISEASE

Pelvic inflammatory disease (PID), or salpingitis, is infection of the uterus, fallopian tubes, and adjacent pelvic structures.[6] Organisms spread to these structures from the cervix and vagina. Most cases are caused by *Chlamydia trachomatis* and/or *N. gonorrhoeae*. *Escherichia coli*, *Bacteroides* species, anaerobic cocci, *Mycoplasma hominis*, and *Ureaplasma urealyticum* have also been found in PID.[7,8,9]

Clinical presentation. The most common presenting symptom is lower abdominal pain, usually bilateral. Gonococcal PID has an abrupt onset with fever and peritoneal irritation. The symptoms of nongonococcal disease are less dramatic. Any of these infections may be asymptomatic. Symptoms are more likely to begin during the first half of the menstrual cycle. Intrauterine devices are a predisposing factor.

Diagnosis. The diagnosis is usually made clinically. Lower abdominal tenderness and pain, adnexal tenderness, and pain on manipulation of the cervix are noted in most cases. Fever, leukocytosis, an elevated erythrocyte sedimentation rate, elevated levels of C-reactive protein, and vaginal discharge may also occur. Endocervical specimens should be examined for *N. gonorrhoeae* and *C. trachomatis*. Direct visualization of inflamed fallopian tubes and other pelvic structures with the laparoscope is the most accurate method of diagnosis, but this procedure is usually not practical. A comprehensive microbiologic evaluation should be performed on specimens obtained through the laparoscope. The differential diagnosis includes acute appendicitis, pelvic endometriosis, hematoma of the corpus luteum, or ectopic pregnancy. Long-term complications (recurrent disease, chronic pain, ectopic pregnancy, infertility) occur from tubal damage and scarring.

Collecting specimens. The following guidelines are recommended for obtaining endocervical specimens:

- Obtain specimens for chlamydia tests after obtaining specimens for Gram-stained smear, *N. gonorrhoeae* culture, or Papanicolaou smear.

TABLE 10-1 Treatment of Sexually Transmitted Diseases

Type or stage	Drug of choice	Dosage	Alternatives
CHLAMYDIA TRACHOMATIS			
Urethritis, cervicitis, conjunctivitis, or proctitis (except lymphogranuloma venereum)			
	Doxycycline[a]	100 mg oral bid for 7 days	Erythromycin[b] 500 mg oral qid for 7 days[c]
OR	Azithromycin	1 gm oral once	Ofloxacin[d] 300mg oral bid for 7 days
Infection in Pregnancy	Erythromycin[b]	500 mg oral qid for 7 days[c]	Amoxicillin 500 mg oral tid for 10 days
			Sulfisoxazole[e] 500 mg oral qid for 10 days
Neonatal			
—Ophthalmia	Erythromycin	12.5 mg/kg oral or IV qid for 14 days	
—Pneumonia	Erythromycin	12.5 mg/kg oral or IV qid for 14 days	Sulfisoxazole[f] 100 mg/kg/day oral or IV in divided doses for 14 days
Lymphogranuloma venereum			
	Doxycycline[a]	100 mg oral bid for 21 days	Erythromycin[b] 500 mg oral qid for 21 days or sulfisoxazole 500 mg orally qid for 21 days or equivalent sulfonamide course
GONORRHEA[g]			
Urethral, cervical, rectal, or pharyngeal			
	Ceftriaxone	125 mg IM once	Cefixime 400 mg oral once[h] Ciprofloxacin[d] 500 mg oral once Ofloxacin[d] 400 mg oral once Spectinomycin 2 gm IM once[i]
Ophthalmia (adults)[j]	Ceftriaxone	1 gm IM once **plus** saline irrigation	Ceftriaxone 1 gm IV or IM daily for 5 days, **plus** saline irrigation
Bacteremia and arthritis[k]	Ceftriaxone	1 gm IV daily for 7 to 10 days, or for 2 to 3 days, followed by cefixime 400 mg oral bid or ciprofloxacin 500 mg oral bid to complete 7 to 10 days total therapy	Ceftizoxime or cefotaxime, 1 gm IV q8h for 2 to 3 days or until improved, followed by cefixime 400 mg oral bid or ciprofloxacin 500 mg oral bid to complete 7 to 10 days total therapy
Meningitis	Ceftriaxone	2 gm IV daily for at least 10 days	Penicillin G at least 10 million U/day IV for at least 10 days[l] Chloramphenicol 4 to 6 gm/day IV for at least 10 days[l]

a. Or tetracycline 500 mg oral qid or minocycline 100 mg bid.
b. Erythromycin estolate is contraindicated in pregnancy.
c. In presence of severe GI intolerance, decrease to 250 mg qid and extend duration to 14 days.
d. Contraindicated in pregnancy. Gonococcal strains with decreased susceptibilities to ciprofloxacin have been isolated.
e. Or another sulfonamide in equivalent dosage; avoid all sulfonamides in the third trimester. Sulfonamides appear to be less effective than other alternatives.
f. Only for infants more than 4 weeks old.
g. Since a high percentage of patients with gonorrhea have coexisting *Chlamydia trachomatis* infection, all patients should also receive a course of treatment effective for *Chlamydia*.
h. Limited data on effectiveness for pharyngeal infection
i. Recommended only for use during pregnancy in patients allergic to beta-lactams. Not effective for pharyngeal infection.
j. An oral fluoroquinolone, such as ciprofloxacin for 3 to 5 days, probably would also be effective, but experience is limited.
k. If the infecting strain of *N. gonorrhoeae* has been tested and is known to be susceptible to penicillin or the tetracyclines, treatment may be changed to penicillin G 10 million U IV daily, amoxicillin 500 mg orally qid, doxycycline 100 mg orally bid, or tetracycline 500 mg orally qid.
l. If infecting strain of *N. gonorrhoeae* has been tested and is known to be susceptible.
m. Not effective for pharyngeal infection.

Continued.

TABLE 10-1, cont'd Treatment of Sexually Transmitted Diseases

Type or stage		Drug of choice	Dosage	Alternatives
Endocarditis		Ceftriaxone	2 gm IV daily for at least 3 to 4 weeks	Penicillin G at least 10 million U/day IV for at least 3 to 4 weeks[l]
Neonatal				
—Ophthalmia		Ceftriaxone	125 mg IM once, **plus** saline irrigation	Penicillin G 100,000 U/kg/day IV in 4 doses[l] for 7 days
	OR	Cefotaxime	25 mg/kg IV or IM q8 to 12 h for 7 days **plus** saline irrigation	**plus** saline irrigation
—Arthritis and septicemia		Cefotaxime	25 to 50 mg/kg IV q8 to 12h for 10 to 14 days	Penicillin G 75,000 to 100,000 U/kg/day IV in 4 doses for 7 days[l]
—Meningitis		Cefotaxime	50 mg/kg IV q8 to 12h for 10 to 14 days	Penicillin G 100,000 U/kg/day IV in 3 or 4 doses for at least 10 days[l]
Children (under 45 kg)				
—Urogenital, rectal, and pharyngeal		Ceftriaxone	125 mg IM once	Spectinomycin[m] 40mg/kg IM once Amoxicillin 50 mg/kg oral once plus probenecid 25 mg/kg (max. 1 gm) oral once[l]
—Arthritis		Ceftriaxone	50 mg/kg/day (max. 2 gm) IV for 7 days	Penicillin G 150,000 U/kg/day IV for 7 days[l]
	OR	Cefotaxime	50 mg/kg/day IV in 2 or 3 doses for 7 days	
—Meningitis		Ceftriaxone	100 mg/kg/day (max. 2 gm) IV for 7 days	Penicillin G 250,000 U/kg/day IV in 6 divided doses for at least 10 days[l]
	OR	Cefotaxime	200 mg/kg/day IV in 2 or 3 doses for at least 10 days	Chloramphenicol 100 mg/kg/day IV for at least 10 days[l]
SEXUALLY ACQUIRED EPIDIDYMITIS				
		Ceftriaxone **followed by** doxycycline[a]	250 mg IM once	Ciprofloxacin 500 mg or ofloxacin 400 mg oral once **followed by** doxycycline[a] 100 mg oral bid for 10 days
			100 mg oral bid for 10 days	Ofloxacin 300 mg oral bid for 10 days
PELVIC INFLAMMATORY DISEASE				
—hospitalized patients		Cefoxitin	2 grams IV q6h	Clindamycin 900 mg IV q8h
	OR	Cefotetan **either one plus**	2 grams IV q12h	**plus** gentamicin 2 mg/kg IV once **followed by** gentamicin 1.5 mg/kg IV
		doxycycline **followed by**	100 mg IV q12h, until improved	q8h until improved **followed by** doxycycline[a] 100 mg
		doxycycline[a]	100 mg oral bid to complete 14 days	oral bid to complete 14 days[n]
—outpatients		Cefoxitin **plus**	2 gm IM once	
		probenecid	1 gm oral once	
	OR	Ceftriaxone **either one followed by**	250 mg IM once	
		doxycycline[a]	100 mg oral bid for 14 days	

n. Or clindamycin 450 mg oral qid to complete 14 days.
o. Metronidazole should be avoided during pregnancy but, for pregnant women with severe symptoms, 2 gm oral (single dose) may be given after the first trimester.
p. Some experts recommend repeating this regimen after 7 days, especially in patients with HIV infection.
q. Treatment with erythromycin is associated with an increased rate of relapse and should be used only if compliance and 12 months' follow-up are assured and other regimens are contraindicated.
r. Patients allergic to penicillin should be desensitized.
s. Single-dose treatment is less effective in HIV-infected patients.
t. Not highly effective for treatment of recurrences, but may help some patients if started early.
u. Some experts suggest that preventive treatment be discontinued for 1 to 2 months once a year to reassess the frequency of recurrence.

TABLE 10-1, cont'd	Treatment of Sexually Transmitted Diseases		
Type or stage	**Drug of choice**	**Dosage**	**Alternatives**
OR	Ofloxacin **plus**	400 mg oral bid	
	clindamycin	450 mg qid for 14 days	
	or metronida-zole	500 mg bid for 14 days	
VAGINAL INFECTION			
Trichomoniasis	Metronidazole[o]	2 gm oral once	Metronidazole 500 mg oral bid for 7 days
Bacterial vaginosis	Metronidazole	500 mg oral bid for 7 days	Clindamycin 300 mg oral bid for 7 days
			Clindamycin cream 2%, one full applicator (5 gm) intravaginally at bedtime for 7 days or metronidazole gel, 0.75% one full applicator (5 gm) intravaginally, twice daily for 5/days
Vulvovaginal candidiasis	Topical butoconazole, clotrimazole, micona-zole, terconazole, or tioconazole		Fluconazole 150 mg oral once
			Topical nystatin, topical nizoral
SYPHILIS			
Early (primary, secondary, or latent less than one year)	Penicillin G benzathine	2.4 million U IM once[p]	Doxycycline 100 mg oral bid for 14 days
			Tetracycline 500 mg oral qid for 14 days
Late (more than 1 year's duration, cardiovascular, gumma, late-latent)	Penicillin G benzathine	2.4 million U IM weekly for 3 weeks	Doxycycline 100 mg oral bid for 4 weeks
Neurosyphilis[r]	Penicillin G	2 to 4 million U IV q4h for 10 to 14 days	Penicillin G procaine 2.4 million U IM daily **plus** probenecid 500 mg qid oral, both for 10 to 14 days
Congenital	Penicillin G	50,000 U/kg IM or IV q8 to 12 h for 10 to 14 days	
OR	Penicillin G procaine	50,000 U/kg IM daily for 10 to 14 days	

Syphilis in pregnancy: see text
Patients with AIDS—see text p. 285

CHANCROID			
OR OR	Erythromycin[b] Ceftriaxone Azithromycin	500 mg oral qid for 7 days 250 mg IM once[s] 1 gram oral once[s]	Ciprofloxacin[d] 500 mg oral bid for 3 days Amoxicillin 500 mg **plus** clavulanic acid 125 mg orally tid for 7 days
HERPES SIMPLEX			
First Episode Genital	Acyclovir	400 mg oral tid for 7 to 10 days	Acyclovir 200 mg oral five times daily for 7 to 10 days
First Episode Proctitis	Acyclovir	800 mg oral tid for 7 to 10 days	Acyclovir 400 mg oral five times daily for 7 to 10 days
Recurrent	Acyclovir[t]	400 mg oral tid for 5 days or 200 mg orally five times daily for 5 days or 800 mg orally bid for 5 days	
Severe (hospitalized patients)	Acyclovir	5 to 10 mg/kg IV q8h for 5 to 7 days	
Prevention of Recurrence[u]	Acyclovir	400 mg oral bid	Acyclovir 200 mg oral 2 to 5 times daily

From *The Medical Letter*, Vol 30 (issue 913), Jan 7, 1994 and *MMWR*: 1993 Sexually Transmitted Diseases Treatment Guidelines, Vol 42, No RR-14, Sep 24, 1993.

- Before obtaining a specimen for a chlamydia test, use a sponge or large swab to remove all secretions and discharge from the cervical os.
- For nonculture chlamydia tests, use the swab supplied or specified by the manufacturer of the test.
- Insert the appropriate swab or endocervical brush 1 to 2 cm into the endocervical canal (i.e., past the squamocolumnar junction). Rotate the swab against the wall of the endocervical canal several times for 10 to 30 seconds. Withdraw the swab without touching any vaginal surfaces and place it in the appropriate transport medium (culture, EIA, or DNA probe testing) or prepare a slide (direct fluorescent antibody [DFA] testing).

Management. Multiple drugs that have activity against gonococci, chlamydiae, facultative gram-negative rods, and anaerobes are usually prescribed. The recommended regimens are found in Table 10-1. Evaluate male sexual partners. Chlamydial and gonococcal infections in these men are often asymptomatic.

RECTAL GONORRHEA

Rectal gonorrhea is acquired by anal intercourse. Women with genital gonorrhea may also acquire rectal gonorrhea from contamination of the anorectal mucosa by infectious vaginal discharge. A history of anal intercourse is the most important clue to the diagnosis, since the symptoms and signs of rectal gonorrhea are in most cases relatively nonspecific.[10]

Anoscopic examination of homosexual men reveals generalized exudate in 54% of culture-positive patients and 37% of culture-negative patients.[11] Many infected patients have normal-appearing rectal mucosae. These figures emphasize what is generally observed—that the specificity of the most common signs and symptoms of rectal gonorrhea is low. Some patients report pain on defecation, blood in the stools, pus on undergarments, or intense discomfort while walking.

Diagnosis. Anal culture should be considered for male homosexuals with symptoms and females with symptoms who have engaged in rectal intercourse. Gonococcal proctitis does not involve segments of bowel beyond the rectum. The area of infection is about 2.5 cm inside the anal canal in the pectinate lining of the crypts of Morgagni. An anoscope is unnecessary to obtain culture material. A sterile cotton-tipped swab is inserted approximately 2.5 cm into the anal canal. (If the swab is inadvertently pushed into feces, another swab must be used to obtain a specimen.) The swab is moved from side to side in the anal canal to sample crypts; 10 to 30 seconds are allowed for absorption of organisms onto the swab.

Gram stain is unreliable because of the presence of numerous other bacteria.

GONOCOCCAL PHARYNGITIS

Gonococcal pharyngitis is acquired by penile-oral exposure and rarely by cunnilingus or kissing. The possibility of infection is increased when the penis is inserted deep into the posterior pharynx as practiced by most homosexuals. Most cases are asymptomatic, and the gonococcus can be carried for months in the pharynx without being detected.[12] In those with symptoms, complaints range from mild sore throat to severe pharyngitis with diffuse erythema and exudates.[13]

Diagnosis. Culture is most productive if exudates are present. *N. meningitidis* is a normal inhabitant of the pharynx; consequently, sugar utilization tests are necessary on *Neisseria* species isolated from the pharynx to determine accurately if infectious organisms are present.

Gram stain is useful only if exudate is present and must therefore be interpreted with caution to avoid confusion with other *Neisseria* species.

DISSEMINATED GONOCOCCAL INFECTION (ARTHRITIS-DERMATITIS SYNDROME)

Disseminated gonococcal infection (DGI) develops in approximately 1% to 3% of patients with mucosal infections. It is the most common form of infectious arthritis. The rate of dissemination may be higher in patients with asymptomatic infection, presumably because of the long period in which the organism can enter the vasculature. Menses exposes the submucosal blood vessels and increases the risk of dissemination. The risk of systemic infection increases during the second and third trimesters of pregnancy. In one study, 71% of women with disseminated infection were diagnosed with the syndrome during pregnancy, during the postpartum period, or within 1 week of the onset of menses.[14] Strains of *Neisseria gonorrhoeae* that disseminate and cause arthritis seem to belong to a subgroup with a unique membrane protein and to have a transparent appearance of the colonies on culture more frequently than strains that do not disseminate.[15]

There is no evidence that dissemination is more likely from the pharynx. Dissemination was formerly much more common in women, but presently men and women in some areas are equally affected.

Initial presentation. Migratory polyarthralgias are the most common presenting symptoms, occurring in up to 80% of patients. Initial signs are tenosynovitis (67%), dermatitis (67%), and fever (63%). Less than 30% have symptoms or signs of localized gonorrhea, such as urethritis or pharyngitis; however, cervical cultures in women with DGI are positive in 80% to 90% of cases and men's urethral cultures are positive in 50% to 75% of cases.

Descriptions of the evolution of DGI vary. Some believe that there are two presentations: a bacteremic phase with positive blood cultures and dermatitis, followed by a joint-localization phase with monoarthritis and positive joint fluid but negative blood cultures. Others find that too much overlap occurs.

TABLE 10-2 Differential Features of Disseminated Gonococcal Infection and Nongonococcal Bacterial Arthritis	
Disseminated gonococcal infection	**Nongonococcal bacterial arthritis**
Generally in young, healthy adults	Often in very young, elderly, or immunocompromised persons
Initial migratory polyarthralgias common	Polyarthralgias rare
Tenosynovitis in majority	Tenosynovitis rare
Dermatitis in majority	Dermatitis rare
>50% polyarthritis	>85% monoarthritis
Positive blood culture result in <10%	Positive blood culture result in 50%
Positive joint fluid culture result in 25%	Positive joint fluid culture result in 85% to 95%

From Goldenberg DL, Reed JI: *N Engl J Med* 312(12):767, 1985. Reprinted by permission of *The New England Journal of Medicine.*

Two presentations. Patients usually exhibit one of two syndromes. The different presentations may result from a difference in gonococcal strains.[16] The features of disseminated gonococcal infection are compared with nongonococcal bacterial arthritis in Table 10-2.

Polyarthralgias, tenosynovitis, dermatitis. Chills (25%) and fever (more than 50%) are accompanied by pain, redness, and swelling of three to six small joints without effusion. This polyarthritis and tenosynovitis occur in the hands and wrists, with pain in the tendons of the wrist and fingers.[17] Toes and ankles may also be affected. These patients are more likely to have positive blood and negative joint cultures. Chills and fever terminate as the rash appears on the extensor surfaces of the hands and dorsal surfaces of the ankles and toes. The total number of lesions is usually less than 10. The skin lesions begin as tiny, red papules or petechiae that either disappear or evolve through vesicular (Figure 10-1, *A*) and pustular stages, developing a grey necrotic and then hemorrhagic center (Figure 10-1, *B*). The central hemorrhagic area is the embolic focus of the gonococcus. These lesions heal in a few weeks.

Purulent arthritis. Usually one or two large joints are affected, most frequently the knee followed by the ankle, wrist, and elbow. The affected joint is hot, painful, and swollen, and movement is restricted.[18] Permanent joint changes may occur. The mean leukocyte count in synovial fluid is often more than 50,000 cells/mm^3. The joints are often sterile, possibly as a result of immunologic mechanisms. Dermatitis is usually absent.

Other less common complications of dissemination include endocarditis, myocarditis, and meningitis.

Figure 10-1 Gonococcal septicemia.

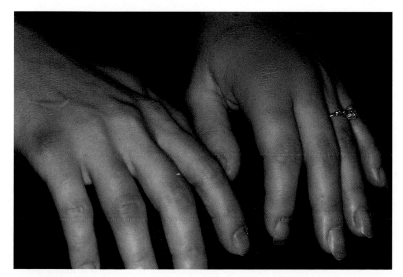

A, There is erythema and swelling of joints on the left hand. A single vesicle is present on the right hand.

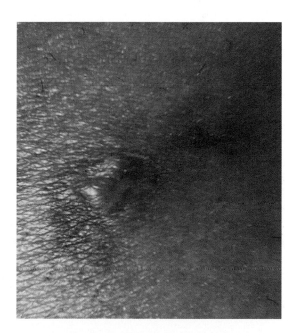

B, More advanced lesion than that shown in *A.* Base has become hemorrhagic and necrotic.

Diagnosis. Gram stain of the skin lesions is performed on the pus obtained by unroofing the pustule. Blood culture results are usually positive only during the first few days and the rate of isolation is low. Mucosal surface cultures of the urethra, endocervix, pharynx, and anus should be done. Gram-stained smears on concentrated sediment of centrifuged synovial fluid show positive results in less than 25%. The diagnosis of septic arthritis is supported by finding an elevated leukocyte count, poor mucin clot, and elevated protein in the aspirated joint fluid. Fewer than 50% of joint culture results are positive for *N. gonorrhoeae*.[14] Fluorescent antibody testing (not available in every laboratory) may be performed on joint exudate and on smears from skin lesions if the diagnosis is suspected, but identification has not been made by other means.

Differential diagnosis. Disseminated gonococcal infection is the most common cause of acute arthritis among sexually active young adults. Other infectious diseases mimic DGI. Hepatitis may present with tenosynovitis, polyarthralgia, and dermatitis. Bacterial endocarditis may be associated with sterile joint effusions and tenosynovitis; skin lesions are embolic. Systemic meningococcal infection is increasing in frequency in this group and can be accompanied by similar findings of joint and skin disease. Patients with meningococcal infection have more skin lesions, high peripheral white blood cell counts, and sterile genital cultures.[19] Reiter's syndrome (urethritis, arthritis, conjunctivitis, and keratoderma blennorrhagica, a psoriasis-like eruption) may be confused with DGI. The arthritis of Reiter's syndrome, however, may be chronic and recurrent and does not respond to antibiotic therapy.

TREATMENT OF GONOCOCCAL INFECTION

Treatment recommendations for gonorrhea are found in Table 10-1, pp. 273 to 274.[20] Ceftriaxone is used for adults with uncomplicated urethral, endocervical, pharyngeal, or rectal infections (see Table 10-1). Ceftriaxone is highly effective against penicillin-resistant strains and can be given in a single, small-volume injection in the deltoid muscle. Ceftriaxone may be effective against incubating syphilis but not against coexisting *C. trachomatis* infection, which is present in up to 45% of women and 25% of heterosexual men with gonorrhea.

Treatment of sexual partners. Men and women exposed to gonorrhea should be examined, cultures should be taken, and the patient should be treated at once with one of the regimens listed in Table 10-1.

Follow-up. Follow-up cultures should be obtained only from persons with persisting symptoms.

Nongonococcal Urethritis

Nongonococcal urethritis (NGU) (nonspecific urethritis) and cervicitis are the most common sexually transmitted diseases in the United States. The diagnosis, as the name implies, used to be one of exclusion; however, routine diagnostic tests for identifying the various infecting organisms are now available. *C. trachomatis* causes 23% to 55% of cases of NGU. *C. trachomatis* is recovered in up to 50% of men with NGU. *C. trachomatis* is isolated in up to 50% of women with mucopurulent cervicitis and approximately 25% to 50% of women with PID. *U. urealyticum* causes 20% to 40% of cases, and *T. vaginalis* causes 2% to 5%.

In many cases a source of infection cannot be identified. Epidemiologic control is difficult because, as is characteristic of gonorrhea, many of those infected have no symptoms. Previously, *C. trachomatis* infections were considered self-limited because most cases became asymptomatic in a few months without treatment. Chlamydial organisms have the ability to exist in the host for years in a latent or subclinical form, and it may be that the individual remains infectious after overt symptoms have resolved.[21] Most women with cervical chlamydial infection, most homosexual men with rectal chlamydial infection, and as many as 30% of heterosexual men with chlamydial urethritis have few or no symptoms.[22]

Nongonococcal urethritis in males. In males urethritis begins with dysuria and urethral discharge. Gonococcal urethritis begins 3 to 5 days after sexual contact and produces a burning, yellow, thick to mucopurulent urethral discharge. NGU begins 7 to 28 days after sexual contact with a smarting sensation while urinating and a mucoid discharge. Table 10-3 compares the two forms of urethritis. *C. trachomatis* causes at least two thirds of the acute "idiopathic" epididymitis in sexually active men under the age of 35 years.[23]

Nongonococcal urethritis in females. The signs and symptoms in females are even more nonspecific. Nongonococcal cervicitis is asymptomatic or begins with a mucopurulent endocervical exudate or a mucoid vaginal dis-

TABLE 10-3 Comparison of Nongonococcal and Gonococcal Urethritis		
	Nongonococcal urethritis	**Gonococcal urethritis**
Incubation period	7-28 days	3-5 days
Onset	Gradual	Abrupt
Dysuria	Smarting feeling	Burning
Discharge	Mucoid or purulent	Purulent
Gram stain of discharge	Polymorphonuclear leukocytes	Gram-negative intracellular diplococci

charge. There is no proof that chlamydiae cause cervical erosions, but cervical erosions may provide more sites for replication of chlamydiae, which apparently cannot infect squamous cells of the vagina or the intact outer or peripheral surfaces of the cervix. *C. trachomatis* has been implicated as a cause of nongonococcal PID and Reiter's syndrome.[24]

Diagnosis. The diagnosis is made by confirming the presence of urethritis, demonstrating the presence of *C. trachomatis*, and excluding gonococcal infection. *C. trachomatis* can be isolated by culture but a variety of nonculture tests are now available. Nonculture tests are less specific than culture tests and may produce false-positive results. All positive nonculture results should be interpreted as presumptive infection until verified by culture or other nonculture tests. The decision to treat and perform additional tests should be based on the specific clinical situation.

First, a Gram stain is made of the urethral discharge. The presence of polymorphonuclear leukocytes confirms the diagnosis of urethritis, and the absence of gram-negative intracellular diplococci suggests urethritis is nongonococcal. Material for Gram stain is most effectively obtained at least 4 hours after urination. For those patients with urethral symptoms but without discharge, polymorphonuclear leukocytes may be seen in material obtained by a Calgiswab inserted approximately 2 cm beyond the urethral meatus.

Second, urethral discharge must be cultured for *N. gonorrhoeae* and culture and/or nonculture diagnostic tests are performed for *C. trachomatis*. These organisms are labile in vitro, and it is difficult to maintain viability during transport. If possible, cultures should be obtained from sexual partners of men with NGU and in pregnant women who may be transmitting the organism to the fetus during birth, causing neonatal conjunctivitis.

Specimen collection. The proper collection and handling of specimens are important in all the methods used to identify *Chlamydia*. Because *Chlamydiae* are obligate intracellular organisms that infect the columnar epithelium, the objective of specimen collection procedures is to obtain columnar epithelial cells from the urethra.

- Delay obtaining specimens until 2 hours after the patient has voided.
- Obtain specimens for *Chlamydia* tests after obtaining specimens for Gram-stain smear or *N. gonorrhoeae* culture.
- For nonculture *Chlamydia* tests, use the swab supplied or specified by the manufacturer.
- Gently insert the urogenital swab into the urethra (females: 1 to 2 cm, males: 2 to 4 cm). Rotate the swab in one direction for at least one revolution for 5 seconds. Withdraw the swab and place it in the appropriate transport medium (culture, EIA, or DNA probe testing) or use the swab to prepare a slide for DFA testing.

Chlamydia cell culture. A major advantage of cell culture is a specificity that approaches 100%. Culture sensitivity is approximately 70% to 90%. Organisms produce intracytoplasmic inclusions. The method is technically difficult, requires 3 to 7 days to obtain a result, and requires stringent transportation and storage temperatures. Nonculture *Chlamydia* tests are easier to perform and provide rapid results.

Nonculture **Chlamydia** *tests.* Laboratory tests (DFA) (Syva), EIA (Abbott), DNA probe, and tests performed in the physician's office (rapid *Chlamydia* tests) are the tests used most often today to diagnosis *Chlamydia* infection.

Treatment. Doxycycline or azithromycin are the drugs of choice (see Table 10-1). Erythromycin is used during pregnancy or for those patients who cannot tolerate tetracycline. Erythromycin is used to treat patients who have persistent symptoms of NGU after having been treated. Persistent disease may indicate the presence of a tetracycline-resistant *U. urealyticum* organism.

Penicillin, ampicillin, cephalosporins, aminoglycosides, and metronidazole are ineffective. Trimethoprim-sulfamethoxazole eradicate *C. trachomatis* but not *U. urealyticum*.

Management of sexual partners. All persons who are sexual partners of patients with NGU should be examined and promptly treated with one of the regimens in Table 10-1.

Follow-up. Patients should be advised to return if symptoms persist or recur. Test-of-cure cultures may not produce positive results until 3 to 6 weeks after treatment.

Persistent or recurrent NGU. Recurrent NGU may result from failure to treat sexual partners. Patients who have persistent or recurrent objective signs of urethritis after they and their partners have received adequate treatment warrant further evaluation for less common causes of urethritis or retreatment with an alternative regimen, such as erythromycin, which ensures treatment of *U. urealyticum* when extended to 14 days.

Syphilis

Syphilis is a human infectious disease caused by the bacterium *Treponema pallidum*. The disease is transmitted by direct contact with a lesion during the primary or secondary stage, in utero by the transplacental route, or during delivery as the baby passes through an infected canal. Like the gonococcus, this bacterium is fragile and dies when removed from the human environment. Unlike the gonococcus, *T. pallidum* may infect any organ, causing an infinite number of clinical presentations; thus the old adage, "he who knows syphilis knows medicine."

Stages defined. Untreated syphilis may pass through three stages, beginning with the infectious cutaneous primary and secondary stages, which may terminate without further sequela or may evolve into a latent stage that lasts for months or years before the now-rare tertiary stage, marked by the appearance of cardiovascular, neurologic, and deep cutaneous complications (Figure 10-2). The Centers for Disease Control defines the stages of syphilis as follows: (1) infectious syphilis includes the stages of primary, secondary, and early latent syphilis of less than 1 year's duration; and (2) latent syphilis is divided into early latent disease of less that 1 year's duration, early latent disease of greater than 1 year's duration, and late latent disease of 4 years' duration or longer.

T. pallidum. *T. pallidum*, the organism responsible for syphilis, is a very small, spiral bacterium (spirochete) whose form and corkscrew rotation motility can be observed only by dark-field microscopy (Figure 10-3). The reproductive time is estimated to be 30 to 33 hours, in contrast to most bacteria, which replicate every 30 minutes. Serum levels of antibiotics must therefore persist for at least 7 to 10 days to expose all replicating organisms. The Gram stain cannot be used, and the bacteria can be grown only with sophisticated tissue culture techniques.

PRIMARY SYPHILIS

Primary syphilis, characterized by a cutaneous ulcer, is acquired by direct contact with an infectious lesion of the skin or the moist surface of the mouth, anus, or vagina. From 10 to 90 days (average, 21 days) after exposure, a primary lesion, the chancre, develops at the site of initial contact. Chancres are usually solitary, but multiple lesions are not uncommon. Extragenital chancres account for 6% to 7% of all chancres, and most occur on the lips and in the oral cavity and are transmitted by kissing or orogenital sex.[25] The lesion begins as a papule that undergoes ischemic necrosis and erodes, forming an 0.3 to 2.0 cm, painless to tender, hard, indurated ulcer; the base is clean, with a scant, yellow, serous discharge. Because the chancre began as a papule, the borders of the ulcer are raised, smooth, and sharply defined (Figure 10-4). The chancre of chancroid is soft and painful. Painless, hard, discrete regional lymphadenopathy occurs in 1 to 2 weeks; the lesions never coalesce or suppurate unless there is a mixed infection. Without treatment the chancre heals with scarring in 3 to 6 weeks. Painless vaginal and anal lesions may never be detected (Figure 10-5). The differential diagnosis includes ulcerative genital lesions such as chancroid, herpes progenitalis, aphthae (Behçet's syndrome), and traumatic ulcers such as occur with biting (Table 10-4).

Course of disease and blood tests

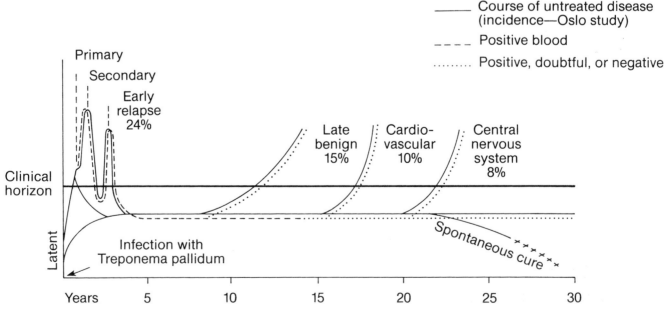

Figure 10-2
Natural history of untreated acquired syphilis. *(From Morgan HJ:* South Med J *26:18, 1933; incidence from Clark EG, Danbolt N:* J Chronic Dis *2:311, 1955.)*

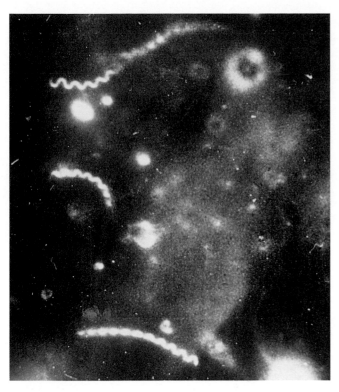

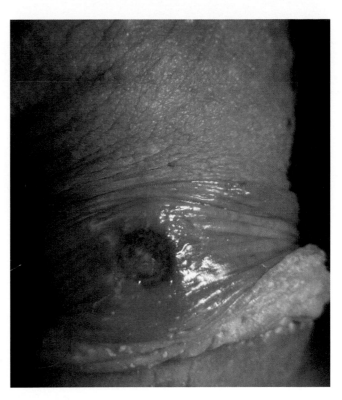

Figure 10-3
Treponema pallidum. Organism responsible for syphilis is seen here photographed through a dark-field microscope.

Figure 10-4
Primary syphilis. Syphilitic chancre is an ulcer with a clean, nonpurulent base and smooth, regular, sharply defined border.

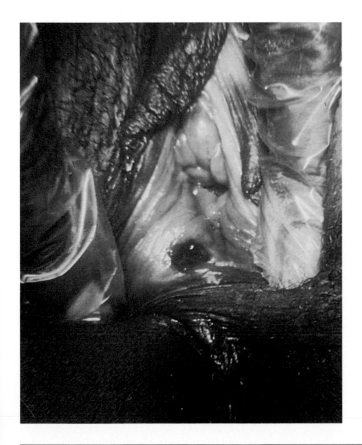

Figure 10-5
Primary syphilis. Chancre in vagina. Lesions are painless and may never be detected.

TABLE 10-4 Differential Diagnosis of Genital Ulcerations

Characteristics and treatment	Chancroid	Granuloma inguinale	Lymphogranuloma venereum (LGV)	Primary syphilis	Herpes simplex
Etiology	*Haemophilus ducreyi*	*Calymmato-bacterium (Donovania) granulomatis*	*Chlamydia*	*Treponema pallidum*	Herpes virus hominis
Incubation period	12 hours to 3 days	3 to 6 weeks	3 days to several weeks	3 weeks	3 to 10 days
Initial lesion	Single or multiple, round to oval, deep ulcers with outlines, ragged and undermined borders, and a purulent base; lesions are tender	Soft, nontender papule(s) that forms irregular ulcer with beefy-red, friable base, and raised, "rolled" border	Evanescent ulcer (rarely seen)	Nontender, eroded papule with clean base and raised, firm, indurated borders; multiple lesions occasionally seen	Primary lesions are multiple, edematous, painful erosions with yellow-white membranous coating; recurrent episodes may have grouped vesicles on an erythematous base
Duration	Undetermined (months)	Undetermined (years)	2 to 6 days	3 to 6 weeks	Primary 2 to 6 weeks; recurrent 7 to 10 days
Site	Genital or peri-anal	Genital, perianal, or inguinal	Genital, perianal, or rectal	Genital, perianal, or rectal	Genital or perianal
Regional adenopathy	Unilateral or bilateral tender, matted, fixed adenopathy that may become soft and fluctuant	Subcutaneous perilymphatic granulomatous lesions that produce inguinal swellings and are not lymphadenitis (pseudobuboes)	Unilateral or bilateral firm, painful inguinal adenopathy with overlying "dusky skin"; may become fluctuant and develop "grooves in the groin"	Unilateral or bilateral firm, movable, nonsuppurative, painless inguinal adenopathy	Bilateral, tender inguinal adenopathy, usually present with primary vulvo-vaginitis and may or may not be present with recurrent genital lesions
Diagnostic tests	Smear, culture, or biopsy of lesion; smear from aspirated unruptured lymph node	Biopsy; touch preparation from biopsy stained with Giemsa	LGV complement fixation test, culture	Dark-field examination, VDRL, FTA-ABS	Tzanck smear; culture

Modified from Margolis RJ, Hood AF: *J Am Acad Dermatol* 6:496, 1982.

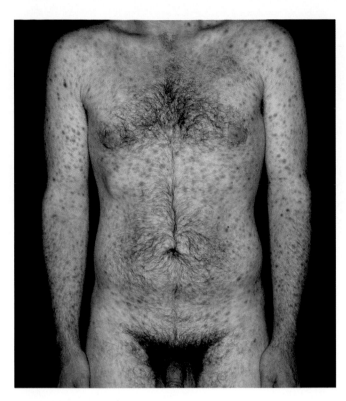

Figure 10-6
Secondary syphilis. Numerous lesions are present on all body surfaces. This is a common presentation with maculopapular and psoriasiform lesions.

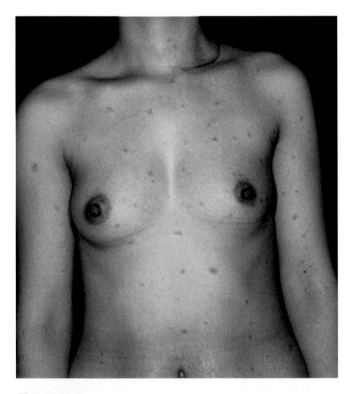

Figure 10-7
Secondary syphilis. Few oval lesions are present on trunk. Initial diagnosis was pityriasis rosea.

SECONDARY SYPHILIS

Secondary syphilis is characterized by mucocutaneous lesions, a flulike syndrome, and generalized adenopathy. Asymptomatic dissemination of *T. pallidum* to all organs occurs as the chancre heals, and the disease then resolves in approximately 75% of cases (see Figure 10-2).[26] In the remaining 25%, the clinical signs of the secondary stage begin approximately 6 weeks (range, 2 weeks to 6 months) after the chancre appears and last for 2 to 10 weeks. Cutaneous lesions are preceded by a flulike syndrome (sore throat, headache, muscle aches, meningismus, and loss of appetite) and generalized, painless lymphadenopathy. Hepatosplenomegaly may be present. In some cases lesions of secondary syphilis appear before the chancre heals. The distribution and morphologic characteristics of the skin and mucosal lesions are varied and may be confused with numerous other skin diseases. As with most other systemic cutaneous diseases, the rash is usually bilaterally symmetric (Figures 10-6 to 10-8).

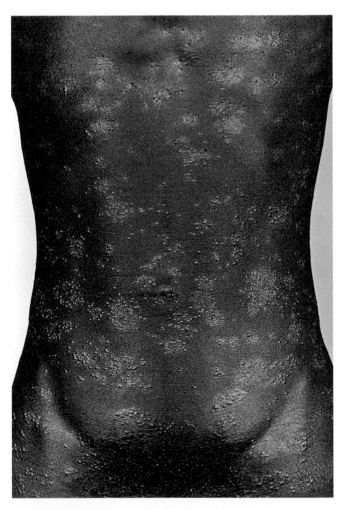

Figure 10-8
Secondary syphilis. This is the uncommon follicular secondary syphilis. *(From Hira S et al:* Int J Dermatol *26:103-106, 1987.)*

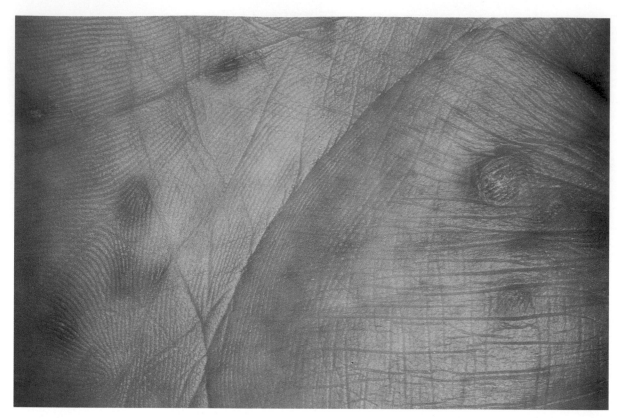

Figure 10-9
Secondary syphilis. Lesions on palms and soles occur in the majority of patients with secondary syphilis. Coppery color resembling that of clean-cut ham is characteristic of secondary syphilis.

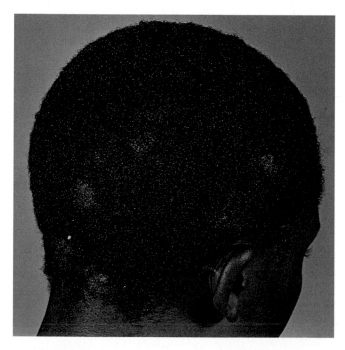

Figure 10-10
Secondary syphilis. Temporary, irregular ("moth eaten") alopecia of the scalp. *(Courtesy Subhash K. Hira M.D.)*

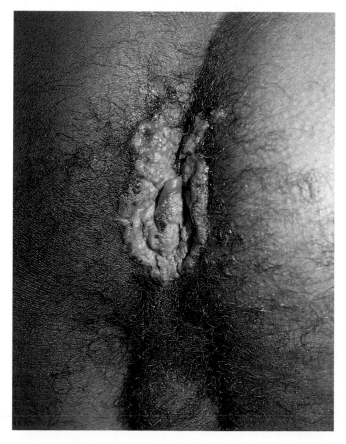

Figure 10-11
Secondary syphilis. Moist, anal, wartlike papules (condylomata lata) are highly infectious.

Lesions. The lesions of secondary syphilis have certain characteristics that differentiate them from other cutaneous diseases.[27,28] There is little or no fever at the onset. Lesions are noninflammatory, develop slowly, and may persist for weeks or months. Pain or itching is minimal or absent. There is a marked tendency to polymorphism, with various types of lesions presenting simultaneously, unlike other eruptive skin diseases in which the morphologic appearance of the lesions is uniform. The color is characteristic, resembling a "clean-cut ham" or having a coppery tint. Lesions may assume a variety of shapes, including round, elliptic, or annular. Eruptions may be limited and discrete, profuse, generalized, or more or less confluent and may vary in intensity.

The types of lesions in approximate order of frequency are maculopapular, papular, macular, annular, papulopustular, psoriasiform, and follicular. The lesions in blacks are marked by the absence of dull-red color.[29] Lesions occur on the palms or soles in most patients with secondary syphilis (Figure 10-9). Unlike the pigmented melanotic macules frequently seen on the palms and soles of older blacks, lesions of secondary syphilis of the palms and soles are isolated, oval, slightly raised, erythematous, and scaly. Temporary irregular ("moth eaten") alopecia of the beard, scalp, or eyelashes may occur (Figure 10-10). Moist, anal, wartlike papules (condylomata lata) are highly infectious (Figure 10-11). Lesions may appear on any mucous membrane. All cutaneous lesions of secondary syphilis are infectious; therefore, if you don't know what it is, don't touch it. The differential diagnosis is vast. The commonly observed diseases that may be confused with secondary syphilis are pityriasis rosea (especially if the herald patch is absent), guttate psoriasis (psoriasis that appears suddenly with numerous small papules and plaques), lichen planus, tinea versicolor, and exanthematous drug and viral eruptions.

The diagnosis is based primarily on clinical and serologic grounds. Histology, in the majority of cases, serves a confirmatory purpose.

Approximately 25% of untreated patients with secondary syphilis may relapse, most of them (approximately 90%) during the first year, a small percentage in the second year, and none after the fourth year.

LATENT SYPHILIS

The concept of latency. A patient has latent disease if a positive serologic result (not a false-positive test) is discovered without evidence of active disease.[30] In latent syphilis, one depends on the accuracy of the patient's history that there were characteristic signs and symptoms or that the blood test, the result of which has been discovered to be positive, was nonreactive at a specific time in the past. Often the physician is unable to confirm the specific time interval.[30] By convention, early latent syphilis is of 1 year or less and late latent syphilis is more than 4 years' duration. The periods of 1 and 4 years were established to help predict a patient's chance of relapsing with signs of secondary infectious syphilis. Approximately 25% of untreated patients in the secondary stage may have a relapse, most of them (approximately 90%) during the first year, a small percentage in the second year, and none after the fourth year. The patient who relapses with secondary syphilis is infectious.

TERTIARY SYPHILIS

In a small number of untreated or inadequately treated patients, systemic disease develops, including cardiovascular disease, central nervous system (CNS) lesions, and systemic granulomas (gummas).[31,32]

SYPHILIS IN THE ERA OF ACQUIRED IMMUNO-DEFICIENCY SYNDROME

Recent reports have documented neurologic relapse after "adequate" penicillin treatment of syphilis in patients with human immunovirus infection.[33,34] *T. pallidum* can invade the CNS during the early months of syphilis infection.[35] Currently recommended penicillin treatment regimens for syphilis result in very low levels of medication in cerebral spinal fluid (CSF). Thus the recommended treatment may not eradicate *T. pallidum* from the CNS, and residual organisms may serve as a reservoir for subsequent relapse. The immunologic response of the patient has an important role in controlling infection. The level of alteration of the immune system in human immunovirus–infected individuals may be enough to allow the standard, marginally adequate treatment regimen to fail. Optimum treatment schedules have not been established. Some authorities have advised treatment with a regimen appropriate for neurosyphilis for all patients coinfected with syphilis and HIV, regardless of the clinical stage of syphilis.[36,37] The regimen of high-dose penicillin recommended for neurosyphilis is not consistently effective in HIV-infected patients with symptomatic neurosyphilis.[37]

CONGENITAL SYPHILIS

T. pallidum can be transmitted by an infected mother to the fetus in utero. In untreated cases stillbirth occurs in 19% to 35% of reported cases, 25% of infants die shortly after birth, 12% are without symptoms at birth, and 40% will have late symptomatic congenital syphilis.[35,38] The treponeme can cross the placenta at any time during pregnancy. Adequate therapy of the infected mother before the sixteenth week of gestation usually prevents infection of the fetus. Treatment after 18 weeks may cure the disease but not prevent irreversible neural deafness, interstitial keratitis, and bone and joint changes in the newborn. The fetus is at greatest risk when maternal syphilis is of less than 2 years' duration. The ability of the mother to infect the fetus diminishes but never disappears in late latent stages.

Early congenital syphilis. Early congenital syphilis is defined as syphilis acquired in utero that becomes symptomatic during the first 2 years of life. The fetal stigmata seen before the age of 2 years include eruptions characteristic of secondary syphilis, such as maculopapular rash and desquamating erythema of the palms and soles; hepatosplenomegaly; and jaundice. Bone and joint symptoms are common. Osteochondritis with the "sawtooth" metaphysis seen on radiographs and periostitis appear with tender limbs and joints. Rhinitis with highly infectious nasal discharge, nontender generalized adenopathy, alopecia, iritis, and failure to thrive occur less frequently.

Late congenital syphilis. Symptoms and signs of late congenital syphilis become evident after age 5 years. The average age at first diagnosis is 30 years. The most important signs are frontal bossae (bony prominences of the forehead) (87%), saddle nose (74%), short maxilla (83%), high arched palate (76%), mulberry molars (more than four small cusps on a narrow first lower molar of the second dentition), Hutchinson's teeth (peg-shaped upper central incisors of the permanent dentition that appear after age 6 years) (63%) (Figure 10-12), Higoumenakis sign (unilateral enlargement of the sternoclavicular portion of the clavicle as an end result of periostitis) (39%), and rhagades (linear scars radiating from the angle of the eyes, nose, mouth, and anus) (8%). Hutchinson's triad (Hutchinson's teeth, interstitial keratitis, and VIIIth nerve deafness) is considered pathognomonic of late congenital syphilis.

SYPHILIS SEROLOGY

The interpretation[39,40] of reactive serologic tests for syphilis is shown in the box on p. 287. Two classes of IgM and IgG antibodies are produced in response to infection with *T. pallidum*; these are nonspecific antibodies measured by the Venereal Disease Research Laboratory (VDRL) and rapid plasma reagin (RPR) tests and specific antibodies measured by the fluorescent treponimal antibody absorption (FTA-ABS) test (Table 10-5).[41] The IgM antibodies are present in the second week of infection, and they disappear 3 months after treatment for early syphilis and 12 months after for late syphilis. They do not pass through the placenta or blood-brain barrier. IgG antibodies reach high levels in 4 to 5 weeks and may persist for life.

Venereal Disease Research Laboratory and rapid plasma reagin tests. The VDRL and RPR are reactive by the seventh day of the chancre. When their results are positive, verification is by the more specific fluorescent treponemal antibody test. All reactive samples are titered to determine the highest reactive dilution. The tests give quantitative as well as qualitative results and can be used to monitor response to therapy. These tests are used for screening purposes and have a high degree of sensitivity (positive in most patients with syphilis) but relatively low specificity (positive in patients without syphilis). A rising titer indicates active disease; the titer falls in response to treatment. Biologic false-positive reactions to nontreponemal tests (range, 3% to 20%) are defined as a positive nontreponemal antibody test result in patients for whom the FTA-ABS finding is negative (see the box on p. 288). Connective tissue disease that forms autoantibodies against nuclear components can produce false-positive reactions.

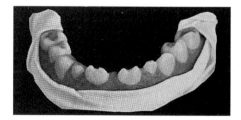

Figure 10-12
Late congenital syphilis. Hutchinson's teeth (peg-shaped upper central incisors of permanent dentition).

TABLE 10-5 Sensitivity of Serologic Tests in the Stages of Syphilis (Percent Positive)*					
Test	**Primary**	**Secondary**	**Latent**	**Tertiary**	**Screening**
VDRL†	72	100	73	77	86
FTA-ABS‡	91	100	97	100	99

*From Griner PF et al: *Ann Intern Med 94*(part 2):585, 1981.
†Specificity variable by stage and proportion of population tested with chronic and autoimmune diseases. Specificity in screening general population approximately 97%.
‡Specificity for all stages probably 98% to 99%, including those with biologic false-positive results on nontreponemal test.

INTERPRETATION OF REACTIVE SEROLOGIC TESTS FOR SYPHILIS

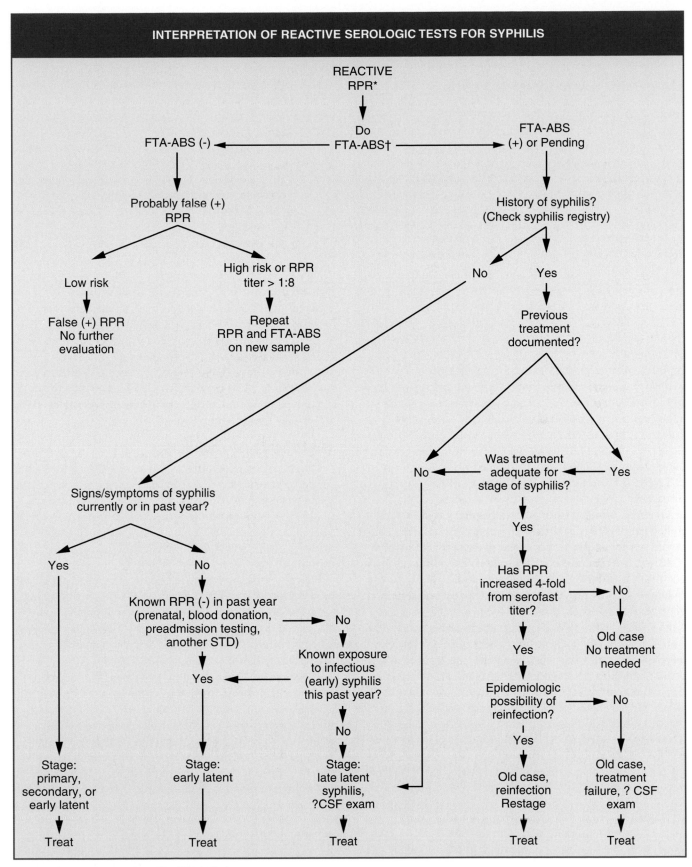

Modified from Coury-Doniger PA: *STD bulletin*.
*Or other nontreponemal serologic test (e.g., VDRL or ART).
†Or other treponemal serologic test (e.g., MHA-TP).

DISEASES THAT RESULT IN POSITIVE REACTIONS TO TESTS ALTHOUGH PATIENTS DO NOT HAVE SYPHILIS (FALSE-POSITIVE REACTIONS)

NONTREPONEMAL TESTS		FTA-ABS
Acute reactor (less than 6 months)	**Chronic reactor (more than 6 months)**	
Pregnancy	Collagen vascular disease	Pregnancy
Drug-induced systemic lupus erythematosus	Senescence	Drug addiction
Acute infection	Leprosy	Herpes genitalis
Infectious mononucleosis	Metastasis to or cirrhosis of the liver	Lupus erythematosus, scleroderma, rheumatoid arthritis (atypical beaded fluorescence pattern)
Malaria	Hashimoto's thyroiditis	Mixed connective tissue disease
Rubeola	Sjögren's syndrome	Alcoholic cirrhosis
Chicken pox	Sarcoidosis	
Atypical pneumonia	Lymphoma	
Smallpox vaccine	Myeloma	
Narcotic addiction	Narcotic addiction	
	Familial false-positive findings	

Undiluted serum containing a high titer of nonspecific antibody, as occurs in secondary syphilis, may result in a negative result on the flocculation test. This is called the *prozone phenomenon* and occurs because the large quantity of antibody occupies all antigen sites and prevents flocculation. The laboratory may perform flocculation tests on diluted serum in anticipation of this problem.

The VDRL test result is uniformly nonreactive in Lyme disease.

Venereal Disease Research Laboratory test in spinal fluid. Neurosyphilis in untreated patients can be detected by the presence of pleocytosis, elevated protein, a positive VDRL finding, or positive FTA test result in CSF. The FTA test result is reactive far more often than the VDRL finding in latent syphilis. The VDRL test on CSF gives a high percentage of false-negative results.[40]

FTA-ABS. The FTA-ABS test is performed when the VDRL or RPR finding is positive and in patients with clinical evidence of syphilis for whom the nontreponemal test result is negative. Its main use is to rule out biologic false-positive reagin test reactions and to detect late syphilis in which the reagin test result may be nonreactive. FTA-ABS measures antibody directed against *T. pallidum* rather than from tissue (reagin), as with the RPR and VDRL tests. False-positive FTA-ABS test results occur most frequently in patients with autoantibodies. A patient who has a reactive treponemal test usually will have a reactive test for a lifetime, regardless of treatment or disease activity (15% to 25% of patients treated during the primary stage may revert to being serologically nonreactive after 2 to 3 years). Treponemal test antibody titers correlate poorly with disease activity and should not be used to assess response to treatment.

FTA-ABS in cerebrospinal fluid. The fluorescent treponemal antibody test can be administered on CSF. A nega-tive result of FTA-ABS-CSF assay can be used to rule out the diagnosis of neurosyphilis. The FTA-ABS-CSF assay has a sensitivity and specificity for neurosyphilis of 100% and 99.2%, respectively.[41]

TREATMENT OF SYPHILIS

Patients to be treated for syphilis should have a baseline serum RPR determination. The best indication of successful therapy is a falling RPR titer.

The drug of choice in the treatment of syphilis is benzathine penicillin G (see Table 10-1).[42] Patients sensitive to penicillin should be treated with the alternative drugs listed in Table 10-1.

Patients with their first attack of primary syphilis will have a nonreactive RPR card test (RPR-CT) result within 1 year. Patients with secondary syphilis will have a nonreactive RPR-CT test result within 2 years.[43] Patients with early latent syphilis of less than 1 year will have negative serologic findings within 4 years.

Patients with a first attack of early latent syphilis of 1 to 4 years' duration treated with the schedules in Table 10-1 will have a nonreactive RPR-CT finding in 5 years. Of patients with late latent syphilis, 45% will have negative serologic test results in 5 years, and the remainder will have reagin fast reactions. CSF examination is not performed unless the patient has neurologic or psychiatric signs and symptoms.

Pregnant patients. Penicillin may be given to pregnant women with syphilis even if they have a history of penicillin allergy provided (1) their skin test reactions of the major and minor penicillin determinants are negative or (2) their skin test reactions are positive, but they are then desensitized to penicillin. Patients can be desensitized and then given standard dosages of this antibiotic. Any pregnant woman with a positive blood test result for syphilis and with no history of treatment should be treated prophylactically, pending the results of a diagnostic workup.

Treatment with erythromycin is not recommended during pregnancy.[44] Erythromycin, although effective for the mother, does not pass to the placenta in sufficient concentration to protect the fetus. Infants born to mothers treated with erythromycin for early syphilis should be treated again with penicillin.

Management of the patient with a history of penicillin allergy. No proven alternatives to penicillin are available for treating neurosyphilis, congenital syphilis, or syphilis in pregnant women. Penicillin is also recommended for use, whenever possible, in the treatment of HIV-infected patients. Only approximately 10% of persons who report a history of severe allergic reactions to penicillin are still allergic. Skin testing with the major and minor determinants can reliably identify persons at high risk for penicillin reactions. Those with positive tests should be desensitized. (See Wendel GD et al: *N Engl J Med* 312[19]:1230, 1985.)

POSTTREATMENT EVALUATION OF SYPHILIS

Frequency of follow-up serologic tests. All patients treated for syphilis must be followed to assess the effectiveness of initial treatment. Quantitative nontreponemal tests (VDRL or RPR) are obtained at certain intervals after treatment (Table 10-6). Repeat treatment should be considered for any patient who has a sustained fourfold increase in titer or when an initially high titer does not show a fourfold decrease within a year.[45]

Serologic responses to treatment

Primary, secondary, and early latent syphilis. All patients with primary syphilis treated with the recommended schedules will have negative serologic findings in 1 year; those with secondary syphilis treated with the recommended schedules will have negative serologic test results in 2 years[45] (Figures 10-13 and 10-14). Persistent low-titer RPR reactivity may occur in 5% of successfully treated patients. The FTA-ABS test indicates past or present exposure and is not related to activity of the disease. Patients treated for early latent syphilis will have negative serum findings within 4 years. The lower the serologic titer before treatment, the quicker the blood test result will revert to normal.[46]

Late latent syphilis. In one study, 44% of patients with late latent syphilis had negative serologic findings within 5 years, and 56% had persistently positive reagin test results.[47] The criteria of effectiveness in the treatment of patients with late latent syphilis are reversion of the reagin blood test for syphilis from reactive to nonreactive, a fourfold or greater decrease in the reagin titer, or a fixed titer with no significant change during the period of observation.

Reinfection in primary, secondary, and latent syphilis. The titers of reagin antibody are higher than those during the first infection, and the serologic responses to treatment are slower, taking about twice the time to become nonreactive compared with the time expected after treatment of a first episode of syphilis.[48]

TABLE 10-6	Use of Nontreponemal Serologic Tests in Follow-Up After Treatment of Syphilis	
Stage	**Follow-up interval**
Early syphilis (less than 1 year)	3, 6, 12 months after treatment
Late syphilis (more than 1 year)	2 years after treatment
Neurosyphilis	Blood and CSF levels every 6 months for 3 years after treatment
Retreatment	CSF level

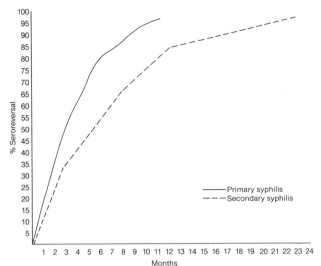

Figure 10-13
Speed of seroreversal of 500 patients with primary syphilis and 522 patients with secondary syphilis: 1977-1981.[43,45,46] *(Graph courtesy Nicholas J. Fiumara, M.D., M.P.H.)*

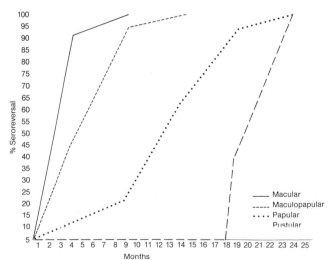

Figure 10-14
Speed of seroreversal of 522 patients with secondary syphilis by type of lesion: 1977-1981. *(Graph courtesy Nicholas J. Fiumara, M.D., M.P.H.)*

Rare Sexually Transmitted Diseases
LYMPHOGRANULOMA VENEREUM

There are 15 serotypes of *C. trachomatis*, three of which (serovars L_1, L_2, or L_3) cause lymphogranuloma venereum (LGV). These serotypes are more invasive and not limited to mucous membranes. LGV is mainly a disease of lymphatic tissue that spreads to tissue surrounding lymphatics.

Primary lesion. After an incubation period of 5 to 21 days, a small papule or viral (herpetiform) vesicle occurs on the penis, fourchette, posterior vaginal wall, or cervix (Figure 10-15). The lesion evolves rapidly to a small, painless erosion that heals without scarring. The lesion may be so innocuous that the patient may not remember it. The primary lesion is rarely seen in women.

Lymphadenopathy. Unilateral or sometimes bilateral inguinal lymphadenopathy accompanied by headache, fever, and migratory polymyalgia and arthralgia appears from 1 to 4 weeks after the primary lesion heals (Figure 10-15). In a short time the lymph nodes become tender and fluctuant and are referred to as *buboes* when they ulcerate and discharge purulent material. Draining buboes may persist for months. Inflammation spreads to adjoining nodes and leads to matting. Abscesses rupture and sinus tracts eventually heal with scarring. Buboes are common in males but occur in only approximately one third of infected females. Enlargement of inguinal nodes above and femoral nodes below Poupart's ligament creates the "groove sign" in approximately one fifth of patients, which is considered pathognomonic for LGV (Figure 10-16).

For unexplained reasons, inflammation of the perineal lymph nodes develops in women and may lead to scarring and ulceration of the labia, rectal mucosa, and vagina. Chronic edema (elephantiasis) of the female external genitals is a late manifestation of lymphatic obstruction.

Diagnosis. The diagnosis of LGV depends mainly on serologic tests; three types of techniques are used: the complement-fixation (CF) test, the single L-type immunofluorescence test, and the microimmunofluorescence test (micro-IF). A fourfold rise of antibody in the course of suspected illness is diagnostic of active infection. However, seroconversion is demonstrated in only a minority of cases since most patients are seen after the acute stage. Moderate or high serum titers may also be caused by other *C. trachomatis* infections and may persist for many years.

Complement fixation test. The result of the LGV complement fixation test (LGV-CFT) becomes positive within 1 to 3 weeks. The antigen used is a genus-specific chlamydial group antigen that is not specific for the LGV organism; therefore the diagnosis cannot be absolute from this test unless rising titers can be demonstrated. Rising titers are difficult to demonstrate because the patient is usually seen after the acute stage, when the initial lesion has healed. Single-point CF titers greater than 1:64 are seen in the majority of patients and are considered indicative of active LGV.

Microimmunofluorescent technique. The most accurate diagnostic serologic assay is the micro-IF test. The micro-IF method is highly sensitive and specific for determining individual serotypes of *C. trachomatis*. Demonstration of a rising titer is difficult, but a single titer of IgM (greater than 1:32) and IgG (greater than 1:512) with the antigen type of the infecting strain provides strong support for the diagnosis of LGV. There is much lower cross-reactivity with other *C. trachomatis* strains in active cases. Micro-IF is only available in a few specialized reference laboratories.

Culture. Culture of *C. trachomatis* is now available in hospital laboratories. *C. trachomatis* can be isolated from bubo pus, genital ulcers and rectal tissue on cycloheximide-treated McCoy cells, but the recovery rate is lower than 50%. Material from the genital ulcers may be inoculated directly into cell tissue culture, but bubo pus and tissues have to be homogenized in tissue culture medium to obtain a 10% and 20% suspension, and 10^{-1} and 10^{-2} dilutions are inoculated into tissue culture. This is necessary to reduce a toxic effect of the pus on the culture cells.

Frei skin test. The Frei skin test is no longer available.
Treatment
Drug regimen. The drug regimen of choice is doxycycline 100 mg orally two times a day for 21 days.

Alternative regimens. Erythromycin 500 mg orally four times a day for 21 days *or* sulfisoxazole 500 mm orally four times a day for 21 days or equivalent sulfonamide course. Persons who have had sexual contact with a patient who has LGV within 30 days before the onset of the patient's symptoms should be examined, tested for urethral or cervical chlamydial infection, and treated.

Lesion management. Fluctuant lymph nodes should be aspirated as needed through healthy, adjacent, normal skin. Incision and drainage or excision of nodes delays healing and is contraindicated. Late sequelae such as stricture or fistula may require surgical intervention.

Figure 10-15
Lymphogranuloma venereum. Primary lesion consists of small, painless erosion that heals in a short time without scarring.

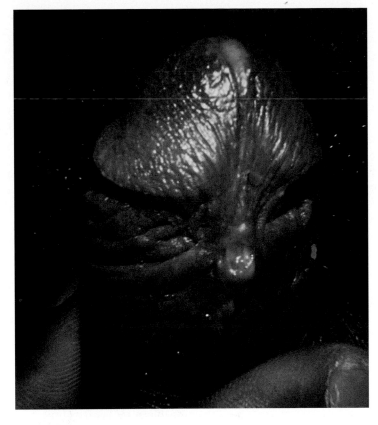

Figure 10-16
Lymphogranuloma venereum. Bilateral inguinal lymphadenopathy that discharges purulent material (buboes). Enlargement of inguinal nodes above and femoral nodes below Poupart's ligament creates the "groove sign."

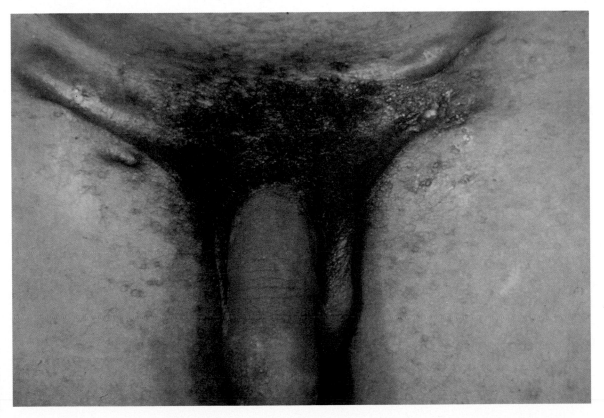

CHANCROID

Chancroid (soft chancre) is the most common of the minor venereal diseases. It is caused by the short gram-negative rod *H. ducreyi*. The male/female ratio of reported cases is approximately 10:1. Chancroid predominantly affects heterosexual men, and most cases originate from prostitutes who are often carriers with no symptoms. The disease is common and endemic in many parts of the world. In the United States chancroid typically occurs in epidemics. A high rate of HIV infection among patients with chancroid has been reported.

Primary state. After an incubation period of 3 to 5 days, a painful, red papule appears at the site of contact and rapidly becomes pustular and ruptures to form an irregular-shaped, ragged ulcer with a red halo. The ulcer is deep, not shallow as in herpes; bleeds easily; and spreads laterally, burrowing under the skin and giving the lesion an undermined edge and a base covered by yellow-gray exudate (Figure 10-17). The ulcers are highly infectious, and multiple lesions appear on the genitals from autoinoculation.

Unlike syphilis, the ulcers may be so painful that some patients refuse the manipulation necessary to obtain culture material. Untreated cases may resolve spontaneously or, more often, progress to cause deep ulceration (Figure 10-18), severe phimosis, and scarring. Systemic symptoms, including anorexia, malaise, and low-grade fever, are occasionally present. Females may have multiple, painful ulcers on the labia and fourchette and, less often, on the vaginal walls and cervix. Autoinoculation results in lesions on the thighs, buttocks, and anal areas. Female carriers may have no detectable lesions and may be without symptoms.

Lymphadenopathy. Unilateral or bilateral inguinal lymphadenopathy develops in approximately 50% of untreated patients, beginning approximately 1 week after the onset of the initial lesion. The nodes then resolve spontaneously or they suppurate and break down.

Diagnosis. The combination of a painful ulcer with tender inguinal adenopathy is suggestive of chancroid and, when accompanied by suppurative inguinal adenopathy, is almost pathognomonic.

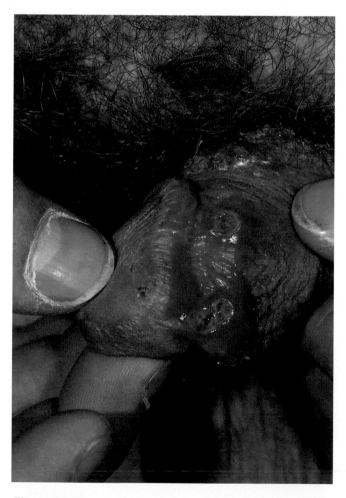

Figure 10-17
Chancroid. Several small, painful ulcers are usually present. Base is purulent, in contrast to the chancre of syphilis.

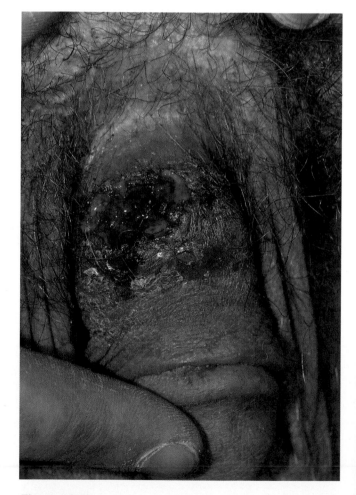

Figure 10-18
Chancroid. Ulcers have coalesced during a 4-week period without treatment.

A probable diagnosis is made in cases of one or more painful genital ulcers and (1) no evidence of *T. pallidum* infection by dark-field examination of ulcer exudate or by a serologic test for syphilis performed at least 7 days after onset of ulcers and (2) the clinical presentation of the ulcers is either not typical of disease caused by herpes simplex virus (HSV) or the HSV test results are negative.

Patients should be tested for HIV infection and tested 3 months later for syphilis and HIV if initial results are negative.

Culture. Accurate diagnosis depends on the ability to culture *H. ducreyi*. Amies' transport medium and all the newly formulated transport media maintain viability of *H. ducreyi* for more than 4 days at 4° C.[50,51,52]

H. ducreyi cannot be cultured on routine medium. Nutritional requirements of *H. ducreyi* seem to be geographically defined. High cultural yield is obtained by using enriched gonococcal agar base and enriched Mueller-Hinton agar in a biplate fashion. Gonococcal agar-base, supplemented with 5% Fildes' extract and unchocolated horse blood, may be used as a single isolation media.[53,54] Most strains are resistant to vancomycin; this antibiotic is routinely added to the culture media. Screening for vancomycin-sensitive organisms is indicated when negative cultures are repeatedly obtained from clinically typical cases originating from the same community.[54-57] More reliable results are obtained if the exudate from the ulcer is inoculated directly onto the plate, not onto transport medium. Incubation is at 33° to 35° C in 5% to 10% CO_2 and a water-saturated atmosphere for 3 to 4 days. The plates are kept for 1 week since the organisms are slow growing.

Gram stain. *H. ducreyi* possesses agglutination properties that account for the clumping of organisms when colonies are dispersed in saline. Agglutination may be responsible for the "school-of-fish" pattern seen on Gram staining. Smears taken from the surface areas are of little use. Material is obtained by drawing the flat surface of a toothpick under the undermined border of the ulcer. The cellular debris is then smeared on a glass slide. Exudate is obtained from the base of a new ulcer with a cotton swab. The swab is rolled in one direction over the slide to preserve the characteristic arrangement of the organisms. The slide is gently fixed with heat and stained with Gram stain. Gram-negative coccobacilli occur in parallel arrays (school-of-fish arrangement). This feature is infrequently seen and other gram-negative bacilli in the smear may result in a false-positive diagnosis. (Figure 10-19). Bacteria may be intracellular. *H. ducreyi* may also be demonstrated with Wright, Giemsa, or Unna-Pappenheim stains.

Herpes simplex genital ulcers can mimic chancroid.[57] A herpes culture and Tzanck smear to look for virus-induced, multinucleated giant cells help to establish the diagnosis. The histologic nature of chancroid is specific, but the biopsy procedure is so painful that other means of confirming the diagnosis should be utilized first.

Treatment. Drug regimens (see Table 10-1) are azithromycin 1 gm orally in a single dose, or ceftriaxone 250 mg intramuscularly in a single dose, erythromycin 500 mg orally four times a day for 7 days. Alternative regimens are oral amoxicillin-clavulanic acid 500/125 mg orally three times a day for 7 days or ciprofloxacin 500 mg orally two times a day for 3 days.[58] A single 2-gm dose of spectinomycin is reported to be effective, but erythromycin is more effective.[59-61]

Trimethoprim-sulfamethoxazole is no longer predictably effective due to the recent emergence of resistance to both sulfonamides and to trimethoprim.[62] Resistance to ceftriaxone has also been reported.

Antimicrobial susceptibility testing should be done on *H. ducreyi* isolated from patients who do not respond to the recommended therapies. Asymptomatic carriage of *H. ducreyi* in males and females has been described,[57,63] therefore aggressive tracing and treatment of sex partners, whether or not they have symptoms, is essential for control.

Fluctuant nodes can be aspirated by needle with the patient under local anesthesia; this is done superior to the abscess rather than from below to prevent continuous dripping.[64] Recent experience showed that suppurative lymphadenopathy responded to appropriate antibiotic regimens. The recommendation was to reserve surgical intervention for buboes that prove recalcitrant to antibiotic therapy.[65]

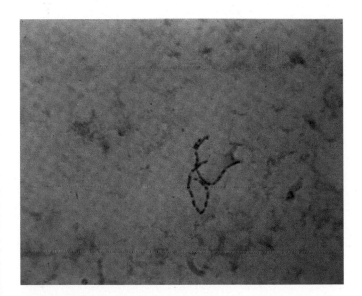

Figure 10-19
Chancroid. Wright's stain of purulent material of base of ulcer shows chain of coccobacilli.

GRANULOMA INGUINALE (DONOVANOSIS)

Granuloma inguinale is a predominantly tropical cause of genital ulcer occurring chiefly in small endemic foci in all continents except Europe. It is a chronic, superficial, ulcerating disease of the genital, inguinal, and perianal areas caused by the gram-negative rod *Calymmatobacterium granulomatis*. The incubation period is unknown, but 14 to 50 days is suspected. The disease begins as a firm papule, nodule, or ulcer on the genitals and then evolves into a painless, broad, superficial ulcer with a rolled border and a friable, beefy-red, granulation tissue-like base raised above the skin surface (Figure 10-20). The ulceration spreads contiguously to the genitocrural and inguinal folds in males and the perineal and perianal areas in females. It remains confined to areas of moist, stratified epithelium, sparing the columnar epithelium of the rectal area.

Women present with genital ulceration (88.5%) and genital tract bleeding (19.7%). The vulva is the most frequent anatomic site involved in both pregnant (88.5%) and nonpregnant (28.6%) women. Multiple sites of infection (vulva, vagina, cervix) occurred only among nonpregnant women.[66] Granuloma inguinale of the cervix presents as a proliferative growth and may mimic carcinoma.[67]

Donovanosis ulcers bleed to the touch and are not usually associated with inguinal lymphadenopathy as with LGV and chancroid.[68] Most regular sexual partners of infected patients have no evidence of co-existent infection with donovanosis.[69]

Diagnosis. Culture of the bacterium in the chicken embryonic yolk sac has been reported but is unsuccessful on artificial culture media. Diagnosis can be confirmed in 1 hour with the following technique.[70] The lesion is washed with saline. Lidocaine ointment is applied, removed in 10 minutes, reapplied, and again removed 10 minutes later. Two scoops are taken as deeply as possible from the lesion with a curet or chalazion spoon. The first is submitted in formalin for histopathologic study. The second is rubbed together between two glass slides to ensure a uniform spread of cells from the material. The slides are taken to the laboratory, immediately air dried, and fixed in methyl alcohol for 5 minutes, followed by staining with 20% Giemsa for 10 minutes. Excess stain is washed off with water. Wright's or Leishman's stain is also suitable. Once dry, 100 × oil-immersion, objective lens microscopic examination reveals bipolar-staining bacilli in vacuoles in the cytoplasm of large histiocytes. The intracellular organisms are called *Donovan bodies* and have a prominent clear capsule when mature (Figure 10-21). If slides cannot be immediately taken to the laboratory, they must be air dried and fixed with an aerosol fixative, such as that used for Papanicolaou smear tests. The RapiDiff technique is suitable for use in the diagnosis of granuloma inguinale (donovanosis) in busy sexually transmitted diseases clinics.[71]

Figure 10-20
Granuloma inguinale. Painless, broad, superficial ulcer with beefy-red texture is raised above the skin surface. *(Courtesy Nicholas J. Fiumara M.D., M.P.H.)*

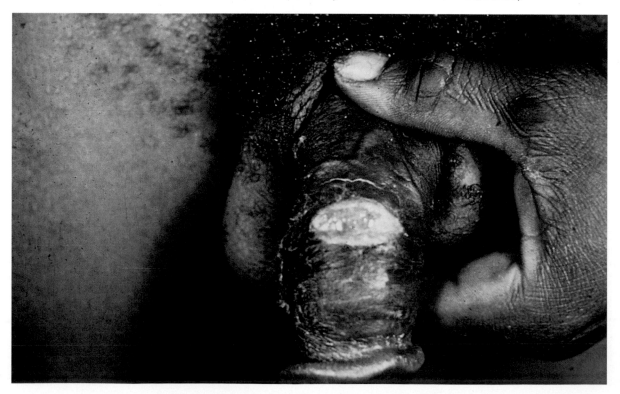

For histopathologic study, the Warthin-Starry silver stains demonstrate the encapsulated bacilli within histiocytes. There is a mixed infiltrate of plasma cells, neutrophils, and histiocytes, but very few lymphocytes.

Treatment. Trimethoprim-sulfamethoxazole and tetracycline are the most effective, but resistance to tetracycline has occurred.[72] The minimum duration of treatment is 21 days; however, treatment should be continued until all lesions have completely healed. The dosages are trimethoprim-sulfamethoxazole (Bactrim-DS, Septra-DS) twice daily[70] or tetracycline 0.5 gm four times a day. Relapses after apparent cure occasionally occur, and such recurrent lesions may become resistant to medication. Under such circumstances switching to another antibiotic generally has been found to be effective. Streptomycin 4 gm per day for 5 days, chloramphenicol 2 gm per day for 10 to 14 days, gentamicin, and erythromycin have all been reported effective.[72] Contacts should be traced for examination but treated only if lesions are found.

REFERENCES

1. Britigan BE, Cohen MS, Sparling PF: Gonococcal infection: a model of molecular pathogenesis, *N Engl J Med* 312:1683-1684, 1985.
2. Hooper RR et al: Cohort study of venereal disease. I. The risk of gonorrhea transmission from infected women to men, *Am J Epidemiol* 108:136-144, 1978.
3. Handsfield HH et al: Asymptomatic gonorrhea in men, *N Engl J Med* 290:117-123, 1974.
4. McCutchan JA: Epidemiology of venereal urethritis: comparison of gonorrhea and nongonococcal urethritis, *Rev Infect Dis* 6:669-688, 1984.
5. Barlow D, Phillips I: Gonorrhea in women: diagnostic, clinical and laboratory aspects, *Lancet* 1:761-764, 1978.
6. McCormack WM: Pelvic inflammatory disease, *N Engl J Med* 330:115-119, 1994.
7. Eschenbach DA et al: Polymicrobial etiology of acute pelvic inflammatory disease, *N Engl J Med* 293:166-171, 1975.
8. Taylor-Robinson D, McCormack WM: The genital mycoplasms, *N Engl J Med* 302:1003-1010, 1980.
9. Mardh PA et al: *Chlamydia trachomatis* infection in patients with acute salpingitis, *N Engl J Med* 296:1377, 1977.
10. Kilpatrick ZM: Gonorrheal proctitis, *N Engl J Med* 287:967-969, 1972.
11. Lebedeff DA, Elliott HB: Rectal gonorrhea in men: diagnosis and treatment, *Ann Intern Med* 92:463-466, 1980.
12. Wiesner PJ et al: Clinical spectrum of pharyngeal gonococcal infection, *N Engl J Med* 228:181-185, 1972.
13. Fiumara NJ: Pharyngeal infection with *Neisseria gonorrhoeae*, *Sex Transm Dis* 6:264-266, 1979.
14. Holmes KK, Counts CW, Beaty HN: Disseminated gonococcal infection, *Ann Intern Med* 74:979-993, 1971.
15. Wiesner PJ, Handsfield HH, Holmes KK: Low antibiotic resistance of gonococci causing disseminated infection, *N Engl J Med* 288:1221-1222, 1973.

Figure 10-21
Granuloma inguinale. The intracellular bipolar-staining bacilli are called *Donovan bodies*.

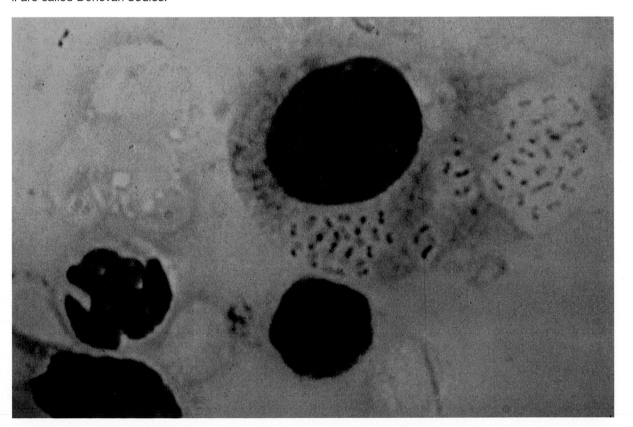

16. O'Brien JP, Goldenberg DL, Rice PA: Disseminated gonococcal infection: a prospective analysis of 49 patients and a review of pathophysiology and immune mechanisms, *Medicine* 62:395-406, 1983.

17. Brogadir SP, Schimmer BM, Myers AR: Spectrum of the gonococcal arthritis dermatitis syndrome, *Semin Arthritis Rheum* 8:177-183, 1979.

18. Goldenberg DL, Reed JI: Bacterial arthritis, *N Engl J Med* 312:764-771, 1985.

19. Rompalo AM et al: The acute arthritis-dermatitis syndrome: the changing importance of *Neisseria gonorrhoeae* and *Neisseria meningitidis*, *Arch Intern Med* 147:281-283, 1987.

20. Antibiotic resistant strains of *Neisseria gonorrhoeae*, *MMWR*, 36 (No. 5S suppl): Sept 11, 1987.

21. Schachter J: Chlamydial infections, *N Engl J Med* 298:428-434, 1978.

22. *Chlamydia trachomatis* infections, Policy guidelines for prevention and control, *MMWR*, 34 (No. 3S suppl): Aug 23, 1985.

23. Berger RE et al: *Chlamydia trachomatis* as a cause of acute "idiopathic" epididymitis, *N Engl J Med* 298:301, 1978.

24. Brunham RC et al: Mucopurulent cervicitis: the ignored counterpart in women of urethritis in men, *N Engl J Med* 311:1, 1984.

25. Allison SD: Extragenital syphilitic chancres, *J Am Acad Dermatol* 14:1094-1095, 1986.

26. Clark EG, Danbolt N: The Oslo study of the natural cause of untreated syphilis, *J Chronic Dis* 2:311, 1955.

27. Gooddard PB: *Ricord's illustrations of venereal disease*, Philadelphia, 1851, A. Hart, Late Carey & Hart.

28. Felman YM, Nikitas JA: Secondary syphilis, *Cutis* 29:322-329, 1982.

29. Hira SK et al: Clinical manifestations of secondary syphilis, *Int J Dermatol* 26:103-107, 1987.

30. Fiumara NJ: Treatment of early latent syphilis under 1 year's duration: serologic response to treatment of 368 patients, *J Am Acad Dermatol* 15:1059-1061, 1986.

31. Kampmeier RH: Late and congenital syphilis. In *Dermatologic Clinics, Symposium on Sexually Transmitted Diseases*, 1(1):23-42, 1983.

32. Luxon LM: Neurosyphilis (review), *Int J Dermatol* 19:310-317, 1980.

33. Tramont EC: Syphilis in the AIDS era, *N Engl J Med* 316:1600-1601, 1987.

34. Lukehart SA et al: Invasion of the central nervous system by *Treponema pallidum*: implications for diagnosis and treatment, *Ann Intern Med* 109:855-862, 1988.

35. Congenital syphilis—United States, 1983-1985, *MMWR* 35:625-628, 1986.

36. Kinloch-de Loës S, Radeff B, Saurat J-H: AIDS meets syphilis: changing patterns of the syphilitic infection and its treatment, *Dermatologica* 177:261-264, 1988.

37. Gordon SM et al: The response of symptomatic neurosyphilis to high-dose intravenous penicillin G in patients with human immunodeficiency virus infection, *N Engl J Med* 331:1469-1473, 1994.

38. Reimer CB et al: The specificity of fetal IgM: antibody or anti-antibody? *Ann NY Acad Sci* 254:77-93, 1975,

39. Griner PF et al: Application of principles, *Ann Intern Med* 94 (part 2):585, 1981.

40. *Interpretive handbook*, Rochester, Minn, 1988, Mayo Medical Laboratories.

41. *1988 test catalogue*, Rochester, Minn, Reference Laboratory of the Mayo Clinic, Mayo Medical Laboratories.

42. Fiumara NJ: Therapy guidelines for sexually transmitted diseases, *J Am Acad Dermatol* 9:600-601, 1983.

43. Fiumara NJ: Treatment of primary and secondary syphilis: serologic response, *J Am Acad Dermatol* 14:487-491, 1986.

44. Hashisaki P et al: Erythromycin failure in the treatment of syphilis in a pregnant woman, *Sex Transm Dis* 10:36-38, 1983.

45. Fiumara NJ: Infectious syphilis. In *Dermatologic clinics, Symposium on Sexually Transmitted Disease*, 1(1):3-21, 1983.

46. Fiumara NJ: Treatment of early syphilis of less than a year's duration, *Sex Transm Dis* 5:85-88, 1978.

47. Fiumara NJ: Serologic responses to treatment of 128 patients with late latent syphilis, *Sex Transm Dis* 6:243-246, 1979.

48. Jaffe HW: Management of the reactive serology. In Holmes KK et al, editors: *Sexually transmitted diseases*, New York, 1984, McGraw-Hill, p 316.

49. Reference deleted in proofs.

50. Sottnek FO et al: Isolation and identification of *Haemophilus ducreyi* in a clinical study, *J Clin Microbiol* 12:170-174, 1980.

51. Borchers SL: Treatment of chancroid, *J Am Acad Dermatol* 8:128-129, 1983 (letter).

52. Dangor Y, Radebe F, et al: Transport media for *Haemophilus ducreyi*, *Sex Transm Dis* 20:5-9, 1993.

53. Dangor Y, Miller SD, et al: A simple medium for the primary isolation of *Haemophilus ducreyi*, *Eur J Clin Microbiol Infect Dis* 11:930-934, 1992.

54. Jones CC, Rosen T: Cultural diagnosis of chancroid, *Arch Dermatol* 127:1823-1827, 1991.

55. Salzman RS et al: Chancroidal ulcers that are not chancroid: cause and epidemiology, *Arch Dermatol* 120:636-639, 1984.

56. Plummer FA et al: Single-dose therapy of chancroid with trimethoprim-sulfametrole, *N Engl J Med* 309:67-71, 1983.

57. Kinghorn GR, Hafiz S, McEntegart MG: Genital colonization with *Haemophilus ducreyi* in the absence of ulceration, *Eur J Sex Transm Dis* 1:89-90, 1983.

58. Tartaglione TA, Hooton TM: The role of fluoroquinolones in sexually transmitted diseases, *Pharmacotherapy* 13:189-201, 1993.

59. Ballard RC, da L'Exposto F, et al: A comparative study of spectinomycin and erythromycin in the treatment of chancroid, *J Antimicrob Chemother* 26:429-434, 1990.

60. Guzman M, Guzman J, et al: Treatment of chancroid with a single dose of spectinomycin, *Sex Transm Dis* 19:291-294, 1992.

61. Traisupa A, Ariyarit C, et al: Treatment of chancroid with spectinomycin or co-trimoxazole, *Clin Ther* 12:200-205, 1990.

62. Knapp JS, Back AF, et al: In vitro susceptibilities of isolates of *Haemophilus ducreyi* from Thailand and the United States to currently recommended and newer agents for treatment of chancroid, *Antimicrob Agents Chemother* 37:1552-1555, 1993.

63. McCarley ME, Cruz PD Jr, Sontheimer RD: Chancroid: clinical variants and other findings from an epidemic in Dallas county, 1986-1987, *J Am Acad Dermatol* 19:330-337, 1988.

64. Gollow MM, Blums M, Haverkort F: Rapid diagnosis of granuloma inguinale, *Med J Aust* 144:502-503, 1986.

65. Rosen T et al: Granuloma inguinale, *J Am Acad Dermatol* 11:433-437, 1984.

66. Bassa AG, Hoosen AA, et al: Granuloma inguinale (donovanosis) in women. An analysis of 61 cases from Durban, South Africa, *Sex Transm Dis* 20:164-167, 1993.

67. Hoosen AA, Draper G, et al: Granuloma inguinale of the cervix: a carcinoma look-alike, *Genitourin Med* 66:380-382, 1990.

68. O'Farrell N, Hoosen AA, et al: Genital ulcer disease: accuracy of clinical diagnosis and strategies to improve control in Durban, South Africa, *Genitourin Med* 70:7-11, 1994.

69. O'Farrell N: Clinico-epidemiological study of donovanosis in Durban, South Africa, *Genitourin Med* 69:108-111, 1993.

70. Lal S, Garg BR: Further evidence of the efficacy of cotrimoxazole in granuloma venereum, *Br J Veneral Dis* 56:412-413, 1980.

71. O'Farrell N, Hoosen AA, et al: A rapid stain for the diagnosis of granuloma inguinale, *Genitourin Med* 66:200-201, 1990.

72. Sehgal VN, Prasad ALS: Donovanosis: current concepts, *Int J Dermatol* 25:8-16, 1986.

CHAPTER ELEVEN

Sexually Transmitted Viral Infections

Additional information about warts, herpes simplex, and molluscum contagiosum can be found in Chapter Twelve.

Genital Warts

The incidence of genital warts is increasing rapidly and exceeds the incidence of genital herpes. The evidence supporting the relationship between genital warts and genital cancer is overwhelming.[1]

Genital warts (condyloma acuminata or venereal warts) are pale pink with numerous, discrete, narrow-to-wide projections on a broad base. The surface is smooth or velvety, moist, and lacks the hyperkeratosis of warts found elsewhere (Figures 11-1 to 11-3). The warts may coalesce in the rectal or perineal area to form a large, cauliflower-like mass.

Another type is seen most often in young, sexually active patients. Multifocal, often bilateral, red- or brown-pigmented, slightly raised, smooth papules have the same virus types seen in exophytic condyloma, but in some instances these papules have histologic features of Bowen's disease. (See discussion of bowenoid papulosis later in this chapter.)

Warts spread rapidly over moist areas and may therefore be symmetric on opposing surfaces of the labia or rectum (Figure 11-4). Common warts can possibly be the source of genital warts, although they are usually caused by different antigenic types of virus. Warts may extend into the vaginal tract, urethra, and rectum, in which case a speculum or sigmoidoscope is required for visualization and treatment. Genital warts frequently recur after treatment. There are two possible reasons. Latent virus exists beyond the treatment areas in clinically normal skin.[2] Warts that are flat and inconspicuous, especially on the penile shaft and urethral meatus,[3] escape treatment; these can be visualized after application of acetic acid.

Oral condyloma in patients with genital human papilloma virus infection. One study showed that 50% of patients with multiple and widespread genital human papilloma virus (HPV) infection who practiced orogenital sex have oral condylomas. All lesions were asymptomatic. Magnification was necessary to detect oral lesions. The diagnosis was confirmed by biopsy. The tongue was the site most frequently affected. Oral condylomas appeared as multiple, small, white or pink nodules, sessile or pedunculate, and as papillary growths with filiform characteristics. The size of oral lesions was greater than 2 mm in more than 50% of lesions, and, in 61% of cases, more than five lesions were present. HPV types 16, 18, 6, and 11 were found.[4]

Pearly penile papules. Dome-shaped or hairlike projections, called *pearly penile papules*, appear on the corona of the penis and sometimes on the shaft just proximal to the corona in up to 10% of male patients. These small angiofibromas are normal variants but are sometimes mistaken for warts. No treatment is required (Figure 11-5).

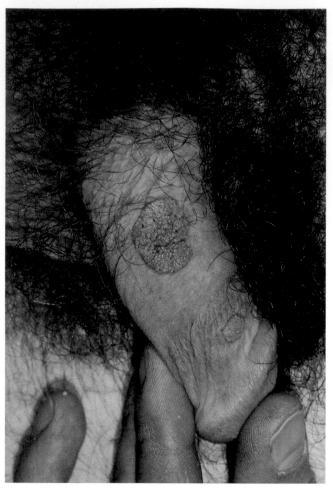

Figure 11-1
Broad-based wart on the shaft of a penis. There are numerous projections on the surface.

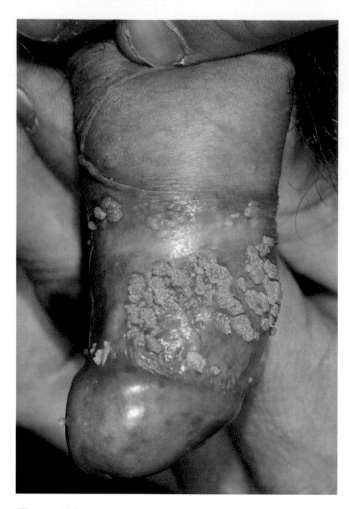

Figure 11-2
Multiple small warts under the foreskin. Multiple inoculations occur on a moist surface. Each wart is made up of many discrete, narrow projections.

Figure 11-3
Wart at the urethral meatus.

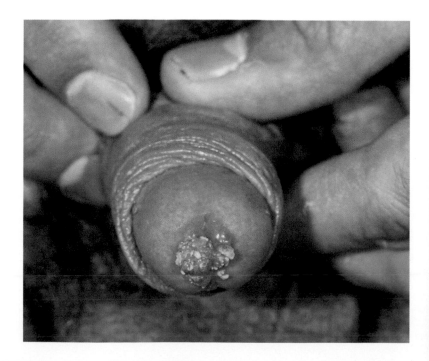

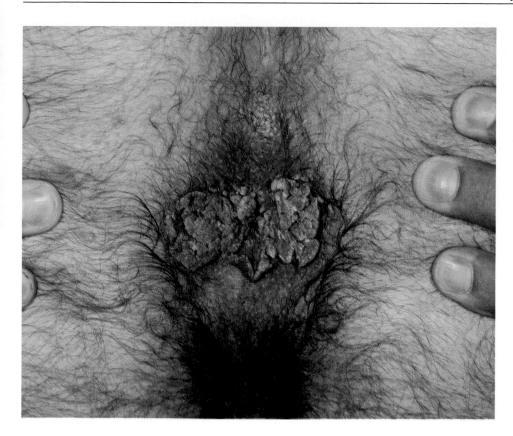

Figure 11-4
Mass of warts on opposing surfaces of the anus.

Figure 11-5 Pearly penile papules.

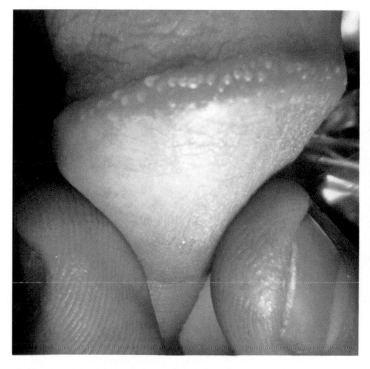

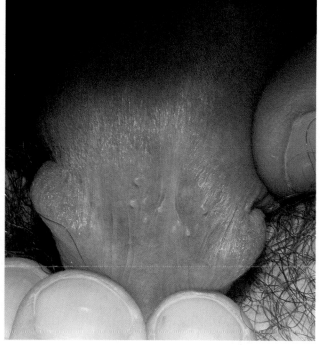

A, An anatomic variant of normal most commonly found on the corona of the penis. They are sometimes mistaken for warts. No treatment is required.

B, A group of papules found just proximal to the corona of the penis is sometimes mistaken for warts.

Genital warts in children. It has been estimated that at least 50% of the cases of condyloma acuminata in children are the result of sexual abuse.[5] In all states there are laws that in effect declare, "If child abuse is recognized or suspected, it has to be reported to authorities." A checklist has been designed to help the clinician determine if child abuse is a possibility:*

1. Physical findings
   A. Fresh bruises
   B. Unusual scars
   C. Burns
2. Medical experience
   A. Past and present medical problems
   B. Prior emergency visits or hospitalizations
   C. Poor compliance with prior medical care; incomplete immunizations for age
   D. Poor mental or physical growth and development
3. Behavior abnormalities
   A. Withdrawal or hyperactivity
   B. Excessive interest in genitals
4. Psychosocial conditions
   A. Disturbed parent-child interaction
   B. Violent interactions in family
   C. Parents were abused as children
   D. Parents were victims of sexual abuse
   E. Family stress—marital discord, unemployment, alcoholism, substance abuse
5. Care of child
   A. Inappropriate custodial care—day care, after school, evenings, weekends
   B. Inappropriate responsibilities for a child
   C. Family isolation—lack of phone, lack of supportive relatives
6. Previous referrals for abuse or neglect

Warts in the genital area can be acquired without sexual abuse.[6] A child with warts on the hands can transfer the warts to the mouth, genitals, and anal area.[7] A mother with hand warts can transfer warts to the child. Sexual play among children is another possible mode of transmission. It is not known whether children can acquire condyloma acuminata from adults with anogenital warts through modes of transmission other than skin-to-skin contact. The incubation period for warts is often many months in duration; this makes it difficult to associate past events.

A study showed what appears to be a relationship between the types of human papilloma virus (HPV-6, HPV-11, and HPV-16) found in condylomas in adults and those seen in children.[8] Other virus types, such as HPV-1, HPV-2, and HPV-3, have also been implicated.[9] These virus types are frequently seen in common, plantar, and plane warts. Thus the finding of identical HPV types in anogenital warts found in a particular adult and child does not prove that anal or vaginal intercourse has occurred. It does support the *possibility* that such an event occurred. Virus typing will be helpful in sorting out these problems when the test becomes more widely available.

Genital warts and cancer. There is strong evidence that several HPV types are associated with genital cancers. Genitoanal warts are predominantly induced by HPV types 6, 11, 16, and 18.[10,11] A strong association has been established between infection by HPV-16 and HPV-18 and the subsequent development of cancer in the uterine cervix. When virus typing becomes generally available, it will be useful to identify patients harboring the high-risk HPV types. HPV-16 was demonstrated in 84% and HPV-18 in 8% of genital tumors.

Seventy-three percent of the nonmalignant, clinically and histologically normal tissue 2 to 5 cm from the tumors contained HPV-16.[12] This implies that HPV can persist latently in tissue that appears normal. Cervical carcinomas and precancerous lesions in women may be associated with genital papilloma virus infection in their male sexual partners. Forty-three percent of male sexual partners of women with genital warts had lesions that could be detected only after application of acetic acid.[13] Homosexual behavior in men is a risk factor for anal cancer. Squamous cell anal cancer is associated with a history of genital warts, which suggests that papilloma virus infection is a cause of anal cancer.[14]

Diagnosis (acetic acid test). Screening men for papilloma virus infection is important in the prevention of cervical neoplasia and in reinfection of female partners.[15] Application of 3% to 5% acetic acid (vinegar is 5% acetic acid) on the penis, cervix, labia, or perianal area makes visible the inconspicuous, flat genital lesions that would otherwise go unnoticed. Dysplastic and neoplastic tissues with large nuclei and scant cytoplasm turn white ("acetowhite"). The acetic acid test offers the sharpest contrast between foci of normal and abnormal tissue. The procedure involves placing a gauze pad moistened with the solution on suspected flat lesions for 5 to 10 minutes. Penile lesions take longer to turn white than lesions on the vulva. When the pad is removed, the full extent of the lesion is sharply delineated by a white opacity. Examination with magnification after application of acetic acid is useful for detecting the smallest areas of infection.[16]

False-positive tests are common. Anything that causes parakeratosis causes acetowhitening. Candidiasis, psoriasis, lichen planus, sebaceous glands, and healing epithelium turn white in acetic acid. Inflammatory processes cause diffuse acetowhitening. An acetowhite genital wart appears as a circumscribed papular or macular lesion with a granular surface and a punctate vascular pattern. False-positive results can be minimized by selective testing. Patients with visible genital warts should be tested to identify the extent of the subclinical disease. Male sexual contacts of women with genital warts or women whose pap smears indicate dysplasia should also be tested.

---

*Adapted from Schachner L, Hankin DE: *J Am Acad Dermatol* 12:157, 1985.

Treatment

Management of sexual partners. Examination of sexual partners is not necessary for the management of genital warts because the role of reinfection is probably minimal. Many sexual partners have obvious warts and may desire treatment. The majority of partners are probably already subclinically infected with HPV, even if they do not have visible warts. The use of condoms may reduce transmission to partners likely to be uninfected, such as new partners. HPV infection may persist throughout a patient's lifetime in a dormant state and become infectious intermittently. Whether patients with subclinical HPV infection are as contagious as patients with exophytic warts is unknown. One study showed that the failure rate of treating women with condylomata acuminata did not decrease if their male sexual partners were also treated.[17]

Pregnancy. The use of podophyllin and podofilox is contraindicated during pregnancy. Genital papillary lesions have a tendency to proliferate and to become friable during pregnancy. Many experts advocate the removal of visible warts during pregnancy. HPV types 6 and 11 can cause laryngeal papillomatosis in infants. The route of transmission is unknown, and laryngeal papillomatosis has occurred in infants delivered by caesarean section. Caesarean delivery should not be performed solely to prevent transmission of HPV infection to the newborn. In rare instances, caesarean delivery may be indicated for women with genital warts if the pelvic outlet is obstructed or if vaginal delivery would result in excessive bleeding.

Podophyllum resin. Moist genital warts are most efficiently treated with 20% podophyllin resin in compound tincture of benzoin applied with a cotton-tipped applicator. The entire surface of the wart is covered with the solution, and the patient remains still until the solution dries in approximately 2 minutes. When lesions covered by the prepuce are treated, the applied solution must be allowed to dry for several minutes before the prepuce is returned to its usual position. Powdering the warts after treatment or applying petrolatum to the surrounding skin may help to avoid contamination of normal skin with the irritating resin. The medicine is removed by washing 1 hour later. The patient is treated again in 1 week. The podophyllum may then remain on the wart for 8 to 12 hours if there was little or no inflammation after the first treatment.

Overenthusiastic initial treatment can result in intense inflammation and discomfort that lasts for days. The procedure is simple and it is tempting to allow home treatment, but in most cases this should be avoided. Very frequently patients overtreat and cause excessive inflammation by applying podophyllum on normal skin. To avoid extreme discomfort, treat only part of a large warty mass in the perineal and rectal area. Warts on the shaft of the penis do not respond as successfully to podophyllum as do warts on the glans or under the foreskin; consequently, electrosurgery or cryosurgery should be used if two or three treatment sessions with podophyllum fail. Many warts disappear after a single treatment. Alternate forms of therapy should be attempted if there is no improvement after five treatment sessions.

WARNING. Systemic toxicity occurs from absorption of podophyllum. Paresthesia, polyneuritis, paralytic ileus, leukopenia, thrombocytopenia, coma, and death have occurred when large quantities of podophyllum were applied to wide areas or allowed to remain in contact with the skin for an extended period.[18] Only limited areas should be treated during each session. Very small quantities should be used in the mouth, vaginal tract, or rectosigmoid.

ALTERATION OF HISTOPATHOLOGY. Podophyllum can produce bizarre forms of squamous cells, which can be mistaken for squamous cell carcinoma. The pathologist must be informed of the patient's exposure to podophyllum when a biopsy of a previously treated wart is submitted.

Podofilox. Podofilox, also known as *podophyllotoxin*, is the main cytotoxic ingredient of podophyllin. Podofilox (Condylox) is available for self-application. Patients are instructed to apply the 0.5% solution to their external genital warts with a drug-dampened applicator twice each day for 3 consecutive days, followed by 4 days without treatment. It is recommended that no more than 10 cm^2 of wart tissue and no more than 0.5 ml of the solution should be used in a day. This cycle is repeated at weekly intervals for a maximum of 4 weeks. Approximately 15% of patients report severe local reactions to the treatment area after the first treatment cycle; this is reduced to 5% by the last treatment cycle. Local adverse effects of the drug, such as pain, burning, inflammation, and erosion, have occurred in more than 50% of patients.[19] Podofilox cleared 74% of warts in one study of women.[20] In another study, therapeutic benefits were enhanced by hydration of the wart and penetration with a grooved needle.[21] The drug is not recommended for use during pregnancy. A 3.5 ml bottle of Condylox with 24 cotton-tipped applicators costs approximately $60.00.

Trichloroacetic acid. Application of trichloroacetic acid (TCA) is effective and less destructive than laser surgery, electrocautery, or liquid nitrogen application. This is an ideal treatment for isolated lesions in pregnant women.[22] Most clinicians use 25% or 50% TCA, but a saturated solution (approximately 85%) may also be used. A very small amount is applied to the wart, which whitens immediately. The acid is then neutralized with water or bicarbonate of soda. The tissue slough heals in 7 to 10 days. Excessive application causes scars.

Electrosurgery. A limited number of warts on the shaft of the penis are best treated with conservative electrosurgery rather than by subjecting the patient to repeated sessions with podophyllum. Large, unresponsive masses of warts around the rectum or vulva may be treated by scissor excision of the bulk of the mass, followed by electrocautery of the remaining tissue down to the skin surface.[23] Removal of a very large mass of warts is a painful procedure and is best performed with the patient under general or spinal anesthesia in the operating room.

Cryosurgery. Liquid nitrogen delivered with a probe, as a spray, or applied with a cotton applicator is very effective for treating smaller genital warts. Warts on the shaft of the penis and vulva respond very well, with little or no scarring. Cryosurgery of the rectal area is painful. Cryotherapy is very effective and safe for both mother and fetus when applied in the second and third trimesters of pregnancy. An intermittent spray technique, using a small spray tip, is used to achieve a small region of cryonecrosis, limiting the run off and scattering of liquid nitrogen.[24] Cervical involvement that requires cervical cryotherapy does not increase the risk to mother or fetus.[25]

Carbon dioxide laser. The CO_2 laser is an ideal method for treating both primary and recurrent condyloma acuminata in men[26] and women because of its precision and the wound's rapid healing without scarring. The laser can be used with an operating microscope to find and destroy the smallest warts. A primary cure rate of 91% was accomplished with the following technique. Gross lesions were vaporized to the level of the surrounding skin surface. A brush technique was then used to superficially coagulate normal-appearing epithelial skin and mucosal surfaces contiguous to warts. This was done to eliminate subclinical virus infection within the normal-appearing epithelium and to avoid destruction of dermis. Extragenital sites were examined and treated to eliminate the most likely location for persistent recurrence. For pregnant women, this is the treatment of choice for large or extensive lesions and for cases that do not respond to repeated applications of trichloroacetic acid. Concern has been expressed about the potential viral contamination from the plumes of smoke generated by carbon dioxide laser treatment.

Interferon alfa-2b recombinant (Intron-A). Warts that do not respond to any form of conventional treatment and patients whose disease is severe enough to impose significant social or physical limitations on their activities may be candidates for treatment with interferon.[27] There are three naturally occurring interferons: alfa, beta, and gamma. Alfa, derived from lymphoblastic tissue, is approved by the FDA for the treatment of condyloma acuminata in patients 18 years of age or older. There are two commercially available preparations available for intralesional injection into the base of the wart. Alferon N injection (Interferon alfa-n3) is available in 1-ml vials; 0.05 ml per wart is administered twice weekly for up to 8 weeks. Intron-A (Interferon alfa-2b, recombinant) is available is several size vials, but the vial of 10 million IU is the only package size specifically designed for use in treatment of condyloma acuminata. Intron-A (0.1 ml of reconstituted Intron-A) is injected into each lesion three times per week on alternate days for 3 weeks. Influenza-like symptoms usually clear within 24 hours of treatment. Total clearing occurs in approximately 40% of treated warts. The medication is very expensive.

Topical 5-fluorouracil. Application of a 5-fluorouracil cream may be considered in cases of genital warts that are resistant to all other treatments. Vaginal warts are treated by inserting an applicator (such as the one supplied by Ortho Pharmaceutical Corporation for the treatment of vaginal *candida*) one-third full of 5% 5-fluorouracil cream (approximately 3 ml) deeply into the vagina at bedtime, once each week for up to 10 consecutive weeks.[28,29] The vulva and urethra are protected with petrolatum. A tampon should be inserted just inside the introitus. In one study, there was no evidence of disease in 85% of patients 3 months after treatment. Resistant cases were treated twice each week. Mild irritation and vaginal discharge may develop. The vulva should be protected with zinc oxide or hydrocortisone ointments if the twice-each-week regimen is used. Application to the keratinized epithelium (vulva, anus, and penis) twice weekly on 2 consecutive days is well tolerated but less effective; such treatment should not be used for pregnant women. Patients should be warned to avoid thick coverage because the excess cream causes inflammation or ulceration in the labiocrural or anal folds. Protective gloves are not necessary, provided that the hands are carefully washed after applying the 5-fluorouracil cream. A single intravaginal dose of 1.5-gm, 5% 5-fluorouracil cream contains only 75 mg of 5-fluorouracil. This is less than 10% of the usual systemic dose and far lower than the toxicity level of the drug even if rapid and complete absorption occurs.

Bowenoid Papulosis

Bowenoid papulosis is an uncommon condition seen in young, sexually active adults. It occurs on the genitals (vulva and circumcised penis) and histologically resembles Bowen's disease.[30] The mean age is 30 years for male patients and 32 years for female patients. Patients have ranged in age from 3 to 80 years. The duration of disease has been from 2 weeks to 11 years.[31] The natural history of the disease is unknown, but the lesions usually follow a benign clinical course and spontaneous regression is observed. Evolution of the lesions to invasive carcinoma is not observed.

The papules are asymptomatic discrete, small (averaging 4 mm in diameter), flat, reddish-violaceous or brown, often coalescent, and usually have a smooth, velvety surface. They may resemble flat warts, psoriasis, or lichen planus (Figure 11-6). In women the lesions are often darkly pigmented and are not as easily confused with other entities. They are located in men on the glans, the shaft, and the foreskin of the penis and in women on the labia majora and minora, on the clitoris, in the inguinal folds, and around the anus. Acetic acid compresses may be necessary to reveal intravaginal lesions. The lesions in women are often bilateral, hyperpigmented, and confluent. Autoinoculation probably explains the bilateral, symmetric distribution in moist areas. Many patients have a history of genital infection with viral warts or herpes simplex. Genital warts are primarily caused by HPV types 6 and 11. HPV type 16 has been found in a high percentage of women with bowenoid papulosis and in cervical and other genital neoplasias.[32,33,34] Therefore the cervix of female patients with bowenoid papulosis and other genitoanal HPV infections should be examined routinely, with careful follow-up. Female partners of patients with bowenoid papulosis should also be followed closely.

Treatment should be conservative. Individual lesions can be adequately treated by electrosurgery, carbon dioxide laser, cryosurgery, or scissor excision, much as ordinary verrucae, without the need for wide surgical margins. Alternatively, lesions may be treated for 3 to 5 weeks with 5% 5-fluorouracil cream until they become inflamed.

Figure 11-6
Bowenoid papulosis. Multiple brown verrucous papules on the shaft of the penis.

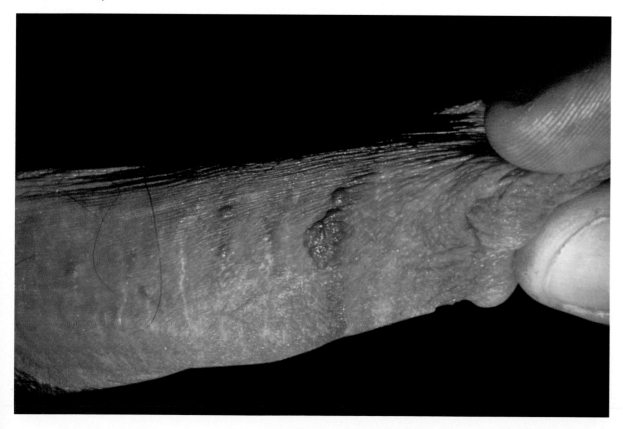

Molluscum Contagiosum

Clinical manifestations. Molluscum contagiosum papules are discrete, 2 to 5 mm in diameter, slightly umbilicated, flesh colored, and dome shaped. They spread by autoinoculation, by scratching, or by touching a lesion. The pubic (Figure 11-7) and genital areas (Figure 11-8) are most commonly involved in adults. Molluscum lesions in other areas are described in Chapter Twelve. They are frequently grouped. There may be few or many covering a wide area. Erythema and scaling at the periphery of a single or several lesions may occur (Figure 11-9). This may be the result of inflammation from scratching, or it may be a hypersensitivity reaction.

The differential diagnosis includes warts and herpes simplex. Molluscum papules are dome shaped, slightly umbilicated, firm, and white. Warts have an irregular, often velvety surface. The vesicles of herpes simplex rapidly become umbilicated (Figure 11-10).

Genital molluscum contagiosum in children may be a manifestation of sexual abuse.

Molluscum contagiosum is a common and at times severely disfiguring eruption in patients with HIV infection. It is often a marker of late-stage disease.[35]

Diagnosis. The patient must be carefully examined, since these discrete white-pink papules are often camouflaged by pubic hair. Most patients have just a few lesions that can be easily overlooked. The focus of examination is the pubic hair, the genitals, anal area, thighs, and trunk. Lesions may appear anywhere except the palms and soles. If necessary, the diagnosis can be easily established by laboratory methods (see Chapter Twelve).

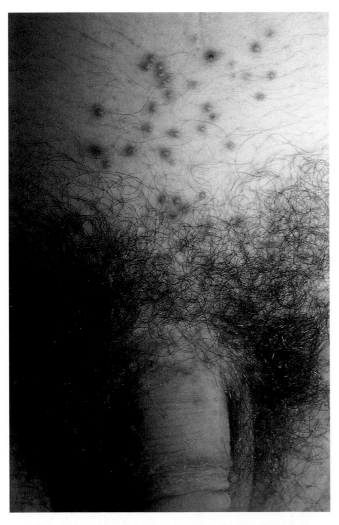

Figure 11-7
Molluscum contagiosum is a sexually transmitted disease in adults. Close observation of individual lesions is necessary to confirm the diagnosis. Lesions are often misdiagnosed as warts or herpes simplex.

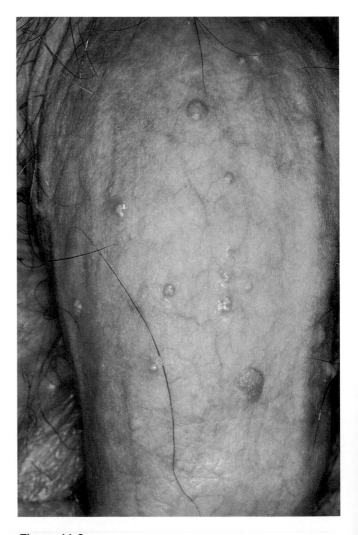

Figure 11-8
Molluscum contagiosum. Lesions are usually discrete, white, and dome shaped. They lack the many small projections found on the surface of genital warts.

Treatment. Genital lesions should be definitively treated to prevent spread through sexual contact. New lesions that were too small to be detected at the first examination may appear after treatment and require attention at a subsequent visit.

Curettage. Small papules can be quickly removed with a curette with or without local anesthesia. Bleeding is controlled with gauze pressure or Monsel's solution. Warn the patient that Monsel's solution is painful. Curettage is useful when there are a few lesions because it provides the quickest, most reliable treatment. A small scar may form; therefore, this technique should be avoided in cosmetically important areas.

Lidocaine/prilocaine (EMLA) cream applied 30 to 60 minutes before treatment effectively prevents the pain of curettage for children.[36]

Cryosurgery. Cryosurgery is the treatment of choice for patients who do not object to the pain. The papule is sprayed or touched lightly with a nitrogen-bathed cotton swab until the advancing, white, frozen border has progressed down the side of the papule to form a 1-mm halo on the normal skin surrounding the lesion. This should take approximately 5 seconds. A conservative approach is necessary because excessive freezing produces hypopigmentation or hyperpigmentation.

Cantharidin. A small drop of Cantharone (cantharidin 0.7%) is applied over the surface of the lesion, while contamination of normal skin is avoided. Lesions blister and may clear without scarring. New lesions occasionally appear at the site of the blister created by cantharidin. An alternate method is to apply a tiny amount of cantharidin or the more potent Verrusol (1% cantharidin, 30% salicylic acid, 5% podophyllin) and cover the area with tape for 1 day. The resulting small blister is treated with polysporin until the reaction subsides.

Laser therapy. In one study, lesions on the vulva cleared after treatment with the carbon dioxide laser. The power setting was 20 W with a spot size of 1.5 mm. The depth of therapy was approximately 3 mm.[37]

Trichloroacetic acid peel. Peels performed with 25% to 50% trichloroacetic acid (average 35%) and repeated every 2 weeks as needed resulted in an average reduction in lesion counts of 40.5% (range 0% to 90%) in HIV patients with extensive molluscum contagiosum. No spread of molluscum lesions, scarring, or secondary infection developed at 2 months' follow-up.[114]

Figure 11-9
Molluscum contagiosum. A single lesion became inflamed and disappeared 10 days later.

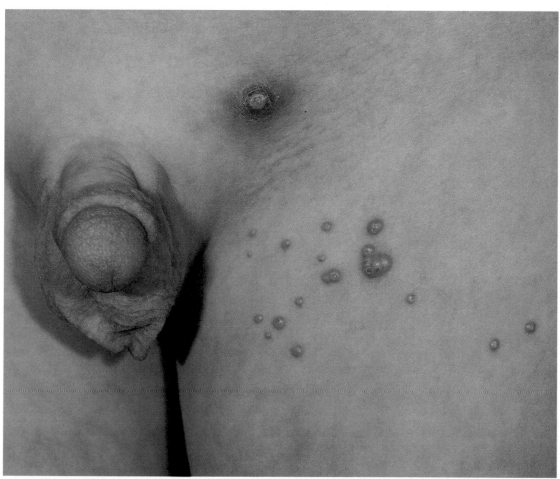

Genital Herpes Simplex

Herpes simplex infection of the penis (herpes progenitalis) (Figures 11-10 to 11-13), vulva (Figure 11-14), and rectum is pathophysiologically identical to herpes infection in other areas. Rarely seen a few decades ago, it has reached epidemic proportions. The public is well informed about the method of transmission, the potential for harm to the infected newborn, and its incurability. Recurrences cannot be predicted, but they often follow sexual intercourse. Sexual encounters are often delayed or avoided for fear of acquiring or transmitting the disease. The psychologic implications are obvious. Herpes simplex virus (HSV) type 2 may not be an important etiologic factor in cervical cancer as was once suspected.

Genital herpes is primarily a disease of young adults. Both antigenic type 1 and type 2 infect the genital area. The virus can be cultured for approximately 5 days from active genital lesions, and the lesions are almost certainly infectious during this time. There is evidence that both males and females who have no symptoms can transmit the disease.[38] Infection can develop in male patients from contact with female carriers who have no obvious disease. The infection may be acquired from an active cervical infection or from cervical secretions of a female who chronically carries the virus, from vulvar ulcers, from fissures, and from anorectal infection.[39]

Psychosocial implications. Herpes is a benign disorder that has a tremendous psychosocial impact.[40] The sensitive physician is aware of the spectrum of symptoms that can evolve and provides emotional support, especially at the time of initial diagnosis. The victim's response usually begins with initial shock and emotional numbing, then a frantic search for a cure. A sense of loneliness and isolation occurs after the patient becomes aware that the disease is chronic and incurable. The anxiety then generalizes to concerns about establishing relationships and that sexual gratification, marriage, and normal reproduction might not be possible. There is diminished self-esteem, social isolation, anxiety, and reluctance to initiate close relationships. Sexual drive persists, but there is a fear of initiating sexual relationships and an inhibition of sexual expression. A minority of patients experience deepening of depression with each recurrence, and all aspects of their lives are affected, including job performance. Recurrent disease can now be controlled by daily oral dosing with antiviral drugs such as acyclovir. This drug has significantly improved the quality of life for many herpes victims.

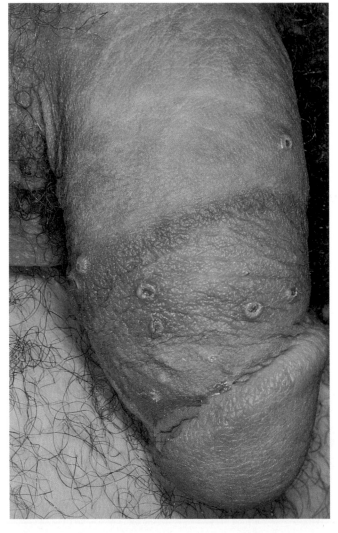

Figure 11-10
Primary herpes simplex. Vesicles are discrete and can be confused with warts and molluscum contagiosum. The primary lesion is a vesicle that rapidly becomes umbilicated.

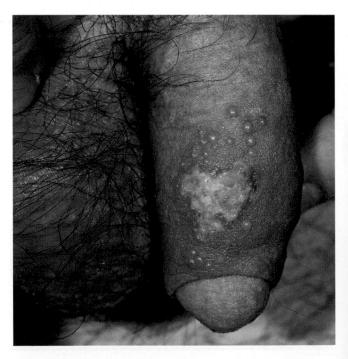

Figure 11-11
Primary herpes simplex. A group of vesicles has ruptured, leaving an erosion. Tense vesicles are at the periphery.

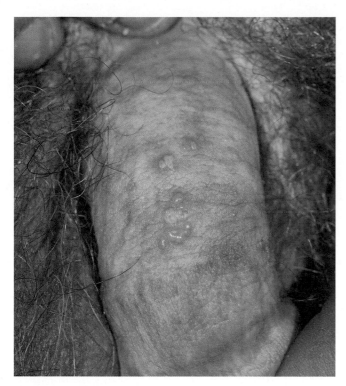

Figure 11-12
Recurrent herpes simplex. A small group of vesicles on an erythematous base. A few smaller vesicles show slight umbilication.

Figure 11-14 Primary herpes simplex.

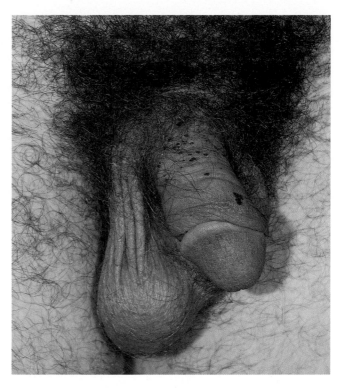

Figure 11-13
Recurrent herpes simplex. Scattered small crusts on the shaft of the penis. The diagnosis should be suspected even though vesicles are absent.

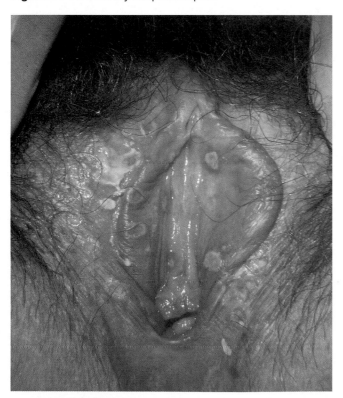

A, Scattered erosions covered with exudate.

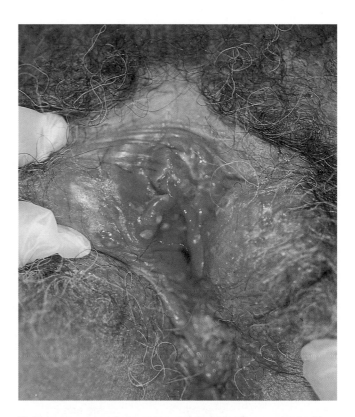

B, Numerous erosions appeared 4 days after contact with an asymptomatic carrier.

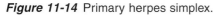

Risk factors for transmission of genital herpes

Rate of transmission. A group of heterosexual couples was studied in which one partner had symptomatic, recurrent genital HSV, and each susceptible partner was without serologic evidence of genital herpes.[41] Herpes simplex is transmitted more efficiently from males to females than from females to males. Seronegative female susceptible partners had the highest risk for acquiring genital herpes infection. The 32% annual risk in seronegative women was significantly higher than the 9% risk in HSV type 1 seropositive women and than the 6% or less risk in susceptible male partners, regardless of previous HSV type 1 infection.

Previous HSV type 1 infection. Previous infection with HSV type 1 reduces the rate of acquisition of genital HSV type 2 infection, reduces the severity of initial HSV type 2 infection, and may increase the proportion of persons acquiring HSV type 2 asymptomatically or subclinically. The presence of HSV type 1 antibody is associated with a decreased likelihood of detecting antibody to HSV type 2 in women.

Asymptomatic transmission. Asymptomatic or subclinical shedding of HSV is a major factor in the transmission of genital herpes infections. One study revealed that 69% of the cases of transmission resulted from sexual contact during periods of asymptomatic excretion of the virus. Thirty-five percent of source partners had no history or signs of genital herpes, and a third of those with symptomatic genital herpes apparently transmitted the infection during periods of asymptomatic shedding.[42] Therefore, highly motivated couples who are aware of the signs and symptoms of genital herpes and attempt to avoid sexual contact with lesions remain at substantial risk for transmission of genital herpes to the uninfected partner. Acyclovir therapy does not totally eliminate symptomatic or asymptomatic viral shedding or the potential for transmission.

Primary and recurrent infections

First-episode infections. First-episode infections include true primary infection and nonprimary first-episode infections. Patients with true primary infections have seronegative test results and have never been infected with any type of herpes virus. Patients with nonprimary first-episode infections have been infected at another site with either type 1 or 2 virus (e.g., the oral area) and have serum antibody and humoral immunity.

First-episode infections are more extensive and have more systemic symptoms. Viral shedding lasts longer (15 to 16 days) in primary first-episode infections.[43] Virus infections spread easily over moist surfaces. Women have more extensive disease and a higher incidence of constitutional symptoms probably because of the larger surface area involved. Wide areas of the female genitals may be covered with painful erosions (see Figure 11-14). The cervix is involved in most cases, and erosive cervicitis is almost always associated with first-episode disease. The virus can be isolated from the cervix in only 10% to 15% of women with recurrent disease. Inflammation, edema, and pain may be so

extreme that urination is interfered with and catheterization is required. The patient may be immobilized and require bed rest at home or in the hospital. A similar pattern of extensive involvement, with edema and possible urinary retention, develops in males, especially if uncircumcised. Crusts do not form under the foreskin (Figure 11-15). The eruption frequently extends onto the pubic area, and it is possibly spread from secretions during sexual contact. The anal area may be involved after anal intercourse.

Ten percent to fifteen percent of patients with first-episode genital herpes are simultaneously infected in the pharynx, probably as a result of orogenital contact.[44] They have extensive genital disease and exudative or ulcerative pharyngitis.

Recurrent infection

Frequency of recurrence. The frequency of recurrence varies with the anatomic site and the virus type.[45] The frequency of recurrences of genital HSV-2 herpes is higher than that of HSV-1 orolabial infection. HSV-1 oral infections recur more often than genital HSV-1 infections. HSV-2 genital infections occur 6 times more frequently than HSV-1 genital infections. The frequency of recurrence is lowest for orolabial HSV-2 infections. Ninety-five percent of patients with primary HSV-2 have recurrences, with a

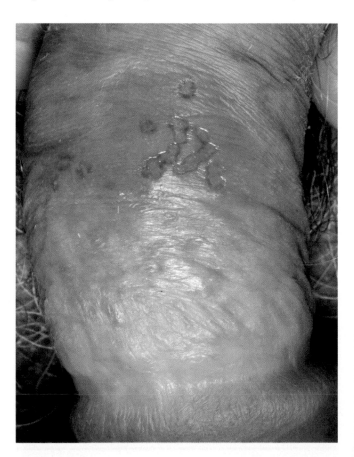

Figure 11-15
Recurrent herpes simplex under the foreskin. A group of discrete erosions is present. Crusts do not form on this moist surface.

median time to the first recurrence of approximately 50 days. Fifty percent of patients with primary HSV-1 have recurrent outbreaks, and the median time to the first recurrence is 1 year. The median number of recurrences during the first year for patients with HSV-2 is four, and 40% to 50% of patients have more than six recurrences per year. The recurrence rate stays at that level for at least 3 years.[45a] A recent study analyzed the recurrence rates in patients with a symptomatic first-episode HSV-2 genital infection (see the box below).[45a]

Recurrent infection in females may be so minor or hidden from view in the vagina or cervix that it is unnoticed. This may explain why some males with primary disease are not aware of the source. Some men transmit the disease when they are without symptoms. The site of asymptomatic shedding is unknown. Virus has not been isolated from the semen or urethra after primary infection.[46]

Prevention. Virus can be recovered from the eroded lesions for approximately 5 days after onset, but sexual contact should be avoided until reepithelialization is complete. Male (urethra) and female (cervix) carriers who have no symptoms can conceivably transmit the infection at any time. The use of spermicidal foams and condoms should be recommended to patients who have a history of recurrent genital herpes. For sexual partners who have both had genital herpes, protective measures are probably not necessary if both carry the same virus type (one partner infected the other) and active lesions are not present. Remember that having herpes in one area is not a protection from acquiring the infection in another location. Contact should be avoided when active lesions are present.

GENITAL HERPES RECURRENCE RATES DURING THE FIRST YEAR AFTER SYMPTOMATIC FIRST-EPISODE HSV-2 INFECTION

89% at least 1 recurrence
38% > 6 recurrences
20% >10 recurrences

NO OR 1 RECURRENCE

26% of women
8% of men

MORE THAN 10 RECURRENCES

14% of women
26% of men

Patients who had severe primary infection had recurrences nearly twice as often and had a shorter time to first recurrence compared with those who had shorter first episodes.

From Benedetti J et al: Recurrence rates in genital herpes after symptomatic first-episode infection, *Ann Intern Med* 121:847-854, 1994.

Laboratory diagnosis

The sensitivity of all laboratory methods depends on the stage of lesions (sensitivity is higher in vesicular than in ulcerative lesions), on whether the patient has a first or a recurrent episode of the disease (higher in first episodes), and on whether the sample is from an immunosuppressed or an immunocompetent patient (more antigen is found in immunosuppressed patients). It is crucial to document genital herpes simplex infection in pregnant women and cutaneous herpes in newborn infants. Consequently, in these instances suspicious vesicular and eroded lesions should be cultured. In all other forms the clinical presentation is usually so characteristic that an accurate diagnosis can be made by inspection. A number of laboratory procedures are available if confirmation is desired.[47]

Culture. The most definitive method for diagnosis is viral culture. Specimens are inoculated into tube cell cultures and monitored microscopically for characteristic morphologic changes (cytopathic effects for up to 5 to 7 days after inoculation for maximum sensitivity). Results may be available in 1 or 2 days. It is essential that the lesion to be sampled is in the vesicular or early ulcerative stage. Resolving lesions (usually 5 days or more) are not generally productive for culture. Vesicles are punctured and the fluid is absorbed into the swab, which is then rubbed onto the base of the lesion. Cervical samples are taken from the endocervix with the swab. From the viewpoint of cost, the insertion of separate swabs from a number of anatomic sites (cervix, vaginal ulcers, vaginal fissures, anus) into one culture vial is the most efficient way to collect genital samples for viral culture.

Tzanck smear. The best results are obtained from intact vesicles. Giant cells with 2 to 15 nuclei are the characteristic finding. Recently infected cells contain a single enlarged nucleus with a thick membrane. Later, the cells begin to fuse and become multinuclear, and the nuclear membrane continues to thicken (Figure 11-16). Characteristic granular, eosinophilic intranuclear inclusions then appear that can be seen only with the Papanicolaou stain.

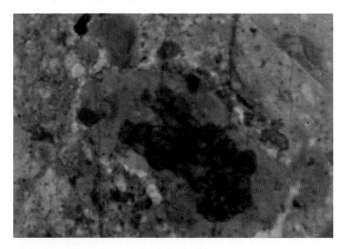

Figure 11-16
Tzanck smear. Multinucleated giant cell.

Specimens are prepared by carefully removing the roof of the vesicle and scraping the underlying moist skin with a #15 surgical blade. Cells are obtained from the base and margins of vesicles or ulcers; vesicular fluid is not to be used. The material is smeared onto a glass slide, fixed for 1 minute with absolute alcohol, and then stained with Giemsa or Wright's stain. An alternate method is to add toluidine blue O 1% wt/vol aqueous solution to an air-dried slide specimen and rinse off with tap water in 15 seconds. Air drying is repeated, and a cover glass is applied over permanent mounting medium. Alternatively, a fast method using a commercially available series of solutions (Diffquik) is used in many laboratories. The material can be stained in approximately 1 minute. Material from lesions of herpes zoster produces identical results.

Papanicolaou smear. This technique is useful for detecting HSV-infected cells in cervical tissue from women without symptoms; routine smears often reveal unsuspected herpes infection. The interpretation of this preparation requires experience. The cells are smeared onto slides, fixed with 95% ethanol or commercial fixative, stained with Papanicolaou's stain, and observed under the microscope. Recently infected cells contain a single enlarged nucleus with a thick membrane. Later, the cells begin to fuse and become multinuclear, and the nuclear membrane continues to thicken. Characteristic granular, eosinophilic intranuclear inclusions then appear.

Histopathology. An intact vesicle should be biopsied. The histologic picture is characteristic but not unique for herpes simplex.

Serology: herpes simplex IgG and IgM serum antibodies. Fifty percent to ninety percent of adults have antibody to HSV. More than 70% of the population have antibody levels ranging from 1:10 to 1:160; only 5% have titers greater than 1:160. Because of the high incidence of antibodies to herpes simplex in the population, assay of a single serum specimen is not of great value. Routine tests do not discriminate between antibodies to herpes types 1 and 2. IgG and IgM are measured in separate tests. Normal titers are less than 1:5 for IgG and IgM. The presence of IgM or a fourfold or greater rise in IgG titer indicates recent infection. The convalescent sample should be drawn 2 to 3 weeks after the acute specimen is drawn. The presence of IgG indicates past exposure.

Subtyping. There are two serotypes of HSV. HSV-1 infections are primarily oropharyngeal; genital infections can also be caused by this serotype. HSV-2 infections are primarily genital but are also detected in the mouth. Subtyping can be helpful for epidemiologic study and patient counseling but is not commonly done in office practice. Typing is done by direct immunofluorescence on cells that have been smeared on a glass slide with saline and dried, or by direct fluorescent antibody testing with monoclonal antibodies on cultured specimens, a highly sensitive test. The newly developed type-specific serologic methods can identify patients with recurrent genital HSV-2 infection, as well as those with unrecognized or subclinical infection.[39]

Treatment (see Table 12-2, p. 339)

Cool compresses. Extensive erosions on the vulva and penis may be treated with silver nitrate 0.5% or Burow's compresses applied for 20 minutes several times daily. This effective local therapy reduces edema and inflammation, macerates and debrides crust and purulent material, and relieves pain. The legs may be supported with pillows under the knees to expose the inflamed tissues and promote drying.

Acyclovir

FIRST CLINICAL EPISODE OF GENITAL HERPES. Primary genital infections of limited extent may be treated with acyclovir ointment (Zovirax) applied every 3 hours six times daily for 7 days. The ointment may be applied before and after wet compresses or may be applied as the only treatment for limited primary infections. Primary genital infections that are severe may be treated intravenously or orally[48] with acyclovir. The intravenous dosage is 5 mg/kg infused at a constant rate over 1 hour every 8 hours for 7 days in adults with normal renal function. The oral dosage is 200 mg five times each day for 7 to 10 days. This schedule decreases the duration of viral excretion, the formation of new lesions, and the duration of vesicle formation, and it promotes rapid healing.

RECURRENT EPISODES. Treatment of recurrent episodes is most effective when instituted during the prodrome or within 2 days of onset of lesions. However, since early treatment can seldom be administered, most immunocompetent patients with recurrent disease do not benefit from acyclovir treatment, and it is not generally recommended. The recommended regimens are acyclovir 200 mg orally five times a day for 5 days, acyclovir 400 mg orally three times a day for 5 days, or acyclovir 800 mg orally two times a day for 5 days. Patients with primary or recurrent herpes genitalis who are immunocompromised may be treated intravenously with Zovirax.

DAILY SUPPRESSIVE THERAPY. Oral acyclovir is effective for the suppression of frequently recurring episodes of genital herpes.[49] The standard dosage is acyclovir 200 mg three to five times per day or acyclovir 400 mg orally two times a day. Treatment is continued for at least 6 to 12 months. Patients should be encouraged to interrupt suppressive treatment periodically to reassess the frequency of episodes and the need for continued treatment. Long-term suppressive therapy (longer than 5 years) appears to be safe.[50] Suppressive therapy does not totally eliminate symptomatic or asymptomatic viral shedding or the potential for transmission.

Lubrication. Occlusive ointments such as petroleum jelly should not be applied to eroded lesions. Light lubricating body lotions are soothing when inflammation subsides and tissues become dry.

Women with multiple eroded lesions on the labia experience great discomfort while urinating. Pain can be avoided by sitting in a bathtub of water and urinating while holding the labia apart.

Neonatal Herpes Simplex Virus Infection

Neonatal infection is serious but rare. It occurs in 1 of every 2500 to 1 of every 10,000 deliveries per year.[51] Boys are affected twice as frequently as girls. Approximately half the infected babies are born prematurely, which raises the question of whether reactivation can trigger early onset of labor. The mortality rate is approximately 50% in the absence of therapy, and many survivors have ocular or neurologic complications. Most infected neonates are exposed to the virus during vaginal delivery, but infection may occur in utero, by transplacental or ascending infection, or postnatally from relatives or attendants. Herpes simplex virus–positive papules may be present on the skin at birth. Infants born to women who have an active primary HSV infection have a risk of approximately 50% of acquiring an infection.[52]

Clinical signs. Clinical signs of infection in the neonate are usually present between 1 and 7 days of life. In one study, the presenting symptoms were neurologic in 79%, cutaneous in 30%, respiratory in 19%, cyanosis/pallor/grayish skin in 16%, irritability in 12%, and fever in 7%. Herpes simplex virus was detected most early and frequently in pharyngeal swabs (in one third on postnatal days 2 to 5). Cerebrospinal fluid (CSF) contained an increased amount of protein, pleocytosis, or both in 72%.[53] Progression to systemic infection from isolated skin vesicles can occur in a matter of days. The mean age at diagnosis is 12.8 days, but at the time of diagnosis these infants have had symptoms for an average of 5 days. This delay in diagnosis puts the infant at great risk of internal disease, which is preventable with antiviral therapy if treatment is started when only skin disease is present.[54] The infection can be limited to the skin, eyes, or mouth or can affect the central nervous system (CNS) or visceral organs, causing hepatitis, pneumonitis, intravascular coagulopathy, or encephalitis.

Prognosis. A large collaborative study showed no deaths among infants with localized HSV infection. The mortality rate was 57% in neonates with disseminated infection and 15% in neonates with encephalitis. Therefore the most important predictor of death is visceral involvement. The risk of death was increased in neonates who were in or near coma, had disseminated intravascular coagulopathy, or were premature. In babies with disseminated disease, HSV pneumonitis was associated with greater mortality. In the survivors, morbidity was most frequent in infants with encephalitis, disseminated infection, seizures, or infection with HSV type 2. With HSV infection limited to the skin, eyes, or mouth, the presence of three or more recurrences of vesicles was associated with an increased risk of neurologic impairment as compared with two or fewer recurrences.[55]

Treatment. The early identification of skin lesions is critical for the outcome of infections that originate in the skin. Ninety percent of infants with initial herpetic skin lesions treated with acyclovir 30 mg/kg/day had no sequelae.[56] A large study showed no differences in outcome between vidarabine (30 mg/kg/day) and acyclovir (30 mg/kg/day) in the treatment of neonatal HSV infection.[57] Death is unusual when disease is limited to the skin but occurs in 15% to 50% of cases of brain and disseminated disease, even with antiviral therapy. Despite antiviral therapy, there is evidence of impairment in approximately 10% of children and debility in more than 50% with CNS and visceral disease.

GENITAL HERPES SIMPLEX DURING PREGNANCY

Neonatal herpes is a well recognized complication of symptomatic maternal primary genital infection at the time of delivery, but most cases are associated with asymptomatic virus shedding and absence of a history of genital herpes.

Infants whose mothers were exposed to herpes virus during pregnancy and in whom a primary infection then develops are at greater risk for morbidity and death than infants whose mothers had herpes before pregnancy and then experienced a recurrence. HSV-2 acquired during pregnancy can infect the products of conception in utero and cause congenital infection that results in spontaneous abortion.[58]

Of the asymptomatic women who shed HSV in early labor, approximately a third have recently acquired genital HSV, and their infants are 10 times more likely to have neonatal HSV than those of women with asymptomatic reactivation of HSV. The presence of maternal antibodies specific to HSV-2 but not to HSV-1 appears to reduce the neonatal transmission of HSV-2.[59] The presence or absence of transplacentally acquired antibody against HSV probably contributes to the difference in neonatal attack rates and morbidity. Neonates born to mothers with a recurrent HSV infection are likely to have HSV antibody at birth, whereas those born to mothers with a primary infection may not.[60]

Fifty to seventy percent of neonates with HSV infection are born to mothers who do not have a history of genital herpes infection during pregnancy.[61,62] Most are probably exposed to HSV as a result of the mother's asymptomatic infection. Asymptomatic shedding of virus from the genitals during pregnancy is more frequent after resolution of primary genital herpes than in nonprimary first-episode infection. Asymptomatic shedding from the cervix is more common after a primary infection, and the labia are more likely to be involved in a recurrent nonprimary infection.

Diagnosis. Laboratory methods rely on culturing herpes simplex virus in living cells in vitro. However, the availability of monoclonal antibodies allows for rapid assays for the confirmation of cultured herpes simplex virus (Kodak SURECELL-herpes test).

Management. Routine antenatal screening in the last trimester of pregnant women with a history of genital herpes before pregnancy is not advised, because the results have been shown to be unreliable in predicting viral shedding and hence the infants' risk of exposure to virus at delivery. The most useful current strategy for management is careful examination of the vulva and cervix for herpes lesions in women coming to labor. All pregnant women, regardless of their history of genital herpes, should be assessed for genital herpes at the time of their hospital admission for labor. The external genitals should be carefully examined for characteristic lesions. Speculum examination of the cervix is not routinely necessary since isolated cervical lesions are unusual.

The virus infects nearly 50% of infants whose mothers have primary genital herpes, whereas less than 5% of infants exposed to recurrent maternal infection at the time of delivery become infected. Therefore women who present with their first clinical episode of genital herpes at delivery should have a caesarean section performed. Even if active lesions are present, in women with a history of recurrent herpes, the risks to the infant are low. The current practice of caesarean delivery for women with a history of genital herpes lesions that recur at delivery is being reevaluated.[63] Staff should be alert to the dangers of postnatal infection and measures should be taken to exclude or reduce virus excretion from staff members or visitors who have orolabial or cutaneous herpes lesions.

Most neonatal exposure to HSV results from the excretion of virus at delivery in mothers without symptoms. Many of these mothers do not have a history of genital herpes. Approximately 1% of women with known recurrent genital herpes shed the virus without showing symptoms on the day of delivery. Sequential cultures of specimens taken late in gestation from women with a history of recurrent genital herpes infection do not predict the infant's risk of exposure to HSV at delivery. It might be worthwhile to obtain a specimen for viral culture at the time of delivery from women with a history of recurrent genital herpes infection. Approximately 1 in 100 of these culture results are positive. The attack rate after such exposure is less than 8%, but such cultures can identify babies who require close observation and can encourage the suspicion of herpes infection if they become ill.[64] The attack rate of neonatal herpes is 50% if the maternal infection at the time of delivery is primary.

Primary herpes simplex virus infection during pregnancy

The rate of complications is high for the fetus after maternal symptomatic primary disease. Whether a similar high rate of complication occurs after asymptomatic primary genital herpes infection requires further study. The greatest risk was observed in women who acquired primary genital herpes during the third trimester of pregnancy. The rate was greater than 40% when infection occurred during the third trimester. Complications included aborted pregnancy, premature labor (36%), and transmission of infection to the infant either in utero or at delivery. When several weeks had elapsed between the primary first episode and delivery, intrauterine growth retardation was observed, the mechanism of which is unknown.[65]

During the first 20 weeks of gestation, primary infection is associated with an increased frequency of spontaneous abortion, stillbirth, and congenital malformations, particularly hydraencephaly and chorioretinitis. However, most infants whose mothers have a primary infection during the first or second trimester are healthy.[65]

Management. If a woman experiences her first attack of genital HSV infection around the time of delivery, the risk that her neonate will acquire an HSV infection is high. In this circumstance a caesarean delivery is probably prudent. If infection occurs during the first, second, or early in the third trimester, the mother must be followed and managed as indicated in the following discussion.

Recurrent herpes simplex virus infection during pregnancy

The risk of symptomatic neonatal HSV infection after vaginal delivery in women with known recurrent genital HSV infections is very low. The frequency of asymptomatic maternal HSV infection during the week before delivery is 1.3%. The frequency at delivery is 1.4%.[66]

Management. Women with a history of genital HSV infection are at risk of asymptomatic viral excretion at delivery. Detection of asymptomatic shedding before delivery does not predict asymptomatic reactivation at the time of delivery. Therefore monitoring pregnant women by means of cultured cervical specimens is inappropriate. Women with a history of genital HSV infection who have no symptoms at the onset of labor should be advised that the risk of exposure to excreted HSV is low and that even if inadvertent exposure occurs, the risk that the neonate will acquire an HSV infection is less than 8%.[64,65] There are no rapid diagnostic methods to detect asymptomatic maternal HSV excretion in the birth canal at the onset of labor. Until these tests become available, vaginal delivery is reasonable for women who have a history of genital herpes but who have no signs or symptoms of recurrence at the onset of labor. The neonatal and maternal morbidity and mortality associated with caesarean delivery must be weighed against the low risk of asymptomatic HSV excretion at delivery and the low rate of HSV infection in infants exposed to recurrent maternal HSV infection. If reactivation occurs late in gestation, serial viral cultures can be useful in demonstrating the cessation of viral shedding. Exposure of infants to HSV should be avoided by caesarean delivery if the mother has herpetic lesions in the genital area at the onset of labor.

Acyclovir for treating pregnant patients

The safety of systemic acyclovir therapy has not been established for pregnant women. In the presence of life-threatening maternal HSV infection (e.g., disseminated infection that includes encephalitis, pneumonitis, and/or hepatitis), intravenously administered acyclovir is probably of value. Among pregnant women without life-threatening disease, systemic acyclovir treatment should not be used for recurrent genital herpes episodes or as suppressive therapy to prevent reactivation near term. Asymptomatic shedding of virus is not prevented by use of oral acyclovir during late gestation in proven recurrent genital herpes even though plasma acyclovir levels are within the normal range.[68,69]

Acquired Immunodeficiency Syndrome

Acquired immunodeficiency syndrome (AIDS) is the end stage of human immunodeficiency virus (HIV) infection. The infection causes a profound defect in cell-mediated immunity, which causes complicating opportunistic infections and neoplastic processes. The initial event is a symptomatic or an asymptomatic HIV infection. The infection may then not be apparent for months or years. In an undetermined number of patients, symptoms emerge and the disease progresses to AIDS. Internal infections[67,70] are the major cause of death. Infections can be controlled but are rarely curable. Most result from reactivation of previously acquired organisms. Concurrent or consecutive infections with a different organism are common. Infections are severe and commonly disseminated.

The virus. HIV is a retrovirus. Retroviruses carry a positive-stranded RNA and use a DNA polymerase enzyme called *reverse transcriptase* to convert viral RNA to DNA. This reverses the usual process of transcription whereby DNA is converted to RNA, thus the term *retrovirus*. HIV attaches to a protein receptor site (CD4) on the surface of CD4+ lymphocytes, penetrates the cell, and exposes its RNA core; then reverse transcriptase converts viral RNA to DNA, which becomes part of the host genome. New viral particles are then produced during normal cellular division, and CD4+ lymphocytes are destroyed.

CD4+ T-lymphocyte destruction leads to infection. HIV selectively attacks helper/inducer CD4+ T lymphocytes, decreases their number, and interferes with their function. CD4+ T lymphocytes are responsible for modulation of essentially the entire immune response. Lymphopenia occurs because of the reduced numbers of CD4+ T lymphocytes. Infections normally controlled by cellular immunity occur with markedly increased frequency.

The initial HIV infection. The incubation period is unknown but has been estimated to be 3 to 6 weeks. An acute mononucleosis-like syndrome develops in 50% to 70% of patients approximately 3 to 6 weeks after initial infection. There is fever, myalgia-arthralgias, pharyngitis, and a diffuse red eruption[71] consisting of macules 0.5 to 2.0 cm in diameter.[72] The symptoms resolve spontaneously within 8 to 12 days. Seroconversion may take place within 1 week to 3 months, and then there is a dramatic decline in viremia. The T-helper cells remain at a normal level of more than 500/mm³, and the patient is without symptoms. After the initial infection viremia may persist for life.

The evolution of disease (Figure 11-17). After primary infection, viral dissemination, and the appearance of HIV-specific immunity, most patients have a period of "clinical latency" that lasts for years. The clinical presentation of patients with HIV infections ranges from asymptomatic, through chronic generalized lymphadenopathy, to subclinical and clinical T-cell deficiency. There is strong association between the development of life-threatening opportunistic illnesses and the absolute number (per microliter of blood) or percentage of CD4+ T lymphocytes. As the number of CD4+ T lymphocytes decreases, the risk and severity of opportunistic illnesses increase. The revised Centers for Disease Control classification system for HIV infection categorizes persons on the basis of clinical conditions associated with HIV infection and CD4+ T-lymphocyte counts. Measures of CD4+ T lymphocytes are used to guide clinical and therapeutic management.

Progression to AIDS Patients have a number of symptoms during disease progression. They exhibit prolonged constitutional symptoms such as chronic fatigue, night sweats, fever, weight loss, and diarrhea. They frequently have clinical manifestations of T-cell dysfunction such as mucous membrane disease (oral candidiasis, hairy leukoplakia) and dermatologic diseases (herpes simplex/zoster, fungal infections).[73]

AIDS is the end stage of HIV infection. It is characterized by a variety of unusual tumors and opportunistic infections. There appears to be a spectrum of disease, and long-term survival may be possible. The probability of survival is 49% at 1 year and 15% at 5 years.

Revised Centers for Disease Control classification and management The revised Centers for Disease Control (CDC) classification system (1993) for HIV-infected adolescents and adults replaces the system published by the CDC in 1986 and is primarily intended for use in public health practice. It categorizes persons on the basis of clinical conditions associated with HIV infection and CD4+ T-lymphocyte counts. The system is based on three ranges of CD4+ T-lymphocyte counts and three clinical categories of conditions associated with HIV infection and is represented by a matrix of nine mutually exclusive categories. The three CD4+ T-lymphocyte categories are defined as follows:

- Category 1: greater than 500 cells/μL
- Category 2: 200 to 499 cells/μL
- Category 3: less than 200 cells/μL

Antimicrobial prophylaxis and antiretroviral therapies have been shown to be most effective within certain levels of immune dysfunction. Antiretroviral therapy should be considered for all persons with CD4+ T-lymphocyte counts of less than 500/μL, and prophylaxis against *Pneumocystis carinii* pneumonia (PCP), the most common serious opportunistic infection diagnosed in men and women with AIDS, is recommended for all persons with CD4+ T-lymphocyte counts of less than 200/μL and for persons who have had prior episodes of PCP. Because of these recommendations, CD4+ T-lymphocyte determinations are an integral part of medical management of HIV-infected persons in the United States.

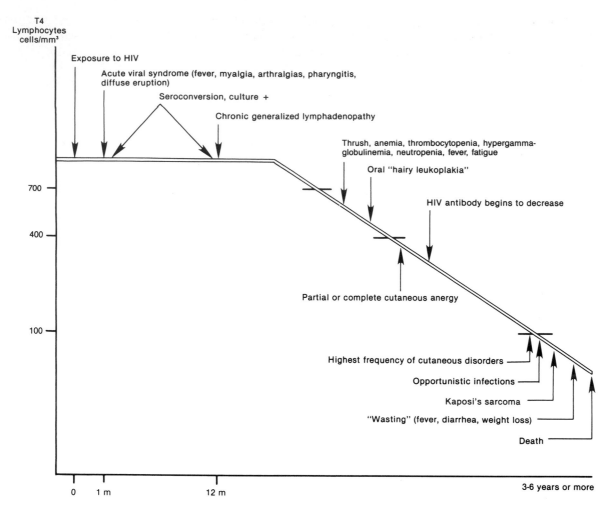

Figure 11-17
AIDS. Evolution of the disease.

ACQUIRED IMMUNODEFICIENCY SYNDROME AND CUTANEOUS DISEASE

Cutaneous diseases are markers for AIDS.[74-78] Their presence may be the first indication of HIV infection, and they can result in significant morbidity. A complete list is found in Table 11-1. Illustrations of these diseases are found in Figures 11-18 to 11-33. The most common skin disorders in HIV disease are caused by infections.

Herpes simplex

Herpes simplex infections are common in patients with AIDS. The herpes virus may unmask and potentiate a subclinical HIV infection. Herpes infections may have an atypical appearance and course and may be severe, disfiguring, and persistent. If left untreated, the ulcers can become deeply erosive and lead to intractable ulcerations. Secondary bacterial infection further distorts the ulcers. Severe progressive perianal and rectal ulcers are seen primarily in

homosexual men.[104] Chronic perianal ulcers caused by herpes simplex virus have been erroneously diagnosed as decubitus ulcers.[105] The infection may be widely distributed and may be confused with other diseases such as impetigo.

Oral acyclovir is usually effective to treat mild mucocutaneous disease in immunocompromised hosts; intravenous therapy (15 mg/kg/day) is required to treat extensive disease. Suppressive therapy is effective and is often necessary because of recurrent disease. Acyclovir-resistant herpes simplex virus infections may become a widespread problem in patients with AIDS.

Herpes zoster

Herpes zoster infection may be an early indicator of HIV disease. It frequently occurs in persons in whom AIDS develops later. The potential for nosocomial transmission with primary varicella and herpes zoster should be kept in mind, particularly in wards where a high proportion of

TABLE 11-1 HIV Infection—Cutaneous Manifestations

Disease	Clinical manifestations	Diagnosis	Treatment
VIRAL INFECTIONS			
Acute HIV exanthema (HIV primary infection)	Fever, myalgias, urticaria Truncal maculopapular eruption Mononucleosis-like syndrome Generalized lymphadenopathy follows later	Time to seroconversion unknown Antibodies found 3 wk to 6 mo after initial infection Low white blood cell count, thrombocytopenia, hypergammaglobulinemia	Zidovudine (AZT) (Retrovir)
Herpes simplex (common)	Persistent erosions and ulcerations Widely disseminated Resembles other infections Intractable perirectal ulcerations Regional lymphadenopathy	HSV culture Tzanck smear for multinucleated giant cells HSV-2 infection is risk factor for subsequent or concurrent HIV infection[79]	200 mg acyclovir 5 times a day until resolved or 15 mg/kg/day intravenously for severe disease Acyclovir ointment Foscarnet (Foscavir)
Herpes zoster Shingles (common sign of AIDS)	Shingles may be severe, resulting in deep scarring Persistent disseminated lesions Intractable herpetic pain	Herpes virus culture Tzanck smear for multinucleated giant cells	25-30 mg/kg/day acyclovir intravenously or 800 mg 5 times orally a day for less severe cases Strict isolation if patient is hospitalized
Chicken pox (uncommon)	Chicken pox with numerous lesions and pneumonia		Same treatment as for herpes zoster
Molluscum contagiosum	Clusters of white umbilicated papules Persistent on face, groin Cutaneous cryptococcus[80,81] can mimic molluscum contagiosum	KOH preparations of soft material in center of lesion show large viral inclusions Biopsy—large viral inclusions	Cryosurgery, curettage Scissor excision with blunt-tipped scissors Trichloroacetic acid peels for extensive cases[114]
Warts/condyloma (common) Human Papilloma Virus (HPV)	Common warts—extensive[82] and persistent Condylomas—increased prevalence, number, size Cervical, anal squamous cell carcinoma (HPV-16,18)	Biopsy or clinical appearance Profound reduction in CD4+ cells	Topical agents, cryosurgery, blunt dissection, excision, surgery
Hairy leukoplakia (Epstein-Barr virus[83]) (common)	Whitish, nonremovable verrucous hairy plaques on sides of tongue[84,85] May resemble fungal tongue infections	Biopsy—acanthosis and parakeratosis with large, pale-staining cells with pyknotic nuclei	Treating oral *Candida* improves appearance Podophyllin resin 25% in ethanol and acetone[115]
FUNGAL INFECTIONS			
Candida albicans (very common)	White plaques on cheeks, tongue Sore throat, dysphagia Deep tongue erosions, thick plaques back of throat Esophageal infection Intractable vaginal infection *Candida* nail infection	Culture Obtain specimen for KOH slide preparation with cotton swab	Nystatin oral suspension Clotrimazole (Mycelex Troche) 10 mg 5x/daily Ketoconazole (200 mg PO qd) Fluconazole 100-200 mg PO qd Amphotericin B (severe cases) 0.3 mg/kg IV qd
Tinea versicolor (common)	Common early and late in HIV infection Thick, scaly hypopigmented or light-brown plaques on trunk	KOH slide preparation shows numerous short hyphae and spores Wood's light accentuates lesions	Topical: selenium sulfide, miconazole, clotrimazole, sodium thiosulfate Oral: ketoconazole (various dosage schedules)

Continued.

TABLE 11-1, cont'd HIV Infection—Cutaneous Manifestations

Disease	Clinical manifestations	Diagnosis	Treatment

Dermatophytes
  Tinea corporis
  Tinea pedis
  Tinea cruris
  Onychomycoses (common)
	Extensive involvement, especially groin and feet
	Thick keratoderma—blennorrhagic-like lesions on feet
	Proximal subungual onychomycosis
		KOH slide preparation shows branched, septated hyphae	Topical: miconazole, clotrimazole, many others
			Oral: griseofulvin, ketoconazole, itraconazole, fluconazole

Cryptococcus neoformans (rare)	White papules that resemble molluscum contagiosum	Assays for antigen in serum or cerebrospinal fluid India ink or Wright stain Culture Biopsy	Amphotericin B 0.5-0.6 mg/kg IV qd or add flucytosine Itraconazole 200 mg PO bid Fluconazole 200-400 mg PO qd
Histoplasma capsulatum (rare)	Multiple papules, nodules, macules and oral and skin ulcers on arms, face, trunk Travel history (South America)	Biopsy—PAS stain Crushed tissue preparation—rapid diagnosis Culture—several weeks required	Amphotericin B 0.5-0.6 mg/kg IV qd Itraconazole 200 mg PO bid
Penicillium marneffei (Southeast Asia)	Fever, anemia, weight loss, molluscum-like papules, cough, lymphadenopathy, hepatomegaly	Culture—skin, blood, bone marrow Skin touch prep Yeast forms with central septae	Amphotericin B, oral imidazoles, lifelong prophylaxis to prevent recurrence
BACTERIAL INFECTIONS			
Staphylococcus aureus (common)	Bullous impetigo—axillae or groin Facial or truncal folliculitis (resembling acne) Impetigo of beard and body	Culture	Dicloxicillin Cefadroxil (many others)
Syphilis (uncommon)	Generalized papulosquamous papules and plaques Can mimic almost any inflammatory cutaneous disorder Incubation period for neurosyphilis may be very brief (months)[86]	VDRL titer may be very high or negative;[87] obtain sequential tests or skin biopsy with special stains	Standard recommended treatment may not be sufficient to prevent central nervous system disease[88,89] See Chapter 10
ARTHROPOD			
Scabies (uncommon)	Generalized crusted papules[90] Norwegian scabies—generalized hyperkeratotic eruption	KOH or oil preparation shows mites	Lindane (Kwell) Premethrin (Elimite)
PROLIFERATIVE DISORDERS			
Seborrheic dermatitis (common)	Red scaling plaques with yellowish, greasy scales and crust Distinct margins, hypopigmentation of scalp, face; sometimes groin, extremities Severity correlates with degree of clinical deterioration	Biopsy differs from ordinary seborrheic dermatitis Parakeratosis is widespread Necrotic keratinocytes Dermoepidermal obliteration by lymphocytes Sparse spongiosis Thick-walled vessels Do KOH to rule out tinea[91]	200-400 mg/day ketoconazole Ketoconazole cream Group V topical steroids
Psoriasis (uncommon)	Activation of previous disease or no history[92]	Biopsy	Treatment-resistant cases may respond to etretinate or zidovudine[93,94] Calcipotriol ontment (Dovonex)

TABLE 11-1, cont'd HIV Infection—Cutaneous Manifestations

Disease	Clinical manifestations	Diagnosis	Treatment
Xeroderma (common) Ichthyosis (uncommon)	Severe dry skin may be associated with erythroderma, seborrheic dermatitis, and dementia Ichthyosiform scaling of legs, keratoderma of palms and soles	Clinical presentation	Lactic acid emollients (Lac-Hydrin)
Pruritic papular eruption (common)	2-5 mm skin-colored papules on head, neck, upper trunk[95] Pruritis and number of papules may wax and wane with time	Biopsy—lymphocytic perivascular infiltrate with numerous eosinophils Follicular damage	Ultraviolet B phototherapy[116,117] Often resistent to topical steroids and oral antihistamines Antipruritic lotions (Sarna) Dapsone 100 mg qd possibly effective
Eosinophilic pustular folliculitis (rare)	Groups of small vesicles and pustules becoming confluent to form irregular pustular lakes and erosions[96] Polycyclic plaques with central hyperpigmentation Severe, intractable pruritus Chronic and persistent Many nonfollicular lesions	Biopsy is diagnostic Eosinophils that invade sebaceous glands and outer root sheaths of hair follicles Moderate eosinophilia and leukocytosis (50%) CD4 counts < 250-300 cells/mm3	Permethrin cream (Elimite) qd until lesions clear Ultraviolet B phototherapy[97] Antihistamines Group I topical steroids Itraconazole 100-400 mg/day Dapsone 100 mg qd possibly effective
VASCULAR DISORDERS			
Telangiectasias of anterior chest wall (uncommon)	Linear telangiectasia in broad, crescent distribution across the chest[98] Associated with erythema in the same distribution	Biopsy shows dilated blood vessels with perivascular small cell infiltrate No endothelial proliferation	None
Bacillary (epithelioid) angiomatosis (rare)	Solitary or multiple dome-shaped friable, bright-red granulation tissue-like papules and subcutaneous nodules (1mm-2 cm)[99] of face, trunk, extremities Visceral angiomatosis Cat bite or scratch[118]	Biopsy—proliferation of small blood vessels lined with plump endothelial cells projecting into lumen *Rochalimaea* bacilli seen with Warthin-Starry silver stain	Erythromycin 500 mg qid × 6 wks Doxycycline 100 mg bid × 6 wks, or trimethoprim/sulfamethoxazole or rifampin
Thrombocytopenic purpura (common)	Petechia	Complete blood count	
NEOPLASTIC DISORDERS			
Kaposi's sarcoma	Pale to deep violaceous, thin, oval plaques Long axis of lesions aligned with skin tension lines Many unusual presentations Numbers vary from few to numerous lesions Any skin surface and mouth, usually palate Visceral lesions Lesions induced by trauma	Biopsy Proliferation of small vessels Proliferation of bundles of interweaving plump spindle cells Slitlike intercellular spaces with extravasated red blood cells	Radiation for individual lesions Intralesional vinblastine (0.1 to 0.5 mg/ml every 4 wks)[119] Liquid nitrogen cryotherapy (keep blister covered to prevent exposure of others to HIV)

Continued.

TABLE 11-1, cont'd HIV Infection—Cutaneous Manifestations

Disease	Clinical manifestations	Diagnosis	Treatment
MISCELLANEOUS			
Cutaneous drug reactions	Morbilliform eruptions predominate Urticaria Much greater incidence than general population	Trimethoprim-sulfamethoxazole Dapsone Aminopenicillins	Stop drug if possible
Pruritus (uncommon)	Intractable pruritus without internal malignancy[100] May be presenting symptom of AIDS	Numerous excoriations Rule out other causes of pruritus (e.g., renal, thyroid, hepatic dysfunction; drugs; malignancy; diabetes; iron deficiency anemia)	Emollients, topical steroids, and prednisone are not effective
Yellow nails	Yellow discoloration of nail plate Many associated with *Pneumocystis carinii* pneumonia[101]	Differentiate from yellow nail syndrome: yellow nail syndrome = yellow nail plate + absent cuticles + diminished growth rate + transverse overcurvature of nail plate + subungual hyperkeratosis	Treat possible aggravating conditions (e.g., *P. carinii* pneumonia)
Dark-blue nails	Darkened bluish appearance at bases of fingernails (black patients > white patients)[102]	Recent history of zidovudine treatment	None
Vitiligo (uncommon) Premature graying of hair (common)	Loss of pigmentation of hair and skin usually follows other AIDS signs and symptoms[103]	Physical examination	None

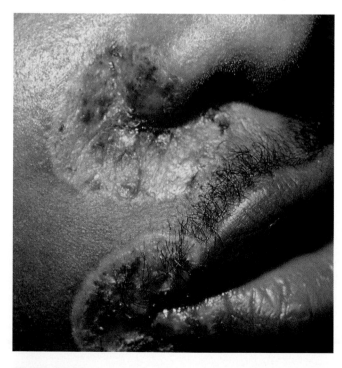

Figure 11-18
Herpes simplex. Erosive. *(Courtesy Neal S. Penneys M.D., Ph.D.)*

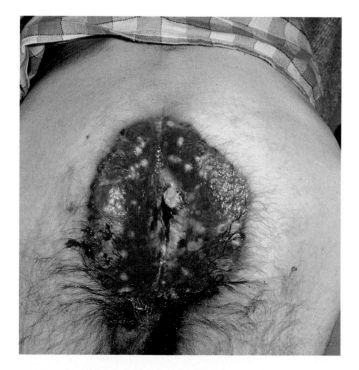

Figure 11-19
Herpes simplex. Erosive. *(Courtesy Benjamin K. Fisher M.D.)*

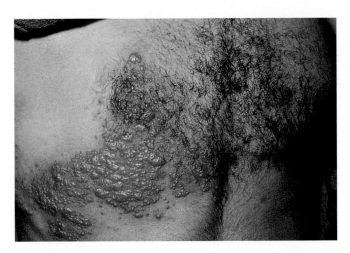

Figure 11-20
Herpes zoster. *(Courtesty Benjamin K. Fisher M.D.)*

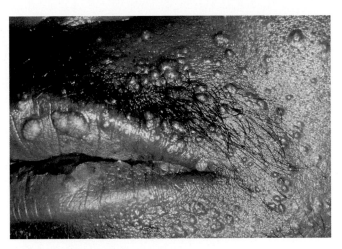

Figure 11-21
Molluscum contagiosum. *(From Redfield RR, James WD, Wright DC:* J Am Acad Dermatol *13:821, 1985.)*

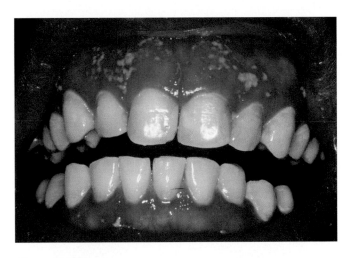

Figure 11-22
Candida albicans. *(Courtesy William D. James M.D.)*

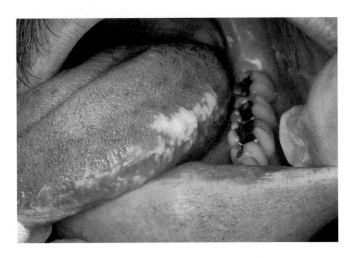

Figure 11-23
Hairy leukoplakia. *(Courtesy Deborah S. Greenspan)*

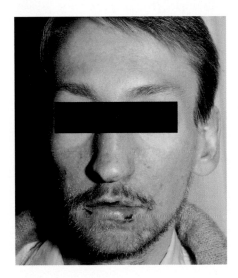

Figure 11-24
Seborrheic dermatitis. *(Courtesy Benjamin K. Fisher M.D.)*

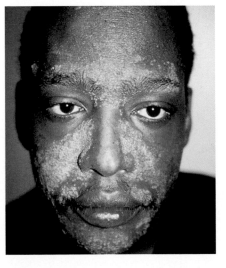

Figure 11-25
Seborrheic dermatitis. *(Courtesy William D. James M.D.)*

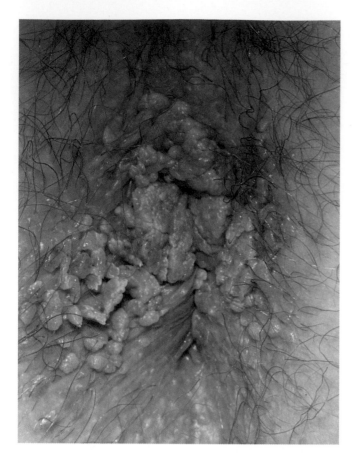

Figure 11-26
Anal warts.

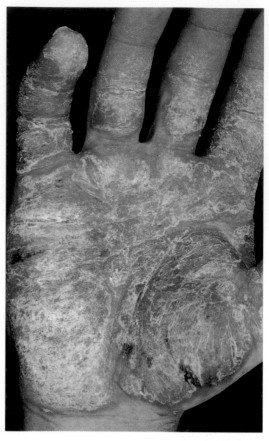

Figure 11-27
Psoriasis. *(Courtesy William D. James M.D.)*

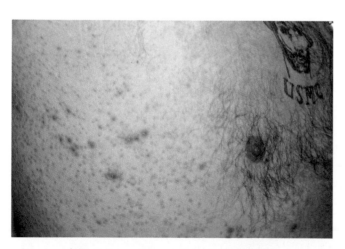

Figure 11-28
Papular eruption. *(Courtesy David Goodman M.D.)*

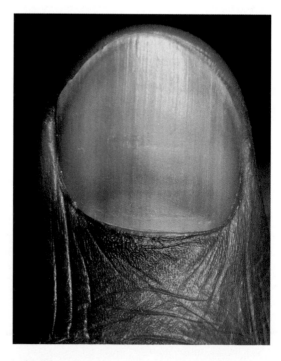

Figure 11-29
Dark-blue nails (after treatment with zidovudine). *(Courtesy William D. James M.D.)*

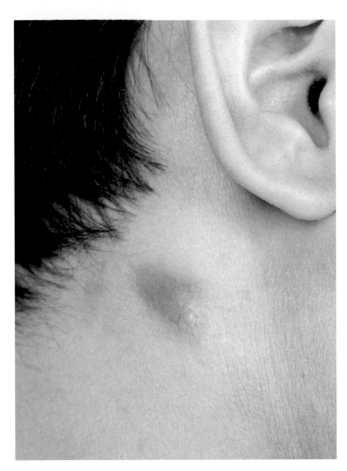

Figure 11-30
Kaposi's sarcoma.*(Courtesy H.J. Hulsebosch M.D.)*

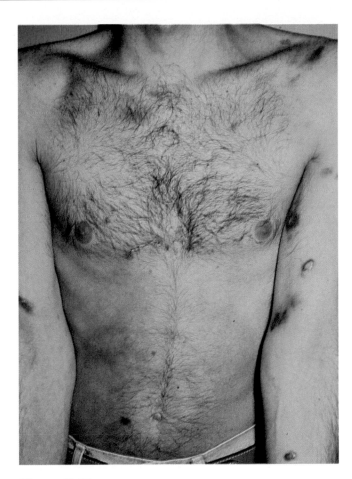

Figure 11-31
Kaposi's sarcoma. *(Courtesy Benjamin K. Fisher M.D.)*

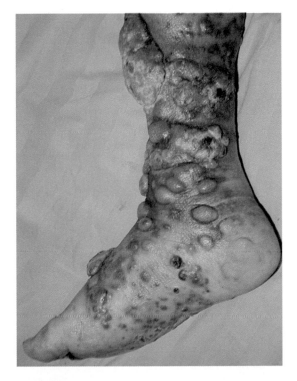

Figure 11-32
Kaposi's sarcoma. *(Courtesy Benjamin K. Fisher M.D.)*

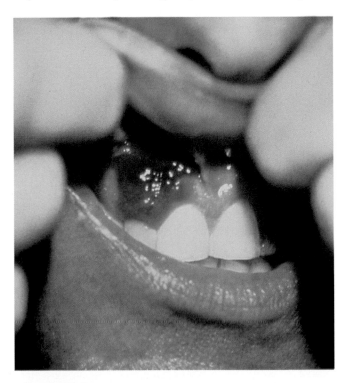

Figure 11-33
Kaposi's sarcoma. *(Courtesy William D. James M.D.)*

patients are immunocompromised.[106] Severe disease should be treated with intravenous acyclovir (30 mg/kg/day).[107]

Candida

Oral candidiasis is the most common fungal infection in HIV-infected patients and is predictive of progressive disease. It may be the initial manifestation of AIDS.[108] Plaques form on the cheeks and tongue and frequently cause sore throat and dysphagia. Infection may descend into the esophagus. Without treatment the disease becomes intractable. Systemic involvement and fungemia are rare. Oral ketoconazole (200 to 400 mg per day) is usually successful, although recurrence is common and intermittent therapy is often necessary. Intravenous miconazole or amphotericin B is necessary in refractory cases.

In children, *Candida* can produce extensive diaper rash, with widespread lesions on the trunk. Vaginal infection can be intractable. *Candida* nail infections occur.

Seborrheic dermatitis

Seborrheic dermatitis is a common occurrence late in the course of disease.[109,110] The severity of the seborrheic dermatitis correlates with the degree of clinical deterioration and with the T-helper cell subset ratio. The inflammation is usually severe, with thick scaling. Generalized involvement of the trunk, groin, and extremities may occur. The patients often have thick, greasy, hyperkeratotic plaques on the scalp that may be associated with nonscarring alopecia. Seborrheic dermatitis associated with AIDS shows a distinctive histologic pattern, indicating that the disease is probably a different clinical entity than typical seborrheic dermatitis.

Kaposi's sarcoma (see p. 733)

Kaposi's sarcoma (KS) probably occurs as a multicentric rather than a metastatic disease in AIDS. Lesions are often multifocal and widespread when first detected. There is strong evidence that KS is induced by a herpes virus. The incidence of the HLA-DR5 antigen is higher in patients with classic and AIDS-associated KS.[111,112] The incidence of KS in AIDS patients declined from 33% in 1981-1983 to 19% in 1986, and to 10% in 1992. The rate of KS was higher among women who acquired HIV infection from bisexual men than among those whose infection was related to intravenous drug use. KS was rare among patients infected by blood transfusions from donors who had KS. Oral involvement is common in HIV-associated KS.

Lesions initially form slightly raised, oval or elongated, poorly demarcated rust-colored infiltrates. Papules and nodules form that may resemble granulation tissue, stasis dermatitis, pyogenic granuloma, or a capillary hemangioma. They are most commonly found on the trunk and the head and neck areas. Lesions may be induced by trauma (Köebner's isomorphic phenomenon) and occur in a dermatome of previously involved herpes zoster, a site of injection, or the site of blunt trauma. Rapid progression to red or purple nodules and plaques follows. Mucous membranes are involved. More than half of the patients have generalized lymphadenopathy at the time of first examination. Eventually most patients have systemic lesions.

Pseudo-Kaposi's sarcoma

True Kaposi's sarcoma must be distinguished from arteriovenous malformations known as *pseudo-Kaposi's sarcoma*. Arteriovenous malformations are vascular abnormalities in which there are one or more direct communications between an artery and vein without any intervening capillary bed. They are either congenital or acquired by trauma. Purple discolorations can appear overlying, or distal to, the malformation and resemble Kaposi's sarcoma.[113] Most are found on a distal extremity. Arteriography confirms the diagnosis.

REFERENCES

1. Chuang T-Y: Condylomata acuminata (genital warts). An epidemiologic view, *J Am Acad Dermatol* 16:376-384, 1987.
2. Ferenczy A et al: Latent papillomavirus and recurring genital warts, *N Engl J Med* 313:784-788, 1985.
3. Rosenberg SK: Subclinical papilloma viral infection of male genitalia, *Urology* 26:554-557, 1985.
4. Panici PB et al: Oral condyloma lesions in patients with extensive genital human papillomavirus infection, *Am J Obstet Gynecol* 167:451-458, 1992.
5. American Academy of Dermatology Task Force on Pediatric Dermatology: genital warts and sexual abuse in children, *J Am Acad Dermatol* 11:529-530, 1984.
6. Cohen BA, Honing P, Androphy E: Anogenital warts in children, *Arch Dermatol* 126:1575-1580, 1990.
7. Obalek S, Jablonska S, et al: Condylomata acuminata in children: frequent association with human papillomaviruses responsible for cutaneous warts, *J Am Acad Dermatol* 23:205-213, 1990.
8. Rock B et al: Genital tract papillomavirus infection in children, *Arch Dermatol* 122:1129-1132, 1986.
9. Krzyzek RA et al: Anogenital warts contain several distinct species of human papillomavirus, *J Virol* 36:236-244, 1980.
10. Reeves WC et al: Human papillomavirus infection and cervical cancer in Latin America, *N Engl J Med* 320:1437-1441, 1989.
11. Von Krogh G, Syrjanen SM, Syrjanen KJ: Advantage of human papillomavirus typing in the clinical evaluation of genitoanal warts, *J Am Acad Dermatol* 18:495-503, 1988.
12. Macnab JCM et al: Human papillomavirus in clinically and histologically normal tissue of patients with genital cancer, *N Engl J Med* 315:1052-1058, 1986.
13. Barrasso R et al: High prevalence of papillomavirus-associated penile intraepithelial neoplasia in sexual partners of women with cervical intraepithelial neoplasia, *N Engl J Med* 317:916-923, 1987.
14. Daling JR et al: Sexual practices, sexually transmitted diseases, and the incidence of anal cancer, *N Engl J Med* 317:973-977, 1987.
15. Sedlacek TV, Cunnane M, Carpiniello V: Colposcopy in the diagnosis of penile condyloma, *Am J Obstet Gynecol* 154:494-496, 1986.
16. Comite SL, Castadot M-J: Colposcopic evaluation of men with genital warts, *J Am Acad Dermatol* 18:1274-1278, 1988.
17. Krebs Hans-B, Helmkamp BF: Treatment failure of genital condylomata acuminata in women: role of the male sexual partner, *Am J Obstet Gynecol* 165:337-340, 1991.
18. Fisher AA: Severe systemic and local reactions to topical podophyllum resin, *Cutis* 28:233, 1981.
19. Baker DA, Douglas J Jr, et al: Topical podofilox for the treatment of condylomata acuminata in women, *Obstet Gynecol* 76:656-659, 1990.
20. Greenberg MD, Rutledge LH, et al: A double-blind, randomized trial

of 0.5% podofilox and placebo for the treatment of genital warts in women, *Obstet Gynecol* 77:735-739, 1991.

21. Kreider JW, Pickel MD: Influence of schedule and mode of administration on effectiveness of podofilox treatment of papillomas, *J Invest Dermatol* 101:614-618, 1993.

22. Schwartz DB et al: The management of genital condylomas in pregnant women, *Obstet Gynecol Clin North Am* 14:589-599, 1987.

23. Robinson JK: Extirpation by electrocautery of massive lesions of condyloma acuminatum in genito-perineo-anal region, *J Dermatol Surg Oncol* 6:733-738, 1980.

24. Damstra RJ, van Vloten WA: Cryotherapy in the treatment of condylomata acuminata: a controlled study of 64 patients, *J Dermatol Surg Oncol* 17:273-276, 1991.

25. Matsunaga J, Bergman A, Bhatia NN: Genital condylomata acuminata in pregnancy: effectiveness, safety and pregnancy outcome following cryotherapy, *Br J Obstet Gynaecol* 94:168-172, 1987.

26. Bar-Am A et al: Treatment of male genital condylomatous lesions by carbon dioxide laser after failure of previous nonlaser methods, *J Am Acad Dermatol* 24:87-89, 1991.

27. Browder JF, Araujo OE, et al: The interferons and their use in condyloma acuminata, *Ann Pharmacother* 26:42-45, 1992.

28. Krebs H-B: Treatment of vaginal condylomata acuminata by weekly topical application of 5-fluorouracil, *Obstet Gynecol* 70:68-71, 1987.

29. Krebs Hans-B: Treatment of genital condylomata with topical 5-fluorouracil, *Dermatol Clin* 9:333-341, 1991.

30. Schwartz RA, Janniger CK: Bowenoid papulosis, *J Am Acad Dermatol* 24:261-264, 1991.

31. Obalek S et al: Bowenoid papulosis of the male and female genitalia: risk of cervical neoplasia, *J Am Acad Dermatol* 14:433-444, 1986.

32. Patterson JW et al: Bowenoid papulosis. A clinicopathologic study with ultrastructural observations, *Cancer* 57:823-836, 1986.

33. Gross G et al: Bowenoid papulosis: presence of human papillomavirus (HPV) structural antigens and of HPV 16-related DNA sequences, *Arch Dermatol* 121:858-863, 1985.

34. Rudlinger R: Bowenoid papulosis of the male and female genital tracts: risk of cervical neoplasia, *J Am Acad Dermatol* 16:625-627, 1987.

35. Schwartz JJ, Myskowski PL: Molluscum contagiosum in patients with human immunodeficiency virus infection. A review of twenty-seven patients, *J Am Acad Dermatol* 27:583-588, 1992.

36. de Waard-van der Spek FB, Oranje AP, et al: Treatment of molluscum contagiosum using a lidocaine/prilocaine cream (EMLA) for analgesia, *J Am Acad Dermatol* 23:685-688, 1990.

37. Amstey MS, Trombetta GC: Laser therapy for vulvar molluscum contagiosum infection, *Am J Obstet Gynecol* 153:800-801, 1985.

38. Rooney JF et al: Acquisition of genital herpes from an asymptomatic sexual partner, *N Engl J Med* 314:1561-1564, 1986.

39. Koutsky LA, Stevens CE, et al: Underdiagnosis of genital herpes by current clinical and viral-isolation procedures, *N Engl J Med* 326:1533-1539, 1992.

40. Luby ED, Klinge V: Genital herpes: a pervasive psychosocial disorder, *Arch Dermatol* 121:494-497, 1985.

41. Mertz GJ, Benedetti J, et al: Risk factors for the sexual transmission of genital herpes, *Ann Intern Med* 116:197-202, 1992.

42. Mertz GJ, Schmidt O, et al: Frequency of acquisition of first-episode genital infection with herpes simplex virus from symptomatic and asymptomatic source contacts, *Sex Transm Dis*, 12:33-39, 1985.

43. Corey L: First-episode, recurrent, and asymptomatic herpes simplex infections, *J Am Acad Dermatol* 18:169-172, 1988.

44. Miller RG et al: Acquisition of concomitant oral and genital infection with herpes simplex virus type 2, *Sex Transm Dis* 14:41-43, 1987.

45. Lafferty WE et al: Recurrences after oral and genital herpes simplex virus infection: influence of site of infection and viral type, *N Engl J Med* 316:1444-1449, 1987.

45a. Benedetti J et al: Recurrence rates in genital herpes after symptomatic first-episode infection, *Am Intern Med* 121:847-854, 1994.

46. McGowan MP et al: Prevalence of cytomegalovirus and herpes simplex virus in human semen, *Int J Androl* 6:331-336, 1983.

47. Solomon AR: New diagnostic tests for herpes simplex and varicella zoster infections, *J Am Acad Dermatol* 18:218-221, 1988.

48. Bryson YJ et al: Treatment of first episodes of genital herpes simplex virus infections with oral acyclovir: a randomized double-blind controlled trial in normal subjects, *N Engl J Med* 308:916, 1983.

49. Mertz GJ et al: Long-term acyclovir suppression of frequently recurring genital herpes simplex virus infection, *JAMA* 260:201-206, 1988.

50. Goldberg LH, Kaufman R, et al: Long-term suppression of recurrent genital herpes with acyclovir. A 5-year benchmark, *Arch Dermatol* 129:582-587, 1993.

51. Sullivan-Bolyai J et al: Neonatal herpes simplex virus infection in King County, Washington: increasing incidence and epidemiologic correlates, *JAMA* 250:3059-3062, 1983.

52. Whitley RJ et al: Changing presentation of herpes simplex virus infection in neonates, *J Infect Dis* 158:109-116, 1988.

53. Koskiniemi M et al: Neonatal herpes simplex virus infection: a report of 43 patients, *Pediatr Infect Dis* J 8:30-35, 1989.

54. Stagno S, Whitley RJ: Herpesvirus infections of pregnancy, Part II. Herpes simplex virus and varicella-zoster virus infection, *N Engl J Med* 313:1327-1330, 1985.

55. Whitley R, Arvin A, et al: Predictors of morbidity and mortality in neonates with herpes simplex virus infections. The National Institute of Allergy and Infectious Diseases Collaborative Antiviral Study Group, *N Engl J Med* 324:450-454, 1991.

56. Arvin AM: Antiviral treatment of herpes simplex infection in neonates and pregnant women, *J Am Acad Dermatol* 18:200-203, 1988.

57. Whitley R, Arvin A, et al: A controlled trial comparing vidarabine with acyclovir in neonatal herpes simplex virus infection. Infectious Diseases Collaborative Antiviral Study Group, *N Engl J Med* 324:444-449, 1991.

58. Monif GRG, Kellner KR, Donnelly W Jr: Congenital herpes simplex type II infection, *Am J Obstet Gynecol* 152:1000-1002, 1985.

59. Brown ZA, Benedetti J, et al: Neonatal herpes simplex virus infection in relation to asymptomatic maternal infection at the time of labor, *N Engl J Med* 324:1247-1252, 1991.

60. Prober CG et al: Low risk of herpes simplex virus infections in neonates exposed to the virus at the time of vaginal delivery to mothers with recurrent genital herpes simplex virus infections, *N Engl J Med* 316:240-244, 1987.

61. Whitley RJ et al: The natural history of herpes simplex virus infection of mother and newborn, *Pediatrics* 66:489-494, 1980.

62. Yeager AS, Arvin AM: Reasons for the absence of a history of recurrent genital infections in mothers of neonates infected with herpes simplex virus, *Pediatrics* 73:188-196, 1984.

63. Randolph AG, Washington AE, et al: Cesarean delivery for women presenting with genital herpes lesions. Efficacy, risks, and costs, *JAMA* 270:77-82, 1993.

64. Prober CG et al: Use of routine viral cultures at delivery to identify neonates exposed to herpes simplex virus, *N Engl J Med* 318:887-891, 1988.

65. Brown ZA et al: Effects on infants of a first episode of genital herpes during pregnancy, *N Engl J Med* 317:1246-1251, 1987.

66. Arvin AM et al: Failure of antepartum maternal cultures to predict the infant's risk of exposure to herpes simplex virus at delivery, *N Engl J Med* 315:796-800, 1986.

67. Glatt AE, Chirgwin K, Landesman SH: Treatment of infections associated with human immunodeficiency virus, *N Engl J Med* 318:1439-1448, 1988.

68. Haddad J, Langer B, et al: Oral acyclovir and recurrent genital herpes during late pregnancy, *Obstet Gynecol* 82:102-104, 1993.

69. Bowman CA, Woolley PD, et al: Asymptomatic herpes simplex virus shedding from the genital tract whilst on suppressive doses of oral acyclovir, *Int J Std Aids* 1:174-177, 1990.

70. Ho DD, Pomerantz RJ, Kaplan JC: Pathogenesis of infection with human immunodeficiency virus, *N Engl J Med* 317:278-286, 1987.

71. Kessler HA et al: Diagnosis of human immunodeficiency virus infection in seronegative homosexuals presenting with an acute viral syndrome, *JAMA* 258:1196-1199, 1987.

72. Rustin MHA et al: The acute exanthem associated with seroconversion to human T-cell lymphotrophic virus III in a homosexual man, *J Infect* 12:161, 1986.

73. Polk BF et al: Predictors of the acquired immunodeficiency syndrome developing in a cohort of seropositive homosexual men, *N Engl J Med* 316:61-66, 1987.

74. Kaplan MH et al: Dermatologic findings and manifestations of acquired immunodeficiency syndrome (AIDS), *J Am Acad Dermatol* 16:485-506, 1987.

75. Coopman SA, Johnson RA, et al: Cutaneous disease and drug reactions in HIV infection, *N Engl J Med* 328:1670-1674, 1993.

76. Matis WL, Triana A, Shapiro R: Dermatologic findings associated with human immunodeficiency virus infection, *J Am Acad Dermatol* 17:746-751, 1987.

77. Valle S-L: Dermatologic findings related to human immunodeficiency virus infection in high-risk individuals, *J Am Acad Dermatol* 17:951-961, 1987.

78. Penneys NS, Hicks B: Unusual cutaneous lesions associated with acquired immunodeficiency syndrome, *J Am Acad Dermatol* 13:845-852, 1985.

79. Holmberg SD et al: Prior herpes simplex virus type 2 infection as a risk factor for HIV infection, *JAMA* 259:1048-1050, 1988.

80. Rico MJ, Penneys NS: Cutaneous cryptococcus resembling molluscum contagiosum in a patient with AIDS, *Arch Dermatol* 121:901-902, 1985.

81. Miller SJ: Cutaneous cryptococcus resembling molluscum contagiosum in a patient with acquired immunodeficiency syndrome, *Cutis* 41:411-412, 1988.

82. Barnett N, Mak H, Winkelstein JA: Extensive verrucosis in primary immunodeficiency disease, *Arch Dermatol* 119:5-7, 1983.

83. Greenspan JS et al: Replication of Epstein-Barr virus within the epithelial cells of oral "hairy" leukoplakia, an AIDS-associated lesion, *N Engl J Med* 313:1564-1571, 1985.

84. Lupton GP et al: Oral hairy leukoplakia, *Arch Dermatol* 123:624-628, 1987.

85. Conant MA: Hairy leukoplakia, *Arch Dermatol* 123:585-587, 1987.

86. Johns DR, Tierney M, Felsenstein D: Alteration in the natural history of neurosyphilis by concurrent infection with the human immunodeficiency virus, *N Engl J Med* 316:1587-1589, 1987.

87. Hicks CB et al: Seronegative secondary syphilis in a patient infected with the human immunodeficiency virus (HIV) with Kaposi sarcoma, *Ann Intern Med* 107:492-495, 1987.

88. Tramont EC: Syphilis in the AIDS era, *N Engl J Med* 316:1600-1601, 1987.

89. Berry CD et al: Neurologic relapse after benzathine penicillin therapy for secondary syphilis in a patient with HIV infection, *N Engl J Med* 316:1587-1589, 1987.

90. Sadick N et al: Unusual features of scabies complicating human T-lymphotropic virus type III infection, *J Am Acad Dermatol* 15:482-486, 1986.

91. Perniciaro C, Peters MS: Tinea faciale mimicking seborrheic dermatitis in a patient with AIDS, *N Engl J Med* 314:315-316, 1986.

92. Johnson TM et al: AIDS exacerbates psoriasis, *N Engl J Med* 313:1415, 1985.

93. Duvis M, Rios A, Brewton GW: Remission of AIDS-associated psoriasis with zidovudine, *Lancet* 2:627, 1987.

94. Ruzicka T et al: Treatment of HIV-induced retinoid-resistant psoriasis with zidovudine, *Lancet* 2:1469, 1987.

95. James WD et al: A papular eruption associated with human T cell lymphotropic virus type III disease, *J Am Acad Dermatol* 13:563-566, 1985.

96. Soeprono FF, Schinella RA: Eosinophilic pustular folliculitis in patients with acquired immunodeficiency syndrome, *J Am Acad Dermatol* 14:1020-1022, 1986.

97. Buchness MR et al: Eosinophilic pustular folliculitis in the acquired immunodeficiency syndrome: treatment with ultraviolet B phototherapy, *N Engl J Med* 318:1183-1186, 1988.

98. Fallon T Jr et al: Telangiectasias of the anterior chest in homosexual men, *Ann Intern Med* 105:679-682, 1986.

99. Cockerell CJ et al: Epithelioid angiomatosis: a distinct vascular disorder in patients with the acquired immunodeficiency syndrome or AIDS-related complex, *Lancet* 2:654, 1987.

100. Shapiro RS, Samorodin C, Hood AF: Pruritus as a presenting sign of acquired immunodeficiency syndrome, *J Am Acad Dermatol* 16:1115-1157, 1987.

101. Chernosky ME, Finley VK: Yellow nail syndrome in patients with acquired immunodeficiency disease, *J Am Acad Dermatol* 13:731-736, 1985.

102. Furth PA, Kazakis AM: Nail pigmentation changes associated with azidothymidine (zidovudine), *Ann Intern Med* 107:350, 1987.

103. Duvic M et al: Human immunodeficiency virus-associated vitiligo: expression of autoimmunity with immunodeficiency? *J Am Acad Dermatol* 17:656-662, 1987.

104. Kalb RE, Grossman ME: Chronic perianal herpes simplex in immunocompromised hosts, *Am J Med* 80:486-490, 1986.

105. Erlish KS et al: Acyclovir-resistant herpes simplex virus infections in patients with the acquired immunodeficiency syndrome, *N Engl J Med* 320:293-300, 1989.

106. Josephson A et al: Airborne transmission of chickenpox from localized zoster, *Am J Infect Control* 14:86, 1986.

107. Balfour HH Jr et al: Acyclovir halts progression of herpes zoster in immunocompromised patients, *N Engl J Med* 308:1448-1453, 1983.

108. Klein RS et al: Oral candidiasis in high-risk patients as the initial manifestation of the acquired immunodeficiency syndrome, *N Engl J Med* 311:354-358, 1984.

109. Eisenstat BA, Wormser GP: Seborrheic dermatitis and butterfly rash in AIDS, *N Engl J Med* 311:189, 1984.

110. Soeprono FF et al: Seborrheic-like dermatitis of acquired immunodeficiency syndrome, *J Am Acad Dermatol* 14:242-248, 1986.

111. Pollack MS, Safai B, Dupont B: HLA-DR5 and DR2 are susceptibility factors for acquired immunodeficiency syndrome with Kaposi's sarcoma in different ethnic subpopulations, *Dis Markers* 1:135-139, 1983.

112. Prince HE et al: HLA studies in acquired immune deficiency syndrome patients with Kaposi's sarcoma, *J Clin Immunol* 4:242-245, 1984.

113. Marshall ME, Hatfield ST, Hatfield DR: Arteriovenous malformations simulating Kaposi's sarcoma (pseudo-Kaposi's sarcoma), *Arch Dermatol* 121:99-101, 1985.

114. Garrett SJ, Robinson JK, et al: Trichloroacetic acid peel of molluscum contagiosum in immunocompromised patients, *J Dermatol Surg Oncol* 18:855-858, 1992.

115. Lozada-Nur F: Podophyllin resin 25% for treatment of oral hairy leukoplakia: an old treatment for a new lesion, *J Acquir Immune Defic Syndr* (letter) 4:543, 1991.

116. Pardp RJ, Bogaert MA, et al: UVB phototherapy of the pruritic papular eruption of the acquired immunodeficiency syndrome, *J Am Acad Dermatol* 26:423-428, 1992.

117. Meola T, Soter NA, et al: The safety of UVB phototherapy in patients with HIV infection, *J Am Acad Dermatol* 29:216-220, 1993.

118. Tappero JW, Mohle-Boetani J, et al: The epidemiology of bacillary angiomatosis and bacillary peliosis, *JAMA* 269:770-775, 1993.

119. Serfling U, Hood AF: Local therapies for cutaneous Kaposi's sarcoma in patients with acquired immunodeficiency syndrome, *Arch Dermatol* 127:1479-1481, 1991.

CHAPTER TWELVE

Warts, Herpes Simplex, and Other Viral Infections

Warts

Warts are benign epidermal neoplasms. Different viruses cause different types of warts. At least 60 distinct types of human papilloma virus (HPV) have been identified by their DNA composition. Each of the HPV types is associated with a particular set of clinical and pathologic entities (Table 12-1). HPV-16 and HPV-18 have been found in cervical cancers.

Warts commonly occur in children and young adults, but may appear at any age. Their course is highly variable. Most resolve spontaneously in weeks or months; others may last years or a lifetime. Warts are transmitted simply by touch; it is not unusual to see warts on adjacent toes ("kissing lesions"). Warts commonly appear at sites of trauma, on the hands, in periungual regions from nail biting, and on plantar surfaces.

Individual variations in cell-mediated immunity may explain differences in severity and duration. Warts occur more frequently, last longer, and appear in greater numbers in patients with AIDS, lymphomas, and those taking immunosuppressive drugs.

Atopic eczema patients may not be at increased risk for viral warts as was once suspected.[1]

Some types of warts respond quickly to routine therapy, whereas others are resistant. It should be explained to patients that warts often require several treatment sessions before a cure is realized. Because warts are confined to the epidermis, they can be removed with little, if any, scarring. In order to avoid scarring, treatment should be conservative. A hand with many scars is not worth trading for lesions that undergo spontaneous resolution.

Warts obscure normal skin lines; this is an important diagnostic feature. When skin lines are reestablished, the wart is gone. Warts vary in shape and location and are managed in several different ways.

TABLE 12-1 Clinical Manifestations and Human Papilloma Virus Types

Clinical manifestation	HPV Types
Bowenoid papulosis	16,18,31,33
Buschke-Lowenstein tumor	6
Cervical squamous cell carcinoma	16,18,31,33
Cervical intraepithelial neoplasia	16,18,31,33
Condylomata acuminata	6,11,16,18
Epidermodysplasia verruciformis	3,5,8,10,14
Papillomaviral infection—subclinical	6,11,16,18
Squamous cell carcinoma—anogenital region	16,18,31,33
Warts—common	1,2,4,7
Warts—flat	3,10
Warts—plantar	1,2,4

Warts: the primary lesion. Viral warts are tumors initiated by a viral infection of keratinocytes. The cells proliferate to form a mass but the mass remains confined to the epidermis. There are no "roots" penetrating into the dermis. Several types of warts form cylindrical projections. These projections are clearly seen in digitate warts that occur on the face (Figure 12-1). The projections become fused together in common warts on thicker skin (Figure 12-2). They form a highly organized mosaic pattern on the surface. This pattern is unique to warts and is a useful diagnostic sign (Figure 12-3). Thrombosed black vessels become trapped in these projections and are seen as black dots on the surface of some warts (Figure 12-4). Although warts remain confined to the epidermis, the growing mass can protrude and displace the dermis. The undersurface of a wart is a smooth round mass (Figure 12-5).

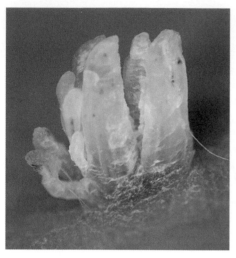

Figure 12-1
Warts form cylindrical projections. They diverge when the wart grows in thin skin.

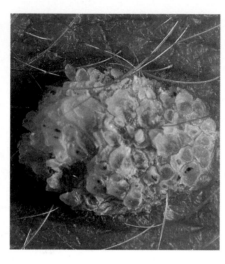

Figure 12-2
The cylindrical projections are partially fused together in this larger wart.

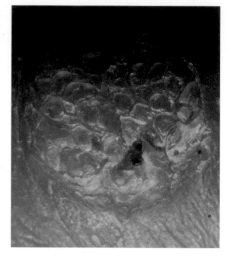

Figure 12-3
The cylindrical projections are tightly packed together, confined by the surrounding skin. This uniform mosaic surface pattern is unique to warts and is a useful diagnostic sign. The pattern can be easily seen with a hand lens.

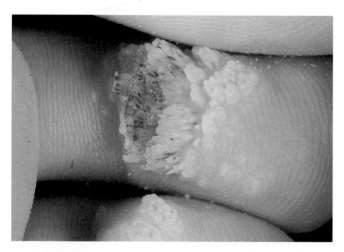

Figure 12-4
Thrombosed black vessels are trapped in the cylindrical projections. Here they are viewed from the side as long, black streaks. They appear as black dots when only the surface of the projections can be seen.

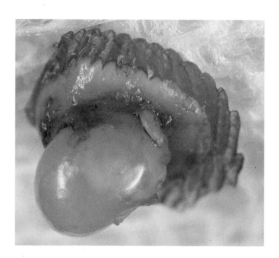

Figure 12-5
The undersurface of a wart. Contrary to popular belief, warts do not have roots. The undersurface is round and smooth. The wart is confined to the epidermis, but it expands and displaces the dermis, giving the impression that it extends into the dermis or subcutaneous tissue.

COMMON WARTS

Common warts (verruca vulgaris) begin as smooth, flesh-colored papules and evolve into dome-shaped, gray-brown, hyperkeratotic growths with black dots on the surface (Figure 12-6). The black dots, which are thrombosed capillaries, are a useful diagnostic sign and may be exposed by paring the hyperkeratotic surface with a #15 surgical blade. The hands are the most commonly involved area, but warts may be found on any skin surface. Generally, the warts are few in number, but it is not unusual for common warts to become so numerous that they become confluent and obscure large areas of normal skin.

Treatment. Topical salicylic acid preparations, liquid nitrogen (Figures 12-7 and 12-8), or very light electrocautery are the best methods for initial therapy. Blunt dissection is used for resistant or very large lesions. (See Chapter Twenty-seven for surgical techniques.) The technique for application of salicylic acid is described in the treatment section for plantar warts.

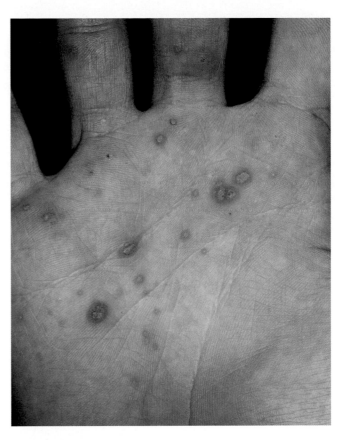

Figure 12-6
Common warts with thrombosed vessels (black dots) on the surface.

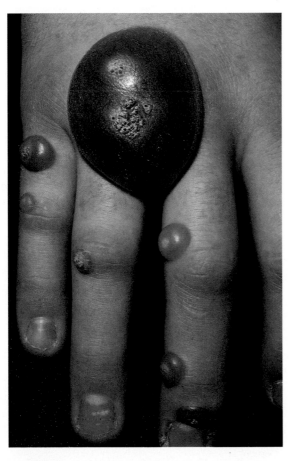

Figure 12-7
Cryosurgery. The virus-infected cells are killed by freezing. The wart, which is localized to the epidermis, is separated from the dermis by freezing. Liquid nitrogen creates a hemorrhagic blister between the dermis and epidermis. The huge blister has been created by excessive freezing. Cryotherapy may cause changes in pigmentation but usually does not scar.

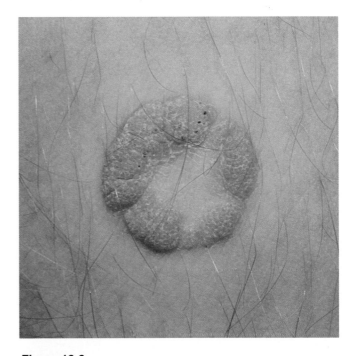

Figure 12-8
Recurrence after cryosurgery. A wart may recur shortly after the blister heals. Virus spreads to the edge of the blister and creates a wart larger than the one that was originally treated.

FILIFORM AND DIGITATE WARTS

These growths consist of a few or several fingerlike, flesh-colored projections emanating from a narrow or broad base. They are most commonly observed about the mouth (Figure 12-9), beard (Figure 12-10), eyes, and ala nasi.

Treatment. These are the easiest warts to treat. Those with a very narrow base do not require anesthesia. A firm base is created by retracting the skin on either side of the wart with the index finger and thumb. A curette is then firmly drawn across the base, removing the wart with one stroke. Bleeding is controlled with gauze pressure rather than by using painful Monsel's solution. This technique is particularly useful for young children who refuse local anesthesia with a needle. Light electrocautery is a useful alternative.

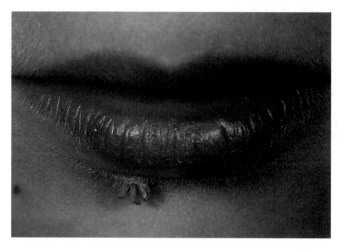

Figure 12-9
Filiform wart with fingerlike projections. These are most commonly observed on the face.

Figure 12-10
Small digitate and filiform warts in the beard area. Shaving spreads the virus over wide areas of the beard. Recurrences are common after cryotherapy or curettage. The infection may last for years.

FLAT WARTS

Flat warts (verruca plana) are pink, light brown, or light yellow, and are slightly elevated, flat-topped papules that vary in size from 0.1 to 0.3 cm. There may be only a few, but generally they are numerous. Typical sites of involvement are the forehead (Figure 12-11), about the mouth (Figure 12-12), the backs of the hands, and shaved areas such as the beard area in men and the lower legs in women. A line of flat warts may appear as a result of scratching these sites.

Treatment. Flat warts present a special therapeutic problem. Their duration may be lengthy and they may be very resistant to treatment. In addition, they are generally located in cosmetically important areas where aggressive, scarring procedures are to be avoided. Treatment may be started with tretinoin cream, 0.025%, 0.05%, or 0.1%, applied at bedtime over the entire involved area. The frequency of application is subsequently adjusted in order to produce a fine scaling with mild erythema. Treatment may be required for weeks or months and often is not effective. Freezing individual lesions with liquid nitrogen or exercising a very light touch with the electrocautery needle may be performed for patients who are concerned with cosmetic appearance and desire quick results. Treatment with 5-fluorouracil cream (Efudex 5%) applied once or twice a day for 3 to 5 weeks may produce dramatic clearing of flat warts; it is worth the attempt if other measures fail.[2,3] Persistent hyperpigmentation may occur following 5-fluorouracil use. This result may be minimized by applying the ointment to individual lesions with a cotton-tipped applicator. Warts may reappear in skin inflamed by 5-fluorouracil.

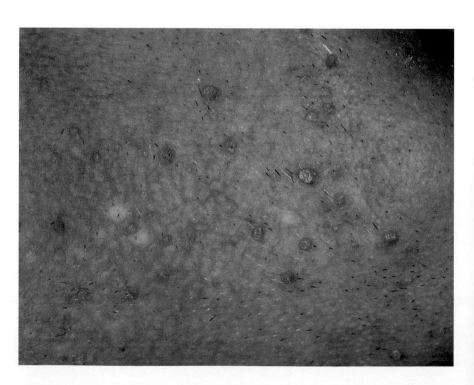

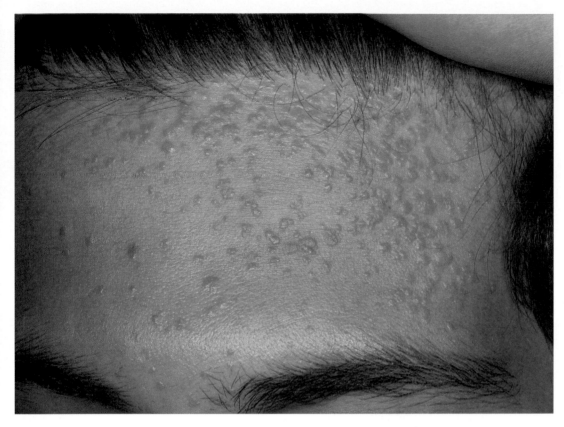

Figure 12-11
Flat warts. The face is a commonly involved site.

Figure 12-12
Flat warts. The wart virus has been inoculated into a scratch line, producing a linear lesion.

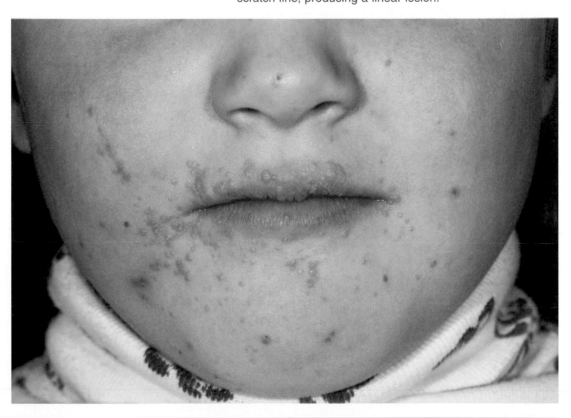

PLANTAR WARTS

Patients may refer to warts on any surface as plantar warts. Plantar warts frequently occur at points of maximum pressure, such as over the heads of the metatarsal bones or on the heels (Figure 12-13). A thick, painful callus forms in response to pressure and the foot is repositioned while walking. This may result in distortion of posture and pain in other parts of the foot, leg, or back. A little wart can cause a lot of trouble.

Warts may appear anywhere on the plantar surface. A cluster of many warts that appears to fuse is referred to as a *mosaic wart* (Figure 12-14).

Differential diagnosis. Corns (clavi) over the metatarsal heads are frequently mistaken for warts. The two entities can be easily distinguished by paring the callus with a #15 surgical blade. Warts lack skin lines crossing their surface and have centrally located black dots that bleed with additional paring. Examination with a hand lens shows a highly organized mosaic pattern on the surface (see Figure 12-3). Clavi or corns also lack skin lines crossing the surface, but they have a hard, painful, well-demarcated, translucent central core (Figure 12-15, *A*). The core or kernel can be removed easily by inserting the point of a #15 surgical blade into the cleavage plane between normal skin and the core, holding the scalpel vertically, and smoothly drawing the blade circumferentially. The hard kernel is freed by drawing the blade horizontally through the base to reveal a deep depression (Figure 12-15, *B*). Pain is greatly relieved by this simple procedure. Lateral pressure on a wart causes pain, but pinching a plantar corn is painless.

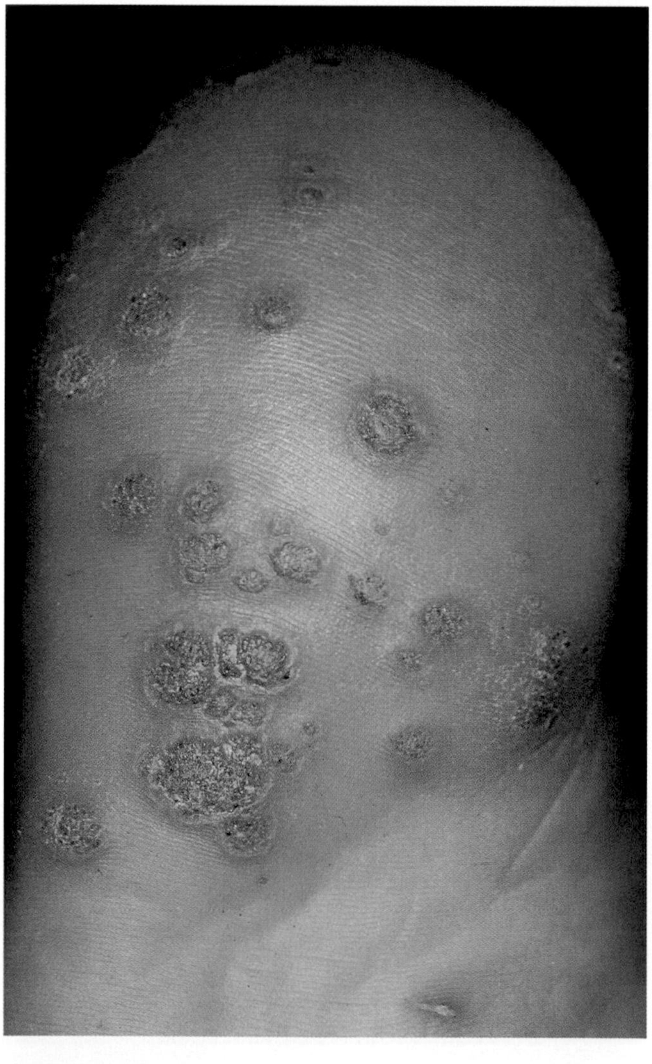

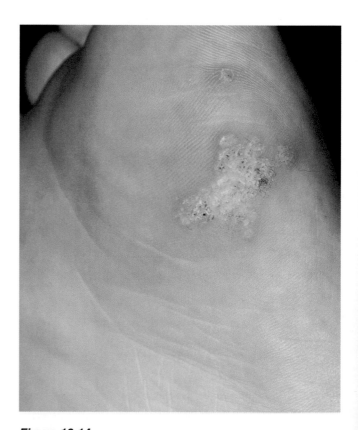

Figure 12-13
Plantar warts. Warts on weight-bearing surfaces accumulate callus and may become painful.

Figure 12-14
Plantar wart. Fusion of numerous small warts to form a mosaic wart. Examination with a hand lens shows a highly organized mosaic pattern on the surface (see Figure 12-3).

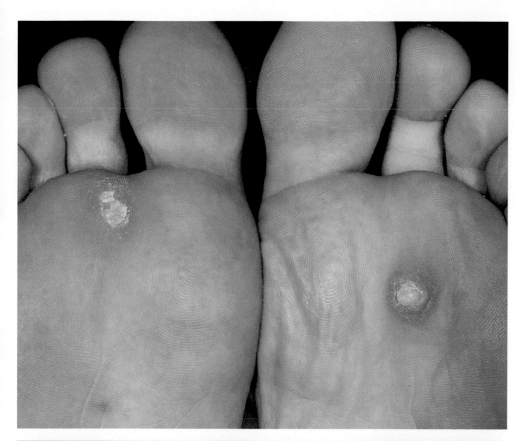

A, Corns (clavi) on the plantar surface are frequently mistaken for warts.

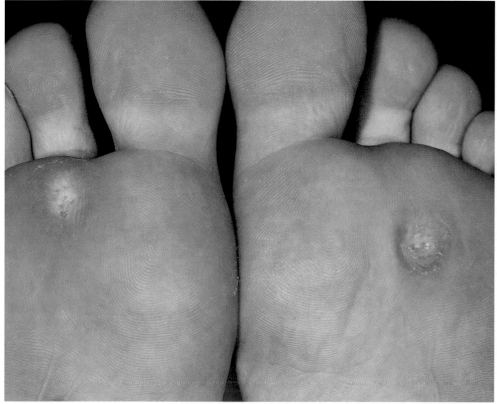

B, Plantar surface depicted in *A* with soft and hard callus removed from corns to reveal a deep depression. Examination with a hand lens shows no organized surface pattern as is seen in a plantar wart.

Figure 12-15

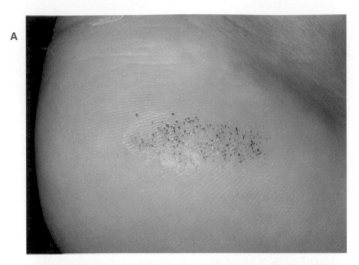

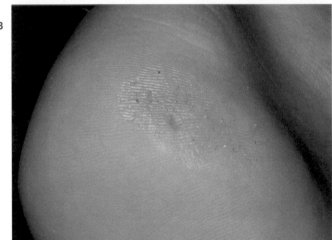

Black heel. A cluster of blue-black dots (ruptured capillaries) may appear on the heel or anywhere on the plantar surface following the shearing trauma of sports that involve sudden stops or position changes (Figure 12-16, *A*). At first glance, this may be confused with a wart, but closer examination reveals normal skin lines, and paring does not cause additional bleeding (Figure 12-16, *B*). The condition resolves spontaneously in a few weeks.

Black warts. Warts in the process of undergoing spontaneous resolution, particularly on the plantar surface, may turn black[4] (Figure 12-17, *A*) and feel soft when pared with a blade (Figure 12-17, *B*). Studies suggest that specific cell-mediated immunity against virus-infected keratinocytes takes place in the process of regression of some warts.[5]

Treatment of plantar warts

Treatment. Plantar warts do not require therapy as long as they are painless. Although their number may increase, it is sometimes best simply to explain the natural history of the virus infection and wait for resolution rather than subject the patient to a long treatment program. Minimal discomfort can be relieved by periodically removing the callus with a blade or pumice stone. Painful warts must be treated. A technique that does not cause scarring should be used; scars on the soles of the feet may be painful and a lasting source of discomfort.

Figure 12-16
A, Black heel. Trauma causes capillaries to shear, resulting in a group of black dots; appearance may be confused with warts. **B**, Paring the skin over the black dots in *A* reveals normal skin lines, proving that a wart is not present.

Figure 12-17 Warts undergoing spontaneous resolution.

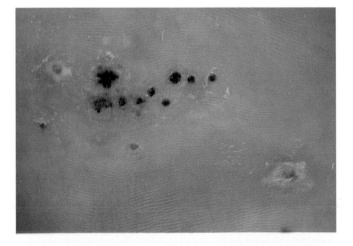

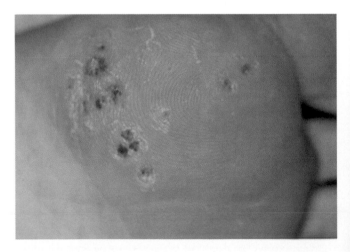

A, Warts in the process of undergoing spontaneous resolution will suddenly turn black.

B, The warts are soft and amorphous and are easily pared with a blade.

Keratolytic therapy (salicylic acid). Keratolytic therapy with salicylic acid (DuoPlant, Occlusal, and many others that are now all available over-the-counter) is conservative initial therapy for plantar warts. The treatment is nonscarring and relatively effective, but it requires persistent application of medication once each day for many weeks.

The wart is pared with a blade, pumice stone, or sand paper (emery board). The affected area is soaked in warm water to hydrate the keratin surface; this facilitates penetration of the medicine. A drop of solution is applied with the applicator and allowed to dry. Solution may be added as needed to cover the entire surface of the wart. Penetration of the acid mixture is enhanced if the treated wart is covered with a piece of adhesive tape. Inflammation and soreness may follow tape occlusion, necessitating periodic interruption of treatment; consequently, the patient may be satisfied with the longer, more comfortable process of simply applying the solution at bedtime. White, pliable keratin forms in a few days and should be pared with a blade or worn away with abrasives such as sandpaper or a pumice stone. Ideally, the white keratin should be removed to expose pink skin. In order to accomplish this, an occasional visit to the office may be necessary.

Keratolytic therapy (40% salicylic acid plasters). This is a safe, nonscarring treatment similar to the previous process, with the exception that in this case the salicylic acid has been incorporated into a pad. Forty percent salicylic acid plasters (Mediplast) are particularly useful in treating mosaic warts covering a large area.

The plaster is cut to the size of the wart. The backing of the plaster is removed and the sticky surface is applied to the wart and secured with tape. The plaster is removed in 24 to 48 hours, the pliable white keratin is reduced in the manner previously described, and another plaster is applied. The treatment requires many weeks, but it is effective and less irritating than salicylic acid and lactic acid paint. Pain is relieved because a large amount of keratin is removed during the first few days of treatment. Forty percent plasters are available in 3- by 4-inch sheets (Mediplast). The cost is approximately $1.00 per sheet.

Blunt dissection. Blunt dissection is a surgical alternative that is fast, effective (90% cure rate), and usually nonscarring. It is superior to both electrodesiccation-curettage and excision because normal tissue is not disturbed.[6] (See Chapter Twenty-seven for surgical techniques.)

Chemotherapy. For years a variety of acids has been successfully employed to treat plantar warts. This technique is occasionally used to treat warts that have recurred following treatment with other techniques; it is sometimes used as initial therapy. Like keratolytic therapy, repeated application is required. Home application of acids is too dangerous; therefore, weekly or biweekly visits to the office are required. A number of acids may be used. (Bichloracetic acid is commercially available.)

Treatment is as follows. The excess callus is pared. The surrounding area is protected with petrolatum. The entire lesion is coated with acid and the acid is worked into the wart with a sharp toothpick. The above procedure is repeated every 7 to 10 days.

Formalin. This may be considered for resistant cases. Mosaic warts or other large involved areas may be treated with daily soaking for 30 minutes in 4% formalin solution. The firm, fixed tissue is pared before subsequent soaking. Lazerformaldehyde solution (10% formaldehyde) is commercially available for direct application to warts. There is a risk of inducing sensitization to formalin.

Cryosurgery. Cryosurgery on the sole may produce a deep, painful blister and interfere with mobility. Repeated light applications of liquid nitrogen are preferred to aggressive treatment.

Contact immunotherapy. Immunotherapy has been reported to be very successful for treatment of resistant warts. This treatment is controversial because, theoretically, the chemical used in the past, dinitrochlorobenzene (DNCB), may be carcinogenic. The mutagenicity of DNCB has been established in experimental models and therefore the safety of this procedure will have to await further studies. The use of other sensitizers such as diphenylcyclopropenone[7] has been suggested as a safer alternative.

Intralesional bleomycin sulfate. Intralesional bleomycin may be considered when all other treatments fail. Five ml bacteriostatic water is added to a 15 U vial of bleomycin sulfate (Blenoxane, Bristol-Myers) to form a 3 U/ml solution; 2 ml of this solution is added to an empty, sterile vial under sterile conditions, followed by the addition of 10 ml of plain lidocaine HCl 1%, thereby forming a final concentration of 0.5 U bleomycin/ml of solution, in a total volume of 12 ml. When reconstituted with 0.9% sodium chloride in a concentration of 3.0 U/ml, it has a utility time of 140 days if stored in polyolefin containers at 4° C . The lidocaine reduces the pain of injection.[8]

With a 30-gauge needle, 0.5 U bleomycin/ml is injected directly into the wart to achieve blanching. In larger warts that require more than one injection, the needle is reinserted into a site already anesthetized by the bleomycin-lidocaine solution. In one study, warts less than 5 mm in diameter received approximately 0.2 ml, warts 5 to 10 mm in diameter received 0.2 to 0.5 ml, and larger warts received up to 1.0 ml, with a maximum of 3 ml (1.5 U) per visit. A multiple puncture technique using a bifurcated vaccination needle to introduce bleomycin sulfate (1 U/ml sterile saline solution) into warts resulted in elimination of 92% of the warts.[9] Leakage of the solution between the projections of some exophytic warts is unavoidable. Follow-up visits are arranged at 2- to 4-week intervals.

The responsive warts show hemorrhagic eschars that heal without scarring. The cure rate is 71% for periungual warts and 48% for plantar warts.[10] The use of bleomycin for the treatment of warts results in significant systemic drug exposure; thus it is prudent to exclude pregnancy before treating women of child-bearing age.[11]

SUBUNGUAL AND PERIUNGUAL WARTS

Subungual and periungual warts (Figure 12-18) are more resistant to both chemical and surgical methods of treatment than are warts in other areas. A wart next to the nail may simply be the tip of the iceberg; much more of the wart may be submerged under the nail. The tips of the fingers and toes are a confined area. Therapeutic measures that cause inflammation and swelling, such as cryosurgery, may produce considerable pain.

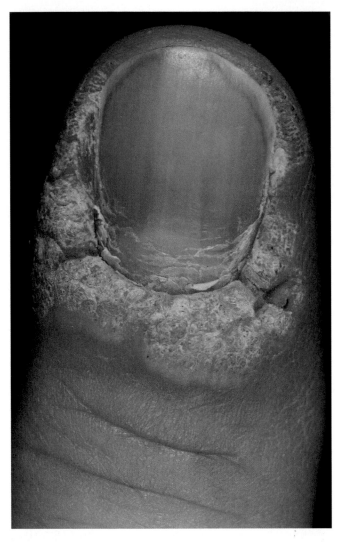

Figure 12-18
Periungual wart. Warts may extend under a nail. Cuticle biting may spread warts.

Treatment

Cryosurgery. Small periungual warts respond to conservative cryosurgery. Warts that extend under the nail do not respond. Aggressive cryosurgery over superficial nerves on the volar or lateral aspects of the proximal phalanges of the fingers has caused neuropathy. Permanent nail changes may occur if the nail matrix is frozen.

Cantharidin. Cantharidin (Cantharone) causes blister formation at the dermoepidermal junction, but does not cause scarring. Adverse effects are postinflammatory hyperpigmentation, painful blistering, and dissemination of warts to the area of blistering.

In treatment, the solution is applied to the surface and allowed to dry. The patient is seen 1 week later for evaluation. Blisters are opened and the remaining wart is retreated. If blistering does not occur, then cantharidin is applied in one to three layers and covered with tape for 48 hours. Each layer should be dry before the next application of cantharidin. The treatment is very effective for some patients, but there are some warts that do not respond to repeated applications.

Keratolytic preparations. The same procedures described for treating plantar warts with salicylic acid and lactic acid paint and salicylic acid plasters are very useful for periungual warts.

Blunt dissection. When conventional measures fail, blunt dissection offers an excellent surgical alternative.[12] (See Chapter Twenty-seven.) Local anesthesia is induced with 2% lidocaine without injection of epinephrine around and under small warts. A digital block is required for larger warts. Hemostasis during the procedure is maintained by firm pressure over the digital arteries or with a rubberband tourniquet. The nail should be removed only if the wart is very large and imbedded. The procedure is exactly the same as described for blunt dissection of plantar warts.

Tape occlusion. This is a technique of unproven efficacy that may be worth attempting for children for whom a conservative approach is desired.[13] To completely cover the wart, the tip of the finger is wrapped with tape. The tape remains in place for 6 days, is removed at home, is then reapplied in a similar manner 12 hours later, and remains in place for another 6 days. The patient is seen 2 weeks after the initial visit and the wart is treated with a drop of liquified phenol, bichloroacetic acid (Kahlenberg), or salicylic acid (Occlusal-HP). The finger is again occluded in the aforementioned manner. The process is repeated until the wart is gone.

GENITAL WARTS

Genital warts are discussed in Chapter Eleven.

Molluscum Contagiosum

Clinical manifestations. Molluscum contagiosum is a virus infection of the skin characterized by discrete, 2- to 5-mm, slightly umbilicated, flesh-colored, dome-shaped papules (Figure 12-19). It spreads by autoinoculation, by scratching, or by touching a lesion. The areas most commonly involved are the face (Figure 12-20), trunk, axillae, extremities in children, and the pubic and genital areas in adults (see Figures 11-7 and 11-8). Lesions are frequently grouped; there may be few or many covering a wide area. Unlike warts, the palms and soles are not involved. It is not uncommon to see erythema and scaling at the periphery of a single or several lesions (see Figure 11-9). This may be the result of inflammation from scratching or may be a hypersensitivity reaction. Lesions spread to inflamed skin, such as areas of atopic dermatitis (Figure 12-21). The individual lesion begins as a smooth, dome-shaped, white-to-flesh colored papule. With time, the center becomes soft and umbilicated. Most lesions are self-limiting and clear spontaneously in 6 to 9 months; however, they may last much longer. Genital molluscum contagiosum may be a manifestation of sexual abuse in children.

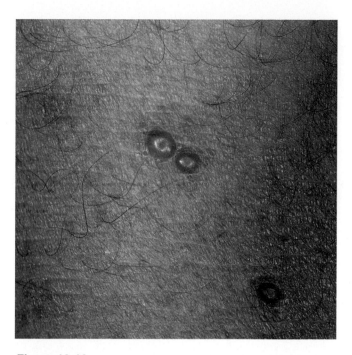

Figure 12-19
Molluscum contagiosum. Individual lesions are 2 to 5 mm, flesh-colored, dome-shaped umbilicated papules.

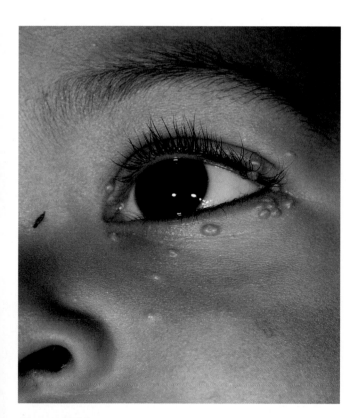

Figure 12-20
Molluscum contagiosum. Inoculation around the eye, a typical presentation for children.

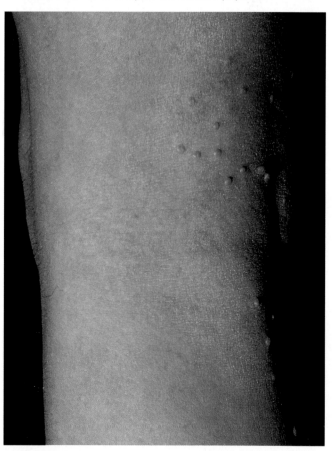

Figure 12-21
Molluscum contagiosum spreads rapidly in eczematous skin. This patient has atopic dermatitis of the popliteal fossa.

Molluscum contagiosum in HIV-infected patients. Molluscum contagiosum is a common and at times severely disfiguring cutaneous viral infection in patients with HIV. Atypical facial lesions with either multiple small papules or giant nodular tumors are common.[14] Cutaneous cryptococcosis may resemble molluscum contagiosum in AIDS patients. Cytologic examination of skin brushing reveals encapsulated budding yeasts.[15] An inverse relation between CD4+ count and the number of mollusum contagiosum lesions is observed.[16]

Diagnosis. If necessary the diagnosis can be established easily by laboratory methods. The virus infects epithelial cells, creating very large intracytoplasmic inclusion bodies and disrupting cell bonds by which epithelial cells are generally held together. This lack of adhesion causes the central core of the lesion to be soft. Rapid confirmation can be made by removing a small lesion with a curette and placing it with a drop of potassium hydroxide between two microscope slides. The preparation is gently heated and then crushed with firm twisting pressure. Larger umbilicated papules have a soft center, the contents of which can be obtained by scooping with a needle. This material contains only infected cells and can be examined directly in a heated potassium hydroxide preparation. The infected cells are dark, round, and disperse easily with slight pressure, whereas normal epithelial cells are flat, rectangular and tend to remain stuck together in sheets. Virions streaming out of the amorphous mass can be seen if Sedi-stain, a supravital stain used to stain urine sediments, is used.[17] Toluidine blue gives the same results. Viral inclusions (large, eosinophilic, round, intracytoplasmic bodies) are easily seen in a fixed and stained biopsy specimen.

Treatment. Treatment must be individualized. Conservative nonscarring methods should be used for children who have many lesions. Genital lesions in adults should be definitively treated in order to prevent spread by sexual contact (see Chapter Eleven). New lesions that are too small to be detected may appear after treatment and may require additional attention.

Curettage. Small papules can be quickly removed with a curette and without local anesthesia in adults. Children can be treated after using a lidocaine/prilocaine cream (EMLA) for analgesia. The cream is applied 30 to 60 minutes before treatment.[18] Bleeding is controlled with gauze pressure. Monsel's solution is too painful to use in an unanesthetized area. Curettage is useful when there are a few lesions because it provides the quickest, most reliable treatment. A small scar may form; therefore, this technique should be avoided in cosmetically important areas.

Cryosurgery. Cryosurgery is the treatment of choice for patients who do not object to the pain. Touch the papule lightly with a nitrogen-bathed cotton swab, or spray until the advancing, white, frozen border has progressed to form a 1-mm halo on the normal skin surrounding the lesion. This should take approximately 5 seconds. This conservative method destroys most lesions in one to three treatment sessions at 1- or 2-week intervals and rarely produces a scar.

Tretinoin. Tretinoin (Retin-A) cream (0.025%, 0.05%, or 0.1%) or gel (0.01% or 0.025%) should be applied once or twice daily to individual lesions. Weeks or months of treatment may be required. This method is useful for children whose parents are anxious for some type of treatment, but it is not very effective.

Salicylic acid. Salicylic acid (Occlusal) applied each day without tape occlusion may cause irritation and encourage resolution.

Cantharidin. Apply a small drop of cantharidin 0.7% (Cantharone) over the surface of the lesion and avoid contaminating normal skin. Lesions blister and may clear without scarring. Occasionally, new lesions appear at the site of the blister created by cantharidin. An alternative method is to apply a tiny bit of cantharidin or the more potent combination of 1% cantharidin, 30% salicylic acid, and 5% podophyllin (Verrusol) and cover with tape for 1 day. The resulting small blister should be treated with polysporin until the reaction subsides.

Laser therapy. Lesions on the vulva cleared after treatment with a carbon dioxide laser in one study. The power setting was 20 watts with a spot size of 1.5 mm. The depth of therapy was approximately 3 mm.[19]

Trichloroacetic acid peel in immunocompromised patients. HIV patients with extensive facial molluscum contagiosum were treated with trichloroacetic acid peels. Peels were performed with 25% to 50% trichloroacetic acid (average 35%) and were repeated every 2 weeks as needed. A total of 15 peels were performed with an average reduction in lesion counts of 40.5% (range 0% to 90%).[20]

Herpes Simplex

Genital herpes simplex virus infections are discussed in Chapter Eleven.

Herpes simplex virus (HSV) infections are caused by two different virus types (HSV-1 and HSV-2) that can be distinguished in the laboratory. HSV-1 is generally associated with oral infections and HSV-2 with genital infections. HSV-1 genital infections and HSV-2 oral infections are becoming more common, possibly as a result of oral-genital sexual contact. Both types seem to produce identical patterns of infection. Many infections are asymptomatic and evidence of previous infection can only be detected by an elevated IgG antibody titer. Herpes simplex virus infections have two phases: the primary infection, after which the virus becomes established in a nerve ganglion; and the secondary phase, characterized by recurrent disease at the same site. The rate of recurrence varies with virus type and anatomic site. Genital recurrences are nearly 6 times more frequent than oral-labial recurrences. Genital HSV-2 infections recur more often than genital HSV-1 infections. Oral-labial HSV-1 infections recur more often than oral HSV-2 infections.[21] Infections can occur anywhere on the skin. Infection in one area does not protect the patient from subsequent infection at a different site. Lesions are intraepidermal and usually heal without scarring.

Primary infection. Many primary infections are asymptomatic and can be detected only by an elevated IgG antibody titer. Like most virus infections, the severity of disease increases with age. The virus may be spread by respiratory droplets, by direct contact with an active lesion, or by virus-containing fluid such as saliva or cervical secretions in patients with no evidence of active disease. Symptoms occur from 3 to 7 or more days after contact. Tenderness, pain, mild paresthesias, or burning occur prior to the onset of lesions at the site of inoculation. Localized pain, tender lymphadenopathy, headache, generalized aching, and fever are characteristic prodromal symptoms. Some patients have no prodromal symptoms. Grouped vesicles on an erythematous base appear and subsequently erode (Figure 12-22). The vesicles in primary herpes simplex are more numerous and scattered than in the recurrent infection (Figures 12-23 and 12-24). The vesicles of herpes simplex are uniform in size in contrast to the vesicles seen in herpes zoster that vary in size. Mucous membrane lesions accumulate exudate, whereas skin lesions form a crust. Lesions last for 2 to 6 weeks unless secondarily infected and heal without scarring. During this primary infection, the virus enters the nerve endings in the skin directly below the lesions and ascends through peripheral nerves to the dorsal root ganglia, where it apparently remains in a latent stage.

Figure 12-22 Herpes simplex—the evolution of lesions.

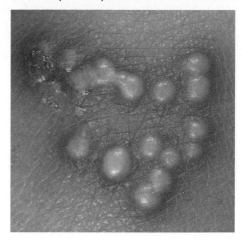

A, Vesicles appear on a red base.

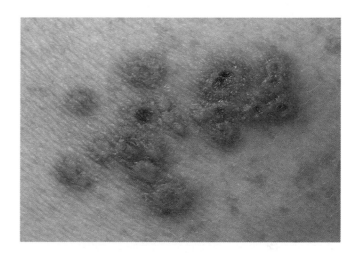

B, The center becomes depressed (umbilicated).

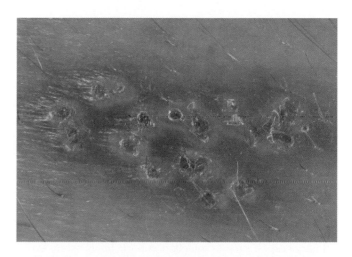

C, Crusts form and the lesions heal with or without scarring.

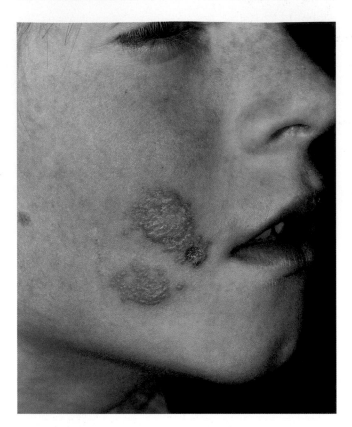

Figure 12-23
Primary herpes simplex infection. Primary infections in children typically begin in or about the oral cavity. Blisters are numerous and confluent.

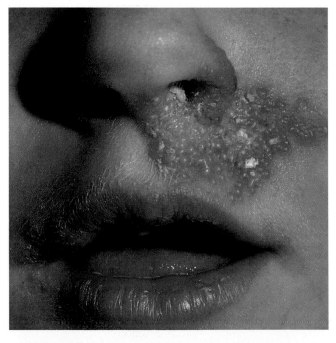

Figure 12-24
Primary herpes simplex infection. A particularly extensive eruption involving the mouths, lips, and nasal orifice.

Recurrent infection. Local skin trauma (e.g., ultraviolet [UV] light exposure, chapping, abrasion) or systemic changes (e.g., menses, fatigue, fever) reactivate the virus, which then travels down the peripheral nerves to the site of initial infection and causes the characteristic focal, recurrent infection. Recurrent infection is not inevitable. Many individuals have a rise in antibody titer and never experience recurrence. The prodromal symptoms, lasting 2 to 24 hours, resemble those of the primary infection. Within 12 hours, a group of lesions evolves rapidly from an erythematous base to form papules and then vesicles. The dome-shaped, tense vesicles rapidly umbilicate. In 2 to 4 days, they rupture, forming aphthaelike erosions in the mouth and vaginal area or erosions covered by crusts on the lips and skin. Crusts are shed in approximately 8 days to reveal a pink, reepithelialized surface. In contrast to the primary infection, systemic symptoms and lymphadenopathy are rare unless there is secondary infection.

The frequency of recurrence varies with anatomic site and virus type.[21] The frequency of recurrence of HSV-2 genital herpes is higher than HSV-1 oral-labial infection. HSV-1 oral infections recur more often than genital HSV-1 infections. HSV-2 genital infections recur 6 times more frequently than HSV-1 genital infections. The frequency of recurrence is lowest for oral-labial HSV-2 infections.

Laboratory diagnosis. The laboratory diagnosis of herpes simplex is covered in Chapter Eleven, which discusses sexually transmitted viral infections.

Treatment. A number of measures can be taken to relieve discomfort and promote healing. These are described in the following sections. Acyclovir (Zovirax), an antiviral drug active against herpes viruses, is available for both topical, oral, and intravenous administration. The appropriate use of this agent is outlined in Table 12-2. The drug decreases the duration of viral excretion, new lesion formation, and vesicles, and it promotes rapid healing. The subsequent recurrence rate is not influenced by acyclovir. Acyclovir-resistant herpes simplex virus infections are becoming a problem in patients with acquired immunodeficiency syndrome. L-lysine is not effective.

TABLE 12-2 Acyclovir Treatment of Herpes Simplex Infections

Type of infection	Treatment	Benefits
First-episode infection (any site)		
Primary first episode (antibodies absent at onset of infection)		
Nonprimary first episode (antibodies already present)		
Mild symptoms (patient refused pills)	Topical: applied every 4 hours, while awake, for 10 days	Decreased symptomatic period; no effect on new vesicle formation
Mild symptoms (immunosuppressed) chronic nonhealing ulcerative lesions	Topical: applied every 4 hours, while awake, for duration of infection	Dramatically speeds healing; rapidly decreases viral shedding and pain
Mild symptoms	Oral: 200 mg 5 times a day, while awake, for 7 to 10 days	50% reduction in duration of pain, healing time, crusting time, and duration of systemic symptoms; reduced incidence of complications
Significant constitutional symptoms	IV: 5 mg/kg every 8 hours for 5 to 7 days	
Recurrent herpes (lips, genitalia, buttocks, fingers)		
Symptomatic infections <6 recurrences/year	Oral: 200 mg 5 times a day for 5 days Or Oral: 400 mg 3 times a day for 5 days Or Oral: 800 mg 2 times a day for 5 days	Patient initiated treatment during the prodrome; decrease in duration of viral shedding and in formation of new lesions; the recurrence rate is not altered.
>6 recurrences/year	Oral: 200 mg 3-5 times a day continually or 400 mg 2 times a day Topically: no substantial benefit	Recurrence rate decreased 60% to 90% Incidence of asymptomatic shedding is reduced Continual treatment for up to 5 or more years
Herpes-associated recurrent erythema multiforme	Oral: 200 mg 3-5 times a day continually or 400 mg 2 times a day	Prevents recurrence of herpes and erythema multiforme

Eczema herpeticum
  Infant
  Children
  Adult
	IV: 10 mg/kg/q8h until resolution
	Oral: 25 to 30 mg/kg/day until resolution
	Oral: 200 mg 5 times a day until resolution
	IV: 5 mg/kg every 8 hours for 7 to 10 days	

Primary genital HSV in pregnant women with disseminated infection	IV: 7.5 mg/kg every 8 hours until resolution	
Disseminated neonatal HSV infection	IV: 10 mg/kg/q8h until resolution	Improved survival from central nervous system infection

ORAL-LABIAL HERPES SIMPLEX

Primary infection. Gingivostomatitis and pharyngitis are the most frequent manifestations of first-episode HSV-1 infection. Infection occurs most commonly in children between ages 1 and 5 years. The incubation period is 3 to 12 days. Although most cases are mild, some are severe. Sore throat and fever may precede the onset of painful vesicles occurring anywhere in the oral cavity. The vesicles rapidly coalesce and erode with a white, then yellow, superficial, purulent exudate. Pain interferes with eating and tender cervical lymphadenopathy develops. Fever subsides in 3 to 5 days and oral pain and erosions are usually gone in 2 weeks; in severe cases, they may last for 3 weeks.

Recurrent infection. Recurrences average 2 to 3 each year but may happen as often as 12 times a year. Oral HSV-1 infections recur more often than oral HSV-2 infections.[21] Recurrent oral herpes simplex can appear as a localized cluster of small ulcers in the oral cavity, but the most common manifestation is eruptions on the vermilion border of the lip (recurrent herpes labialis) (Figure 12-25). Fever (fever blisters), upper respiratory infections (cold sores), and exposure to UV light, among other things, may precede the onset. The course of the disease in the oral-labial area is the same as it is in other areas. Immunosuppressed patients are at greater risk of developing lesions on the lips, in the oral cavity, and on surrounding skin (Figure 12-26). The recurrence rate and long-term natural history are not well defined. Many people experience a decrease in the frequency of recurrences, but others experience an increase.

Treatment. A number of treatment modalities have been tried for herpes on the vermilion border. Oral acyclovir can be used to treat the primary infection and to prevent recurrent disease (see Table 12-2). Measures can be taken to delay recurrence and promote rapid healing.

The lips should be protected from sun exposure with opaque creams such as zinc oxide or with sun-blocking agents incorporated into a lip balm (Chapstick 15). A cool water or Burow's compress decreases erythema and debrides crusts to promote healing.

Lubricating creams may be applied if lips become too dry, but petrolatum-based ointments applied directly to an erosion may delay healing.

Figure 12-25
Herpes simplex labialis. Typical presentation with tense vesicles appearing on the lips and extending onto the skin.

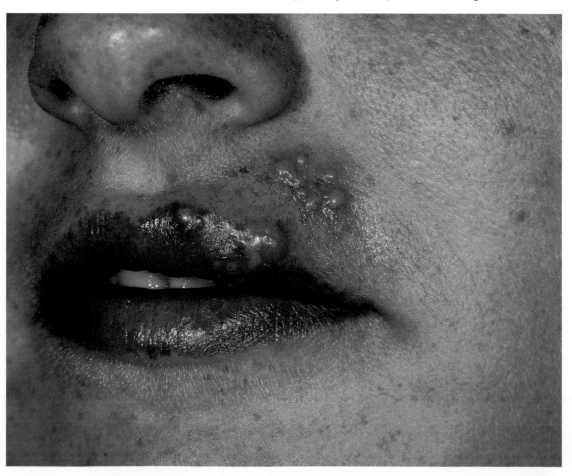

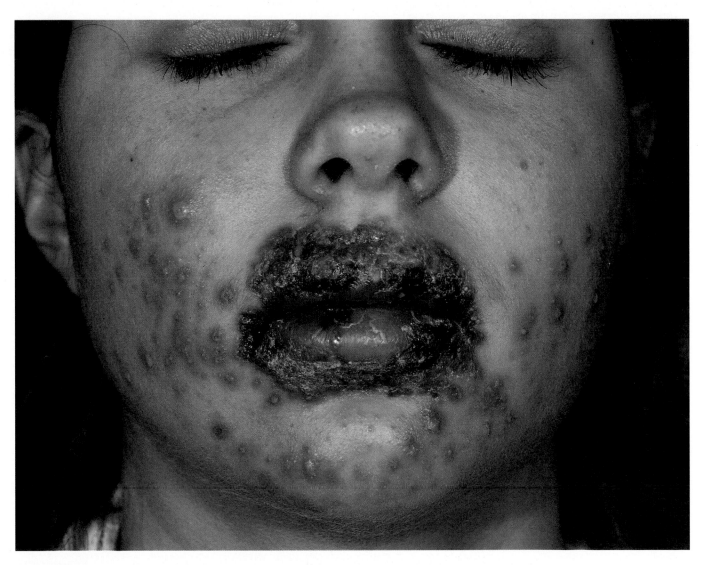

Figure 12-26
Herpes simplex labialis. Extensive involvement in an
immunosuppressed patient.

CUTANEOUS HERPES SIMPLEX

Herpes simplex may appear on any skin surface (Figures 12-27 and 12-28). It is important to identify all of the characteristic features when attempting to differentiate cutaneous herpes from other vesicular eruptions.

Herpetic whitlow. Herpes simplex of the fingertip (herpetic whitlow) (Figure 12-29) can resemble a group of warts or a bacterial infection. Health care professionals who had frequent contact with oral secretions used to be the most commonly affected group; the incidence has decreased, probably as a result of heightened awareness of the condition and stricter infection-control precautions. Today, herpetic whitlow is most often reported in pediatric patients with gingivostomatitis and in adult women with genital herpes.[22]

Herpes gladiatorum (cutaneous herpes in athletes involved in contact sports) is transmitted by direct skin-to-skin contact. This is a recognized health risk for wrestlers.[23] Prompt identification and exclusion of wrestlers with skin lesions may reduce transmission.

Herpes simplex of the buttock. Herpes simplex of the buttock area seems to be more common in women (Figure 12-30).

Herpes simplex of the trunk. Herpes simplex of the lumbosacral region or trunk may be very difficult to differentiate from herpes zoster; the diagnosis becomes apparent only at the time of recurrence.

Oral acyclovir is useful for suppressive therapy, particularly for recurrent fingertip and buttock infection.[24]

Figure 12-27
Herpes simplex of the skin: vesicular stage. The uniform size of the vesicles helps differentiate this from herpes zoster, in which vesicles vary in size.

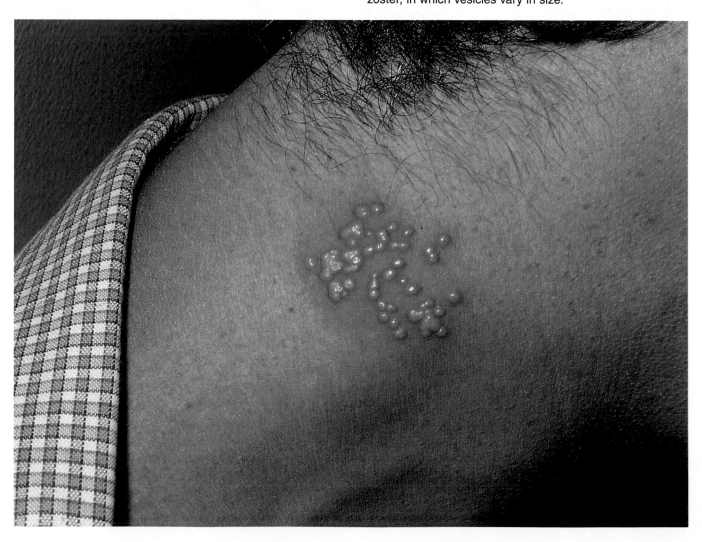

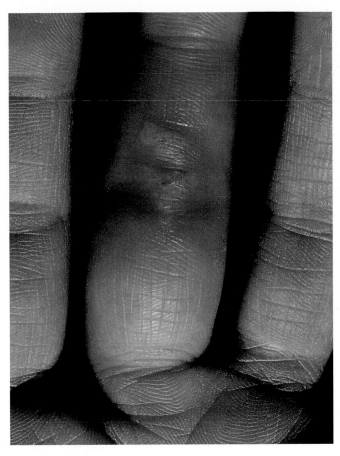

Figure 12-28
Recurrent herpes simplex of the finger. Infections in this area are unusual and mimic other blistering eruptions such as poison ivy or bites.

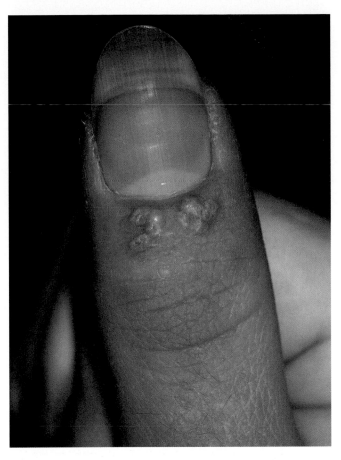

Figure 12-29
Herpes simplex of the finger (herpetic whitlow). Inoculation followed examination of a patient's mouth.

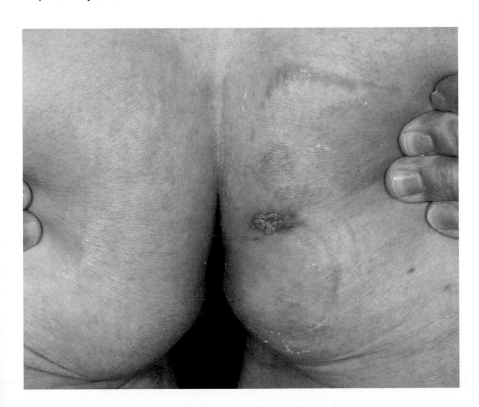

Figure 12-30
Herpes simplex of the buttocks. Infection of this location is seen more frequently in women.

ECZEMA HERPETICUM

Eczema herpeticum (Kaposi's varicelliform eruption) is the association of two common conditions: atopic dermatitis and herpes simplex virus infection. Certain atopic infants and adults may develop the rapid onset of diffuse cutaneous herpes simplex. The severity of infection ranges from mild and transient to fatal. The disease is most common in areas of active or recently healed atopic dermatitis, particularly the face, but normal skin can be involved. The disease in most cases is a primary herpes simplex infection. In one third of the patients in a particular study, there was a history of herpes labialis in a parent in the previous week.[25] Recurrences are uncommon and usually limited. Approximately 10 days after exposure, numerous vesicles develop, become pustular, and umbilicate markedly (Figure 12-31). Secondary staphylococcal infection commonly occurs. New crops of vesicles may appear during the following weeks. The most intense viral dissemination is located in the areas of dermatitis, but normal-appearing skin may ultimately be involved. High fever and adenopathy occur 2 to 3 days after the onset of vesiculation. The fever subsides in 4 to 5 days in uncomplicated cases, and the lesions evolve in the typical manner (Figure 12-32). Viremia with infection of internal organs can be fatal. Recurrent disease is milder and usually without constitutional symptoms.

Treatment. Eczema herpeticum of the young infant is a medical emergency. Early treatment with acyclovir can be life saving.[26,27] Eczema herpeticum is managed with cool, wet compresses, similar to the management of diffuse genital herpes simplex. Oral dosages of acyclovir 25 to 30 mg/kg/day have been effective.[28] Infants were successfully treated with intravenous acyclovir, 1500 mg/m²/day, administered over a 1-hour period three times a day.[29,30] Oral antistaphylococcal antibiotics are an important part of treatment. Minor relapses do not require a second course of acyclovir. Adults respond to the standard intravenous acyclovir dosage of 250 mg three times a day. Oral acyclovir 200 mg five times a day is expected to be equally effective.

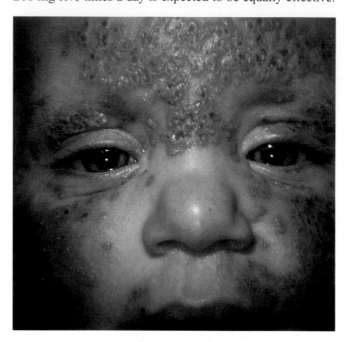

Figure 12-31
Eczema herpeticum. Numerous umbilicated vesicles of the face.

Figure 12-32
Eczema herpeticum. First crop of lesions has formed crusts; a new lesion has appeared on the ear.

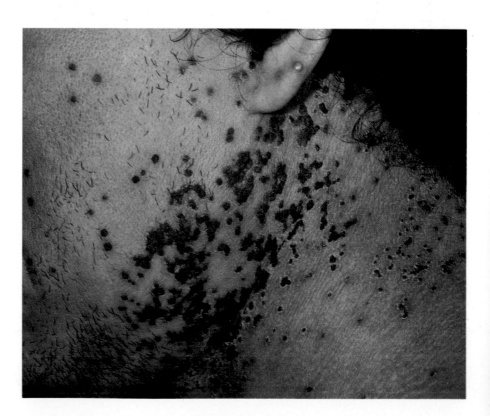

Varicella

Varicella, or chicken pox, is a highly contagious viral infection that, during epidemics, affects the majority of urban children before puberty. The incidence peaks sharply in March, April, and May in temperate climates. Transmission is by airborne droplets or vesicular fluid. Patients are contagious from 2 days before onset of the rash until all lesions have crusted. The systemic symptoms, extent of eruption, and complications are greater in adults; thus some parents intentionally expose their young children. Patients with defective, cell-mediated immunity or those using immunosuppressive drugs, especially systemic corticosteroids, have a prolonged course with more extensive eruptions and a greater incidence of complications. An attack of chicken pox usually confers lifelong immunity. Varicella vaccine is now available in the U.S. from Merck, Inc. It is approved for use in children and adults.

Clinical course. The incubation period averages 14 days, with a range of 9 to 21 days; in the immunosuppressed host, the incubation period can be shorter. The prodromal symptoms in children are absent or consist of low fever, headache, and malaise, which appear directly before or with the onset of the eruption. In adults, symptoms consist of fever, chills, malaise, and backache, which are more severe, and occur 2 to 3 days before the eruption.

Eruptive phase. The rash begins on the trunk (centripetal distribution) (Figure 12-33) and spreads to the face (Figure 12-34) and extremities (centrifugal spread). The extent of involvement varies considerably. Some children have so few lesions that the disease goes unnoticed. Older children and adults have a more extensive eruption involving all areas, sometimes with lesions too numerous to count.

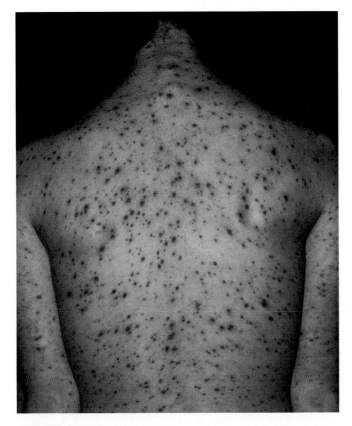

Figure 12-33
Chicken pox. Numerous lesions on the trunk (centripetal distribution).

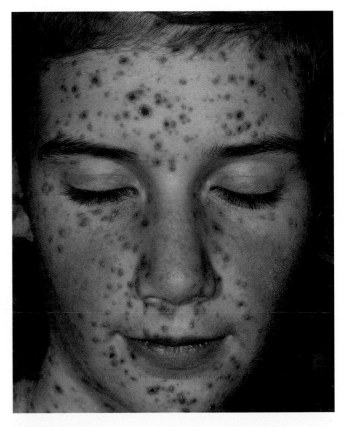

Figure 12-34
Chicken pox. Lesions present in all stages of development.

Figure 12-35 Chicken pox—the evolution of lesions.

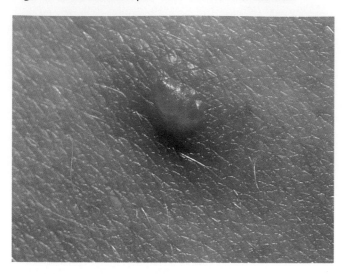

A, "Dew drop on a rose petal": a thin-walled vesicle with clear fluid forms on a red base.

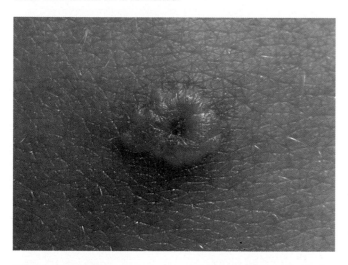

B, The vesicle becomes cloudy and depressed in the center (umbilicated), the border is irregular (scalloped).

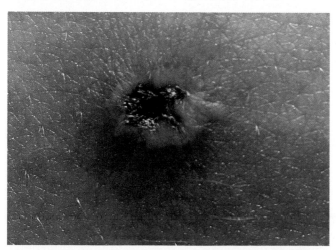

C, A crust forms in the center and eventually replaces the remaining portion of the vesicle at the periphery.

Lesions of different stages are present at the same time in any given body area. New lesion formation ceases by day 4 and most crusting occurs by day 6; the process lasts longer in the immunosuppressed patient. The lesion starts as a 2- to 4-mm red papule, which develops an irregular outline (rose petal) as a thin-walled clear vesicle appears on the surface (dew drop) (Figure 12-35). This lesion, "dew drop on a rose petal," is highly characteristic. The vesicle becomes umbilicated and cloudy and breaks in 8 to 12 hours to form a crust as the red base disappears. Fresh crops of additional lesions undergoing the same process occur in all areas at irregular intervals during the following 3 to 5 days, giving the characteristic picture of intermingled papules, vesicles, pustules, and crusts (Figure 12-34). Moderate to intense pruritis is usually present during the vesicular stage. The degree of temperature elevation parallels the extent and severity of the eruption and varies from 101° to 105° F. The temperature returns to normal when the vesicles have disappeared. Crusts fall off in 7 days (with a range of 5 to 20 days) and heal without scarring. Secondary infection or excoriation extends the process into the dermis, producing a craterlike, pockmark scar. Vesicles often form in the oral cavity and vagina and rupture quickly to form multiple, aphthaelike ulcers.

Complications

Skin infection. The most common complication in children is bacterial skin infection. Secondary infection should be suspected when the vesiculopustules develop large, moist, denuded areas, and particularly when the lesions become painful.

Neurologic complications. Encephalitis and Reye's syndrome are the next most common complications of chicken pox.[31] There are two forms of encephalitis. The cerebellar form seen in children is self-limited and complete recovery occurs. There is ataxia with nystagmus, headache, nausea, vomiting, and nuchal rigidity. Adult encephalitis patients have altered sensorium, seizures, and focal neurologic signs with a mortality rate of up to 35%.[32] Reye's syndrome is an acute, noninflammatory encephalopathy associated with hepatitis or fatty metamorphosis of the liver; 20% to 30% of Reye's syndrome cases are preceded by varicella.[33] The fatality rate is 20%. Salicylates used during the varicella infection may increase the risk of developing Reye's syndrome.

Pneumonia. Pneumonia is rare in normal children, but it is the most common serious complication in normal adults. Viral pneumonia develops 1 to 6 days after onset of the rash. In most cases it is asymptomatic and can only be detected by a chest x-ray examination.[34] Cough, dyspnea, fever, and chest pain can occur. Fatalities are rare.

Other. Hepatitis is the most common complication in immunosuppressed patients. Mild degrees of thrombocytopenia can accompany routine cases.

CHICKEN POX IN THE IMMUNOCOMPROMISED PATIENT

Patients with cancer or patients who are taking immunosuppressive drugs, particularly systemic and intranasal[35] corticosteroids,[36] have extensive eruptions and more complications. The mortality rate for immunosuppressed children or children with leukemia is 7% to 14%.[37] Adults with malignancy and varicella have a mortality rate as high as 50% (Figure 12-36). Hemorrhagic chicken pox, also called *malignant chicken pox*, is a serious complication in which the lesions are numerous, often bullous, and bleeding occurs in the skin at the base of the lesion.[38] The bullae turn dark brown and then black as blood accumulates in the blister fluid. Patients are usually toxic, have high fever and delirium, and may develop convulsions and coma. They frequently bleed from the gastrointestinal tract and mucous membranes. Pneumonia with hemoptysis commonly occurs. The mortality rate was 71% in one series.[37]

CHICKEN POX AND HIV INFECTION

Many children with HIV infection who acquire varicella have an uncomplicated clinical course and have a significant antibody response to varicella-zoster virus.[39] Some, however, have chronic, recurrent, or persistent varicella.[40,41] Varicella in adult HIV-infected patients is a potentially severe infection, but these patients respond well to acyclovir therapy. Immune status to varicella does not correlate with the declining CD4 counts and is well preserved, even in patients with fewer than 200 CD4 cells/mm^3.[42]

CHICKEN POX DURING PREGNANCY

Varicella during pregnancy poses a risk for both the mother and the unborn child. In a study of 43 pregnant women, 4 developed symptomatic pneumonia and 1 died of the infection.[43] Smoking is a possible risk factor. Pregnant women with pneumonitis who received high-dose intravenous acyclovir, ranging from 10 to 18 mg/kg every 8 hours, showed rapid improvement. Lower dosages may not be effective.[44]

Figure 12-36
Hemorrhagic chicken pox. Numerous vesicular and bullous lesions with hemorrhage at the base.

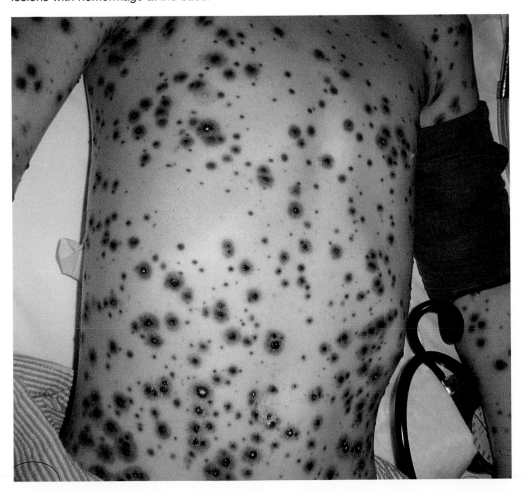

CONGENITAL AND NEONATAL CHICKEN POX
Maternal varicella

First trimester. Infection with the varicella-zoster virus during pregnancy can produce an embryopathy characterized by limb hypoplasia, chorioretinitis, cortical atrophy, and cutaneous scars (congenital varicella syndrome).[43,45] The risk is greatest when infection occurs during the first 20 weeks of pregnancy. The absolute risk of embryopathy after maternal varicella infection in the first 20 weeks of pregnancy is approximately 2%.[46,47]

Second trimester. Maternal varicella in the middle months of pregnancy may result in undetected fetal chicken pox. The newborn child who has already had chicken pox is at risk for developing herpes zoster (shingles). This may explain why some infants and children develop herpes zoster without the expected history of chicken pox.

Near birth. The time of onset of maternal lesions correlates directly with the frequency and severity of neonatal disease (Figure 12-37). If the mother has varicella 2 to 3 weeks before delivery, the fetus may be infected in utero and be born with or develop lesions 1 to 4 days after birth. Transplacental maternal antibody protects the infant and the course is usually benign. The risk of infection and complications is greatest when the maternal onset of varicella is from 5 days before to 2 days after delivery. When maternal infection appears more than 5 days before delivery, maternal antibody can develop and transfer via the placenta. Maternal infection that develops more than 2 days after delivery is associated with onset of disease in a newborn approximately 2 weeks later, at which point the immune system is better able to respond to the infection.

There is a high incidence of disseminated varicella in the infant when the mother's eruption appears 1 to 4 days before delivery or the child's eruption appears 5 to 10 days after birth. When the maternal rash appears within 5 days before delivery, approximately one third of infants become infected. After 5 days, transmission occurs in approximately 18%.[48] When the rash appears in infants between 5 and 10 days old, the mortality rate may be as high as 20%.[49] In this situation, the virus is either acquired transplacentally or from contact with maternal lesions during birth; there is insufficient time to receive adequate maternal antibody. The infant is immunologically incapable of controlling the infection and is at great risk of developing a disseminated disease. These infants should be given zoster immune globulin (ZIG), varicella-zoster immune globulin (VZIG) (see the box below), or gamma globulin if ZIG or VZIG are not available.

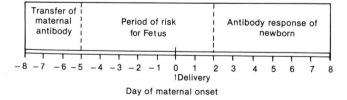

Figure 12-37
Varicella in newborns. For neonates, the risk of varicella infection and its associated complications is greatest when maternal onset of disease occurs in a 7-day period from 5 days before delivery to 2 days after delivery. *(From Straus SE et al: Ann Intern Med 108:221, 1988.)*

GUIDELINES FOR USE OF VZIG

EXPOSURE CRITERIA

One of the following exposures to persons with chicken pox or zoster:
Continuous household contact
Playmate contact (generally more than 1 hour of indoor play)
Hospital contact (in same two- to four-bed room or adjacent beds of large ward, or prolonged face-to-face contact with infectious staff member)
Newborn contact (newborn of mother who had onset of chicken pox less than 6 days before or less than 2 days after delivery)
Time elapsed after exposure is such that varicella-zoster immune globulin can be administered within 96 hours.

PERSONS FOR WHOM USE IS INDICATED

Susceptible to varicella
Significant exposure
One of these underlying illnesses or conditions:
Leukemia or lymphoma
Cellular immune deficiency
Immunosuppressive treatment
Newborn of mother who had onset of chicken pox less than 6 days before or less than 2 days after delivery
Premature infant (greater than 28 weeks gestation) whose mother lacks previous history of chicken pox
Premature infant (less than 28 weeks gestation or less than 1000 gm) regardless of maternal history
Pregnant women
Normal adults on an individual basis

From Strauss SE et al: *Ann Intern Med* 108:221-237, 1988.
Recommendations of the Immunization Practices Advisory Committee, Centers for Disease Control, Atlanta, Georgia.

Laboratory diagnosis

Culture. In questionable cases, virus can be cultured from vesicular fluid. See the section on herpes virus in Chapter Eleven for culture technique.

Serologic testing. The main value of serologic testing is the assessment of the immune status of immunocompromised patients (such as children with neoplastic diseases) who are at risk of developing severe disease with varicella-zoster virus infection. There are qualitative and quantitative tests.[50] The quantitative test measures IgG and IgM antibodies. The presence of IgM antibodies or a fourfold or greater rise in paired sera IgG titer indicates recent infection. The presence of IgG indicates past exposure and immunity. The qualitative screening test uses the same method but IgG is measured at only a single dilution (1:10).

Tzanck smear. Cytologic smear (Tzanck smear), as described for the diagnosis of herpes simplex, is a valuable tool for rapid diagnosis. Eighty percent of patients with zoster had a positive smear.[51] The test does not differentiate herpes simplex from varicella.

A chest x-ray examination should be obtained if respiratory symptoms develop. The white blood cell count (WBC) is variably elevated, but it is necessary to obtain a count only if the disease progresses.

Treatment

Bland antipruritic lotions (e.g., Sarna [menthol]) provide symptomatic relief. Antihistamines (hydroxyzine) may help control excoriation. Oral antibiotics active against *Streptococcus* and *Staphylococcus* are indicated for secondarily infected lesions.

Acyclovir and Vidarabine

CHILDREN AND ADOLESCENTS. Oral acyclovir therapy initiated within 24 hours of illness for otherwise healthy children with varicella typically results in a 1-day reduction of fever and approximately a 15% to 30% reduction in the severity of cutaneous and systemic signs and symptoms. Therapy has not been shown to reduce the rate of acute complications, pruritus, spread of infection, or duration of absence from school.

The American Academy of Pediatrics Committee on Infectious Diseases has published recommendations for the use of oral acyclovir in otherwise healthy children with varicella. Recommendations: (1) Oral acyclovir therapy is not routinely recommended for the treatment of uncomplicated varicella in otherwise healthy children. (2) For certain groups at increased risk of severe varicella or its complications, oral acyclovir therapy for varicella should be considered if it can be initiated within the first 24 hours after the onset of rash. These groups include the following: otherwise healthy, nonpregnant individuals 13 years of age or older;[52] children older than 12 months with a chronic cutaneous or pulmonary disorder; and those receiving long-term salicylate therapy, although in the latter instance a reduced risk for Reye's syndrome has not been shown to result from oral acyclovir therapy nor from milder illness with varicella.

ADULTS. Early therapy with oral acyclovir decreases the time to cutaneous healing of adult varicella, decreases the duration of fever, and lessens symptoms. Initiation of therapy after the first day of illness is of no value in uncomplicated cases of adult varicella.[53]

IMMUNOCOMPROMISED PATIENTS. Studies show that immunosuppressed patients treated with vidarabine or acyclovir had decreased morbidity from visceral dissemination; there was a modest effect on the cutaneous disease (Table 12-3).[54,55] The recommended schedules are vidarabine 10 mg/kg/day intravenously for 5 to 10 days or acyclovir 500 mg/m^2 or 10 mg/kg every 8 hours intravenously for 7 to 10 days.[56] Treatment of varicella in the normal host decreased the duration of fever but did not alter viral shedding or lesion healing. There is a high morbidity rate even in normal nonimmunosuppressed patients with clinically evident varicella pneumonia; intravenous acyclovir (500 mg/m^2/day for 7 days) may help.

Varicella-zoster immune globulin. Varicella-zoster immune globulin (VZIG), a more readily available preparation than ZIG, has been used to modify the course of varicella. It is indicated for immunosuppressed patients and certain nonimmunosuppressed patients as outlined in the box on p. 348. VZIG must be administered as early as possible after the presumed exposure but may be effective when given as late as 96 hours after exposure. VZIG is not known to be useful in treating clinical varicella or zoster or in preventing disseminated zoster. The duration of protection is estimated to be 3 weeks. Patients exposed again more than 3 weeks after a dose of VZIG should receive another full dose. VZIG is given intramuscularly.[57]

Gammaglobulin. Intravenous gammaglobulin may be an acceptable substitute if VZIG is not available.[58]

Varicella vaccine. Varicella vaccine has been extensively investigated for years. Studies show that protection against varicella seems to last at least 6 years.[59] The incidence of zoster in children with leukemia is no greater than in children who have had natural varicella infection.[60] The vaccine has been approved for use in the U.S. and is available from Merck, Inc. It is approved for children and adults. The live attenuated vaccine should not be given to patients with HIV infection or to other immunosuppressed patients.

TABLE 12-3 Acyclovir Treatment of Herpes Zoster Infections

Type of infection	Treatment	Benefits
Herpes zoster		
Normal patient	Oral: 800 mg 5 times a day for 7 to 10 days IV: 500 mg/m² or 10 mg/kg every 8 hours for 7 days	Prompt resolution of skin and viral shedding; marked reduction in incidence of episcleritis, keratitis, and iritis
Immunosuppressed	IV: 500 mg/m² or 10 mg/kg every 8 hours for 7 days	Prompt healing of skin lesions; diminished duration of pain if administered within 72 to 96 hours of onset; possible reduction in incidence of postherpetic neuralgia if treatment begins within 4 days of the onset of pain or 48 hours of onset of rash[75]
Immunocompromised	Topical: ointment applied 4 times a day	Significantly shortened time to complete healing
Varicella		
Normal adult	Oral: 800 mg 5 times a day for 5 days IV: 500 mg/m² or 10 mg/kg every 8 hours for 5 to 7 days	
Immunocompromised children (congenital and neonatal chicken pox)	IV: 500 mg/m² or 10 mg/kg every 8 hours for 7 days	Much lower frequency of visceral complications
Immunocompromised adults including pregnant women	IV: 500 mg/m² every 8 hours for 7 to 10 days or 10 mg/kg every 8 hours for 7 to 10 days	Substantial effect in prevention of cutaneous and visceral dissemination

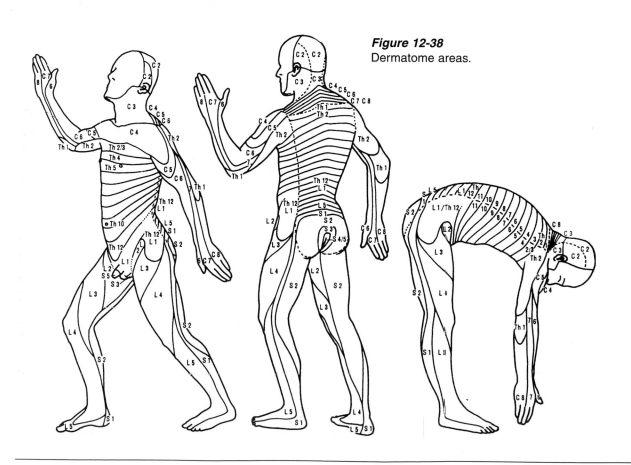

Figure 12-38
Dermatome areas.

Herpes Zoster

Herpes zoster, or shingles, a cutaneous viral infection generally involving the skin of a single dermatome (Figure 12-38), occurs during the lifetime of 10% to 20% of all persons. People of all ages are afflicted; it occurs regularly in young individuals,[61] but the incidence increases with age. There is an increased incidence of zoster in normal children who acquire chicken pox when younger than 2 months.[62] Patients with zoster are not more likely to have an underlying malignancy.[63,64] Zoster may be the earliest clinical sign of the development of the acquired immunodeficiency syndrome in high-risk individuals.[65]

Zoster results from reactivation of varicella virus that entered the cutaneous nerves during an earlier episode of chicken pox, travelled to the dorsal root ganglia, and remained in a latent form. Age, immunosuppressive drugs, lymphoma,[66] fatigue, emotional upsets, and radiation therapy have been implicated in reactivating the virus, which subsequently travels back down the sensory nerve infecting the skin. Some patients, particularly children with zoster, have no history of chicken pox. They may have acquired chicken pox by the transplacental route. Although reported, herpes zoster acquired by direct contact with a patient having active varicella or zoster is rare. Following contact with such patients, infections are more inclined to result from reactivation of latent infection.

Varicella zoster virus can be cultured from vesicles during an eruption. It may also cause chicken pox in those not previously infected.

The predisposition in the elderly for the development of herpes zoster is considered to be a consequence of diminishing immunologic function. The elderly are also at greater risk to develop segmental pain, which can continue for months after the skin lesions have healed.

Clinical presentation. Preeruptive pain (preherpetic neuralgia), itching, or burning, generally localized to the dermatome, precedes the eruption by 4 to 5 days. An extended period of pain (7 to 100 days) has been reported.[67] The pain may simulate pleurisy, myocardial infarction, abdominal disease, or migraine headache, and may present a difficult diagnostic problem until the characteristic eruption provides the answer. Preeruptive tenderness or hyperesthesia throughout the dermatome is a useful predictive sign. "Zoster sine herpete" refers to segmental neuralgia without a cutaneous eruption and is rare. Constitutional symptoms of fever, headache, and malaise may precede the eruption by several days. Regional lymphadenopathy may be present. Segmental pain and constitutional symptoms gradually subside as the eruption appears. Prodromal symptoms may be absent, particularly in children.

Eruptive phase. Although generally limited to the skin of a single dermatome (Figures 12-39 and 12-40), the eruption may involve one or two adjacent dermatomes (Figures 12-41 and 12-42). Occasionally, a few vesicles appear across the midline. Eruption is rare in bilaterally symmetric or asymmetric dermatomes. Approximately 50% of patients with uncomplicated zoster have a viremia, with the appearance of 20 to 30 vesicles scattered over the skin surface outside the affected dermatome. Possibly because chicken pox is centripetal (located on the trunk), the thoracic region is affected in two thirds of herpes zoster cases. An attack of herpes zoster does not confer lasting immunity, and it is not abnormal to have two or three episodes in a lifetime.

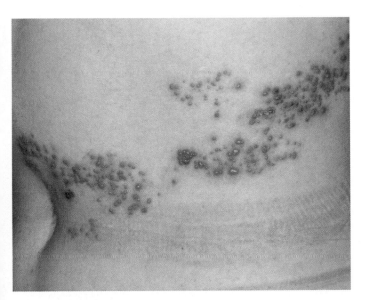

Figure 12-39
Herpes zoster. A common presentation with involvement of a single thoracic dermatome.

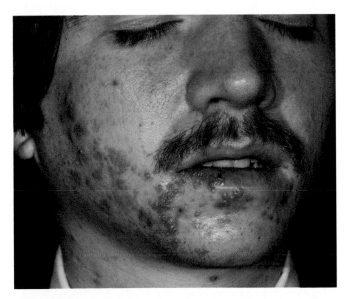

Figure 12-40
Herpes zoster. Unilateral single-dermatome distribution involving the mandibular branch of the fifth nerve.

The eruption begins with red, swollen plaques of various sizes and spreads to involve part or all of a dermatome. The vesicles arise in clusters from the erythematous base and become cloudy with purulent fluid by day 3 or 4. In some cases vesicles do not form or are so small that they are difficult to see (Figure 12-43). The vesicles vary in size, in contrast to the cluster of uniformly sized vesicles noted in herpes simplex (Figure 12-44). Successive crops continue to appear for 7 days. Vesicles either umbilicate (Figure 12-45) or rupture before forming a crust, which falls off in 2 to 3 weeks. The elderly or debilitated patients may have a prolonged and difficult course. For them, the eruption is typically more extensive and inflammatory, occasionally resulting in hemorrhagic blisters, skin necrosis, secondary bacterial infection, or extensive scarring (Figure 12-46), which is sometimes hypertrophic or keloidal (Figure 12-47).

Herpes zoster and HIV infection. Zoster may be the earliest clinical sign of the development of the acquired immunodeficiency syndrome in high-risk individuals. The incidence of herpes zoster is significantly higher among HIV-seropositive patients. The risk of herpes zoster is not associated with duration of HIV infection and is not predictive of faster progression to AIDS.[68]

Zoster during pregnancy. Herpes zoster during pregnancy, whether it occurs early or late in the pregnancy, appears to have no deleterious effects on either the mother or infant.[69]

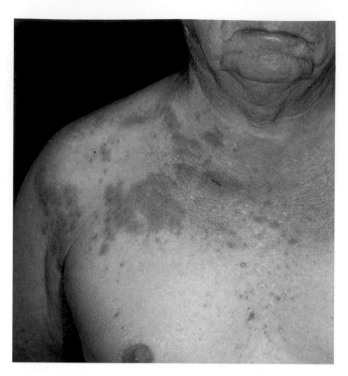

Figure 12-41
Herpes zoster. Lesions may involve several dermatomes.

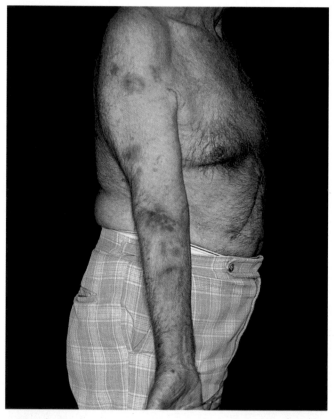

Figure 12-42
Herpes zoster. Lesions often involve more than one dermatome. Many patients do not understand that shingles can appear on any body surface and attribute lesions in this distribution to an allergy or bacterial infection.

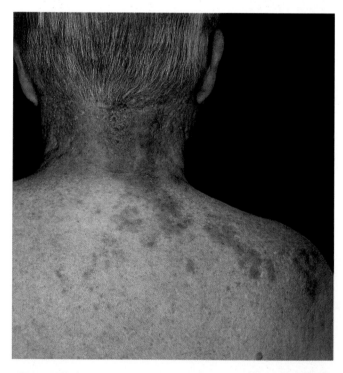

Figure 12-43
Herpes zoster. An early eruption without blisters. Blisters arise from an inflamed or urticarial base. Sometimes blisters do not occur.

HERPES ZOSTER—THE EVOLUTION OF LESIONS

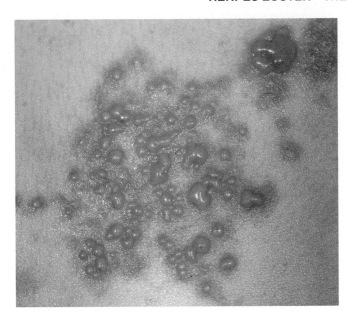

Figure 12-44
Herpes zoster. A group of vesicles that vary in size. Vesicles of herpes simplex are of uniform size.

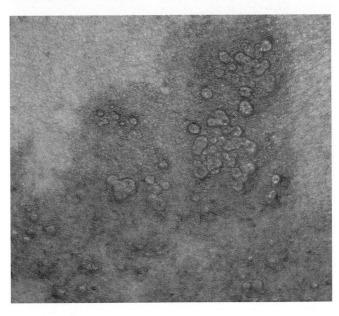

Figure 12-45
Herpes zoster. Vesicles become umbilicated and then form crusts.

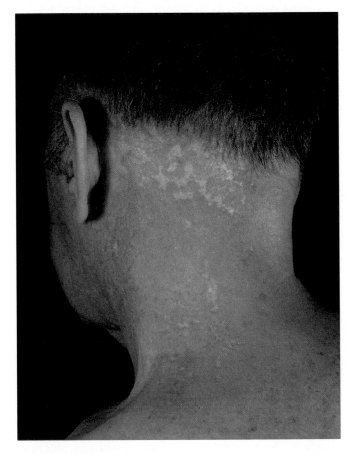

Figure 12-46
Herpes zoster. Several scars localized to a dermatome.

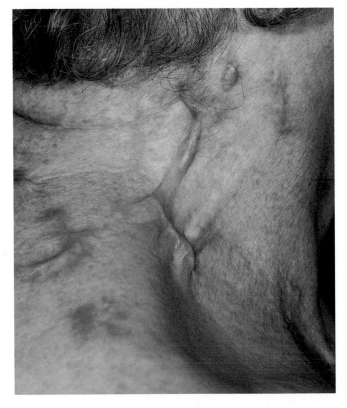

Figure 12-47
Herpes zoster. Hypertrophic scars. Plastic surgery was required to improve mobility of the neck.

TABLE 12-4	Ocular Complications in 86 Patients with Herpes Zoster Ophthalmicus*	
Complication		**No. of patients**
Lid involvement		11
Corneal involvement		66
Scleral involvement		4
Canalicular scarring		2
Uveitis		37
Glaucoma (secondary)		10
Persistent		2
Cataract		7
Neuroophthalmic involvement		7
Postherpetic neuralgia		15

Modified from Womack LW, Liesegang TJ: *Arch Ophthalmol* 101:44, 1983. By permission of Mayo Foundation.
*Some patients had more than one manifestation of involvement.

Syndromes

Ophthalmic zoster. The fifth cranial, or trigeminal, nerve has three divisions: the ophthalmic, maxillary, and mandibular. The ophthalmic division further divides into three main branches: the frontal, lacrimal, and nasociliary nerves. The frontal nerve separates into the supraorbital and supratrochlear nerves. Involvement of any branch of the ophthalmic nerve is called *herpes zoster ophthalmicus.* It is involved in 8% to 56% in various series, with 20% to 72% developing ocular complications. Anterior uveitis and the various varieties of keratitis are commonest, affecting 92% and 52% of patients with ocular involvement, respectively. Sight-threatening complications include neuropathic keratitis, perforation, secondary glaucoma, posterior scleritis/orbital apex syndrome, optic neuritis, and acute retinal necrosis (Table 12-4). Twenty-eight percent of initially involved eyes develop long-term ocular disease (6 months), with chronic uveitis, keratitis, and neuropathic ulceration being the commonest. With ophthalmic zoster, the rash

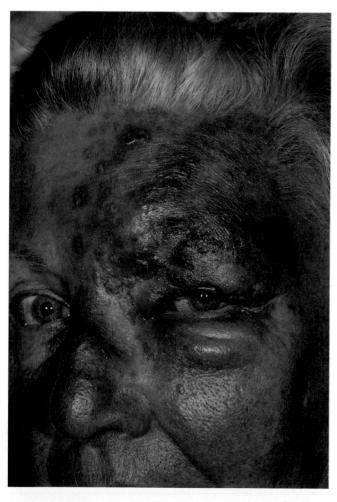

Figure 12-48
Herpes zoster (ophthalmic zoster). Involvement of the first branch of the fifth nerve. Vesicles on the side of the nose are associated with the most serious ocular complications.

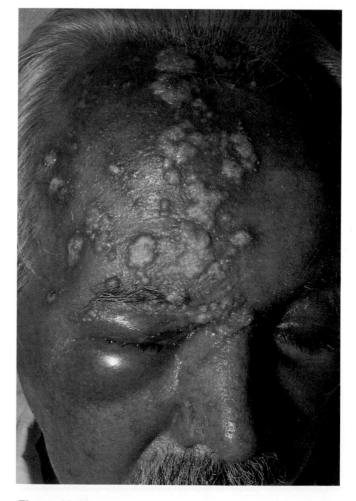

Figure 12-49
Herpes zoster (ophthalmic zoster). A virulent infection of the skin and eye.

extends from eye level to the vertex of the skull, but does not cross the midline (Figure 12-48 and 12-49). Herpes zoster ophthalmicus may be confined to certain branches of the trigeminal nerve. The tip and side of the nose and eye are innervated by the nasociliary branch of the trigeminal nerve. Vesicles on the side or tip of the nose (Hutchinson's sign) that occur during an episode of zoster are associated with the most serious ocular complications, including conjunctival, corneal, scleral, and other ocular diseases, although this is not invariable. Involvement of the other sensory branches of the trigeminal nerve is most likely to yield periocular involvement but spare the eyeball. Acute pain occurs in 93% of patients and remains in 31% at 6 months. Of patients aged 60 and over, pain persists in 30% for 6 months or longer, and this rises to 71% in those aged 80 and over.

Prompt treatment with oral acyclovir (800 mg five times daily for 7 days) reduces the severity of the skin eruption, the incidence and the severity of late ocular manifestations, and the intensity of postherpetic neuralgia. It is not useful to treat with acyclovir for more than 7 days.[70] At 6 months, late ocular inflammatory complications are seen in 29.1% of acyclovir-treated patients vs. 50% to 71% of untreated patients. Ophthalmic 3% acyclovir ointment may be used for established ocular complications.[71]

Ramsay Hunt's syndrome. Varicella zoster of the geniculate ganglion is called *Ramsay Hunt's syndrome*. The clinical definition is herpes zoster oticus, facial nerve paralysis, and auditory symptoms.[72] There is involvement of the sensory portion and motor portion of the seventh cranial nerve. There may be unilateral loss of taste on the anterior two thirds of the tongue and vesicles on the tympanic membrane, external auditory meatus, concha, and pinna. Involvement of the motor division of the seventh cranial nerve causes unilateral facial paralysis. Auditory nerve involvement occurs in 37.2% of patients, resulting in hearing deficits and vertigo.[73] Recovery from the motor paralysis is generally complete, but residual weakness is possible.

Sacral zoster (S2, S3, or S4 dermatomes). A neurogenic bladder with urinary hesitancy or urinary retention has reportedly been associated with zoster of the sacral dermatome S2, S3, or S4 (Figure 12-50).[74] Migration of virus to the adjacent autonomic nerves is responsible for these symptoms.

Figure 12-50 Ilioinguinal and sacral zoster.

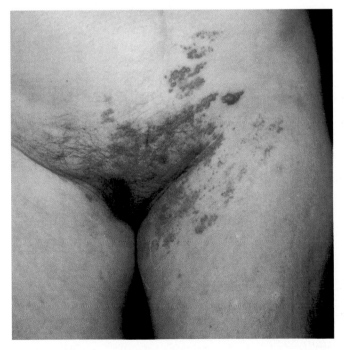

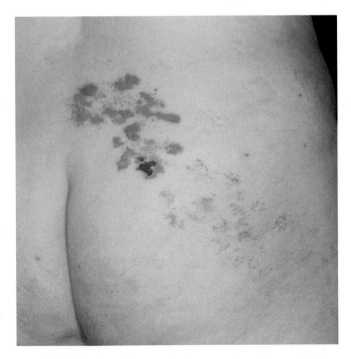

A, Zoster of T12, L1-L2, and S2-S4 dermatomes can occasionally cause a neurogenic bladder. Acute urinary retention and polyuria are the most common symptoms.

B, Lesions cover the entire dermatome, from the groin to the buttock.

Complications

Postherpetic neuralgia. Pain is the major cause of morbidity in zoster. There is an increasing incidence and duration of pain with age. Pain can persist in a dermatome for months or years after the lesions have disappeared. The pain is often severe, intractable, and exhausting. The patient protects areas of hyperesthesia to avoid the slightest pressure, which activates another wave of pain. There is a yearning for a few hours of sleep, but sharp paroxysms of lancinating pain invade the mind and the patient is again awakened. Despair and sometimes suicide occur if hope and encouragement are not provided.

The majority of patients under 30 years of age experience no pain. By age 40, the risk of prolonged pain lasting longer than 1 month increases to 33%. By age 70, the risk increases to 74%. Postherpetic neuralgia is more common and persists longer in cases of trigeminal nerve involvement. The degree of pain is not related to the extent of involvement, nor to the number of vesicles or degree of inflammation or fibrosis in peripheral nerves.[75] The mechanism of pain has not been explained. The absence of pain at the onset of cutaneous herpes zoster does not preclude its later development.

Dissemination. Patients with Hodgkin's disease are uniquely susceptible to herpes zoster. Furthermore, 15% to 50% of zoster patients with active Hodgkin's disease have disseminated disease involving the skin, lungs, and brain; 10% to 25% of those patients die.[76] In patients with other types of cancer, death from zoster is unusual.

Motor paresis. Muscle weakness in the muscle group associated with the infected dermatome may be observed before, during, or after an episode of herpes zoster. The weakness results from the spread of the virus from the dorsal root ganglia to the anterior root horn. Patients in the sixth to eighth decade of life are most commonly involved. Motor neuropathies are usually transient and approximately 75% of patients recover. They occur in approximately 5% of all cases of zoster but in up to 12% of patients with cephalic zoster. Ramsay Hunt's syndrome accounts for more than half of the cephalic motor neuropathies.[77]

Necrosis, infection, and scarring. Elderly, malnourished, debilitated, or immunosuppressed patients tend to have a more virulent and extensive course of disease. The entire skin area of a dermatome may be lost following diffuse vesiculation. Large adherent crusts promote infection and increase the depth of involvement (Figure 12-51). Scarring, sometimes hypertrophic or keloidal (see Figures 12-46 and 12-47), follows.

Encephalitis. Neurologic symptoms characteristically appear within the first 2 weeks of onset of the skin lesions. It is possible that encephalitis is immune-mediated rather than a result of viral invasion. Patients at greatest risk are those with trigeminal and disseminated zoster, as well as the immunosuppressed. The mortality rate is 10% to 20%; most survivors recover completely. The diagnosis is hampered by the fact that the virus is rarely isolated from the spinal fluid. Cell counts and protein concentration of the spinal fluid are elevated in encephalitis and in approximately 40% of typical zoster patients.

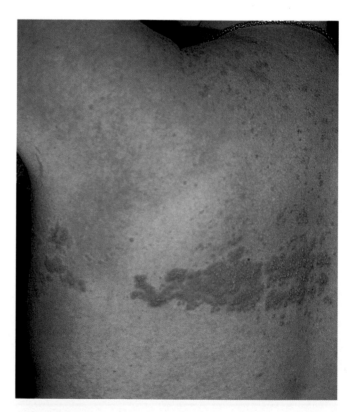

Figure 12-52
Herpes zoster mimicking poison ivy. A group of blisters on a broad base is often mistaken for an acute eczematous eruption.

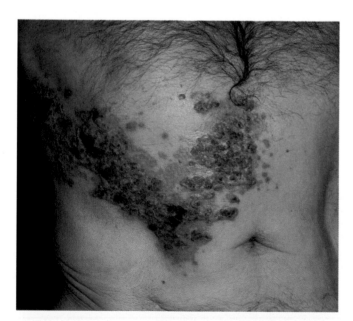

Figure 12-51
Herpes zoster. Massive involvement of a dermatome: numerous vesicles have been replaced by large crusts.

Differential diagnosis

Herpes simplex. The diagnosis of herpes zoster is usually obvious. Herpes simplex can be extensive, particularly on the trunk. It may be confined to a dermatome and possess many of the same features as zoster (zosteriform herpes simplex). The vesicles of zoster vary in size, whereas those of simplex are uniform within a cluster. A later recurrence proves the diagnosis.

Poison ivy. A group of vesicles on a red, inflamed base may be mistaken for poison ivy (Figure 12-52).

"Zoster sine herpete." Neuralgia within a dermatome without the typical rash can be confusing. A concurrent rise in varicella zoster complement–fixation titers has been demonstrated in a number of such cases.

Cellulitis. The eruption of zoster may never evolve to the vesicular stage. The red, inflamed, edematous or urticarial-like plaques may appear infected, but they usually have a fine, cobblestone surface indicative of a cluster of minute vesicles. A skin biopsy shows characteristic changes.

Laboratory diagnosis

The laboratory methods for identification are the same as for herpes simplex. Tzanck smears, skin biopsy (Figures 12-53 and 12-54), complement-fixation titers, vesicular-fluid immunofluorescent antibody stains, electron microscopy, and culture of vesicle fluid are some of the studies to consider.

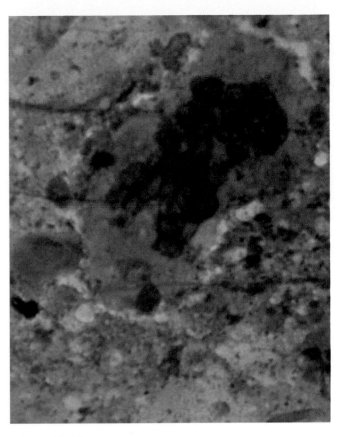

Figure 12-53
Tzanck smear. A cytologic smear of the base of a herpetic blister. The multinucleated giant cells are characteristic of herpes simplex and herpes zoster.

Figure 12-54
Herpes zoster. A skin biopsy showing multinucleated giant cells at the base of a vesicle.

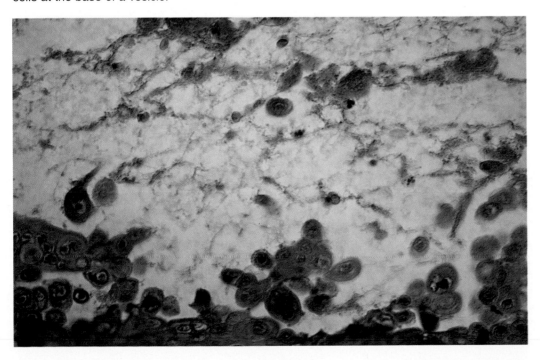

Treatment
Suppression of inflammation, pain, and infection

TOPICAL THERAPY. Burow's solution or cool tap water can be used in a wet compress. The compresses, applied for 20 minutes several times a day, macerate the vesicles, remove serum and crust, and suppress bacterial growth. A whirlpool with betadine solution is particularly helpful in removing the crust and serum that occurs with extensive eruptions in the elderly.

ORAL STEROIDS. Pain reduction is greater during the acute phase of disease in patients treated with steroids; however, there are no significant differences between steroid-treated and nonsteroid-treated patients in the time to a first or a complete cessation of pain. Steroid recipients report more complications.[78]

INTRALESIONAL STEROIDS AND XYLOCAINE. Attenuation or elimination of pain in the eruptive stage and for postherpetic neuralgia may be accomplished with the following simple technique.[79] Lidocaine (Xylocaine) 0.5% to a total of 4 to 5 ml is injected into the subcutaneous tissue at the most painful sites. For patients with intolerable pain and/or necrotic herpes zoster, 2 ml of 1% lidocaine is injected deep into the proximal area, innervating the herpes zoster lesions. Injections are repeated every 4 to 5 days as needed. Others have claimed substantial relief with a similar schedule using subcutaneous injections through the affected skin with a combination of lidocaine and triamcinolone acetonide (Kenalog).[80] The mixture is prepared by diluting triamcinolone acetonide (10 mg/5 ml) with equal parts 1% lidocaine. Diluting Kenalog with bacteriostatic saline makes the injection less painful.

SYMPATHETIC BLOCKS. Sympathetic blocks (stellate ganglion or epidural) with 0.25% bupivacaine terminates the pain of acute herpes zoster[81] and prevents or relieves postherpetic neuralgia in more than 80% of patients treated within 2 months of onset of the acute phase of the disease. Three injections are made on alternate days. When thoracic dermatomes are involved, an epidural catheter is left in place for the 5 days of therapy to avoid having to replace the needle each time. Epidural injections are made at or just above the highest dermatome of the rash. There is prompt relief of pain and all symptoms are usually gone after the second injection.[82] Sympathetic blockade applied within the first 2 months after the onset of acute herpes zoster terminates[83] the acute phase of the disease, probably by restoring intraneural blood flow, thus preventing the death of the large fibers and avoiding the development of postherpetic neuralgia. After 2 months, the damage to the large fibers is irreversible.

Attenuation of the acute phase (see the box below)

ORAL AND INTRAVENOUS ACYCLOVIR. Intravenous and high-dose oral acyclovir decrease acute pain, inflammation, vesicle formation, and viral shedding. The median duration of pain in acyclovir recipients is 20 days vs. 62 days for their placebo counterparts.[84] Several studies show no effect on the subsequent development of postherpetic neuralgia, even in patients who experience immediate pain relief.[85,86] A study showed a possible reduction of the incidence of postherpetic neuralgia if treatment began within 4 days of the onset of pain or within 48 hours of the onset of rash.[87] Acyclovir appears to change the nature of postherpetic neuralgia.[88] Its use should be considered for immunosuppressed, debilitated patients who appear to be developing extensive cutaneous disease and for patients with ophthalmic zoster who are at increased risk of ocular complications.[89] Treatment is most effective when started within the first 48 hours of infection. The recommended oral dosage for adults is 800 mg five times daily for 5 to 10 days (see Table 12-3), usually for 7 days.[90] Proper hydration and urine flow must be maintained. The recommended intravenous dosage is 500 mg/m^2 or 10 mg/kg every 8 hours in 1-hour infusions for 7 days. Intravenous drugs at these dosages must be given with great care to patients with impaired renal function. Hydration and urine flow must be maintained and the mental status of the patient must be monitored.

TREATMENT OPTIONS FOR ACUTE HERPES ZOSTER (DOSAGE)

ACYCLOVIR
800 mg
5×/day for 7 days

VALACYCLOVIR
1000 mg
3×/day for 7 days

FAMCICLOVIR
500 mg
3×/day for 7 days

Acyclovir-resistant infection. Persons with AIDS who have CD4+ counts less than 100, and transplant patients, especially bone marrow allograft recipients, may experience infections with acyclovir-resistant varicella-zoster virus. This may be associated with the appearance of atypical hyperkeratotic papules.[91] Patients who have received prior repeated acyclovir treatment appear to be at the highest risk of harboring acyclovir-resistant strains. Treatment with foscarnet (40 mg/kg IV every 8 hours) should be initiated within 7 to 10 days in patients suspected to have acyclovir-resistant varicella-zoster virus infections. Foscarnet therapy should be continued for at least 10 days or until lesions are completely healed.[92]

Disseminated herpes zoster in the immunocompromised host. Acyclovir (30 mg/kg/day at 8-hour intervals) and vidarabine (continuous 12-hour infusion at 10 mg/kg/day) for 7 days (longer if resolution of cutaneous or visceral disease is incomplete) are equally effective for the treatment of disseminated herpes zoster. The resultant mortality is low.[93]

TOPICAL ACYCLOVIR. Topical acyclovir ointment applied four times a day for 10 days to immunocompromised patients significantly shortened complete-healing time.

VALACYCLOVIR (VALTREX—500 MG CAPLETS). Valacyclovir is converted to acyclovir after absorption. It is absorbed 3 to 5 times better than acyclovir. Studies demonstrate a significant advantage of Valtrex compared to Zovirax on decreasing the duration and incidence of pain, including both acute pain and postherpetic neuralgia. The dosage for acute herpes zoster is 1 gm PO tid for 7 days. Patients who may have trouble complying with five times daily dosing of oral Zovirax and patients at highest risk for postherpetic neuralgia (e.g., older patients and those with prodromal pain) may benefit from valacyclovir.

FAMCICLOVIR (FAMVIR—500 MG TABLETS). Famciclovir is available for oral treatment of acute uncomplicated herpes zoster. The recommended dosage beginning within 72 hours after the onset of rash is 500 mg tid for 7 days. The benefits appear to be similar to acyclovir.

Prevention of postherpetic neuralgia. The use of systemic steroids during the early acute phases of herpes zoster to prevent postherpetic neuralgia has been controversial. A recent double-blind, controlled trial showed that prednisolone therapy initiated at a dose of 40 mg per day and tapered over a three-week period does not reduce the frequency of postherpetic neuralgia.[78] Systemic corticosteroids have no effect on postherpetic neuralgia when the lesions have healed.

Treatment of postherpetic neuralgia

CAPSAICIN. Capsaicin is a chemical that depletes the pain impulse transmitter substance P and prevents its resynthesis within the neuron. Substantial relief of pain follows the application (three to five times daily) of this chemical in the form of a white cream (Zostrix and Zostrix-HP).[94] Substantial pain relief occurs in 4 weeks in most patients. Maximum benefit occurs when capsaicin cream is applied for many weeks. Capsaicin is available without prescription.

ANALGESICS. Oral analgesics (e.g., Tylenol with codeine, Percodan, Percocet) should be used as needed.

ANTIDEPRESSANTS AND TRANQUILIZERS. Amitriptyline (75 mg/day) provided good to excellent pain relief for 16 of 24 patients in a double-blind, crossover study.[95] There is a strong correlation between pain relief and the interval between the occurrence of herpes zoster and the initiation of treatment with amitriptyline—early treatment is almost twice as likely to be successful as late treatment.[88] Tricyclic antidepressants alone or in conjunction with other drugs have been advocated for patients with chronic pain.[96]

TOPICAL LIDOCAINE GEL. In one study lidocaine gel was applied for 8 hours, without occlusion in cranial neuralgia, and for 24 hours under Tegaderm occlusion in patients with limb or torso neuralgia. Significant pain relief was provided with both techniques.[97]

SURGERY. Rhizotomy, or surgical separation of pain fibers by a neurosurgeon, may be considered in extreme cases where no therapy has been helpful and the pain is intolerable and persistent.

EMOTIONAL SUPPORT. Patients with postherpetic neuralgia can be miserable for several months. Emotional support is as important as other therapeutic measures.

REFERENCES

1. Williams H, Pottier A, et al: Are viral warts seen more commonly in children with eczema? *Arch Dermatol* 129:717-720, 1993.
2. Lockshin NA: Flat facial warts treated with fluorouracil, *Arch Dermatol* 115:929-1030, 1979.
3. Lee S, Kim J-G, Chun SI: Treatment of verruca plana with 5% 5-fluorouracil ointment, *Dermatologica* 160:383-389, 1980.
4. Berman A, Domnitz JM, Winkelmann RK: Plantar warts recently turned black, *Arch Dermatol* 118:47-51, 1982.
5. Iwatsuki K, Tagami H, Takigawa M, et al: Plane warts under spontaneous regression, *Arch Dermatol* 122:655-659, 1986.
6. Pringle WM, Helms BC: Treatment of plantar warts by blunt dissection, *Arch Dermatol* 108:79-82, 1973.
7. Naylor MF et al: Contact immunotherapy of resistant warts, *J Am Acad Dermatol* 19:679-683, 1988.
8. Manz LA, Pelachyk JM: Bleomycin-lidocaine mixture reduces pain of intralesional injection in the treatment of recalcitrant verrucae, *J Am Acad Dermatol* 25:524-526, 1991.
9. Shelley WB, Shelley ED: Intralesional bleomycin sulfate therapy for warts. A novel bifurcated needle puncture technique, *Arch Dermatol* 127:234-236, 1991.
10. Amer M et al: Therapeutic evaluation for intralesional injection of bleomycin sulfate in 143 resistant warts, *J Am Acad Dermatol* 18:1313-1316, 1988.
11. James MP, Collier PM, et al: Histologic, pharmacologic, and immunocytochemical effects of injection of bleomycin into viral warts, *J Am Acad Dermatol* 28:933-937, 1993.
12. Habif TP, Graf FA: Extirpation of subungual and periungual warts by blunt dissection, *J Dermatol Surg Oncol* 7:553-555, 1981.
13. Litt JZ: Don't excise—exorcise: treatment for subungual and periungual warts, *Cutis* 22:673-676, 1978.
14. Petersen CS, Gerstoft J: Molluscum contagiosum in HIV-infected patients, *Dermatology* 184:19-21, 1992.
15. Ghigliotti G, Carrega G, et al: Cutaneous cryptococcosis resembling molluscum contagiosum in a homosexual man with AIDS. Report of a case and review of the literature, *Acta Derm Venereol* 72:182-184, 1992.
16. Schwartz JJ, Myskowski PL: Molluscum contagiosum in patients with human immunodeficiency virus infection. A review of twenty-seven patients, *J Am Acad Dermatol* 27:583-588, 1992.
17. Shelley WB, Burmeister V: Office diagnosis of molluscum contagiosum by light microscopic demonstration of virions, *Cutis* 465, 1985.
18. de Waard-van der Spek FB, Oranje AP, et al: Treatment of molluscum contagiosum using a lidocaine/prilocaine cream (EMLA) for analgesia, *J Am Acad Dermatol* 23:685-688, 1990.
19. Amstey MS, Trombetta GC: Laser therapy for vulvar molluscum contagiosum infection, *Am J Obstet Gynecol* 153:800-801, 1985.
20. Garrett SJ, Robinson JK, et al: Trichloroacetic acid peel of molluscum contagiosum in immunocompromised patients, *J Dermatol Surg Oncol* 18:855-858, 1992.
21. Lafferty WE et al: Recurrences after oral and genital herpes simplex virus infection: influence of site of infection and viral type, *N Engl J Med* 316:1444-1449, 1987.
22. Gill MJ, Arlette J, Buchan K: Herpes simplex virus infection of the hand: a profile of 79 cases, *Am J Med* 84:89-93, 1988.
23. Belongia EA, Goodman JL, et al: An outbreak of herpes gladiatorum at a high-school wrestling camp, *N Engl J Med* 325:906-910, 1991.
24. Laskin OL: Acyclovir and suppression of frequently recurring herpetic whitlow, *Ann Intern Med* 102:494-495, 1985.
25. Novelli VM, Atherton DJ, Marshall WC: Eczema herpeticum: clinical and laboratory features, *Clin Pediatr* 27:231-233, 1988.
26. Ingrand D et al: Eczema herpeticum of the child, *Clin Pediatr* 24:660-663, 1985.
27. Sanderson IR, Brueton LA, Savage MO, et al: Eczema herpeticum: a potentially fatal disease, *Br Med J* 294:693-694, 1987.
28. Muelleman PJ, Doyle JA, House RF Jr: Eczema herpeticum treated with oral acyclovir, *J Am Acad Dermatol* 15:716-717, 1986.
29. Jawitz JC, Hines HC, Moshell AN: Treatment of eczema herpeticum with systemic acyclovir, *Arch Dermatol* 121:274-275, 1985.
30. Taieb A, Fontan I, Maleville J: Acyclovir therapy for eczema herpeticum in infants, *Arch Dermatol* 121:1380-1381, 1985.
31. Jackson MA, Burry VF, et al: Complications of varicella requiring hospitalization in previously healthy children, *Pediatr Infect Dis J* 11:441-445, 1992.
32. Preblud SR: Varicella: complications and costs, *Pediatrics* 78:728-735, 1986.
33. Hurwitz ES et al: National surveillance for Reye syndrome: a five-year review, *Pediatrics* 70:895-900, 1982.
34. Triebwasser JH et al: Varicella pneumonia in adults; report of seven cases and a review of the literature, *Medicine* 46:409, 1967.
35. Abzug MJ, Cotton MF: Severe chickenpox after intranasal use of corticosteroids, *J Pediatr* 123:577-579, 1993.
36. Dowell SF, Bresee JS: Severe varicella associated with steroid use, *Pediatrics* 92:223-228, 1993.
37. Feldman S, Hughes WT, Daniel CB: Varicella in children with cancer: seventy-seven cases, *Pediatrics* 56:388-397, 1975.
38. Miller HC, Stephan M: Hemorrhagic varicella: a case report and review of the complications of varicella in children, *Am J Emerg Med* 11:633-638, 1993.
39. Kelley R, Mancao M, et al: Varicella in children with perinatally acquired human immunodeficiency virus infection, *J Pediatr* 124:271-273, 1994.
40. Leibovitz E, Cooper D, et al: Varicella-zoster virus infection in Romanian children infected with the human immunodeficiency virus, *Pediatrics* 92:838-842, 1993.
41. Srugo I, Israele V, et al: Clinical manifestations of varicella-zoster virus infections in human immunodeficiency virus–infected children, *Am J Dis Child* 147:742-745, 1993.
42. Wallace MR, Hooper DG, et al: Varicella immunity and clinical disease in HIV-infected adults, *South Med J* 87:74-76, 1994.
43. Paryani SG, Arvin AM: Intrauterine infection with varicella-zoster virus after maternal varicella, *N Engl J Med* 314:1542-1546, 1986.
44. Boyd K, Walker E: Use of acyclovir to treat chicken pox in pregnancy, *Br Med J* 296:393, 1988.
45. Wheller TH: Varicella and herpes zoster: changing concepts of the natural history, control, and importance of a not-so-benign virus, *N Engl J Med* 309:1434, 1983.
46. Pastuszak AL, Levy M, et al: Outcome after maternal varicella infection in the first 20 weeks of pregnancy, *N Engl J Med* 330:901-905, 1994.
47. Balducci J, Rodis JF, et al: Pregnancy outcome following first-trimester varicella infection, *Obstet Gynecol* 79:5-6, 1992.
48. Meyers JD: Congenital varicella in term infants: risk reconsidered, *J Infect Dis* 129:215-217, 1974.
49. Stagno S, Whitley RJ: Herpesvirus infections of pregnancy. Part II. Herpes simplex virus and varicella-zoster virus infections, *N Engl J Med* 313:1327-1330, 1985.
50. Leavelle DE, editor: *Mayo Medical Laboratories interpretive handbook,* Rochester, Minn., 1989, Mayo Medical Laboratories.
51. Solomon AR, Rasmussen JE, Weiss JS: A comparison of the Tzanck smear and viral isolation in varicella and herpes zoster, *Arch Dermatol* 122:282-285, 1986.
52. Balfour H Jr, Rotbart HA, et al: Acyclovir treatment of varicella in otherwise healthy adolescents. The Collaborative Acyclovir Varicella Study Group, *J Pediatr* 120:627-633, 1992.
53. Wallace MR, Bowler WA, et al: Treatment of adult varicella with oral acyclovir. A randomized, placebo-controlled trial, *Ann Intern Med* 117:358-363, 1992.
54. Whitley R et al: Vidarabine therapy of varicella in immunosuppressed patients, *J Pediatr* 101:125-131, 1982.
55. Prober CG, Kirk LE, Keeney RE: Acyclovir therapy of chicken pox in immunosuppressed children: a collaborative study, *J Pediatr* 101:622-625, 1982.

56. Straus SE, moderator, NIH conference: Varicella-zoster virus infections: biology, natural history, treatment, and prevention, *Ann Intern Med* 108:221-237, 1988.

57. Varicella-zoster immune globulin for the prevention of chicken pox: recommendations of the immunization practices advisory committee. Centers for Disease Control, Department of Health and Human Services, Atlanta, Ga, *Ann Intern Med* 100:859-865, 1984.

58. Paryani SG et al: Varicella zoster antibody titers after the administration of intravenous immune serum globulin or varicella zoster immune globulin, *Am J Med* 76:124-127, 1984.

59. Watson B, Gupta R, et al: Persistence of cell-mediated and humoral immune responses in healthy children immunized with live attenuated varicella vaccine, *J Infect Dis* 169:197-199, 1994.

60. Lawrence R et al: The risk of zoster after varicella vaccination in children with leukemia, *N Engl J Med* 318:543-548, 1988.

61. Funaki B, Elpern DJ: Herpes zoster incidence in younger age groups, *J Am Acad Dermatol* 16:883-884, 1987.

62. Baba K, Yabuuchi H, Takahashi M, et al: Increased incidence of herpes zoster in normal children infected with varicella zoster virus during infancy: community-based follow-up study, *J Pediatr* 108:372-377, 1986.

63. Ragozzino MW et al: Risk of cancer after herpes zoster: a population-based study, *N Engl J Med* 307:393-397, 1982.

64. Fueyo MA, Lookingbill DP: Herpes zoster and occult malignancy, *J Am Acad Dermatol* 11:480-482, 1984.

65. Friedman-Kien AE et al: Herpes zoster: a possible early clinical sign for development of acquired immunodeficiency syndrome in high-risk individuals, *J Am Acad Dermatol* 14:1023-1028, 1986.

66. Rusthoven JJ et al: Varicella zoster infection in adult cancer patients: a population study, *Arch Intern Med* 148:1561-1566, 1988.

67. Gilden DH, Dueland AN, et al: Preherpetic neuralgia, *Neurology* 41:1215-1218, 1991.

68. Buchbinder SP, Katz MH, et al: Herpes zoster and human immunodeficiency virus infection, *J Infect Dis* 166:1153-1156, 1992.

69. McKinlay WJD: Herpes zoster in pregnancy, *Br Med J* 280:561-562, 1980.

70. Hoang-Xuan T, Buchi ER, et al: Oral acyclovir for herpes zoster ophthalmicus, *Ophthalmology* 99:1062-1070, 1992.

71. Harding SP: Management of ophthalmic zoster, *J Med Virol* 1:97-101, 1993.

72. Sato K, Nakamura S, et al: A case of Ramsey Hunt syndrome with multiple cranial nerve paralysis and acute respiratory failure, *Nippon Kyobu Shikkan Gakkai Zasshi* 29:1037-1041, 1991.

73. Scott MJ Sr, Scott MJ Jr: Ipsilateral deafness and herpes zoster ophthalmicus, *Arch Dermatol* 119:235-236, 1983.

74. Weaver SM, Kelly AP: Herpes zoster as a cause of neurogenic bladder, *Cutis* 29:611-612, 1982.

75. Watson PN, Evans RJ: Postherpetic neuralgia: a review, *Arch Neurol* 43:836-840, 1986.

76. Mazur MH, Dolin R: Herpes zoster at the NIH: a 20-year experience, *Am J Med* 65:738-744, 1978.

77. Reichman RC: Neurologic complications of varicella-zoster infections, *Ann Intern Med* 89:379-380, 1978.

78. Wood MJ, Johnson RW, et al: A randomized trial of acyclovir for 7 days or 21 days with and without prednisolone for treatment of acute herpes zoster, *N Engl J Med* 330:896-900, 1994.

79. Ogata A et al: Local anesthesia for herpes zoster, *J Dermatol* 7:161, 1980.

80. Epstein E: Treatment of herpes zoster and postzoster neuralgia by subcutaneous injection of triamcinolone, *Int J Dermatol* 20:65-68, 1981.

81. Riopelle JM, Naraghi M, Grush KP: Chronic neuralgia incidence following local anesthetic therapy for herpes zoster, *Arch Dermatol* 120:747-750, 1984.

82. Burney RG, Peeters-Asdourian C: Herpetic neuralgia, *Semin Anesth* 4:275-280, 1985.

83. Winnie AP, Hartwell PW: Relationship between time of treatment of acute herpes zoster with sympathetic blockade and prevention of postherpetic neuralgia: clinical support for a new theory of the mechanism by which sympathetic blockade provides therapeutic benefit, *Reg Anesth* 18:277-282, 1993.

84. Huff JC, Drucker JL, et al: Effect of oral acyclovir on pain resolution in herpes zoster: a reanalysis, *J Med Virol* 1:93-96, 1993.

85. Bean B, Braun C, Balfour HH: Acyclovir therapy for acute herpes zoster, *Lancet* 2:118-121, 1982.

86. Peterslund NA et al: Acyclovir in herpes zoster, *Lancet* 2:827-830, 1981.

87. Klenerman P et al: Antiviral treatment and postherpetic neuralgia, *Br Med J* 298:832, 1989.

88. Bowsher D: Acute herpes zoster and postherpetic neuralgia: effects of acyclovir and outcome of treatment with amitriptyline, *Br J Gen Pract* 42:244-246, 1992.

89. Cobo LM et al: Oral acyclovir in the therapy of acute herpes zoster ophthalmicus: an interim report, *Ophthalmology* 92:1574-1583, 1985.

90. Wassilew SW, Reimlinger S, Nasemann T, et al: Oral acyclovir for herpes zoster: a double-blind controlled trial in normal subjects, *Br J Dermatol* 117:495-501, 1987.

91. Jacobson MA, Berger TG, et al: Acyclovir-resistant varicella zoster virus infection after chronic oral acyclovir therapy in patients with the acquired immunodeficiency syndrome (AIDS), *Ann Intern Med* 112:187-191, 1990.

92. Balfour H Jr., Benson C, et al: Management of acyclovir-resistant herpes simplex and varicella-zoster virus infections, *J Acquir Immune Defic Syndr* 7:254-260, 1994.

93. Whitley RJ, Gnann J Jr., et al: Disseminated herpes zoster in the immunocompromised host: a comparative trial of acyclovir and vidarabine. The NIAID Collaborative Antiviral Study Group, *J Infect Dis* 165:450-455, 1992.

94. Bernstein JE, Bickers DR, Dahl MV, et al: Treatment of chronic postherpetic neuralgia with topical capsaicin, *J Am Acad Dermatol* 17:93-96, 1987.

95. Watson CP et al: Amitriptyline vs. placebo in postherpetic neuralgia, *Neurology* 32:671-673, 1982.

96. Rosenblatt RM, Reich J, Dehring D: Tricyclic antidepressants in treatment of depression and chronic pain, *Anesth Analg* 63:1025-1031, 1984.

97. Rowbotham MC et al: Topical lidocaine gel relieves postherpetic neuralgia, *Ann Neurol* 37:246-253, 1995.

CHAPTER THIRTEEN

Superficial Fungal Infections

Dermatophyte Fungal Infections

The dermatophytes include a group of fungi (ringworm) that under most conditions have the ability to infect and survive only on dead keratin; that is, the top layer of the skin (stratum corneum or keratin layer), the hair, and the nails. They cannot survive on mucosal surfaces such as the mouth or vagina where the keratin layer does not form. Very rarely dermatophytes undergo deep local invasion and multivisceral dissemination in the immunosuppressed host. Dermatophytes are responsible for the vast majority of skin, nail, and hair fungal infections. Lesions vary in presentation and closely resemble other diseases; therefore laboratory confirmation is often required. There is evidence that genetic susceptibility may predispose a patient to dermatophyte infection. Studies show that although several blood-related members of a family may share similar manifestations of disease,[1] spouses, despite prolonged exposure, do not become infected. Patients with chronic dermatophytosis have a relatively specific defect in delayed hypersensitivity to *Trichophyton*, but their cell-mediated responses to other antigens are somewhat depressed. There is also a greater frequency of atopy in chronically infected patients.[1]

Classification. Dermatophytes are classified in several ways. The ringworm fungi belong to three genera: *Microsporum*, *Trichophyton*, and *Epidermophyton*. There are several species of *Microsporum* and *Trichophyton* and one species of *Epidermophyton*.

Place of origin. The anthropophilic dermatophytes grow only on human skin, hair, or nails. The zoophilic varieties originate from animals, but may infect humans. Geophilic dermatophytes live in soil but may infect humans.

Type of inflammation. The inflammatory response to dermatophytes varies. In general, zoophilic and geophilic dermatophytes elicit a brisk inflammatory response on skin and in hair follicles. The inflammatory response to anthropophilic fungi is usually mild.

Type of hair invasion. Some species are able to infect the hair shaft. Microscopic examination of infected hairs show fungal spores and hyphae either inside the hair shaft or both inside and on the surface. The endothrix pattern consists of fungal hyphae inside the hair shaft, whereas the ectothrix pattern consists of fungal hyphae inside and on the surface of the hair shaft.

Spores of fungi are either large or small. The type of hair invasion is further classified as large- or small-spored ectothrix or large-spored endothrix.

Clinical classification. Tinea means fungal infection. Clinically, dermatophyte infections are classified by body region. The dermatophytes, or ringworm fungi, produce a variety of disease patterns that vary with the location and species. Learning the numerous patterns of disease produced by each species is complicated and unnecessary because all dermatophytes respond to the same topical and oral agents. It is important to be familiar with the general patterns of inflammation in different body regions and to be able to interpret accurately a potassium hydroxide wet mount preparation of scale, hair, or nails. Species identification by culture is necessary only for scalp infections, inflammatory skin infections, and some nail infections.

The active border. One very characteristic pattern of inflammation is the active border of infection. The highest numbers of hyphae are located in the active border, and this is the best area to get a sample for a potassium hydroxide examination. Typically the active border is scaly, red, and slightly elevated (Figure 13-1). Vesicles appear at the active border when inflammation is intense (Figure 13-2). This pattern is present in all locations except the palms and soles.

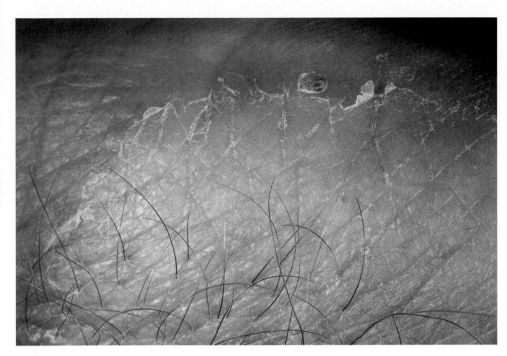

Figure 13-1
Tinea infection. Active border (classic presentation). The border is red, scaly, and slightly raised. The central area is often lighter than the surrounding normal skin.

Diagnosis

Potassium hydroxide wet mount preparation. The single most important test for the diagnosis of dermatophyte infection is direct visualization under the microscope of the branching hyphae in keratinized material.

SAMPLING SCALE. Scale is obtained by holding a #15 surgical blade perpendicular to the skin surface and smoothly but firmly drawing the blade with several short strokes against the scale. If an active border is present, the blade is drawn along the border at right angles to the fringe of the scale. If the blade is drawn from the center of the lesion out and parallel to the active border, some normal scale may also be included.

WET MOUNT PREPARATION. The small fragments of scale are placed on a microscope slide, gently separated, and a coverslip is applied. Potassium hydroxide (10% or 20% solution) is applied with a toothpick or eye dropper to the edge of the coverslip and allowed to run under by capillary action. The preparation is gently heated under a low flame and then pressed to facilitate separation of the epithelial cells and fungal hyphae. Potassium hydroxide dissolves material binding cells together, but does not distort the epithelial cells or fungi. Lowering the condenser of the microscope and dimming the light enhances contrast, making hyphae easier to identify.

Nail-plate keratin is thick and difficult to digest. The nail plate can be adequately softened by leaving the fragments along with several drops of potassium hydroxide in a watch glass covered with a petri dish for 24 hours. Hair specimens require no special preparation or digestion and can be examined immediately.

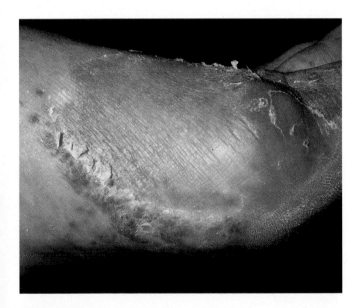

Figure 13-2
Tinea infection. Active border, which contains vesicles that indicate acute inflammation.

MICROSCOPY. The preparation is studied carefully by scanning the entire area under the coverslip at low power. The presence of hyphae should be confirmed by examination with the 40 × objective. Slight back-and-forth rotation of the focusing knob aids visualization of the entire segment of the hyphae, which may be at different depths. It is not uncommon to find one small fragment of scale containing many hyphae and the rest of the preparation free of hyphae. The entire preparation should be studied carefully.

INTERPRETATION. The interpretation of potassium hydroxide wet mounts takes experience. Dermatophytes appear as translucent, branching, rod-shaped filaments (hyphae) of uniform width, with lines of separation (septa) spanning the width and appearing at irregular intervals (Figures 13-3 and 13-4). The uniform width and characteristic bending and branching distinguish hyphae from hair and other debris. Hair tapers at the tip. Lines that intersect across cell walls at different planes of the scale are viewed using the microscope's fine adjustment knob. Some hyphae contain a single-file line of bubbles in their cytoplasm. Hyphae may frag-ment into round or polygonal fragments that look like spores. Hyphae may be seen in combination with scale or floating free in the potassium hydroxide.

ARTIFACT. Confusion may arise with the so-called mosaic artifact produced by lipid droplets appearing in a single-file line between cells, especially from specimens taken from the palms and soles (Figure 13-5). These disappear when the cells are separated further by additional heating and pressure. Although spores and branching and short, nonbranching hyphae are seen in superficial *Candida* infections and tinea versicolor, only branching hyphae are seen in dermatophyte infections. Longitudinal, rod-shaped potassium hydroxide crystals that simulate hyphae may appear if the wet mount is heated excessively.

Special stains. Hyphae may be difficult to find in a potassium hydroxide wet mount. Chlorazol Fungal Stain,[2] Swartz Lamkins Fungal Stain, or Parker's blue ink[3] clearly stain hyphae, rendering them visible under low power. The specialized stains are available from Dermatologic Lab and Supply, Inc, Council Bluffs, IA, 1-800-831-6273.

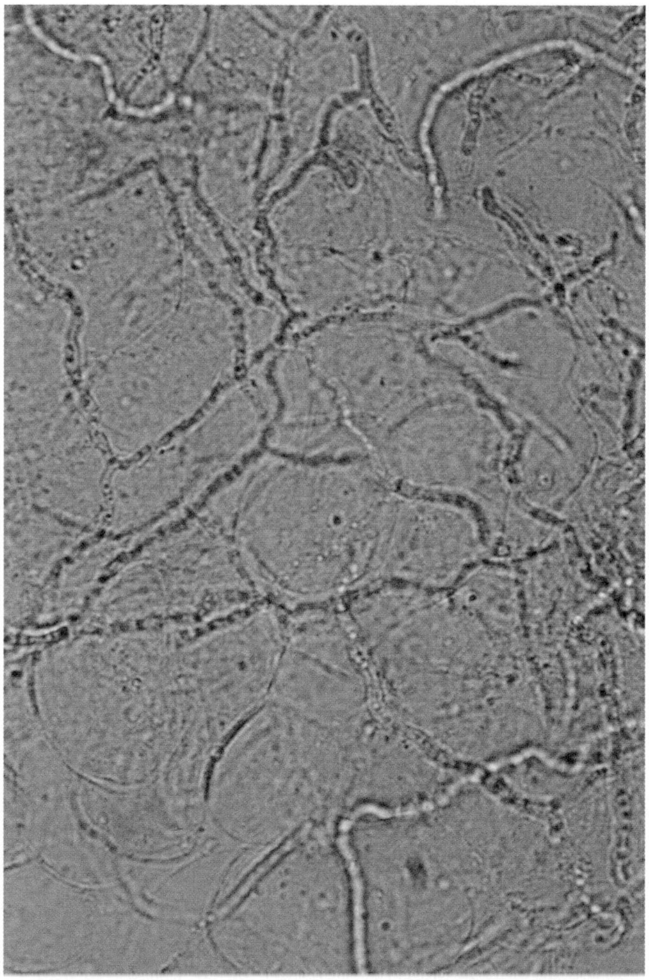

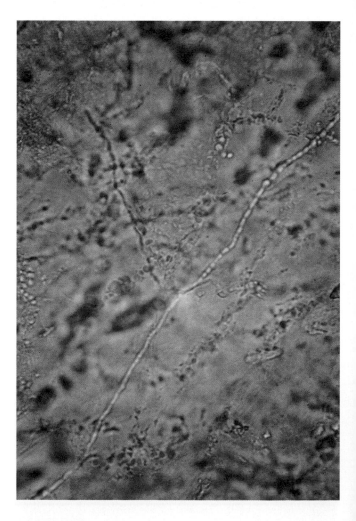

Figure 13-3
Fungal hyphae in a potassium hydroxide wet mount. The identifying characteristic is the branching, filamentous structure that is uniform in width.

Figure 13-4
A drop of ink added to the potassium hydroxide wet mount accentuates hyphae. *(Courtesy Dr. Leanor Haley, Centers for Disease Control.)*

Culture. It is usually not necessary to know the species of dermatophyte infecting skin in most cases because the same oral and topical agents are active against all of them. Fungal culture is necessary for hair and nail fungal infections. Scalp hair infections in children may originate from an animal that carries a typical species of dermatophyte. The animal can then be traced and treated or destroyed to prevent further infection of other humans. Nail plate, especially of the toenails, may be infected with nondermatophytes, such as the saprophytic mold *Scopulariopsis*, which do not respond to treatment. Identification of the genus of fungus responsible for nail-plate infection is therefore necessary before embarking on a long course of treatment.

COTTON SWAB TECHNIQUE FOR CULTURE. A sterile cotton swab that is moistened with sterile water or on an agar plate and rubbed vigorously over the lesion produces results comparable to those obtained by scraping with a scalpel blade.[4] A light sweep over the lesion does not collect sufficient material, therefore the swab must be rubbed vigorously over the active part of the lesion and then over the surface of the agar. The swab is useful in areas that are difficult to scrape, such as the scalp, eyelids, ears, nose, and between the toes. The sterile swab is less threatening than a blade, and it is safer in situations in which the sudden movement of a child could lead to a painful stab or cut.

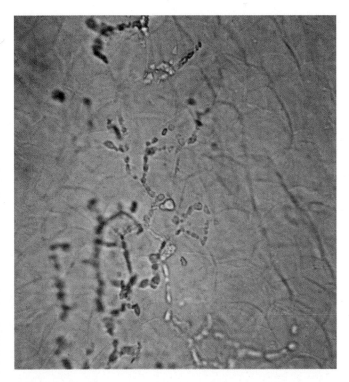

Figure 13-5
Mosaic artifact. Lipid droplets appearing in a single-file line between epithelial cells simulate fungal hyphae in potassium hydroxide wet mounts. Heat encourages cell separation and the artifact disappears. *(Courtesy Dr. Leanor Haley, Centers for Disease Control.)*

CULTURE MEDIA FOR TINEA. Dermatophytes are aerobic and grow on the surface of media. The three types of culture media used most often for isolation and identification are Dermatophyte Test Medium, Mycosel agar, and Sabouraud's dextrose agar. Many hospital laboratories lack the experience to interpret fungal cultures and send them to outside laboratories for analysis. Material to be cultured can be sent directly to a laboratory because, unlike many bacteria, fungi remain viable for days in scale and hair without being inoculated onto media. Alternatively, many hospitals and individual practitioners now rely on Dermatophyte Test Medium for faster but slightly less accurate results.

Dermatophyte Test Medium is a commercially available medium supplied in vials that are ready for direct inoculation. The yellow medium, which contains the indicator phenol red, turns pink in the presence of the alkaline metabolic products of dermatophytes in approximately 6 or 7 days, but remains yellow in the presence of the acid metabolic products of nonpathogenic fungi. It must be discarded after 2 weeks because saprophytes can induce a similar color change from this time on. Species identification is possible with Dermatophyte Test Medium but is more accurately determined with Mycosel agar and Sabouraud's agar because the dye in Dermatophyte Test Medium media may interfere with interpretation.

Mycosel agar is a modification of Sabouraud's medium that contains cycloheximide and chloramphenicol to prevent the growth of bacteria and saprophytic fungi; the dextrose content of Mycosel agar has been lowered and the pH has been raised to allow for better growth of dermatophytes.

Sabouraud's agar, which does not contain antibiotics, allows the growth of most fungi, including nondermatophytes. This may be useful for nail infections because the detection of nondermatophytes is desirable in nail infections; but the more selective Mycosel agar is best for evaluation of hair tinea because only dermatophytes cause hair tinea. Cultures usually become positive in 1 to 2 weeks.

CULTURE MEDIA FOR YEAST. Yeast may be isolated on plates obtained from the hospital laboratory. Acu-Nickerson is a commercially available medium in a slant for use in the isolation and identification of *Candida* species.

Wood's light examination. Light rays with a wavelength above 365 nm are produced when ultraviolet light is projected through a Wood's filter. Hair, but not the skin of the scalp, fluoresces with a blue-green color if infected with *M. canis* or *M. audouinii*. The rarer *T. schoenleinii* produces a paler green fluorescence of infected hair. No other dermatophytes that infect hair produce fluorescence. Fungal infections of the skin do not fluoresce, except for tinea versicolor, which produces a pale white-yellow fluorescence. Erythrasma, a noninflammatory, pale brown, scaly eruption of the toe webs, groin, and axillae caused by the bacteria *Corynebacterium minutissimum*, shows a brilliant coral-red fluorescence with the Wood's light. Wood's light examination should be performed in a dark room with a high-intensity instrument. The fluorescence of hair may be caused by tryptophan metabolites.

TINEA

Clinically, dermatophyte infections have traditionally been classified by body region. Tinea means fungus infection. The term *tinea capitis*, for example, indicates dermatophyte infection of the scalp.

TINEA OF THE FOOT

The feet are the most common area infected by dermatophytes (tinea pedis, "athlete's foot"). Shoes promote warmth and sweating, which encourage fungal growth. Fungal infections of the feet are common in adult males and uncommon in women. Although uncommon, tinea pedis does occur in prepubertal children. Tinea should be considered in the differential diagnosis of children with foot dermatitis.[5,6] The occurrence of tinea pedis seems to be inevitable in immunologically predisposed individuals regardless of elaborate precautions taken to avoid the infecting organism. Locker-room floors contain fungal elements and the use of communal baths may create an ideal condition for repeated exposure to infected material.[7] White socks do nothing to prevent tinea pedis. Once established, the individual becomes a carrier and is more susceptible to recurrences. There are many different clinical presentations of tinea pedis.

Clinical presentations. Tinea of the feet may present with the classic "ringworm" pattern (Figure 13-6), but most infections are found in the toe webs or on the soles.

Interdigital tinea pedis (toe web infection). Tight-fitting shoes compress the toes, creating a warm, moist environment in the toe webs; this environment is suited to fungal growth. The web between the fourth and fifth toes is most commonly involved, but all webs may be infected. The web can become dry, scaly, and fissured (Figure 13-7) or white, macerated, and soggy. Itching is most intense when the shoes and socks are removed. The bacterial flora is unchanged when the tinea-infected webs demonstrate scale and peeling without maceration. Overgrowth of the resident bacterial population determines the severity of interdigital toe web infection. The macerated pattern of infection occurs from an interaction of bacteria and fungus.[8] Dermatophytes initiate the damage to the stratum corneum and, by the production of antibiotics, influence the selection of a more antibiotic-resistant bacterial population.[9] The prevalence of *Staphylococcus aureus*, gram-negative bacteria, *C. minutissimum*, *S. epidermidis*, and *Micrococcus sedentarius* increases. Extension out of the web space onto the plantar surface or the dorsum of the foot is common and occurs with the typical, chronic, ringworm type of scaly, advancing border or with an acute, vesicular eruption (Figures 13-8 and 13-9). Identification of fungal hyphae in the macerated skin of the toe webs may be difficult.

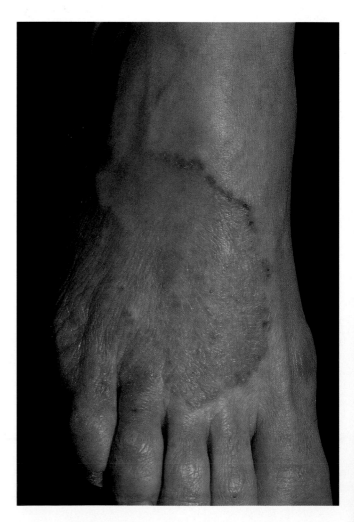

Figure 13-6
Tinea pedis. The classic "ringworm" pattern of tinea can appear on any body surface.

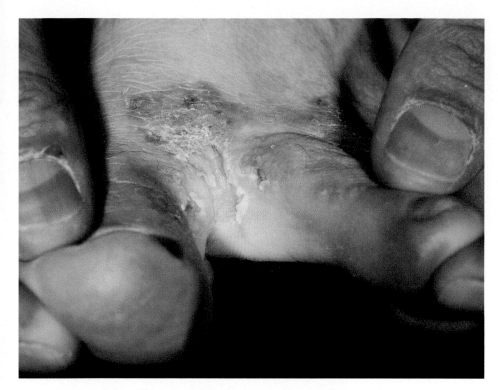

Figure 13-7
Tinea pedis (toe web infection). The toe web space contains macerated scale. Inflammation has extended from the web area onto the dorsum of the foot.

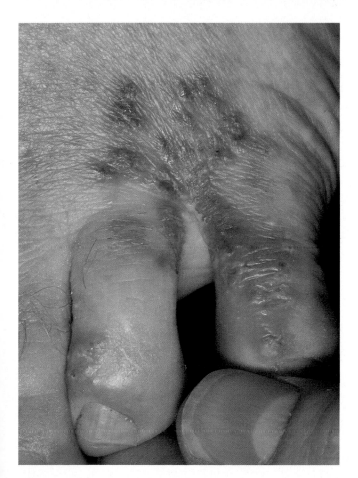

Figure 13-8
Tinea pedis. The infection has spread out of the toe web.

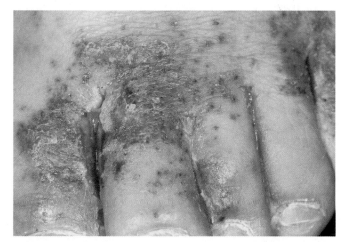

Figure 13-9
Tinea pedis. A chronic toe web and dorsal foot fungal infection have become secondarily infected with *staphylococci*.

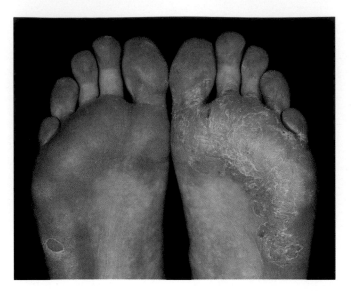

Figure 13-10
Tinea pedis. Web spaces and plantar surfaces of one foot
have been inflamed for years; the other foot remains clear.

Chronic scaly infection of the plantar surface. Plantar
hyperkeratotic or moccasin-type tinea pedis is a particularly
chronic form of tinea that is resistant to treatment. The entire
sole is usually infected and covered with a fine, silvery
white scale (Figures 13-10 to 13-12). The skin is pink, tender, and/or pruritic. The hands may be similarly infected. It
is rare to see both palms and soles infected simultaneously;
rather, the pattern is infection of two feet and one hand or of
two hands and one foot. *T. rubrum* is the usual pathogen.
This pattern of infection is difficult to eradicate. *T. rubrum*
produce substances that diminish the immune response and
inhibit stratum corneum turnover.

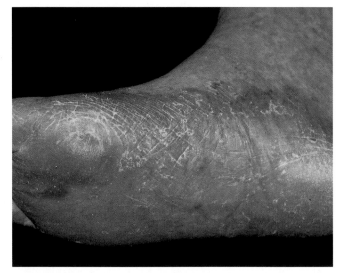

Figure 13-12
Tinea pedis. This patient has chronic inflammation of the
soles that periodically flares on the dorsum and ankle.

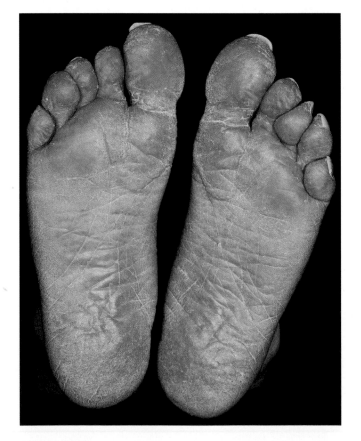

Figure 13-11
Tinea pedis. The entire plantar surface of both feet is
thickened, tan colored, and covered with a fine, white scale.

Acute vesicular tinea pedis. A highly inflammatory fungal infection may occur, particularly in people who wear occlusive shoes. This acute form of infection often originates from a more chronic web infection. A few or many vesicles evolve rapidly on the sole or on the dorsum of the foot. The vesicles may fuse into bullae (Figure 13-13) or remain as collections of fluid under the thick scale of the sole and never rupture through the surface. Secondary bacterial infection occurs commonly in eroded areas after bullae rupture. Fungal hyphae are difficult to identify in severely inflamed skin. Specimens for potassium hydroxide examination should be taken from the roof of the vesicle. A second wave of vesicles may follow shortly in the same areas or at distant sites such as the arms, chest, and along the sides of the fingers. These itchy sterile vesicles represent an allergic response to the fungus and are termed a *dermatophytid* or *id reaction*.[9] They subside when the infection is controlled. At times the id reaction is the only clinical manifestation of a fungus infection. Careful examination of these patients may show an asymptomatic fissure or area of maceration in the toe webs.

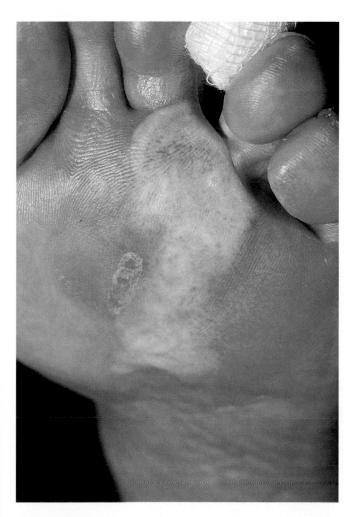

Figure 13-13
Acute vesicular tinea pedis. Inflammation appeared abruptly in a patient with chronic toe web infection after wearing heavy wet boots for several hours.

Treatment. The newest class of antifungal agents, the allylamines (e.g., terbinafine cream), have been shown to produce higher cure rates and more rapid responses in dermatophyte infections than older agents. Terbinafine is a fungicidal that brings about more rapid and persistent clearing. Naftifine (Naftine), a fungicidal cream that requires 4 weeks of treatment, produced a significantly higher cure rate and significantly lower relapse rate than the antifungal/corticosteroid combination (Lotrisone).[10]

Fluconazole is effective when taken once a week (see Table 13-2). In one study, patients with tinea pedis were treated with a once-weekly dose of oral fluconazole 150 mg. A mean of three doses was administered; 28 to 30 days after the last dose, 77% patients were clinically cured. The number of doses received did not correlate with either the mycologic response or relapse rates at long-term follow-up.[11]

Toe web infections respond to the various topical creams and lotions listed in the Formulary (see p. 839). Terbinafine 1% cream applied twice daily for 1 week results in a high cure rate in interdigital tinea pedis. In one series, terbinafine gave progressive mycologic improvement; at 5 weeks after treatment, 88% of the patients were clear of infection.[12] Effective short-course therapy with potent fungicidal drugs such as terbinafine[13] may avoid treatment failure caused by noncompliance with fungistatic agents, such as clotrimazole, that require 4 weeks of treatment.[14] Econazole nitrate (Spectazole) has activity against several bacterial species associated with severely macerated interdigital interspaces.[15] Recurrence is prevented by wearing wider shoes and expanding the web space with a small strand of lamb's wool (Dr. Scholls' Lamb's Wool). Powders, not necessarily medicated, absorb moisture. The powders should be applied to the feet rather than to the shoes. Wet socks should be changed.

Hyperkeratotic, moccasin-type tinea of the plantar surface responds slowly to conventional therapy. Oral terbinafine 250 mg twice a day,[16] 250 mg once a day,[17] or 125 mg twice a day[18] for 2 to 6 weeks produced sustained cure rates of 71% to 94%. Griseofulvin 250 to 500 mg twice a day for 6 weeks resulted in a 27% to 35% cure rate.

Acute vesicular tinea pedis responds to wet Burow's compresses applied for 30 minutes several times each day. Griseofulvin should be started and topical antifungal agents applied once the macerated tissue has been dried. Secondary bacterial infection is treated with oral antibiotics. A vesicular id reaction sometimes occurs at distant sites during an inflammatory foot infection. Wet dressings, group V topical steroids, and, occasionally, prednisone 20 mg two times a day for 8 to 10 days are required for control of id reactions.

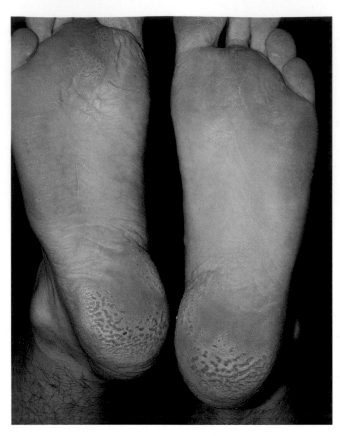

Figure 13-14
Pitted keratolysis. Deep longitudinal furrows are located primarily on weight-bearing surfaces.

PITTED KERATOLYSIS

Pitted keratolysis, a disease mimicking tinea pedis, is an eruption of the weight-bearing surfaces of the soles. The disease is bacterial in origin but is often misinterpreted as a fungal infection. It is characterized by many circular or longitudinal, punched-out depressions in the skin surface (Figures 13-14 and 13-15). Most cases are asymptomatic, but painful, plaquelike lesions may occur in both adults and children.[19] The eruption is limited to the stratum corneum and causes little or no inflammation. Hyperhidrosis, moist socks, or immersion of the feet favors its development. There may be a few circular pits that remain unnoticed, or the entire weight-bearing surface may be covered with annular furrows. Several bacteria have been implicated, including *Dermatophilus congolensis* and *M. sedentarius*. These bacteria produce and excrete exoenzymes (keratinase) that are able to degrade keratin and produce pitting in the stratum corneum when the skin is hydrated and the pH rises above neutrality.[20] These organisms are not easily cultured, but the filamentous and coccoid microorganisms can be demonstrated by H & E staining of a formalin-fixed section of shaved stratum corneum prepared for histopathology. The clinical presentation is so characteristic that laboratory confirmation is usually not necessary.

Treatment. Treatment consists of promoting dryness. Socks should be changed frequently. Rapid clearing occurs with application of 20% aluminum chloride (Drysol) twice a day. For resistant cases, 20% aluminum chloride is applied to the feet at bedtime and covered with a plastic bag. The bag is removed each morning and the feet, if dry, are lubricated with a light lotion (e.g., Nutraderm). This is repeated each evening until clearing. Treatment can then be employed periodically when necessary. Application twice a day of alcohol-based benzoyl peroxide (Panoxyl 5) may also be useful. Treatment with topical erythromycin is also curative.

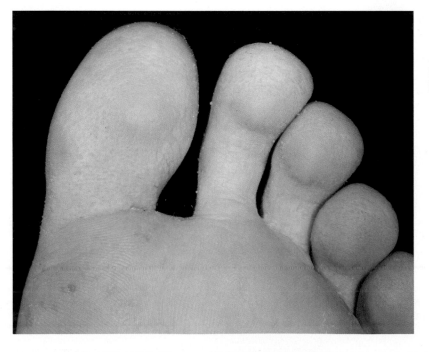

Figure 13-15
Pitted keratolysis. The skin around the deep pits is often wet and macerated.

TINEA OF THE GROIN

Tinea of the groin (tinea cruris, jock itch) occurs often in the summer months after sweating or wearing wet clothing and in the winter months after wearing several layers of clothing. The predisposing factor, as with many other types of superficial infection, is the presence of a warm, moist environment. Men are affected much more frequently than women. Children rarely develop tinea of the groin. Itching becomes worse as moisture accumulates and macerates this intertriginous area.

The lesions are most often bilateral and begin in the crural fold. A half moon–shaped plaque forms as a well-defined scaling, and sometimes a vesicular border advances out of the crural fold onto the thigh (Figure 13-16). The skin within the border turns red-brown, is less scaly, and may develop red papules. Acute inflammation may appear after a person has worn occlusive clothing for an extended period. The infection occasionally migrates to the buttock and gluteal cleft area. Involvement of the scrotum is unusual—unlike *Candida* reactions, in which it is common. Specimens for potassium hydroxide examination should be taken from the advancing scaling border.

Topical steroid creams are frequently prescribed for inflammatory skin disease of the groin and modify the typical clinical presentation of tinea. The eruption may be much more extensive, and the advancing, scaly border may not be present. Red papules sometimes appear at the edges and center of the lesion (Figure 13-17; see Figure 13-33). This modified form (tinea incognito) may not be immediately recognized as tinea; the only clue is the history of a typical, half moon–shaped plaque treated with cortisone cream. Scale, if present, contains numerous hyphae.

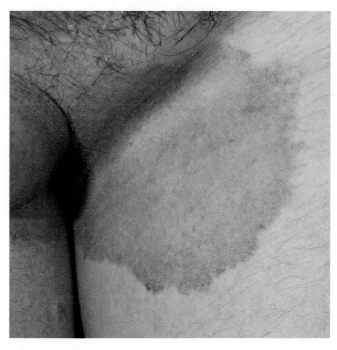

Figure 13-16
Tinea cruris. A half moon–shaped plaque has a well-defined, scaling border.

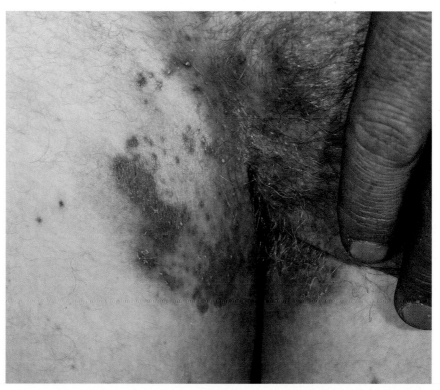

Figure 13-17
Tinea incognito. Red papules and pustules appeared suddenly in the groin after application of a topical steroid to an area infected with dermatophytes.

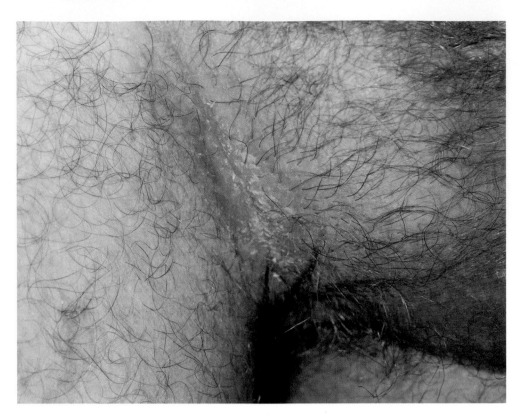

Figure 13-18
Intertrigo. A tender, red plaque with a moist macerated surface extends to an equal extent onto the scrotum and thigh.

Figure 13-19
Intertrigo. An advanced case with deep longitudinal fissuring in the crural fold.

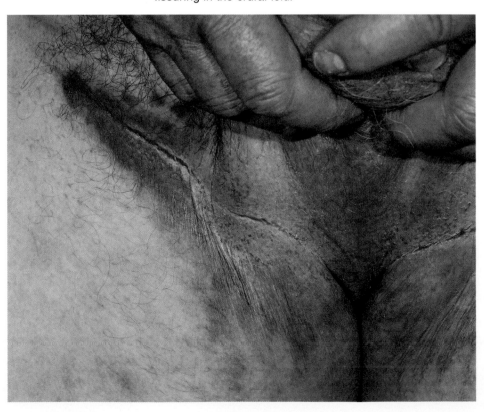

Differential diagnosis

Intertrigo. A red, macerated, half moon–shaped plaque, resembling tinea of the groin and extending to an equal extent onto the groin and down the thigh, forms after moisture accumulates in the crural fold (Figure 13-18). The sharp borders touch where the opposed skin surfaces of the skin folds of the groin and thigh meet. Obesity contributes to this inflammatory process, which may be infected with a mixed flora of bacteria, fungi, and yeast. Painful, longitudinal fissures occur in the crease of the crural fold (Figure 13-19). Groin intertrigo recurs after treatment unless weight and moisture are controlled. Psoriasis and seborrheic dermatitis of the groin may mimic intertrigo (see the section on *Candida* intertrigo).

Erythrasma. This bacterial infection (*C. minutissimum*) may be confused with tinea cruris because of the similar, half moon–shaped plaque (Figure 13-20). Erythrasma differs in that it is noninflammatory, it is uniformly brown and scaly, it has no advancing border, and it fluoresces coral-red with the Wood's light. Tinea of the groin does not fluoresce. Erythrasma of the vulva may be misinterpreted as a candidal infection, especially if the Wood's light examination is negative.[21] Gram stain of the scale shows gram-positive, rodlike organisms in long filaments. However, the scale is difficult to fix to a slide for Gram stain. One technique is stripping the scale with clear tape and then carefully staining the taped-scale preparation. A biopsy demonstrates rods and filamentous organisms in the keratotic layer. Erythrasma responds equally well to erythromycin[22] orally (250 mg four times a day for 2 weeks) or topically (A/T/S, Staticin, or EryDerm twice a day for 2 weeks). The topical erythromycins contain alcohol and may be irritating when applied to the groin.

Treatment. Tinea of the groin responds to any of the topical antifungal creams listed in the Formulary (see p. 839). Lesions may appear to respond quickly, but creams should be applied twice a day for at least 10 days. Moist intertriginous lesions may be contaminated with dermatophytes, other fungi, or bacteria. Antifungal creams with activity against *Candida* and dermatophytes (e.g., miconazole) are applied and covered with a cool wet Burow's compress for 20 to 30 minutes two to six times daily until macerated, wet skin has been dried. The wet dressings are discontinued when the skin is dry, but the cream is continued for at least 14 days or until all evidence of the fungal infection has disappeared. Any residual inflammation from the intertrigo is treated with a group V through VII topical steroid twice a day for a specified length of time (e.g., 10 days). A limited amount of topical steroid cream is prescribed to discourage long-term use. Absorbent powders, not necessarily medicated (e.g., Z- Sorb), help to control moisture, but should not be applied until the inflammation is gone. Resistant infections respond to any of the oral agents listed in Table 13-1.

Lotrisone cream (betamethasone dipropionate/clotrimazole) may be used for initial treatment if lesions are red, inflamed, and itchy. A pure antifungal cream should be used once symptoms are controlled. Prolonged use of this steroid, antifungal cream may not cure the infection and may cause striae in this intertriginous area.

Figure 13-20
Erythrasma: a bacterial infection (*Corynebacterium minutissimum*). The diffuse brown, scaly plaque resembles tinea cruris.

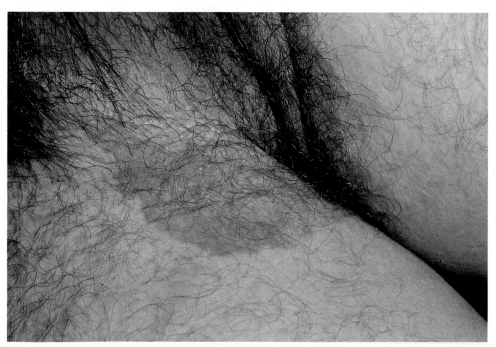

TINEA OF THE BODY AND FACE

Tinea of the face (excluding the beard area in men), trunk, and limbs is called *tinea corporis* (ringworm of the body). The disease can occur at any age and is more common in warm climates. There is a broad range of manifestations, with lesions varying in size, degree of inflammation, and depth of involvement. This variability is explained by differences in host immunity and the species of fungus. An epidemic of tinea corporis caused by *T. tonsurans* was reported in student wrestlers.[25]

Round annular lesions. In classic ringworm, lesions begin as flat, scaly spots that then develop a raised border that extends out at variable rates in all directions. The advancing, scaly border may have red, raised papules or vesicles. The central area becomes brown or hypopigmented and less scaly as the active border progresses outward (Figures 13-21 and 13-22). However, it is not uncommon to see several red papules in the central area (Figures 13-23 and 13-24). There may be just one ring that grows to a few centimeters in diameter and then resolves or several annular lesions that enlarge to cover large areas of the body surface (Figure 13-25). These larger lesions tend to be mildly itchy or asymptomatic. They may reach a certain size and remain for years with no tendency to resolve. Clear, central areas of the larger lesions are yellow-brown and usually contain several red papules. The borders are serpiginous or annular and very irregular.

Pityriasis rosea and multiple small annular lesions of ringworm may appear to be similar. However, the scaly ring of pityriasis rosea does not reach the edge of the red border as it does in tinea. Other distinguishing features of pityriasis rosea include rapid onset of lesions and localization to the trunk. Tinea from cats may appear suddenly as multiple round-to-oval plaques on the trunk and extremities.

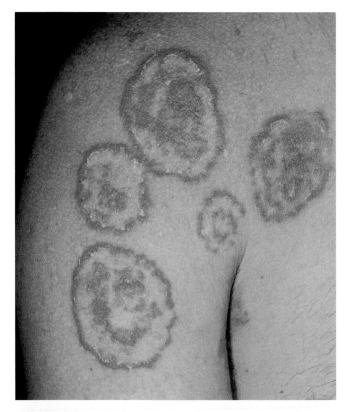

Figure 13-21
Tinea corporis. A classic presentation with an advancing red, scaly border. The reason for the designation "ringworm" is obvious.

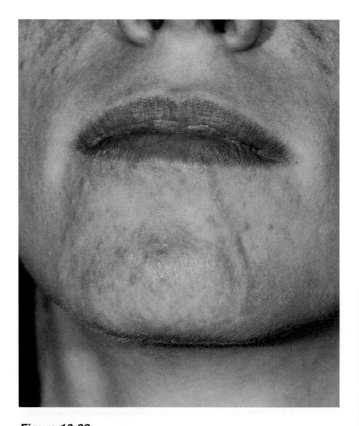

Figure 13-22
Tinea of the face. Sharply defined borders extend from the lip to the chin. The central area is hypopigmented.

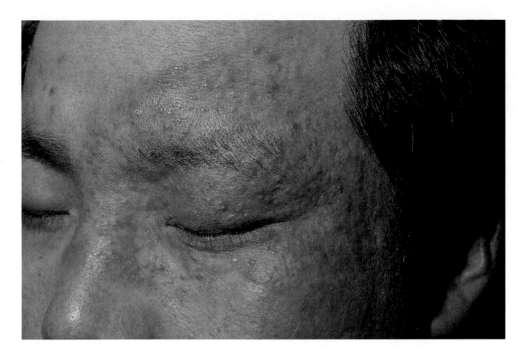

Figure 13-23
Tinea of the face. The fungal infection has extended deep into the follicles, creating a papular surface. Topical antifungal agents may not penetrate deep enough to adequately treat this process.

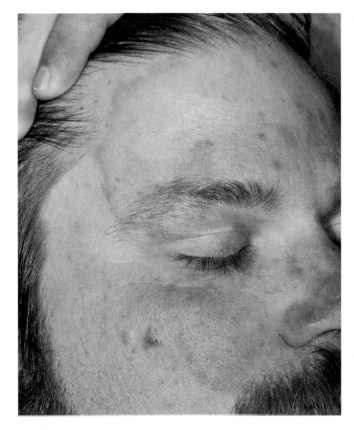

Figure 13-24
Tinea of the face. The plaque involves the forehead and central portion of the face. A sharp border occurs on the temple, across the lateral aspect of the eyebrow, and across the midportion of the cheek.

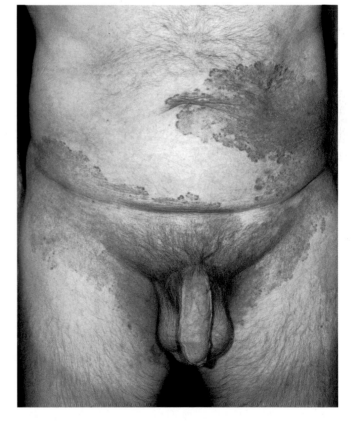

Figure 13-25
Tinea corporis. The border areas are fairly distinct and contain red papules. The central area is light brown and scaly.

Deep inflammatory lesions. Zoophile fungi such as *T. verrucosum* from cattle may produce a very inflammatory skin infection.[26] The infection is more common in the North, where cattle are confined in close quarters during the winter. The round, intensely inflamed lesion has a uniformly elevated, red, boggy, pustular surface. The pustules are follicular and represent deep penetration of the fungus into the hair follicle (Figure 13-26). Secondary bacterial infection can occur. The process ends with brown hyperpigmentation and scarring (Figure 13-27). A fungal culture helps to identify the animal source of the infection.

A distinctive form of inflammatory tinea called *Majocchi's granuloma*[27] and caused by *T. rubrum* and other species[28] was originally described as occurring on the lower legs of women who shave, but it is also seen at other sites on men and children. The primary lesion is a follicular papulopustule or inflammatory nodule. Intracutaneous and subcutaneous granulomatous nodules arise from these initial inflammatory tinea infections. Lesions have necrotic areas containing fungal elements; they are surrounded by epithelioid cells, giant cells, lymphocytes, and polymorphonuclear leukocytes, and they are believed to result from the rupturing of infected follicles into the dermis and subcutis: thus the term *granuloma*. There is marked variation from the usual hyphal forms. These include yeast forms, bizarre hyphae, and mucinous coatings. These variations may be a factor in allowing the dermatophytes to persist and grow in an abnormal manner.[28] Lesions are single or multiple and discrete or confluent. The area involved covers a few to 10 cm and may be red and scaly, but it is not as intensely inflamed as the *T. verrucosum* infection described above. The border may not be well defined. Skin biopsy with special stains for fungi are required for diagnosis if hyphae cannot be demonstrated in scale or hair.

Treatment. The superficial lesions of tinea corporis respond to the antifungal creams described in the Formulary (see p. 839). Lesions usually respond after 2 weeks of twice-a-day application, but treatment should be continued for at least 1 week after resolution of the infection. Extensive superficial lesions or those with red papules respond more predictably to oral therapy (see Table 13-1). The recurrence rate is high for those with extensive superficial infections. Deep inflammatory lesions require 1 to 3 or more months of oral therapy. Inflammation can be reduced with wet Burow's compresses, and bacterial infection is treated with the appropriate oral antibiotics. Some authors feel that oral or topical antifungal agents do not alter the course of highly inflammatory tinea (e.g., tinea verrucosum), because the intense inflammatory response destroys the organisms. However, griseofulvin is safe, and few physicians would withhold such therapy. As with tinea capitis kerion infections, a short course of prednisone may be considered for patients who have highly inflamed kerions, such as the patient in Figure 13-26.[29]

Invasive dermatophyte infection. Dermatophytes are typically confined within the keratinized, epithelial layer of the skin. The pathogenic potential is dependent, however, on a variety of local and systemic factors affecting the natural host resistance to dematophytic infection. Underlying systemic conditions that cause depressed cellular immunity, such as malignant lymphomas and Cushing's disease, as well as the administration of exogenous steroids or immunosuppressive agents, can lead to atypical, generalized, or invasive dermatophyte infection. Invasive dermatophyte infection should be included in the differential diagnosis of nodular, firm, or fluctuant masses (particularly on the extremities).[30] Several dermatophyte species have caused a deep, generalized infection in which the organism invaded various visceral organs.[31]

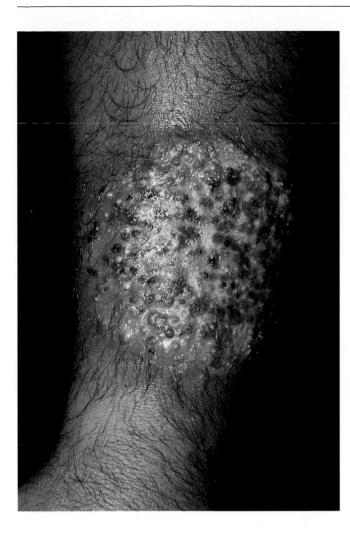

Figure 13-26
Trichophyton verrucosum. A zoophilic fungi from cattle that causes intense inflammation in humans.

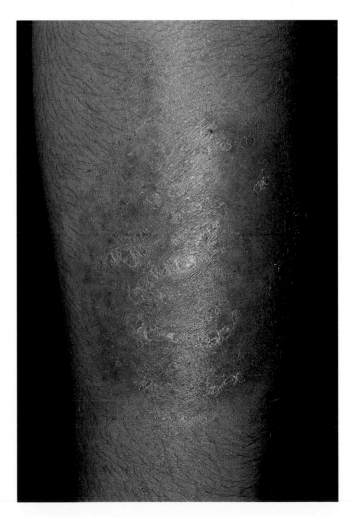

Figure 13-27
Trichophyton verrucosum. The deep Inflammatory Infectlon has caused brown hyperpigmentation and scarring. The hair follicles were destroyed.

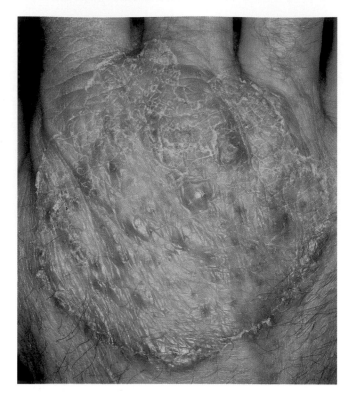

Figure 13-28
Tinea of the hand. The classic "ringworm" pattern of infection with a prominent scaling border.

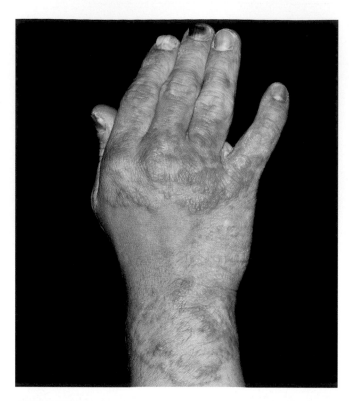

Figure 13-29
Tinea of the hand and wrist. The infected areas are red with little or no scale. Note infection of the fingernails.

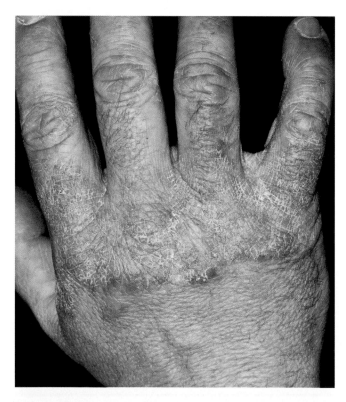

Figure 13-30
Tinea of the hand. There is a well-defined red border. Scaling is present, in contrast to the case illustrated in Figure 13-29.

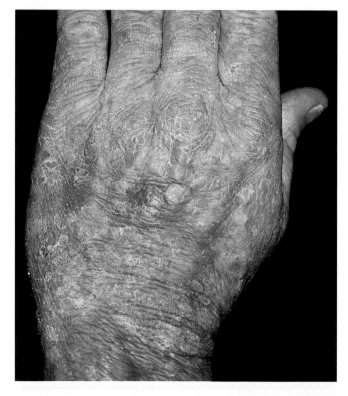

Figure 13-31
Tinea of the hand. There is diffuse erythema and scaling, simulating contact dermatitis. Compare this presentation with the case of tinea pedis in Figure 13-11.

TINEA OF THE HAND

Tinea of the dorsal aspect of the hand (tinea manuum) has all of the features of tinea corporis; tinea of the palm has the same appearance as the dry, diffuse, keratotic form of tinea on the soles (Figures 13-28 to 13-31). The dry keratotic form may be asymptomatic and the patient may be unaware of the infection, attributing the dry, thick, scaly surface to hard physical labor (Figure 13-32). Tinea of the palms is frequently seen in association with tinea pedis. The usual pattern of infection is involvement of one foot and two hands or of two feet and one hand. Fingernail infection often accompanies infection of the dorsum of the hand or palm. Treatment is the same as for tinea pedis and, as with the soles, a high recurrence rate can be expected for palm infection.

Figure 13-32
Tinea of the palm. The involved palm is thickened, very dry, and scaly. The patient is often unaware of the infection and feels that these changes are secondary to dry skin or hard physical labor.

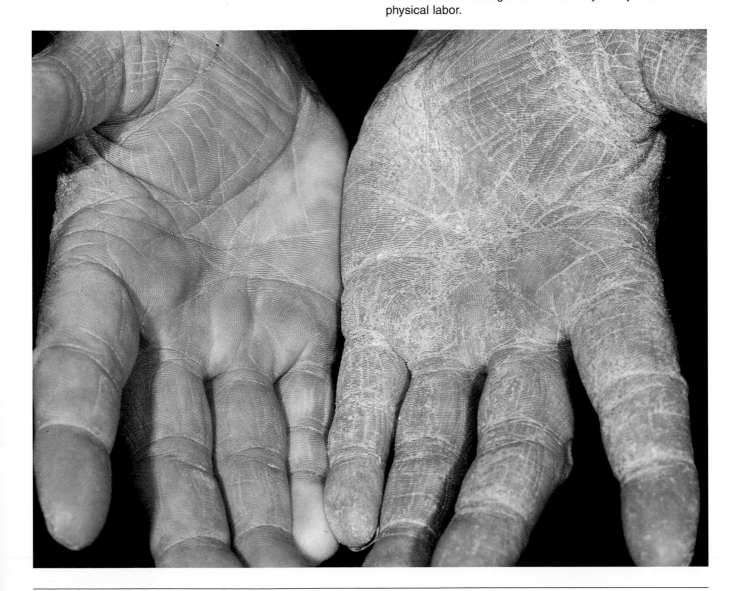

TINEA INCOGNITO

Fungal infections treated with topical steroids often lose some of their characteristic features. Topical steroids decrease inflammation and give the false impression that the rash is improving while the fungus flourishes secondary to cortisone-induced immunologic changes. Treatment is stopped, the rash returns, and memory of the good initial response prompts reuse of the steroid cream, but by this time the rash has changed. Scaling at the margins may be absent. Diffuse erythema, diffuse scale, scattered pustules (Figure 13-33) or papules, and brown hyperpigmentation may all result. A well-defined border may not be present and a once-localized process may have expanded greatly. The intensity of itching is variable. Tinea incognito is most often seen on the groin, on the face, and on the dorsal aspect of the hand. Tinea infections of the hands are often misdiagnosed as eczema and treated with topical steroids. Hyphae are easily demonstrated, especially a few days after discontinuing use of the steroid cream when scaling reappears.

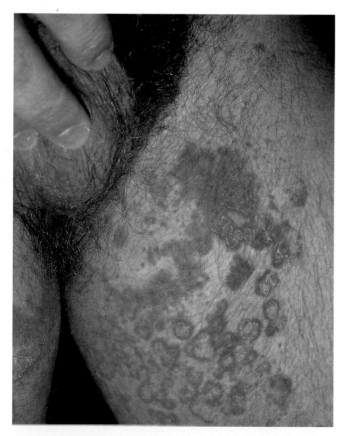

Figure 13-33
Tinea incognito. A group IV topical steroid was applied to the area of tinea cruris for 3 weeks. Characteristic features of tinea are missing.

TINEA OF THE SCALP

Tinea of the scalp (tinea capitis) occurs most frequently in prepubertal children. The infection has several different presentations.[32] The species of dermatophyte likely to cause tinea capitis varies from country to country, but anthropophilic species predominate in all areas. Tinea capitis is most common in areas of poverty and crowded living conditions. A species will be common in a geographic area for years only to be replaced or eradicated.

Most tinea capitis in the United States is caused by *T. tonsurans*, which does not fluoresce, but prior to the 1950s fluorescent tinea capitis caused by *M. canis* and *M. audouinii* predominated. Therefore, years ago, physicians relied on the Wood's light to make or confirm the diagnosis, but since the 1960s the majority of cases have been nonfluorescent. *T. tonsurans* is also found in Africa, along with *T. schoenleinii* and *T. violaceum*; *M. canis* is found in the United Kingdom, South America, and Saudi Arabia,[33] and *T. megninii* is found in Portugal. The infection originates from contact with a pet or an infected person. Each animal is associated with a limited number of fungal species. Therefore, an attempt should be made to identify the fungus by culture to help locate and treat a possible animal source.[34] Spores are shed in the air in the vicinity of the patient. Therefore, direct contact is not necessary to spread infection. Unlike other fungal infections, tinea of the scalp may be contagious by direct contact or from contaminated clothing; this provides some justification for briefly isolating those with proven infection.

Hair shaft invasion and infection. Hair shaft infection is preceded by invasion of the stratum corneum of the scalp. (See diagram of hair anatomy on p. 740.) The fungus grows down through this dead protein layer into the hair follicle and gains entry into the hair in the lower intrafollicular zone, just below the point where the cuticle of the hair shaft is formed. Because of the cuticle, the fungi cannot cross over from the perifollicular stratum corneum into the hair but must go deep into the hair follicle to circumvent the cuticle.[35] This may explain why topical antifungal agents are ineffective for treating tinea capitis. The fungi then invade the keratinized, outer root sheath, enter the inner cortex, and digest the keratin contained inside the hair shaft. The growth of hyphae occurs within the hair above the zone of keratinization of the hair shaft and keeps pace with the growth of hair. Distal to this zone of active growth, arthrospores are formed within or on the surface of the hair, depending on the species of dermatophytes. In black dot tinea capitis caused by *T. tonsurans* and *T. violaceum*, the hair cortex is almost completely replaced by spores and swells at the infundibular level, impeding further exit of the growing hair and causing the already weakened hair to coil up inside the infundibulum, forming a black dot.[36] The spores remain in the hair shaft and produce the endothrix pattern of invasion. Some of the *M. canis* hyphae break through the surface of the hair shaft (cuticle) and invade the keratinized inner root sheath and are there transformed into arthrospores. The spores are therefore located both on the inside of the hair shaft and on the outer surface to produce the ectothrix pattern seen under the microscope.[37]

Patterns of hair invasion. There are three patterns of hair invasion; small-spored ectothrix, large-spored ectothrix, and large-spored endothrix. Infection originates inside the hair shaft in all patterns. Hyphae grow inside and fragment into short segments called *arthrospores*. The arthrospores remain inside the hair shaft in the endothrix pattern (Figure 13-34).

In the ectothrix type, they dislodge (Figure 13-35), obscure and penetrate the surface cuticle on the hair-shaft surface, and form a sheath of closely packed spheres. The arthrospores are either large (6 to 10 μm) or small (2 to 3 μm). Large spores can be seen as separate structures with the low-power microscope objective. Higher power is needed to see the small spores.

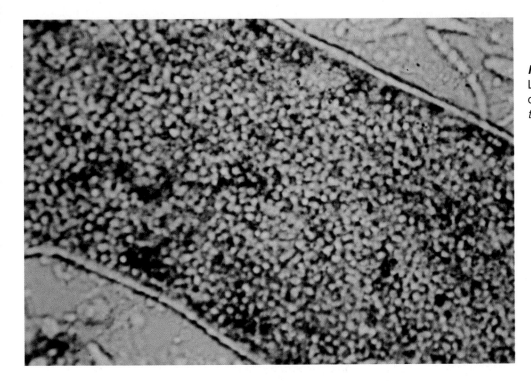

Figure 13-34
Large spore endothrix pattern of hair invasion. *Trichophyton tonsurans* ("a sack of marbles").

Figure 13-35
Large spore ectothrix pattern of hair invasion. *Trichophyton verrucosum.*

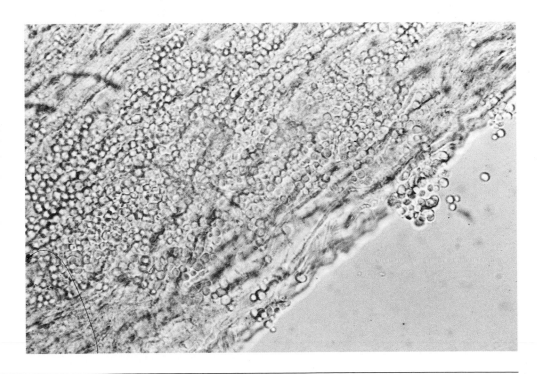

SYSTEMATIC APPROACH TO INVESTIGATION OF TINEA CAPITIS

DETERMINE CLINICAL PRESENTATION

Most forms of tinea capitis begin with one or several round patches of scale or alopecia.

Inflammatory lesions, even if untreated, tend to resolve spontaneously in a few months; the noninflammatory infections are more chronic.

Patchy alopecia + fine dry scale + no inflammation
    Short stubs of broken hair ("gray patch ringworm")
        M. audouinii
    Hairs broken off at surface ("black dot ringworm")
        T. tonsurans (most common), *T. violaceum*
    Patchy alopecia + swelling + purulent discharge
        M. canis, T. mentagrophytes (granular), *T. verrucosum*

Kerion is a severe inflammatory reaction with boggy induration. Any fungus, but especially *M. canis, T. mentagrophytes* (granular), *T. verrucosum* (see Figures 13-37 and 13-38)

WOOD'S LIGHT EXAMINATION

Blue-green fluorescence of hair—only *M. canis* and *M. audouinii* have this feature. Scale and skin do not fluoresce.

POTASSIUM HYDROXIDE WET MOUNT OF PLUCKED HAIRS

The pattern of hair invasion is characteristic for each species of fungus. Hairs that can be removed with little resistance are best for evaluation.

Large-spored endothrix pattern-chains of large spores (densely packed) within the hair, "like a sack full of marbles."
    T. tonsurans, T. violaceum (see Figure 13-34)

Large-spored ectothrix pattern-chains of large spores inside and on the surface of the hair shaft and visible with the low power objective
    T. verrucosum, T. mentagrophytes (see Figure 13-35)

Small-spored ectothrix—small spores randomly arranged in masses inside and on the surface of the hair shaft, not visible with the low-power objective. Looks like a stick dipped in maple syrup and rolled in sand.
    M. canis, M. audouinii

IDENTIFICATION OF SOURCE AFTER SPECIES IS VERIFIED BY CULTURE

Anthropophilic (parasitic on humans)—infection from other humans
    M. audouinii, T. tonsurans, T. violaceum

Zoophilic (parasitic on animals)—infection from animals or other infected humans
    M. canis—dog, cat, monkey
    T. mentagrophytes (granular)—dog, rabbit, guinea pig, monkey
    T. verrucosum—cattle

Clinical patterns of infection. A systematic approach for the clinical and laboratory investigations of tinea capitis is presented in the box at left. The inflammatory response to infection is variable. Noninflammatory tinea of the scalp is illustrated in Figure 13-36. A severe, inflammatory reaction with a boggy, indurated, tumorlike mass that exudes pus is called a *kerion* (Figure 13-37). It represents a hypersensitivity reaction to fungus and heals with scarring and some hair loss (Figure 13-38). The hair loss is less than would be expected from the degree and depth of inflammation.

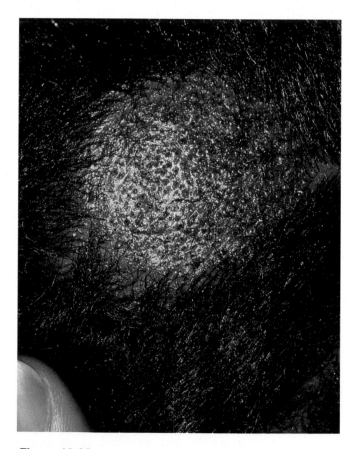

Figure 13-36
Trichophyton tonsurans. Black dot ringworm. There are areas of alopecia with scale but no inflammation. Arthrospores inside the shafts of infected hairs weaken the hair and cause it to break off at or below the scalp surface, resulting in the "black dot" appearance of the surface. *(From Solomon LM et al:* Current Concepts *2(3):224, 1985; reproduced by permission of Blackwell Scientific Publications.)*

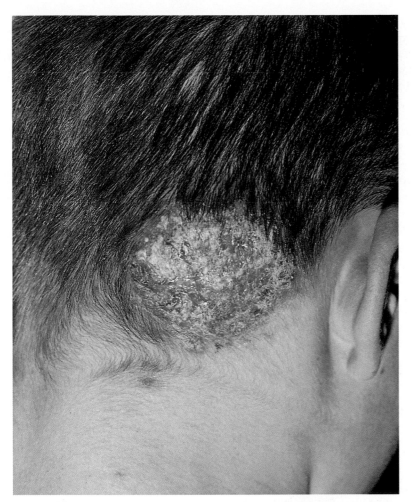

Figure 13-37
Tinea capitis. A severely inflammatory, boggy, indurated, tumor-like mass (kerion).

Figure 13-38
Tinea capitis. A huge kerion healed after 2 months of treatment with griseofulvin. The scalp is scarred, and hair follicles have been destroyed.

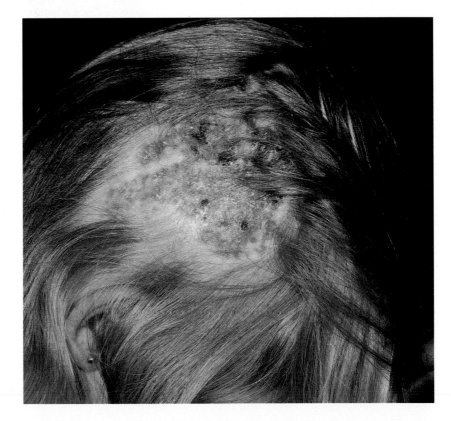

Trichophyton tonsurans

Since the 1950s, *T. tonsurans* (large-spored endothrix) has been responsible for more than 90% of the scalp ringworm in the United States, but *M. canis* (small-spored ectothrix) is still a major cause in some parts of the United States. The occurrence rate is equal in boys and girls, and most cases are seen in the crowded inner cities in blacks or Hispanics.[38] Tinea capitis prior to the 1950s was caused by *M. audouinii*, which spontaneously clears in adolescence and fluoresces green with the Wood's light. *T. tonsurans* does not fluoresce and infects people of all ages. It can remain viable for long periods on inanimate objects such as combs, brushes, blankets, and telephones.[39] *T. tonsurans* lesions may occur outside of the scalp in patients, their families, and their close friends. These lesions serve as a reservoir for reinfection. Therefore, all siblings or close contacts within the family should be examined. The peak incidence of infection occurs at ages 3 through 9 years. This fungal infection does not tend to resolve spontaneously at puberty, resulting in a large population of infected carriers.

Four patterns of infection. *T. tonsurans* has four different clinical infection patterns. There may be multiple cases within a family, and each person may have a different infection pattern. The clinical presentation may be related to specific host T-lymphocyte response. This dermatophytosis is most frequently incurred from contact with an infected child, either directly or via a variety of fomites. Current studies indicate that an asymptomatic adult carrier state exists and may provide a source for continued reinfection in children.[40,41]

Noninflammatory black dot pattern. This is the most distinctive pattern and occurs in approximately 5% of patients. Large areas of alopecia are present without inflammation. There is a mild-to-moderate amount of scalp scale. Occipital adenopathy may be present. Lack of inflammation may be explained by the fact that cell-mediated immunity to *Trichophyton* antigen skin tests is negative in these patients. The infected hairs of *T. tonsurans* have arthrospores inside the hair shaft; the arthrospores weaken the hair and cause it to break off at or below the scalp surface, resulting in a "black dot" appearance of the scalp surface (see Figure 13-36). Broken hairs are typically less than 2 mm long. Hairs long enough to be pulled are generally not infected.

Culture techniques. The short hairs are traditionally collected with forceps—a tedious, time-consuming method. A better method is to firmly rub a tap water–moistened gauze[42] or a toothbrush over the involved area. Tightly woven gauze is the most effective (Topper dressing sponge). Each hair is lifted off the gauze with a needle or forceps and placed on a slide for potassium hydroxide preparation. The brush-culture method involves gently rubbing a previously sterilized toothbrush in a circular motion over areas where scale is present or over the margins of patches of alopecia.[43] The brush fibers are then pressed into the culture media and the brush is discarded. Cultures turn positive significantly faster when the sample is obtained with the brush technique. (Figure 13-39). Heating the slide may burst the hair and make it difficult to differentiate the endothrix pattern from the ectothrix pattern.

Figure 13-39

Trichophyton tonsurans. Culture technique for sampling dry scale in the scalp. *(From Solomon LM et al:* Current Concepts *2(3):224, 1985; reproduced by permission of Blackwell Scientific Publications.)*

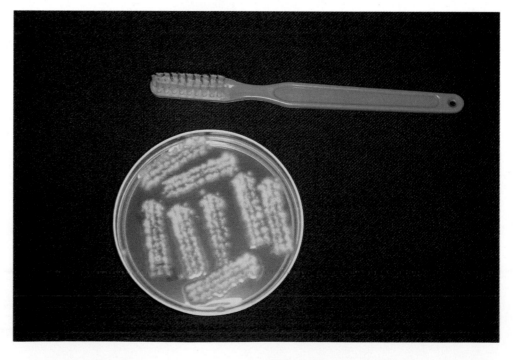

Inflammatory tinea capitis (kerion). Most patients with this infection pattern have a positive skin test to *Trichophyton* antigen, suggesting that the patient's immune response may be responsible for intense inflammation. Approximately 35% of patients infected with *T. tonsurans* have this pattern. There are one or multiple inflamed, boggy, tender areas of alopecia with pustules on and/or in surrounding skin (see Figure 13-37). Fever, occipital adenopathy, leukocytosis, and a diffuse, morbilliform rash may occur. Potassium hydroxide wet mounts and fungal cultures are often negative because of destruction of fungal structures by inflammation, and treatment may have to be initiated based on clinical appearance.[44] Scarring alopecia may occur (see Figure 13-38).

Seborrheic dermatitis type. This type is common and the most difficult to diagnosis because it resembles dandruff. There is diffuse or patchy, fine, white, adherent scale on the scalp. Close examination shows tiny, perifollicular pustules and/or hair stubs that have broken off at the level of the scalp: the black dot pattern. Less commonly, there is patchy or diffuse hair loss.[45] Adenopathy is often present. Culture is often necessary to make the diagnosis because only 29% of affected patients have a positive potassium hydroxide examination.[46]

Pustular type. There are discrete pustules or scabbed areas without scaling or significant hair loss. Pustules suggest bacterial infection, and patients with pustules may receive several courses of antibiotics before the correct diagnosis is made. The pustules may be sparse or numerous. As with kerions, the cultures and potassium hydroxide wet mounts may be negative.

Differential diagnosis. Seborrheic dermatitis and psoriasis may be confused with tinea of the scalp. Tinea amiantacea, a form of seborrheic dermatitis that occurs in children, is frequently misdiagnosed as tinea. Tinea amiantacea is a localized 2- to 8-cm patch of large, brown, polygonal-shaped scales that adheres to the scalp and mats the hair. The matted scale grows out, attached to the hair (see Figure 8-27). There is little or no inflammation.

Management (Table 13-2)

Griseofulvin. Griseofulvin (15 mg/kg/day ultramicrosized) administered once as a single dose or divided into two doses is effective. Griseofulvin is absorbed more efficiently with a fatty meal; children can be given the medicine with ice cream or whole milk. Ketoconazole is less effective at dosages recommended by the manufacturer.[47] Some children require larger dosages of medication to eradicate the infection. Patients are reexamined in 3 or 4 weeks. If the potassium hydroxide wet mount or culture is still positive, or if there is little clinical improvement, treatment should be continued. Patients with tinea capitis should be treated 2 weeks beyond the time that cultures and potassium hydroxide preparations become negative. This generally requires at least 6 to 12 weeks of treatment. Continuous daily treatment is desirable, but unreliable patients can be treated with a single, 4 gm dose of microsized griseofulvin that has been pulverized and mixed with food. This single-dose schedule gives a high cure rate in noninflammatory tinea capitis.[48] A few authors have suggested suppressing the inflammation of a kerion with topical,[49] oral, or intralesional steroids. Prednisone 1 to 2 mg/kg/day may hasten resolution and reduce or prevent scarring. Although this seems reasonable, there has been little experience with this practice.

Terbinafine. Patients with dry, noninflammatory tinea capitis were given oral terbinafine for 6 weeks (3 to 6 mg/kg/day): 80% were completely cured, 10% were mycologically cured and showed minimal signs and symptoms, and another 10% showed improvement (negative mycology, but persistent clinical signs and symptoms).[50]

Itraconazole. Fifty patients with tinea capitis were treated with itraconazole 25 to 100 mg/day (3 to 5 mg/kg/day) for 20 to 73 days: 76% completely healed and 18% showed marked improvement. The primary organisms reported were *M. canis* and *T. tonsurans.*[51]

Prevention of recurrence. *T. tonsurans* spores may remain viable on furniture, combs, and brushes. Scrupulous cleaning of all possibly contaminated objects helps to prevent reinfection. All family members should be examined carefully for tinea capitis and tinea corporis.

TINEA OF THE BEARD

Fungal infection of the beard area (tinea barbae) should be considered when inflammation occurs in this area. Bacterial folliculitis and inflammation secondary to ingrown hairs (pseudofolliculitis) are common. However, it is not unusual to see patients who have finally been diagnosed as having tinea after failing to respond to several courses of antibiotics. A positive culture for staphylococcus does not rule out tinea, in which purulent lesions may be infected secondarily with bacteria. Like tinea capitis, the hairs are almost always infected and easily removed. The hairs in bacterial folliculitis resist removal.

Superficial infection. This pattern resembles the annular lesions of tinea corporis. The hair is usually infected.

Deep follicular infection. This pattern clinically resembles bacterial folliculitis except that it is slower to evolve and is usually restricted to one area of the beard. Bacterial folliculitis spreads rapidly over wide areas after shaving. Tinea begins insidiously with a small group of follicular pustules. The process becomes confluent in time with the development of a boggy, erythematous, tumorlike abscess covered with dense, superficial crust similar to fungal kerions seen in tinea capitis (Figures 13-40 and 13-41). Hairs may be painlessly removed at almost any stage of the infection and examined for hyphae. Zoophilic *T. mentagrophytes* and *T. verrucosum* are the most common pathogens. Species identification by culture helps to identify the possible animal reservoir of infection.

Treatment. Treatment is the same as that for tinea capitis. Oral agents (see Table 13-1) are usually required because creams do not penetrate to the depths of the hair follicle.

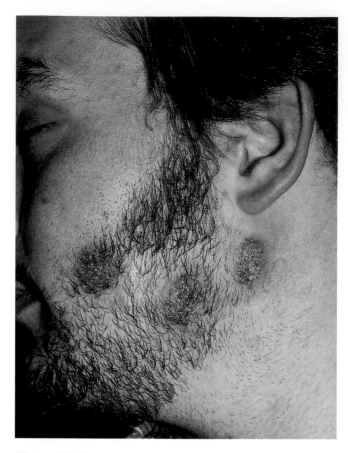

Figure 13-40
Tinea barbae. Inflamed areas are indurated and eroded on the surface. Hairs may be painlessly removed. Removal of beard hair in bacterial infections is usually painful.

Figure 13-41
Tinea of the beard. A deep boggy infection of the follicles. Oral antifungal agents are required.

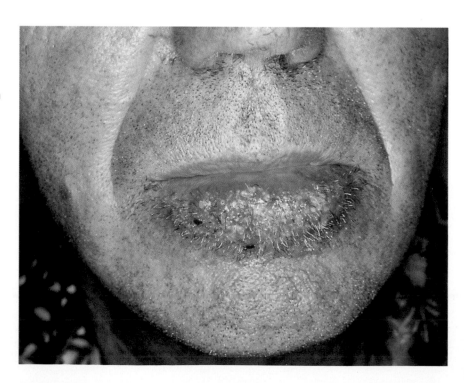

TREATMENT OF FUNGAL INFECTIONS

Topical preparations. A variety of preparations are commercially available. Studies have shown that undecylenic acid (e.g., Desenex) may be almost as effective for treating dermatophyte infections as all of the newer agents.[52] Most of the medicines are available as creams or lotions; some are available as powders or aerosols. They are effective for all dermatophyte infections except for deep, inflammatory lesions of the body and scalp. They have no effect on tinea of the nail. Creams or lotions should be applied twice a day until the infection is clear. (See the Formulary, p. 839, for a list of the available topical agents.)

Systemic agents (see Tables 13-1 and 13-2)

Griseofulvin. Griseofulvin is active only against dermatophytes; yeast infections, including those caused by *Candida* organisms and *Pityrosporum* organisms (tinea versicolor), and deep fungi do not respond. The drug has been available for more than 20 years and has been proven safe. Griseofulvin has a fungistatic effect, therefore it works best on actively growing dermatophytes in which it may inhibit fungal cell-wall synthesis. Griseofulvin probably diffuses into the stratum corneum from the extracellular fluid and sweat. Increased sweating may increase the concentration in the stratum corneum, thereby enhancing the drug's effect. Griseofulvin produces a sustained blood level so that a once- or twice-a-day schedule is adequate. Absorption varies from person to person; individual patients attain consistently high or low levels of the drug. Taking the drug with fatty foods may enhance absorption.

Two preparations are available: microsize and ultramicrosize. The newer, ultramicrosized forms are better absorbed and require approximately 50% to 70% of the dosage of the microsized form. Many brands are available in both forms. In microsize, the drug is supplied as 125-mg, 250-mg, and 500-mg tablets; in ultramicrosize, it is supplied as 125-mg, 250-mg, and 330-mg tablets. The recommended dosage and duration of therapy are listed in Table 13-2. The dosage should be adequate. Reported treatment failures are probably the result of using too small a dosage rather than resistant organisms.

ADVERSE REACTIONS. Griseofulvin is a safe drug. Headaches and GI symptoms are the most common side effects. The dosage can be temporarily lowered to see if they clear, but sometimes the drug must be discontinued. Hepatotoxicity, leukopenia, and photosensitivity rarely occur.[53] Therefore, routine blood studies are not necessary[24] unless treatment is to last for many months or the dosage is exceptionally high. If a headache occurs, it usually does so during the first few days of treatment and may disappear as treatment is continued. A trial at a lower dosage level is warranted for those with headaches lasting more than 48 hours. Patients with persistent headaches after a lower dosage trial need alternative treatment. Bone marrow suppression, once attributed to griseofulvin, probably never occurs, and routine CBCs are not necessary. GI upset, urticaria, photosensi-

tivity, and morbilliform skin eruptions have been reported. Griseofulvin activates hepatic enzymes that cause degradation of warfarin and other drugs. Appropriate steps should be taken if combined treatment is used.

One article suggests that griseofulvin may have decreased the effectiveness of the estrogen that was being used as part of a contraceptive pill.[54]

Imidazoles

Ketoconazole. Ketoconazole is an oral imidazole with a wider spectrum of action than griseofulvin. It is effective against dermatophytes, yeasts, and *P. orbiculare* and *P. ovale*. The drug alters fungal cell-membrane permeability by inhibiting the synthesis of ergosterol. Cell-membrane dysfunction leads to cell lysis. It has not been determined whether ketoconazole is absorbed more effectively with food or on an empty stomach. Ketoconazole requires gastric acidity for absorption, and variations in plasma levels often relate to gastric acidity. Absorption may be reduced in some patients with achlorhydria. H_2 blockers (e.g., cimetidine) markedly reduce absorption, particularly in conjunction with antacid administration. If H_2 blockers are needed, they should be given at least 2 hours after ketoconazole administration. Ketoconazole appears in eccrine sweat, where it binds to the stratum corneum, hair, and nails. It is metabolized in the liver and excreted primarily in the feces. Because renal elimination is relatively unimportant, ketoconazole may be used in patients with renal impairment without the need for dosage adjustment.

INDICATIONS. Ketoconazole is indicated for the treatment of systemic candidiasis; chronic mucocutaneous candidiasis; oral thrush; blastomycosis; coccidioidomycosis; histoplasmosis; chromomycosis; paracoccidioidomycosis; and severe, recalcitrant, cutaneous dermatophyte infections.

ADVERSE REACTIONS. Idiosyncratic hepatotoxicity, primarily of the hepatocellular type, may occur. The most serious side effect of ketoconazole is hepatitis, which has proved fatal in seven reported cases; one patient survived after a successful liver transplant.[55] The reported incidence of hepatotoxicity has been approximately 1:10,000 exposed patients. The true incidence of symptomatic hepatic injury may be closer to 1 in 2000.[56] The median duration of therapy is 2 months (range 3 to 365 days).[57] Jaundice is the most common symptom; anorexia, nausea, vomiting, and malaise are the next most frequent complaints. Since these reactions are idiosyncratic rather than immunoallergic or toxic, they are unrelated to daily dosage, cumulative total dose, or duration of therapy; therefore monitoring liver enzyme levels and stopping ketoconazole therapy may not help to prevent the progression of hepatitis. Serious hepatic reactions occur more often in patients previously treated over the long term with griseofulvin.

Hepatic injury is usually reversible and self-limited, and it resolves in weeks or months when therapy is stopped. Corticosteroids may help accelerate recovery.[58] Hepatitis has been reported in children. Liver function tests (such as SGGT, alkaline phosphatase, SGPT, SGOT, and bilirubin)

TABLE 13-1 Oral Antifungal Drugs

	Griseofulvin	Ketoconazole (Nizoral)	Fluconazole (Diflucan)	Itraconazole (Sporanox)	Terbinafine (Lamisil)
Dosage forms	125, 250, 333 mg ultramicronized tablet 125 mg/5 ml food enhances absorption	200 mg tablet taken with breakfast with an acidic fruit juice	50, 100, 200 mg tablets Water soluble, well absorbed	100 mg capsule food enhances absorption[23]	250 mg
Fungicidal	No	No	No	No	Yes
Persistent in plasma after Rx	2 weeks	2 days	—	1 week	4 to 6 weeks
Persistent in skin and nails after Rx	1 to 2 weeks	Unknown	3 months	6 to 9 months	4 to 6 weeks
Laboratory monitoring	Rx 6 weeks complete blood count (CBC) liver function test (LFT)	Baseline CBC, LFT; repeat each month	Baseline CBC, LFT; repeat each month	Baseline CBC, LFT; repeat each month	CBC, repeat each month
Adverse reactions	8% to 15%	13%	7%	7%	5%
Safety profile	Multiple uncommon side effects	Fulminant hepatotoxicity in 1/10,000	Less hepatotoxicity than ketoconazole	Less hepatotoxicity than ketoconazole	Few side effects; minor GI disturbances
Adverse reactions	Abdominal pain, erythema multiforme, headache, mixed drug reactions, nausea and vomiting, photosensitivity, urticaria	Abdominal pain, nausea and vomiting, dizziness, fever, headache, pruritus, inhibition of testicular and adrenal steroidogenesis	Abdominal pain, nausea and vomiting, headache, rash	Nausea and vomiting, abdominal pain, hypokalemia, increased aminotransferase activity, dizziness, headache, pruritus, rash, sleepiness	Nausea and vomiting, abdominal pain, dizziness, headache, pruritus, rash, taste loss
Potential drug interaction	Alcohol, barbiturates, coumarin, oral contraceptives, warfarin	Alcohol, antacids, astemizole, coumarin, cyclosporine, erythromycin, H$_2$ antagonists, isoniazid, phenytoin, rifampin, sulfonylureas, terfenadine	Coumarin, cyclosporine, hydrochlorothiazids, isoniazid, oral contraceptives, phenytoin, rifampin, sulfonylureas, valproic acid	Astemizole, carbamazepine, coumarin, cyclosporine, digoxin, erythromycin, H$_2$ antagonists, isoniazid, phenobarbital, phenytoin, rifampin, sulfonylureas, terfenadine	H$_2$ antagonists, rifampin, cyclosporine
Cost to pharmacist/pill	$90/100 pills	$232/100 pills	$173/30 pills (100 mg)	$139/30 pills	Available in 1995 or 1996 in the United States

TABLE 13-2 Oral Antifungal Drug Dosages[64-79]

	Griseofulvin (ultramicrosize)	Ketoconazole (Nizoral)	Fluconazole (Diflucan)	Itraconazole (Sporanox)	Terbinafine (Lamisil)
Tinea corporis and cruris	500 mg/qd—adult 5-7 mg/kg/day— child 2-6 weeks	200-400 mg/day 2 weeks	150 mg once a week 3-4 weeks	200 mg qd 1-2 weeks	250 mg qd 2 weeks
Tinea capitis	15 mg/kg/day 4-12 weeks	NR	50 mg qd 3 weeks	3-5 mg/kg/day 4-6 weeks	125 mg qd (3-6 mg/kg/day) 4 weeks
Onychomycosis	500-1000 qd 6 to 18 months	NR	150 mg once a week 9 months	200 mg qd Fingernails 6 weeks Toenails 12 weeks Pulse dosing 200 mg bid— 1 week on, 3 weeks off, Toenails 3-4 months, Fingernails 2-3 months	250 mg qd Fingernails 6 weeks Toenails 12 weeks
Tinea pedis	500 mg/qd—adult 5-7 mg/kg/day— child 6-12 weeks	NR	150 mg once a week 3-4 weeks	400 mg qd 4 weeks	250 mg qd 6 weeks
Tinea versicolor	Not effective	400 mg single dose or 200 mg/day 5-10 days	400 mg single dose	200 mg qd 5 or 7 days	Studies ongoing
Vaginal candidiasis	Not effective	200-400 mg qd 5 days	150 mg single dose	200 mg tid one day or 200 mg qd 3 days	Studies ongoing

NR, Not recommended.

are frequently assessed before and at frequent intervals during treatment.

Elevations of transaminase levels during treatment are common (6% estimated) and considered harmless. These elevations usually resolve during continued therapy. Some authors suggest that periodic liver function screening may serve no clinical purpose, since it probably would not help to avoid serious hepatic side effects.[59,60] Millions of patients have taken ketoconazole with a low incidence of hepatic reactions; however, periodic laboratory and clinical evaluations may not avoid fulminant hepatic reactions.

Symptomatic, life-threatening ventricular arrhythmias have been reported with the concomitant use of terfenadine (Seldane) and ketoconazole. Similar cardiovascular consequences have also occurred in patients treated concurrently with a macrolide antibiotic, such as erythromycin, and ketoconazole. Simultaneous treatment with rifampin and ketoconazole is contraindicated. By inducing hepatic microsomal enzymes, rifampin drastically lowers the serum concentration of ketoconazole. Given with ketoconazole, levels of rifampin also drop.[61]

Ketoconazole can cause oligospermia, gynecomastia, a decrease in serum testosterone, a loss of libido, a loss of potency, and adrenal insufficiency. The drug blocks testicular and adrenal steroid synthesis in a dose-dependent, time-dependent manner by blocking key P450 enzymes. These effects are relatively transient at dosages of 200 to 400 mg daily.

DOSAGE. The dosage is 200 mg daily, increasing to 400 mg daily after 1 month for slow responders. Ketoconazole is given once each morning in order to have the least impact on adrenal hormone concentration.[62] Ketoconazole is indicated for the treatment of patients with severe, recalcitrant, cutaneous dermatophyte infections who have not responded to topical therapy or oral griseofulvin, or who are unable to take griseofulvin. Minimum treatment for recalcitrant tinea corporis is 4 weeks. Palmar and plantar infections may respond more slowly. Successful therapy requires adequate duration of treatment because premature discontinuation of medication results in persistent infection and recurrence of clinical symptoms.[63]

Triazoles. Triazoles are similar to imidazoles in chemical structure and mechanism of action.

Fluconazole (Diflucan). Fluconazole is much more specific and effective at inhibiting cytochrome P450 than the imidazole agents. The characteristics of fluconazole are shown in Table 13-1. Fluconazole is highly water soluble and is transported to the skin through sweat and concentrated by evaporation. It achieves high concentrations in the epidermis and nails.

Itraconazole (Sporanox). Itraconazole, like the other antifungal azoles, inhibits fungal cytochrome P450–dependent enzymes, blocking the synthesis of ergosterol, the principal sterol in the fungal cell membrane. The characteristics of itraconazole are shown in Table 13-1. The concentration in the stratum corneum remains detectable for 4 weeks after therapy. Itraconazole levels in sebum are 5 times higher than in plasma and remain high for as long as 1 week after therapy. This suggests that secretion in sebum may account for the high concentrations found in skin. Itraconazole reaches high levels in the nails that persist for at least 6 months after therapy is stopped.

Allylamines. Allylamines, like the azoles, inhibit ergosterol synthesis, but do so at an earlier point. The result, as with the azoles, is membrane disruption and cell death.

Terbinafine. Terbinafine is well absorbed and is lipophilic. This results in accumulation in the dermis, epidermis, and adipose tissues, from which it is slowly released into circulation. Plasma levels are detectable at low levels for 4 to 8 weeks after therapy. Terbinafine remains in the skin and nails for 4 to 6 weeks after therapy.

Persistence of the drug in plasma is of concern when side effects are experienced. Terbinafine appears to reach the skin by diffusion through the dermis and epidermis and via secretion in sebum. It has not been detected in sweat. Terbinafine levels in keratin decline parallel to plasma levels, which may indicate a lack of affinity for keratinized tissues and no long-term accumulation in nail.

Candidiasis (Moniliasis)

The yeastlike fungus *C. albicans* and a few other *Candida* species are capable of producing skin, mucous membrane, and internal infections. The organism lives with the normal flora of the mouth, vaginal tract, and gut, and it reproduces through the budding of oval yeast forms. Pregnancy, oral contraception, antibiotic therapy, diabetes, skin maceration, topical steroid therapy, certain endocrinopathies, and factors related to depression of cell-mediated immunity may allow the yeast to become pathogenic and produce budding spores and elongated cells (pseudohyphae) or true hyphae with septate walls. The pseudohyphae and hyphae are indistinguishable from dermatophytes in potassium hydroxide preparations (Figure 13-42). Culture results must be interpreted carefully because the yeast is part of the normal flora in many areas.

The yeast infects only the outer layers of the epithelium of mucous membrane and skin (the stratum corneum). The primary lesion is a pustule, the contents of which dissect horizontally under the stratum corneum and peel it away. Clinically, this process results in a red, denuded, glistening surface with a long, cigarette paper–like, scaling, advancing border. The infected mucous membranes of the mouth and vaginal tract accumulate scale and inflammatory cells that develop into characteristic white or white-yellow, curdy material.

Yeast grows best in a warm, moist environment; therefore, infection is usually confined to the mucous membranes and intertriginous areas. The advancing infected border usually stops when it reaches dry skin.

CANDIDIASIS OF NORMALLY MOIST AREAS

Candidiasis affects normally moist areas such as the vagina, the mouth, and the uncircumcised penis. In the vagina, it causes vulvovaginitis; in the mouth, it causes thrush; and in the uncircumcised penis, it causes balanitis.

Vulvovaginitis

Vaginal candidiasis is the most common cause of vaginal discharge. Infection is usually due to *C. albicans*. The incidence of infections due to yeasts other than *C. albicans* has increased in the last few years. Of these nonalbicans species, *C. tropicalis* and *C. glabrata* are the most important. Currently used drug therapies (e.g., imidazoles) do not adequately eradicate nonalbicans species. A possible explanation for the recent increased selection of these species may be the shortened antifungal therapies (1- to 3-day regimens) that suppress *C. albicans*, but create an imbalance of flora that facilitates an overgrowth of nonalbicans species.[80]

Candida is present in the normal flora of the vaginal tract and rectum in 10% of women.[81] *Candida* vaginitis develops in approximately one fourth of women in their child-bearing years. Heat and moisture are increased under large folds of fat and occlusive undergarments. Symptoms may worsen a few days prior to menstruation. One study showed that 30% of women treated with antibiotics developed candidal vaginitis.[82] *Candida* usually begins with vaginal itching and/or a white, thin-to-creamy discharge. Symptoms may resolve spontaneously after several days, or they may progress. The vaginal mucous membranes and external genitalia become red, swollen, and sometimes eroded and painful. They are covered with a thick, white, crumbly discharge, which becomes more copious during pregnancy. The infection may spread onto the thighs and anus, producing a tender, red skin surface with discrete pustules, called *satellite lesions*, which appear outside the edges of the advancing border. The diagnosis is confirmed by a potassium hydroxide preparation of the discharge.

Recurrent disease. Patients with chronic and recurrent candidal vaginitis rarely have recognizable precipitating or causal factors.[83] Appearance of nonalbicans *Candida* species is possible but unusual. Resistance to azoles is not a causal factor. Relapse is due to persistent yeast in the vagina rather than to frequent vaginal reinfection. Attempts to reduce the number of attacks by treating sexual partners and

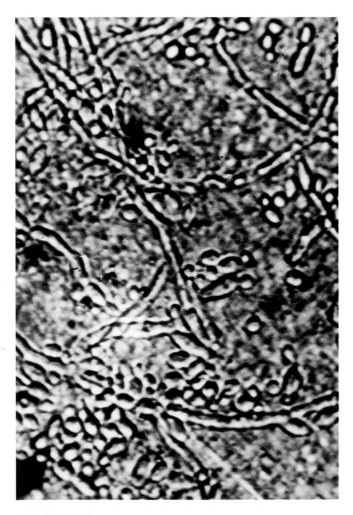

Figure 13-42
Candida albicans. A potassium hydroxide wet mount of skin scrapings showing both elongated pseudohyphae and budding spores.

suppressing a GI tract focus have failed. There is no definitive cure for recurrent candidal vaginitis, but many therapeutic maintenance regimens with azoles are available that effectively control symptomatic infection. Women with recurrent candidal vaginitis are more likely to use contraceptive pills and commercially available solutions for vulvoperineal cleansing or vaginal douching. Increasing frequency of sexual intercourse correlates with recurrent infection.[84] Recurrence of vaginal candidiasis is not usually related to the development of drug resistance to topical or oral imidazoles.[85] Frequent yeast infections could be an early sign of HIV infection.

Management

Topical antifungals. There are a large variety of topical medications in many forms including tablets, creams, and tampons (see the Formulary, p. 839). Clotrimazole and miconazole are the most widely used. The cure rate with polyenes (nystatin) is 70% to 80%. The cure rate with azole derivatives is 85% to 90%. Topical antimycotic therapy is free of systemic side effects. The initial application may cause local burning especially if inflammation is severe. The burning is a local irritant reaction rather than an allergy.

Topical azole therapy of vaginal candidiasis. Treatment schedules are listed in the Formulary (p. 858). The course should be repeated if symptoms have not subsided. Cream is useful if the external areas are also infected. The cream runs out and coats the vulva. Cream may also be applied directly from the tube. There is enough cream supplied for both external and internal application.

Nystatin (Mycostatin). One tablet is placed with the applicator high in the vaginal tract twice a day for 2 weeks. The duration of treatment is extended if signs or symptoms persist. Although nystatin must be used longer than the azoles, it is still an effective and safe medicine.

Gentian violet. This purple dye has been used for years and is a safe, effective agent that has both antiyeast and antibacterial activity. A sanitary napkin prevents staining of clothing. Gentian violet may be useful in resistant cases that require long periods of treatment. Gentian violet should be used one to two times a day for at least 7 days or until symptoms have cleared.

Boric acid. One study demonstrated that boric acid was effective in curing 98% of the patients who did not respond to the most commonly used antifungal agents, and it was indicated as the treatment of choice for prophylaxis.[86]

Oral antifungals. Oral preparations include ketoconazole, fluconazole, and itraconazole. A recent literature review compared oral fluconazole with conventional treatment regimens. Most of the trials used single-dose fluconazole. Fluconazole was shown to be as effective as other oral and intravaginal regimens, with minimal adverse effects.[87] Studies have shown oral ketoconazole (Nizoral 200 mg oral tablet) to be as effective as miconazole vaginal creams in eradicating the yeast. The recurrence rate, however, may be higher with ketoconazole.

Acute vaginal candidiasis. The imidazoles and triazoles are the first choice of treatment for vulvovaginal candidiasis (Table 13-3). There is a lack of clear superiority of one azole agent or dosing regimen. Most patients are treated with a short course of intravaginal therapy (1 to 3 days) for acute, uncomplicated candidal vaginitis. The physician's judgment and the patient's preference determine the specific antifungal agent and route of administration. Cost, distribution of inflammation, and medicine vehicle characteristics are factors in the decision. Many patients prefer oral treatment. Oral and vaginal medication are almost equally effective in treating acute disease.

Chronic recurrent vaginal candidiasis. Recurrent cases may require longer topical therapy (6 to 14 days). Patients with multiple recurrences may benefit from long-term suppression with oral or topical programs (Table 13-4). Therapeutic goals include elimination of the yeast and correction of predisposing factors. Patients with recurrent disease should be advised to lose excess weight and wear loose-fitting, cotton undergarments. Reduction of the number of yeast in the GI tract with nystatin and an attempt to restore normal flora with *Lactobacillus* preparations may be useful in resistant cases. Daily ingestion of 8 ounces of yogurt containing *L. acidophilus* decreased both candidal colonization and infection in one study.[97] The efficacy of yeast elimination diets is unknown. *Candida* should be documented by culture for any patient who has recurrent or persistent disease and a negative potassium hydroxide (KOH) slide.

TABLE 13-3 Oral Therapy for Acute *Candida* Vaginitis

Medication	Treatment schedule	Percentage Cured
Itraconazole	200 mg/day for 3 days	96%—1 week post-Rx[88,89,90]
Fluconazole	150 mg, single dose	75%[91] to 92%[92]—1 and 6 weeks
		75%—4 months post-Rx
Ketoconazole	400 mg/day for 5 days	83%—1 and 6 weeks[92]

Patient preference. Half the patients prefer oral medication; only 5% prefer intravaginal therapy, and the others have no clear preference. Before treating vaginal candidiasis, the physician should ask the patient about her preference.

Partner treatment. Vaginal candidiasis is usually not a sexually transmitted disease and routine treatment of male partners is not necessary. One study showed that treatment of male partners with a brief course of ketoconazole was not of value in reducing the incidence of relapse in women with recurrent vaginal candidiasis.[98] Partner treatment is indicated for men with balanoposthitis or for chronic recurrent cases.

Side effects. Side effects of treatment for vaginal candidiasis are rare.

Pregnancy. Oral therapy should not be given to pregnant patients or to patients who are not using reliable contraceptive measures. Topical therapy during pregnancy may require longer therapy (6 to 14 days). Women who use no reliable contraception should use oral treatment only during the first 10 days of the menstrual cycle.

Candida strains can be cultured from the vagina in 10% to 20% of pregnant women. The incidence of vaginal candidiasis in pregnancy is twice as high as in the nonpregnant state. The incidence is higher late in pregnancy. In 80% to 90% of the cases, candidiasis is caused by *C. albicans*. Treatment of vaginal candidiasis in pregnancy is indicated not only to make the woman symptom-free, but also to protect the fetus from a life-threatening *Candida* sepsis. Itraconazole cannot be used for oral treatment of vaginal candidiasis in pregnant women because of possible teratogenic effects.

Treating resistant cases. Some women have repeated or ongoing infection even after several courses of intravaginal antiyeast therapy. The pathogenesis is poorly understood and the majority of patients have no recognizable predisposing factors. Elimination of risk factors is sometimes helpful. Recontamination from the rectal area may be the cause. The yeast in the GI tract can be reduced in number by giving one or two tablets of nystatin (Mycostatin 500,000 U oral tablet) three times a day for 2 weeks. Intravaginal antiyeast creams or tablets are used simultaneously. *Lactobacillus* preparations (Lactinex tablets or granules or Bacid capsules) given during and after the treatment period may help to restore the normal flora. Other predisposing factors for recurrence should be ruled out. Oral contraceptives may have to be discontinued. Some patients claim a yeast-free diet is helpful.

Long-term maintenance therapy schedules are listed in Table 13-4.

Resistant organisms. Vaginal candidiasis due to *C. glabrata* may not respond to any of the azole drugs. Vaginal nystatin or local application of 1% gentian violet may eradicate this species. Recurrent infections after treatment may be with more common *Candida* species.[100]

TABLE 13-4 Long-term Suppression for Multiple Recurrences of *Candida* Vaginitis		
Medication	**Treatment schedule**	**Percentage Cured**
Itraconazole	200 mg a month on days 5 and 6 of menstrual cycle for 6 months[93]	65%
	200 mg daily for 5 days, then 200 mg twice weekly for 6 months[94]	33% recurred during suppressive therapy; 48% recurred within 6 months after completion of therapy
	400 mg at the beginning of each menstrual period	
Clotrimazole	500 mg topically once a month postmenstrual	30%[95] to 70%[96] during suppressive therapy; 85% recurred
	200 mg ovules for 5 days, then 200 mg twice weekly for 6 months	0% recurred during suppressive therapy; 64% recurred within 6 months after completion of therapy[94]
Ketoconazole	400 mg qd for 2 weeks, then 100 mg qd for 6 months[99]	4.8% recurred during treatment; 48% recurred at end of 12 months of follow-up

Oral candidiasis

C. albicans may be transmitted to the infant's oral cavity during passage through the birth canal. It is part of the normal mouth flora in many adults.

Infants. Oral candidiasis in children is called *thrush*. Healthy, newborn infants, especially if premature, are susceptible. In older infants, thrush usually occurs in the presence of predisposing factors such as antibiotic treatment or debilitation. In the healthy newborn, thrush is a self-limited infection, but it should be treated to avoid interference with feeding. The infection appears as a white, creamy exudate or white, flaky, adherent plaques. The underlying mucosa is red and sore. The mother should be examined for vaginal candidiasis.

Adults. In the adult, oral candidiasis occurs for several reasons; clinically, it is found in a variety of acute and chronic forms. Extensive oral infection may occur in diabetics, patients with depressed cell-mediated immunity, the elderly, and patients with cancer, especially leukemia. Prolonged corticosteroid, immunosuppressive or broad-spectrum antibiotic therapy, and inhalant steroids may also cause infection. Oral candidiasis in high-risk patients may be the initial manifestation of the acquired immunodeficiency syndrome.[101]

The acute process in adults is similar to the infection in infants. The tongue is almost always involved (Figure 13-43). Infection may spread into the trachea or esophagus and cause very painful erosions, appearing as dysphagia, or it may spread onto the skin at the angles of the mouth (perlèche). A specimen may be taken by gently scraping with a tongue blade. Pseudohyphae are easily demonstrated. In other cases, the oral cavity may be red, swollen, and sore, with little or no exudate (Figure 13-44). In this instance, pseudohyphae are often difficult to find and treatment may have to be started without laboratory verification.

Chronic infection appears as localized, firmly adherent plaques with an irregular, velvety surface on the buccal mucosa. They may occur from the mechanical trauma of cheek biting, poor hygiene of dental prostheses, pipe smoking, or irritation from dentures. A biopsy is indicated to rule out leukoplakia and lichen planus if organisms cannot be demonstrated.

Localized erythema and erosions with minimal white exudate may be caused by candidal infection beneath dentures and is commonly called "denture sore mouth." The border is usually sharply defined. Hyperplasia with thickening of the mucosa occurs if the process is long lasting. The gums and hard palate are most frequently involved. Organisms may be difficult to find.

Treatment

Nystatin (Mycostatin) oral suspension. For infants, the dosage is 2 ml of nystatin (Mycostatin) oral suspension four times a day, 1 ml in each side of the mouth. For adults, the dosage is 4 to 6 ml, with one half of the dose in each side of the mouth retained as long as possible before swallowing. Treatment is continued for 48 hours after symptoms have disappeared; a 10-day course is typical. The oral suspension is useful for infants, but less effective for adults, probably because the liquid may not come in contact with the entire surface of the oral cavity. The medication is very expensive.

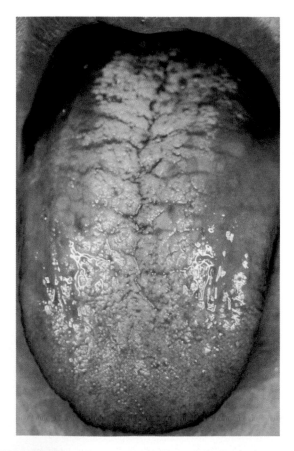

Figure 13-43
Oral candidiasis. A chronic infection with white debris covering the surface of the tongue.

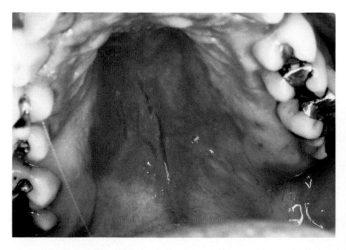

Figure 13-44
Oral candidiasis. The hard palate is red and swollen.

Clotrimazole (Mycelex) troche. Children and adults are effectively treated by slowly dissolving a clotrimazole (Mycelex) troche in the mouth 5 times a day for 14 days.

Gentian violet. Gentian violet, a purple solution, (available from Purepac as a 1% or 2% aqueous solution in a 1-oz bottle) is used to paint the oral cavity of infants or adults twice a day. The medicine lasts longer than nystatin when applied directly to the affected areas, and it is probably more effective than nystatin. Unfortunately, it spreads easily to clothing and produces stains. Irritation may occur if gentian violet is swallowed, therefore the 1% solution should be used in children.

Ketoconazole (Nizoral). Ketoconazole (Nizoral 200 mg oral tablet) given once a day may be the drug of choice in resistant cases of oral thrush. In a large study in which over half the patients had concomitant neoplastic disease, 94% of patients were clinically healed or had only mild residual lesions in a median time of 2 weeks.[102]

Candida balanitis

The uncircumcised penis provides the warm, moist environment ideally suited for yeast infection, but the circumcised male is also at risk. *Candida* balanitis sometimes occurs after intercourse with an infected female. Tender, pinpoint, red papules and pustules appear on the glans and shaft of the penis. The pustules rupture quickly under the foreskin and may not be noticed (Figure 13-45). Typically, 1- to 2-mm, white, doughnut-shaped, possibly confluent rings are seen after the pustules break. In some cases pustules never evolve, and the multiple red papules may be transient, resolving without treatment. White exudate similar to that seen in *Candida* vaginal infections may be present (Figure 13-46). The infection may occur and persist without sexual exposure.

Treatment. The eruption responds quickly with twice-a-day application for 10 days of miconazole, clotrimazole, or several of the other medications listed in the Formulary. Relief is almost immediate, but treatment should be continued for 10 days. Preparations containing topical steroids give temporary relief by suppressing inflammation, but the eruption rebounds and worsens, sometimes even before the cortisone cream is discontinued.

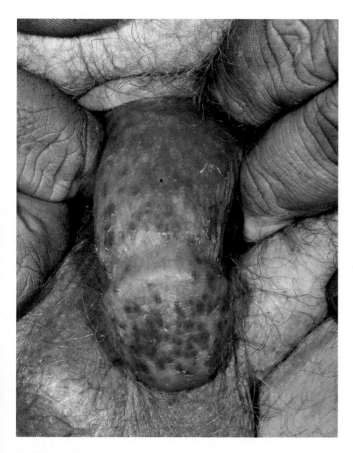

Figure 13-45
Candida balanitis. Multiple red, round erosions are present on the glans and shaft of the penis. There is a white exudate.

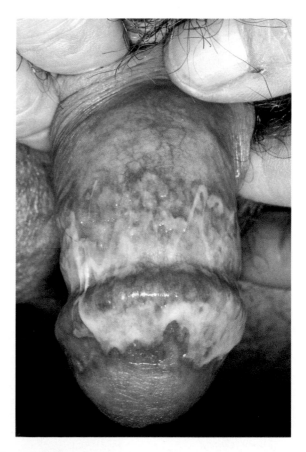

Figure 13-46
Candida balanitis. The moist space between the skin surfaces of the uncircumcised penis is an ideal environment for *Candida* infection. This thick white exudate is typical of a severe acute infection.

CANDIDIASIS OF LARGE SKIN FOLDS

Candidiasis of large skin folds (*Candida* intertrigo) occurs under pendulous breasts, between overhanging abdominal folds, in the groin and rectal area, and in the axillae. Skin folds (intertriginous areas where skin touches skin) contain heat and moisture, providing the environment suited for yeast infection. Hot, humid weather; tight or abrasive underclothing; poor hygiene; and inflammatory diseases occurring in the skin folds, such as psoriasis, make a yeast infection more likely.

There are two presentations. In the first type, pustules form but become macerated under apposing skin surfaces and develop into red papules with a fringe of moist scale at the border. Intact pustules may be found outside the apposing skin surfaces (Figure 13-47). The second type consists of a red, moist, glistening plaque that extends to or just beyond the limits of the apposing skin folds (Figure 13-48). The advancing border is long, sharply defined, and has an ocean wave–shaped fringe of macerated scale (Figure 13-49). The characteristic pustule of candidiasis is not observed in intertriginous areas because it is macerated away as soon as it forms. Pinpoint pustules do appear outside the advancing border and are an important diagnostic feature when present (Figure 13-50). There is a tendency for painful fissuring in the skin creases.

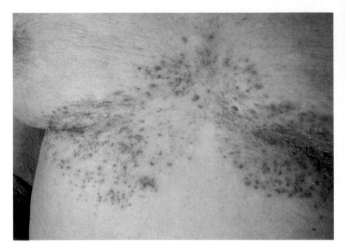

Figure 13-47
Candidiasis under the breast. There are several moist, red papules with a fringe of white scale.

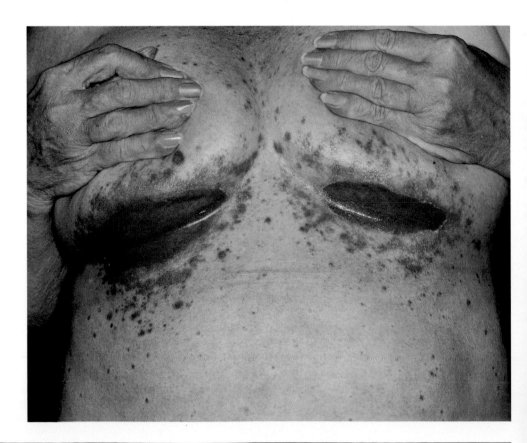

Figure 13-48
Candida intertrigo. An acute infection. The fringe of scale is present on the opposing borders. There are numerous satellite pustules beyond the intertriginous area.

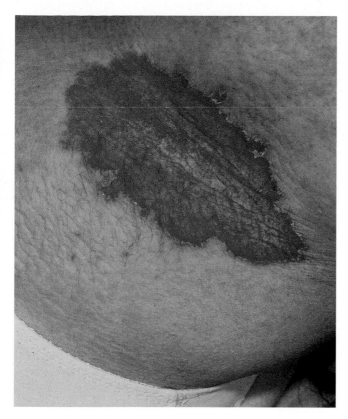

Treatment. Eradication of the yeast infection must be accompanied by maintained dryness of the area. A cool, wet Burow's compress is applied for 20 to 30 minutes several times each day to promote dryness. Antifungal cream is applied in a thin layer twice a day until the rash clears. Some of these medicines are also available in lotion form, but the liquid base may cause stinging when applied to intertriginous areas. Miconazole nitrate (Monistat-Derm lotion) is the least irritating. Application of compresses should be continued until the skin remains dry. Heat from a gooseneck lamp held several inches away from the involved site is sometimes useful to enhance drying. An absorbent powder, not necessarily medicated, such as Z-Sorb, may be applied after the inflammation is gone. The powder absorbs a small amount of moisture and acts as a dry lubricant, allowing skin surfaces to slide freely, thus preventing moisture accumulation in a potentially stagnant area.

Figure 13-49
Candidiasis of the axillae. A prominent fringe of scale is present at the border.

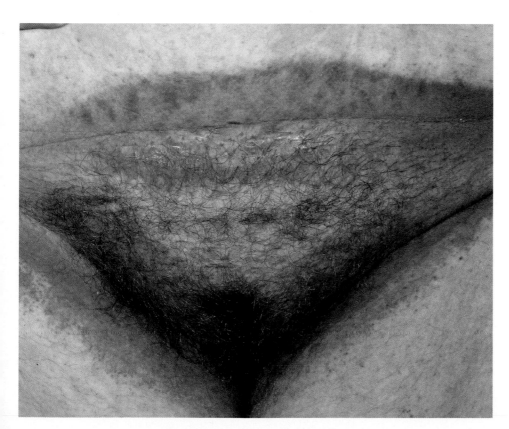

Figure 13-50
Candida intertrigo. The overhanging abdominal fold and groin area are infected in this obese patient.

Diaper candidiasis

An artificial intertriginous area is created under a wet diaper, predisposing the area to a yeast infection with the characteristic red base and satellite pustules as described above (Figure 13-51). Diaper dermatitis is often treated with steroid combination creams that contain antibiotics. Although these creams may contain the antiyeast agent, clotrimazole, its concentration may not be sufficient to control the yeast infection. The cortisone component may alter the clinical presentation and prolong the disease. A nodular, granulomatous form of candidiasis in the diaper area, appearing as dull, red, irregularly shaped nodules, sometimes on a red base, has been described and may represent an unusual reaction to *Candida* organisms or to a *Candida* organism infection modified by

steroids (Figure 13-52). Although dermatophyte infections are unusual in the diaper area, they do occur.[103] Every effort should be made to identify the organism and treat the infection appropriately.

Treatment. Dryness should be maintained by changing the diaper frequently or leaving it off for short periods. Antifungal creams should be applied twice a day until the eruption is clear, in approximately 10 days. Some erythema from irritation may be present after 10 days; this can be treated by alternately applying 1% hydrocortisone cream followed in a few hours by creams active against yeasts (see the Formulary). Apply each agent twice a day. Baby powders may help prevent recurrence by absorbing moisture.

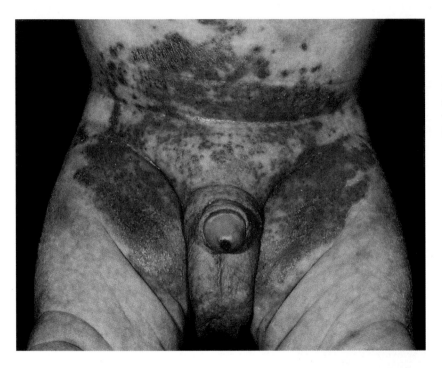

Figure 13-51
Diaper candidiasis, an advanced case. The skin folds are deeply erythematous. The urethral meatus is infected and numerous satellite pustules are on the lower abdominal area.

Figure 13-52
Nodular candidiasis of the diaper area. Red nodules are present on a red base and beyond the diffusely inflamed area. The patient had been treated with a cream containing corticosteroids and antifungal agents.

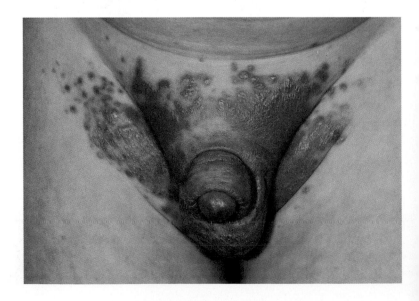

CANDIDIASIS OF SMALL SKIN FOLDS
Finger and toe webs

Web spaces are like small intertriginous areas. Cooks, bartenders, dishwashers, dentists, and others who work in a moist environment are at risk. White, tender, macerated skin erodes, revealing a pink, moist base (Figures 13-53 and 13-54). Candidiasis of the toe webs occurs most commonly in the narrow interspace between the fourth and fifth toes, where it may coexist with dermatophytes and gram-negative bacteria. Clinically and in potassium hydroxide preparations, infection by *Candida* and dermatophytes may appear to be identical. Macerated, white scale becomes thick and adherent. Diffuse candidiasis of the webs and feet is unusual. Both areas are treated with any of the antifungal creams or lotions listed in the Formulary (see p. 839). Strands of lamb's wool (Dr. Scholl's Lamb's Wool) can be placed between the toe webs to separate and promote dryness.

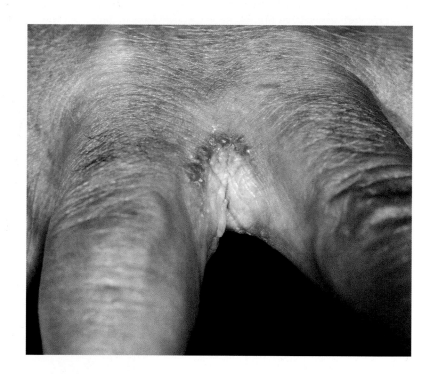

Figure 13-53
Candidiasis of the finger web. The acute phase with maceration of the web. Pustules are present at the border.

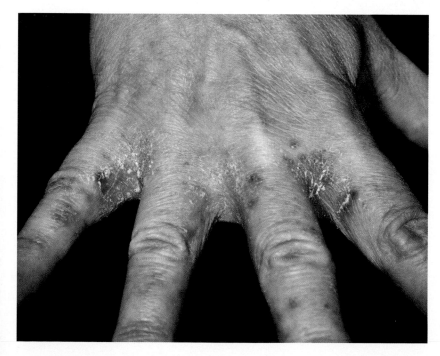

Figure 13-54
Candidiasis of the finger webs. All webs are infected except the wide space between the thumb and index finger.

Angles of the mouth

Angular cheilitis or perlèche, an inflammation at the angles of the mouth, can occur at any age. Patients may have the misconception that they have a vitamin B deficiency. Yeast and bacteria may be involved in the process. Lip licking, biting the corners of the mouth, or thumb sucking causes perlèche in the young. Continued irritation may lead to eczematous inflammation. The presence of saliva at the angles of the mouth is the most important factor. Excess saliva occurs as a result of mouth breathing secondary to nasal congestion and of malocclusion resulting from poorly fitting dentures and compulsive lip licking. Aggressive use of dental floss may cause mechanical trauma to mouth angles.[104] A moist, intertriginous space forms in skin folds at the angles of the mouth as a result of advancing age, congenital excessive-angle skin folds, sagging that occurs with weight loss, or abnormal vertical shortening of the lower one third of the face from loss of teeth and resultant resorption of the alveolar bone. Capillary action draws fluid from the mouth into the fold, creating maceration, chapping, fissures, erythema, exudation, and secondary infection with *Candida* organisms and/or staphylococci.

The infection starts as a sore fissure in the depth of the skin fold (Figure 13-55). Erythema, scale, and crust form at the sides of the fold. Patients lick and moisten the area in an attempt to prevent further cracking. This attempt at relief only aggravates the problem and may lead to eczematous inflammation, staphylococcal infection, or hypertrophy of the skin fold.

Treatment. Treatment consists of applying antifungal creams (see the Formulary, p. 839), followed in a few hours by a group V steroid cream with a nongreasy base (such as triamcinolone acetonide [Aristocort A] 0.1%) until the area is dry and free of inflammation. As an alternative, Lotrisone may be applied twice a day until symptoms resolve. Patients should discontinue topical steroids when inflammation has resolved. Thereafter, a thick, protective lip balm (e.g., ChapStick) is applied frequently. Zyplast collagen injected at the mouth angles can decrease the depth of the grooves[105] and fill the depression that often occurs below the lateral lower lip, thereby correcting the anatomic defect causing the problem.

Figure 13-55
Angular cheilitis (perlèche). Skin folds at the angles of the mouth are red and eroded.

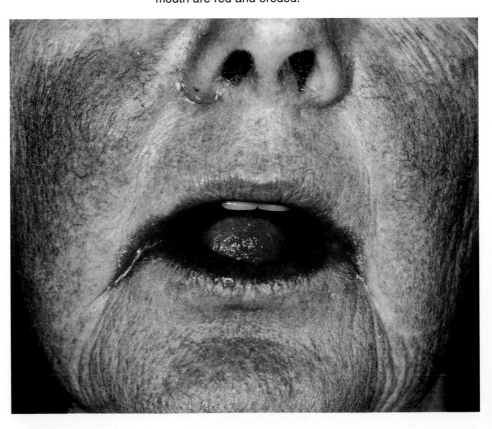

CHRONIC MUCOCUTANEOUS CANDIDIASIS

Chronic mucocutaneous candidiasis (CMC) is a syndrome that is characterized by recurrent and persistent *Candida* infection of the skin, nails, and mucous membranes without disseminated candidiasis. There are three categories based on the age of the patient at onset:[106] (1) The early onset syndromes usually have autosomal dominant CMC or CMC associated with immunodeficiency and endocrinopathy syndromes. The two major groups of endocrine abnormalities are hypoparathyroidism with hypoadrenocorticalism, and hypothyroidism. Autoimmune abnormalities include ovarian failure, pernicious anemia, and vitiligo. These associated abnormalities may not occur until the fifth decade. The term *autoimmune polyglandular syndrome*[107] has been used to describe these patients. There are many subtypes of this syndrome. (2) *Candida* infections that begin around puberty: these patients usually have autosomal recessive CMC, and (3) late-onset disease that develops after the fourth decade of life and is associated with underlying neoplasm (pancreatic islet cell carcinoma, oral carcinoma, lymphoma), and, most commonly, thymoma. CMC may be a minor component of another more severe disease, such as severe combined immunodeficiency or agammaglobulinemia. These severely affected patients have many other infections. The reason for the marked susceptibility to mucocutaneous candidiasis without systemic candidiasis in all of these patients is unknown. The exact immunologic deficiency in these syndromes has not been defined, but most have defects in cell-mediated immunity. These may be limited to antigens of *C. albicans*, but in some patients they are more extensive and involve the T-lymphocyte–mediated responses to all antigens.

The early-onset syndrome usually begins in early childhood with yeast infections of the fingernails, mouth, vagina, and skin. The hypertrophic fingernail infection with dystrophic changes and chronic swelling of the nailfolds is characteristic and is rarely seen as an isolated phenomenon without the other stigmata of this syndrome (see Chapter Twenty-five). Thick, yeast-infected, crusted masses (*Candida* granulomas) occur on the scalp and sometimes on the skin. Brown-red, asymptomatic, slowly expanding plaques with a sharp margin and soft scale occur on the back of the hands, feet, intertriginous skin, trunk, and around the mouth. The entire oral cavity is lined with white, adherent debris. Systemic candidiasis is rare. Recurrent or severe infections with organisms other than *Candida* were seen in 80% of the patients.[108] These may result in serious morbidity or death.

The late-onset syndromes are also associated with infection of the skin, nails, and oral mucosa, but involvement is not as extensive. Itraconazole,[109] fluconazole,[110] and ketoconazole are effective. Mucosal lesions heal within days, skin lesions within weeks to a few months, and nail lesions after a variable period of up to several months. Relapse is common once therapy is stopped.

SYSTEMIC CANDIDIASIS IN HEROIN ADDICTS

Oculocutaneous candidiasis. Systemic candidiasis in heroin addicts is a new syndrome characterized by skin (96.6%), eye (57.6%), and bone (27.1%) lesions.[111] A sudden occurrence of elevated temperature, reaching 39° to 40° C with chills; severe, diffuse headache; myalgia; and profuse sweating occurs 2 to 8 hours after intravenous injection of brown heroin. This initial, febrile, septicemic syndrome lasts between 1 and 3 days and is followed by the appearance of painful papules, nodules, and pustules in the beard and hair-bearing areas of the scalp. Nodules are the most common characteristic and are pathognomonic of the disease; 10 to 100 painful, deep-seated nodules appear suddenly and may be so numerous that they feel like a sack of marbles. Nodules may open and drain pus. Painful follicular and nonfollicular pustules on an inflamed base occur on the scalp,[112] face, and hairy zones of the chest, axillae, pubic region, and thighs.

Untreated cases resolve in 2 to 4 weeks, leaving areas of alopecia.[113] Eye and bone lesions occur concomitantly or after the skin lesions are cured. Chorioretinitis, anterior uveitis, and hyalitis are the most common eye characteristics and occur 3 to 20 days after the septic syndrome. Eye disease is most often unilateral. Firm costochondral tumors of varying size appear between 15 days and 5 months after the cutaneous signs. The vertebrae, knee, sacroiliac joint, costal cartilage, and other sites are sometimes infected. The diagnosis is established by finding *C. albicans* in the blood, skin, eye, or costochondral lesions. Culture of biopsy specimens has been more accurate than isolation from pus smears or histologic studies for organism identification.[111] Blood cultures are negative in most cases. The source of infection has never been discovered. It was postulated that *C. albicans*–contaminated lemon juice[114] used to dissolve the brown heroin is the source of the infection. Others have found patients who were unusually colonized by *C. albicans* on their skin (particularly on hairy zones). They hypothesize that the skin may constitute the reservoir for *C. albicans* in oculocutaneous candidiasis.[115] Cutaneous disease is treated with ketoconazole 400 mg/day for 15 to 30 days. Surgery or administration of amphotericin B or flucytosine may be required to effectively manage eye and bone disease.

Tinea Versicolor

Tinea versicolor is a common fungal infection of the skin caused by the lipophilic yeast *P. orbiculare* (round form) and *P. ovale* (oval form). Some authors believe these are different forms of the same organism. (Both were previously called *Malassezia furfur*.) The organism is part of the normal skin flora and appears in highest numbers in areas with increased sebaceous activity. Excess heat and humidity, adrenalectomy, Cushing's disease, pregnancy, malnutrition, burns, corticosteroid therapy, immunosuppression, and oral contraceptives may lower the patient's resistance, allowing this normally nonpathogenic resident to proliferate in the upper layers of the stratum corneum. Whether the disease is contagious or not is unknown. The disease may occur at any age, but it is much more common during the years of higher sebaceous activity (i.e., adolescence and young adulthood). Some individuals, especially those with oily skin, may be more susceptible.

Clinical presentation. The individual lesions and their distribution are highly characteristic. Lesions begin as multiple small, circular macules of various colors (white, pink, or brown) that enlarge radially (Figures 13-56 to 13-58). Tinea versicolor infections produce a spectrum of clinical presentations and colors that include (1) red to fawn-colored macules, patches, or follicular papules that are predominantly caused by a hyperemic inflammatory response; (2) hypopigmented lesions that are caused by alterations in melanosome formation and transfer to keratinocytes; and (3) tan to dark brown macules and patches that are caused by alterations in melanosome formation and distribution.[116] The lesions may be hyperpigmented in blacks. The color is uniform in each individual. The lesions may be inconspicuous in fair-complected individuals during the winter. White hypopigmentation becomes more obvious as unaffected skin tans. The upper trunk is most commonly affected, but it is not unusual for lesions to spread to the upper arms, neck, and abdomen. Involvement of the face, back of the hands, and legs can occur. Facial lesions are more common in children; the forehead is the site of facial involvement usually affected. The eruption may itch if it is inflammatory, but it is usually asymptomatic. The disease may vary in activity for years, but it diminishes or disappears with advancing age. The differential diagnosis includes vitiligo, pityriasis alba, seborrheic dermatitis, secondary syphilis, and pityriasis rosea.

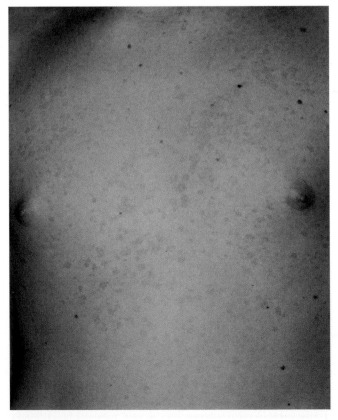

Figure 13-56
Tinea versicolor. Numerous circular, scaly lesions. The eruption is light brown or fawn colored in fair-complected, untanned skin.

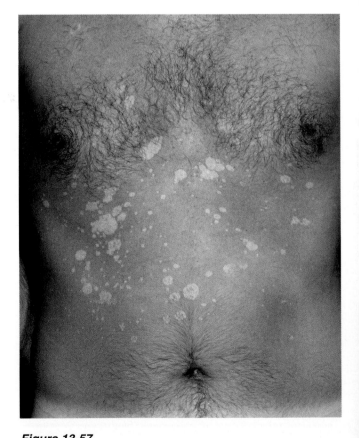

Figure 13-57
The classic presentation of tinea versicolor with white, oval or circular patches on tan skin.

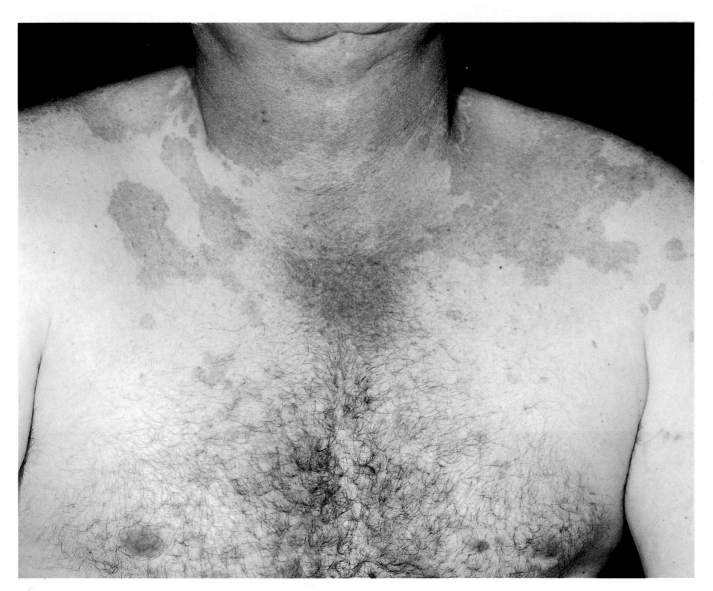

Figure 13-58
Tinea versicolor. Broad confluent scaly patches in a
fair-skinned individual.

Diagnosis. A powdery scale that may not be obvious on inspection can easily be demonstrated by scraping lightly with a #15 surgical blade (Figure 13-59). Potassium hydroxide examination of the scale shows numerous hyphae that tend to break into short, rod-shaped fragments intermixed with round spores in grapelike clusters, giving the so-called spaghetti-and-meatballs pattern (Figure 13-60). Wood's light examination shows irregular, pale, yellow-to-white fluorescence that fades with improvement. Some lesions do not fluoresce. Culture is possible but rarely necessary.

Treatment. Griseofulvin is not active against tinea versicolor. A variety of medicines eliminates the fungus, but relief is usually temporary and recurrences are common (40% to 60%). Patients must understand that the hypopigmented areas will not disappear immediately after treatment. Sunlight accelerates repigmentation. The inability to produce powdery scale by scraping with a #15 surgical blade indicates the fungus has been eradicated. Fungal elements may be retained in frequently worn garments that are in contact with the skin; discarding or boiling such clothing might decrease the chance of recurrence. Patients without obvious involvement who have a history of multiple recurrences might consider repeating a treatment program just before the summer months to avoid uneven tanning.

Topical treatment. Topical treatment is indicated for limited disease. Recurrence rates are high.

Medication (see the Formulary, p. 840)

Selenium sulfide suspension 2.5%. When applied for 10 minutes every day for 7 consecutive days, the suspension (available as Selsun or Exsel) resulted in an 87% cure rate at a 2-week follow-up evaluation.[117] Blood and urine levels done during this study showed that no significant absorption of selenium took place.[118] The suspension is applied to the entire skin surface from the lower posterior scalp area down to the thighs. Another commonly recommended schedule is to apply the lotion and wash it off in 24 hours. This is repeated once each week for a total of 4 weeks. There are many suggested variations of this treatment schedule.

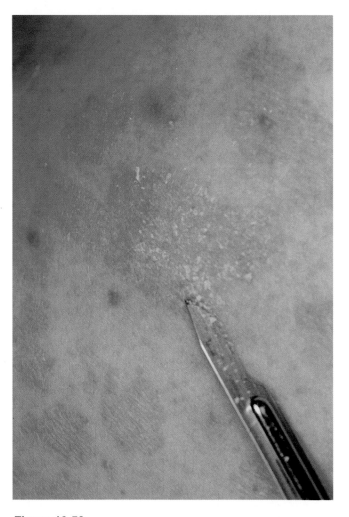

Figure 13-59
Tinea versicolor. The central area was scraped with a #15 surgical blade to demonstrate white, powdery scale.

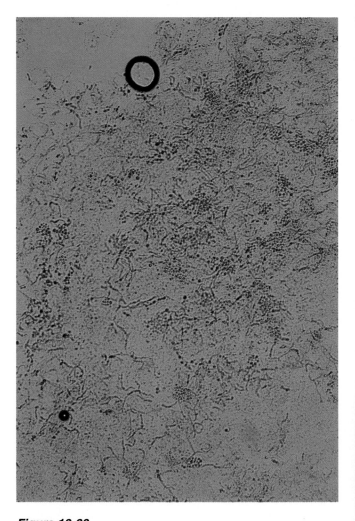

Figure 13-60
Tinea versicolor. A potassium hydroxide wet mount. A low power view showing numerous short, broad hyphae and clusters of budding cells, which have been described as having the appearance of "spaghetti and meatballs."

Sodium thiosulfate 25%. Sodium thiosulfate (Tinver lotion, 5 oz bottle) is applied twice a day to the entire involved area for 2 to 4 weeks. This preparation is effective and inexpensive, but most patients object to the odor.

Antifungal antibiotics. Miconazole, clotrimazole, econazole, or ciclopirox olamine is applied to the entire affected area one to two times a day for 2 to 4 weeks. The creams are odorless and nongreasy but expensive.

Ketoconazole. Ketoconazole cream is applied once daily for 2 weeks.

Sulfur-salicylic shampoo. Sulfur-salicylic shampoo (Sebulex shampoo) is applied as a lotion at bedtime and washed off in the morning for 1 week.[119]

Zinc pyrithione shampoo. Zinc pyrithione shampoo 1% is applied to a wet bathtub brush with a long handle, and the trunk, arms, and thighs are lathered for 5 minutes before showering. This procedure is repeated every day for 2 weeks.[120] There are suggested variations of this treatment.

Keratolytic soaps. Sal acid soap (Stiefel) may be useful to prevent recurrences for patients who can tolerate the drying effect.

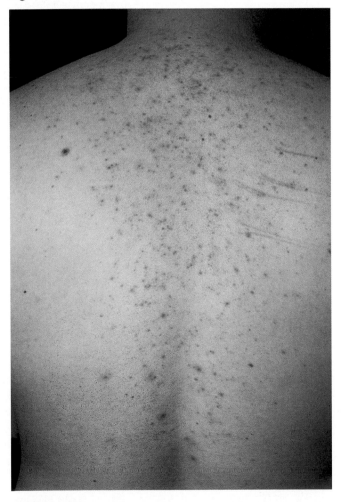

Figure 13-61
Pityrosporum folliculitis. Asymptomatic or slightly itchy follicular papules and pustules located on the upper back. It is frequently diagnosed as acne.

Oral treatment (see Table 13-2)

Ketoconazole. Ketoconazole may be used in patients with extensive disease and those who do not respond to conventional treatment or have frequent recurrences. Once the potential side effects have been explained, one of the following schedules may be tried: 400 mg in a single dose or 200 mg a day for 5 days. The cure rate is greater than 90%.[80] Retreat patients with recurrences. Prophylactic treatment may be considered for immunocompromised patients. Efficacy can be enhanced by refraining from antacids and taking the drug at breakfast with a fruit juice. The patient should not bathe for at least 12 hours after treatment. Refraining from bathing allows the medication to accumulate in the skin.

Itraconazole. A number of studies have shown that itraconazole is effective. The total dose required for effective treatment is 1000 mg, and it has been given as 200 mg for 5 days.[82] The cure rate is greater than 90%.

Fluconazole. Fluconazole 400 mg given as a single dose in one study resulted in a 74% cure rate 3 weeks after treatment.[81]

PITYROSPORUM FOLLICULITIS

Pityrosporum folliculitis is an infection of the hair follicle caused by the yeast *P. orbiculare*, the same organism that causes tinea versicolor. The typical patient is a young woman with asymptomatic or slightly itchy follicular papules and pustules localized to the upper back and chest, upper arms, and neck.[121] Occlusion and greasy skin may be important predisposing factors. It is frequently diagnosed as acne (Figure 13-61). Diabetes mellitus and administration of broad-spectrum antibiotics or corticosteroids are predisposing factors. Follicular occlusion may be a primary event, with yeast overgrowth as a secondary occurrence.[122] Hodgkin's disease may predispose to pityrosporum folliculitis.[123] These patients complain of severe generalized pruritis; the eruption may involve the trunk and extremities.

Pityrosporum is very common in the tropics, where it presents as a polymorphous eruption with the following characteristics.[124] The primary lesion is a keratinous plug that underlies four clinical types of lesion: follicular papules (dome-shaped papules with a central depression), pustules, nodules, and cysts. The lesions evolve from follicular plugs colonized by *Pityrosporum*. The face is often affected—this is the most common site in female patients and the second most common in males. The lesions are localized to the mandible, chin, and sides of the face. This is in contrast to the usually more central facial location of acne vulgaris. Lesions also are found on the nape of the neck, abdomen, buttocks, and thighs. Both young men and young women are equally affected. Their active sebaceous glands presumably provide the lipid-rich environment required by the yeast.

A potassium hydroxide examination reveals abundant round, budding yeast cells and sometimes hyphae. Treatment is the same as for tinea versicolor. Lesions respond rapidly to oral ketoconazole.[124] Salicylic acid wash (Sal Ac) is keratolytic and is effective against yeast.[125]

REFERENCES

1. Sorensen GW, Jones HE: Immediate and delayed hypersensitivity in chronic dermatophytosis, *Arch Dermatol* 112:40-42, 1976.
2. Burke WA, Jones BE: A simple stain for rapid office diagnosis of fungus infection of the skin, *Arch Dermatol* 120:1519-1520, 1984.
3. Brodell RT, Helms SE, et al: Office dermatologic testing: the KOH preparation, *Am Fam Physician* 43:2061-2065, 1991.
4. Head ES, Henry JC, MacDonald EM: The cotton swab technic for the culture of dermatophyte infections: its efficacy and merit, *J Am Acad Dermatol* 11:797-801, 1984.
5. Kearse HJ, Miller OF: Tinea pedis in prepubertal children: does it occur? *J Am Acad Dermatol* 19:619-622, 1988.
6. McBride A, Cohen BA: Tinea pedis in children, *Am J Dis Child* 146:844-847, 1992.
7. Svejgaard E, Christophersen J, Jelsdorf HM: Tinea pedis and erythrasma in Danish recruits: clinical signs, prevalence, incidence, and correlation to atopy, *J Am Acad Dermatol* 14:993-999, 1986.
8. Kates SG, Nordstrom KM, et al: Microbial ecology of interdigital infections of toe web spaces, *J Am Acad Dermatol* 22:578-582, 1990.
9. Dahl MV: Suppression of immunity and inflammation by products produced by dermatophytes, *J Am Acad Dermatol* 28:S19-S23, 1993.
10. Smith EB et al: Double-blind comparison of naftifine cream and clotrimazole/betamethasone dipropionate cream in the treatment of tinea pedis, *J Am Acad Dermatol* 26:125-127, 1992.
11. Del Aguila R, Gei FM, et al: Once-weekly oral doses of fluconazole 150 mg in the treatment of tinea pedis, *Clin Exp Dermatol* 17:402-406, 1992.
12. Berman B, Ellis C, et al: Efficacy of a 1-week, twice-daily regimen of terbinafine 1% cream in the treatment of interdigital tinea pedis. Results of placebo-controlled, double-blind, multicenter trials, *J Am Acad Dermatol* 26:956-960, 1992.
13. Smith EB: Topical antifungal drugs in the treatment of tinea pedis, tinea cruris, and tinea corporis, *J Am Acad Dermatol* 28:S24-S28, 1993.
14. Bergstresser PR, Elewski B, et al: Topical terbinafine and clotrimazole in interdigital tinea pedis: a multicenter comparison of cure and relapse rates with 1- and 4-week treatment regimens, *J Am Acad Dermatol* 28:648-651, 1993.
15. Kates SG et al: The antibacterial efficacy of econazole nitrate in interdigital toe web infections, *J Am Acad Dermatol* 22:583-586, 1990.
16. Hay RJ et al: A comparative study of terbinafine versus griseofulvin in "dry-type" dermatophyte infections, *J Am Acad Dermatol* 24:243-246, 1991.
17. White JE, Perkins PJ, et al: Successful 2-week treatment with terbinafine (Lamisil) for moccasin tinea pedis and tinea manuum, *Br J Dermatol* 125:260-262, 1991.
18. Savin RC: Oral terbinafine versus griseofulvin in the treatment of moccasin-type tinea pedis, *J Am Acad Dermatol* 23:807-809, 1990.
19. Shah AS, Kamino H, et al: Painful, plaque-like, pitted keratolysis occurring in childhood, *Pediatr Dermatol* 9:251-254, 1992.
20. Hanel H, Kalisch J, et al: Quantification of keratinolytic activity from *Dermatophilus congolensis*, *Med Microbiol Immunol* 180:45-51, 1991.
21. Mattox TF, Rutgers J, et al: Nonfluorescent erythrasma of the vulva, *Obstet Gynecol* 81:862-864, 1993.
22. Hamann K, Thorn P: Systemic or local treatment of erythrasma? A comparison between erythromycin tablets and Fucidin cream in general practice, *Scand J Prim Health Care* 9:35-39, 1991.
23. Barone JA, Koh JG, et al: Food interaction and steady-state pharmacokinetics of itraconazole capsules in healthy male volunteers, *Antimicrob Agents Chemother* 37:778-784, 1993.
24. Sherertz EF: Are laboratory studies necessary for griseofulvin therapy? *J Am Acad Dermatol* 22:1103, 1990.
25. Stiller MJ, Klein WP, et al: Tinea corporis gladiatorum: an epidemic of *Trichophyton tonsurans* in student wrestlers, *J Am Acad Dermatol* 27:632-633, 1992.
26. Powell FC, Muller SA: Kerion of the glabrous skin, *J Am Acad Dermatol* 7:490-494, 1982.
27. Janniger CK: Majocchi's granuloma, *Cutis* 50:267-268, 1992.
28. Smith KJ, Neafie RC, et al: Majocchi's granuloma, *J Cutan Pathol* 18:28-35, 1991.
29. Weksberg F, Fisher BF: Unusual tinea corporis caused by *Trichophyton verrucosum*, *Int J Dermatol* 25:653-655, 1986.
30. Barson WJ: Granuloma and pseudogranuloma of the skin due to microsporum canis, *Arch Dermatol* 121:895-897, 1985.
31. Hironaga M, Okazaki N, Saito K, et al: *Trichophyton mentagrophytes* granulomas: unique systemic dissemination to lymph nodes, testes, vertebrae, and brain, *Arch Dermatol* 119:482-490, 1983.
32. Albert AA: Tinea capitis, *Arch Dermatol* 124:1554-1557, 1988.
33. Venugopal PV, Venugopal TV: Tinea capitis in Saudi Arabia, *Int J Dermatol* 32:39-40, 1993.
34. Jacobs PH: Dermatophytes that infect animals and humans, *Cutis* 42:330-331, 1988.
35. Shelley WB, Shelley ED, Burneister V: The infected hairs of tinea capitis due to *Microsporum canis*: demonstration of uniqueness of the hair cuticle by scanning electron microscopy, *J Am Acad Dermatol* 16:354-361, 1987.
36. Lee JY, Hsu ML: Pathogenesis of hair infection and black dots in tinea capitis caused by *Trichophyton violaceum*: a histopathological study, *J Cutan Pathol* 19:54-58, 1992.
37. Okuda C, Ito M, et al: Fungus invasion of human hair tissue in tinea capitis caused by *Microsporum canis*: light and electron microscopic study, *Arch Dermatol Res* 281:238-246, 1989.
38. Bronson DM, Desai DR, Barsky S, et al: An epidemic of infection with *Trichophyton tonsurans* revealed in a 20-year survey of fungal infections in Chicago, *J Am Acad Dermatol* 8:322-330, 1983.
39. Hebert AA, Head ES, MacDonald EM: Tinea capitis caused by *Trichophyton tonsurans*, *Pediatr Dermatol* 2:219-223, 1985.
40. Babel DE, Baughman SA: Evaluation of the adult carrier state in juvenile tinea capitis caused by *Trichophyton tonsurans*, *J Am Acad Dermatol* 21:1209-1212, 1989.
41. Babel DE, Rogers AL, et al: Dermatophytosis of the scalp: incidence, immune response, and epidemiology, *Mycopathologia* 109:69-73, 1990.
42. Borchers SW: Moistened gauze technic to aid in diagnosis of tinea capitis, *J Am Acad Dermatol* 13:672-673, 1985.
43. Hubbard TW, de Triquet JM: Brush-culture method for diagnosing tinea capitis, *Pediatrics* 90:416-418, 1992.
44. Frieden IL: Diagnosis and management of tinea capitis, *Pediatr Ann* 16:39-48, 1987.
45. Rippon JW: Tinea capitis: current concepts. Special symposia. Identification of dermatophytes in the clinical office, *Pediatr Dermatol* 2:224-237, 1985.
46. Gan VN, Petruska M, Ginsburg CM: Epidemiology and treatment of tinea capitis: ketoconazole vs. griseofulvin, *Pediatr Infect Dis* J 6:46-49, 1987.
47. Tanz RR, Hebert AA, Esterly NB: Treating tinea capitis: should ketoconazole replace griseofulvin? *J Pediatr* 112:987-991, 1988.
48. Stritzler C et al: Tinea capitis treated with griseofulvin, *Arch Dermatol* 85:99, 1962.
49. Stephens CJ, Hay RJ, et al: Fungal kerion—total scalp involvement due to *Microsporum canis* infection, *Clin Exp Dermatol* 14:442-444, 1989.
50. Haroon TS, Hussain I, et al: An open clinical pilot study of the efficacy and safety of oral terbinafine in dry non-inflammatory tinea capitis, *Br J Dermatol* 126:47-50, 1992.
51. Legendre R, Esola-Macre J: Itraconazole in the treatment of tinea capitis, *J Am Acad Dermatol* 23:559-560, 1990.
52. Landau JW: Commentary: undecylenic acid and fungus infections, *Arch Dermatol* 119:351-353, 1983.
53. Blank H: Commentary: treatment of dermatomycoses with griseofulvin, *Arch Dermatol* 118:835-836, 1982.
54. Catalano PM, Blank H: Griseofulvin-oral contraceptive interaction, *Arch Dermatol* 121:1381, 1985.

55. Knight TE, Shikuma CY, Knight J: Ketoconazole-induced fulminant hepatitis necessitating liver transplantation, *J Am Acad Dermatol* 25:398-400, 1991.

56. Stricker BH, Block APR, et al. Ketoconazole-associated hepatic injury, *J Hepatol* 3:399-406, 1986.

57. Lewis JH, Zimmerman HJ, Benson GD, et al: Hepatic injury associated with ketoconazole therapy: analysis of 33 cases, *Gastroenterology* 86:503-513, 1984.

58. Rollman O, Loof L: Hepatic toxicity of ketoconazole (letter). *Br J Dermatol* 108:376-378, 1983.

59. Duarte PA, Chow CC, et al: Fatal hepatitis associated with ketoconazole therapy, *Arch Intern Med* 144:1069-1070, 1984.

60. Svedhem A: Toxic hepatitis following ketoconazole treatment, *Scand J Infect Dis* 16:123-125, 1984.

61. Engelhard D, Statman HR, Marks MI: Interaction of ketoconazole with rifampin and isoniazid, *N Engl J Med* 311:1681-1683, 1986.

62. Lesher JL, Smith JG Jr: Antifungal agents in dermatology, *J Am Acad Dermatol* 17:383-394, 1987.

63. Robertson MH et al: Ketoconazole in griseofulvin-resistant dermatophytosis, *J Am Acad Dermatol* 6:224-229, 1982.

64. Panagiotidou D, Kousidou T, et al: A comparison of itraconazole and griseofulvin in the treatment of tinea corporis and tinea cruris: a double-blind study, *J Int Med Res* 20:392-400, 1992.

65. del Palacio Hernandez A, Lopez Gomez S, et al: A comparative double-blind study of terbinafine (Lamisil) and griseofulvin in tinea corporis and tinea cruris, *Clin Exp Dermatol* 15:210-216, 1990.

66. Suchil P, Gei FM, et al: Once-weekly oral doses of fluconazole 150 mg in the treatment of tinea corporis/cruris and cutaneous candidiasis, *Clin Exp Dermatol* 17:397-401, 1992.

67. Montero-Gei F, Perera A: Therapy with fluconazole for tinea corporis, tinea cruris, and tinea pedis, *Clin Infect Dis* 14:S77-S81, 1992.

68. Gatti S et al: Treatment of kerion with fluconazole, *Lancet* 338:157, 1991.

69. Piepponen T, Blomqvist K, et al: Efficacy and safety of itraconazole in the long-term treatment of onychomycosis, *J Antimicrob Chemother* 29:195-205, 1992.

70. Willemsen M, De Doncker P, et al: Posttreatment itraconazole levels in the nail. New implications for treatment in onychomycosis, *J Am Acad Dermatol* 26:731-735, 1992.

71. Goodfield MJ, Andrew L, et al: Short-term treatment of dermatophyte onychomycosis with terbinafine, *Br Med J* 304:1151-1154, 1992.

72. van der Schroeff JG, Cirkel PK, et al: A randomized treatment duration finding study of terbinafine in onychomycosis, *Br J Dermatol* 126:36-39, 1992.

73. Goodfield MJ: Short-duration therapy with terbinafine for dermatophyte onychomycosis: a multicentre trial, *Br J Dermatol* 126:33-35, 1992.

74. Zaias N: Management of onychomycosis with oral terbinafine, *J Am Acad Dermatol* 23:829-832, 1990.

75. Lachapelle JM, De Doncker P, et al: Itraconazole compared with griseofulvin in the treatment of tinea corporis/cruris and tinea pedis/manus: an interpretation of the clinical results of all completed double-blind studies with respect to the pharmacokinetic profile, *Dermatology* 184:45-50, 1992.

76. Saul A, Bonifaz A: Itraconazole in common dermatophyte infections of the skin: fixed treatment schedules, *J Am Acad Dermatol* 23:559-560, 1990.

77. Goodless DR, Ramos-Caro FA, et al: Ketoconazole in the treatment of pityriasis versicolor: international review of clinical trials, *Drug Intell Clin Pharm* 25:395-398, 1991.

78. Faergemann: Treatment of pityriasis versicolor with a single dose of fluconazole, *Acta Derm Venereol* (Stockh) 72:74-75, 1992.

79. Delescluse J: Itraconazole in tinea versicolor: a review, *J Am Acad Dermatol* 23:551-554, 1990.

80. Horowitz BJ, Giaquinta D, et al: Evolving pathogens in vulvovaginal candidiasis: implications for patient care, *J Clin Pharmacol* 32:248-255, 1992.

81. de Oliveira JM, Cruz AS, et al: Prevalence of *Candida albicans* in vaginal fluid of asymptomatic Portuguese women, *J Reprod Med* 38:41-42, 1993.

82. Bluestein D, Rutledge C, et al: Predicting the occurrence of antibiotic-induced candidal vaginitis (AICV), *Fam Pract Res J* 11:319-326, 1991.

83. Sobel JD: Pathogenesis and treatment of recurrent vulvovaginal candidiasis, *Clin Infect Dis* 14:S148-S153, 1992.

84. Spinillo A, Pizzoli G, et al: Epidemiologic characteristics of women with idiopathic recurrent vulvovaginal candidiasis, *Obstet Gynecol* 81:721-727, 1993.

85. Fong IW, Bannatyne RM, et al: Lack of in vitro resistance of *Candida albicans* to ketoconazole, itraconazole and clotrimazole in women treated for recurrent vaginal candidiasis, *Genitourin Med* 69:44-46, 1993.

86. Jovanovic R, Congema E, et al: Antifungal agents vs. boric acid for treating chronic mycotic vulvovaginitis, *J Reprod Med* 36:593-597, 1991.

87. Patel HS, Peters M II, et al: Is there a role for fluconazole in the treatment of vulvovaginal candidiasis? *Ann Pharmacother* 26:350-353, 1992.

88. Stein GE, Mummaw N: Placebo-controlled trial of itraconzole for treatment of acute candidiasis, *Antimicrob Agents Chemother* 37:89-92, 1993.

89. Silva-Cruz A, Andrade L, et al: Itraconazole versus placebo in the management of vaginal candidiasis, *Int J Gynaecol Obstet* 36:229-232, 1991.

90. Tobin JM, Loo P, et al: Treatment of vaginal candidosis: a comparative study of the efficacy and acceptability of itraconazole and clotrimazole, *Genitourin Med* 68:36-38, 1992.

91. Slavin MB, Benrubi GI, et al: Single dose oral fluconazole vs. intravaginal terconazole in treatment of *Candida* vaginitis. Comparison and pilot study, *J Fla Med Assoc* 79:693-696, 1992.

92. Mazziotti F, Cirillo L, et al: Comparative clinical study of a new imidazole molecule (fluconazole) and ketaconazole in the treatment of *Candida albicans* vulvovaginitis, *Minerva Ginecol* 44:653-659, 1992.

93. Merkus JM, Van Heusden AM: Chronic vulvovaginal candidosis: the role of oral treatment, *Br J Clin Pract Symp* 71 (Suppl):81-84, 1990.

94. Fong IW: The value of chronic suppressive therapy with itraconazole versus clotrimazole in women with recurrent vaginal candidiasis, *Genitourin Med* 68:374-377, 1992.

95. Sobel JD, Schmitt C, et al: Clotrimazole treatment of recurrent and chronic *Candida* vulvovaginitis, *Obstet Gynecol* 73:330-334, 1989.

96. Roth AC, Milsom I, et al: Intermittent prophylactic treatment of recurrent vaginal candidiasis by postmenstrual application of a 500 mg clotrimazole vaginal tablet, *Genitourin Med* 66:357-360, 1990.

97. Hilton E, Isenberg HD, et al: Ingestion of yogurt containing *Lactobacillus acidophilus* as prophylaxis for candidal vaginitis, *Ann Intern Med* 116:353-357, 1992.

98. Fong IW: The value of treating the sexual partners of women with recurrent vaginal candidiasis with ketoconazole, *Genitourin Med* 68:174-176, 1992.

99. Sobel JD: Recurrent vulvovaginal candidiasis: a prospective study of the efficacy of maintenance ketoconazole therapy, *N Engl J Med* 315:1455-1458, 1986.

100. Whitc DJ, Johnson EM, et al: Management of persistent vulvo vaginal candidosis due to azole-resistant *Candida glabrata*, *Genitourin Med* 69:112-114, 1993.

101. Klein RS et al: Oral candidiasis in high-risk patients as the initial manifestation of the acquired immunodeficiency syndrome, *N Engl J Med* 311:354-358, 1984.

102. Loukas DF et al: Multicenter evaluation of Nizoral (ketoconazole) in the treatment of oral thrush, *Ir Med J* 7:78-89, 1986.

103. Jacobs AH, O'Connell BM: Tinea in tiny tots, *Am J Dis Child* 140:1034-1038, 1986.

104. Kahana M, Yahalom R, Schewach-Miller M : Recurrent angular cheilitis caused by dental flossing, *J Am Acad Dermatol* 15:113-114, 1986.

105. Chernosky, ME: Collagen implant in management of perlèche (angular cheilosis), *J Am Acad Dermatol* 12:493-496, 1985.

106. Kirpatrick CH, Windhorst DB: Mucocutaneous candidiasis and thymoma, *Am J Med* 66:939-945, 1979.

107. Ahonen P et al: Clinical variation of autoimmune polyendocrinopathy-candidiasis-ectodermal dystropy (APECED) in a series of 68 patients, *N Engl J Med* 322:1829-1836, 1990.

108. Herrod HG: Chronic mucocutaneous candidiasis in childhood and complications of non-*Candida* infection: a report of the Pediatric Immunodeficiency Collaborative Study Group, *J Pediatr* 116:377-382, 1990.

109. Burke WA: Use of itraconazole in a patient with chronic mucocutaneous candidiasis, *J Am Acad Dermatol* 21:1309-1310, 1989.

110. Hay RJ: Overview of studies of fluconazole in oropharyngeal candidiasis, *Rev Infect Dis* 12:S334-S337, 1990.

111. Bielsa I et al: Systemic candidiasis in heroin abusers, *Int J Dermatol* 26:314-319, 1987.

112. Leclerc G, Weber M, Contet-Audonneau N, et al: *Candida* folliculitis in heroin addicts, *Int J Dermatol* 25:100-102, 1986.

113. Dupont B, Drouhet E: Cutaneous, ocular, and osteoarticular candidiasis in heroin addicts: new clinical and therapeutic aspects in 38 patients, *J Infect Dis* 152:577-591, 1985.

114. Shankland GS, Richardson MD: Possible role of preserved lemon juice in the epidemiology of *Candida* endophthalmitis in heroin addicts, *Eur J Clin Microbiol Infect Dis* 8:87-89, 1989.

115. Elbaze P, Lacour JP, et al: The skin as the possible reservoir for *Candida albicans* in the oculocutaneous candidiasis of heroin addicts, *Acta Derm Venereol* 72:180-181, 1992.

116. Dotz WI, Henrikson DM, Gloria SM, et al: Tinea versicolor: a light and electron microscopic study of hyperpigmented skin, *J Am Acad Dermatol* 12:37-44, 1985.

117. Sanchez JL, Torres VM: Double-blind efficacy study of selenium sulfide in tinea versicolor, *J Am Acad Dermatol* 11:235-238, 1984.

118. Sanchez JL, Torres VM: Selenium sulfide in tinea versicolor: blood and urine levels, *J Am Acad Dermatol* 11:238-241, 1984.

119. Bamford JTM: Treatment of tinea versicolor with sulfur-salicylic shampoo, *J Am Acad Dermatol* 8:211-213, 1983.

120. Fredriksson T, Faergemann J: Double-blind comparison of a zinc pyrithione shampoo and its shampoo base in treatment of tinea versicolor, *Cutis* 31:436-437, 1981.

121. Back O, Faergemann J, Hornqvist R: *Pityrosporum* folliculitis: a common disease of the young and middle-aged, *J Am Acad Dermatol* 12:56-61, 1985.

122. Hill MK, Goodfield MJ, et al: Skin surface electron microscopy in *Pityrosporum* folliculitis. The role of follicular occlusion in disease and the response to oral ketoconazole, *Arch Dermatol* 126:1071-1074, 1990.

123. Helm KF, Lookingbill DP: *Pityrosporum* folliculitis and severe pruritus in two patients with Hodgkin's disease (letter), *Arch Dermatol* 129:380-381, 1993.

124. Jacinto-Jamora S, Tamesis J, et al: *Pityrosporum* folliculitis in the Philippines: diagnosis, prevalence, and management, *J Am Acad Dermatol* 24:693-696, 1991.

125. Hartmann AA: The influence of various factors on the human resident skin flora, *Semin Dermatol* 9:305-308, 1990.

CHAPTER FOURTEEN

Exanthems and Drug Eruptions

The word *exanthem* means a skin eruption that bursts forth or blooms. Exanthematous diseases are characterized by widespread, symmetric, erythematous, discrete or confluent macules and papules that initially do not form scale. Exanthematous disease is one of the few diseases for which the term *maculopapular* is an appropriate descriptive term. Other lesions such as pustules, vesicles, and petechiae may form, but most of the exanthematous diseases begin with red macules or papules. Widespread red eruptions such as guttate psoriasis or pityriasis rosea may have a similar beginning and are often symmetric, but these conditions have typical patterns of scale and are, therefore, referred to as *papulosquamous eruptions*. Diseases that begin with exanthems may be caused by bacteria, viruses, or drugs. Most have a number of characteristic features such as a common primary lesion, distribution,[1] duration, and systemic symptoms. Some are accompanied by oral lesions that are referred to as *enanthems*.

Exanthems were previously consecutively numbered according to their historical appearance and description: first disease, measles; second disease, scarlet fever; third disease, rubella; fourth disease, "Dukes' disease" (probably coxsackievirus or echovirus); fifth disease, erythema infectiosum; and sixth disease, roseola infantum.

Measles

Measles (rubeola or morbilli) is a highly contagious viral disease transmitted by contact with droplets from infected individuals who cough. These droplets may remain suspended in the air in nonventilated doctors' waiting rooms and infect patients even after the infected patient has left.[2] Most cases have a benign course, but encephalitis occurs in 1 of 2000 individuals; survivors frequently have permanent brain damage and mental retardation. Death, predominantly from respiratory and neurologic causes, occurs in 1 of every 3000 reported measles cases. The risk of death is known to be greater for infants and adults than for children and adolescents. Measles occurring during pregnancy may affect the fetus. Most commonly, this involves premature labor, moderately increased rates of spontaneous abortion, and low birth-weight infants. Measles infection in the first trimester of pregnancy may be associated with an increased rate of congenital malformation.[3] In the prevaccine era, most measles cases affected preschool and young school-age children. In 1980, more than 60% of cases in which the age was known occurred among persons 10 years or older.

Lifelong immunity is established with a single injection of live measles virus vaccine given at approximately 15 months of age. From 1963 to 1967, both live and inactivated measles vaccines were in use; since 1968 only the live vaccine has been used. Susceptible persons include those who were vaccinated between 1963 and 1967 with inactivated vaccine, patients given live measles virus vaccine before their first birthdays, and those patients who have never had measles. Prior recipients of killed measles vaccine may develop atypical measles syndrome when exposed to natural measles and should be revaccinated with live measles virus.

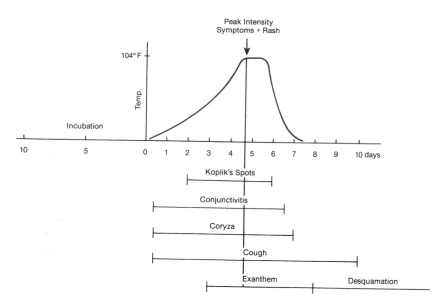

Figure 14-1
Measles. Evolution of the signs and symptoms.

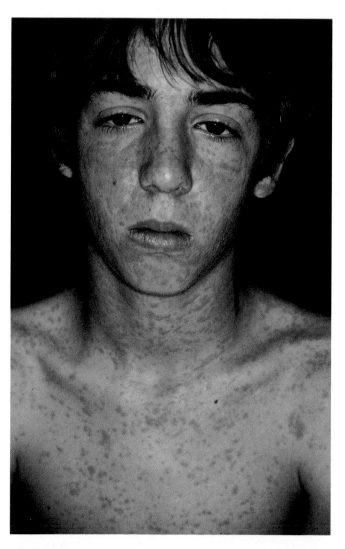

Figure 14-2
Measles. Early eruptive stage with involvement of the face and trunk. Eruption has become confluent on the face.

Typical measles

Typical measles (Figure 14-1) has an incubation period of 10 or 11 days, with a range from 7 to 14 days. The disease is spread by respiratory droplets and can be communicated from slightly before the beginning of the prodromal period to 4 days after appearance of the rash; communicability is minimal after the second day of the rash. Prodromal symptoms of severe, brassy cough; coryza; conjunctivitis; photophobia; and fever appear 3 to 4 days before the exanthem and increase daily in severity. The nose and eyes run continuously: the classic sign of measles. Koplik's spots (blue-white spots with a red halo) appear on the buccal mucous membrane opposite the premolar teeth 24 to 48 hours before the exanthem and remain for 2 to 4 days.

Eruptive phase. The rash begins on the fourth or fifth day on the face and behind the ears, but in 24 to 36 hours, it spreads to the trunk and extremities (Figure 14-2). It reaches maximum intensity simultaneously in all areas in approximately 3 days and fades after 5 to 10 days. The rash consists of slightly elevated maculopapules that vary in size from 0.1 to 1.0 cm and vary in color from dark red to a purplish hue. They are frequently confluent on both the face and body, a feature that is such a distinct characteristic of measles that eruptions of similar appearance in other diseases are termed *morbilliform*. The early rash blanches on pressure; the fading rash is yellowish-brown with a fine scale, and it does not blanch. Supportive treatment is the only necessity unless complications, such as bacterial infection or encephalitis, appear.

Atypical measles

Prior recipients of killed measles vaccine given between 1963 and 1967 (and in other countries in the early 1970s) may develop severe atypical measles syndrome when exposed to natural measles. Atypical measles therefore occurs in young adults. As with typical measles, there is a prodromal period accompanied by conjunctivitis, coryza, cough, and Koplik's spots. After a 3- to 5-day prodromal period, the rash begins on the wrists and ankles as a mildly pruritic, maculopapular rash. It extends to the palms and soles, and the hands and feet are often swollen. The temperature rises to 41° C and within 2 to 5 days the rash gradually spreads centripetally to involve the extremities and torso.[4] The face is usually spared. The rash may become vesicular, purpuric, and hemorrhagic. Pulmonary consolidation and pleural effusions may occur. The illness is self-limited and clears in 2 weeks. Mild desquamation of the palms and soles may follow. Such patients should receive two doses of live vaccine separated by no less than 1 month.

Management of measles

Vitamin A treatment. Vitamin A, retinol-binding protein (RBP), and albumin are significantly reduced early in the exanthem. Treatment with vitamin A reduces morbidity[5] and mortality in measles, and all children with severe measles should be given vitamin A supplements whether or not they are thought to have a nutritional deficiency.[6,7] Vitamin A–treated children recover more rapidly from pneumonia and diarrhea, have less croup, and spend fewer days in the hospital.[8] Treated patients have an increase in the total number of lymphocytes and measles IgG antibody.[9] The risk of death or a major complication during a hospital stay is half that of untreated patients. One study treated patients with 150,000 U of vitamin A palmitate IM on day 1 followed by 15,000 U orally for 7 days;[10] another recommends a total dose of 400,000 IU of retinol palmitate given orally.[7]

Vaccination

Measles immunity. Persons are considered immune to measles if they (1) were born before 1957, (2) have documentation of physician-diagnosed measles, (3) have laboratory evidence of immunity to measles, or (4) have documentation of adequate vaccination. Persons with measles-specific antibody, detectable by any test, are considered immune.

Persons who received inactivated vaccine, available in the United States from 1963 to 1967 (early 1970s in other countries) are at risk of developing severe atypical measles syndrome when exposed to the natural virus. They should receive two doses of live vaccine separated by no less than 1 month (Table 14-1).

The initial dose of measles vaccine is given at 12 months of age, with a second dose at 11 to 12 years. Infants in underdeveloped countries are at an increased risk of developing measles before 12 months of age, and case fatality rates of 2% to 10% are common. The World Health Organization recommends administration of measles vaccine in underdeveloped countries immediately after 9 months of age, regardless of nutritional status or the presence of minor illnesses.[11]

Approximately 5% to 30% of those vaccinated may develop malaise and fever to 39.4° C (103° F) 4 to 10 days after vaccination: symptoms last 2 to 5 days but cause little disability. Rash, coryza, mild cough, and Koplik's spots occasionally occur.

Outbreaks

Sporadic epidemics of measles continue to appear, especially among adolescents and unimmunized, young children.[12]

Outbreak control. A measles outbreak exists when one case of measles is confirmed. Preventing the dissemination of measles depends on the vaccination of susceptible persons. Serologic confirmation should be attempted for every suspected case that cannot be linked to a confirmed case (Table 14-2). The diagnosis can be made by demonstrating the presence of IgM antibody in a single specimen. IgM antibody peaks approximately 10 days after rash onset and is usually undetectable 30 days after rash onset.

USE OF VACCINE. Exposure to measles is not a contraindication to vaccination. If live measles vaccine is given within 72 hours of measles exposure, it may provide some protection. This approach is preferable to using immune globulin for persons more than 12 months of age.

TABLE 14-1 1989 Recommendations for Measles Vaccination*	
Routine childhood schedule (United States)	
Most areas	Two doses • first dose at 12 months • second dose at 11 to 12 years (entry to kindergarten or first grade)
High-risk areas (counties reporting more than five cases of measles among preschool-age children during each of the previous 5 years.)	Three doses • first dose (monovalent) at 9 months • second dose at 15 months • revaccinate at 4 to 6 years (entry to kindergarten or first grade)
Colleges and other educational institutions post–high school OR Medical personnel beginning employment	Documentation of receipt of doses of measles vaccine after the first birthday or other evidence of measles immunity

*From Measles prevention: Recommendations of the immunization practices advisory committee (ACIP), *MMWR* Vol 38/No.S- Dec 29,

USE OF IMMUNE GLOBULIN (Ig). Ig can prevent or modify measles. It may be used within 6 days of exposure. Ig given later than the third day of the incubation period for passive protection may extend the incubation to 21 days instead of preventing the disease. Ig is not recommended for outbreak control. The recommended dose of Ig is 0.25 ml/kg (0.11 ml/lb); 0.5 ml/kg for immunocompromised patients (maximum dose of 15 ml). Ig may be especially indicated for susceptible household contacts, particularly contacts less than 1 year of age; pregnant women; or immunocompromised persons, for whom the risk of complications is increased. Live measles vaccine should be given 3 months later (when passively acquired measles antibodies should have disappeared) if the individual is then at least 15 months old.

Serology. The presence of IgM antibodies or a fourfold or greater rise in paired sera IgG titer indicates recent infection. The presence of IgG generally indicates past exposure and immunity.

TABLE 14-2 Recommendations for Measles Outbreak Control (Use two-dose regimen)	
Outbreaks in preschool-aged children	Lower age for vaccination to as young as 6 months of age in outbreak areas if cases occur in children less than 1 year of age
Outbreaks in institutions: day-care centers, K through 12th grades, colleges, and other institutions	Revaccination of all students and their siblings and of school personnel born in 1957 or after who do not have documentation of immunity to measles (use two-dose regimen).
Outbreaks in medical facilities	Revaccination of all medical workers born in 1957 or after who have direct patient contact and who do not have proof of immunity to measles. Vaccination may also be considered for workers born before 1957.
	Susceptible personnel who have been exposed should be relieved from direct patient contact from the 5th to the 21st day after exposure regardless of whether they received measles vaccine or Ig or—if they become ill—for 7 days after they develop a rash.

*From Measles prevention: Recommendations of the immunization practices advisory committee (ACIP), *MMWR* Vol 38/No.S- Dec 29, 1989. (See this report for complete details.)

Hand, Foot, and Mouth Disease

Hand, foot, and mouth disease, which has no relation to hoof-and-mouth disease in cattle, is one of the most distinctive disease complexes caused by *Coxsackie* virus. This contagious disease may occur as an isolated phenomenon, or it may occur in epidemic form. It is more common among children.

Clinical presentation. The incubation period is 4 to 6 days. There may be mild symptoms of low-grade fever, sore throat, and malaise for 1 or 2 days. Twenty percent of patients develop submandibular and/or cervical lymphadenopathy.

Eruptive phase. Oral lesions, present in 90% of cases, are generally the initial sign. Aphthaelike erosions varying from a few to 10 or more appear anywhere in the oral cavity and are most frequently small and asymptomatic (Figure 14-3). The cutaneous lesions, which occur in approximately two thirds of patients, appear less than 24 hours after the enanthem. They begin as 3- to 7-mm, red macules that rapidly become pale, white, oval vesicles with a red areola (Figure 14-4). There may be a few inconspicuous lesions or there may be dozens. The vesicles occur on the palms, soles (Figure 14-5), dorsal aspects of the fingers and toes, and occasionally on the face, buttocks, and legs. They heal in approximately 7 days, usually without crusting or scarring.

Differential diagnosis. When cutaneous lesions are absent, the disease may be confused with aphthous stomatitis. The oral erosions of hand, foot, and mouth disease are usually smaller and more uniform. The vesicles of herpes appear in clusters, and those of varicella endure longer and always crust. Both varicella and herpes have multinucleated, giant cells in smears taken from the moist skin exposed when a vesicle is removed (Tzanck smear). Giant cells are not present in lesions of hand, foot, and mouth disease.

Treatment. Symptomatic relief and reassurance are all that is required.

HAND, FOOT, AND MOUTH DISEASE

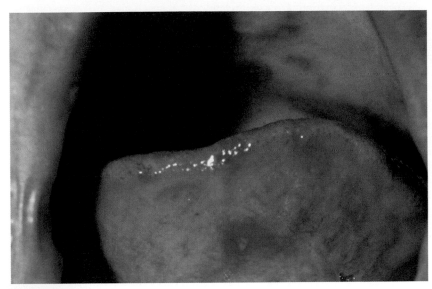

Figure 14-3
Hand, foot, and mouth disease. Aphthae-like erosions may appear anywhere in the oral cavity.

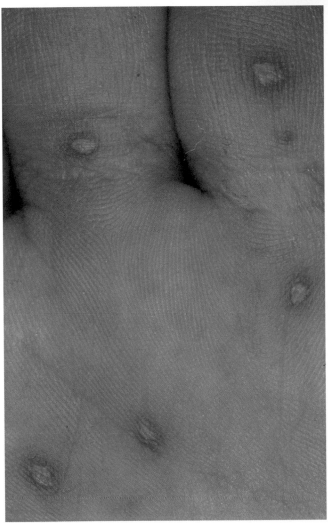

Figure 14-4
Hand, foot, and mouth disease. Cloudy vesicles with a red halo are highly characteristic of this disease.

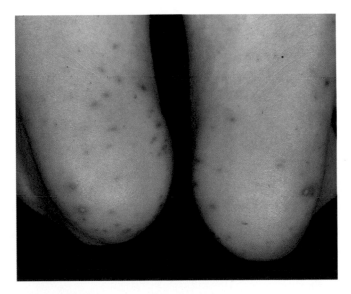

Figure 14-5
Hand, foot, and mouth disease. A cluster on the soles of a young boy. The pale, white, oval vesicles with a red areola are a distinguishing feature of this disease.

Scarlet Fever

Scarlet fever (scarlatina) is an endemic, contagious disease produced by a streptococcal, erythrogenic toxin. The circulating toxin is responsible for the rash and systemic symptoms. The infection may originate in the pharynx or skin and is most common in children who lack immunity to the toxin. Scarlet fever was a feared disease in the nineteenth and early twentieth centuries, when it was more virulent, but presently scarlet fever is usually benign. Virulent strains may appear in the future. New waves of scarlet fever are associated with an increase in frequency of *Streptococcus pyogenes* clones carrying variant gene alleles encoding streptococcal pyrogenic exotoxin A (scarlet fever toxin). The occurrence of new epidemics can be predicted by comprehensive monitoring of the frequency of *S. pyogenes* clones with variant toxin alleles.[13,14]

Incubation period. The incubation period of scarlet fever (Figure 14-6) is 2 to 4 days.

Prodromal and eruptive phase. The sudden onset of fever and pharyngitis is followed shortly by nausea, vomiting, headache, and abdominal pain. The entire oral cavity may be red and the tongue is covered with a yellowish-white coat through which red papillae protrude. Diffuse lymphadenopathy may appear just prior to the onset of the eruption. The systemic symptoms continue until the fever subsides. The rash begins about the neck and face and spreads in 48 hours to the trunk and extremities; the palms and soles are spared (Figure 14-7). The face is flushed except for circumoral pallor, while all other involved areas exhibit a vivid scarlet hue with innumerable pinpoint papules that give a sandpaper quality to the skin (Figure 14-8). The rash is more limited and less dramatic in milder cases. Linear petechiae (Pastia's sign) are characteristic; they are found in skin folds, particularly the antecubital fossa and inguinal area. The tongue sheds the white coat to reveal a red, raw, glazed surface with engorged papillae (Figure 14-9).

Figure 14-6
Scarlet fever. Evolution of signs and symptoms.

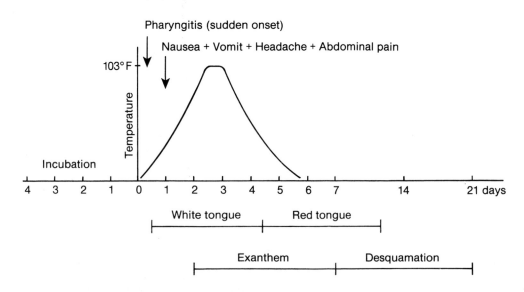

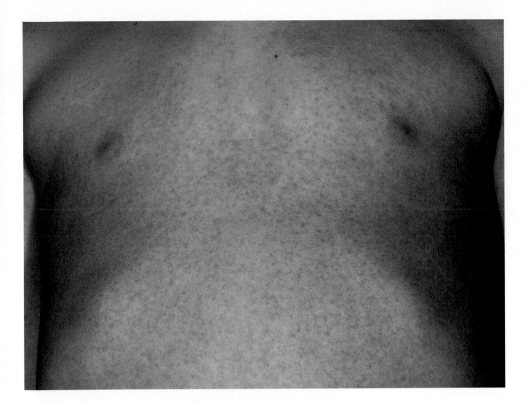

Figure 14-7
Scarlet fever. Early eruptive stage on the trunk showing numerous pinpoint, red papules.

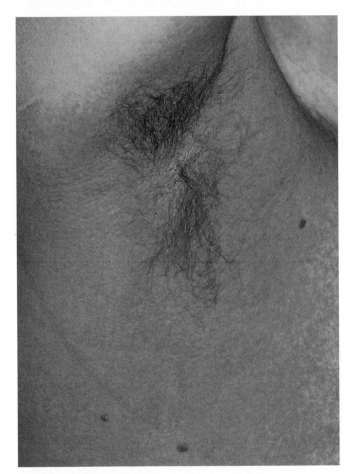

Figure 14-8
Scarlet fever. Fully evolved eruption. Numerous papules giving a sandpaper-like texture to the skin.

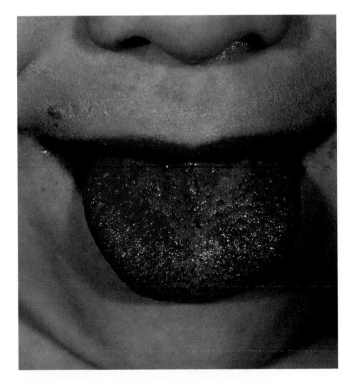

Figure 14-9
Scarlet fever. Portions of the white coat remain in the center, but the remainder of the tongue is red with engorged papillae ("strawberry tongue").

The fever and rash subside and desquamation appears, more pronounced than in any of the eruptive fevers. It begins on the face, where it is sparse and superficial; progresses to the trunk, often with a circular, punched-out appearance; and finally spreads to the hands (Figure 14-10) and feet (Figure 14-11), where the epidermis is the thickest. Clinically, the hands and feet appear normal during the initial stages of the disease. Large sheaths of epidermis may be shed from the palms and soles in a glovelike cast, exposing new and often tender epidermis beneath. A transverse groove may be produced in all of the nails (Beau's lines) (Figure 14-12). The pattern of desquamation of the palms and soles and grooving of the nails is such a distinct characteristic of scarlet fever that it is helpful in making a retrospective diagnosis in cases where the eruption is minimal. A rising antistreptolysin-O titer constitutes additional supporting evidence for a recent infection. Desquamation is generally complete in 4 weeks, but it may last for 8 weeks.

Treatment. Various drugs are available for treatment. They include (1) penicillin G benzathine (single injection): for patients weighing less than 60 lbs, 600,000 U; for patients weighing more than 60 lbs, 1.2 million U, (2) penicillin V (10-day oral course): for patients weighing less than 60 lbs, 125 mg four times a day; for patients weighing more than 60 lbs, 250 mg four times a day, and (3) oral erythromycin; children, 40 mg/kg/day; adults, 250 mg four times a day.

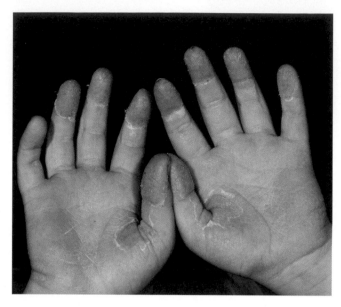

Figure 14-10
Scarlet fever. Desquamation of the hands.

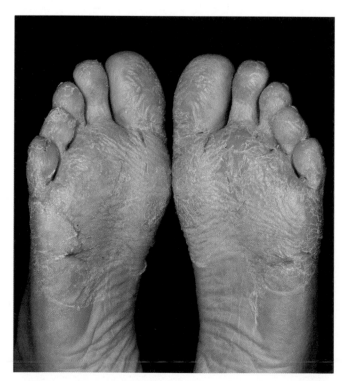

Figure 14-11
Scarlet fever. Desquamation of the feet.

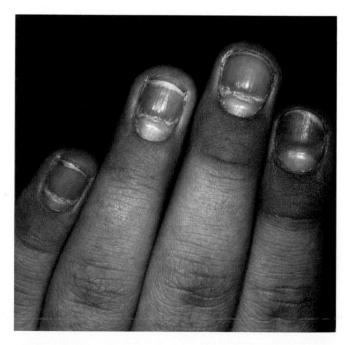

Figure 14-12
Scarlet fever. Beau's lines: transverse grooves on all nails several weeks after skin signs of scarlet fever have cleared.

Rubella

Rubella (German measles, 3-day measles), a benign, contagious, viral disease spread by the respiratory route, is most common in children and young adults. The incidence has decreased since the introduction of rubella vaccine, which is given with mumps and measles vaccines in a single injection at the age of 15 months.

Pregnant women who have rubella early in the first trimester may transmit the disease to the fetus, which may consequently develop a number of congenital defects (congenital rubella syndrome). The number of women susceptible to rubella is substantial.[15,16] The incidence of the congenital rubella syndrome is increasing. Presently, most women who plan a pregnancy have rubella titers measured. Many women have had a subclinical infection and already have an adequate titer. Women with no evidence of previous infection should be immunized and warned that pregnancy must be avoided for 2 months, during which time attenuated virus may be present in the tissues. Women of unknown immune status who conceive and are subsequently exposed to rubella or develop an exanthem that in any way resembles rubella should have a titer measured immediately and again 7 to 14 days later. If infection is likely and therapeutic abortion is unacceptable, then passive immunization with immune serum globulin (0.25 mg/lb) should be given. The value of this prophylactic treatment is unknown.

Reinfection with rubella. Reinfection with rubella during pregnancy is rare. It may occur in previously immunized or infected women whose hemagglutinin titers are lower than 1/64. The disease is asymptomatic in some of these women. In general, reinfection does not result in fetal injury,[17] but cases have been described in which babies of mothers infected during pregnancy were born suffering from various degrees of congenital rubella syndrome.[18,19] In questionable cases, perform cordocentesis or amniocentesis[20] for culture and antibody titers before making a decision on interruption of pregnancy.[21] The measurement of IgG avidity (avidity-ELISA) can differentiate between acute or recent primary rubella (low IgG avidity) from pre-existing rubella immunity (high IgG avidity), including rubella reinfections.[22,23]

Incubation period. The incubation period of rubella (Figure 14-13) is 18 days, with a range of 14 to 21 days.

Prodromal phase. Mild symptoms of malaise, headache, and moderate temperature elevation may precede the eruption by a few hours or a day. Children are usually asymptomatic. Lymphadenopathy, characteristically postauricular, suboccipital, and cervical, may appear 4 to 7 days before the rash and be maximal at the onset of the exanthem. In 2% of cases, petechiae on the soft palate occur late in the prodromal phase or early in the eruptive phase.

Eruptive phase. The eruption begins on the neck or face and spreads in hours to the trunk and extremities. The lesions are pinpoint to 1 cm, round or oval, pinkish or rosy red, macules or maculopapules. The color is less vivid than that of scarlet fever and lacks the blue or violaceous tinge seen in measles (Figure 14-14). The lesions are usually discrete, but may be grouped or coalesced on the face or trunk. The rash fades in 24 to 48 hours in the same order in which it appeared and may be followed by a fine desquamation. Arthritis, affecting primarily the phalangeal joints of women, may occur in the prodromal period and may last for 2 to 3 weeks after the rash has disappeared.[24] No treatment is required.

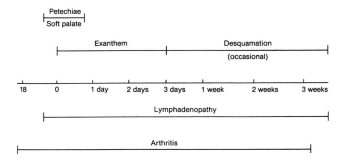

Figure 14-13
Rubella. Evolution of signs and symptoms.

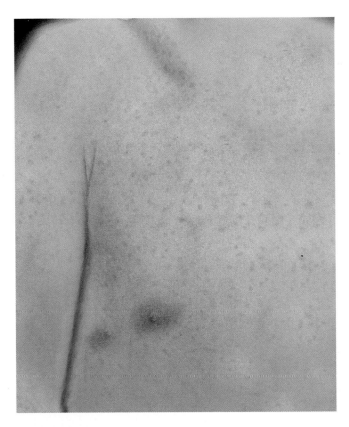

Figure 14-14
Rubella. Pink, oval maculopapules lack the rich color of scarlet fever and measles.

Erythema Infectiosum

Erythema infectiosum (fifth disease) is caused by the B19 parvovirus. It is relatively common, mildly contagious, and appears sporadically or in epidemics. Peak attack rates occur in children between 5 and 14 years of age; more than 50% of adults have serologic evidence of past infection. Asymptomatic infection is common. Parvovirus B19 infection can cause severe complications in pregnant women, individuals with hemolytic anemia, and those who are immunocompromised. People who do not have erythrocyte *Parvovirus* antigen, which is the cellular receptor for parvovirus B19, are naturally resistant to infection with this virus.[25]

Incubation period. The incubation period of erythema infectiosum (Figure 14-15) is 13 to 18 days.[26] The period of communicability is unknown.

Prodromal symptoms. Symptoms are usually mild or absent. Pruritus, low-grade fever, malaise, and sore throat precede the eruption in approximately 10% of cases. Lymphadenopathy is absent. Older individuals may complain of joint pain.

Eruptive phase. There are three distinct, overlapping stages.

Facial erythema ("slapped cheek"). Red papules on the cheeks rapidly coalesce in hours, forming red, slightly edematous, warm, erysipelas-like plaques that are symmetric on both cheeks and spare the nasolabial fold and the circumoral region (Figure 14-16). The "slapped cheek" appearance fades in 4 days.

Net pattern erythema. This unique characteristic eruption—erythema in a fishnetlike pattern—begins on the extremities approximately 2 days after the onset of facial erythema and extends to the trunk and buttocks, fading in 6 to 14 days (Figure 14-17). At times, the exanthem begins with erythema and does not become characteristic until irregular clearing takes place. Livedo reticularis has a similar netlike pattern, but it does not fade quickly.

Recurrent phase. The eruption may fade and then reappear in previously affected sites on the face and body during the next 2 to 3 weeks. Temperature changes, emotional upsets, and sunlight may stimulate recurrences. The rash fades without scaling or pigmentation. There may be a slight lymphocytosis or eosinophilia.

The petechial glove and sock syndrome. A recently described febrile dermatosis characterized by (1) fever, (2) pruritic edema, followed by pain and petechial involvement of hands and feet with sharp demarcation at the wrists and ankles, and (3) an enanthem of petechiae and oral erosions may be caused by human parvovirus B19.[27]

Figure 14-15
Erythema infectiosum. Evolution of signs and symptoms.

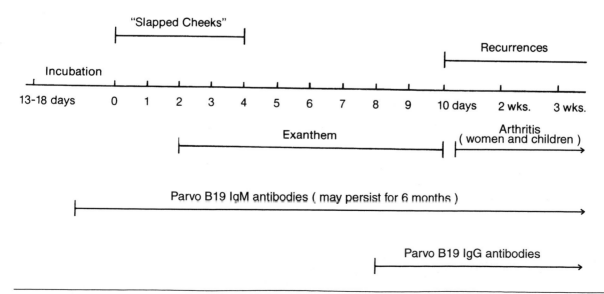

Arthritis and pruritus

Adults. Women exposed to the parvovirus during outbreaks may develop itching and arthritis.[28] The itching varies from mild to intense and is localized or generalized. In most cases a nonspecific macular eruption occurs without the appearance of the typical netlike pattern before the arthritis. Women develop moderately severe, symmetric polyarthritis that evolves to a form that is often indistinguishable from rheumatoid arthritis.[29] It lasts 2 weeks to 4 years. Most have involvement of the knees and other joints, as well as migratory arthritis.[30,31] The differential diagnosis includes acute rheumatoid arthritis, seronegative arthritis, and Lyme disease.[32] Men are not affected. Parvovirus infection should be considered when an adult woman has acute polyarthropathy associated with pruritus, especially if she has been exposed to children with erythema infectiosum. Adult flulike symptoms and arthropathies begin coincident with IgG antibody production in 18 to 24 days after exposure and are probably immune-complex mediated.

Children. Both male and female children may develop joint symptoms. Most cases have acute arthritis of brief duration; a few have arthralgias. Two patterns are seen: polyarticular, affecting more than five joints; and pauciarticular, affecting four or fewer joints. Large joints are affected more often than small joints. The knee is the most common joint affected (82%). Laboratory findings are normal. The duration of joint symptoms is usually less than 4 months, but some have persistent arthritis for 2 to 13 months, which fulfills the criteria for the diagnosis of juvenile rheumatoid arthritis.[33]

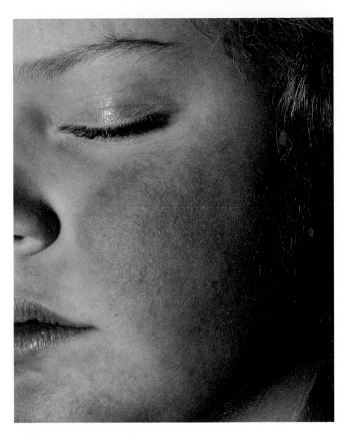

Figure 14-16
Erythema infectiosum. Facial erythema "slapped cheek." The red plaque covers the cheek and spares the nasolabial fold and the circumoral region.

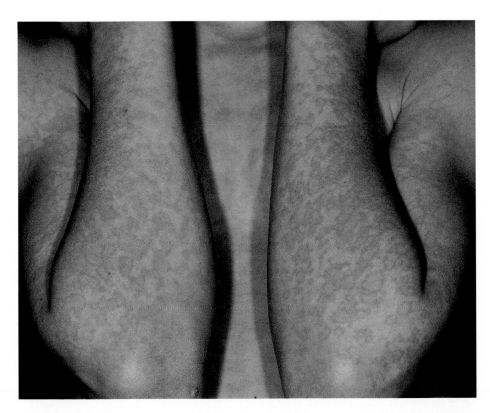

Figure 14-17
Erythema infectiosum. Netlike pattern of erythema.

Infection in the pregnant woman (intrauterine infection and spontaneous abortion). In pregnant women, infection can, but usually does not, lead to fetal infection (refer to the box below). Fetal infection sometimes causes severe anemia, congestive heart failure, generalized edema (fetal hydrops), and death. The fetus has a high rate of red-cell production; its immature immune system may not be able to mount an adequate immune response. Parvovirus has been implicated as a cause of spontaneous abortion (from severe fetal anemia and hydrops fetalis).[34,35] The overall risk of fetal loss following maternal exposure may be less than 3% in the first 20 weeks of gestation or approximately 10% if the mother is actually infected.[36] Approximately 17% to 50% of adults of child-bearing age are already immune to the parvovirus. Those in daily contact with school-age children have a fivefold increased annual occupational risk for B19 infection.[37] Approximately 15% of patients who are not immune may become infected in the setting of a school outbreak. Thus the risk to a pregnant teacher who does not know her immune status appears to be less than 1%. B19-associated congenital abnormalities have not been reported among several hundred liveborn infants of B19-infected mothers. The polymerase chain reaction is a sensitive and rapid method for the diagnosis of intrauterine infection.[38]

Anemia. The virus has the propensity to infect and lyse erythroid precursor cells and interrupt normal red-cell production. In a person with normal hematopoiesis, B19 infection produces a self-limited red-cell aplasia that is clinically inapparent. In patients who have increased rates of red-cell destruction or loss and who depend on compensatory increases in red cell production to maintain stable red-cell indices, B19 infection may lead to transient aplastic crisis. Patients at risk for transient aplastic crisis include those with hemoglobinopathies (sickle cell disease, thalassemia, hereditary spherocytosis, and pyruvate kinase deficiency) and those with anemias associated with acute or chronic blood loss. B19 infection accounts for most if not all aplastic crises in sickle cell disease, but at least 20% of infections do not result in aplasia.[39,40] Up to 30% of hospital staff members may be infected when exposed to infected sickle cell patients.[41] In immunodeficient persons and those with AIDS,[42] B19 may persist, causing chronic red cell aplasia, which results in chronic anemia. Some of these patients may be cured with immune globulin therapy.[43]

Laboratory. IgM antibodies are the most sensitive indicator of acute B19 infection in immunologically normal persons and can persist for up to 6 months.[44] Circulating B19 DNA can often be detected by polymerase chain reaction up to 6 months after onset of illness even in immunologically normal hosts and might be a useful adjunct test for diagnosis of acute B19 infection.[45]

Management. Parents need only to be assured that this unusual eruption will fade and does not require treatment. Most health departments do not recommend exclusion from school for children with fifth disease. Many infections are inapparent, and exposure may occur in the community as well as in school. Because the major immune response appears to be humoral, patients with chronic infection have been treated with immune globulin.

FACTS AND RECOMMENDATIONS FOR PREGNANT WOMEN EXPOSED TO B19 PARVOVIRUS

RISK OF MATERNAL INFECTION DURING AN EPIDEMIC: 30% TO 65%

Infected women may be asymptomatic.

NURSES AND SCHOOL TEACHERS: HIGH RATE OF INFECTION IF EXPOSED

People with fifth disease are contagious before they develop the rash, therefore exposure at the onset of an outbreak cannot be avoided.
Pregnant personnel should remain at home until 2 to 3 weeks after the last identified case.

LABORATORY TESTS

IgM tests for symptomatic exposed women
Fetal ultrasonography for confirmed or suspected cases.
Polymerase chain reaction testing (if available) of amniotic fluid and fetal serum—a sensitive and rapid method for diagnosis of intrauterine infection
Monitor alpha-fetoprotein* in exposed and infected women.
Ultrasonography when alpha-fetoprotein levels are increased
Abnormal ultrasound: fetal blood sampling as a guide for possible fetal transfusion

Teratogenic effects not demonstrated
Therapeutic abortion not indicated

Adapted from Levy M, Stanley ER: *Can Med Assoc J* 143:849-858, 1990.
*Maternal serum alpha-fetoprotein is a marker for fetal aplastic crisis during intrauterine human parvovirus infection.

Roseola Infantum

Roseola infantum (exanthem subitum, "sudden rash," sixth disease, rose rash of infants, 3-day fever) is caused by human herpes virus 6 (HHV-6), which is epidemiologically and biologically similar to cytomegalovirus.[46] Two genotypes of HHV-6 (type Λ and type B) have been distinguished. As with other herpes viruses, HHV-6 shows persistent and intermittent or chronic shedding in the normal population, making the unusually early infection of children (seroconversion in the first year of life in up to 80% of all children) understandable. It is probably latent in salivary glands and blood. Virus may infect infants through the saliva mainly from mother to child. A severe, infectious mononucleosis–like syndrome in adults may be caused by a primary infection with HHV-6.[47] HHV-6 has also been implicated in idiopathic pneumonitis in immunocompromised hosts.[48]

Most cases are asymptomatic or present with fever of unknown origin and occur without a rash.[49,50] The disease is sporadic, and the majority of cases occur between the ages of 6 months and 4 years. HHV-6 antibody is present in 90% to 100% of the population over age 2. The development of high fever, as is seen in roseola, is worrisome, but the onset of the characteristic rash is reassuring. In infants and young children HHV-6 is a major cause of visits to the emergency department, febrile seizures, and hospitalizations.[50]

Incubation period. The incubation period of roseola infantum (Figure 14-18) is 12 days, with a range of 5 to 15 days.

Prodromal symptoms. There is a sudden onset of high fever of 103° to 106° F with few or minor symptoms. Most children appear inappropriately well for the degree of temperature elevation, but they may experience slight anorexia or one or two episodes of vomiting, running nose, cough, and hepatomegaly. Seizures (but more frequently general cerebral irritability) may occur before the eruptive phase. Most recover without sequelae.[51] Cases of encephalitis/encephalopathy with abnormal electroencephalograms and cerebral computed tomograms have been reported; epilepsy developed in one case and another died.[52] HHV-6 DNA has been detected in the cerebrospinal fluid (CSF); this suggests that HHV-6 may invade the brain during the acute phase.[53] HHV-6 infection should be suspected in infants with febrile convulsions, even those without the exanthem.[54] Mild-to-moderate lymphadenopathy, usually in the occipital regions, begins at the onset of the febrile period and persists until after the eruption has subsided.

Eruptive phase. The rash begins as the fever subsides. The term *exanthem subitum* indicates the sudden "surprise" of the blossoming rash after the fall of the fever. Numerous pale pink, almond-shaped macules appear on the trunk and neck, become confluent, and then fade in a few hours to 2 days without scaling or pigmentation (Figures 14-19 and 14-20). The exanthem may resemble rubella or measles, but the pattern of development, distribution, and associated symptoms of these other exanthematous diseases are different.

Laboratory evaluation. Leukocytosis develops at the onset of fever, but leukopenia with a granulocytopenia and relative lymphocytosis appears as the temperature increases and persists until the eruption fades.[55] Seroconversion during the convalescent phase can be detected with immunofluorescence or enzyme immunoassays.

Treatment. Control temperature with aspirin and provide reassurance.

Figure 14-18
Roseola infantum. Evolution of signs and symptoms.

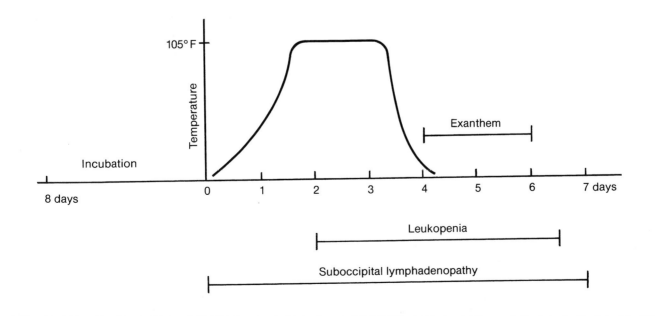

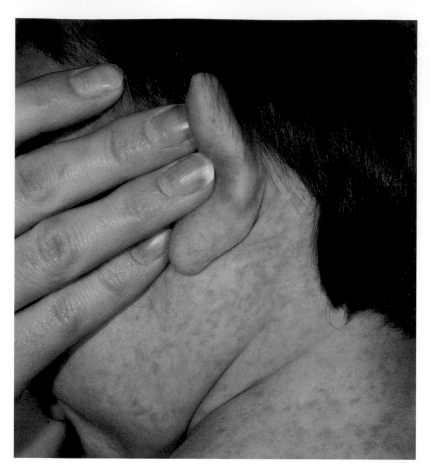

Figure 14-19
Roseola infantum. Pale pink macules may appear first on the neck.

Figure 14-20
Roseola infantum. Numerous pale pink, almond-shaped macules.

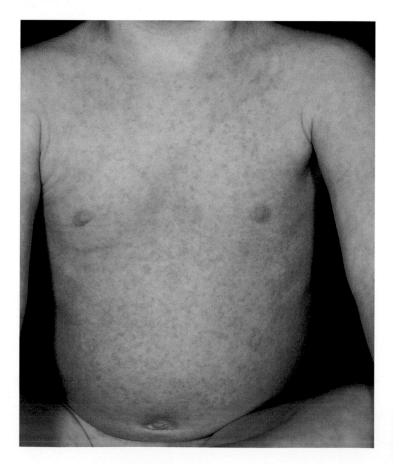

Infectious Mononucleosis

In approximately 3% to 15% of cases, infectious mononucleosis caused by the Epstein-Barr virus may appear with a morbilliform eruption indistinguishable from that of other viral exanthems. Most infections are probably subclinical. Transmission appears to occur by direct contact. The incubation period is from 33 to 49 days.

Clinical features. In the clinical course (Figure 14-21), headache and malaise are followed by fever of 101° to 104° F. Sore throat (80% of cases) and membranous tonsillitis (20% of cases) develop a few days later, followed shortly by petechiae of the soft and hard palate (25% of cases), cervical or generalized lymphadenopathy and splenomegaly. Hepatomegaly and icteric hepatitis may occur. The exanthem, if it occurs, appears on the fourth to sixth day. A macular or maculopapular morbilliform eruption appears on the trunk and/or upper arms and may involve the face and, less frequently, the distal extremities. Sometimes the eruption resembles scarlet fever or it may be urticarial. The exanthem fades in a few days. Most symptoms subside in 3 weeks, but fatigue lasting for several more weeks may occur, especially in adults. The majority of patients with infectious mononucleosis who are treated with ampicillin develop a generalized morbilliform eruption 5 to 8 days after starting ampicillin ("typical ampicillin rash").

Laboratory diagnosis. A heterophile antibody titer of greater than 1:128 is considered significant. In one study, 38% of patients showed a significant level at 1 week, 60% showed a significant level by 2 weeks, and 80% showed a significant level by 3 weeks. A rapid slide test has a low incidence of false reactions and a high degree of specificity. There is usually a white blood cell count (WBC) of 10,000, but it may be greater than 40,000 with lymphocytosis and atypical lymphocytes. A throat culture rules out streptococcal pharyngitis.

Treatment. Treatment is symptomatic. Use of ampicillin should be avoided because of the high incidence of skin eruptions. The patient should be protected from abdominal trauma during the next 6 months in order to prevent possible damage to an enlarged spleen.

Figure 14-21
Infectious mononucleosis. Evolution of signs and symptoms.

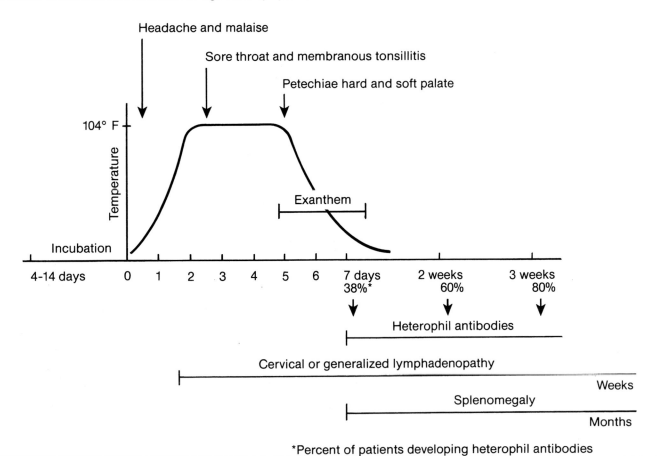

*Percent of patients developing heterophil antibodies

Enteroviruses: Echovirus and Coxsackievirus Exanthems

The previously described diseases characteristically display a predictable set of signs and symptoms. Roseola and erythema infectiosum are relatively common. Many physicians never see measles, German measles, or scarlet fever. The most common exanthematous eruptions are caused by the enteroviruses, echovirus and coxsackievirus. A large number of these viruses may begin with a skin eruption. Some of these eruptions are characteristic of the virus type, but in most cases one must be satisfied with the diagnosis of "viral rash." In many cases, drug eruptions cannot be distinguished from the nonspecific exanthems of these enteroviruses.

Systemic symptoms. Many are possible, such as fever, nausea, vomiting, and diarrhea, along with typical viral symptoms of photophobia, lymphadenopathy, sore throat, and possibly encephalitis.

Exanthem. The rash may appear at any time during the course of the illness, and it is usually generalized. Lesions are erythematous maculopapules with areas of confluence, but they may be urticarial, vesicular, or sometimes petechial (Figure 14-22). The palms and soles may be involved. The eruptions are more common in children than in adults. In most cases, the rash fades without pigmentation or scaling.

Treatment. Treatment consists of relieving symptoms.

Figure 14-22
Viral exanthem. Symmetric erythematous maculopapular eruption.

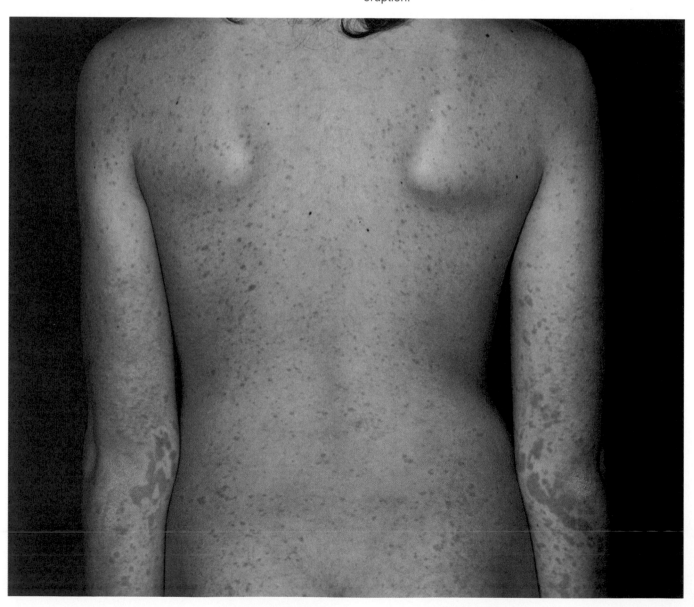

Kawasaki Syndrome

Kawasaki syndrome, or mucocutaneous lymph node syndrome, was first described in Japan in 1967, but now is reported in both endemic and epidemic forms worldwide. Patients' ages range from 7 weeks to 12 years (mean 2.6 years); rare adult cases are reported.[56] Kawasaki disease is an acute multisystem vasculitis of unknown etiology that is associated with marked activation of T cells and monocyte/macrophages.[57,58] An infectious agent[59,60] is strongly suggested by its occurrence primarily in young children (who apparently lack immunity) and by the existence of outbreaks. The agent may trigger genetically influenced immune responses.[61] Recurrences are rare. The major causes of short- and long-term morbidity are the cardiovascular manifestations. The histopathologic features of vasculitis involving arterioles, capillaries, and venules appear in the earliest phase of the disease.

Clinical manifestations. There is no single clinical finding or laboratory test that is diagnostic, but the diagnosis should be considered in children with rash and fever of unknown origin. The Centers for Disease Control (CDC) definition is shown in Table 14-3. There are a number of other clinical findings in Kawasaki syndrome (Table 14-4). The evolution of signs and symptoms is shown in Figure 14-23. Children have high fever for 1 to 2 weeks, rash, and edema of the extremities that is painful and interferes with walking, and they are extremely irritable.

Major diagnostic features

Fever. The fever, without chills or sweats, is a constant feature (range 5 to 30 days, mean 8.5 days) in untreated patients. It begins abruptly and spikes from 101° to 104° F and does not respond to antibiotics or antipyretics.

Conjunctival injection. Self-limited, bilateral congestion of the bulbar and sometimes the palpebral conjunctivae is an almost constant feature. Typically, the inflammation spares the area of the conjunctiva around the limbus. Uveitis occurs in 70% of cases. There is no discharge or ulceration as seen in Stevens-Johnson syndrome.

Oral mucous membrane changes. The lips and oral pharynx become red 1 to 3 days after the onset of the fever. The lips become dry, fissured, cracked, and crusted (Figure 14-24). Secondary infection of the lips can occur. Hypertrophic tongue papillae result in the "strawberry tongue" typically seen in scarlet fever. There is no sore throat but small ulcerations may form. Cough occurs in 25% of patients.

Extremity changes. Within 3 days of the onset of fever, the palms and soles become red, and the hands and feet become edematous (Figure 14-25, *A*). The edema is nonpitting. The tenderness can be severe enough to limit walking and use of the hands. The edema lasts for approximately 1 week. Peeling of the hands and feet occurs 10 to 14 days after the onset of fever (Figure 14-25, *B*). The peeling is similar to that seen in scarlet fever. Generalized desquamation of the skin is uncommon. The skin peels off in sheets, beginning about the nails and fingertips and progressing down to the palms and soles. The skin of children with diaper area inflammation peels at the margins of the rash and on the labia and scrotum. Beau's lines appear in the nails weeks later.

TABLE 14-3 Kawasaki Syndrome CDC Diagnostic Criteria	
Symptom	**Percentage of occurrence**
Fever lasting longer than 5 days plus at least four of the following:	100%
1. Bilateral conjunctival injection	92%
2. Mucous membrane changes (1 or more)	100%
Red or fissured lips	84%
Red pharynx	72%
"Strawberry" tongue	32%
3. Lower extremity changes (1 or more)	
Erythema of palms or soles	72%
Edema of hands or feet	48%
Desquamation (generalized or periungual)	56%
4. Rash—erythematous exanthem	100%
5. Cervical lymphadenopathy (At least 1 node larger than 1.5 cm)	72%

Data from Velez-Torres R, Callen JP: *Intern J Dermatol* 26:96-102, 1987.

TABLE 14-4 Kawasaki Syndrome Other Clinical Findings	
Symptom	**Percentage of occurrence**
Arthralgias	24%
Cough	25%
Urethritis—sterile pyuria	75%
Aseptic meningitis and irritability	25%
Hepatitis—jaundice	20%
Diarrhea	28%
Hydrops of the gallbladder	5%
Vomiting	60%
Cardiac involvement	33%
Myocarditis	6%-24%
Pericarditis	4%
Coronary artery aneurysms	17%-31%

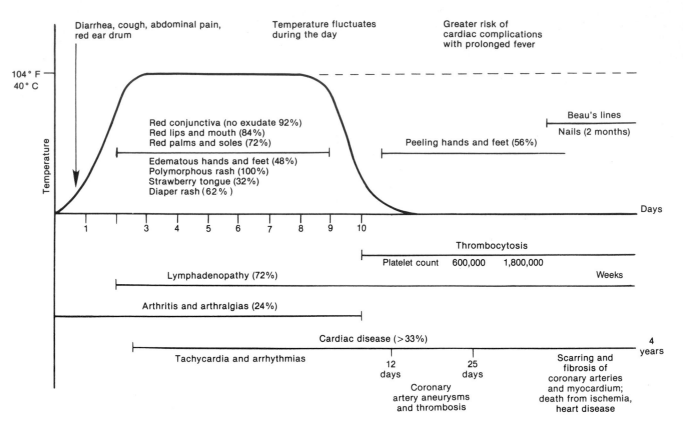

Figure 14-23
Kawasaki syndrome. Evolution of signs and symptoms.

Figure 14-24
Kawasaki syndrome. Nonpurulent conjunctival injection and "cherry red" lips with fissuring and crusting are early signs of the disease. *(Courtesy Anne W. Lucky M.D.)*

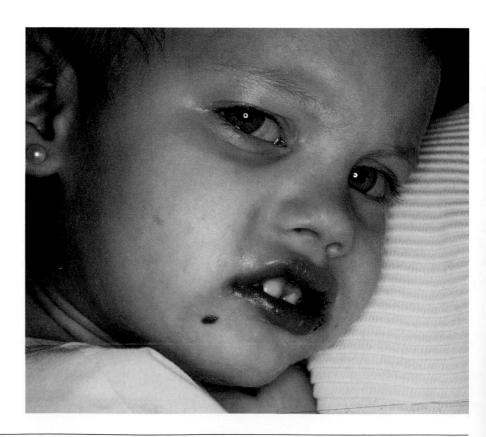

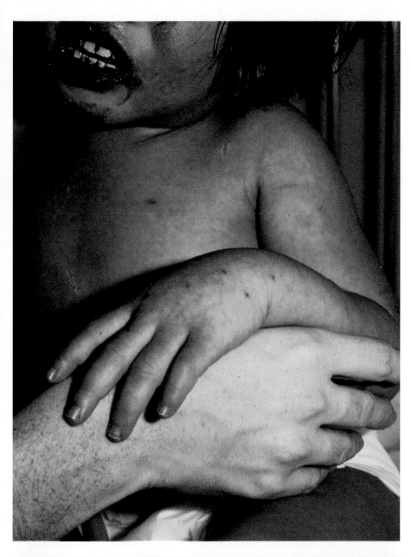

Figure 14-25 Kawasaki syndrome—
Evolution of hand lesions. *(Courtesy Nancy B. Esterly M.D.)*

A, The hands become red and swollen.

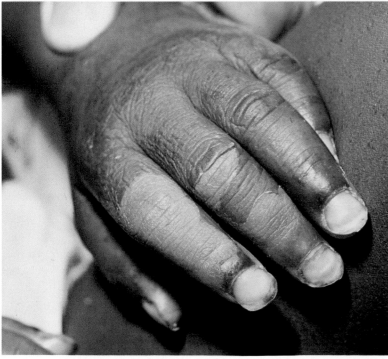

B, The hands peel approximately 2 weeks after the onset of fever.

Rash. A rash appears soon after the onset of fever. Several symptoms have been described. The most common forms are urticarial and a diffuse, deep red, maculopapular eruption (Figure 14-26, *A*). Less often the rash resembles erythema multiforme, scarlet fever, or the erythema marginatum seen in rheumatic fever. Dermatitis in the diaper area is common. The perineal rash usually occurs in the first week of the onset of symptoms. Red macules and papules become confluent (Figure 14-26, *B*). Desquamation occurs within 5 to 7 days. Perineal desquamation occurs 2 to 6 days before desquamation of the fingertips and toes (Figure 14-26, *C*). Vesiculopustules may develop over the elbows and knees.

Figure 14-26 Kawasaki syndrome—erythematous exanthem rash.

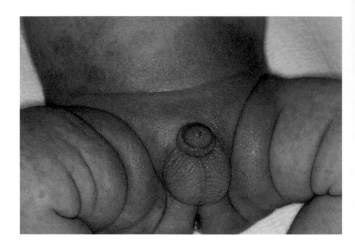

B, Red macules and papules appear in the perineal area 3 to 4 days after the onset of the illness. The rash becomes confluent and desquamates within 5 to 7 days. Desquamation of the fingertips and toes occurs 2 to 6 days later.

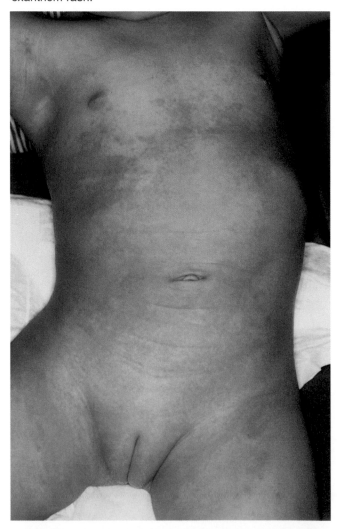

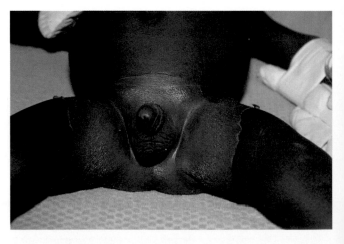

A, Diffuse, blanching, erythematous, macular exanthem. The eruption is frequently concentrated in the perineal area.

C, The skin of children with diaper-area inflammation peels at the margin of the rash. *(Courtesy Anne W. Lucky M.D.)*

Cervical lymphadenopathy. Firm, nontender, nonsuppurative lymphadenopathy is often limited to a single node and occurs in only 50% of patients.

Other clinical features

Abdominal symptoms. Hydrops of the gallbladder[62] can occur with right upper quadrant pain and jaundice in the first or second week of the illness. It resolves in a few days without surgery.

Urethritis. Inflammation of the mucosa of the urethra causes sterile pyuria and is seen in more than 75% of patients.

Arthritis and arthralgias. A polyarticular arthritis or arthralgia of the feet and hands often develops in the first 10 days. This process may evolve to a pauciarticular arthritis that involves the larger joints such as the knees and hips.

Aseptic meningitis. Approximately 25% have irritability or severe lethargy and stiff neck. Lumbar puncture reveals WBCs (mostly lymphocytes) ranging from 8 to 40/mm^3.[63] The sugar is normal and the protein is not elevated.

Cardiac and other organ vessel involvement. Kawasaki disease is the major cause of acquired heart disease in children in the United States. Clinical cardiac involvement occurs in 16.3% of patients.[64] It is probable that some degree of cardiac involvement occurs in all patients. The prevalence of cardiac sequelae is particularly high in males, infants younger than 1 year, and children older than 5 years of age. Boys under the age of 1 year[65] who have prolonged fever, elevated platelet count, and high erythrocyte sedimentation rate are at greatest risk for coronary involvement.[66] Arterial changes are seen at various other sites and organs as part of systemic arteritis. Aneurysms may be found in the axillary, common iliac, celiac, and mesenteric arteries. Arterial involvement of organs such as the kidney is well documented.

Acute phase. During the acute phase, myocarditis with tachycardia and gallop rhythms are seen in more than 50% of patients. They occur from myocarditis, arteritis, or pericarditis. Congestive heart failure may occur as a result of myocarditis.

Subacute phase. Aneurysms and thrombi form in the subacute phase (between 12 and 25 days after onset),[67] resulting in congestive heart failure, pericardial effusions, arrhythmias, and death from myocardial ischemia or aneurysmal rupture. Dilation or stenosis of coronary arteries, myocardial infarction, and valvular lesions occur 1 month or more after onset in 15% to 25% of patients. The walls of the coronary arteries and other medium-sized muscular arteries may show evidence of focal segmental destruction, with coronary-artery aneurysms or ectasia. The abnormalities peak in the third week and often resolve thereafter.

Chronic phase. The ultimate fate of involved vessels is unknown. Scarring and fibrosis of the coronary arteries and myocardium occur in the late phase (between 28 days and 4 years after onset) and may result in death from ischemic heart disease. Among those in whom coronary artery abnormalities develop, angiography 1 to 2 years later reveals persistent aneurysms in approximately half the affected children. In one large study, 13.7% had coronary artery involvement.[68] Approximately 80% of small or moderate-sized aneurysms regressed within 5 years. Giant aneurysms (maximum diameter of 8 mm) were found in 4% of children. Giant aneurysms did not regress during the follow-up period. Myocardial infarction occurred in 1.5% of all patients. All of these children had giant aneurysms. Therefore the severity of coronary artery involvement during the initial stages of Kawasaki disease influences the regression of these lesions. Giant coronary-artery aneurysms were not observed among patients treated with a single-infusion gamma globulin regimen.[69]

Imaging studies. Echocardiography is used for studies of ventricular function, proximal coronary arteries, and pericardial effusions.[65] Coronary artery dilatation may be detected 7 days after the onset of fever and usually peaks in 3 to 4 weeks. Coronary arteriography is used to study patients with distal coronary artery lesions, patients with persistently abnormal echocardiograms, or patients with symptoms of myocardial ischemia.[70]

Fatalities. Death is caused by cardiac complications. Case fatality percentages of 1% to 2.8%[71] are reported. Early myocarditis with normal coronary arteries appears to be the cause of death in approximately 12% of cases. Most deaths are the result of myocardial infarction in children with thrombosis of large coronary-artery aneurysms.[72] The mortality rate of boys with Kawasaki disease in Japan is twice that of healthy boys of the same age; most deaths occur within 2 months of diagnosis. The mortality rate of girls with the disease is similar to that of healthy girls.[71]

Laboratory evaluation. The acute phase is characterized by marked inflammation and immune activation. Leukocytosis (20,000 to 30,000) with a shift to the left (80%), thrombocytosis, anemia, and T-cell and monocyte-macrophage activation occur. Acute-phase reactants, such as erythrocyte sedimentation rate (90%), C-reactive protein, and serum alpha$_1$-antitrypsin, are elevated with the onset of fever and persist for up to 10 weeks after onset of illness. Other findings include elevated aspartate aminotransferase (92%), abnormal urinalysis consisting of sterile pyuria (68%), and CSF pleocytosis (25%). Thrombocytosis is a distinctive sign of this disease. The platelet count begins to rise on the tenth day of the illness, peaks at 600,000 to 1.6 million, and returns to normal by the thirtieth day of the illness.

RECOMMENDED THERAPY FOR KAWASAKI DISEASE

ACUTE PHASE

Aspirin: 100 mg/kg/day in four divided doses until approximately the fourteenth day of illness

Intravenous gammaglobulin: 2 gm/kg as a single dose given over 12 hours (schedule of choice); or 400 mg/kg once daily for 4 consecutive days

Digitalis and diuretics as needed for congestive heart failure

CONVALESCENT PHASE (AFTER THE FOURTEENTH DAY OF ILLNESS IN AN AFEBRILE PATIENT)

Aspirin: 3 to 5 mg/kg/day in a single dose; discontinue 6 to 8 weeks after onset of illness after verifying that there are no coronary abnormalities

CHRONIC THERAPY FOR PATIENTS WITH CORONARY ARTERY ABNORMALITIES

Aspirin: 3 to 5 mg/kg/day in a single dose, with or without dipyridamole

Coumadin or heparin with antiplatelet therapy in patients with particularly severe coronary findings or past evidence of coronary thrombosis

ACUTE CORONARY THROMBOSIS

Prompt fibrinolytic therapy with streptokinase, urokinase, or tissue plasminogen activator

CHRONIC MYOCARDIAL ISCHEMIA

Transluminal coronary angioplasty
Coronary artery bypass graft surgery
Cardiac transplantation

From Leung DY: *Curr Opin Rheumatol* 5:41-50, 1993.

Treatment

Aspirin. High dosages of aspirin have a marked effect on the clinical findings related to acute inflammatory changes. They shorten the duration of fever and positive serum C-reactive protein and may lower the incidences of coronary arterial involvement. Maximum benefit is achieved when serum salicylate concentrations are 150 μg/ml.[73] Aspirin 100 mg/kg/day administered every 6 hours provides these dosage levels. This is continued through the 14th day of the illness or until the patient is afebrile. Aspirin is then continued for a minimum of 6 to 8 weeks at a dosage of 3 to 5 mg/kg/day (administered as a single daily dose) to inhibit platelet aggregation (refer to the box at left).

Gamma globulin. Iveegam (currently $488.00 for a single 10-gm dose) is approved in the United States for treating Kawasaki disease. The most common side effects are headache, back or abdominal pain, and nausea and vomiting. High-dose intravenous gamma globulin (400 mg/kg/day) given with aspirin for 4 consecutive days significantly reduces the prevalence of coronary artery abnormalities when administered early in the course of the disease.[74,75] A single large dose of intravenous gamma globulin (2 gm/kg given over 10 hours) is more effective than this conventional regimen of four smaller daily doses and is equally safe.[65,69] In one study, fever resolved and laboratory indexes of systemic inflammation returned to normal more quickly than those treated with the 4-day regimen. Consider using the four-dose regimen or slower rates of infusion for children with evidence of myocardial dysfunction. The efficacy of gamma globulin when started after the tenth day of illness has not been demonstrated.

It appears reasonable to retreat children who remain febrile 72 hours after 2 gm/kg of intravenous gammaglobulin and aspirin or who, after being afebrile for at least 24 hours, develop recurrent fever that is associated with at least one criterion of acute Kawasaki disease.[76]

The treatment significantly reduces fever and laboratory-measured levels of acute-phase reactants, suggesting a rapid, generalized, antiinflammatory effect, possibly from cytokine depression.[77] Aspirin is used for its antiinflammatory and thrombasthenia-inducing effects (important because of the thrombocytosis associated with this disorder).

Toxic Shock Syndrome

Toxic shock syndrome (TSS) (Figure 14-27) is a rare, potentially fatal, multisystem illness associated with *Staphylococcus aureus* infection and production of toxins. There is speculation that this is the same disease described by Thucydides as the plague of Athens between 430 and 427 BC,[78] therefore TSS is also called *the Thucydides syndrome*. Since 1981 there has been an estimated incidence of two to four cases per 100,000 women. The overall case-fatality rate is 3.7%, with a higher case-fatality rate for male patients (12.2%) than female patients (2.6%).[79] Most reported cases occur in menstruating women using high-absorbency tampons. Nonmenstrual *S. aureus* infections account for 20% to 30% of reported cases of TSS. Approximately 5% occur in men, and 40% of these occur between the ages of 15 and 24 years.[80] Cases of TSS resulting from nonsurgical skin infection, influenza, childbirth and abortion, surgical wound infections, use of nasal packing, and use of contraceptive sponges have been reported. The disease has several features in common with Kawasaki syndrome and scarlet fever.

Staphylococcus aureus. Five distinct enterotoxins are elaborated by staphylococci (SE A to E) plus toxic shock syndrome toxin-1 (TSS toxin-1). They cause centrally mediated gastrointestinal (GI) symptoms, rash, desquamation, and many other signs and symptoms of severe damage to almost all organ systems. Staphylococci isolated from patients with TSS can produce several other toxins (e.g., enterotoxin B) in addition to TSS toxin-1.[81] Isolation of staphylococcal TSS toxin-1 has occurred in 90% of menstrual cases and in 62% of nonmenstrual cases.[82] A passive latex agglutination test can rapidly detect if the strain of *S. aureus* is TSS toxin-1–producing.

Streptococcal toxic shock syndrome (STSS). Serious infections due to group A beta-hemolytic streptococcus have been reported with increasing frequency in recent years. The new more virulent strains have a greater tendency to produce potent exotoxins than prior strains.[83] The erythrogenic toxins A, B, and C are now more properly designated *streptococcal pyrogenic exotoxins* in recognition of their diverse biologic effects. In addition to inducing the rash of scarlet fever, these toxins cause fever, changes in the blood-brain barrier, organ damage, and lethal shock. They exert profound effects on the immune system, including alteration in T-cell function. Erythrogenic toxins (pyrogenic exotoxins) A, B, and C produced by group A beta-hemolytic streptococci (*S. pyogenes*) and, rarely, group B[84] may cause a disease with all the defining criteria for TSS. Generalized erythroderma with or without bullae may occur before or concomitant with the onset of the full syndrome. Patients may have fever, hypotension, cerebral dysfunction, renal failure, respiratory distress syndrome, toxic cardiomyopathy, hepatic dysfunction, and hypocalcemia. Desquamation follows the rash. STSS differs from that due to *S. aureus* in two ways. A focus of infection in soft tissue and skin[85] is usually present in STSS, and many patients have bacteremia. A

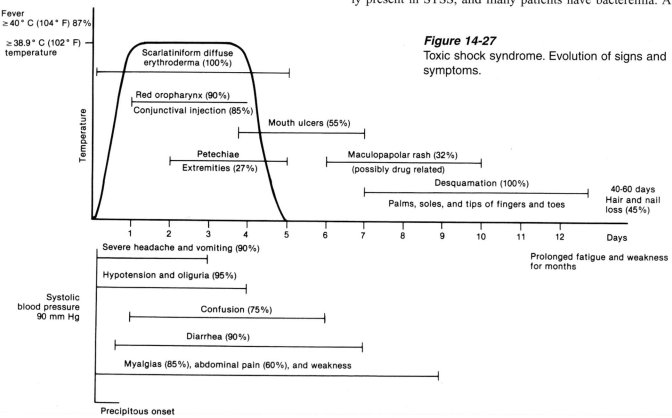

Figure 14-27
Toxic shock syndrome. Evolution of signs and symptoms.

case following streptococcal pharyngitis was reported.[86] In one series, a portal of entry was present in 65%, and 60% had bacteremia; the mortality rate was 30%.[87] STSS probably does not make up a single syndrome, but rather many clinical subtypes that reflect different characteristics of individual *S. pyogenes* isolates.[88] Early diagnosis, treatment with antibiotics, and operative debridement are required.[89]

Menstrual toxic shock syndrome (MTSS). Most cases reported in the late 1970s occurred in women using tampons. Menstruating women become ill within 4 days of onset of their menstrual periods. Women who used high-absorbency tampons had a greater relative risk of developing TSS than women who used low-absorbency tampons.[90] It appears that a tampon can lower the magnesium concentration in the vagina by a process of ion exchange, thus creating an environment that favors the production of TSS toxin-1 by *S. aureus*. The tampon characteristics responsible for the associated risk of TSS are poorly understood. Tampon manufacturers have removed chemicals used to enhance absorbency. The reported number of menstrually related cases

related cases of TSS has dropped substantially,[91] although they continue to account for 50% to 70% of all cases of TSS in women of reproductive age.[92]

Nonmenstrual toxic shock syndrome (NMTSS). In contrast to patients with MTSS, those with NMTSS comprise a heterogeneous group with varying host factors and clinical presentations. The nonmenstrual cases are frequently observed in children and may be associated with a wide variety of staphylococcal infections. Infected burn wounds in hospitalized children and bacterial tracheitis (in some cases following influenza B infection) are relatively high-risk settings for pediatric TSS.[93] NMTSS patients experience delayed onset of TSS symptoms after a precipitating injury or event, more frequent CNS manifestations, less frequent musculoskeletal involvement, and higher degrees of anemia than patients with MTSS.[94]

Influenza. Many cases of TSS associated with influenza have been reported. In one study, a series of nine patients with influenza developed TSS, and five deaths occurred. The initial clinical presentation is suggestive of nonsuppura-

---

TOXIC SHOCK SYNDROME CASE DEFINITION

MAJOR CRITERIA (ALL FOUR MUST BE MET)

Fever: Temperature >38.9° C (102° F)

Rash: Diffuse or palmar erythroderma progressing to subsequent peripheral desquamation (hands and feet)

Mucous membrane: Nonpurulent conjunctival hyperemia, or oropharyngeal hyperemia, or vaginal hyperemia or discharge

Hypotension: Systolic blood pressure (BP) less than 90 mm Hg for an adult (over 16 years of age) or less than 5th percentile for age for a child; or orthostatic hypotension as shown by a drop in diastolic BP greater than 15 mm Hg from recumbent to sitting; or history of orthostatic dizziness

MULTISYSTEM INVOLVEMENT (THREE OR MORE MUST BE PRESENT)

Gastrointestinal: History of vomiting or diarrhea at onset of illness

Muscular: Creatinine phosphokinase (CPK) more than 2 times the upper limit of normal for laboratory values 4 to 20 days after onset

CNS: Disorientation or alteration in consciousness without focal signs at a time when patient is not in shock or hyperpyrexic

Renal: BUN or serum creatinine clearance levels more than 2 times the upper limit of normal; and abnormal findings on urinalysis (>5 WBCs per HPF; >1 RBC per HFP; protein >1+); or oliguria defined as urine output <1 ml/kg/hr for 24 hr

Hepatic: Total serum bilirubin level greater than 1.5 times the upper limit of normal or SGPT levels more than 2 times the upper limit of normal

Hematologic: Thrombocytopenia (platelet: less than 100,000/mm³)

Cardiopulmonary: Adult respiratory distress syndrome; or pulmonary edema; or new onset 2 or 3 heart block; or ECG criteria for myocarditis decreased voltage and ST-T wave changes; or heart failure shown by new onset of gallop rhythm, or by increase in size of cardiac silhouette from one chest roentgenogram to another during the course of the illness, or diagnosed by cardiologist

Metabolic: Serum calcium level less than 7.0 mg/dl with serum phosphate level less than 2.5 mg/dl, and total serum protein level less than 5.0 mg/dl

EVIDENCE FOR ABSENCE OF OTHER CAUSES

When obtained: Negative blood, throat, urine, or CSF cultures

When obtained: Absence of serologic evidence of leptospirosis, rickettsial disease, or rubeola

Evidence for absence of Kawasaki syndrome; no unilateral lymphadenopathy or fever lasting more than 10 days

From Chesney PJ et al. Clinical manifestations of toxic shock syndrome, *JAMA* 246:741-748, 1981.

tive tracheitis or viral pneumonia. Cultures of respiratory secretions show *S. aureus*, which produces either TSS toxin-1 or enterotoxin B. It is postulated that patients are likely to be nasopharyngeal carriers of toxigenic strains of *S. aureus* before the onset of illness. Patients subsequently developed tracheitis in association with influenza or other viral illness. A mucosal injury allows increased proliferation of *S. aureus* strains, producing TSS toxin-1 or enterotoxin B and leading to TSS in susceptible hosts (i.e., those without protective antibody, particularly children[96] and adolescents).[95]

Clinical manifestations. The criteria for diagnosis are listed in the box on p. 432. The evolution of signs and symptoms is illustrated in Figure 14-27. The Centers for Disease Control definition of TSS requires a temperature greater than 38.9° C, hypotension with a systolic blood pressure less than 90 mm Hg, or postural dizziness, rash, desquamation, evidence of multiple organ system involvement, and exclusion of other reasonable pathogens.

Dermatologic manifestations. The dermatologic manifestations are listed in the box below, left. A diffuse scarlatiniform erythroderma, bulbar conjunctiva hyperemia, and palmar edema are highly characteristic early signs. Desquamation of the tips of the fingers and toes occurs 1 to 2 weeks after the onset in exactly the same manner as is seen in scarlet fever and Kawasaki syndrome.

Diagnosis. The diagnosis is made when the clinical criteria mentioned in the box on p. 432 are met. The important laboratory findings are listed in the box below, right. A biopsy may be helpful in the early stages to establish the diagnosis. The diagnostic features are a superficial perivascular and interstitial, mixed-cell infiltrate that contains neutrophils and sometimes eosinophils, foci of spongiosis that contain neutrophils, and scattered necrotic keratinocytes that sometimes are arranged in clusters within the epidermis. Assays for toxin and antibody can be performed. The differential diagnosis of TSS is listed below:

Drug eruptions
Kawasaki syndrome
Scarlet fever
Staphylococcal scalded skin syndrome
Toxic epidermal necrolysis
Viral exanthems

Treatment. Beta-lactamase–resistant, antimicrobial antibiotics (oxacillin, nafcillin, cefoxitin, vancomycin, and clindamycin) are given intravenously. Conversion to oral therapy should be instituted after resolution of the acute illness (which usually occurs in 3 to 5 days). The total duration of therapy should be at least 2 weeks. Patients require intravenous fluids with or without dopamine or dobutamine to maintain blood pressure.

DERMATOLOGIC MANIFESTATIONS OF TOXIC SHOCK SYNDROME

ERYTHRODERMA (100%)

Diffuse scarlatiniform involving chest, abdomen or back, and extremities

DESQUAMATION (100%)

Palms, soles, tips of fingers and toes without scarring

EDEMA OF THE HANDS AND FEET (50%)

Nonpitting edema not associated with synovitis

PETECHIAE (27%)

Primarily on the extremities

CONJUNCTIVAL INJECTION (85%)

Bilateral, nonpurulent palpebral and bulbar conjunctivitis

OROPHARYNGEAL HYPEREMIA (90%)

Beefy red without exudate or membrane formation, strawberry tongue; some have multiple, punctate, nonpurulent buccal ulcerations

VAGINAL HYPEREMIA (100%)

Frequently tender external genitalia

LOSS OF HAIR AND NAILS (45%)

Telogen effluvium occurs 2½ months after onset

Data from Chesney PJ et al: Clinical manifestations of toxic shock syndrome, *JAMA* 246:741-748, 1981.

TOXIC SHOCK SYNDROME: IMPORTANT LABORATORY ABNORMALITIES

PRESENT IN MORE THAN 85% OF PATIENTS IN THE FIRST 2 DAYS OF HOSPITALIZATION

Coagulase—positive staphylococci cultured from specific sites, not from blood
Immature and mature polys greater than 90% of WBC
Total lymphocyte count less than 650/mm³
Total serum protein level less than 5.6 gm/dl
Serum albumin level less than 3.1 gm/dl
Serum calcium level less than 7.8 mg/dl
Serum creatinine clearance greater than 1.0 mg/dl
Serum bilirubin value greater than 1.5 mg/dl
Serum cholesterol level less than 120 mg/dl
Prothrombin time greater than 12 sec

PRESENT IN MORE THAN 70% OF PATIENTS IN THE FIRST 2 DAYS OF HOSPITALIZATION

Platelet count less than 150,000/mm³
Pyuria of greater than 5 WBC per high-power field
Proteinuria greater than 2+
BUN greater than 20 mg/dl
SGOT greater than 41 U/L

From Chesney PJ et al: Clinical manifestations of toxic shock syndrome, *JAMA* 246:741-748, 1981.

Cutaneous Drug Reactions

Rashes are among the most common adverse reactions to drugs. They occur in many forms and mimic many dermatoses. They occur in 2% to 3% of hospitalized patients (Table 14-5)[97-99]; in those patients there is no correlation between the development of an adverse reaction and the patients's age, diagnosis, or survival. Drugs may be taken for weeks or years without ill effect, but once sensitization occurs, a reaction may occur within minutes to 24 to 48 hours, depending on the type of allergic reaction precipitated. A particular drug may cause different reactions in different patients, and a drug may cause different reactions in the same patient at different times. Chemically related drugs may cross-react in a patient sensitized to one agent. Some life-threatening cutaneous drug eruptions are exfoliative erythroderma and toxic epidermal necrolysis. Two groups of mechanisms are involved in the pathogenesis of drug reactions: immunologic, with all four types of hypersensitivity reactions described; and nonimmunologic, accounting for at least 75% of all drug reactions. Toxic epidermal necrolysis and other severe cutaneous adverse drug reactions may be linked to an inherited defect in the detoxification of drug metabolites. In a few predisposed patients a drug metabolite may bind to proteins in the epidermis and trigger an immune response leading to immunoallergic cutaneous adverse drug reactions. The drugs most often responsible for the eruptions are antimicrobial agents and antipyretic/antiinflammatory analgesics.[98]

Clinical characteristics. The most common types of reactions are maculopapular (exanthematous eruptions),

urticarial, and fixed drug eruptions.[99] Toxic epidermal necrolysis, erythema multiforme, and fixed drug eruptions share similar pathologic features and are caused by many of the same drugs. Photoallergic drug reactions require the interaction of drugs, UV irradiation, and the immune system. Eruptions seen in serum sickness include exanthem, urticaria, vasculitis, urticarial vasculitis, and erythema multiforme.[101]

The typical patient seen by the dermatologist is a hospitalized patient who is on several medications. A fever occurs and hours later a diffuse maculopapular rash, hives, and/or generalized pruritus develop; the attending physician stops all medications and consults the dermatologist. Although maculopapular and urticarial eruptions are the most common examples of a drug eruption, several other patterns occur:

Acneiform	Photosensitivity
Alopecia	Pigmentation
Eczema	Pityriasis rosea–like
Erythema multiforme	Purpura
Erythema nodosum	Seborrheic dermatitis–like
Exanthems (maculopapular, morbilliform)	Toxic epidermal necrolysis
Exfoliative erythroderma	Urticarial vasculitis
Fixed eruption	Vesiculobullous (pemphigus-like)
Lichenoid (lichen planus–like)	
Lupus erythematosus–like	

Knowledge of these patterns and the drugs that commonly cause them helps to solve what is often a difficult problem when patients take many drugs simultaneously.

Diagnosis. The pattern of eruption should be determined. Maculopapular and urticarial eruptions are the most frequent patterns. Maculopapular eruptions occur suddenly, often with fever, 7 to 10 days after the drug is first taken. They are generalized, symmetric, and often pruritic. Drug eruptions are always suspected when hives are present. One must be familiar with the many other patterns of skin eruptions and the types of eruptions caused by specific drugs in order to diagnose drug-related disease. Knowledge of the frequency with which certain drugs cause allergic drug reactions also helps to identify offending agents. The clinical characteristics of each type of reaction are described below.

Clinical evaluation. A flow sheet documenting time of onset of eruption, drugs, dosages, duration, and interruptions in the use of drugs should be prepared. Suspected offending agents should be discontinued. The decision to rechallenge a patient with a specific drug must be made on an individual basis. Rechallenge in patients who have had urticarial-, bullous-, or erythema multiforme–like eruptions can be very dangerous.

Treatment. The offending drug should be stopped. Maculopapular and eczematous eruptions will dissipate. Symptomatic relief is provided with antihistamines and group V topical steroids.

TABLE 14-5 Rates of Allergic Skin Reactions to Specific Drugs (Urticaria, Generalized Maculopapular Eruption, Generalized Pruritus)

Drug or substance	Percentage of reactions
Platelet	45%
Amoxicillin	5%
Trimethoprim-sulfamethoxazole	3%
Ampicillin	3%
Ipodate	3%
Blood	2%
Penicillin	2%
Cephalosporins	2%
Erythromycin	2%
Dihydralazine hydrochloride	2%
Cyanocobalamin	2%
Quinidine	1%
Hyoscine butylbromide	1%
Cimetidine	1%
Phenylbutazone	1%

Data from Bigby M, Jick S, Jick H, et al: *JAMA* 256:3358-3363, 1986.

DRUG ERUPTIONS: CLINICAL PATTERNS AND MOST FREQUENTLY CAUSAL DRUGS
Exanthems (maculopapular)

Maculopapular eruptions, the most frequent of all cutaneous drug reactions, are often indistinguishable from viral exanthems. They are the classic ampicillin and amoxicillin drug rashes, but several other drugs also cause this pattern (see the box on pp. 436 and 437). Red macules and papules become confluent in a symmetric, generalized distribution that often spares the face. Itching is common. Mucous membranes, palms, and soles may be involved. Fever may be present from the onset. These eruptions are identical in appearance to a viral exanthem and routine laboratory tests usually fail to differentiate the two diseases. Onset is 7 to 10 days after starting the drug but may not occur until after the drug is stopped. The rash lasts for 1 to 2 weeks and fades in some cases even if the drug is continued. The pathogenesis is unknown.

Ampicillin rashes. Two types of skin reactions occur; they are an urticarial reaction mediated by skin-sensitizing antibody and a much more common exanthematous maculopapular reaction for which no allergic basis can be established. Ampicillin and other penicillins should not be given to patients who have had previous urticarial reactions while taking ampicillin. Ampicillin may safely be given to patients who have previously had a maculopapular ampicillin rash. The exanthematous reaction occurs in 50% to 80% of patients with infectious mononucleosis who take ampicillin. One study reported a high rate of drug exanthems in patients taking ampicillin in combination with allopurinol, but another study found no increased rate.[100]

Clinical presentation. The rash begins 5 to 10 days (range, 1 day to 4 weeks) after beginning ampicillin and may occur after the drug is terminated. The rash starts on the trunk as a mildly pruritic, red, maculopapular, sometimes confluent eruption and spreads in hours in a symmetric fashion to the face and extremities (Figure 14-28). The palms, soles, and mucous membranes are spared. The rash begins to fade in 3 days and is gone in 6 days, even if ampicillin is continued.

Management. No treatment is required for the maculopapular eruption. If the nature of a previous reaction is unknown and there is no adequate substitute drug, then skin tests with ampicillin, major determinants penicilloyl-polylysine (PPL: Pre-Pen), and a minor determinant (diluted penicillin G or sodium penicilloate) should be undertaken.

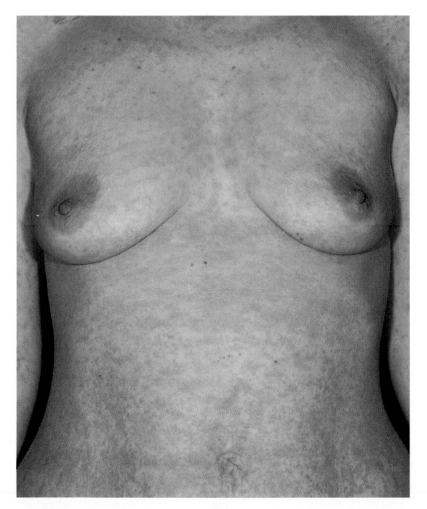

Figure 14-28
Drug eruption (ampicillin). Asymmetric, confluent maculopapular eruption.

DRUG REACTIONS AND THE DRUGS THAT CAUSE THEM

MACULOPAPULAR (EXANTHEMATOUS) ERUPTIONS

Ampicillin
Barbiturates
Diflunisal (Dolobid)
Gentamicin
Gold salts
Isoniazid
Meclofenamate (Meclomen)
Phenothiazines
Phenylbutazone
Phenytoin
   (5% of children—dose dependent)
Quinidine
Sulfonamides
Thiazides
Thiouracil
Trimethoprim-sulfamethoxazole
   (in patients with AIDS)

ANAPHYLACTIC REACTIONS

Aspirin
Penicillin
Radiographic dye
Sera (animal derived)
Tolmetin (Tolectin)

SERUM SICKNESS

Aspirin
Penicillin
Streptomycin
Sulfonamides
Thiouracils

ACNEIFORM (PUSTULAR) ERUPTIONS

Bromides
Hormones
   ACTH
   Androgens
   Corticosteroids
   Oral contraceptives
Iodides
Isoniazid
Lithium
Phenobarbital (aggravates acne)
Phenytoin

ALOPECIA

Allopurinol
Anticoagulants
Antithyroid drugs
Chemotherapeutic agents
   Alkylating agents
   Antimetabolites
   Cytotoxic agents
Colchicine
Hypocholesteremic drugs
Indomethacin
Levodopa
Oral contraceptives
Propranolol
Quinacrine
Retinoids
Thallium
Vitamin A

ERYTHEMA NODOSUM

Iodides
Oral contraceptives
Sulfonamides

EXFOLIATIVE ERYTHRODERMA

Allopurinol
Arsenicals
Barbiturates
Captopril
Cefoxitin
Chloroquine
Cimetidine
Gold salts
Hydantoins
Isoniazid
Lithium
Mercurial diuretics
Paraaminosalicylic acid
Phenylbutazone
Sulfonamides
Sulfonylureas

FIXED DRUG ERUPTIONS

Aspirin
Barbiturates
Methaqualone
Phenazones
Phenolphthalein
Phenylbutazone
Sulfonamides
Tetracyclines
Trimethoprim-sulfamethoxazole
Many others reported

LICHEN PLANUS–LIKE ERUPTIONS

Antimalarials
Arsenicals
Beta-blockers
Captopril
Furosemide
Gold salts
Methyldopa
Penicillamine
Quinidine
Sulfonylureas
Thiazides

ERYTHEMA MULTIFORME–LIKE ERUPTIONS

Allopurinol
Barbiturates
Carbamazepine
Hydantoins
Minoxidil
Nitrofurantoin
Nonsteroidal anti-
   inflammatory agents
Penicillin
Phenolphthalein
Phenothiazines
Rifampin
Sulfonamides
Sulfonylureas
Sulindac

LUPUS–LIKE ERUPTIONS

Common
   Hydralazine
   Procainamide
Uncommon
   Chlorpromazine
   Hydrochlorothiazide
   Isoniazid
   Methyldopa
   Quinidine

Probable
   Acebutolol
   Carbamazepine
   Ethosuximide
   Lithium carbonate
   Penicillamine
   Phenytoin
   Propylthiouracil
   Sulfasalazine

PHOTOSENSITIVITY

Amiodarone
Carbamazepine
Chlorpropamide
Furosemide
Griseofulvin
Lomefloxacin
Methotrexate (sunburn reactivation)
Nalidixic acid
Naproxen
Phenothiazines
Piroxicam (Feldene)
Psoralens
Quinine
Sulfonamides
Tetracyclines
   Demeclocycline
   Doxycycline
   (less frequently with tetracycline and minocycline)
Thiazides
Tolbutamide

SKIN PIGMENTATION

ACTH (brown as in Addison's disease)
Amiodarone (slate-gray)
Anticancer drugs
   Bleomycin (30%—brown, patchy, linear)
   Busulphan (diffuse as in Addison's disease)
   Cyclophosphamide (nails)
   Doxorubicin (nails)
Antimalarials (blue-gray or yellow)
Arsenic (diffuse, brown, macular)
Chlorpromazine (slate-gray in sun-exposed areas)
Clofazimine (red)
Heavy metals (silver, gold, bismuth, mercury)
Methsergide maleate (red)
Minocycline (patchy or diffuse blue-black)
Oral contraceptives (chloasma-brown)
Psoralens
Rifampin—very high dose (red man syndrome)

PITYRIASIS ROSEA–LIKE ERUPTIONS

Arsenicals
Barbiturates
Bismuth compounds
Captopril
Clonidine
Gold compounds
Methoxypromazine
Metronidazole
Pyribenzamine

TOXIC EPIDERMAL NECROLYSIS

Large areas of skin become bright red, then slough at
   the dermoepidermal border. This is a life-threatening
   reaction (see Chapter Eighteen)
Allopurinol
Phenylbutazone
Phenytoin
Sulfonamides
Sulindac

SMALL-VESSEL CUTANEOUS VASCULITIS

Allopurinol
Diphenylhydantoin
Hydralazine
Penicillin
Piroxicam (Feldene) (Henoch-Schönlein purpura)
Propylthiouracil
Quinidine
Sulfonamides
Thiazides

VESICLES AND BLISTERS

Barbiturates (pressure areas—comatose patients)
Bromides
Captopril (pemphigus–like)
Cephalosporins (pemphigus–like)
Clonidine (cicatricial pemphigoid–like)
Furosemide (phototoxic)
Iodides
Nalidixic acid (phototoxic)
Naproxen (like porphyria cutanea tarda)
Penicillamine (pemphigus foliaceus–like)
Phenazones
Piroxicam (Feldene)
Sulfonamides

OCULAR PEMPHIGOID

Demecarium bromide
Echothiophate iodide
Epinephrine
Idoxuridine
Pilocarpine
Timolol

CHEMOTHERAPY-INDUCED ACRAL ERYTHEMA

Cyclophosphamide
Cytosine arabinoside
Doxorubicin
Fluorouracil
Hydroxyurea
Mercaptopurine
Methotrexate
Mitotane

Urticaria

Aspirin, penicillin, and blood products are the most frequent causes of urticarial drug eruptions, but almost any drug can cause hives. Pruritic red wheals vary in size from small papules to huge plaques. The hives typically fade in less than 24 hours only to recur in another area. Angioedema refers to urticarial swelling of deep dermal and subcutaneous tissues and mucous membranes; the reaction may be life-threatening. There are three mechanisms of drug-induced urticaria: anaphylactic and accelerated reactions, serum sickness, and nonimmunologic histamine release.

Anaphylactic and accelerated reactions. These IgE-dependent reactions occur within minutes (immediate reactions) to hours (accelerated reactions) of drug administration. Penicillin and its derivatives are the most common causes. Scratch testing can be used to diagnose this pattern. Scratch testing for penicillin allergy is now a routine procedure. Radioallergosorbent (RAST) tests for IgE may be helpful in difficult cases. They are not as reliable as scratch testing.

Serum sickness. Circulating immune complexes cause serum sickness. Urticaria occurs 4 to 21 days after drug ingestion. The drug is ingested, antibody is formed over the next few days, and drug and antibody combine to form circulating immune complexes. Fever, hematuria, lymphadenopathy, and arthralgias follow. (See Chapter Six.)

Nonimmunologic histamine releasers. Reaction can occur in minutes. The drug may exert a direct action on the mast cell or on other pathways. Nonimmunologic histamine releasers include the following:

Morphine
Codeine
Polymyxin B
Lobster
Strawberries

Acneiform (pustular) eruptions

These pustular eruptions mimic acne but comedones are absent.

Eczema

A patient who develops contact dermatitis with a topical agent develops either a focal flare at sites of previous inflammation or a generalized cutaneous eruption if exposed orally to the same or chemically related medication (the so-called external-internal sensitization) (Table 14-6). Continued use of the medication can intensify the reaction and lead to generalization of the eruption.

Erythema multiforme and toxic epidermal necrolysis

Reactions may be limited to skin or mucous membranes or generalized with classic target lesions or bullae or loss of a major portion of the cutaneous surface (toxic epidermal necrolysis). Severe forms are often caused by medications. Less severe forms are caused by mycoplasmal pneumonia, herpes simplex infections, and medication. Toxic epidermal necrolysis is severe and is fatal in up to 30% of cases. The cause of death is loss of large areas of skin, resulting in fluid loss and sepsis. See the box on pp. 436 and 437 and Chapter Eighteen.

Exfoliative erythroderma

Generalized erythema and scaling may occur if an offending agent is not withdrawn (see the box on pp. 436 and 437). The reaction is potentially life-threatening.

TABLE 14-6 Eczematous Eruptions (External-Internal Sensitization*)

Topical medication	Oral medication
Aminophylline suppositories	Ethylenediamine antihistamines
Benadryl cream	Benadryl, Dramamine
Caladryl lotion	Benadryl, Dramamine
Formaldehyde	Methenamine
Neomycin sulfate	Streptomycin, kanamycin, gentamicin
Thiuram and disulfiram (rubber and insecticide compounds)	Antabuse
Benzocaine, glyceryl PABA sunscreens (paraamino compounds)	Azo dyes in foods and drugs, acetohexamide, tolbutamide, chlorpropamide, chlorothiazide, paraaminosalicylic acid

Adapted from Fisher AA: *Contact dermatitis*, ed 3, Philadelphia, 1986, Lea & Febiger.
*Patients allergic to certain topical medications develop focal or generalized eruptions when exposed to a chemically related oral medication.

Fixed drug eruptions

Fixed drug eruptions are a unique form of drug allergy which produce red plaques or blisters that recur at the same cutaneous site each time the drug is ingested[102] (see the box on pp. 436 and 437). The reaction may represent a cell-mediated immunologic response to a variety of antigens.[103] The clinical pattern and distribution of lesions may be influenced by the drug in question, and the study of the pattern may provide useful information in selecting the most likely causative drug. Tetracycline[104] and co-trimoxazole commonly cause lesions limited to the glans penis.[105] Cases of familial occurrence suggest that a genetic predisposition might be an important causal factor.[106,107]

Clinical manifestations. Single or multiple, round, sharply demarcated, dusky red plaques appear soon after drug exposure and reappear in exactly the same site each time the drug is taken (Figure 14-29). The lesions are generally preceded or accompanied by itching and burning, the intensity of which is usually proportionate to the severity of the inflammatory changes. Pruritus and burning may be the only manifestations of reactivation in an old patch. The area often blisters and then erodes; desquamation or crusting (after bullous lesions) follows and brown pigmentation (Figure 14-30) forms with healing. Nonpigmenting reactions have been documented.[108-110] Lesions can occur on any part of the skin or mucous membrane,[111] but the glans penis (Figure 14-31) is the most common site. Regional lymphadenopathy is absent.

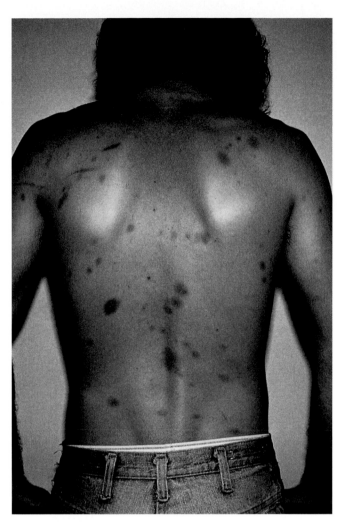

Figure 14-30
Fixed drug eruption. Multiple round, sharply demarcated plaques appeared shortly after methaqualone (Quaalude) was taken. The plaques healed with brown hyperpigmentation. *(Courtesy David W. Knox M.D.)*

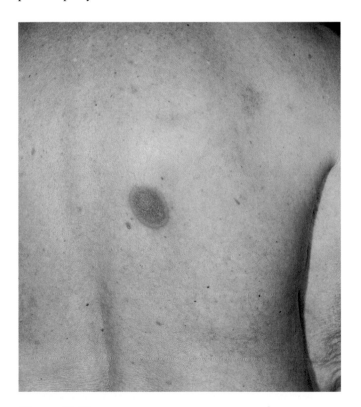

Figure 14-29
Fixed drug eruption. A single sharply demarcated, round plaque appeared shortly after trimethoprim was taken.

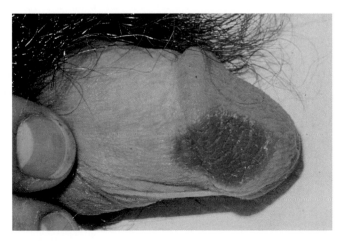

Figure 14-31
Fixed drug eruption. The glans penis is the most common site.

Reactivation and refractory phase. The length of time from the reexposure to a drug and the onset of symptoms is 30 minutes to 8 hours (mean, 2.1 hours).[112] Following each exacerbation, some patients demonstrate a refractory period (weeks to several months),[113] during which the offending drug does not activate the lesions.

Cross-sensitivity. Ingestion of a drug with a similar chemical structure may precipitate exacerbations. This phenomenon has been reported with tetracycline derivatives and sulfonamides. One report suggests that there is a lack of cross-sensitivity between tetracycline, doxycycline, and minocycline in patients that reacted to tetracycline.[114] Drugs of different chemical structures also can precipitate exacerbations; this reaction is polysensitivity.[115]

Diagnosis. A careful history is important because patients often do not relate their complaints to the use of a drug that they may be taking as a laxative (phenolphthalein)[116] or headache remedy. Provoking the lesion with the suspected drug confirms the diagnosis, prevents recurrences, and allays the anxiety of the patient regarding venereal origin of the disease. The challenge dose should be smaller than the normal therapeutic dose,[117] but it can be cautiously increased up to the normal therapeutic dose until the reaction is elicited. In some cases 2 to 3 times the original dose may be required to elicit a repeat reaction. Some authors do not recommend these tests because of the possible risk of generalized bullous eruptions. Topical and intradermal[118] provocation tests have been used as an alternative to systemic provocation tests. Patch tests are performed on the patient's normal and prelesional skin with the drug in a petrolatum base. In one study, a positive reaction occurred only at the previously lesional site.[119]

A biopsy shows hydropic degeneration of the epidermal basal cells and pigmentary incontinence.

Lichenoid (lichen planus–like drug eruptions)

Clinically and histologically these mimic generalized lichen planus. There are multiple flat-topped, itchy violaceous papules; oral lesions may be present. The mean age of patients with lichen planus is approximately 50 years; the mean age for lichenoid drug eruptions is approximately 60 years. The latent period between the beginning of administration of a drug and the eruption is between 3 weeks and 3 years.[120] The lesions are chronic and persist for weeks or months after the offending drug is stopped. Lesions heal with brown pigmentation. Gold and antimalarials are most often associated with drug-induced lichen planus (see the box on pp. 436 and 437).

Lupus erythematosus–like drug eruptions

The reaction has been reported with a number of drugs,[121] but most frequently with procainamide and hydralazine (see the box on pp. 436 and 437). The reaction is dose related. A variety of skin signs can occur, including erythema with a "butterfly" rash, urticaria, livedo reticularis, and vasculitis, but they all are infrequently seen in drug-induced lupus. Clinical presentation includes arthritis, arthralgias, and elevated erythrocyte sedimentation rate. Fever, renal involvement, and CNS disease are rare. The ratio of females to males is 4:1. The antinuclear antibody (ANA), antihistone, and anti–single stranded DNA antibodies are markers for lupus-like drug eruptions. The predominant nuclear antibodies are directed against histone proteins.[122,123] In one study ANAs occurred in 83% of patients receiving procainamide for cardiac arrhythmias; they had no symptoms of a connective tissue disease. Significant elevation of antibody binding to single-stranded DNA and double-stranded DNA was seen; 65.4% had antibodies to total histones.[124] Serum complement levels remained normal. Dermoepidermal junction immunofluorescence, as measured by the "lupus-band test" was positive in 6% of patients with procainamide-induced lupus, compared with positive test results in 54% of patients with idiopathic systemic lupus erythematosus (SLE).[125] A genetic predisposition exists. Both drugs are inactivated by acetylation; most patients have the slow acetylation phenotype. The combination of HLA-DRW-4, female sex, slow acetylator status, and a minimum dosage of 200 mg/day of hydralazine inevitably leads to the syndrome.[126] Susceptible patients may be identified by determination of acetylator type and DR status. Stopping the drug results in rapid clinical improvement and gradual (months) disappearance of autoantibodies.

Photosensitivity

Both systemic and topical medications can induce photosensitivity. There are two main types: phototoxicity and photoallergy.

Phototoxic reactions are related to drug concentration and can occur in anyone. There is erythema within 24 hours of light exposure; brown pigmentation occurs after resolution. The eruption is confined to sun-exposed areas. The reaction can occur on first administration and subsides when the drug is stopped.

Photoallergic reactions are less common and are not concentration related. They occur in only a small fraction of people exposed and may spread to involve areas that have not been exposed to the sun. Typically there is a delay of 48 hours after exposure before the eruption appears. On rare occasions, the reaction can persist for years, even without further drug exposure.

Onycholysis (separation of the nail plate from the nail bed) may occur from drug photosensitivity and has occurred with tetracyclines, psoralens, and fluoroquinolones.

Pigmentation

Pigmentation can result from deposition of melanin, drug, or a combined product within the skin.

Vasculitis

Small vessel necrotizing vasculitis (palpable purpura) may be precipitated by drugs. Lesions are most often concentrated on the lower legs but may be generalized and involve the kidneys, joints, and brain.

Vesiculobullous eruptions

Blisters may develop alone, as part of other eruptions (e.g., erythema multiforme, toxic epidermal necrolysis, and fixed drug eruptions), or with exanthemic drug eruptions.[127]

Chemotherapy-induced acral erythema

Chemotherapy-induced acral erythema occurs most commonly with cytosine arabinoside, fluorouracil, doxorubicin, and, less often, with other drugs (see the box on p. 437).[128] It appears to be dose dependent, and a direct toxic effect of the drug is likely. The time of onset (24 hours to 10 months) and the severity is variable. Tingling on the palms and soles is followed in a few days by painful, symmetric, well-defined swelling and erythema. The hands are more severely affected than the feet and are sometimes the only area involved. During the next several days areas of pallor develop that blister, desquamate, and reepithelialize. Cytosine arabinoside has a predilection to progress to blisters; doxorubicin and fluorouracil are much less likely to cause blisters.[129] The progression takes 1 to 2 weeks once chemotherapy is stopped. The desquamation may be more dramatic and obvious than the erythema. Acute graft-vs.-host reaction has a similar appearance. Treatment is supportive, with elevation and cold compresses. Systemic steroids have been used with variable success. Cooling the hands and feet during treatment to decrease blood flow may attenuate the reaction. Modification of the dosage schedule may also help. Pyridoxine appears to decrease the intensity and pain caused by fluorouracil infusions.[130]

Drug-induced ocular pemphigoid

Drug-induced pemphigoid with progressive conjunctival shrinking and scarring has been documented from patients using topical glaucoma medications for extended periods. The disease may progress after the medication is discontinued. The diagnosis can be missed unless the fornices are inspected for shortening in patients using long-term topical medications. Immunofluorescent studies have not demonstrated IgG or C3.

Skin eruptions associated with specific drugs

Gold. Gold compounds are used primarily for the treatment of rheumatoid arthritis, but they have recently been proven effective for pemphigus[131,132] and psoriatic arthritis. There are many different forms of gold rashes. The most common type is a nonspecific, eczematous, papular, itchy eruption with no specific distribution or histologic features. Twenty-five percent of gold rashes resemble lichen planus, but the distribution is atypical and the oral cavity is rarely involved. Unlike idiopathic lichen planus, there are parakeratoses, eosinophils, neutrophils, and plasma cells with a diminished granular zone in the biopsy specimen. Patients who develop dermatitis following treatment with gold have T cells that proliferate in an HLA-DR–restricted manner. This observation may lead to more accurate diagnosis and treatment.[133] A pityriasis rosea–like eruption occurs, but dyskeratotic cells do not appear within the epidermis.[134] Gold therapy is stopped when a rash develops. All forms of dermatitis resolve at similar rates—the rate of resolution correlates with the extent of the rash and not with the specific morphologic form. The median duration to resolution is 10 weeks; the range is 10 days to 2 years. Unless the patient has erythema nodosum,[135] there is no increased risk of developing the rash when gold therapy is resumed.[136] Group V topical steroids provide symptomatic relief but do not hasten resolution. Systemic steroids may be required for severe reactions.

Cutaneous complications of chemotherapeutic agents. Cancer chemotherapeutic agents adversely affect rapidly dividing cells. Stomatitis, alopecia, onychodystrophy, chemical cellulitis, phlebitis, and hyperpigmentation occur with several agents. Self-limited palmar-plantar erythema, occasionally with bulla formation, has been reported (see above).

Anticonvulsant hypersensitivity syndrome. This syndrome has a variable spectrum of clinical and laboratory findings. There are fever, rash, lymphadenopathy, and hepatitis (hepatomegaly and increase in serum aminotransferase), with leukocytosis and eosinophilia. The three most commonly used anticonvulsants—phenytoin, phenobarbital, and carbamazepine—can each produce the reaction. Cutaneous reactions to phenytoin occur in up to 19% of patients. These vary from morbilliform eruptions to erythroderma, erythema multiforme, and toxic epidermal necrolysis. A small percentage of patients develop a hypersensitivity syndrome that presents with a macular or papular rash or erythroderma and, rarely, pustules.[137] The outcome depends on the severity of the hepatic injury and the presence of other complications. The reaction is serious and may result in death.

REFERENCES

1. Sison-Fonacier L, Bystryn J-C: Regional variations in antigenic properties of skin: a possible cause for disease-specific distribution of skin lesions, *J Exp Med* 164:2125-2130, 1986.
2. Remington PL et al: Airborne transmission of measles in a physician's office, *JAMA* 253:1574-1577, 1985.
3. Jespersen CS, Littauer J, Sagild U: Measles as a cause of fetal defects, *Acta Paediatr Scand* 66:367-372, 1977.
4. Martin DB et al: Atypical measles in adolescents and young adults, *Ann Intern Med* 90:887, 1979.
5. Frieden TR, Sowell AL, et al: Vitamin A levels and severity of measles. New York City, *Am J Dis Child* 146:182-186, 1992.
6. Fawzi WW, Chalmers TC, et al: Vitamin A supplementation and child mortality. A meta-analysis, *JAMA* 269:898-903, 1993.
7. Hussey GD, Klein M: A randomized, controlled trial of vitamin A in children with severe measles, *N Engl J Med* 323:160-164, 1990.
8. Caballero B, Rice A: Low serum retinol is associated with increased severity of measles in New York City children, *Nutr Rev* 50:291-292, 1992.
9. Coutsoudis A, Kiepiela P, et al: Vitamin A supplementation enhances specific IgG antibody levels and total lymphocyte numbers while improving morbidity in measles, *Pediatr Infect Dis J* 11:203-209, 1992.
10. Bluhm DP, Summers RS: Plasma vitamin A levels in measles and malnourished pediatric patients and their implications in therapeutics, *J Trop Pediatr* 39:179-182, 1993.
11. Halsey NA et al: Response to measles vaccine in Haitian infants 6 to 12 months old: influence of maternal antibodies, malnutrition, and concurrent illnesses, *N Engl J Med* 313:544-549, 1985.
12. Markowitz L et al: Patterns of transmission in measles outbreaks in the United States, 1985-1986, *N Engl J Med* 320:75-81, 1989.
13. Musser JM, Nelson K, et al: Temporal variation in bacterial disease frequency: molecular population genetic analysis of scarlet fever epidemics in Ottawa and in eastern Germany, *J Infect Dis* 167:759-762, 1993.
14. Knoll H, Sramek J, et al: Scarlet fever and types of erythrogenic toxins produced by the infecting streptococcal strains, *Int J Med Microbiol* 276:94-106, 1991.
15. Kelley PW, Petruccelli BP, et al: The susceptibility of young adult Americans to vaccine-preventable infections. A national serosurvey of US Army recruits, *JAMA* 266:2724-2729, 1991.
16. Lee SH, Ewert DP, et al: Resurgence of congenital rubella syndrome in the 1990s. Report on missed opportunities and failed prevention policies among women of childbearing age, *JAMA* 267:2616-2620, 1992.
17. Zolti M, Ben-Rafael Z, et al: Rubella-specific IgM in reinfection and risk to the fetus, *Gynecol Obstet Invest* 30:184-185, 1990.
18. Best JM, Banatvala JE, et al: Fetal infection after maternal reinfection with rubella: criteria for defining reinfection, *Br Med J* 299:773-775, 1989.
19. Miron D, On A: Congenital rubella syndrome after maternal immunization, *Harefuah* 122:291-293, 1992.
20. Skvorc-Ranko R, Lavoie H, et al: Intrauterine diagnosis of cytomegalovirus and rubella infections by amniocentesis, *Can Med Assoc J* 145:649-654, 1991.
21. Schoub BD, Blackburn NK, et al: Symptomatic rubella re-infection in early pregnancy and subsequent delivery of an infected but minimally involved infant. A case report, *S Afr Med J* 78:484-485, 1990.
22. Enders G, Knotek F: Rubella IgG total antibody avidity and IgG subclass-specific antibody avidity assay and their role in the differentiation between primary rubella and rubella reinfection, *Infection* 17:218-226, 1989.
23. Hedman K, Rousseau SA: Measurement of avidity of specific IgG for verification of recent primary rubella, *J Med Virol* 27:288-292, 1989.
24. Judelson RG, Wyll SA: Rubella in Bermuda: termination of an epidemic by mass vaccination, *JAMA* 223:401, 1973.
25. Brown KE et al: Resistance to parvovirus B19 infection due to lack of virus receptor (erythrocyte *P.* antigen), *N Engl J Med* 330:1192-1196, 1994.
26. Joseph PR: Incubation period of fifth disease, *Lancet* 2:1390-1391, 1986.
27. Halasz CL, Cormier D, et al: Petechial glove and sock syndrome caused by parvovirus B19, *J Am Acad Dermatol* 27:835-838, 1992.
28. Jacks TA: Pruritus in parvovirus infection, *J R Coll Gen Pract* 37:210, 1987.
29. Naides SJ: Parvovirus B19, *Rheum Dis Clin North Am* 19:457-475, 1993.
30. White DG et al: Human parvovirus arthropathy, *Lancet* 1:419-421, 1985.
31. Naides SJ et al: Rheumatologic manifestations of human parvovirus B19 infection in adults, *Arthritis Rheum* 33:1297-1309, 1990.
32. Mayo DR, Vance DW Jr: Parvovirus B19 as the cause of a syndrome resembling Lyme arthritis in adults, *N Engl J Med* 324:419-420, 1991.
33. Nocton JJ, Miller LC, et al: Human parvovirus B19-associated arthritis in children, *J Pediatr* 122:186-190, 1993.
34. Kovacs BW, Carlson DE, et al: Prenatal diagnosis of human parvovirus B19 in nonimmune hydrops fetalis by polymerase chain reaction, *Am J Obstet Gynecol* 167:461-466, 1992.
35. Sheikh AU, Ernest JM, et al: Long-term outcome in fetal hydrops from parvovirus B19 infection, *Am J Obstet Gynecol* 167:337-341, 1992.
36. Berry PJ, Gray ES, et al: Parvovirus infection of the human fetus and newborn, *Semin Diagn Pathol* 9:4-12, 1992.
37. Adler SP, Manganello AM, et al: Risk of human parvovirus B19 infections among school and hospital employees during endemic periods, *J Infect Dis* 168:361-368, 1993.
38. Torok TJ, Wang QY, et al: Prenatal diagnosis of intrauterine infection with parvovirus B19 by the polymerase chain reaction technique, *Clin Infect Dis* 14:149-155, 1992.
39. Serjeant GR, Serjeant BE, et al: Human parvovirus infection in homozygous sickle cell disease, *Lancet* 341:1237-1240, 1993.
40. Rao SP, Miller ST, et al: Transient aplastic crisis in patients with sickle cell disease. B19 parvovirus studies during a 7-year period, *Am J Dis Child* 146:1328-1330, 1992.
41. Bell LM et al: Human parvovirus B19 infection among hospital staff members after contact with infected patients, *N Eng J Med* 321:485-491, 1989.
42. Naides SJ, Howard EJ, et al: Parvovirus B19 infection in human immunodeficiency virus type 1–infected persons failing or intolerant to zidovudine therapy, *J Infect Dis* 168:101-105, 1993.
43. Kurtzman G et al: Pure red-cell aplasia of 10 years' duration due to persistent parvovirus B19 infection and its cure with immunoglobulin therapy, *N Eng J Med* 321:519-523, 1989.
44. Erdman DD, Usher MJ, et al: Human parvovirus B19 specific IgG, IgA, and IgM antibodies and DNA in serum specimens from persons with erythema infectiosum, *J Med Virol* 35:110-115, 1991.
45. Patou G, Pillay D, et al: Characterization of a nested polymerase chain reaction assay for detection of parvovirus B19, *J Clin Microbiol* 31:540-546, 1993.
46. Okada K, Ueda K, et al: Exanthema subitum and human herpesvirus 6 infection: clinical observations in fifty-seven cases, *Pediatr Infect Dis J* 12:204-208, 1993.
47. Akashi K et al: Brief report: severe infectious mononucleosis-like syndrome and primary human herpesvirus 6 infection in an adult, *N Engl J Med* 329:168-169, 1993.
48. Cone RW et al: Human herpesvirus 6 in lung tissue from patients with pneumonitis after bone marrow transplantation, *N Engl J Med* 329:156-161, 1993.
49. Pruksananonda P et al: Primary human herpesvirus 6 infection in young children, *N Eng J Med* 326:1445-1450, 1992.
50. Breese C et al: Human herpes virus-6 infection in children, *N Engl J Med* 331:432-438, 1994.
51. Hayashi M, Hasegawa T, et al: Long-term neurological outcome in children with convulsions during exanthema subitum, *No To Hattatsu* 25:53-58, 1993.

52. Suga S, Yoshikawa T, et al: Clinical and virological analyses of 21 infants with exanthem subitum (roseola infantum) and central nervous system complications, *Ann Neurol* 33:597-603, 1993.

53. Kondo K, Nagafuji H, et al: Association of human herpesvirus 6 infection of the central nervous system with recurrence of febrile convulsions, *J Infect Dis* 167:1197-1200, 1993.

54. Segondy M et al: Herpesvirus 6 infection in young children, *N Eng J Med* 327:1099-1100, 1992.

55. Wiersbitzky S, Abel E, et al: The blood picture in exanthema subitum (Zahorsky): critical 3-day fever-exanthema in young children, *Kinderarztl Prax* 59:258-261, 1991.

56. Meade RH III, Brandt L: Manifestations of Kawasaki disease in New England outbreak of 1980, *Pediatrics* 97:780, 1980.

57. Abe J, Kotzin BL, et al: Characterization of T cell repertoire changes in acute Kawasaki disease, *J Exp Med* 177:791-796, 1993.

58. Sato N, Sagawa K, et al: Immunopathology and cytokine detection in the skin lesions of patients with Kawasaki disease, *J Pediatr* 122:198-203, 1993.

59. Akiyama T, Yashiro K: Probable role of *Streptococcus pyogenes* in Kawasaki disease, *Eur J Pediatr* 152:82-92, 1993.

60. Leung DYM et al: Toxic shock syndrome toxin-secreting *staphylococcus aureus* in Kawasaki syndrome, *Lancet* 342:1385, 1995.

61. Shulman ST, Melish M, et al: Immunoglobulin allotypic markers in Kawasaki disease, *J Pediatr* 122:84-86, 1993.

62. Bishop WP, Kao SC: Prolonged postprandial abdominal pain following Kawasaki syndrome with acute gallbladder hydrops: association with impaired gallbladder emptying, *J Pediatr Gastroenterol Nutr* 13:307-311, 1991.

63. Morens DM, Anderson LJ, Hurwitz ES: National surveillance of Kawasaki disease, *Pediatrics* 65:21-25, 1980.

64. Nakamura Y, Fujita Y, et al: Cardiac sequelae of Kawasaki disease in Japan: statistical analysis, *Pediatrics* 88:1144-1147, 1991.

65. Wu JR, Hwang KP, et al: Study on coronary artery lesions in patients with Kawasaki disease: recent 9 years' experience, *Kao Hsiung I Hsueh Ko Hsueh Tsa Chih* 9:27-38, 1993.

66. Newburger JW et al: The treatment of Kawasaki syndrome with intravenous gamma globulin, *N Engl J Med* 315:341-347, 1986.

67. Naoe S, Takahashi K, et al: Kawasaki disease, with particular emphasis on arterial lesions, *Acta Pathol Jpn* 41:785-797, 1991.

68. Akagi T, Rose V, et al: Outcome of coronary artery aneurysms after Kawasaki disease, *J Pediatr* 121:689-694, 1992.

69. Newburger JW et al: A single intravenous infusion of gamma globulin as compared with four infusions in the treatment of acute Kawasaki syndrome, *N Eng J Med* 324:1633-1639, 1991.

70. Kondo C, Nakanishi T, et al: Scintigraphic monitoring of coronary artery occlusion due to Kawasaki disease, *Am J Cardiol* 71:681-685, 1993.

71. Nakamura Y, Yanagawa H, et al: Mortality among children with Kawasaki disease in Japan, *N Engl J Med* 326:1246-1249, 1992.

72. Fujiwara T, Fujiwara H, Hamashima Y: Frequency and size of coronary arterial aneurysm at necropsy in Kawasaki disease, *Am J Cardiol* 59:808-811, 1987.

73. Umezawa T, Matsuo N, et al: Treatment of Kawasaki disease using the intravenous aspirin anti-inflammatory effect of salicylate, *Acta Paediatr Jpn* 34:584-588, 1992.

74. Feigin RD, Barron KS: Treatment of Kawasaki syndrome, *N Engl J Med* 315:388-390, 1986.

75. Hsu CH, Chen MR, et al: Efficacy of plasmin-treated intravenous gamma-globulin for therapy of Kawasaki syndrome, *Pediatr Infect Dis J* 12:509-512, 1993.

76. Shulman ST: Recommendations for intravenous immunoglobulin therapy of Kawasaki disease, *Pediatr Infect Dis J* 11:985-986, 1992.

77. Dwyer JM: Manipulating the immune system with immune globulin, *N Engl J Med* 326:107-116, 1992.

78. Markowitz LE, Hightower AW, Broome CV, et al: Toxic shock syndrome: evaluation of national surveillance data using a hospital discharge survey, *JAMA* 258:75-78, 1987.

79. Reingold AL: Epidemiology of toxic shock syndrome, United States, 1960-1984, *MMWR* 33:19SS-22SS, 1984.

80. Reingold AL et al: Nonmenstrual toxic shock syndrome: a review of 130 cases, *Ann Intern Med* 96:871-874, 1982.

81. Garbe PL et al: *Staphylococcus aureus* isolates from patients with nonmenstrual toxic shock syndrome: evidence for additional toxins, *JAMA* 253:2538-2542, 1985.

82. Berkley SF, Hightower AW, Broome CV, et al: The relationship of tampon characteristics to menstrual toxic shock syndrome, *JAMA* 258:917-920, 1987.

83. Hoge CW, Schwartz B, et al: The changing epidemiology of invasive group A streptococcal infections and the emergence of streptococcal toxic shock-like syndrome. A retrospective population-based study, *JAMA* 269:384-389, 1993.

84. Schlievert PM, Gocke JE, et al: Group B streptococcal toxic shock-like syndrome: report of a case and purification of an associated pyrogenic toxin, *Clin Infect Dis* 17:26-31, 1993.

85. Torres-Martinez C, Mehta D, et al: Streptococcus associated toxic shock, *Arch Dis Child* 67:126-130, 1992.

86. Chapnick EK, Gradon JD, et al: Streptococcal toxic shock syndrome due to noninvasive pharyngitis, *Clin Infect Dis* 14:1074-1077, 1992.

87. Stevens DL et al: Severe group A streptococcal infections associated wtih a toxic shock–like syndrome and scarlet fever toxin A, *N Engl J Med* 321:1-7, 1989.

88. Talkington DF, Schwartz B, et al: Association of phenotypic and genotypic characteristics of invasive *Streptococcus pyogenes* isolates with clinical components of streptococcal toxic shock syndrome, *Infect Immun* 61:3369-3374, 1993.

89. Wood TF, Potter MA, et al: Streptococcal toxic shock-like syndrome. The importance of surgical intervention, *Ann Surg* 217:109-114, 1993.

90. Wolfe SM: Dangerous delays in tampon absorbency warnings, *JAMA* 258:949-951, 1987.

91. Schuchat A, Broome CV: Toxic shock syndrome and tampons, *Epidemiol Rev* 13:99-112, 1991.

92. Reingold AL: Toxic shock syndrome: an update, *Am J Obstet Gynecol* 165:1236-1239, 1991.

93. Resnick SD: Staphylococcal toxin-mediated syndromes in childhood, *Semin Dermatol* 11:11-18, 1992.

94. Kain KC, Schulzer M, et al: Clinical spectrum of nonmenstrual toxic shock syndrome (TSS): comparison with menstrual TSS by multivariate discriminant analyses, *Clin Infect Dis* 16:100-106, 1993.

95. Hurwitz RM, Ackerman AB: Cutaneous pathology of the toxic shock syndrome, *Am J Dermatopathol* 7:563-578, 1985.

96. Tolan R Jr: Toxic shock syndrome complicating influenza A in a child: case report and review, *Clin Infect Dis* 17:43-45, 1993.

97. Bigby M, Jick S, Jick H, et al: Drug-induced cutaneous reactions: a report from the Boston collaborative drug surveillance program on 15,438 consecutive inpatients, 1975 to 1982, *JAMA* 256:3358-3363, 1986.

98. Roujeau JC, Stern RS: Severe adverse cutaneous reactions to drugs, *N Engl J Med* 331:1272-1285, 1994.

99. Alanko K, Stubb S, Kauppinen K: Cutaneous drug reactions—clinical types and causative agents: a five-year survey of in-patients (1981-1985), *Acta Derm Venereol* (Stockh) 69:223-226, 1989.

100. Hoigne R et al: Occurrence of exanthems in relation to aminopenicillin preparations and allopurinol, *N Engl J Med* 316:1217, 1987.

101. Bigby M, Stern RS, et al: Allergic cutaneous reactions to drugs, *Prim Care* 16:713-727, 1989.

102. Sehgal VH, Gangwani OP: Genital fixed drug eruptions, *Genitourin Med* 62:56-58, 1986.

103. Smoller BR, Luster AD, et al: Fixed drug eruptions: evidence for a cytokine-mediated process, *J Cutan Pathol* 18:13-19, 1991.

104. Thankappan TP, Zachariah J: Drug-specific clinical pattern in fixed drug eruptions, *Int J Dermatol* 30:867-870, 1991.

105. Gaffoor PM, George WM: Fixed drug eruptions occurring on the male genitals, *Cutis* 45:242-244, 1990.

106. Hatzis J, Noutsis K, et al: Fixed drug eruption in a mother and her son, *Cutis* 50:50-52, 1992.

107. Pellicano R, Silvestris A, et al: Familial occurrence of fixed drug eruptions, *Acta Derm Venereol* 72:292-293, 1992.
108. Roetzheim RG, Herold AH, et al: Nonpigmenting fixed drug eruption caused by diflunisal, *J Am Acad Dermatol* 24:1021-1022, 1991.
109. Desmeules H: Nonpigmenting fixed drug eruption after anesthesia, *Anesth Analg* 70:216-217, 1990.
110. Benson PM, Giblin WJ, et al: Transient, nonpigmenting fixed drug eruption caused by radiopaque contrast media, *J Am Acad Dermatol* 23:381-385, 1990.
111. Jain VK, Dixit VB, et al: Fixed drug eruption of the oral mucous membrane, *Ann Dent* 50:9-11, 1991.
112. Korkij W, Soltani K: Fixed drug eruption: a brief review, *Arch Dermatol* 120:520-524, 1984.
113. Sehgal VN, Gangwani OP: Fixed drug eruption: current concepts, *Int J Dermatol* 26:67-74, 1987.
114. Bargman H: Lack of cross-sensitivity between tetracycline, doxycycline, and minocycline with regard to fixed drug sensitivity to tetracycline, *J Am Acad Dermatol* 11:900-901, 1984.
115. Kauppinen K, Stubb S: Fixed eruptions: causative drugs and challenge tests, *Br J Dermatol* 112:575-578, 1985.
116. Zanolli MD, McAlvany J, et al: Phenolphthalein-induced fixed drug eruption: a cutaneous complication of laxative use in a child, *Pediatrics* 91:1199-1201, 1993.
117. Kanwar AJ, Bharija SC, et al: Ninety-eight fixed drug eruptions with provocation tests, *Dermatologica* 177:274-279, 1988.
118. Osawa J, Naito S, et al: Evaluation of skin test reactions in patients with non-immediate type drug eruptions, *J Dermatol* 17:235-239, 1990.
119. Lee AY, Lee YS: Provocation tests in a chlormezanone-induced fixed drug eruption, *Drug Intell Clin Pharm* 25:604-605, 1991.
120. Halevy S, Shai A: Lichenoid drug eruptions, *J Am Acad Dermatol* 29:249-255, 1993.
121. Hess EV: Drug-related lupus, *Curr Opin Rheumatol* 3:809-814, 1991.
122. Monestier M, Kotzin BL: Antibodies to histones in systemic lupus erythematosus and drug-induced lupus syndromes, *Rheum Dis Clin North Am* 18:415-436, 1992.
123. Adams LE, Balakrishnan K, et al: Genetic, immunologic and biotransformation studies of patients on procainamide, *Lupus* 2:89-98, 1993.
124. Mongey AB, Donovan-Brand R, et al: Serologic evaluation of patients receiving procainamide, *Arthritis Rheum* 35:219-223, 1992.
125. Batchelor JR et al: Hydralazine-induced systemic lupus erythematosus: influence of HLA-DB and sex on susceptibility, *Lancet* 1:1107, 1980.
126. Kauppinen K, Stubb S: Drug eruptions: causative agents and clinical types—series of inpatients during a 10-year period, *Acta Derm Venereol* (Stockh) 64:320-324, 1984.
127. Fiore PM, Jacobs IV, Goldberg DB: Drug-induced pemphigoid: a spectrum of diseases, *Arch Ophthalmol* 105:1660-1663, 1987.
128. Baack BR, Burgdorf WHC: Chemotherapy-induced acral erythema, *J Am Acad Dermatol* 24:457-461, 1991.
129. Waltzer JF, Flowers FP: Bullous variant of chemotherapy-induced acral erythema, *Arch Dermatol* 129:43-45, 1993.
130. Vukelja SJ et al: Pyridoxine for the palmar-plantar erythrodysesthesia syndrome, *Ann Intern Med* 111:688-689, 1989.
131. Walton S, Keczkes K: Pemphigus foliaceus: successful treatment with adjuvant gold therapy, *Clin Exper Dermatol* 12:364-365, 1987.
132. Tumiati B, Baricchi R, Bellelli A: Psoriatic arthritis: long term treatment with auranofin, *Clin Rheumatol* 5:124-125, 1986.
133. Verwilghen J, Kingsley GH, et al: Activation of gold-reactive T lymphocytes in rheumatoid arthritis patients treated with gold, *Arthritis Rheum* 35:1413-1418, 1992.
134. Okamoto H et al: Dyskeratotic degeneration of epidermal cells in pityriasis rosea: light and electron microscopic studies, *Br J Dermatol* 107:189, 1982.
135. Stone RL, Claflin A, Penneys NS: Erythema nodosum following gold sodium thiomalate therapy, *Arch Dermatol* 107:602-604, 1972.
136. Klinefelter HF: Reinstitution of gold therapy in rheumatoid arthritis after mucocutaneous reaction, *J Rheumatol* 2:21-27, 1975.
137. Kleier RS, Breneman DL, et al: Generalized pustulation as a manifestation of the anticonvulsant hypersensitivity syndrome, *Arch Dermatol* 127:1361-1364, 1991.

CHAPTER FIFTEEN

Infestations and Bites

Scabies

Human scabies is a contagious disease caused by the mite *Sarcoptes scabiei* var. *hominis*. Dogs and cats may be infested by almost identical organisms; these sometimes may be a source for human infestation.[1] In the past, scabies was attributed to poor hygiene. Most contemporary cases, however, appear in individuals with adequate hygiene who are in close contact with numbers of individuals, such as schoolchildren. Blacks rarely acquire scabies; the reason is unknown.

Anatomic features, life cycle, and immunology

ANATOMIC FEATURES. The adult mite is $1/3$ mm long and has a flattened, oval body with wrinklelike, transverse corrugations and eight legs (Figure 15-1). The front two pairs of legs bear claw-shaped suckers and the two rear pairs end in long, trailing bristles. The digestive tract fills a major portion of the body and is readily observed when the mite is seen in cross-section of histologic specimens (Figure 15-2, *A*).

INFESTATION AND LIFE CYCLE. Infestation begins when a fertilized female mite arrives on the skin surface. Within an hour, the female excavates a burrow in the stratum corneum (dead, horny layer) (Figure 15-2, *B*). During the mite's 30-day life cycle, the burrow extends from several millimeters to a few centimeters in length. The burrow does not enter the underlying epidermis except in the case of hyperkeratotic Norwegian scabies, a condition in which retarded, immunosuppressed, or elderly patients develop scaly, thick skin in the presence of thousands of mites. Eggs laid at the rate of 2 or 3 a day (Figure 15-3) and fecal pellets (scybala) are deposited in the burrow behind the advancing female. Scybala are dark, oval masses that are seen easily with the eggs when burrow scrapings are examined under a microscope. Scybala may act as an irritant and may be responsible for some of the itching. The larvae hatch, leaving the egg casings in the burrow, and reach maturity in 14 to 17 days. The adult mites copulate and repeat the cycle. Therefore, 3 to 5 weeks after infestation, there are only a few mites present. This life cycle explains why patients experience few if any symptoms during the first month after contact with an infested individual. After a number of mites (usually less than 20) have reached maturity and have spread by migration or the patient's scratching, the initial, minor, localized itch evolves into intense, generalized pruritis.

IMMUNOLOGY. A hypersensitivity reaction rather than a foreign-body response may be responsible for the lesions, which may delay recognition of symptoms of scabies. Some patients infested with scabies develop elevated IgE titers, eosinophilia, and an immediate-type hypersensitivity reaction to an extract prepared from female mites.[2] IgE levels fall within a year after infestation. Eosinophilia returns to normal shortly after treatment. The fact that patients develop symptoms much more rapidly when reinfested supports the claim that the symptoms and lesions of scabies are the result of a hypersensitivity reaction.

Clinical manifestations.

Transmission of scabies occurs during direct skin contact with an infected person. Whether or not the mite can be acquired from infested clothing or bed linen is not known. A mite can possibly survive for days in normal home surroundings after leaving human skin.[3] Mites survive up to 7 days in mineral oil microscopic slide mounts.

SYMPTOMS. The disease begins insidiously. Symptoms are minor at first and are attributed to a bite or dry skin. Scratching destroys burrows and removes mites, providing initial relief. The patient remains comfortable during the day

Figure 15-1
Sarcoptes scabiei in a potassium hydroxide wet mount (× 40).

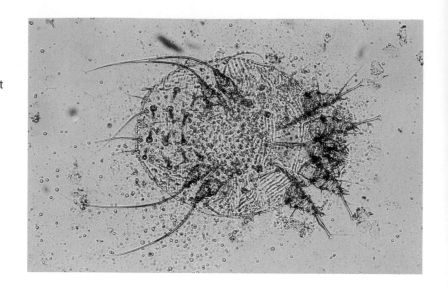

Figure 15-2 *Sarcoptes scabiei.*

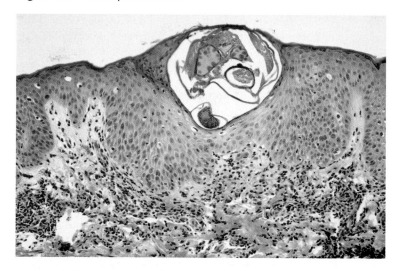

A, Cross-section of a mite in the stratum corneum.

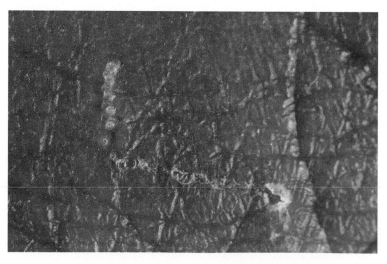

B, Burrow. The mite excavates a burrow in the stratum corneum (the dead, horny layer of the epidermis).

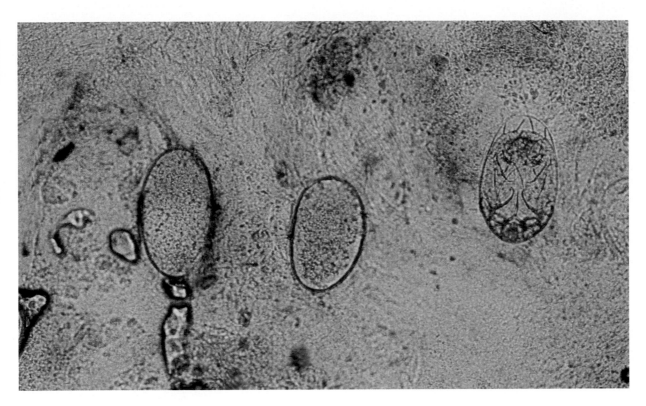

Figure 15-3
Sarcoptes scabiei. Eggs containing mites. A potassium
hydroxide wet mount (× 40).

but itches at night. Nocturnal pruritis is highly characteristic
of scabies. Scratching spreads mites to other areas and after
6 to 8 weeks the once localized area of minor irritation has
become a widespread, intensely pruritic eruption.

The most characteristic features of the lesions are pleo-
morphism and a tendency to remain discrete and small.
Primary lesions are soon destroyed by scratching.

Primary lesions. Mites are found in burrows and at the
edge of vesicles, but rarely in papules.

Burrow. The linear, curved, or S-shaped burrows are
approximately as wide as #2 suture material and are 2 to 15
mm long (Figure 15-2, *B*). They are pink-white and slightly
elevated. A vesicle or the mite, which may look like a black
dot at one end of the burrow, often may be seen. Scratching
destroys burrows, therefore they do not appear in some
patients. Burrows are most likely to be found in the finger
webs, wrists, sides of the hands and feet, penis, buttocks,
scrotum, and the palms and soles of infants.

Vesicles and papules. Vesicles are isolated, pinpoint,
and filled with serous rather than purulent fluid. The fact
that they remain discrete is a key point in differentiating scabies from other vesicular diseases such as poison ivy. The
finger webs are the most likely area to find intact vesicles
(Figure 15-4). Infants may have vesicles or pustules on the
palms and soles. Small, discrete papules may represent a
hypersensitivity reaction and rarely contain mites.

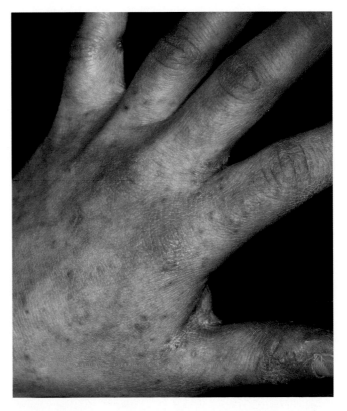

Figure 15-4
Scabies. Tiny vesicles and papules in the finger webs and
back of the hand.

Secondary lesions. Secondary lesions result from infection or are caused by scratching. They often dominate the clinical picture. Pinpoint erosions are the most common secondary lesions. Pustules are a sign of secondary infection (Figure 15-5). Scaling, erythema, and all stages of eczematous inflammation occur as a response to excoriation or to irritation caused by overzealous attempts at self-medication.

Nodules occur in covered areas such as the buttocks, groin, scrotum, penis, and axillae. The 2- to 10-mm indolent, red papules and nodules sometimes have slightly eroded surfaces, especially on the glans penis (Figure 15-6). Nodules may persist for weeks or months after the mites have been eradicated. They may result from persisting antigens of mite parts.[4]

Figure 15-5
Scabies. Pustules on the palms of an infant. Note the papular lesions on the wrist.

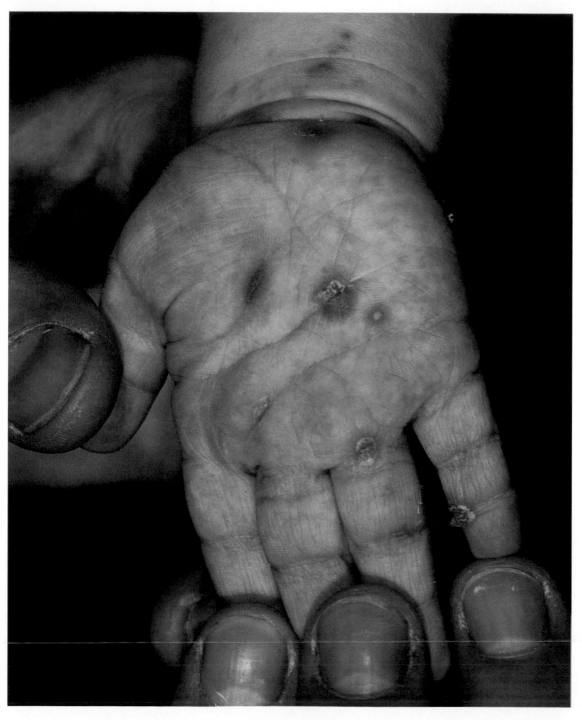

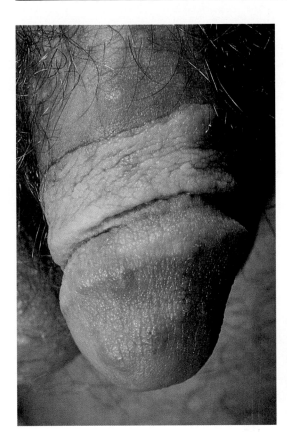

Figure 15-6 Scabies of the penis and scrotum.

A, Eroded papules on the glans is a highly characteristic sign of scabies.

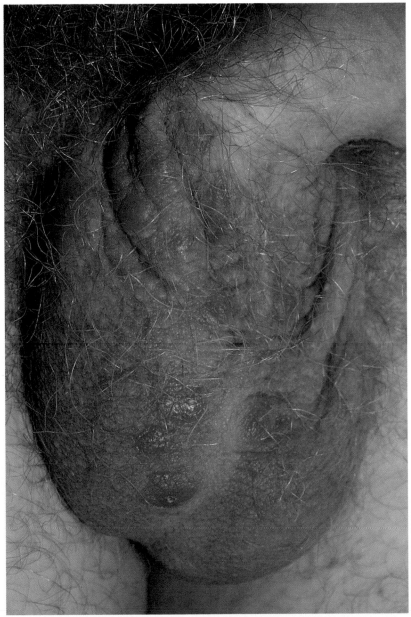

B, An established infestation of the penis and scrotum. Large papules may remain after appropriate therapy and sometimes require treatment with intralesional steroids.

Distribution. Lesions of scabies are typically found in the finger webs, wrists, extensor surfaces of the elbows and knees, sides of the hands and feet, axillary areas, buttocks, waist area, and ankle area (Figures 15-7 and 15-8). In men, the penis and scrotum are usually involved; in women, the breast, including the areola and nipple, may be infested. Lesions, often vesicular or pustular, may be most numerous on the palms and soles of infants. The scalp and face, rarely involved in adults, occasionally are infested in infants.

The number and type of lesions and the extent of involvement vary greatly among patients. Some patients have a few itchy vesicles in the finger webs early in the course of their disease. Many patients in these early stages attempt self-treatment and are encouraged by the relief obtained from over-the-counter, antipruritic lotions. Topical steroids offer greater relief, but mask the progressive disease by suppressing inflammation. Delay of proper treatment allows the eruption to extend into all of the characteristic areas, as well as onto the trunk, arms, legs, and occasionally the face. Extensive involvement is often accompanied by erythema, scaling, and infection. Infants and children have diffuse scabies more often than do adults. Symptoms vary from periods of nocturnal pruritis to constant, frantic itching. Untreated scabies can last for months or years.

Infants. Infants, more frequently than adults, have widespread involvement. This may occur because the diagnosis is not suspected and proper treatment is delayed while medication is given for other suspected causes of itching, such as dry skin, eczema, and infection. Infants occasionally are infested on the face and scalp, something rarely seen in adults. Vesicles are common on the palms and soles; this is a highly characteristic sign of scabies in infants (Figure 15-9). Secondary eczematization and impetiginization are common, but burrows are difficult to find. Nodules may be seen in the axillae and diaper area.

The elderly. Elderly patients may have few cutaneous lesions, but itch severely. The decreased immunity associated with advanced age may allow the mites to multiply and survive in great numbers. These patients have few cutaneous lesions other than excoriations, dry skin, and scaling, but they experience intense itching. Eventually papules and nodules appear and may become numerous. Entire nursing home populations may be infested (see treatment section). A skin scraping from any scaling area may show numerous mites at all stages of development.

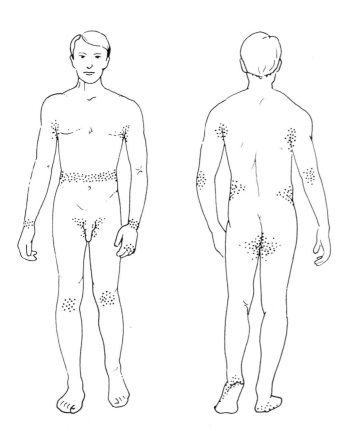

Figure 15-7
Scabies. Distribution of lesions.

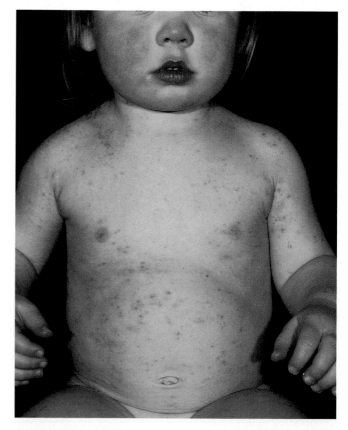

Figure 15-8
Diffuse scabies on an infant. The face is clear. The lesions are most numerous around the axillae, chest, and abdomen.

Crusted (Norwegian) scabies. The term *Norwegian scabies* was first used in 1848 to describe an overwhelming scabies infestation of patients with Hansen's disease. In patients with crusted scabies, lesions tend to involve hands and feet with asymptomatic crusting rather than the typical inflammatory papules and vesicles. There is thick, subungual, keratotic material and nail dystrophy. Digits and sites of trauma may show wartlike formations. Gray scales and thick crusts may be present over the trunk and extremities. Desquamation of the facial skin may occur. The hair may shed profusely. Crusted scabies occurs in people with neurologic or mental disorders (especially Down's syndrome), senile dementia, nutritional disorders, infectious diseases, leukemia, and immunosuppression (such as patients with AIDS).[3,5,6] Itching may be absent or severe. A lack of immunity and indifference to pruritis have been suggested as reasons for the development of this distinct clinical picture. A mineral oil or potassium hydroxide examination of crusts shows numerous mites at all stages of development.

Diagnosis. The diagnosis is suspected when burrows are found or when a patient has typical symptoms with characteristic lesions and distribution (see the box at right).

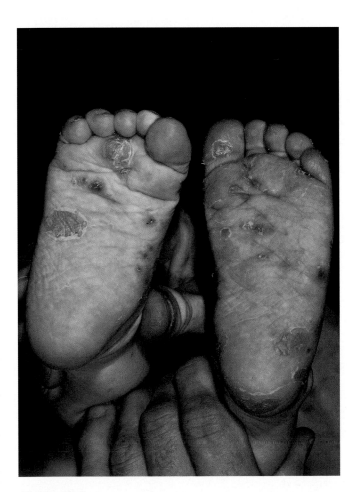

Figure 15-9
Scabies. Infestation of the palms and soles is common in infants. The vesicular lesions have all ruptured.

SIGNS AND SYMPTOMS OF SCABIES
Nodules on the penis and scrotum
Rash present for 4 to 8 weeks has suddenly become worse
Pustules on the palms and soles of infants
Nocturnal itching
Generalized, severe itching
Pinpoint erosions and crusts on the buttocks
Vesicles in the finger webs
Diffuse eruption sparing the face
Patient becomes better, then worse, after treatment with topical steroids
Rash is present in several members of the same family
Patient (especially an infant) develops more extensive rash despite treatment with antibiotics and topical medications

A definite diagnosis is made when any of the following products are obtained from burrows or vesicles and identified microscopically: mites, eggs, egg casings (hatched eggs), or feces (scybala).

Burrow identification. Initially, the areas most apt to contain burrows are observed. To enhance burrows for better viewing, the surface should be touched with a drop of mineral or immersion oil or a blue or black fountain or felt-tip pen (the ink method dyes the burrow; surface ink may be removed with an alcohol swab). The burrow absorbs the ink and is highlighted as a dark line (Figure 15-10). The accentuated lesions are smoothly scraped away with a curved #15 scalpel blade and transferred to a glass microscope slide for examination.

Papules and vesicles. Nonexcoriated papules and vesicles may be sampled, but do not usually contain the eggs and egg casings found in an established burrow.

Sampling techniques and slide mount preparation. Various techniques are available for obtaining diagnostic material. In most cases the suspected lesion can be sampled easily if it is shaved or scraped with a #15 surgical blade and the material is transferred to a microscope slide for direct examination.

MINERAL OIL MOUNTS. A drop of mineral oil may be placed over the suspected lesion prior to removal. Skin scrapings adhere, feces are preserved, and the mite remains alive and motile in clear oil. Squamous cells do not separate when heated in a clear oil mount and mites under a clump of squamous cells may be missed.

POTASSIUM HYDROXIDE WET MOUNTS. The scrapings are transferred directly to a glass side, a drop of potassium hydroxide is added, and a cover slip is applied. If diagnostic material is not found, the preparation is gently heated and the cover slip is pressed to separate squamous cells. Feces remain intact for short periods, but may be dissolved quickly when the mount is heated. Skin biopsy is rarely necessary to make the diagnosis.

Treatment and management

Permethrin. Permethrin (Elimite cream) is a synthetic pyrethrin that demonstrates extremely low mammalian toxicity.[7] Many clinicians feel that this is now the scabicide of choice. A large study compared 5% permethrin cream with 1% lindane lotion. Complete resolution occurred in 91% of patients treated with permethrin and in 86% of patients given lindane. Pruritis persisted in 14% of the permethrin group and in 25% of the lindane group.[8] Permethrin is safe and effective, even in areas such as Panama[9] where this disease has become resistant to lindane.[10] One application is highly effective for treating scabies and is a safe alternative to lindane.[11]

Lindane. Lindane is the generic name for the chemical gamma benzene hexachloride, a compound chemically similar to an agricultural pesticide also referred to as lindane. Kwell is one brand name for lindane. Generic lindane is available. Lindane is available as a cream, shampoo, and lotion. Some dermatologists feel that the cream is the most reliable form of medication for scabies. Lotion dispensed from bulk containers may not be agitated, therefore the concentration of lindane may be inadequate. When used properly, lindane is an effective scabicide and may be used for children of all ages and pregnant and nursing mothers. Reports of lindane-resistant scabies are beginning to appear.[10,12]

Controversy exists about the safety of lindane because of reports of neurotoxicity in infants following systemic absorption through the skin.[13] Further evaluation of these few case reports revealed that lindane had been misused substantially. Children with severe, underlying, cutaneous disease may be at greater risk for developing toxicity. This is also true for premature, emaciated, or malnourished children and those with a history of seizure disorders.[14]

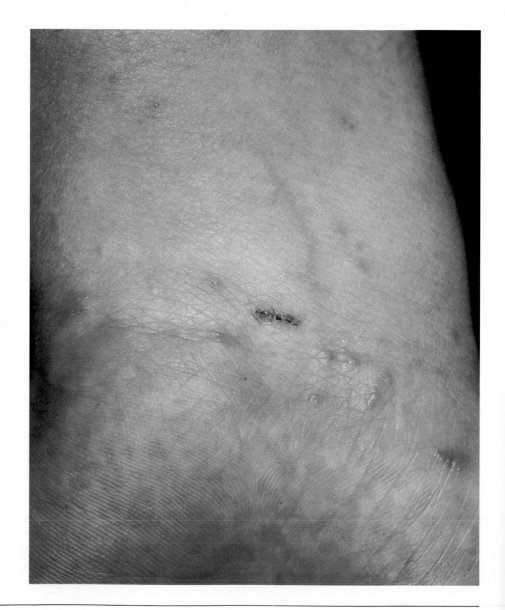

Figure 15-10
Felt-tipped ink pen has penetrated and highlighted a burrow. The ink is retained after the surface is wiped clean with an alcohol swab.

Ivermectin. In one study the anthelmintic agent ivermectin (6 mg tablets), given in a single oral dose (200 μg per kilogram), was found to be an effective and safe treatment for scabies in otherwise healthy patients and in patients with HIV infection.[15] The average adult dose was 9 to 18 mg depending on body weight. Pruritus was rapidly controlled. Patients with thick crusted lesions would be expected to do better with a combination of ivermectin and topical treatment such as permethrin cream. Ivermectin may prove useful for the treatment of large groups, such as in nursing homes.

Sulfur. Sulfur has been used to treat scabies for more than 150 years. The pharmacist mixes 6% (5% to 10% range) precipitated sulfur in petrolatum or a cold cream base. The compound is applied to the entire body below the neck once each day for 3 days. The patient is instructed to bathe 24 hours after each application. Sulfur applied in this manner is highly effective, but these preparations are messy, have an unpleasant odor, stain, and cause dryness.[16] Sulfur in petrolatum was thought to be safer than lindane for treating infants, but the safety of topical sulfur has never been established.[17]

APPLICATION TECHNIQUE FOR PERMETHRIN AND LINDANE. The cream or lotion is applied to all skin surfaces below the neck and the face in children. Patients with relapsing scabies and the elderly should be treated from head (including the scalp) to toe. One ounce is usually adequate for adults. Reapply medicine to the hands if hands are washed. The nails should be cut short and medication applied under them vigorously with a toothbrush.[18,19] A hot, soapy bath is not necessary prior to application. Moisture increases the permeability of the epidermis and increases the chance for systemic absorption. Infants should have lindane applied during the day and be fully clothed and observed to prevent licking of treated sites. If licking cannot be prevented, sulfur or permethrin should be used. Adults wash 12 hours after application and infants should be washed 8 to 12 hours[20] after application. One application of either medicine is considered adequate. The *Physicians' Desk Reference* recommends one application of lindane, but one expert recommends two applications 1 week apart.[14]

Patients should be told that it is normal to continue to itch for days or weeks after treatment and that further application of medication is usually not necessary and worsens itching by causing irritation. Bland lubricants may be applied to relieve itching.

Crotamiton (Eurax lotion). A study of children with scabies showed an 89% cure rate after 4 weeks with permethrin 5% cream (Elimite) and a 60% cure rate with crotamiton cream.[21] The toxicity of crotamiton is unknown. Reported cure rates for once-a-day application for 5 days range from 50% to 100%.[14] Crotamiton may have antipruritic properties, but this has been questioned.

MANAGEMENT OF SCABIES EPIDEMIC IN AN EXTENDED-CARE FACILITY

1. Educate patients, staff, family, and frequent visitors about scabies and the need for cooperation in treatment.
2. Apply scabicide to all patients, staff, contact staff, and frequent visitors, symptomatic or not. Treat symptomatic family members of staff and visitors.
3. Launder all bedding and clothes worn in the last 48 hours in hot water (or dry clean).
4. Clean beds and floors with routine cleaning agents just before scabicide is removed.
5. Reexamine for treatment failures in 1 week and 4 weeks.

Eradication program for nursing homes. Scabies is a problem in nursing homes.[22,23] The severity is greater than in an ambulatory population. The face and scalp can be involved, and multiple treatments may be necessary. The first problem is proper diagnosis. The elderly have an atypical presentation with few lesions other than excoriations, dry skin, and scaling, but they experience intense itching. Lesions are located on the back and buttocks rather than the web spaces, axilla, and groin. A plan for eradication of scabies in nursing homes is outlined in the box above.

Management of complications

Eczematous inflammation and pyoderma. Although there is little evidence that lindane is absorbed in greater quantity through inflamed skin, it seems prudent to control secondary changes prior to the application of this scabicide. Patients with signs of infection should be started on appropriate oral antibiotics. A group V topical steroid may be applied three times a day to all red, scaling lesions for 1 or 2 days prior to the application of lindane.

Postscabietic pruritis. Itching usually decreases substantially 24 hours after treatment with lindane and then gradually decreases during the following week or two. Patients with persistent itching may be treated with oral antihistamines, and, if inflammation is present, they may be treated with topical steroids.

Nodular scabies. Persistent nodular lesions, most commonly found on the scrotum, are treated with intralesional steroids (e.g., triamcinolone acetonide [Kenalog] 10 mg/ml).

Environmental management. Intimate contacts and all family members in the same household should be treated. Clothing that has touched infected skin probably plays a minimal role in the transmission of scabies; however, it is difficult to convince patients of that fact. Patients should wash all clothing, towels, and bed linen (in a normal washing machine cycle) that have touched the skin. It is not necessary to rewash clean clothing that has not yet been worn. Emphasize that coats, furniture, rugs, floors, and walls do not need to be cleaned in any special manner.

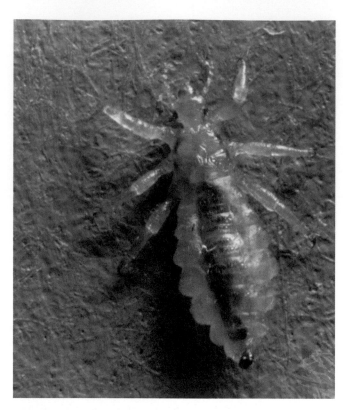

Figure 15-11
Body louse. The largest of three lice infesting humans.
(Courtesy Ken Gray, Oregon State University Extension Services.)

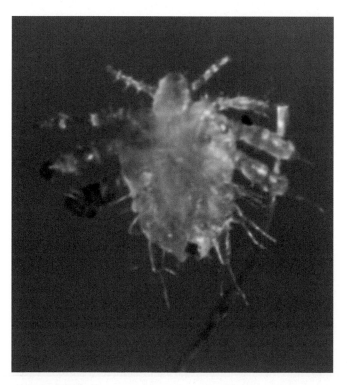

Figure 15-12
Crab louse has a short body and large claws used to grasp hair. *(Courtesy Ken Gray, Oregon State University Extension Services.)*

Pediculosis

Infestation with lice is called *pediculosis*. Lice are transmitted by close personal contact and contact with objects such as combs, hats, clothing, and bed linen. Diagnosis is made by seeing the lice or their eggs. Treatment with lindane, permethrin, or pyrethrins is effective.

Biology and life cycle. Lice are obligate human parasites that cannot survive off their host for more than 10 days (adults) to 3 weeks (fertile eggs). Actual survival rates may be shorter than this. Lice are called *ectoparasites* because they live on, rather than in, the body. They are classified as insects because they have six legs. Three kinds of lice infest humans: *Pediculus humanus* var. *capitis* (head louse), *Pediculus humanus* var. *corporis* (body louse), and *Pthirus pubis* (pubic or crab louse). All three have similar anatomic characteristics. Each is a small (less than 2 mm), flat, wingless insect with three pairs of legs located on the anterior part of the body directly behind the head. The legs terminate in sharp claws that are adapted for feeding and permit the louse to grasp and hold firmly on to hair or clothing. The body louse is the largest and is similar in shape to the head louse (Figure 15-11). The crab louse is the smallest, with a short, oval body and prominent claws resembling sea crabs (Figure 15-12).

Lice feed approximately five times each day by piercing the skin with their claws, injecting irritating saliva, and sucking blood. They do not become engorged like ticks, but, after feeding, they become rust colored from the ingestion of blood; their color is an identifying characteristic. Lice feces can be seen on the skin as small, rust-colored flecks. Saliva and, possibly, fecal material can induce a hypersensitivity reaction and inflammation. Lice are active and can travel quickly, which explains why they can be transmitted so easily. The life cycle from egg to egg is approximately 1 month. The female lays approximately six eggs, or nits, each day. The louse incubates, hatches in 8 to 10 days, and reaches maturity in approximately 18 days. Nits are 0.8 mm long and are firmly cemented to the bases of hair shafts close to the skin to acquire adequate heat for incubation (Figure 15-13). Nits are very difficult to remove from the hair shaft.

Clinical manifestations

Pediculosis capitis. Lice infestation of the scalp is most common in children.[24] More girls than boys are afflicted and American blacks rarely have head lice.[25] Head lice can be found anywhere on the scalp, but are most commonly seen on the back of the head and neck and behind the ears (Figure 15-14). Scratching causes inflammation and secondary bacterial infection, with pustules, crusting, and cervical adenopathy. Posterior cervical adenopathy without obvious disease is characteristic of lice. The eyelashes may be involved, causing redness and swelling. Examination of the posterior scalp shows few adult organisms, but many nits. Nits are cemented to the hair, whereas dandruff scale is easily moved along the hair shaft.

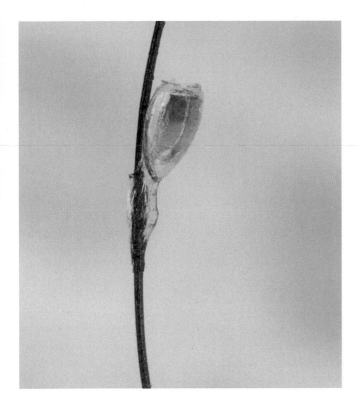

Figure 15-13
Louse egg (nit) is cemented to a hair shaft.

Pediculosis corporis. Infestation by body lice is uncommon. Typhus, relapsing fever, and trench fever are spread by body lice during wartime and in underdeveloped countries. Pediculosis corporis is a disease of the unclean. Body lice live and lay their nits in the seams of clothing and return to the skin surface only to feed. They run and hide when disturbed and are rarely seen. Body lice induce pruritis that leads to scratching and secondary infection.

Eyelash infestation. Infestation of the eyelashes is seen almost exclusively in children. The lice are acquired from other children or from an infested adult with pubic lice. Eyelash infestation may induce blepharitis with lid pruritus, scaling, crusting, and/or purulent discharge. Eyelash infestation may be a sign of childhood sexual abuse.

Pediculosis pubis. Pubic lice are the most contagious sexually transmitted problem known. Up to 30% of patients infested with pubic lice have at least one other sexually transmitted disease. The chance of acquiring pubic lice from one sexual exposure with an infested partner is more than 90%, whereas the chance of acquiring syphilis or gonorrhea from one sexual exposure with an infected partner is approximately 30%. Blacks are affected with the same frequency as whites. The pubic hair is the most common site of infestation, but lice frequently spread to the hair around the anus. On hairy persons, lice may spread to the upper thighs, abdominal area, axillae (Figure 15-15), chest, and beard. Infested adults may spread pubic lice to the eyelashes of children.

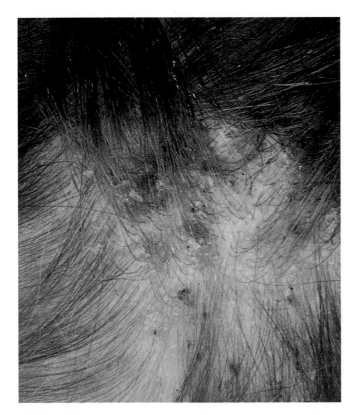

Figure 15-14
Pediculosis capitis. A heavy infestation with secondary pyoderma.

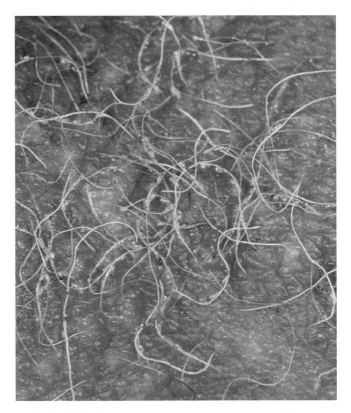

Figure 15-15
Pediculosis pubis. A heavy infestation with numerous nits and lice on the scrotum.

The majority of patients complain of pruritis. Many patients are aware that something is crawling on the groin, but are not familiar with the disease and have never seen lice. Approximately 50% of patients have little inflammation, but those who delay seeking help may develop widespread inflammation and infection of the groin with regional adenopathy. Occasionally, gray-blue macules (maculae ceruleae)[26] (Figure 15-16) varying in size from 1 to 2 cm are seen in the groin and at sites distant from the infestation. Their cause is not known, but they may represent altered blood pigment.

Diagnosis. Lice are suspected when a patient complains of itching in a localized area without an apparent rash. Scalp and pubic lice will be apparent to those who carefully examine individual hairs; they are not apparent with only a cursory examination. Lice and nits can be seen easily under a microscope. Live nits fluoresce and can be detected easily by Wood's light examination, a technique that is especially useful for rapid examination of a large group of children. Nits that contain an unborn louse fluoresce white. Nits that are empty fluoresce gray.

Treatment

Head, body, and pubic lice. Lindane (Kwell), synergized pyrethrins[27] (RID, A-200, R & C), and permethrin (Nix Creme Rinse) are effective for treating lice.[28] Lindane and pyrethrins are available as shampoos or lotions and are equally effective.[29] The shampoos are applied, lathered, and washed off in 5 minutes. Lotions are used for treating body and pubic hair infestation. They are applied over the entire affected area and washed off in 10 minutes. Treatment should be repeated in 7 to 10 days. Permethrin is approved for treating head lice. A sufficient amount is used to saturate the hair and scalp (25 to 50 ml) and rinsed out after 10 minutes.[30] Pyrethrins are chemicals extracted from certain flowers and plants. Of the available insecticides, they are the least toxic to humans. They induce nervous system paralysis in insects.

CO-TRIMOXAZOLE. A rare patient with severe hair matting and dense infestation may not respond to topical medicine. The two remaining options are shaving the head or treatment with co-trimoxazole. One study of 20 females with pediculosis capitis showed that one tablet of co-trimoxazole (Bactrim or Septra: 80 mg of trimethoprim plus 400 mg of sulfamethoxazole) twice daily for 3 days resulted in a cure. Within 12 to 48 hours after treatment, the lice migrated to the bed linen and died.[31] Co-trimoxazole has no effect on nits, therefore a second course must be given 7 to 10 days later.

Nit removal. All preparations kill lice, but some studies show that some nits may survive,[29] therefore the child with nits may have lice hatch and be transmitted.[32] Even dead nits remain attached to the hair until removed. A product called *Step 2 Creme Rinse* that contains formic acid appears to loosen the chitin bond attaching nits to the hair. The cream rinse is applied to wet hair after the pediculicidal shampoo has been rinsed out with water. The cream rinse should remain on the hair for 10 minutes; the hair should be rinsed with water, dried, and then combed with the metal nit removal comb that is provided with the product. The cement holding nits to the hair shaft may be dissolved with vinegar compresses applied to the hair for 15 minutes. Many pyrethrin products are sold with a plastic nit comb. Metal nit combs are more effective and can be purchased separately. As many nits as possible should be removed to prevent reinfestation. A close haircut may be considered for patients with hundreds of nits.

Eye infestation. Several methods are used for treating eye infestation. The most practical and effective method is to place petrolatum (Vaseline) on the fingertips, close the eyes, and rub the petrolatum slowly into the lids and brows three times each day for 5 days. A simple alternative is to close the eyes and apply baby shampoo to the lashes and brows with a cotton swab three times each day for 5 days. Some patients are so mortified by the presence of lice close to their eyes that they demand immediate removal. To do so, the reclining patient closes the eyes and the lice are plucked from the eyelashes with forceps. Older children tolerate this simple procedure. Fluorescein drops (10% to 20%) applied to the lids and lashes produce an immediate toxic effect on the lice.[33] Yellow oxide of mercury, which was used in the past, is no longer available.

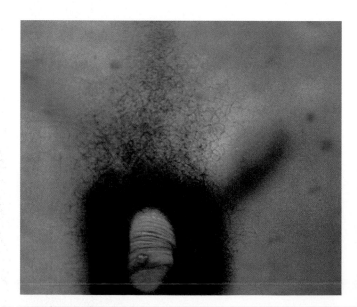

Figure 15-16
Pediculosis pubis (*Maculae ceruleae*). Blue-gray macules can be seen with lice infestation.

Caterpillar Dermatitis

Caterpillars are the larvae of butterflies or moths. Many species of caterpillars possess short hairs (setae) that can irritate the skin (Figure 15-17). Outbreaks of caterpillar dermatitis are seasonal; they occur shortly after the young caterpillars have appeared. Contact with the setae occurs by direct exposure to the caterpillar or windblown setae. Whether the pruritic cutaneous reaction that follows contact is secondary to mechanical irritation, the injection of vasoactive substances, or a hypersensitivity reaction remains unclear.[34]

The brown tail moth and the gypsy moth are found in the northeastern states. Gypsy moth caterpillars hang from trees on long threads. Suspension in the air allows setae to float away on the wind and land on skin or clothing hung out to dry. The puss caterpillar, also known as the wooly slug, is found in the southeastern states. It is approximately 1 inch long and its back and sides are completely covered with fine bristles.[35] The Io moth caterpillar is found east of the Rocky Mountains. It is 2 to 3 inches long and pale green with reddish stripes. Each body segment is armed with tufts of spines. The saddleback caterpillar is found east of Texas and south of Massachusetts. It is approximately 1 inch long, green, and fleshy. The characteristic marking is a brown or purple saddle-shape on the midback. Stout spines are located at each end and along the sides; these spines are hollow and contain a toxin.

Caterpillars (larvae of the buck moth) caused an epidemic of painful dermatitis in West Virginia.[36] An outbreak of dermatitis occured in 12% of the residents and 20% of the employees of a tourist hotel in Cozumel, Mexico. The moth *Hylesia alinda Druce*, which has nettling hairs on its abdomen that excrete a histamine-like substance, was responsible. This moth is normally present in small numbers, but the passage of hurricane Gilbert killed its natural predators (wasps and bees), allowing its population to overgrow. The moth's natural predators returned the next spring and dramatically reduced the moth population. No further outbreaks of dermatitis occurred.

Clinical manifestations. Erythema, papules, and vesicles may appear shortly after contact. Irritation may result from mechanical stimulation or from release of irritating substances on the hairs (Figure 15-18). The sting of the puss caterpillar produces an immediate, severe, shooting, burning pain in practically all cases. Some patients experience delayed symptoms such as itching and may develop papules and vesicles similar to insect bites 12 hours after exposure. Closed patch testing with gypsy moth caterpillar hairs has revealed that these patients develop a delayed hypersensitivity response similar to that in poison ivy contact dermatitis.[37]

Figure 15-17
Gypsy moth caterpillar. The caterpillar is covered with numerous hairlike structures. *(Courtesy Kathleen Shields, Ph. D., United States Department of Agriculture, Hamden, Conn.)*

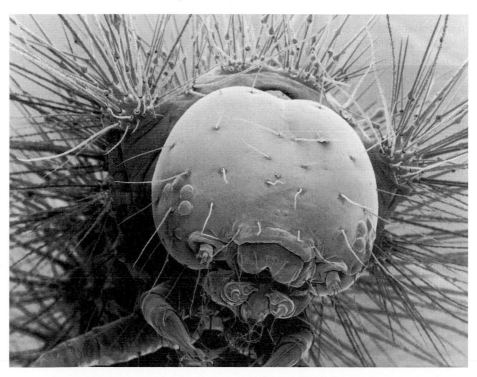

Distribution. Linear lesions are noted where caterpillars crawl on the skin. Eruptions secondary to windblown hairs that become embedded in clothing are localized around the collar region, the inside surfaces of the arms and legs, the abdominal flank, and the feet. A unique, gridlike track may be left on the skin after contact with the puss caterpillar. In addition to cutaneous signs, some patients develop rhinitis, conjunctivitis, and wheezing. No deaths from caterpillar contact have been reported in the United States.

DIAGNOSIS. The diagnosis is suspected when a rash of the above description is seen in the early spring. The diagnosis can be confirmed by demonstrating caterpillar hairs on the skin surface. The technique is as follows. The sticky side of a strip of clear tape is applied to the affected area of skin. The tape is then turned sticky side down onto a microscope slide and observed under low power. Short, straight, thread-like hairs are diagnostic of caterpillar dermatitis.[38]

Treatment. Most cases resolve spontaneously within a few days to 2 weeks. For puss caterpillar stings, the immediate, gentle application of adhesive or clear tape helps to remove remaining spines. Calamine lotion may be helpful, and antihistamines sometimes bring relief if used immediately. Group V topical steroids are useful for persistent or pruritic lesions. Puss caterpillar stings often produce severe pain, which may require potent analgesics. Clothing should not be hung out to dry when thread-suspended caterpillars such as the gypsy moth caterpillar appear in the spring.

Figure 15-18
Gypsy moth dermatitis. A group of papules and vesicles occurred shortly after a gypsy moth caterpillar was dropped on the neck of this young boy.

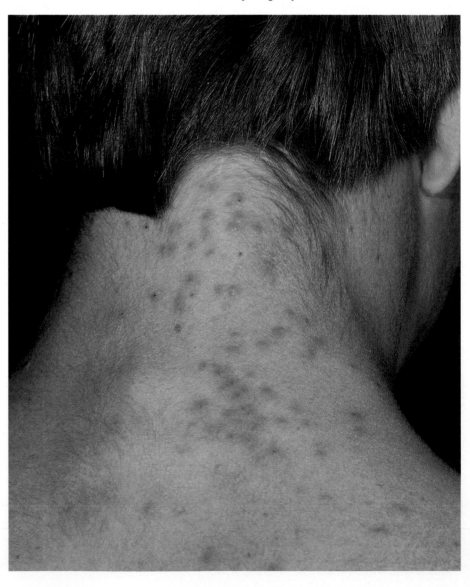

Spiders

Spiders are carnivorous arthropods that have fangs and venom, which they use to catch and immobilize or kill their prey. Most spiders are small and their fangs are too short to penetrate human skin. Spiders are not aggressive and bite only in self-defense. Spider bites may not be felt at the instant they occur. Localized pain, swelling, itching, erythema, blisters, and necrosis may occur. Most spider venoms are composed of the harmless, enzyme-spreading factor hyaluronidase and a toxin that is distributed by the spreading factor. Most toxins simply cause pain, swelling, and inflammation; however, brown recluse spider toxin causes necrosis, and black widow spider toxin causes neuromuscular abnormalities. Spider bites are common, but of the 50 species of spiders in the United States that have been known to bite humans, only the black widow and the brown recluse spider are capable of producing severe reactions.[39] The diagnosis of a spider bite cannot be made with certainty unless the act is witnessed or the spider is recovered.

COMMON SPIDER BITES

Most spider bites cause pain at the instant they occur. A hivelike swelling (raised above the surface) appears at the bite site and expands radially, usually for just a few centimeters; however, the swelling can sometimes reach gigantic proportions. Occasionally, two puncta or fang marks can be found on the skin surface. The warmth and deep erythema of a bite may resemble bacterial cellulitis, but the hivelike swelling and small, satellite hives are not characteristic of bacterial infection. A biopsy, although usually not necessary for diagnosis, may show mouth parts and intense inflammation. The lesion resolves spontaneously, but itching and swelling can be controlled with cool compresses and antihistamines.

BLACK WIDOW SPIDER

The black widow spider, *Latrodectus mactans* ("shoe-button spider"), is so named because the female attacks and then consumes her mate shortly after copulation. The black widow is found in every state except Alaska and is especially numerous in the rural South.

The spider. The female has a smooth, black body; a globose abdomen that resembles an old-fashioned shoe button; long, slender legs; and a red hourglass marking on the underside of the abdomen. This marking may appear as triangles, spots, or an irregular blotch. Adult females have a total length of 4 cm (Figure 15-19) and are the only spiders capable of envenomation. The venom contains a neurotoxin, alpha-latrotoxin, that acts as a calcium ionophore that results in release of acetylcholine from neuromuscular junctions of both sympathetic and parasympathetic nerves. Males are smaller and retain the bright colors of immaturity. Black widow spiders place their webs close to the ground in protected places near logs, dark sheltered areas such as crevices in old barns, lumber piles, and privies. They usually do not bite when away from the web because they are clumsy and need the web for support.

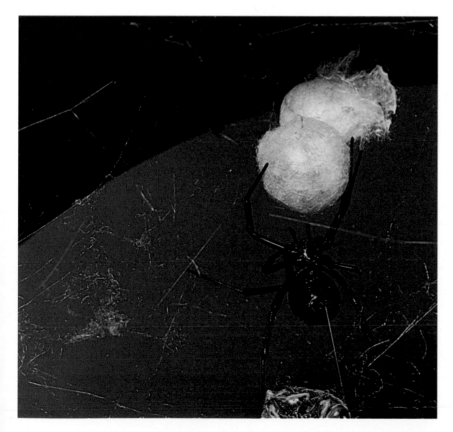

Figure 15-19
Female black widow spider with a red hourglass marking on the underside of her abdomen. Note the haphazard, randomly arranged threads of the web. *(Courtesy Ken Gray, Oregon State University Extension Services.)*

Clinical manifestations. The bite may produce an immediate, sharp pain or may be painless. The subsequent reaction is minimal, with slight swelling and the appearance of a set of small, red fang marks. The symptoms that follow are caused by lymphatic absorption and vascular dissemination of the neurotoxin and are collectively known as *latrodectism*. The most common presenting complaints are generalized abdominal, back, and leg pain. Fifteen minutes to 2 hours after the bite, a dull muscle cramping or severe pain with numbness gradually spreads from the inoculation site to involve the entire torso but is usually more severe in the abdomen and legs. Any or all of the skeletal muscles may be involved. Severe abdominal pain and spasm simulating a surgical abdomen are the most prominent and distressing features of latrodectism (Figure 15-20). The abdominal muscles assume a boardlike rigidity, but tenderness and distension usually do not occur. There is a generalized increase in the deep tendon reflexes. Other symptoms include dizziness, headache, sweating, nausea, and vomiting. The symptoms increase in severity for several hours (up to 24 hours), slowly subsiding and gradually decreasing in severity in 2 or 3 days.[40-42] Residual symptoms such as weakness, tingling, nervousness, and transient muscle spasm may persist for weeks or months after recovery from the acute stage. Recovery from one serious attack usually offers complete systemic immunity to subsequent bites. Convulsions, paralysis, shock, and death occur in approximately 5% of cases, usually in the young or the debilitated elderly.[43]

Treatment

Immediate first aid. If the patient is seen within a few minutes of being bitten, ice may be applied to the bite site to help restrict the spread of venom. Pain relief is achieved with either black widow spider–specific antivenin alone or a combination of IV opioids and muscle relaxants.

Antivenin. The use of antivenin significantly shortens the duration of symptoms in severe envenomations. *Latrodectus mactans* or black widow spider antivenin (Merck & Co., Inc.) is effective regardless of which species of *Latrodectus* causes the bite. The dose consists of the entire contents of one vial (2.5 ml) given intramuscularly or, in severe cases when the patient is under 12 years old or in shock, intravenously in 10 to 50 ml of saline over a 15-minute period. Antivenin may be given intramuscularly for 1 or 2 days. The antivenin is prepared from horse serum and is therefore supplied with a 1-ml vial of normal horse serum for eye-sensitivity testing. The symptoms usually subside in 30 minutes to 3 hours after treatment; occasionally, a second dose is necessary. Hospitalization and treatment with antivenin are indicated for patients who are less than 16 years of age, older than 60 to 65 years of age, are pregnant, or who have hypertensive heart disease, respiratory distress, or symptoms and signs of severe latrodectism. One ampule is sufficient and relieves most of the symptoms within 1 to 2 hours. Healthy patients between ages 16 and 60 years of age usually respond to muscle relaxants and recover spontaneously. In emergencies, the local or state poison center or the Department of Public Health may be called for information about the closest source of antivenin.

Muscle relaxants. Although calcium gluconate was once the first-line treatment of severe envenomations, it was found in one large series to be ineffective for pain relief compared with a combination of IV opioids and benzodiazepines.[44] Calcium gluconate (10%; 10 ml given intravenously) acts as a muscle relaxant. The administration is repeated only once if pain persists or recurs after 1 to 2 hours.[45] Intravenous Valium may be used and later replaced with Valium pills. Alternatively, diazepam or 1 or 2 gm of methocarbamol (100 mg/ml of Robaxin in 10-ml vials) may be administered undiluted over a 5- to 10-minute period. Oral doses may be used thereafter, and they usually sustain the relief initiated by the injection.

Analgesics. Aspirin or, if pain is severe, intravenous morphine may be given. Morphine should be used with caution, since the venom is a neurotoxin and may cause respiratory paralysis.

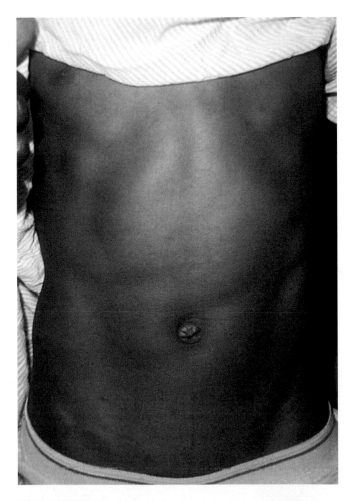

Figure 15-20
Latrodectism. Severe abdominal muscle spasms occurring hours after a black widow spider bite.

BROWN RECLUSE SPIDER

The spider. The brown recluse spider, *Loxoscelidae reclusus* ("fiddle-back spider"), is small, approximately 1.5 cm in overall length. Its color ranges from yellowish-tan to dark brown. A characteristic, dark, violin- or fiddle-shaped marking is located on the spider's back. The broad base of the violin is near the head and the violin stem points toward the abdomen (Figure 15-21). The spider is a timid recluse, avoiding light and disturbances and living in dark areas (under woodpiles and rocks and inside human habitations, often in closets, behind picture frames, under porches, and in barns and basements). Its web is small, haphazard, and woven in cracks, crevices, or corners. It bites only when forced into contact with the skin, such as when a person puts on clothing in which the spider is residing or rummages through stored material harboring the spider. The brown recluse is usually found in the southern half of the United States, but some have been found as far north as Connecticut.[46]

Clinical manifestations. The bite produces a minor stinging or burning or an instantaneous sharp pain resembling a bee sting. Most bite reactions are mild and cause only minimal swelling and erythema (Figure 15-22). Site location seems to be a factor in the severity of the local bite reaction; fatty areas such as the proximal thigh and buttocks show more cutaneous reaction. Severe bites may become necrotic within 4 hours.

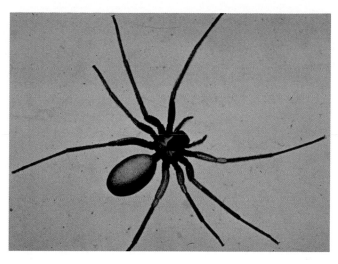

Figure 15-21
The brown recluse spider. A dark, violin-shaped marking is located on the spider's back.

Figure 15-22
Brown recluse spider bite. Most bite reactions are mild and cause only minimal swelling and erythema.

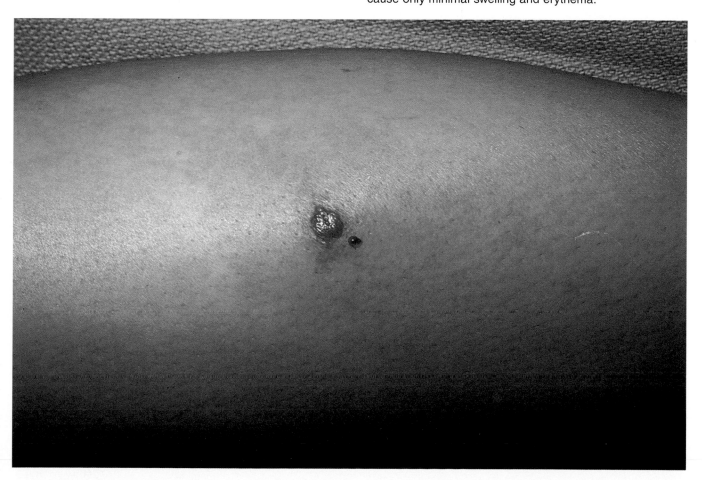

The first and most characteristic cutaneous change in necrotic arachnidism, or loxoscelism, is the development and rapid expansion of a blue-gray, macular halo around the puncture site; this halo represents local hemolysis. A cyanotic pustule or vesicle/bulla may also appear at the bite site. The lesion may have an oblong, irregular configuration area at the bite site and a sudden increase in tenderness. At this stage, the superficial skin may be rapidly infarcting and the pain is severe. The necrotizing, blue macule widens and the center sinks below the normal skin surface ("sinking infarct") (Figure 15-23). The extent of the infarct is variable. Most patients experience localized reactions, but the depth of the necrotic tissue may extend to the muscle and over broad areas of skin, sometimes involving most of an extremity. The dead tissue sloughs, leaving a deep, indolent ulcer with ragged edges. Ulcers take weeks or months to heal; scarring is significant.

A few people develop a severe progressive reaction that begins with moderate to severe pain at the bite site. Within 4 hours, the pain is unbearable and the initial erythema gives way to pallor. Within 12 to 14 hours after the bite, the victims often experience fever, chills, nausea, vomiting, weakness, joint and muscle pains, and hives or measle-like rashes. The toxin may produce severe systemic reactions such as thrombocytopenia or hemolytic anemia with generalized hemolysis, disseminated intravascular coagulation, renal failure, and sometimes death. Severe systemic reactions are rare and occur most frequently in children.

Management. Experience has shown that most bites should be treated conservatively with the following measures:
1. Bite sites are treated with ice bags and elevation.
2. Strenuous exercise is avoided.
3. Localized heat and immediate surgery are avoided.
4. Antibiotics (erythromycin) or cephalosporins and aspirin are given.[40]
5. Tetanus toxoid is given if necessary.

The application of cold packs to bite sites markedly reduces inflammation, slows lesion evolution, and improves all other combinations of therapy. The application of heat to brown recluse bite sites makes lesions much worse.[47] Secondary infection increases localized skin temperature; therefore, routine use of antibiotics is suggested.

Serious bites are usually obvious within the first 24 to 48 hours and need medical, but not surgically aggressive, treatment. Early excision of necrotic areas was once thought to help prevent both the spread of the toxin and further necrosis. This practice is probably ineffective and should be discouraged.[48] If a proven or suspected brown recluse spider bite does not become clinically necrotic within 72 hours, a serious wound healing problem rarely develops.

Immediate surgical excision of brown recluse bite sites induced more complications than did the use of dapsone with or without delayed excision and/or repair.[49] Dapsone 50 to 100 mg/day may be helpful in severe cutaneous reactions to prevent extensive necrosis, even if it is administered 48 hours after the bite.[50,51] Dapsone may help prevent the venom-induced perivasculitis with polymorphonuclear leukocyte infiltration that occurs with extensive cutaneous necrosis.[52]

There is little evidence that oral and intralesional steroids decrease the severity of the progressive reaction. Patients should be treated with systemic corticosteroids for 14 to 21 days when lesions show a necrotic area greater than 2 cm.[53] Patients with necrosis greater than 1 cm should be tested to see if progressive hemolytic anemia, manifested by an increasing level of free serum hemoglobin or thrombocytopenia, has developed. Severe systemic loxoscelism may be treated with prednisone (1 mg/kg) given as early as possible in the development of systemic symptoms in order to treat hematologic abnormalities. Surgery is reserved for debridement of necrotic lesions. A specific antivenom to *L. reclusa* has been developed but is not yet commercially available. A series of 147 cases of spider bites were treated with high-voltage, direct-current shocks; they arrested venom damage to tissue and improved pain and systemic symptoms usually within 15 minutes.[54]

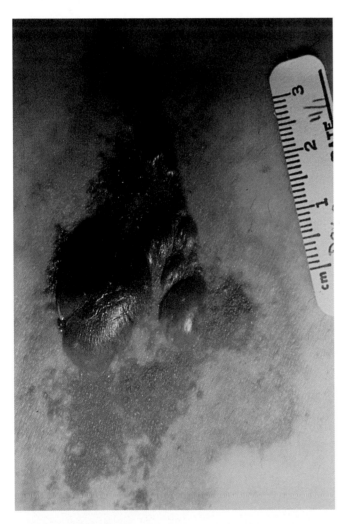

Figure 15-23
Brown recluse spider bite. A severe reaction in which infarction, bleeding, and blistering have occurred.

Ticks

Ticks are blood-sucking ectoparasites that act as vectors for rickettsial, spirochetal, bacterial, and parasitic infections.

Ticks. Adult ticks of some species can reach 1 cm in length; they have eight legs, the front two are curved forward, as in crabs. The large oval or teardrop-shaped body is flat and saclike and has a leathery outer surface. There are two families of ticks: hard-bodied (*Ixodidae*) and soft-bodied ticks (*Argasidae*). They are distinguished by the consistency of their bodies. Hard (ixodid) ticks are of greatest concern because they are vectors for most of the serious tick-borne diseases. They can inflict local reaction such as pain, erythema, and nodules, and they are more difficult to remove than the soft (argasid) ticks. Ticks should be removed from the host as soon as possible after they are discovered to reduce the chance of infection. Proper removal of the tick, however, is just as important in reducing the chance of infection as timely removal (see box on p. 475).

Tick bites. Ticks perch on grass tips and bushes and wait for a warm-blooded host to pass by. They insert their recurved teeth into the skin, produce a gluelike secretion that tightens their grip, suck blood (Figure 15-24), and become engorged, sometimes tripling in size. Hard ticks may remain attached to the host for up to 10 days, whereas soft ticks release in a few hours. The bite itself is painless, but within hours an urticarial wheal appears at the puncture site and may cause itching. Ticks may go unnoticed, particularly in children, for several hours after attachment to an inconspicuous area such as the scalp.

Types of ticks. Ticks and their associated diseases are listed in Table 15-1. The deer tick (*Ixodes dammini*) transmits human babesiosis and Lyme disease; it is found in areas such as Massachusetts, Connecticut, New Jersey, and the islands of coastal New England. This tick is common in many areas of southern Connecticut, where it parasitizes three different host animals during its 2-year life cycle. Larval and nymphal ticks have parasitized 31 different

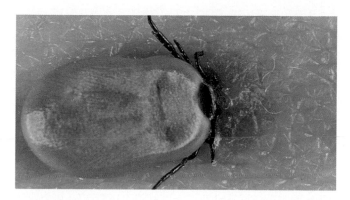

Figure 15-24
Tick. Mouth parts are deeply imbedded in the skin and the tick is fully engorged with blood.

species of mammals and 49 species of birds. White-tailed deer appear to be crucial hosts for adult ticks. All three feeding stages of the tick parasitize humans, although most infections are acquired from feeding nymphs in May through early July. Reservoir hosts for the spirochete include rodents, other mammals, and even birds. White-footed mice are particularly important reservoirs, and, in parts of southern Connecticut where Lyme disease is prevalent in humans, *Borrelia* are universally present during the summer in these mice. Prevalence of infected ticks has ranged from 10% to 35%. Isolates of *B. burgdorferi* from humans, rodents, and *I. dammini* are usually indistinguishable, but strains of *B. burgdorferi* with different major proteins have been identified.[55] The recent expansion of the geographic range has been attributed to the proliferation of deer in North America. The spotted fever tick (*Dermacentor variabilis*) is found in sections of the United States other than the Rocky Mountain region. Most *Dermacentor* ticks have white anterodorsal ornamentation. The Rocky Mountain wood tick (*Dermacentor andersoni*) is the vector for Rocky Mountain spotted fever in the west.

TABLE 15-1 Major Tick-borne Diseases in the United States				
Disease	Causative agent	Classification	Major vector	Region
Lyme disease	*Borrrelia burgdorferi*	Bacteria (spirochete)	Ixodes	Northeast, Wisconsin, Minnesota, California
Relapsing fever	*Borrelia* species	Bacteria (spirochete)	Ornithodoros	West
Tularemia	*Francisella tularensis*	Bacteria	Dermacentor, amblyomma	Arkansas, Missouri, Oklahoma
Rocky Mountain spotted fever	*Rickettsia rickettsii*	Rickettsia	Demacentor	Southeast, West south central
Ehrlichiosis	*Ehrlichia chaffeensis*	Rickettsia	Dermacentor, amblyomma?	South central, south Atlantic
Colorado tick fever	Coltivirus species	Virus	Dermacentor	West
Babesiosis	Babesia species	Protozoa	Ixodes	Northeast
Tick paralysis	Toxin	Neurotoxin	Dermacentor, amblyomma	Northwest, South

From Spach DH et al: *N Engl J Med* 329:936, 1993.

Lyme Disease and Erythema Migrans

Lyme disease and erythema migrans (EM), which means "chronic migrating red rash," are caused by the spirochete *Borrelia burgdorferi* and are transmitted by the bite of certain ixodes ticks of the *Iiricinus* complex and possibly by other ticks. *Ixodes* ticks have *B. burgdorferi* in their gastrointestinal systems. Lyme disease is named after Lyme, Connecticut, where the initial cluster of children with arthritis (brief but recurrent attacks of asymmetric swelling and pain in a few large joints, especially the knee, over a period of years) was reported in 1975. Like syphilis, the disease affects many systems, occurs in stages, and mimics other diseases. Cases have since been reported from all parts of the country and people of all ages are affected. A disproportionate number of children contract Lyme disease since they spend more time in wooded areas than adults. The rapid emergence of focal epidemics is possible.[56] There are now approximately 8000 cases reported annually in the United States.[57] Antigenic differences between European and American strains of the organism may explain some of the minor differences in the clinical presentation of the disease, such as the more prominent skin involvement in European cases.

Geographic distribution. Lyme disease is now recognized on six continents and in at least 20 countries. Most cases in the United States are clustered in three regions (Figure 15-25): the Northeast coastal regions; Minnesota and Wisconsin; and parts of California, Oregon, Utah, and Nevada. The geographic distribution suggests that *Borrelia* spreads when infested ticks are transported by migratory birds. *Ixodes dammini* (Figures 15-26 and 15-27) is the vector of disease in the Northeast and Midwest, *Ixodes pacificus* in the West, *Iiricinus* in Europe, and *Ixodes persulcatus* in Asia. The disease is reported throughout Europe. Most cases occur in the summer or early fall when people are outdoors, wearing shorts, and walking barefoot through the woods and grass. In the Northeast, they infest the white-tailed deer and white-footed mouse.

Figure 15-25
Reported cases of Lyme disease, 1993. *(From MMWR 43(31), 1994.)*

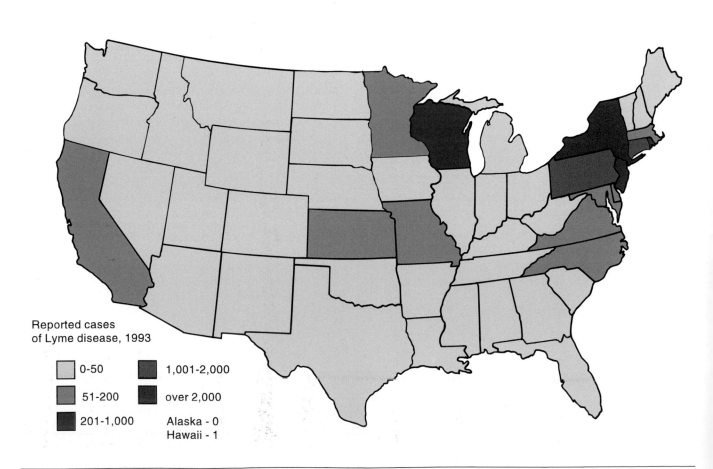

Reported cases
of Lyme disease, 1993

☐ 0-50   ☐ 1,001-2,000

☐ 51-200   ☐ over 2,000

☐ 201-1,000   Alaska - 0
Hawaii - 1

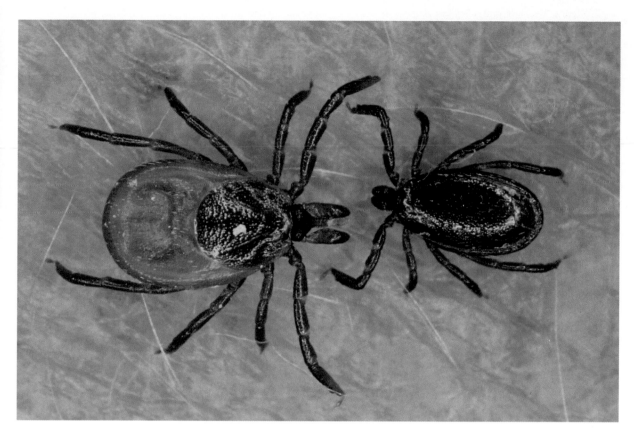

Figure 15-26
The deer tick (*Ixodes dammini*), partly engorged (left) and
unengorged (right).

Figure 15-27
The deer tick *(Ixodes dammini)*, one of the vectors for
transmitting Lyme disease. This tick is very small and
can easily go unnoticed when fixed to the skin in an
unengorged state.

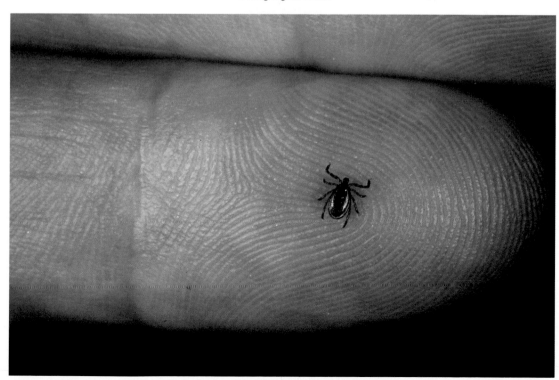

Clinical manifestations

Lyme disease has its onset 3 to 21 days after the bite of the *Ixodes* tick.

Cutaneous manifestations. There are three cutaneous lesions associated with Lyme disease: erythema migrans (formally referred to as *erythema chronicum migrans*), *Borrelia* lymphocytoma, and acrodermatitis chronica atrophicans. There is some evidence that several other cutaneous diseases are associated with *Borrelia burgdorferi* infection.[58,59]

Erythema migrans. The skin lesion erythema migrans (EM) is the most characteristic aspect of Lyme disease, but it is not present in all cases. EM may occur as an isolated phenomenon. It is a spontaneously healing erythematous lesion occurring at the site of *Borrelia* inoculation. The average interval between the infectious bite and the appearance of the skin lesion is approximately 9 days (range: 1 to 28

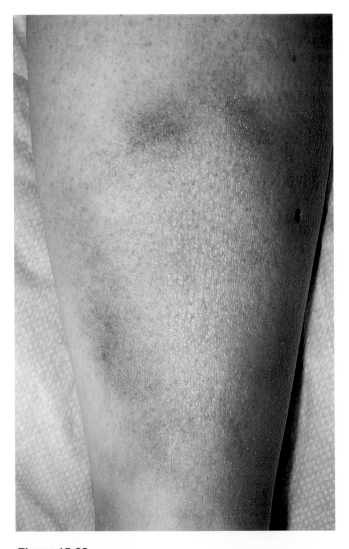

Figure 15-28
Erythema migrans. Broad oval area of erythema has slowly migrated from the central area.

days). The lesion begins as a small papule at the bite site. The papule forms into a slowly enlarging ring, while the central erythema gradually fades and leaves a surface that is usually normal, but may be slightly blue. The ring remains flat, blanches with pressure, and does not desquamate, vesiculate, or have scale at the periphery, as ringworm does. The most common configuration of the lesion is circular, but as migration proceeds over skin folds, distortions of the configuration occur. The border of the lesion may be slightly raised.[60] Some patients complain of burning or itching. Over several days, the erythema expands rapidly away from the central bite puncture, centrifugally forming a broad, round-to-oval area of erythema measuring 5 to 10 cm (Figure 15-28). Within 1 week, it clears centrally, leaving a red, 1- to 2-cm ring that advances for days or weeks and may reach a diameter of 50 cm; 20% to 50% of cases have multiple concentric rings. Tenderness is present and itching is minimal. Even in untreated patients, EM lesions usually fade within 3 to 4 weeks. During early infection, secondary EM lesions or *Borrelia* lymphocytoma may occur. Multiple EM-like lesions, occurring as a result of hematogenous spread, are the cutaneous markers of disseminated disease.[61]

Borrelia lymphocytoma. *Borrelia* lymphocytoma (BL) generally presents as a bluish-red nodule during the early stages of infection. It most commonly appears on the earlobe or nipple. Histologically there is a dense polyclonal lymphocytic infiltrate, which may appear after EM or as the first manifestation of Lyme borreliosis. EM and BL are early, localized cutaneous manifestations, but sometimes extracutaneous signs or symptoms of disseminated disease may appear simultaneously with either of these lesions. BL is rare; the prevalence ranges from 0.6% to 1.3% of cases of Lyme disease.[62]

Acrodermatitis chronica atrophicans. During late infection, acrodermatitis chronica atrophicans, an erythematous, atrophic plaque unique to Lyme disease, may appear. It has been described in approximately 10% of patients with Lyme disease in Europe, but it is rarely seen in the United States. It starts with an early inflammatory phase with localized edema and bluish-red discoloration on the extensor surfaces of the hands, feet, elbows, and knees. Years to decades later there may be an atrophic phase where the skin becomes atrophic and dull red and may have a cigarette paper–like appearance.[63]

Early and late disease. Early Lyme borreliosis includes localized infection, entailing erythema migrans and *Borrelia* lymphocytoma without signs or symptoms of disseminated infection (see the box on p. 467); regional lymphadenopathy and/or minor constitutional symptoms may be present; early disseminated infection, entailing multiple erythema migrans–like skin lesions and early manifestations of neuroborreliosis, arthritis, carditis, or other organ involvement. Late Lyme borreliosis includes chronic infection, entailing acrodermatitis chronica atrophicans; neurologic, rheumatic, or other organ manifestations that are persistent or remit for at least 12 (or 6) months.[64,65]

CLINICAL MANIFESTATIONS OF LYME BORRELIOSIS (LB)

EARLY MANIFESTATIONS: 3 TO 4 WEEKS (RANGE, 1 DAY TO 14 MONTHS)

Erythema migrans (72% to 80%)

Begins as a red papule at the tick bite site 3 to 32 days (median 7 days) after the tick is noted. An expanding, ringed (10- to 50-cm) lesion with partial central clearing. Multiple smaller, annular, secondary lesions may appear within days at other sites (25% to 50% of cases).

Minor constitutional symptoms

Typically intermittent and changing. Influenza-like symptoms of headache (64%), stiff neck (48%), fever (59%), chills, regional lymphadenopathy. Malaise, lethargy, and fatigue (80%) may be constant and incapacitating.

Disseminated disease

Meningeal irritation and mild encephalopathy—episodic attacks of excruciating headaches, neck pain, stiffness, or pressure typically lasting hours (no spinal fluid pleocytosis or objective neurologic deficit). Migratory musculoskeletal pain, hepatitis, generalized lymphadenopathy, splenomegaly, sore throat, nonproductive cough, and testicular swelling.

Laboratory

Elevated ESR (53%), total serum IgM (33%), SGOT (19%), lymphopenia during the acute phase.

LATER MANIFESTATIONS

Nervous system (15%)

Occurs weeks to months after initial symptoms.[65] Meningitis (89%), encephalitis (29%), cranial neuropathy (particularly Bell's palsy), and peripheral radiculoneuropathy. In highly endemic areas, LB may be responsible for 25% of cases of Bell's palsy.[66] Acute peripheral facial palsy is the most frequent manifestation of LB in childhood (55% of all cases).[67] Ultrasonography of the parotid gland in patients with Lyme induced acute facial paralysis shows enlarged lymph nodes in the caudal portion of the parotid gland around the stylomastoid foramen.[68]

Symptoms lasts for months, usually resolving completely. Months to years after the initial infection, patients may have chronic encephalopathy, polyneuropathy, psychiatric disorders, and incapacitating fatigue, or, less commonly, leukoencephalitis. These chronic neurologic abnormalities usually improve with antibiotic therapy.[69,70]

Intrathecal antibody determinations are the most specific diagnostic test currently available for Lyme neuroborreliosis.[71] Many patients with early or late neurologic involvement have intrathecal antibody production to *B. burgdorferi*, usually IgG or IgA, in their cerebrospinal fluid (CSF).[72] They may lack diagnostic serum levels of antibody to *B. burgdorferi*.[73]

Heart (8%)

Occurs within several weeks after initial symptoms in adults and children (29%).[74] Fluctuating degrees of atrioventricular block is most frequent manifestation of Lyme carditis[75] (distribution in all patients: 49% third degree, 16% second degree, and 12% first degree),[76] Wenckebach, or complete heartblock, may require a temporary pacemaker. Electrocardiogram changes of acute myopericarditis, and radionuclide evidence of mild left ventricular dysfunction. ECG changes may occur before symptoms. Duration is brief (3 days to 6 weeks), overall prognosis is good, rarely recurs, most patients respond to antibiotics.

Joints (60%)

Occurs within a few weeks to 2 years after onset.

Arthralgia alone (18%) occurs early in illness. Migratory musculoskeletal pain in joints, tendons, bursae, muscle, and bone often without joint swelling. Pain affects one or two sites at a time, lasting a few hours to several days.

Intermittent episodes of arthritis (50%) occur months after onset. Intermittent attacks of joint swelling and pain, primarily in large joints, especially the knees. Knees are commonly much more swollen than painful, often hot, and, rarely, red. Baker's cysts sometimes form and rupture early.

Chronic arthritis (10%) attacks, lasting weeks to months, may recur for several years. Fever is unusual. In adults, Lyme arthritis is most like Reiter's syndrome or reactive arthritis, and in children, it is most similar to the pauciarticular form of juvenile rheumatoid arthritis.[77]

Chronic Lyme arthritis appears to have an immunogenetic basis—89% of patients with chronic arthritis had the HLA-DR4 or HLA-DR2 specificities, compared with 27% with arthritis of short duration. The combination of the HLA-DR4 specificity and strong IgG responses to both OspA and OspB (*B. burgdorferi* outer surface proteins) are associated with chronic arthritis and the lack of response to antibiotic therapy.[78] Therefore, particular class II major histocompatibility genes determine a host immune response to *B. burgdorferi* that results in chronic arthritis and lack of response to antibiotic therapy.[79]

Joint fluid WBC—500 to 110,000 cells/mm^3 (mostly polys); total protein—3 to 8 gm/dl; C3, C4 levels greater than 1/3 serum; and glucose levels greater than 1/3 serum. Rheumatoid factor is negative.

Long-term course in children of initially untreated Lyme disease may include acute infection followed by attacks of arthritis that become less frequent and less severe with time and then by keratitis, subtle joint pain, or chronic encephalopathy.[80]

LYME BORRELIOSIS
3 STAGES WITH REMISSIONS AND EXACERBATIONS

	STAGE 1	STAGE 2	STAGE 3
	LOCALIZED INFECTION	DISSEMINATED INFECTION	PERSISTENT INFECTION

IXODES TICK
(Attached at least
48 hours)
Transmits
spirochete,
Borrelia burgdorferi

**SYSTEMIC
SYMPTOMS
+
HEART**

STAGE 1
LOCALIZED INFECTION
Begins 7 days
(range 3 to 32 days)

Low-grade fever
Profound fatigue
Regional adenopathy (41%)
Generalized adenopathy (20%)

— Months —

Cardiac involvement (8%)
Fluctuating degrees of AV block
Myopericarditis
Left ventricular dysfunction
Begins several weeks after Stage 1

— 3 days to 6 weeks —

Symptoms
subside

JOINTS

Myalgias and arthralgias
Migratory pain—no swelling
Hours or days—one or two locations

— Months —

Arthritis (80%)
Brief attacks of swelling and pain
Lasts hours to days, then months
One or two locations
Few large joints (especially knee)
Episodes of arthralgia or periarticular
involvement—tendinitis, bursitis between
attacks of arthritis

— During second or
third year —

Chronic arthritis (10%)
Joint inflammation > 1 year
Erosion cartilage + bone
Knees
Longer episodes—lasting months

SKIN

Erythema migrans (60% to 80%)
(lasts for several weeks)

— Days —

Multiple annular secondary lesions (50%)
All lesions fade in 3 to 4 weeks (range 1 day to 14 months)

— Years —

Acrodermatitis chronica atrophicans
(rare in U.S.)

**NERVOUS
SYSTEM**

Sx of meningeal irritation and mild
encephalopathy
(attacks of severe headache,
stiff neck)

— Weeks or months —

Neurologic abnormalities (15%)
Fluctuating Sx of meningitis with superimposed cranial
or peripheral radiculoneuropathy
Facial or Bell's palsy
CSF—lymphs 100 cells/mm³ + elevated protein

— Months to years —

Chronic neurologic Sx
Subtle encephalopathy affecting
memory, mood, or sleep
CSF—elevated protein
Distal paresthesias or spinal or
radicular pain
EMG—proximal and distal nerve
segment abnormalities

Three stages of infection. Lyme disease has three stages that can overlap or occur alone: stage 1 (early disease)—expanding skin lesion (erythema migrans) and flulike symptoms; stage 2—cardiac and neurologic disease; stage 3—arthritis and chronic neurologic syndromes. The infection remains localized to the skin during stage 1. Within days or weeks, the spirochete may spread in the blood or lymph (stage 2). The infection can persist for years in areas such as the joints and nervous system (stage 3). The acute illness begins with malaise, fatigue, fever up to 105° F, the EM skin lesion, headache, stiff neck, myalgias, and arthralgias. Influenza will be suspected at this stage if the EM rash is absent. The complete blood count and erythrocyte sedimentation rate are normal. The electrocardiogram may show signs of carditis. Approximately 1 month after the acute symptoms, some patients develop one or more swollen, warm (but not red), and painful joints; it is usually the knee that is affected. Inflammation typically lasts for 1 week and may recur.[81] The sedimentation rate, serum cryoglobulins, and serum IgM are elevated in many patients with acute joint symptoms. The signs and symptoms of the three stages are listed in the box on p. 468.

The most frequent manifestation in one study of Lyme neuroborreliosis in childhood was acute peripheral facial palsy, found in 55%.[67]

The Lyme disease spirochete may spread transplacentally to organs of the fetus. Women who acquire Lyme disease while pregnant should be treated promptly.[82]

Laboratory diagnosis. Lyme disease can be reliably diagnosed in the presence of erythema migrans, but diagnosis without the rash may be difficult. Routine laboratory studies are not helpful in confirming the diagnosis. Serology is currently the only practical laboratory aid in diagnosis,[83] but the insensitivity of the assays and the interlaboratory variability are frequent problems.[84,85] Borderline-positive results have often been used to confirm the diagnosis in patients at low risk for Lyme disease who have only nonspecific symptoms. In such situations it is statistically more likely that the serologic result is a false positive and the symptoms have some other cause. The use of polymerase chain reactions may be the most useful and accurate way of detecting *B. burgdorferi*.

Serology. Following infection there is an early T-cell response and a more slowly evolving B-cell response to *B. burgdorferi* antigens. In untreated patients, the IgM antibody response appears first, peaking 3 to 6 weeks after infection and gradually waning.[86] IgG antibody is detectable for at least 16 months by immunoblot and enzyme-linked immunosorbent assay (ELISA).[87] Up to 90% have an elevated titer between the EM phase and convalescence. In patients with later manifestations, 94% have elevated titers.[88] The early administration of antibiotics may abolish the antibody response, but therapy later does not appear to have a significant effect on antibody levels. Chronic Lyme disease may subsequently develop without diagnostic levels of antibodies.[89] High titers of either IgG or IgM antibodies indicate disease, but lower titers can be misleading. The IgM antibodies may remain after the initial infection, and IgG antibodies may remain for years. Antibiotic therapy early in the infection may interfere with antibody production. ELISA is generally used to detect IgM and IgG antibodies to the Lyme spirochete. Western blot analysis may be used to confirm results.[83,90] The diagnosis of Lyme neuroborreliosis can be made by ELISA when an increased concentration of anti-Bb antibodies are demonstrated in the CSF relative to the serum. The CSF and serum samples should be assayed at the same time.

False positive tests. False positive ELISA titers occur with syphilis, infectious mononucleosis, Rocky Mountain spotted fever, autoimmune diseases, and in 7% of normal blood bank donors.[91] Syphilis serologic tests for *Treponema pallidum*, such as rapid plasma reagin, venereal disease research laboratory (VDRL), or microhemagglutination assays are usually negative in Lyme disease, but the fluorescent *Treponema* antibody absorption test may be frequently positive.[92] Some false positive reactions may be due to prior subclinical infections with *B. burgdorferi*.

Culture and biopsy. The culture or direct visualization of *B. burgdorferi* from patient specimens is possible but difficult. Skin biopsies performed in patients with EM and cultured for *B. burgdorferi* in modified Barbour-Stoenner-Kelly medium at 33° C were positive in 72% of patients prior to treatment but in none during or after completion of a course of antimicrobial therapy.[93] The ability to recover *B. burgdorferi* from skin biopsy cultures of untreated patients with EM lesions wanes with increasing duration of EM, suggesting that this organism may also be spontaneously cleared from skin over time. Heparinized blood or serum specimens are also cultured on modified Barbour-Stoenner-Kelly medium.[94] With Warthin-Starry silver stain, the *Ixodes dammini* spirochete was found, usually in the papillary dermis, in 86% of EM lesions.[95]

The overdiagnosis of Lyme disease. In areas where anxiety about the disease is high, patients and physicians often ascribe clinical concerns to Lyme disease. Incorrect diagnosis often leads to unnecessary antibiotic treatment (often prolonged or repeated intravenous therapy). Anxiety about possible late manifestations of Lyme disease has made Lyme disease a "diagnosis of exclusion" in many endemic areas. Persistence of mild to moderate symptoms after adequate therapy and misdiagnosis of fibromyalgia and fatigue may incorrectly suggest persistence of infection, leading to further antibiotic therapy. Attention to patients' anxiety and increased awareness of these musculoskeletal problems after therapy should decrease unnecessary therapy of previously treated Lyme disease.[96-98]

Treatment. Serologic testing has poor sensitivity in early disease. The presence of erythema migrans offers physicians the best opportunity for diagnosis. Aggressive antibiotic treatment may be initiated solely on the basis of this early clinical finding. The optimum treatment for Lyme disease has not been determined. The most recent recommendations[99,100] are listed in Table 15-2. For adults, early in the illness, oral doxycycline or amoxicillin may be the treatment of choice.[101] These two antibiotics were found to be extremely effective for treatment and for preventing late sequelae. Oral azithromycin 500 mg on the first day, followed by 250 mg once a day for 4 days, was found to be as effective as amoxicillin and doxycycline for the treatment of early Lyme disease.[102] Minocycline 100 mg twice a day may

TABLE 15-2 Treatment of Lyme Disease[a]

	Drug	Adult dosage	Pediatric dosage[b]
ERYTHEMA MIGRANS	Doxycycline[c] (*Vibramycin* and others)	100 mg orally bid	
OR	amoxicillin (*Amoxil* and others)	250 to 500 mg orally tid	25 to 50 mg/kg/day divided tid
OR	azithromycin	500 mg first day then 250 mg qd for 4 days	
Alternative:	cefuroxime axetil (*Ceftin*)	500 mg bid	250 mg bid
NEUROLOGIC DISEASE			
Bell's palsy	Doxycycline[c]	100 mg orally bid	
OR	amoxicillin	250 to 500 mg orally tid	25 to 50 mg/kg/day divided tid
More serious CNS disease[d]	ceftriaxone (*Rocepin*)	2 gm/day IV	75 to 100 mg/kg/day IV
OR	penicillin G	20 to 24 million U/day IV	300,000 U/kg/day IV
CARDIAC DISEASE			
Mild	Doxycyline[c]	100 mg orally bid	
OR	amoxicillin	250 to 500 mg orally tid	25 to 50 mg/kg/day divided tid
More serious[e]	ceftriaxone	2 gm/day IV	75 to 100 mg/kg/day IV
OR	pencillin G	20 to 24 million U/day IV	300,000 U/kg/day IV
ARTHRITIS[d]			
Oral	Doxycycline[c]	100 mg orally bid	
OR	amoxicillin	500 mg orally tid	50 mg/kg/day divided tid
Parenteral	ceftriaxone	2 gm/day IV	75 to 100 mg/kg/day IV
OR	penicillin G	20 to 24 million U/day IV	300,000 U/kg/day IV

From *The Medical Letter* 35(881), 1992.
a. Recommendations are based on limited data and should be considered tentative. The duration of treatment is not well established for any indication; it is usually based on severity of disease and rapidity of response. Clinicians generally recommend 10 to 30 days for oral drugs and 14 to 21 days for intravenous treatment.
b. Should not exceed adult dosage.
c. Or tetracycline HCl (*Achromycin*, and others), 250 to 500 mg qid or minocycline 100 mg bid. Doxycycline, tetracycline, and minocycline should not be used for children less than 8 years old or for pregnant or lactating women.
d. In late disease, the response to treatment may be delayed for several weeks or months.
e. A temporary pacemaker may be necessary.

be considered as an alternative.[103] It is well absorbed after oral ingestion, rarely produces GI symptoms or photosensitivity, and vertigo is now uncommon with the new sustained-release preparation. Amoxicillin is used to treat children. The duration of therapy is guided by the clinical response. A few patients require re-treatment with oral or intravenous therapy. A study showed that recommended treatment schedules are successful in preventing late sequelae in children; new episodes of erythema migrans were, however, reported in 11% of those patients 1 to 4 years after the initial episode.[104] Other studies show that major late manifestations of Lyme disease are unusual after appropriate early antibiotic therapy.[105-107]

Persistent infection. Some authors have documented persistent infection after treatment with currently recommended schedules. Several months of treatment was required to cure their patients.[108] Approximately half the patients continue to experience minor symptoms, such as headache, musculoskeletal pain, and fatigue, after antibiotic treatment. Patients with severe cardiac involvement who do not respond quickly to antibiotic therapy may respond to steroids. Ceftriaxone is recommended for treatment of disseminated Lyme disease. Ceftriaxone is excreted in the urine and bile. Biliary precipitation of ceftriaxone as a calcium salt is a known cause of pseudocholelithiasis (sludging), cholelithiasis, biliary colic, and cholecystitis. Upper abdominal ultrasonography is used for patients who develop biliary colic while receiving ceftriaxone.[109]

JARISCH-HERXHEIMER–LIKE REACTION. Fourteen percent of patients, generally those with more severe disease, have an intensification of symptoms during the first 24 hours after the start of therapy. This Jarisch-Herxheimer–like reaction[110] (severe chills, myalgias, headache, fever, increased heart and respiratory rate lasting for hours, and increased visibility of the rash) usually occurs a few hours after treatment is begun. The reaction occurs more often with penicillin and tetracycline than with erythromycin, presumably because penicillin and tetracyline kill larger numbers of organisms more quickly than does erythromycin.[111] Regardless of the antibiotic agent given, nearly half of the patients experience minor late complications—recurrent episodes of lethargy and headache or pain in joints, tendons, bursae, or muscles.

Asymptomatic patients with an elevated Lyme disease antibody titer. Lyme disease antibody titers are sometimes ordered for patients with a history of Lyme disease–like symptoms but who are currently asymptomatic. The proper management of asymptomatic patients with an elevated Lyme disease antibody titer has not been defined. Until studies are completed, these patients may be treated with the schedule for erythema migrans outlined in Table 15-2.

Prevention of Lyme disease after tick bites. There is controversy about whether or not persons bitten by a deer tick in an area in which Lyme disease is endemic routinely should receive antimicrobial prophylaxis. The risk of Lyme disease after a recognized deer tick bite is very low, even in areas in which the disease is endemic. Erythema migrans develops in the overwhelming majority of persons who become infected with *B. burgdorferi*. Asymptomatic infection in a person with a tick bite is rare, and the risk of late sequelae of Lyme disease is small, therefore, serologic tests in such persons are not routinely indicated. On the basis of these facts authors conclude that the routine use of antimicrobial prophylaxis for persons with a recognized deer tick bite is not indicated.[112]

Prevention. Tick repellents are divided into those applied to the skin and those applied to clothing. The insect repellent *N,N*-diethyl-meta-toluamide (deet) used on the skin repels a variety of insects, including ticks; 2-ethyl-1,3-hexanediol, and dimethyl phthalate are also effective. Permethrin in an aerosol is the most effective clothing repellent for protection against ticks. DEET plus a permethrin-containing clothing repellent offers the best overall protection. Tréo and Avon's Skin-So-Soft Moisturizing Suncare Plus lotion contain the insect repellent oil of citronella (a natural component of plants). They are safe, effective, non-DEET repellents. Physical measures to prevent tick bites include avoiding tick-infested areas, wearing light-colored clothing for easy identification of crawling ticks, regularly checking the body and pets for ticks, wearing protective garments and closed-toed shoes, and removing attached ticks promptly.[113] It is especially important to detect and to remove ticks as soon as possible, since transmission of *B. burgdorferi* is unlikely if a deer tick is removed within 48 hours of attachment.[114,115]

Rocky Mountain Spotted and Spotless Fever

The name *Rocky Mountain spotted fever* was coined to describe a disease that was first observed in the Bitter Root Valley of western Montana. The disease occurs in many areas of the United States but is most common in Oklahoma and the South Atlantic states (Figure 15-29). Ninety-five percent of patients report onset of illness between April 1 and September 30, the period when ticks are most active. Rocky Mountain spotted fever is caused by *Rickettsia rickettsii* and is transmitted by tick bites. *Rickettsiae* are released from tick salivary glands during the 6 to 10 hours they are attached to the host. The principal vector in the eastern United States is *Dermacentor variabilis* (the American dog tick); in the West South Central states it is *Amblyomma americanum* (the Lone Star tick) and the American dog tick; and in the West it is *Dermacentor andersoni*.

Clinical manifestations. After the tick bites, organisms disseminate via the bloodstream and multiply in vascular endothelial cells, resulting in multisystem manifestations. One week (with a range of 3 to 21 days) after the bite, there is abrupt onset of fever (94%), severe headache (88%), myalgia (85%), and vomiting (60%). Rickettsia infect the endothelium and vessel wall, not the cerebral tissue.

The rash is reported in 83% of cases and typically begins on the fourth day, erupting first on the wrists and ankles. In hours it involves the palms and soles (73%), then it becomes generalized.[116] The rash is discrete, macular, and blanches with pressure at first; it becomes petechial in 2 to 4 days (Figure 15-30). The rash is very difficult to see in blacks, which may explain the higher fatality rate for blacks (16%) as compared with whites (3%). In approximately 15% of cases, the rash does not appear; the disease is then referred to as *Rocky Mountain spotless fever*.[117] Rashless disease is much more common in adults.

Rocky Mountain spotted fever should be suspected in residents or visitors to endemic areas who report fever, headache, and myalgias without a rash. Symptoms and signs referable to the pulmonary system (cough or rales), the GI system (nausea, vomiting, abdominal pain), or the CNS (stupor, meningismus) are seen with Rocky Mountain spotted fever and should not delay diagnosis or treatment.[118,119] Splenomegaly is present in one half of the cases. The fever subsides in 2 to 3 weeks, and the rash, if present, fades with residual hyperpigmentation. Although the overall mortality rate fluctuates between 3% and 7%, the mortality rate for untreated persons may exceed 30%. The case mortality rate is higher for individuals 40 years of age or older (9%) than for individuals under the age of 40 years (2%). Death usually results from visceral and CNS dissemination leading to irreversible shock.[120] Many of those who die have a fulminant course and are dead in 1 week. Interstitial nephritis is found at autopsy in most cases.

Figure 15-29
Reported cases and incidence rates of Rocky Mountain spotted fever, 1990. *(From MMWR 40(27), 1991.)*

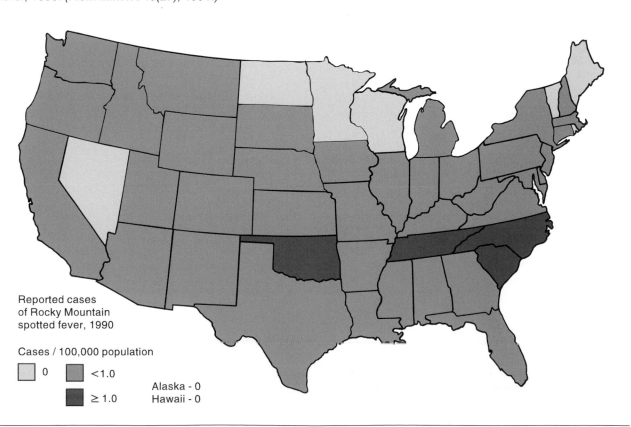

Reported cases
of Rocky Mountain
spotted fever, 1990

Cases / 100,000 population

☐ 0   ▨ <1.0

■ ≥ 1.0

Alaska - 0
Hawaii - 0

Diagnosis. The diagnosis must rely on clinical (fever, headache, rash, myalgia) and epidemiologic (tick exposure) criteria since laboratory confirmation cannot occur before 10 to 14 days after the onset of illness. The leukocyte count is normal or low. There is thrombocytopenia, elevated serum hepatic aminotransferase and hyponatremia. The blood urea nitrogen (BUN) may be elevated, indicating prerenal azotemia or interstitial nephritis.

Cases can be confirmed by serologic testing with a four-fold increase in antibody titer between acute- and convalescent-phase serum specimens by complement fixation (CF), indirect fluorescent antibody (IFA), indirect hemagglutination, latex agglutination, or microagglutination; or by a single convalescent titer 1:16 or higher (CF) or 1:64 or higher (IFA) in a clinically compatible case. Diagnosis can also be confirmed by blood or tissue culture isolation of spotted fever group rickettsiae or by fluorescent antibody staining of biopsy or autopsy specimens, but this is not practical and is rarely performed. False positive latex agglutination assays occur during pregnancy. The incidence increases with the duration of pregnancy and reaches 12.1% in the third trimester.[121]

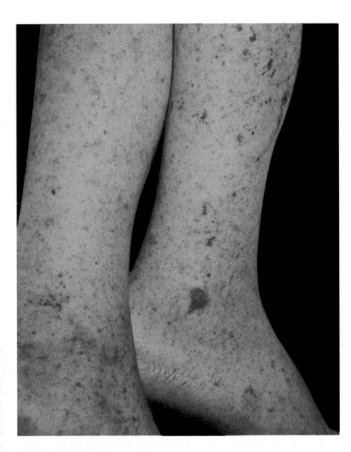

Figure 15-30
Rocky Mountain spotted fever. A generalized petechial eruption that involves the entire cutaneous surface, including the palms and soles.

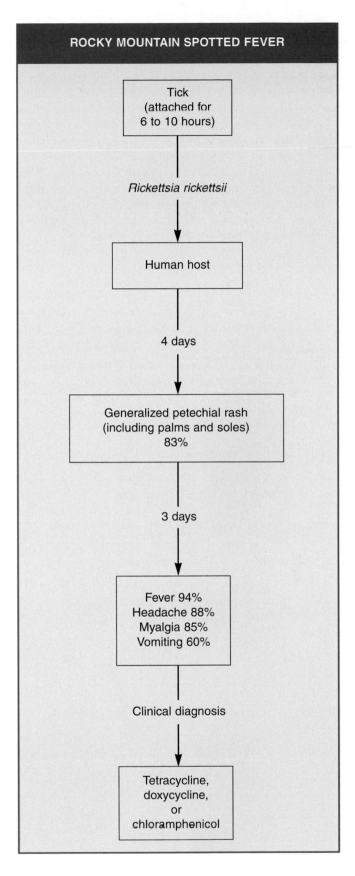

Treatment. Tetracycline, doxycycline,[122] and chloramphenicol are very effective and should be given in full dosages early in the course of the disease (see the box on p. 473). Persons over 8 years of age, except pregnant women, should be treated with tetracycline. Other causes of central nervous system infections such as *Neisseria meningitidis* or *Haemophilus influenzae* should be considered in the differential diagnosis, especially in the young. In these cases when diagnosis is uncertain, initial empirical therapy with chloramphenicol is indicated. Chloramphenicol is used for pregnant women and for children 8 years of age and under. A therapeutic trial of tetracycline should be considered for any adult in an endemic geographic area during the summer months who has fever, myalgia, and headache.

Tick bite paralysis

Tick bite paralysis[123] probably results from a neurotoxin[124] in tick saliva that is injected while the tick is feeding. The disease is most common in children, especially girls with long, thick hair. The tick, which hides on the scalp, groin, or other inconspicuous areas, must be attached for approximately 5 days before symptoms appear. The patient complains of fatigue, irritability, and leg paresthesias, followed by loss of coordination and an ascending paralysis within 24 hours. There is no pain or fever in the early stages. Death from respiratory failure can occur if the tick is not found and removed. Recovery occurs 24 hours after the tick is detached. Tick bite paralysis is most commonly seen in the Pacific Northwest and is caused by *Dermacentor andersoni*.

Figure 15-31
TICKED OFF. A plastic tool used to extract ticks. The entire tick, including the mouth parts, is removed.

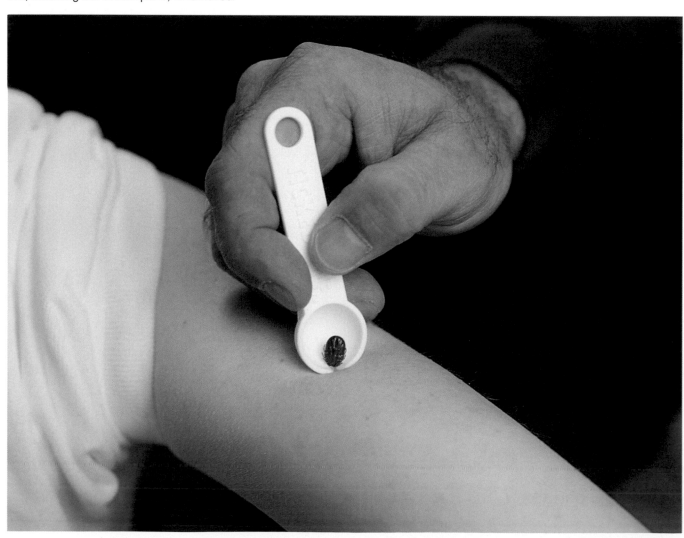

Removing ticks

TICKED OFF. A simple plastic tool called TICKED OFF removes ticks, including the mouth parts (Figure 15-31). Crawling or embedded ticks are removed completely, in one motion, while the bowl contains the tick for disposal. The tool can be used in any direction to remove ticks from the front, back, or side. TICKED OFF is held vertically. Applying slight pressure downward on the skin pushes the tick remover forward so it surrounds the tick on three sides, the small part of the "V" framing the tick. Continuous sliding motion of the notched area releases the tick. These inexpensive tools are now generally available.

Another technique for removing ticks is described in the box below. *Ixodid* ticks are difficult to remove because they cement their mouth parts into the skin (Figure 15-32). Mechanical removal may or may not remove the cement. If no cement, or "fleshlike" material, is attached to the mouth parts after extraction, the cement is still in the skin and attempts should be made to remove it to prevent subsequent irritation and infection. Ticks continue to salivate after extraction and must be disposed of immediately. In one study the application of petroleum jelly, fingernail polish, isopropyl alcohol, or a hot kitchen match failed to induce detachment of ticks. Hot objects may induce the ticks to salivate or regurgitate infected fluids into the wound.[125]

Ticks should not be removed by direct finger contact because of the danger of contracting a rickettsial infection. *Dermacentor* ticks are removed by gentle, steady, firm traction; the mouth parts usually come away attached to the tick. *Ixodes dammini* can rarely be removed intact by manual extraction. If detached, the mouth parts remain below the skin surface. The residual parts may be walled off and cause little harm or they may produce chronic irritation or stimulate a foreign-body reaction, resulting in a nodule known as a *tick-bite granuloma*. Twisting or jerking the tick during removal may break off the mouth parts. Manipulating a tick's body may cause infectious fluids to escape and enter the skin of the host or of the person removing the tick. The body of the tick should not be squeezed because additional fluid may be injected into the skin.

RECOMMENDED PROCEDURE FOR TICK REMOVAL

Use blunt curved forceps, tweezers, or a thread. If fingers are used, shield them with a rubber glove or thick cloth.

Grasp the tick with forceps as close to the skin surface as possible and pull upward with steady, even pressure.

Do not twist or jerk the tick, because this may cause the mouth parts and cement to be left embedded in the skin. Alternatively, take a thread (out in the woods find a loose thread in the seam of clothing), make a loop knot, pull it over the tick, and draw it tight around the smallest part of the tick at the skin surface. Pull both ends hard enough to lift up the skin. Hold this tension with thread or forceps for 3 or 4 minutes and the tick will slowly back out. Take care not to squeeze, crush, or puncture the body of the tick because its fluids (saliva, hemolymph, and gut contents) may contain infective agents.

Do not handle the tick with bare hands, because infectious agents may enter via mucous membranes or breaks in the skin. This precaution is particulary directed to individuals who "detick" domestic animals using unprotected fingers. Children should not be permitted to perform this procedure. After removing the tick, thoroughly disinfect the bite site and wash hands with soap and water.

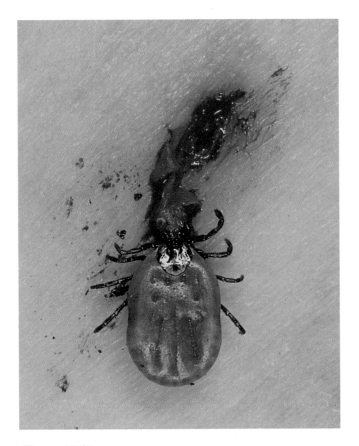

Figure 15-32
This tick was improperly extracted by grasping and pulling on the body. A large piece of tissue was torn away by the embedded mouth parts.

Cat-Scratch Disease

Cat-scratch disease is usually a benign, self-limited disease. The incidence in adults may be higher than previously reported.[126] Cat contact is documented in 99% of cases, and in most cases the cat is immature. Cat-scratch disease is not easily acquired. Usually just one member of a family is affected and adults rarely show symptoms even when all family members are exposed to the same animal. Cats do not have to scratch to transmit the disease. *Rochalimaea henselae* (order Rickettsiales) has been implicated as the cause.[127,128] Cats thought to be involved in cases of cat-scratch disease do not appear to be ill, but a study showed they may have become infected with *R. henselae* and be carriers of that organism. The natural reservoir is unknown, but fleas may be involved.[126]

Clinical manifestations. In one study, the primary inoculation site was observed in 93% of cases.[129] A red macule appears at the contact site and evolves into a nonpruritic papule (insect bites itch, but the papule of cat-scratch disease does not) 3 to 5 days after exposure to a cat; later the papule evolves into a vesicle filled with sterile fluid. The papule evolves through the vesicular and crust stage in 2 to 3 days. Regional lymphadenopathy appears in 1 or 2 weeks. Location of lymphadenopathy depends on the site of inoculation and is seen most often in the axilla, neck, jaw, and groin. The papule may go unnoticed or be attributed to injury, and lymphadenopathy may not be appreciated. The lesion persists for 1 to 3 weeks, with a few persisting for 3 months, and ends with a scar resembling chicken pox. The enlarged nodes may persist for months with gradual resolution. In 12% of the cases, the lymph nodes undergo focal necrosis within 5 weeks. Consider the possibility of cat-scratch disease in adults with chronic lymphadenopathy who own cats.

Most patients experience mild symptoms of generalized aching, malaise, and anorexia. The temperature is usually normal, but in approximately one third of cases it is elevated above 39° C (102° F). Inoculation within the confines of the eyelids or on the lids themselves causes a nonpainful palpebral conjunctivitis, preauricular lymphadenopathy, and fever, which characterizes the most common variant of cat-scratch disease (the oculoglandular syndrome of Parinaud).[130,131]

Severe systemic disease, including hepatosplenomegaly, osteolytic lesions, splenic abscesses and granulomas,[132] mediastinal masses, encephalopathy, and neuroretinitis, are uncommon. The majority of patients recover without sequelae.

Neurologic complications. A large study characterized the neurologic complications of cat-scratch disease. Encephalopathy occurred in 80% of patients; 20% had cranial and peripheral nerve involvement with facial nerve paresis, neuroretinitis, or peripheral neuritis. The average age of encephalopathy patients was 10.6 years (range, 1 to 66 years). Almost twice as many males as females were affected. Fifty percent were afebrile and only 26% had temperatures higher than 39° C. Convulsions occurred in 46% and combative behavior in 40%. Lethargy with or without coma was accompanied by variable neurologic signs. Results of laboratory studies, including imaging of the CNS, were inconsistent and nondiagnostic. All patients recovered within 12 months; 78% recovered within 1 to 12 weeks. There were no neurologic sequelae. Treatment consisted of control of convulsions and supportive measures.

Bacillary angiomatosis. A more severe form of systemic cat-scratch disease has been reported. There is prolonged fever, arthralgia, weight loss, and splenomegaly of 2 or more weeks' duration.[133] Multiple and widely distributed angiomatous nodules resembling Kaposi's sarcoma accompanied by symptoms of systemic cat-scratch disease were first reported in patients with AIDS.[134-136] There are three characteristic lesions: pyogenic granuloma–like papules, erythematous indurated plaques, and subcutaneous nodules. They vary from 1 mm to several cm in diameter and may be painful.[137] The pyogenic granuloma–like papules bleed easily. Cutaneous and parenchymal lesions also occur in immunocompromised cardiac and renal transplant recipients.[138] Immunocompetent persons can also develop cutaneous bacillary angiomatosis.

Diagnosis. The diagnosis can be established by finding a primary lesion site in the presence of lymphadenopathy and a history of intimate exposure to cats. Lymph node biopsy may not be necessary if the above are present. An indirect fluorescent antibody test for detection of humoral response to *R. henselae* has a high sensitivity (88%) and specificity (96%).[126,139] Lymph node histopathology varies with time. A Warthin-Starry silver stain of lymph nodes and skin at the primary site of inoculation shows small pleomorphic bacilli.[140] The gram-negative pleomorphic bacilli are found within cells and are most abundant in areas of necrosis in skin and lymph nodes. The primary lesion should be carefully sought in young patients experiencing unilateral lymphadenopathy. It may be remembered as a bump or pimple, or it may be hidden on the scalp, within the earlobe, or between the fingers. A skin test has been described for years but is not standarized or approved for general use. The bacillus can be cultured in biphasic brain-heart infusion media; culture is not routinely performed.[140] The differential diagnosis includes nontuberculous mycobacterial disease.

Treatment. Conservative, symptomatic treatment is recommended for the majority of patients with mild or moderate disease. Antibiotics are prescribed for severe disease. Many commonly used antibiotics are of little or no value. A recent review claims that erythromycin (500 mg four times daily) is the drug of choice. Excellent responses were also obtained with doxycycline.[141] A study showed that four antimicrobials were efficacious. Efficacy of the three oral drugs in decreasing order was rifampin 87%, ciprofloxacin 84%,[142] and trimethoprim-sulfamethoxazole 58%. Gentamicin sulfate intramuscular was 73% effective.[143] Suppurating lymph nodes should be aspirated with a 16- to 18-gauge needle. Resistance to first-generation cephalosporins correlated with clinical failure of therapy.

Animal and Human Bites

Animal bites. Animal bites, especially from dogs and cats, are common injuries. Most wounds heal with conservative therapy designed to cleanse and disinfect the bite site. Bite wound infections may be caused by *S. aureus*, *S. intermedius*, alpha-hemolytic streptococci, *Capnocytophaga canimorsus*, and other members of the oral flora. Anaerobic bacteria are present in approximately one third of bite wounds and cause abscesses and relatively serious infections. Animal bite wounds contain *Pasteurella multocida* (25% of dog bites and 50% of cat bites).[144,145] One study of animal and human bite wounds showed that 88% of recent animal bite wounds harbored potential bacterial pathogens in significant numbers.[146] It is difficult from a clinical perspective to predict which wounds will become infected.

Human bites. Anaerobic and aerobic bacteria infect human bite wounds. Humans harbors more pathogens than animals. Human bites have a higher incidence of serious infections and complications.[147] There are two types of human bites. Occlusional wounds occur when the teeth are sunk into the skin. Clenched-fist injuries occur when a tooth penetrates the hand. These require radiographic and surgical evaluation because severe complications result if a joint or bone is penetrated. Bacteria is carried beyond the penetration site beneath the skin when tendons are moved. The wound is usually 5 mm long. The hand becomes painful and swollen in 6 to 8 hours. *S. aureus*, *Eikenella corrodens*, *Haemophilus* species, and (in more than 50% of cases) anaerobic bacteria infect human bites. Residual disability and complications are frequent after clenched-fist injuries. Abscesses, osteomyelitis,[148] tendinitis, tendon rupture caused by infection, and residual stiffness of the joint may occur.

Management

Irrigation and debridement. Culture infected wounds before irrigation or debridement. Irrigation of the wound decreases the risk of infection. Tear wounds are copiously irrigated with sterile normal saline solution. Puncture wounds are irrigated using normal saline solution in a 20-ml syringe with an 18-gauge needle as a high-pressure jet. Devitalized tissue in human bite wounds predisposes to infection. Elimination of the crushed devitalized tissue by debridement of wound edges is the key to control infection and to ensure a successful outcome following surgical reconstruction.[149]

Immunization. Tetanus toxoid is given to patients requiring a booster. Determine the local prevalence of rabies. The decision to use a rabies vaccination must be made early.[150] Rabies prophylaxis is indicated for bites by carnivorous wild animals (skunks, raccoons), bats, and unvaccinated domestic dogs and cats. Vaccination is prophylactic, not therapeutic. Once signs of rabies occur survival is rare. Rabies Ig is also injected into the wound at various sites on the first day of treatment. Injecting a properly cleansed bite wound with rabies Ig is a safe practice and should be performed whenever there is a possibility that the biting animal might have rabies.[151] The vaccine is then given on days 3, 7, 14, and 28.

Suturing. One large study showed that human bite wounds did not have to be singled out as examples of wounds that should be left open.[152] Another author recommends initial approximation with adhesive strips and delayed closure in appropriate cases of animal bites.[153] Proper wound preparation with irrigation and debridement of devitalized tissue is the key to success.

Antibiotics. One study suggests that prophylactic oral antibiotics in low-risk dog bite wounds are not indicated.[154] Another study showed that even uncomplicated early human bites of the hand should be treated with antibiotics.[155] Others believe that antimicrobial therapy is indicated for all moderate to severe wounds, crush injuries, puncture wounds, wounds to the hands or near a bone, and wounds that may have penetrated a joint, even if clinically uninfected at the time of presentation.[153,156] Elevate edematous body parts. Infection responds in most cases to amoxicillin/clavulanic acid or penicillin, which are active against most potential bite pathogens. Many isolates of *P. multocida* are resistant to dicloxacillin, cephalexin, cefaclor, cefadroxil, and erythromycin.[157,158] Cefuroxime is active against *P. multocida*. Doxycycline and minocycline may be used for those allergic to penicillin. Ciprofloxacin is active against many potential pathogens but has not been studied.

Stinging Insects

Honeybees, wasps, hornets, and yellow jackets sting when confronted. A wasp, for example, will vigorously pursue nest intruders. Insect repellents, (e.g., deet) offer no protection. A firm, sharp stinger is imbedded in the skin, followed immediately by secretion of venom. The honey bee stings once and dies. Its barbed stinger, glands, and viscera remain in the victim. Imbedded honey bee stingers should be flicked away with a knife or fingernail. If the stinger is grasped with fingertips, the venom glands will compress and make the sting worse. Stingers of other stinging insects are not barbed and remain intact, ready to be used again. The injected venom can cause a localized or generalized reaction. Reactions are classified as toxic or allergic.

Toxic reactions. Hymenoptera stings cause cutaneous local reactions of limited size and duration in most individuals. This nonallergic local reaction is a toxic response to venom constituents. There is a sharp, pinprick sensation at the instant of stinging, followed by moderate burning pain at the site. A red papule or wheal appears and enlarges if scratched (Figure 15-33). The reaction subsides in hours. Multiple stings can produce a systemic toxic reaction with vomiting, diarrhea, headache, fever, muscle spasm, and loss of consciousness. More than 500 stings at one time may be fatal.

Allergic reactions. Allergic reactions are mediated by IgE antibodies directed at venom constituents. Reactions are localized or generalized.

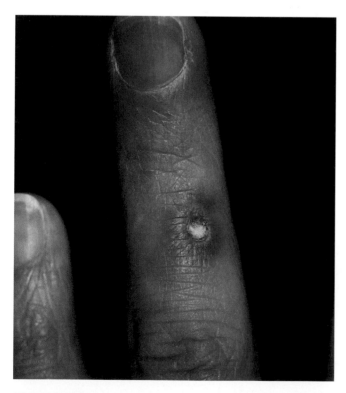

Figure 15-33
Bee sting. Severe local reaction with necrosis and ulceration at the sting site.

Localized reactions. Like the toxic reaction, the local allergic reaction begins with immediate pain, but the urticarial response is exaggerated. Swelling is thick and hard, as in angioedema. The urticarial plaque may be small or huge (Figure 15-34). Swelling lasts 1 to several days. Allergic local reactions greater than 10 cm in diameter are called *large local reactions*. They last for up to 5 days. Forty percent of patients with generalized allergic reactions have previously had large localized reactions.

Generalized reactions. The prevalence of generalized reactions to stings is approximately 0.4%. There are 40 fatalities from stings each year in the United States. Generalized reactions begin 2 to 60 minutes after the sting. Reactions vary from generalized itching with a few hives to anaphylaxis. Anaphylactic symptoms are typical of those occurring from any cause. They include generalized itching and hives, followed by shortness of breath, wheezing, nausea, and abdominal cramps. The reaction usually subsides spontaneously, but, in the unfortunate few, it progresses, with edema of the upper airway causing obstruction and death. Following sting anaphylaxis, approximately 50% of patients continue to have allergic reactions to subsequent stings, but up to 42% have an improved response.[159]

Most reactions in children are mild, with just hives. Children with dermal reactions only have a benign course and are unlikely to have recurrent reactions. The more severe reactions, such as shock and loss of consciousness, are more common in adults. Adults whose reactions include urticaria, obstruction of the upper or lower airway, or hypotension, and children whose reactions include obstruction of the upper or lower airway or hypotension, have an increased risk of future systemic reactions to stings.[160] Patients may develop delayed-onset allergic symptoms up to a week after the sting that range from typical anaphylaxis to serum sickness and are mediated by venom-specific IgE. Immunotherapy is recommended for patients with these reactions.[161] The possibility of a fatal insect sting should be considered in unwitnessed deaths occurring outdoors in summer.

The prognosis of patients with urticarial reactions to insect stings cannot be predicted by the immunologic tests presently available. One study found that 14% of patients with an urticarial reaction to previous insect stings had a systemic reaction with urticaria and angioedema with the next bite.[162]

Diagnosis. A diagnostic workup is not recommended for local reactions or for persons who have not experienced a systemic reaction. Patients who have large localized or generalized eruptions should be tested with venom extracts from honeybees, yellow jackets, yellow hornets, white-faced hornets, or wasps. Skin testing with species-specific, pure venom is the procedure of choice for determining sensitivity. Up to 15% of the general population may have positive results to such tests. The absolute titers of serum venom-specific IgE appear to be unrelated to a specific feature of stinging insect sensitivity.[163] Negative RAST may have more clinical validity than a positive RAST. Low venom-specific

IgG levels are associated with an elevated risk of treatment failure during the first 4 years of immunotherapy with yellow jacket or mixed vespid venoms.[164]

Venom immunotherapy. Venom immunotherapy is highly effective and confers 98% to 99% protection in patients who have experienced previous systemic reactions to insect stings. A 2- to 5-hour regimen of rapid venom immunotherapy is a safe, alternative method of venom administration for patients who are at immediate risk for re-sting anaphylaxis.[165] Venom immunotherapy is effective in preventing recurrences of large local reactions but is not usually recommended for either adults or children.[166]

A large study demostrated a surprisingly low rate of reactions among untreated children. No characteristics could be identified that were predictive of repeat reactions. Only 9.2% of stings in untreated children led to a systemic reaction, and, since there was no progression to a more severe reaction, it was concluded that venom immunotherapy was unnecessary for most children who are allergic to insect stings.[167]

For most patients, 3 years of therapy appear to be adequate, despite persistence of positive venom skin tests.[168] Well-tolerated honeybee venom immunotherapy may be stopped after at least 3 years, provided its efficacy has been documented by a sting challenge without a systemic reaction.[169] Venom immunotherapy should be continued for 5 years in patients with pre-venom immunotherapy field-sting reactions of grade IV (maximum) severity. Venom skin tests and venom-specific antibody results do not reli-ably predict the outcome of deliberate sting challenges or the subsequent clinical course of individual patients who stop venom immunotherapy.[170]

Treatment. Localized nonallergic stings are treated with ice or a paste made by mixing 1 teaspoon of meat tenderizer with 1 teaspoon of water. Localized allergic reactions are treated with cool, wet compresses and antihistamines.

Treatment of severe generalized reactions for adults includes aqueous epinephrine 1:1000 in a dosage of 0.3 to 0.5 ml administered subcutaneously and repeated once or twice at 20-minute intervals if needed. Epinephrine may be given intramuscularly if shock is imminent. If the patient is hypotensive, intravenous injections of 1:10,000 dilution may be necessary. If a severe reaction is feared, epinephrine should be administered immediately; to wait for symptoms to develop can be a dangerous practice.

Kits with preloaded epinephrine syringes are available (e.g., Epipen Auto-Injector, Anakit). Highly sensitive patients should have these kits available at home and during travel. For practice, one injection of physiologic saline should be self-administered under the supervision of a physician. Shortly after administration of epinephrine, antihistamines such as diphenhydramine (Benadryl 25 to 50 mg) are given orally or intramuscularly depending on the severity of the reaction.

Patients with a history of insect sting anaphylaxis and positive venom skin tests should have epinephrine available.

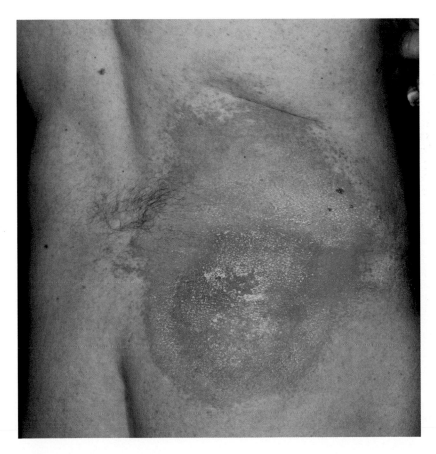

Figure 15-34
Bee sting. A huge, urticarial plaque occurred within hours in this patient with a known history of bee-sting allergy.

Biting Insects

Biting insects such as fleas, flies, and mosquitoes do not bite in the literal sense; rather, they stab their victims with a sharp stylet covered with saliva. The sharp pain is caused by the stab; the reaction depends on the degree of sensitivity to the saliva. All of these insects are capable of transmitting infectious diseases. Biting insects seem to prefer some individuals to others. They are attracted by the warmth and moisture of humans. The patient's individual sensitivity determines the type and severity of the bite reaction. Patients who have not had previous exposure or those who have had numerous bites may show little or no response. Those who are sensitive develop localized urticarial papules and plaques immediately following the bite. The papules and plaques proceed to fade in hours and are replaced by red papules that last for days.

Papular urticaria. Papular urticaria refers to hypersensitivity bite reactions in children.[171,172] Young children who are left outside unattended in the summer months may receive numerous bites. They soon become sensitized, and subsequent bites show red, raised, urticarial papules that itch intensely (Figure 15-35). The young child who was initially indifferent to bites may habitually excoriate newly evolved lesions, creating crusts and infection. Chronically excoriated lesions may last for months, eventually leaving white, round scars.

Fleas. Fleas are tiny, red-brown, hard-bodied, wingless insects that are capable of jumping approximately 2 feet. They have distinctive, laterally flattened abdomens that allow them to slip between the hairs of their hosts (Figure 15-36). They live in rugs and on the bodies of animals and may jump onto humans.

Flea bites occur in a cluster or group (Figure 15-37). A tiny, red dot or bite punctum may be seen at times. Most lesions are grouped around the ankles or lower legs, areas within easy leaping distance of the floor. Adult men are infrequently affected because their socks and pants protect them. Fleas reside on cats, dogs, the animal's bedding, and in the entire house. All sources must be treated for effective flea control.

Methoprene is an important new chemical for management of flea infestation. This is a synthetic equivalent of a natural insect hormone essential for growth regulation. Methoprene prevents flea larvae from maturing, and if used early in the year on carpets and animals' bedding should afford effective control. Methoprene (Siphotrol) is available in a spray and fogger. These products are claimed to protect against infestation for 4 months.[173] Bubonic plague was spread throughout Europe in the Middle Ages by fleas that had fed on infected rats.

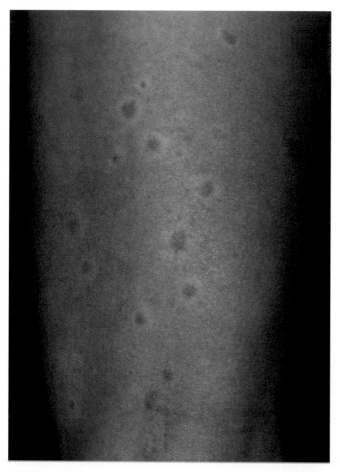

Figure 15-35
Papular urticaria. A hypersensitivity reaction to insect bites seen in children. A wheal develops at the site of each bite.

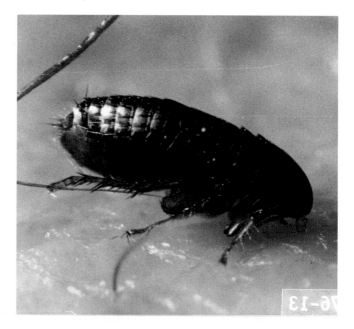

Figure 15-36
Flea. Thin wingless insects with very hard bodies and large hind legs adapted for jumping. *(Courtesy Ken Gray, Oregon State University Extension Services.)*

Myiasis. Flies such as the horsefly, deerfly, and black fly can inflict a painful bite. The common housefly does not bite or sting. The invasion of live human or animal tissue by fly larvae (maggots) is termed *myiasis*. Many organs can be involved[174] but the skin is the most common site.

Larvae species. Many species of flies around the world cause myiasis. Most cases are seen in returning travelers from Central or South America (*Dermatobia hominis*, the human botfly) or from Africa (*Cordylobia anthropophaga*, the tumbu fly).[175,176]

Infestation. Flies of several different species deposit their eggs on skin. Young children who fall asleep outside are likely victims. Larvae may be acquired from petting or kissing dogs or cats contaminated with larvae. Larvae adhere and enter the nose, eyes, mouth, anus, or they penetrate skin. Larvae in the eyes, nose, or trachea of humans may attempt migration through deep organs. Those that penetrate skin develop at the site of penetration. Larvae enter the skin and reach the underlying subcutaneous tissue, where they feed and grow.[177] The time required for mature larvae to develop is species specific. At maturity they enlarge the central pore and prepare to exit.

Clinical presentation. Most patients presented in late August or early September. Lesions are found on the face, scalp, chest, arms, or legs. A red papule 2 to 4 mm in diameter develops (Figure 15-38). The lesion resembles a furuncle or inflamed cyst and is called a *warble*, the maggot is called a *bot*. Flies that cause furuncular myiasis are called *botflies*. The head of the larva rises to the surface for air about once a minute through a small central pore. Movement of the larval spiracle (respiratory apparatus) may be observed. Serous or seropurulent exudate flows from the central punctum. Symptoms range from a mild itching or stinging to intense pain leading to agitation and insomnia. An intense inflammatory reaction occurs in the tissue surrounding the larvae. Infection by *Tunga penetrans* may resemble myiasis. *T. penetrans* is a flea that invades the skin and produces a furuncular nodule. Tungiasis is almost always on the feet, whereas myiasis on the feet is rare. Tungiasis is aquired in South America and Africa.

Treatment. In most cases the larva can be forced through the central hole with manual pressure. *D. hominis* is attached to the skin by hooklets. Application of petroleum jelly over the pore may force the larva out for air. Another method involves the injection of lidocaine hydrochloride under the nodule. The pressure of the injection is sufficient to push the larva out.[178] Bacon therapy is another noninvasive technique. The fatty parts of raw bacon are placed over the opening of the skin lesion. The fly larva crawls far enough into the bacon and can be removed with forceps within 3 hours.[179] It is usually not necessary to enlarge the hole, but if the larva does not emerge, a #11 blade may be used to enlarge the hole slightly (Figure 15-38). There is usually only one maggot in each mass.

Mosquitoes. Mosquito saliva is the source of antigens that produce the bite reactions in humans. Cutaneous reactions to mosquito bites are usually pruritic wheals and delayed papules. The rate of immediate reaction increases from early childhood to adolescence and decreases with age from adulthood. The appearance and intensity of the delayed reaction decreases with age. Arthus-type local and systemic symptoms can occur, but anaphylactic reactions are very rare.

A characteristic sequence of events takes place in all subjects exposed to mosquito bites over time. The initial bite causes no reaction, but with subsequent bites a delayed cutaneous lesion appears several hours after the bite and lasts 1 to 3 days or longer. After repeated bites for approximately 1 month, an immediate wheal develops that varies from 2 to 10 mm. Then, with further exposure for several months, the delayed reaction disappears. After repeated bites, the old bite sites may show flare-ups. Blisters can occur on the lower legs. In England, the condition known as *seasonal bullous eruption* was shown to be caused by mosquitoes. Patients with chronic lymphocytic leukemia may exhibit severe, delayed bite reactions that can appear before the malignancy has been diagnosed.[180] Patients with acquired

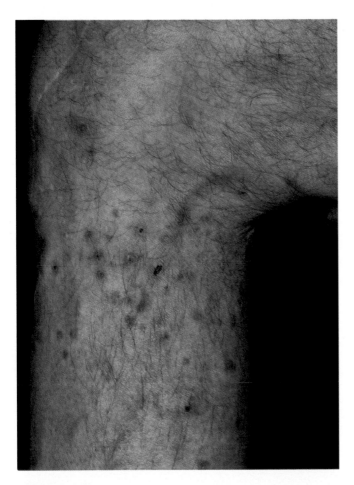

Figure 15-37
Flea bites. A cluster of bites in the knee area. This is a common site because a flea can jump no higher than approximately 2 feet.

immunodeficiency syndrome who had pruritus and chronic, nonspecific-appearing skin eruptions showed increased antibody titers to mosquito salivary gland antigens. This represents a form of chronic "recall" reaction. The increase may be a consequence of nonspecific B-cell activation, a feature of AIDS.[181] No desensitization treatment is generally available for mosquito allergy.

Prevention and management. Biting insects are attracted to human body odor.

DEET. The most effective insect repellent available is diethyltoluamide (deet). It is especially active against mosquitoes, but it also repels biting flies, gnats, chiggers, ticks, and other insects. It is an effective repellent for most biting insects and ticks, but it does not repel stinging insects. Deet blocks the ability of some biting insects to track the victim's vapor trail. It is provided in most commercially available insect repellents, either alone or in combination with other chemicals that may enhance its effectiveness. Products containing deet in concentrations above 75% are the most effective. Repellents are available as liquids, sticks, sprays, and saturated pads. The sprays contain the lowest concentration of deet and are the most expensive. All exposed skin surfaces must be covered with repellent; insects seek out even small areas of skin that have not been covered. When insects begin to land on the skin, it is time for another application of deet. Repellent may have to be applied every 2 hours in hot, humid weather, or it may protect up to 6 hours when the air is dry and cool.

OIL OF CITRONELLA. Oil of citronella is a natural component of plants. It is an effective non-DEET repellent. Avon's Skin-So-Soft Moisturizing Suncare Plus and Tréo 3-way Outdoor Protection lotion contain oil of citronella.

ANTIHISTAMINES. In mosquito-sensitive subjects, prophylactically administered cetirizine (10 mg), a new nonsedating antihistamine, is an effective drug against both immediate and delayed mosquito-bite symptoms.[182]

PERMETHRIN. Permethrin, a pesticide used for the treatment of lice, is also effective as a clothing spray for protection against mosquitoes and ticks. The aerosol is available as Permanone Tick Repellent.

THIAMINE. A few reports claim that 75 to 150 mg of thiamine hydrochloride taken orally each day during the summer months protects against insect bites.[183] Others think that it is not effective. Thiamine hydrochloride is safe and may be worth trying, especially for children who are bitten often.

Insect bite symptoms are treated with cool, wet compresses, topical steroids, and oral antihistamines. A paste made of 1 teaspoon of meat tenderizer and 1 teaspoon of water provides symptomatic relief and discourages children from excoriating bites.

Rarely, a patient may develop a generalized reaction to fly bites. Whole-body fly extracts are available for desensitization for the rare patient who develops a generalized reaction to fly bites.

Figure 15-38 Myiasis (extraction of the larva).

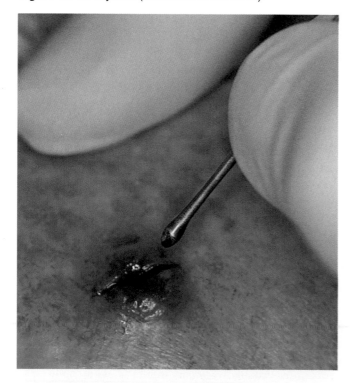

A, An incision is made across the central hole.

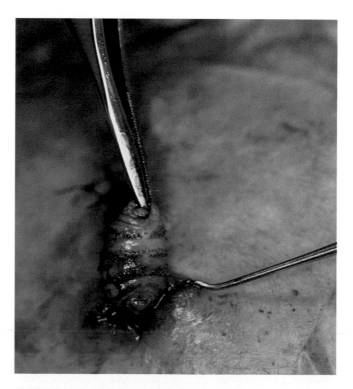

B, The larva is extracted intact with forceps.

Creeping Eruption

Creeping eruption (cutaneous larva migrans) is a unique cutaneous eruption caused by the aimless wandering of the hookworm larvae through the skin. *Ancylostoma braziliense* is the most common species. Infection is most frequent in warmer climates such as the Caribbean (especially Jamaica), Africa, South America, Southeast Asia, and the Southeastern United States. Adult nematodes thrive in the intestines of dogs and cats, where they deposit ova that are carried to the ground in feces. The ova hatch into larvae and lie in ambush in the soil waiting for a cat or dog. In their haste to complete their growth cycle, these indiscriminate parasites may penetrate the skin of a human at the point where skin touches the soil. Workers who crawl on their backs under houses may acquire a diffuse infiltration with numerous lesions. The hookworms soon learn that they have preyed on the wrong host. The larva penetrates the skin in hopes of eventually reaching the intestines; however, physiologic limitations in humans prevent invasion deeper than the basal area of the epidermis. The trapped larva struggles a few millimeters to a few centimeters each day laterally through the epidermis in a random fashion, creating a tract reminiscent of the trail of a sea snail wandering aimlessly over the sand at low tide (Figure 15-39). Many larvae may be present in the same area, creating several closely approximated wavy lines.

Symptoms begin days to 3 weeks after exposure to infested soil. During larval migration, a local inflammatory response is provoked by release of larval secretions consisting largely of proteolytic enzymes. Itching is moderate to intense and secondary infection or eczematous inflammation occurs (Figure 15-40). Eosinophilia may approach 30% in some cases. The 1-cm larva stays concealed directly ahead of the advancing tip of the wavy, twisted, red-to-purple, 3 mm tract. If untreated, larvae usually die within 2 to 8 weeks, but occasionally persist for up to a year. The dead worm is eventually sloughed away as the epidermis matures.[184]

Löffler's syndrome, which is a transitory, patchy infiltration of the lung, may develop with an accompanying eosino-

CUTANEOUS LARVA MIGRANS

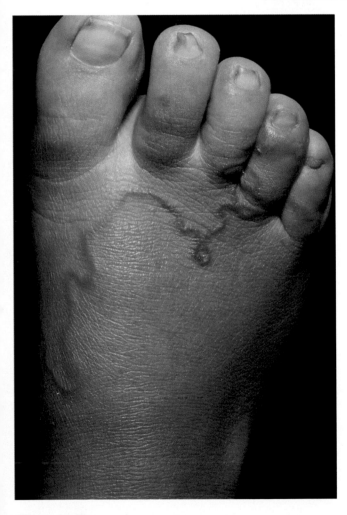

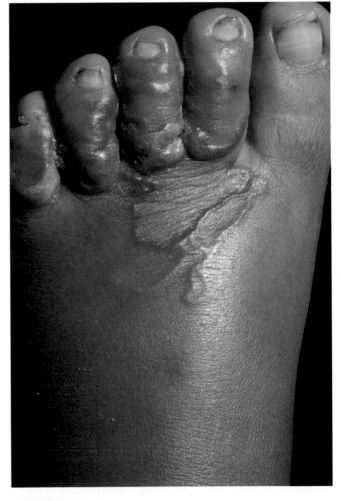

Figure 15-39
Elevated tracks that change position and shape as the larvae migrate through the epidermis.

Figure 15-40
A severe infestation with multiple tracts and secondary infection of the toe webs.

philia of the blood and sputum.[185,186] This occurs with dermal penetration and subsequent larval invasion of the bloodstream. This is most common in patients with severe cutaneous infestation.

Management. Children are advised not to sit, lie, or walk barefoot on wet soil or sand. The ground should be covered with impenetrable material when sitting or lying on the ground. Thiabendazole (Mintezol) is a vermicidal effective against hookworm larvae. It is available in chewable tablets (500 mg) and oral suspension (500 mg/5 ml).

Topical application of thiabendazole is the treatment of choice.[187] It is available as a 15% liquid, or a 15% cream may be compounded. The topical medicine is applied generously two to three times a day for 5 days; 98.1% of patients treated in this way were cured. The cream is prepared by crushing 500-mg thiabendazole tablets and formulating it in a water-soluble cream base. Resolution of pruritus and cessation of larval track migration occurs within 48 hours. The cream is applied to affected areas and 2 cm past the advancing border, since the parasite has often migrated well beyond the site of visible skin change. Albendazole, given either as a single dose of 400 mg or 200 mg twice a day for 3 days cured six (85.7%) patients[188-190]. Albendazole can be obtained through the Centers for Disease Control and Prevention (Atlanta, Ga). Two hundred micrograms per kilogram of oral ivermectin in a single dose also cures the disease.[191,192] This new avermectin B derivative is available in some parts of Europe. Oral antibiotics and topical steroids are prescribed if secondary infection and eczematous inflammation are present.

Oral thiabendazole is effective, but albendazole is better tolerated. Thiabendazole is associated with nausea, vomiting, and dizziness in 40% of cases, and patient noncompliance is high. The usual dose for patients weighing less than 150 lb is 10 mg/lb. For patients weighing over 150 lb, the dose is 1.5 gm. Each dose is taken twice a day after meals for 2 days and repeated after 2 days if the lesions remain active. Freezing the advancing tip of the tract is not very effective and causes unnecessary tissue destruction. The larval track represents an allergic reaction and does not correlate with the exact location of the worm. Therefore the use of liquid nitrogen on the leading edge of the track is an imprecise treatment method.

Ants

FIRE ANTS

The fire ant entered the United States from South America circa 1920 and spread quickly to several states in the southeast. They have no natural enemies and may ultimately infest one quarter of the United States.[193] Between 30% and 60% of the population in infested areas are stung each year. Stings are most frequent during the summer; the legs of children are the most common target. Fire ants are small ($\frac{1}{16}$ to $\frac{1}{4}$ inch long) and yellow-to-red or black with a large head containing prominent incurved jaws and a beelike stinger on the tail. They build large mounds (1 to 3 feet in diameter) in playgrounds, yards, and open fields in concentrations as high as 200 per acre. Colonies are formed at ground level in sandy areas. The grass at the periphery of the mound remains undisturbed and unharvested, unlike the mound of the harvester ant. The venom is made up almost entirely of piperidine alkaloids, in contrast to the venoms of other *Hymenoptera*, such as the wasp, which is up to one half polypeptide proteins, measured by weight. The small fraction of proteins in fire-ant venom induces the IgE response.

The sting reaction. Sting reactions range from local pustules and large, late-phase responses to life-threatening anaphylaxis. The fire ant is aggressive and vicious. When provoked, they attack in numbers. In an instant, the fire ant grasps the skin with its jaws, which establishes a pivot point. It arches its body, injects venom through a distal abdominal stinger, then, if undisturbed, rotates and stings repeatedly, inflicting as many as 20 stings. This often results in a circle of stings with two tiny, red dots in the center where the jaws were attached. The pain is immediate and sharp, like a bee sting. Pain subsides in minutes and is replaced by a wheal and flare that resolves in 30 to 60 minutes;[194] 8 to 24 hours later a sterile vesicle forms and later becomes umbilicated. The contents of the vesicle rapidly become purulent (Figure 15-41). Pustules resolve in approximately 10 days. A large, local, late-phase reaction occurs in 17% to 56% of patients and lasts 24 to 72 hours. The plaque is red, edematous, indurated, and extremely pruritic. Eosinophils, neutrophils, and fibrin are present. Edema may be severe and compress nerves and blood vessels.

Patients who are allergic to fire ants may present with anaphylaxis.[168] This life-threatening reaction may occur hours after a sting. Check for stings on the lower extremity, especially between the toes, when a patient presents with anaphylaxis.

Treatment. The bite is treated with cool compresses, followed by application of a paste made with baking soda. Sarna lotion (0.5% camphor + 0.5% menthol) is soothing, especially if it is refrigerated. Application of meat tenderizer is of no value.[195] Oral antihistamines (e.g., hydroxyzine) provide some relief. A short course of prednisone is used for severe local reactions.

Immunotherapy. Consider immunotherapy for patients with severe hypersensitivity to the venom or those who have had a previous anaphylactic reaction. The optimum technique for skin testing and desensitization has not been determined.[196] Because of the lack of availability of venom, whole-body extracts are routinely used for desensitization.[197] The recommended desensitization schedule is weekly subcutaneous injections of the extract, with the dosage increased until an empirically determined maintenance dosage, usually 0.5 ml of a 1:10 dilution of commercially available whole-body extract, is reached. This maintenance dose is then given approximately once a month.[198]

HARVESTER ANTS

Harvester ants are large ($\frac{1}{4}$ to $\frac{1}{2}$ inch long), red-brown, and sometimes winged. They are found in the southeastern United States, where they build flat-topped, raised mounds surrounded by a zone that has been harvested or cleared of grass. The harvester ant destroys crops. When disturbed, they attack in numbers and inflict vicious stings. The red bite clears in days and does not form a pustule, unlike the bite of the fire ant.

Figure 15-41
Fire ant stings. Multiple pustules in a cluster.

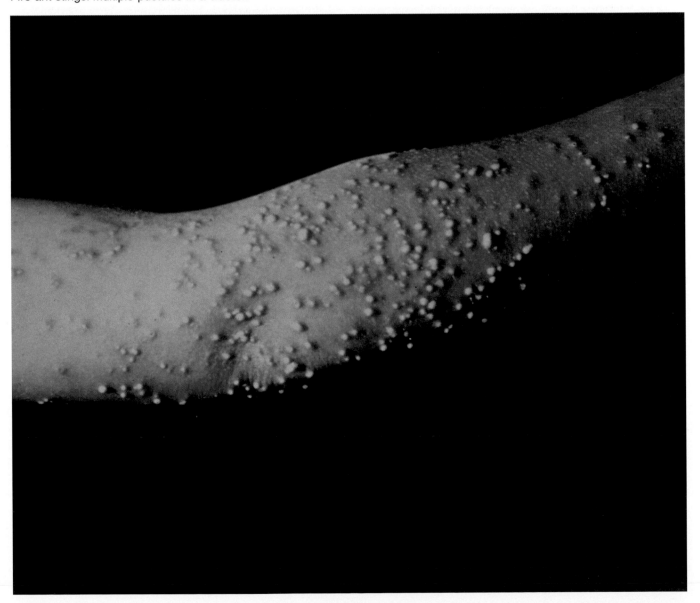

Dermatitis Associated with Swimming

There is increasing human contact with marine life. As more people travel to oceans for sports diving and other marine-related activities, the incidence of marine envenomations rises. Serious injury from a number of common sea creatures is possible (see the boxes on pp. 488 and 489).[199-201]

SWIMMER'S ITCH (FRESH WATER)

Swimmer's itch (schistosome cercarial dermatitis) occurs on uncovered skin and is a transient, pruritic dermatitis caused by the epidermal penetration of cercariae, a larval form of animal schistosomes. The microscopic larvae of the parasitic flatworm schistosomes, after being released from snails, swim in the water seeking a warm-blooded host, such as a duck. The indiscriminant larvae may accidently penetrate a human and do not develop further. Schistosomes of humans cause systemic disease, but animal schistosome cercariae die after epidemal penetration, resulting in a rash. The disease is found throughout the world and restricted primarily to fresh water, although salt water infestations have been reported.[202] In the United States, the states surrounding the Great Lakes have the highest incidence. Outbreaks are episodic and determined by snail maturation. Shedding occurs on bright, warm days in early or midsummer, with the highest incidence of infestation occurring near the shore.

Symptoms. The intensity of the eruption depends on the degree of sensitization. Some people do not develop a rash, whereas others swimming in the same water develop intense eruptions. Initial symptoms are minor after the first exposure and papules occur only after sensitization is acquired, approximately 5 to 13 days later. The typical eruption occurs with subsequent exposures. It begins as bathing water evaporates from the skin surface and cercariae begin penetrating the skin.[203] Itching occurs for approximately 1 hour and is followed hours later by the development of discrete, highly pruritic papules and, occasionally, pustules surrounded by erythema at the points of contact. They reach maximum intensity in 2 to 3 days and subside in a week. Secondary infection occurs following excoriation.

Treatment. Treatment consists of relieving symptoms while the eruption fades. Itching is controlled with antihistamines, cool compresses, and shake lotions such as calamine lotion. Intense inflammation may be suppressed with group II through V topical steroids. Towel drying immediately after leaving the water is an effective preventative measure, since most larvae penetrate the skin as water is evaporating.

NEMATOCYST STINGS

Nematocysts are unique structures found on animals in the phylum Cnidaria. Nematocyst stings are responsible for the vast majority of skin problems in people who visit the reefs. Nematocysts are microscopic capsules used for both capturing prey and defense. They contain a toxin-covered, flexible, barbed whip that is uncoiled and discharged when touched (see diagram above).

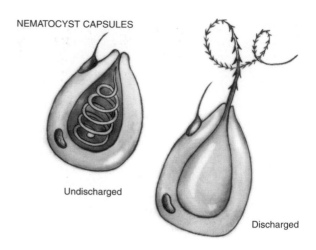

NEMATOCYST CAPSULES

Undischarged

Discharged

Cnidarians are either fixed to the reef or free swimming. Most are tiny individual animals that group together by the thousands to form fixed colonies, such as the corals and hydroids that make up most of a coral reef's structure. Jellyfish and anemones live as individuals. All of these animals have tentacles that contain nematocysts on their surfaces. The stings of most cnidarians are not harmful, but a few are quite toxic.

It is advisable to bring a plastic bottle of vinegar to the beach, because rubbing the affected area or washing with fresh water can cause nematocysts to discharge. Saturating the area with vinegar immobilizes unspent nematocysts.

Seabather's Eruption

Seabather's eruption occurs under bathing suits and is predominant in Mexico, Bermuda, Florida, the Gulf states, and as far north as Long Island, New York. Larvae of members of the phylum Cnidaria (formerly Coelenterata), such as jellyfish,[204] and sea anemones,[205] have been implicated. Outbreaks occur when jellyfish or anemone larvae are transported to shore by ocean currents. The sea thimble is the jellyfish responsible for seabather's eruption in the Caribbean (Figure 15-42). Each larva has more than 200 nematocysts, tiny organs that uncoil a threadlike, hollow stinger. When activated by skin contact, pressure, or contact with fresh water, the nematocysts are activated and toxin is forcefully injected into the swimmer's skin. Larvae are trapped under the bathing suit. Stinging is noted when the bather comes into shallow water or leaves the water. Prolonged wearing of a contaminated suit, strenuous exercise, and exposure to showers or fresh-water pools activate nematocysts and make the symptoms much worse. Red, itchy papules or wheals resembling insect bites occur minutes to several hours later. The papules may coalesce to cover wide areas (Figure 15-43). The rash lasts for 3 to 7 days; severe cases last 6 weeks. Headache, chills, and fever are present in extensive cases. The rash may recur if a suit contaminated with nematocysts is reworn. Treatment is symptomatic, with cooling lotions (e.g., Sarna), antihistamines, topical steroids, and, in severe cases, prednisone.

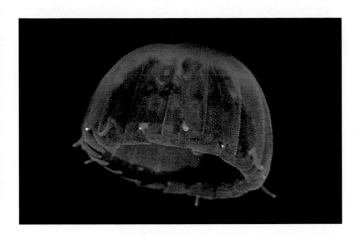

Figure 15-42
Sea thimble. The larva of this tiny jellyfish (½ to ¾ inches) is responsible for most cases of seabather's eruption in the Caribbean. *(Courtesy Reid E. McNeal, Grand Cayman, BWI.)*

Figure 15-43
Seabather's eruption. A common problem in the Caribbean. Nematocyst-bearing larvae may be trapped under the bathing suit and produce an intensely itching and painful papular eruption.

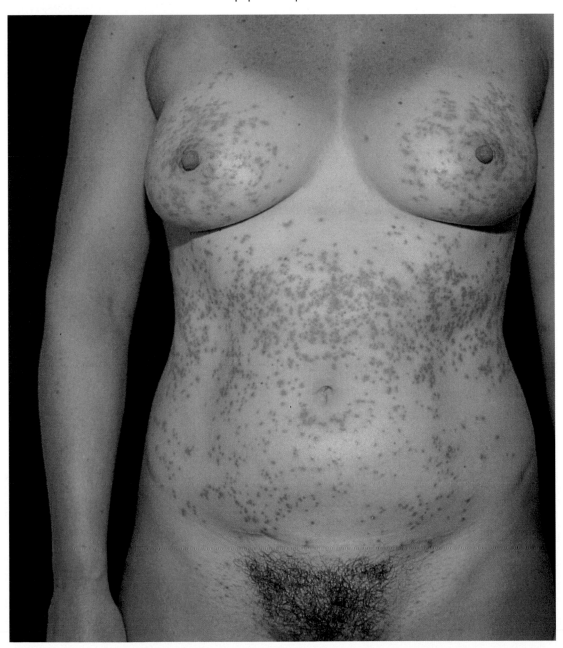

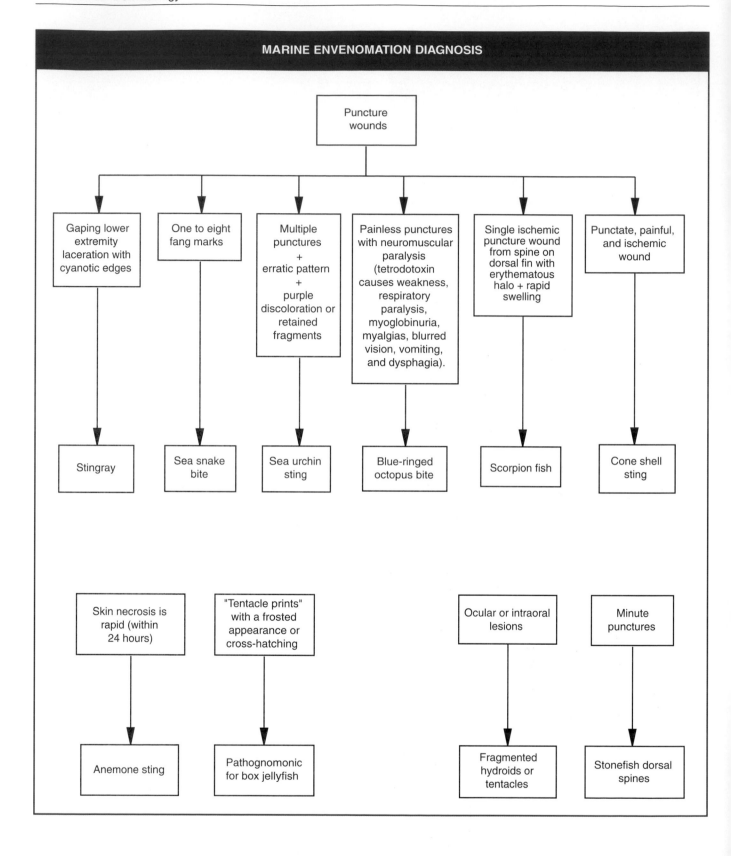

MARINE ENVENOMATION DIAGNOSIS

Puncture wounds

- Gaping lower extremity laceration with cyanotic edges → Stingray
- One to eight fang marks → Sea snake bite
- Multiple punctures + erratic pattern + purple discoloration or retained fragments → Sea urchin sting
- Painless punctures with neuromuscular paralysis (tetrodotoxin causes weakness, respiratory paralysis, myoglobinuria, myalgias, blurred vision, vomiting, and dysphagia). → Blue-ringed octopus bite
- Single ischemic puncture wound from spine on dorsal fin with erythematous halo + rapid swelling → Scorpion fish
- Punctate, painful, and ischemic wound → Cone shell sting

- Skin necrosis is rapid (within 24 hours) → Anemone sting
- "Tentacle prints" with a frosted appearance or cross-hatching → Pathognomonic for box jellyfish
- Ocular or intraoral lesions → Fragmented hydroids or tentacles
- Minute punctures → Stonefish dorsal spines

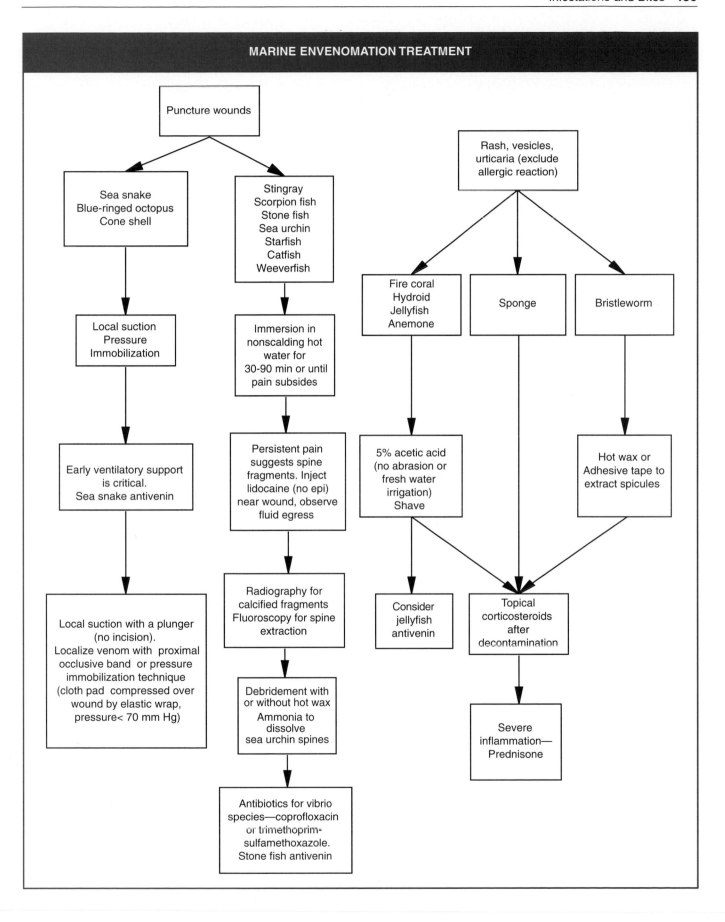

MARINE ENVENOMATION TREATMENT

Puncture wounds

Sea snake
Blue-ringed octopus
Cone shell

Stingray
Scorpion fish
Stone fish
Sea urchin
Starfish
Catfish
Weeverfish

Local suction
Pressure
Immobilization

Immersion in
nonscalding hot
water for
30-90 min or until
pain subsides

Early ventilatory support
is critical.
Sea snake antivenin

Persistent pain
suggests spine
fragments. Inject
lidocaine (no epi)
near wound, observe
fluid egress

Local suction with a plunger
(no incision).
Localize venom with proximal
occlusive band or pressure
immobilization technique
(cloth pad compressed over
wound by elastic wrap,
pressure< 70 mm Hg)

Radiography for
calcified fragments
Fluoroscopy for spine
extraction

Debridement with
or without hot wax
Ammonia to
dissolve
sea urchin spines

Antibiotics for vibrio
species—coprofloxacin
or trimethoprim-
sulfamethoxazole.
Stone fish antivenin

Rash, vesicles,
urticaria (exclude
allergic reaction)

Fire coral
Hydroid
Jellyfish
Anemone

Sponge

Bristleworm

5% acetic acid
(no abrasion or
fresh water
irrigation)
Shave

Hot wax or
Adhesive tape to
extract spicules

Consider
jellyfish
antivenin

Topical
corticosteroids
after
decontamination

Severe
inflammation—
Prednisone

FLORIDA, CARIBBEAN, BAHAMAS

Seabather's eruption (sea itch) is the most common marine-related problem in the waters south of the United States. Swimmers and divers are affected by the nematocyst-bearing tiny larvae of the sea thimble (a jellyfish). Itchy papules occur under or at the edge of bathing suits and wet suits. The eruption used to be seasonal but is now reported year-round. Areas with a high concentration of larvae change with the wind and tides.

Most sea animals are defensive. Divers who do not touch the fragile reef or handle fish are safe. Some of the sponges, corals, and anemones are toxic. Injuries to the feet caused by sea urchin spines are now uncommon because divers wear protective foot gear. Shuffling the feet in the water, rather than walking like on land, scares up sting rays buried in the sand. Sting rays are not aggressive, but stepping on a submerged ray's back can result in a deep, gaping wound. The floating Portuguese man-of-war is seen in Florida but is not common in the Caribbean. Becoming wrapped in its tentacles can result in severe swelling and blistering of an entire extremity. Box jellyfish (sea wasps) have a 2- to 3-inch cuboidal dome with 3-inch tentacles. These small creatures are occasionally seen in shallow water at night and are attracted to light. They are one of the most toxic animals on earth and can produce severe stings and shock. The erect dorsal spines of the odd-shaped, bottom-dwelling spotted scorpion fish are covered with a toxin that can penetrate rubber and skin (Figure 15-44).

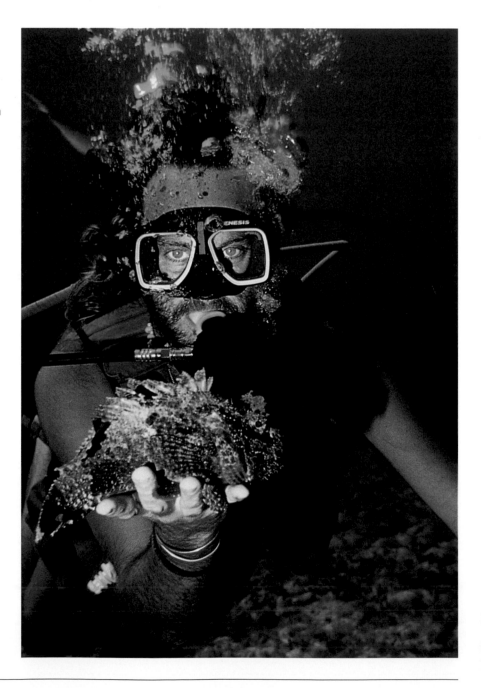

Figure 15-44
Spotted scorpion fish. These ugly fish lie motionless on the coral reef and blend in with the background. Their spines are very sharp and when erected can cause penetrating wounds. *(Courtesy Mike Nelson, South Africa.)*

Jellyfish and Portuguese Man-Of-War

There are two groups of stinging jellyfish found in the coastal waters of North America: the Portuguese man-of-war and the sea nettle (Figure 15-45). The dreaded Portuguese man-of-war has a large, purple air float up to 12 cm long that rides high out of the water and is carried by the wind across the ocean. Tentacles, with their attached stinging structure, the nematocysts, trail out several feet into the water. The red or white jellyfish seen floating in large groups or washed up on the beaches of the Atlantic coast are called *sea nettles*. They, too, have nematocyst-bearing tentacles, which measure up to 4 feet in length. Nematocysts are also found on the inferior surface of the body of the jellyfish. The southeast Pacific box jellyfish contains the most potent marine venom known.

The sting. When a small organism or a human brushes against an outstretched tentacle, the object is stung. Each tentacle has numerous rings of projecting stinging cells, and each cell contains a shiny oval body, the nematocyst. A tiny projecting trigger is on the outer surface of each nematocyst. On tactile stimulation, the nematocyst fires a threadlike whip with a hollow poisonous tip and recurved hooks on a nodelike swelling at the base. The hooks hold the prey while the poisonous contents of the nematocyst are discharged through the thread into the body. The force of discharge is great enough to penetrate the upper dermis where the venom diffuses to enter the circulation.

Stings produce immediate burning, numbness, and paresthesias. Linear papules or wheals occur where a tentacle has brushed against the skin (Figure 15-46). Lesions either fade in hours or blister and become necrotic.[206] Systemic toxic reactions (e.g., nausea, vomiting, headache, muscle spasms, weakness, ataxia, dizziness, low-grade fever) occur with severe or widespread stings. Movement of the envenomated part, such as a limb, leads to increased mobilization of the venom from the inoculation site. Fatalities may occur. It has been estimated that at least 50 feet of box jellyfish tentacles must touch the skin of an adult to deliver a fatal dose.[207] Anaphylactic reactions may occur in victims who are allergic to jellyfish venom.[208,209]

Recurrent linear eruptions after a sole primary envenomation have been reported.[210] Most patients have only one recurrence, which takes place 5 to 30 days later, but some have multiple recurrences. In multiple recurrences, the duration of succeeding episodes become shorter and the symptom-free intervals lengthen with successive recurrences.[211] The recurrent eruption may be more severe. An immunologic reaction to intracutaneous sequestered antigen may explain this phenomenon.

Treatment. The envenomated part is immobilized to prevent mobilization of the venom. It is important to remove or inactivate the nematocysts as rapidly as possible. As long as the tentacles remain in contact with the skin, the nematocysts continue to discharge venom. If washed with fresh water or towel dried, unfired nematocysts on tentacles are activated. Tentacles and toxin are washed off by gently pouring sea water over the affected area. Remaining nematocysts and toxin on the skin are inactivated with alcohol (rubbing alcohol or liquor) or hot sea water. Any remaining tentacles are gently lifted off with a gloved hand. Remaining structures are removed after covering the area with a paste made of baking soda, flour, or talcum and sea water; this paste coalesces the tentacles. The dried paste is scraped off with a knife. Nematocysts of the Portuguese man-of-war can also be deactivated with vinegar. A good general rule for treatment is as follows: for areas on the East Coast north of North Carolina, baking soda should be used; for all other coastal areas of the continental United States, vinegar should be used.[212] Moist beach sand is applied to soothe the irritation. Cool compresses and topical steroid creams suppress inflammation.

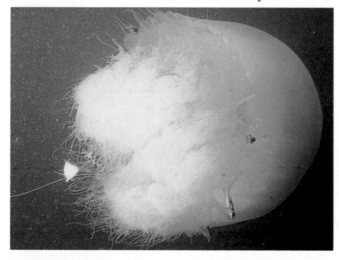

Figure 15-45
Jellyfish. Tentacles of varying lengths project from the base and trail in the water. Each tentacle contains hundreds of nematocysts. *(Courtesy Mike Nelson, South Africa.)*

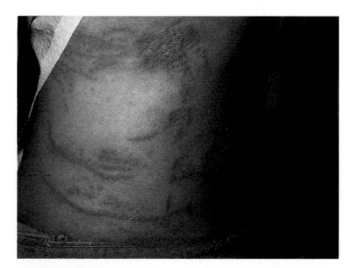

Figure 15-46
Portuguese man-of-war stings. Linear papules produced by nematocysts on tentacles that brushed against the skin.

Coral, Hydroids, and Anemones

Coral. Coral is formed by limestone-secreting polyps that become fused, forming sharp, stonelike structures of various shapes and sizes. Coral is encountered in the Caribbean area, including Florida, Bermuda, the Bahamas, the West Indies, and in the Coral Sea extending from Australia to Hawaii and the Philippines. Like jellyfish, coral has nematocysts, but these are few in number and produce minor symptoms. The most important injuries are cuts. Itchy, red wheals ("coral poisoning") occur around the wound. Minor wounds are painful, slow to heal, and often become infected. Retained bits of calcium may cause a delayed, foreign-body reaction. Wounds should be cleansed thoroughly to remove bits of debris and treated with hydrogen peroxide.

Hydroids. Stinging hydroids have a branched skeleton that grows in patterns resembling feathers or ferns (Figure 15-47). Tiny tentacles with stinging nematocysts project from the branches.

Sea anemones. Sea anemones are solitary soft polyps with a slitlike central mouth (Figure 15-48). Tentacles covered with nematocysts project from their surface. The nematocysts are mildly toxic.

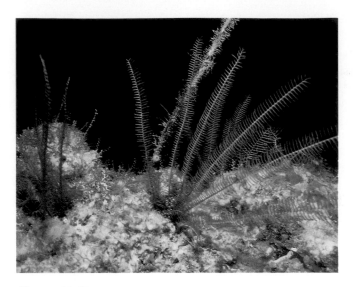

Figure 15-47
Feather hydroid. Nematocysts are present on the tips of the branches. *(Courtesy Mike Nelson, South Africa.)*

Figure 15-48
Sea anemone. Tentacles covered with nematocysts project from their surface. *(Courtesy Reid E. McNeal, Grand Cayman, BWI.)*

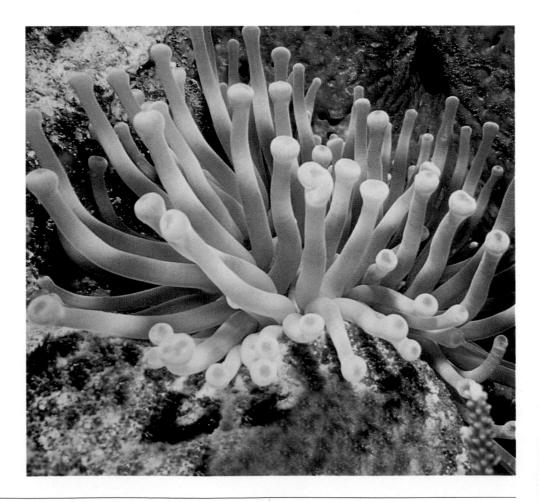

ECHINODERMS (SEA URCHINS AND STARFISH)

Sea urchins are attached to rocks on the ocean floor. They are encased in a spheric hard shell with numerous brittle, sharp, calcified spines projecting from their surface (Figure 15-49). Pedicellariae are triple-jawed, pincerlike structures that are intermingled with the spines of some tropical species. Stepping or falling on the urchin results in penetrating wounds from spines or pedicellariae. The spines may break off and become imbedded in the wound. The spines or pedicellariae are venomous in some species (e.g., *Toxopneustes pileolus*). Venom-bearing spines are long, slender, and sharp, and are covered with a thin skin. Certain starfish produce wounds similar to those of sea urchins. Glandular tissue located beneath the skin produces slime that is released when the epidermal sheath is torn.

Reactions are immediate and delayed.[213] Contact with spines produces an immediate burning sensation with redness and edema that may persist for hours. Wounds from venomous urchins cause immediate, excruciating pain and severe muscle aching. The wound area may be violet-black because of pigments located in the spines. Venomous species may cause the rapid onset of systemic symptoms such as paresthesias, muscular cramps and paralysis, hypotension, nausea, syncope, ataxia, and respiratory distress. Spines that enter joints may induce severe synovitis. Penetration over a metacarpal bone can cause a severe fusiform, reactive, distal swelling of the finger. Retained spines, if not spontaneously discharged or easily removed, may be dissolved with ammonia. An old native treatment is to pour hot wax on the skin and allow it to cool. The wax is then peeled off with the spines in it. Deep spines may have to be surgically excised. X-ray examination is important prior to surgical exploration. Delayed reactions are most commonly foreign-body granulomatous nodules that occur weeks or months later. They are less than 5 mm in diameter and are pink to purple.[214] These may represent a hypersensitivity reaction. They respond to intralesional injections of triamcinolone acetonide (10 mg/ml) and to the surgical removal of spines. Chemicals present on the sea urchin's spines are apparently responsible for a delayed reaction that occurs in some individuals; this reaction consists of induration about the fingers and toes. It lasts for weeks, may cause joint deformity, and responds to systemic antibiotics and corticosteroids.

BRISTLEWORMS (FIRE WORMS)

Bristleworms are segmented marine worms that are covered with silky or bristlelike setae, which become erect on contact (Figure 15-50). The hollow, venom-filled setae penetrate and break off in the victim's skin. Contact with a bristleworm is followed by intense burning and pain. Red papules and local swelling follow. The tiny bristles are removed by tape stripping. Cool water compresses relieve pain. Severe, localized, soft-tissue edema and intense itching may develop. Stings from bristleworms occur mainly in Florida and Caribbean waters.

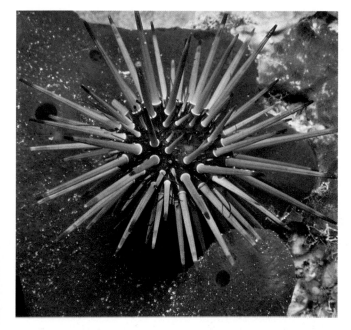

Figure 15-49
Reef urchin; body 1½ to 2 inches, spines 1 to 1½ inches. Pointed spines can cause puncture wounds. The spines crumble and remain lodged in the wound. *(Courtesy Steven F. Bennett, Grand Cayman, BWI.)*

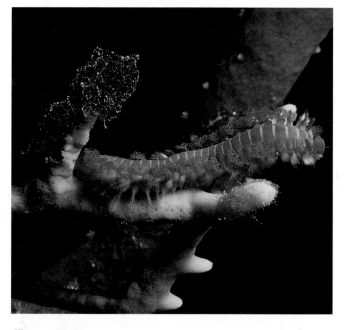

Figure 15-50
Bearded-tipped fireworm; size 4 to 6 inches. The worm displays bristles when disturbed, which penetrate and break off in the skin and cause a painful burning sensation. *(Courtesy Mike Nelson, South Africa.)*

SPONGES

Sponges are the simplest of the multicellular animals. Sponges come in many sizes, colors, and shapes. The touch-me-not sponge and the fire sponge ("dread red") (Figure 15-51) are orange to red or dark brown encrusting sponges that take the shape of whatever they overgrow. Variations of color within the same species make correct identification difficult. Skin contact causes burning and pain. Allergic reactions can be more severe. Irritation occurs 5 minutes to 2 hours after contact ("like glass has been rubbed into the skin"). Paresthesia may be noted. Erythema with or without vesicles can last more than a week. Skin lesions can recur for months. Avoid wetting the area. Calamine lotion and group II topical steroids provide some relief.

MOLLUSKS (CONE SHELLS, OCTOPUS)

Mollusks are soft-bodied invertebrates, most of which secrete protective shells. Certain species of cone shells and octopus are dangerous.

Cone shells. Venomous species of cone shell are found in shallow tropical and subtropical waters of Australia, New Guinea, California, and possibly Florida. Great care must be exercised in handling live cone shells; the soft underportion of the animal must be avoided. Collectors of the 4-inch shells are stung by a detachable dartlike "radular tooth" that causes the puncture wound. Local and systemic reactions occur, depending on the species encountered. The degree of pain varies from mild to excruciating.

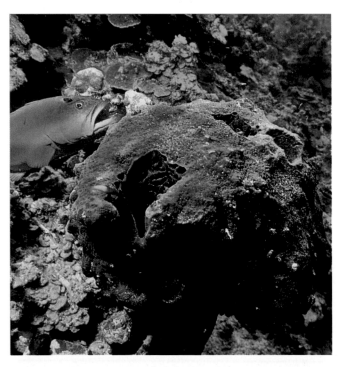

Figure 15-51
Touch-me-not sponge. Contact with this massive red sponge may cause a severe allergic reaction. *(Courtesy Steven F. Bennett, Grand Cayman, BWI.)*

The venom has curarelike effects that block peripheral-nerve conduction. Edema, ischemia, numbness, and paresthesias occur at the bite site.[215] Paresthesias may become widespread; the lips and mouth are commonly affected. Muscular paralysis may progress to generalized weakness with respiratory distress and cardiopulmonary failure. Diplopia, blurred vision, dysphagia, slurred speech, numbness, muscular weakness, paralysis (respiratory paralysis), and terminal coma may progress to death in 6 hours.[216] There is no antivenin. The victim should be kept at rest, and the sting area kept dependent and immobilized. Compression restricts lymphatic and venous spread.[217] The mortality rate is as high as 15% to 20%. A respirator and oxygen may be lifesaving.

Octopus. Two species, the blue-ringed and the spotted octopus, can inflict fatal bites. Caribbean octopi bites are not fatal. The 3- to 4-inch blue-ringed octopus is found in Australia and the Indo-Pacific region. Salivary glands produce the venom that is delivered through a powerful beak.[218] Local symptoms include pain, swelling, erythema, intense pruritus, and profuse bleeding. A paralytic octopus bite results in one or two painless punctures, followed by rapid paralysis. Cardiac arrest can occur as a result of respiratory insufficiency and anoxia. Systemic symptoms include giddiness, visual disturbances, difficulty in speech and swallowing, muscular paralysis, and death from hypoxia, which may occur within 90 minutes of the bite. The venom contains tetrodotoxin, which inhibits sodium transport across neuronal membranes, causing conduction failure. There is no antivenin. Compression bandages on the bite site and splinting of the affected limb prevent rapid lymphatic spread or vascular absorption.

SEA SNAKES

Sea snakes are found in the Pacific and Indian oceans. Most attacks occur in Southeast Asia, the Persian Gulf, and Malaysia. Potent neurotoxins are delivered by two to four hollow fangs. The pinprick-size puncture wounds (usually 1 to 8 wounds) are not very painful, and there is little or no local reaction. Symptoms usually begin within 2 to 3 hours of the bite, and always within 8 hours. There is painful muscle movement, ascending paralysis, blurred vision, ptosis, slurred speech, muscular incoordination and fasciculation, increased salivation, convulsions, respiratory arrest, and myoglobinuria. Death is rare, but reactions may include bulbar paralysis, myonecrosis, hepatic and respiratory insufficiency, and renal and cardiac failure.

First aid consists of application of a compression bandage and immobilization by splinting. A cloth pad is compressed over the wound by an elastic wrap that circles[219] the extremity at a pressure of 70 mm Hg or less. The centripetal flow of venom is impeded. Sea snake antivenin[220] is available from Commonwealth Serum Laboratories, Melbourne, Australia; Haffkine Institute, Bombay, India; Health Services Department, Sea World, San Diego; Sea World, Aurora, Ohio; and the Steinhart Aquarium, San Francisco.

REFERENCES

1. Chakrabarti A: Human notoedric scabies from contact with cats infected with *Notoedres cati*, *Int J Dermatol* 25:646-648, 1986.
2. Falk ES: Serum IgE before and after treatment for scabies, *Allergy* 36:167, 1981.
3. Arlian LG, Estes SA, Vyszenski-Moher DL: Prevalence of *Sarcoptes scabiei* in the homes and nursing homes of scabietic patients, *J Am Acad Dermatol* 19:806-811, 1988.
4. Liu HN, Sheu WJ, et al: Scabietic nodules: a dermatopathologic and immunofluorescent study, *J Cutan Pathol* 19:124-127, 1992.
5. Barnes L, McCallister RE, Lucky AW: Crusted (Norwegian) scabies, *Arch Dermatol* 123:95-97, 1987.
6. Rau RC, Baird IM: Crusted scabies in a patient with acquired immunodeficiency syndrome, *J Am Acad Dermatol* 15:1058-1059, 1986.
7. Taplin D, Meinking TL: Pyrethrins and pyrethroids in dermatology, *Arch Dermatol* 126:213-221, 1990.
8. Schultz MW, Gomez M, et al: Comparative study of 5% permethrin cream and 1% lindane lotion for the treatment of scabies, *Arch Dermatol* 126:167-170, 1990.
9. Taplin D, Porcelain SL, et al: Community control of scabies: a model based on use of permethrin cream, *Lancet* 337:1016-1018, 1991.
10. Purvis RS, Tyring SK: An outbreak of lindane-resistant scabies treated successfully with permethrin 5% cream, *J Am Acad Dermatol* 25:1015-1016, 1991.
11. Taplin D et al: Permethrin 5% dermal cream: a new treatment for scabies, *J Am Acad Dermatol* 15:995-1001, 1986.
12. Judd LE: Gamma benzene hexachloride resistant scabies, *N Z Med J* 106:61-63, 1993.
13. Solomon LM, Fahrner L, Dennis PW: Gamma benzene hexachloride toxicity: a review, *Arch Dermatol* 113:353-357, 1977.
14. Rasmussen JE: Lindane: a prudent approach, *Arch Dermatol* 123:1008-1009, 1987.
15. Meinking TL: The treatment of scabies with ivermectin, *N Engl J Med* 333:26-30, 1995.
16. Avila-Romay A, Alvarez-Franco M, et al: Therapeutic efficacy, secondary effects, and patient acceptability of 10% sulfur in either pork fat or cold cream for the treatment of scabies, *Pediatr Dermatol* 8:64-66, 1991.
17. Maibach HI, Surber C, Orkin M: Sulfur revisited, *J Am Acad Dermatol* 23:154-155, 1990.
18. Scher RK: Subungual scabies, *Am J Dermatopathol* 5:187-189, 1983.
19. Witkowski JA, Parish LC: Case reports. Scabies: subungual areas harbor mites, *JAMA* 252:1318-1319, 1984.
20. Shacter B: Treatment of scabies and pediculosis with lindane preparations: an evaluation, *J Am Acad Dermatol* 5:517-527, 1981.
21. Taplin D, Meinking TL, et al: Comparison of crotamiton 10% cream (Eurax) and permethrin 5% cream (Elimite) for the treatment of scabies in children, *Pediatr Dermatol* 7:67-73, 1990.
22. Holness DL, De Koven JG, et al: Scabies in chronic health care institutions, *Arch Dermatol* 128:1257-1260, 1992.
23. Yonkosky D, Ladia L, et al: Scabies in nursing homes: an eradication program with permethrin 5% cream, *J Am Acad Dermatol* 23:1133-1136, 1990.
24. The efficacy of pediculicides in Israel, *Isr J Med Sci* 27:562-565, 1991.
25. Kanof NM: Of lice and man, *J Am Acad Dermatol* 3:91, 1980.
26. Miller RAW: Maculae ceruleae, *Int J Dermatol* 25:383-384, 1986.
27. Newsom JH, Flore JL Jr, Hackett E: Treatment of infestation with *Phthirius pubis*: comparative efficacies of synergized pyrethrins and gamma-benzene hexachloride, *Sex Trans Dis* 6:203, 1975.
28. Rasmussen JE: Pediculosis and the pediatrician, *Pediatr Dermatol* 2:74-79, 1984.
29. Meinking TL, Taplin D, Kalter DC, et al: Comparative efficacy of treatments for pediculosis capitis infestations, *Arch Dermatol* 122:267-271, 1986.
30. Taplin D, Meinking TL, Castillero PM, et al: Permethrin 1% creme rinse for the treatment of *Pediculus humanus* var *capitis* infestation, *Pediatr Dermatol* 3:344-348, 1986.
31. Shashindran CH, Gandhi IS, Krishnasamy S, et al: Oral therapy of pediculosis capitis with cotrimoxazole, *Br J Dermatol* 98:699-700, 1978.
32. Altschuler DZ, Kenney LR: Pediculicide performance, profit, and public health, *Arch Dermatol* 122:259-261, 1986.
33. Matthew M, DiSouza P, Mehta DK: A new treatment of phthiriasis palpebrarum, *Ann Ophthalmol* 14:439-441, 1982.
34. Allen VT, Miller OF, et al: Gypsy moth caterpillar dermatitis—revisited, *J Am Acad Dermatol* 24:979-981, 1991.
35. Pinson RT, Morgan JA: Envenomation by the puss caterpillar (*Megalopyge opercularis*), *Ann Emerg Med* 20:562-564, 1991.
36. Walker RB, Thomas T, et al: An epidemic of caterpillar sting dermatitis in a rural West Virginia community, *WV Med J* 58-60, 1993.
37. Beaucher WN, Farnham JE: Gypsy-moth-caterpillar dermatitis, *N Engl J Med* 306:1301-1302, 1982.
38. Shama SK et al: Gypsy-moth-caterpillar dermatitis, *N Engl J Med* 306:1300-1301, 1982.
39. Wong RC, Hughes SE, Voorhees JJ: Spider bites: review in depth, *Arch Dermatol* 123:98-104, 1987.
40. Maretic Z: Latrodectism: variations in clinical manifestations produced by *Latrodectus* species of spiders, *Toxicon* 21:457, 1983.
41. Miller TA: Latrodectism: bite of the black widow spider, *Am Fam Physician* 45:181-187, 1992.
42. Zukowski CW: Black widow spider bite, *J Am Board Fam Pract* 6:279-281, 1993.
43. Schuman SH, Caldwell ST: 1990 South Carolina physician survey of tick, spider and fire ant morbidity, *J S C Med Assoc* 87:429-432, 1991.
44. Clark RF, Wethern-Kestner S, et al: Clinical presentation and treatment of black widow spider envenomation: a review of 163 cases, *Ann Emerg Med* 21:782-787, 1992.
45. Key GF: A comparison of calcium gluconate and methocarbamol (Robaxen) in the treatment of lactrodectism (black widow spider) envenomation, *Am J Trop Med Hyg* 30:273, 1981.
46. Alario A, Price G, Stahl R, et al: Cutaneous necrosis following a spider bite: a case report and review, *Pediatrics* 79:618-621, 1987.
47. King LE Jr, Rees R: Brown recluse spider bites: keep cool, *JAMA* 254:2895-2896, 1985.
48. Anderson PC: Necrotizing spider bites, *Am Fam Pract* 26:198-203, 1982.
49. Rees RS et al: Brown recluse spider bites: a comparison of early surgical excision versus dapsone and delayed surgical excision, *Ann Surg* 202:659-663, 1985.
50. King LE, Rees RS: Dapsone treatment of a brown recluse bite, *JAMA* 250:648, 1983.
51. Futrell JM: Loxoscelism, *Am J Med Sci* 304:261-267, 1992.
52. Smith CW, Micks DW: The role of polymorphonuclear leukocytes in the lesion caused by the venom of the brown spider, *Loxosceles reclusa*, *Lab Invest* 22:90-93, 1976.
53. Ingber A, Trattner A, et al: Morbidity of brown recluse spider bites. Clinical picture, treatment and prognosis, *Acta Derm Venereol* 71:337-340, 1991.
54. Osborn CD: Treatment of spider bites by high voltage direct current, *J Okla State Med Assoc* 84:257-260, 1991.
55. Anderson JF: Ecology of Lyme disease, *Conn Med* 53:343-346, 1989.
56. Lastavica CC et al: Rapid emergence of a focal epidemic of Lyme disease in coastal Massachusetts, *N Engl J Med* 320:133-137, 1989.
57. Lyme disease surveillance—United States, 1989-1990, *MMWR* 40:417-421, 1991.
58. Malane MS, Grant-Kels JM, et al: Diagnosis of Lyme disease based on dermatologic manifestations, *Ann Intern Med* 114:490-498, 1991.
59. Asbrink E: Cutaneous manifestations of Lyme borreliosis. Clinical definitions and differential diagnoses, *Scand J Infect Dis Suppl* 77:44-50, 1991.
60. Berger BW: Erythema chronicum migrans of Lyme disease, *Arch Dermatol* 120:1017-1021, 1984.

61. Melski JW et al: Primary and secondary erythema migrans in central Wisconsin, *Arch Dermatol* 129:709-716, 1993.

62. Albrecht S et al: Lymphadenosis benigna cutis resulting from *Borrelia* infection (*Borrelia* lymphocytoma), *J Am Acad Dermatol* 24:621-625, 1991.

63. Buechner SA, Rufli T, Erb P: Acrodermatitis chronica atrophicans: a chronic T-cell–mediated immune reaction against *Borrelia burgdorferi*? *J Am Acad Dermatol* 28:399-405, 1993.

64. Asbrink E, Hovmark A: Comments on the course and classification of Lyme borreliosis, *Scand J Infect Dis Suppl* 77:41-43, 1991.

65. Kristoferitsch W: Neurological manifestations of Lyme borreliosis: clinical definition and differential diagnosis, *Scand J Infect Dis Suppl* 77:64-73, 1991.

66. Halperin JJ, Golightly M: Lyme borreliosis in Bell's palsy. Long Island Neuroborreliosis Collaborative Study Group, *Neurology* 42:1268-1270, 1992.

67. Christen HJ, Hanefeld F, et al: Epidemiology and clinical manifestations of Lyme borreliosis in childhood. A prospective multicentre study with special regard to neuroborreliosis, *Acta Paediatr* 82:1-75, 1993.

68. Mann WJ, Amedee RG, et al: Ultrasonography for the diagnosis of Lyme disease in cases of acute facial paralysis, *Laryngoscope*, 102:525-527, 1992.

69. Logigian EL, Kaplan RF, et al: Chronic neurologic manifestations of Lyme disease, *N Engl J Med* 323:1438-1444, 1990.

70. Logigian EL, Steere AC: Clinical and electrophysiologic findings in chronic neuropathy of Lyme disease, *Neurology* 42:303-311, 1992.

71. Halperin JJ: North American Lyme neuroborreliosis, *Scand J Infect Dis Suppl* 77:74-80, 1991.

72. Halperin JJ, Luft BJ, et al: Lyme neuroborreliosis: central nervous system manifestations, *Neurology* 39:753-759, 1989.

73. Steere AC, Berardi VP, et al: Evaluation of the intrathecal antibody response to *Borrelia burgdorferi* as a diagnostic test for Lyme neuroborreliosis, *J Infect Dis* 161:1203-1209, 1990.

74. Woolf PK, Lorsung EM, et al: Electrocardiographic findings in children with Lyme disease, *Pediatr Emerg Care* 7:334-336, 1991.

75. Cox J, Krajden M: Cardiovascular manifestations of Lyme disease, *Am Heart J* 122:1449-1455, 1991.

76. van der Linde MR: Lyme carditis: clinical characteristics of 105 cases, *Scand J Infect Dis Suppl* 77:81-84, 1991.

77. Steere AC: Clinical definitions and differential diagnosis of Lyme arthritis, *Scand J Infect Dis Suppl* 77:51-54, 1991.

78. Kalish RA, Leong JM, et al: Association of treatment-resistant chronic Lyme arthritis with HLA-DR4 and antibody reactivity to OspA and OspB of *Borrelia burgdorferi*, *Infect Immun* 61:2774-2779, 1993.

79. Steere AC, Dwyer E, et al: Association of chronic Lyme arthritis with HLA-DR4 and HLA-DR2 alleles [published erratum appears in *N Engl J Med* 1991 Jan 10; 324(2):129], *N Engl J Med* 323:219-223, 1990.

80. Szer IS, Taylor E, et al: The long-term course of Lyme arthritis in children, *N Engl J Med* 325:159-163, 1991.

81. Steere AC et al: Erythema chronicum migrans and Lyme arthritis: the enlarging clinical spectrum, *Ann Inter Med* 86:685-698, 1977.

82. Schlesinger PA et al: Maternal-fetal transmission of the Lyme disease spirochete, *Borrelia burgdorferi*, *Ann Inter Med* 103:67-68, 1985.

83. Berg D, Abson KG, Prose NS: The laboratory diagnosis of Lyme disease, *Arch Dermatol* 127:866-870, 1991.

84. Luger SW, Krauss E: Serologic tests for Lyme disease. Interlaboratory variability, *Arch Intern Med* 150:761-763, 1990.

85. Corpuz M, Hilton E, et al: Problems in the use of serologic tests for the diagnosis of Lyme disease, *Arch Intern Med* 151:1837-1840, 1991.

86. Shrestha M, Grodzicki RL, Steere AC: Diagnosing early Lyme disease, *Am J Med* 78:235-240, 1985.

87. Feder H Jr, Gerber MA, et al: Persistence of serum antibodies to *Borrelia burgdorferi* in patients treated for Lyme disease, *Clin Infect Dis* 15:788-793, 1992.

88. Steere AC et al: The spirochetal etiology of Lyme disease, *N Engl J Med* 308:733-740, 1983.

89. Dattwyler RJ et al: Seronegative Lyme disease, *N Engl J Med* 319:1441-1446, 1988.

90. Magnarelli LA: Serologic testing for Lyme disease, *Postgrad Med* 87:149-150, 1990.

91. Craft JE, Grodzicki RL, Steere AC: Antibody response in Lyme disease: evaluation of diagnostic tests, *J Infect Dis* 149:789-795, 1984.

92. Carlsson B, Hanson HS, et al: Evaluation of the fluorescent treponemal antibody-absorption (FTA-Abs) test specificity, *Acta Derm Venereol* 71:306-311, 1991.

93. Nadelman RB, Nowakowski J, et al: Failure to isolate *Borrelia burgdorferi* after antimicrobial therapy in culture-documented Lyme borreliosis associated with erythema migrans: report of a prospective study, *Am J Med* 94:583-588, 1993.

94. Nadelman RB, Pavia CS, et al: Isolation of *Borrelia burgdorferi* from the blood of seven patients with Lyme disease, *Am J Med* 88:21-26, 1990.

95. Berger BW et al: Cultivation of *Borrelia burgdorferi* from blood of two patients with erythema migrans lesions lacking extracutaneous signs and symptoms of Lyme disease, *J Am Acad Dermatol* 30:48-51, 1994.

96. Sigal LH: Summary of the first 100 patients seen at a Lyme disease referral center, *Am J Med* 88:577-581, 1990.

97. Burdge DR, O'Hanlon DP: Experience at a referral center for patients with suspected Lyme disease in an area of nonendemicity: first 65 patients, *Clin Infect Dis* 16:558-560, 1993.

98. Steere AC, Taylor E, et al: The overdiagnosis of Lyme disease, *JAMA* 269:1812-1816, 1993.

99. Sigal LH: Current recommendations for the treatment of Lyme disease, *Drugs* 43:683-699, 1992.

100. Treatment of Lyme disease, *Med Lett Drugs Ther* 34:95-97, 1992.

101. Dattwyler RJ, Volkman DJ, et al: Amoxycillin plus probenecid versus doxycycline for treatment of erythema migrans borreliosis, *Lancet* 336:1404-1406, 1990.

102. Massarotti EM, Luger SW, et al: Treatment of early Lyme disease, *Am J Med* 92:396-403, 1992.

103. Liegner KB: Minocycline in Lyme disease, *J Am Acad Dermatol* 26:263-264, 1992.

104. Salazar JC, Gerber MA, et al: Long-term outcome of Lyme disease in children given early treatment, *J Pediatr* 122:591-593, 1993.

105. Steere AC, Pachner AR, Malawista SE: Neurologic abnormalities of Lyme disease: successful treatment with high-dose intravenous penicillin, *Ann Intern Med* 99:767-772, 1983.

106. Steere AC et al: Successful parenteral penicillin therapy of established Lyme arthritis, *N Engl J Med* 312:869-874, 1985.

107. Treatment of Lyme disease, *Med Lett Drugs Ther* 30(769):65-66, 1988.

108. Liegner KB et al: Recurrent erythema migrans despite extended antibiotic treatment with minocycline in a patient with persisting *Borrelia burgdorferi* infection, *J Am Acad Dermatol* 28:312-314, 1993.

109. Ceftriaxone-associated biliary complications of treatment of suspected disseminated Lyme disease—New Jersey, 1990-1992, *MMWR* 42:39-42, 1993.

110. Moore JA: Jarisch-Herxheimer reaction in Lyme disease, *Cutis* 39:397-398, 1987.

111. Berger BW: Treating erythema chronicum migrans of Lyme disease, *J Am Acad Dermatol* 15:459-463, 1986.

112. Shapiro ED et al: A controlled trial of antimicrobial prophylaxis for Lyme disease after deer-tick bites, *N Engl J Med* 327:1769-1773, 1992.

113. Couch P, Johnson CE: Prevention of Lyme disease, *Am J Hosp Pharm* 49:1164-1173, 1992.

114. Piesman J, Mather TN, et al: Duration of tick attachment and *Borrelia burgdorferi* transmission, *J Clin Microbiol* 25:557-558, 1988.

115. Piesman J, Maupin GO, et al: Duration of adult female *Ixodes dammini* attachment and transmission of *Borrelia burgdorferi*, with description of a needle aspiration isolation method, *J Infect Dis* 163:895-897, 1991.

116. Rocky mountain spotted fever—United States, 1985. Reports of 700 cases, Viral and Rickettsial Zoonoses Br Div of Viral Diseases, Center for Infectious Diseases, CDC, *MMWR* 35:247-249, 1986.

117. Sexton DJ, Corey GR: Rocky Mountain "spotless" and "almost spotless" fever: a wolf in sheep's clothing, *Clin Infect Dis* 15:439-448, 1992.

118. Woodward TE: Rocky Mountain spotted fever: epidemiological and early clinical signs are key to treatment and reduced mortality, *J Infect Dis* 150:465-468, 1984.

119. Kirk JL, Fine DP, et al: Rocky Mountain spotted fever. A clinical review based on 48 confirmed cases, 1943-1986, *Medicine* 69:35-45, 1990.

120. Green WR, Walker DH, Cain BG: Fatal viscerotrophic Rocky Mountain spotted fever, *Am J Med* 64:523-528, 1978.

121. Welch KJ, Rumley RL, et al: False-positive results in serologic tests for Rocky Mountain spotted fever during pregnancy, *South Med J* 84:307-311, 1991.

122. Fischer JJ: Rocky Mountain spotted fever. When and why to consider the diagnosis, *Postgrad Med* 87:109-118, 1990.

123. Garin C, Bujadoux A: Paralysis by ticks. 1922 [classical article], *Clin Infect Dis* 16:168-169, 1993.

124. Harwood RF, James MT: *Entomology in human and animal health*, New York, 1979, Macmillan.

125. Needham GR: Evaluation of five popular methods for tick removal, *Pediatrics* 75:997-1002, 1985.

126. Zangwill KM, Hamilton DH, et al: Cat scratch disease in Connecticut. Epidemiology, risk factors, and evaluation of a new diagnostic test, *N Engl J Med* 329:8-13, 1993.

127. Margileth AM, Hayden GF: Cat scratch disease. From feline affection to human infection, *N Engl J Med* 329:53-54, 1993.

128. Dolan MJ, Wong MT, et al: Syndrome of *Rochalimaea henselae*, adenitis suggesting cat scratch disease, *Ann Intern Med* 118:331-336, 1993.

129. Carithers HA: Cat-scratch disease: an overview based on a study of 1,200 patients, *Am J Dis Child* 139:1124-1133, 1985.

130. Jawad AS, Amen AA: Cat-scratch disease presenting as the oculoglandular syndrome of Parinaud: a report of two cases, *Postgrad Med J* 66:467-468, 1990.

131. Jackson MA, Tyson M, et al: Antimicrobial therapy for Parinaud's oculoglandular syndrome, *Pediatr Infect Dis J* 11:130-132, 1992.

132. Delahoussaye PM, Osborne BM: Cat-scratch disease presenting as abdominal visceral granulomas, *J Infect Dis* 161:71-78, 1990.

133. Margileth AM et al: Systemic cat-scratch disease: report of 23 patients with prolonged or recurrent severe bacterial infection, *J Infect Dis* 155:390, 1987.

134. Schwartzman WA, Marchevsky A, et al: Epithelioid angiomatosis or cat scratch disease with splenic and hepatic abnormalities in AIDS: case report and review of the literature, *Scand J Infect Dis* 22:121-133, 1990.

135. Relman DA, Loutit JS, et al: The agent of bacillary angiomatosis. An approach to the identification of uncultured pathogens, *N Engl J Med* 323:1573-1580, 1990.

136. Tappero JW, Mohle-Boetani J, et al: The epidemiology of bacillary angiomatosis and bacillary peliosis, *JAMA* 269:770-775, 1993.

137. Koehler JE et al: Cutaneous vascular lesions and disseminated cat-scratch disease in patients with the acquired immunodeficiency syndrome (AIDS) and AIDS-related complex, *Ann Intern Med* 109:449, 1988.

138. Kemper CA, Lombard CM, et al: Visceral bacillary epithelioid angiomatosis: possible manifestations of disseminated cat scratch disease in the immunocompromised host: a report of two cases, *Am J Med* 89:216-222, 1990.

139. Regnery RL, Olson JG, et al: Serological response to "*Rochalimaea henselae*" antigen in suspected cat-scratch disease, *Lancet* 339:1443-1445, 1992.

140. English CK et al: Cat-scratch disease: isolation and culture of the bacterial agent, *JAMA* 259:1347, 1988.

141. Adal KA et al: Cat scratch disease, bacillary angiomatosis, and other infections due to *Rochalimaea*, *N Engl J Med* 330:1509-1515, 1994.

142. Holley H Jr.: Successful treatment of cat-scratch disease with ciprofloxacin, *JAMA* 265:1563-1565, 1991.

143. Margileth AM: Antibiotic therapy for cat-scratch disease: clinical study of therapeutic outcome in 268 patients and a review of the literature, *Pediatr Infect Dis J* 11:474-478, 1992.

144. Goldstein EJ: Bite wounds and infection, *Clin Infect Dis* 14:633-638, 1992.

145. Holst E, Rollof J, et al: Characterization and distribution of *Pasteurella* species recovered from infected humans, *J Clin Microbiol* 30:2984-2987, 1992.

146. Goldstein EJC, Reinhardt JF, Murray PM, et al: Outpatient therapy of bite wounds, *Int J Dermatol* 26:123-127, 1987.

147. Brook I: Human and animal bite infections, *J Fam Pract* 28:713-718, 1989.

148. Gonzalez MH, Papierski P, et al: Osteomyelitis of the hand after a human bite, *J Hand Surg* [Am] 18:520-522, 1993.

149. Agrawal K, Mishra S, et al: Primary reconstruction of major human bite wounds of the face, *Plast Reconstr Surg* 90:394-398, 1992.

150. Frenia ML, Lafin SM, et al: Features and treatment of rabies, *Clin Pharm* 11:37-47, 1992.

151. Wilde H, Bhanganada K, et al: Is injection of contaminated animal bite wounds with rabies immune globulin a safe practice? *Trans R Soc Trop Med Hyg* 86:86-88, 1992.

152. Lindsey D et al: Natural course of the human bite wound: incidence of infection and complications in 434 bites and 803 lacerations in the same group of patients, *J Trauma* 27:45-48, 1987.

153. Goldstein EJC: Management of human and animal bite wounds, *J Am Acad Dermatol* 21:1275-1279, 1989.

154. Dire DJ, Hogan DE, et al: Prophylactic oral antibiotics for low-risk dog bite wounds, *Pediatr Emerg Care* 8:194-199, 1992.

155. Zubowicz VN, Gravier M: Management of early human bites of the hand: a prospective randomized study, *Plast Reconstr Surg* 88:111-114, 1991.

156. Anderson CR: Animal bites. Guidelines to current management, *Postgrad Med* 92:134-136, 1992.

157. Goldstein EJC, Goodhart GL, Moore JE: *Pasteurella multocida* infection after animal bites, *N Eng J Med* 315:460, 1986.

158. Goldstein EJC, Citron DM, Richwald GA: Lack of in vitro efficacy of oral forms of certain cephalosporins, erythromycin and oxacillin against *Pasteurella multocida*, *Antimicrob Agents Chemother* 32:213-215, 1988.

159. Settipane GA, Boyd GK: Natural history of insect sting allergy: the Rhode Island experience, *Allergy Proc* 10:109-113, 1989.

160. Li JT, Yunginger JW: Management of insect sting hypersensitivity, *Mayo Clin Proc* 67:188-194, 1992.

161. Reisman RE, Livingston A: Late-onset allergic reactions, including serum sickness, after insect stings, *J Allergy Clin Immunol* 84:331-337, 1989.

162. Engel T, Heinig JH, Weeke ER:*Allergy* 43:289-293, 1988.

163. Reisman RE, De Masi JM: Relationship of serum venom–specific IgE titers to clinical aspects of stinging insect allergy, *Int Arch Allergy Appl Immunol* 89:67-70, 1989.

164. Golden DB, Lawrence ID, et al: Clinical correlation of the venom-specific IgG antibody level during maintenance venom immunotherapy, *J Allergy Clin Immunol* 90:386-393, 1992.

165. Bernstein DI, Mittman RJ, et al: Clinical and immunologic studies of rapid venom immunotherapy in *Hymenoptera*-sensitive patients, *J Allergy Clin Immunol* 84:951-959, 1989.

166. Wright DN, Lockey RF: Local reactions to stinging insects (*Hymenoptera*), *Allergy Proc* 11:23-28, 1990.

167. Valentine MD, Schuberth KC, et al: The value of immunotherapy with venom in children with allergy to insect stings, *N Engl J Med* 323:1601-1603, 1990.

168. Reisman RE: Stinging insect allergy, *Med Clin North Am* 76:883-894, 1992.

169. Muller U, Berchtold E, et al: Honeybee venom allergy: results of a sting challenge 1 year after stopping successful venom immunotherapy in 86 patients, *J Allergy Clin Immunol* 87:702-709, 1991.

170. Keating MU, Kagey-Sobotka A, et al: Clinical and immunologic follow-up of patients who stop venom immunotherapy, *J Allergy Clin Immunol* 88:339-348, 1991.

171. Alexander JO: Papular urticaria and immune complexes, *J Am Acad Dermatol* 12:374-375, 1985.

172. Heng MCY, Kloss SG, Haberfelde GC: Pathogenesis of papular urticaria, *J Am Acad Dermatol* 10:1030-1034, 1984.

173. Burns DA: The investigation and management of arthropod bite reactions acquired in the home, *Clin Exp Dermatol* 12:114-120, 1987.

174. Singh I, Gathwala G, et al: Myiasis in children: the Indian perspective, *Int J Pediatr Otorhinolaryngol* 25:127-131, 1993.

175. Schiff TA: Furuncular cutaneous myiasis caused by *Cuterebra* larva, *J Am Acad Dermatol* 28:261-263, 1993.

176. Baird JK, Baird CR, et al: North American cuterebrid myiasis. Report of seventeen new infections of human beings and review of the disease, *J Am Acad Dermatol* 21:763-772, 1989.

177. Arosemena R, Booth SA, et al: Cutaneous myiasis, *J Am Acad Dermatol* 28:254-256, 1993.

178. Loong PT, Lui H, et al: Cutaneous myiasis: a simple and effective technique for extraction of *Dermatobia hominis* larvae, *Int J Dermatol* 31:657-659, 1992.

179. Brewer TF et al: Bacon therapy and furuncular myiasis, *JAMA* 270:2087, 1993.

180. Weed RI: Exaggerated delayed hypersensitivity to mosquito bites in chronic lymphocytic leukemia, *Blood* 26:257-268, 1993.

181. Penneys NS, Nayar JK, et al: Chronic pruritic eruption in patients with acquired immunodeficiency syndrome associated with increased antibody titers to mosquito salivary gland antigens, *J Am Acad Dermatol* 21:421-425, 1989.

182. Reunala T, Brummer-Korvenkontio H, et al: Treatment of mosquito bites with cetirizine, *Clin Exp Allergy* 23:72-75, 1993.

183. Marks MB: Stinging insects: allergy implications, *Pediatr Clin North Am* 16:177-191, 1969.

184. Katz R, Ziegler J, Blank H: The natural course of creeping eruption and treatment with thiabendazole, *Arch Dermatol* 91:420-424, 1965.

185. Guill MA, Odom RB: Larva migrans complicated by Loeffler's syndrome, *Arch Dermatol* 114:1525-1526, 1978.

186. Ambrus J, Klein E: Loffler syndrome and *ancyclostoma braziliense*, *N Y State J Med* 88:498-499, 1988.

187. Edelglass JW et al: Cutaneous larva migrans in northern climates, *J Am Acad Dermatol* 7:353-358, 1982.

188. Davies HD, Sakuls P, et al: Creeping eruption. A review of clinical presentation and management of 60 cases presenting to a tropical disease unit, *Arch Dermatol* 129:588-591, 1993.

189. Jones SK, Reynolds NJ, et al: Oral albendazole for the treatment of cutaneous larva migrans, *Br J Dermatol* 122:99-101, 1990.

190. Sturchler D, Schubarth P, et al: Thiabendazole vs. albendazole in treatment of toxocariasis: a clinical trial, *Ann Trop Med Parasitol* 83:473-478, 1989.

191. Caumes E, Datry A, et al: Efficacy of ivermectin in the therapy of cutaneous larva migrans [letter], *Arch Dermatol* 128:994-995, 1992.

192. Louis FJ, de Quincenet G, et al: Value of single-dose ivermectin in the treatment of cutaneous larva migrans syndrome (letter), *Presse Med* 21:1483, 1992.

193. de Shazo RD, Soto-Aguilar M: Reactions to imported fire ant stings, *Allergy Proc* 14:13-16, 1993.

194. Ginsburg CM: Fire ant envenomation in children, *Pediatrics* 73:689-692, 1984.

195. Ross EV Jr, Badame AJ, Dale SE: Meat tenderizer in the acute treatment of imported fire ant stings, *J Am Acad Dermatol* 16:1189-1192, 1987.

196. Stafford CT, Wise SL, et al: Safety and efficacy of fire ant venom in the diagnosis of fire ant allergy, *J Allergy Clin Immunol* 90:653-661, 1992.

197. Freeman TM, Hylander R, et al: Imported fire ant immunotherapy: effectiveness of whole body extracts, *J Allergy Clin Immunol* 90:210-215, 1992.

198. deShazo RD, Butcher BT, Banks WA: Reactions to the stings of the imported fire ant, *N Eng J Med* 323:462-466, 1990.

199. Gurry D: Marine stings, *Aust Fam Physician* 21:26-34, 1992.

200. McGoldrick J, Marx JA: Marine envenomations; Part 1: vertebrates, *J Emerg Med* 9:497-502, 1991.

201. Auerbach PS: Marine envenomations, *N Engl J Med* 325:486-493, 1991.

202. Cercarial dermatitis outbreak at a state park—Delaware, 1991, *MMWR* 41:225-228, 1992.

203. Mulvihill CA, Burnett JW: Swimmer's itch: A cercarial dermatitis, *Cutis* 46:211-213, 1990.

204. Tomchik RS, Russell MT, et al: Clinical perspectives on seabather's eruption, also known as 'sea lice,' *JAMA* 269:1669-1672, 1993.

205. Freudenthal AR, Joseph PR: Seabathers' eruption, *N Engl J Med* 329:542-544, 1993.

206. Ioannides G, Davis JH: Portuguese man-of-war stinging, *Arch Dermatol* 91:448-451, 1965.

207. Burnett JW, Calton GJ, Burnett HW: Jellyfish envenomation syndromes, *J Am Acad Dermatol* 14:100-106, 1986.

208. Togias AG, Lichtenstein LM, Kagey-Sobotka A, et al: Anaphylaxis following contact with a jellyfish, *J Allergy Clin Immunol* 75:672-675, 1985.

209. Burnett JW, Calton GJ, Burnett HW, et al: Local and systemic reactions from jellyfish stings, *Clin Dermatol* 5:14-28, 1987.

210. Mansson T et al: Recurrent cutaneous jellyfish eruptions without envenomation, *Acta Derm Venereol* 65:72-75, 1985.

211. Burnett JW et al: Recurrent eruptions following unusual solitary coelenterate envenomations, *J Am Acad Dermatol* 17:86-92, 1987.

212. Burnett JW, Calton GJ, Morgan RJ: Venomous coelenterates, *Cutis* 39:191-192, 1987.

213. Fisher AA: *Atlas of aquatic dermatology*, New York, 1978, Grune & Stratton.

214. Burnett JW, Calton GJ, Morgan RJ: Venomous sea urchins, *Cutis* 38:151, 1986.

215. Kizer KW: Marine envenomations, *J Toxicol Clin Toxicol* 21:527, 1983.

216. Burnett JW et al: Cone snails, *Cutis* 39:107, 1980

217. Halstead BW, Auerbach PS, (editors): *Dangerous aquatic animals of the world: a color guide, with prevention, first aid, and emergency treatment procedures*, Princeton NJ, 1990, Darwin Press.

218. Williamson JAH: The blue-ringed octopus and envenomation syndrome, *Clin Dermatol* 5:127, 1987.

219. Sutherland SK et al: Simple method to delay the movement from the site of injection of low molecular weight substances, *Med J Aust* 1:81 1980.

220. Madhusudana SN, Aggarwal P: Snake bites in India and its management, *J Indian Med Assoc* 88:235-236, 1990.

CHAPTER SIXTEEN

Vesicular and Bullous Diseases

Vesicles and bullae are the primary lesions in many diseases. Some are of short duration and are quite characteristic, such as those in poison ivy and herpes zoster. In other diseases, such as erythema multiforme and lichen planus, a blister may or may not occur during the course of the disease. Finally, there is a group of disorders in which bullae are present almost continuously during the period of active disease. These diseases tend to be chronic, and many are associated with tissue-bound or circulating antibodies. This chapter deals with those disorders.

A blister occurs when fluid accumulates at some level in the skin. The histologic classification of bullous disorders is based on the level in the skin at which that separation occurs (Figure 16-1). Subcorneal blisters are not commonly seen intact; the very thin roof has little structural integrity and collapses. Intraepidermal blisters have a thicker roof and are more substantial, whereas subepidermal blisters have great structural integrity and can remain intact even when firmly compressed.

Diagnosis of Bullous Disorders

The diagnosis of many chronic bullous disorders can often be made clinically. These diseases have such important implications that the diagnosis should be confirmed by histology and, in many instances, immunofluorescence (see the box on p. 500, Figure 16-2, and Table 16-1).

Biopsy

For light microscopy. A biopsy specimen must be taken from the proper area to demonstrate the level of blister formation and the nature of the inflammatory infiltrate (Figure 16-2). Small, early vesicles or inflamed skin provide the most diagnostic features. Ruptured or excoriated lesions are of little value and should not be sampled. A small portion of the intact skin should be included in the biopsy specimen. Punch biopsies done through the center of a large blister are of little value.

For immunofluorescence. In most cases the first biopsy specimen should be taken from the edge of a fresh lesion. A second biopsy is often desirable to establish the diagnosis. One should sample skin near the lesion, preferably from a nonedematous, normal, or red area. The best site for obtaining a biopsy specimen is shown in Table 16-1 and Figure 16-2.

Level of blister formation. For blisters occurring above the basement membrane zone, the level of blister formation can be determined easily with routine studies. Blisters occurring in the dermoepidermal junction (basement membrane zone) area (see Figure 16-1) were once considered subepidermal in location. With the electron microscope it has been shown that blisters may occur at different levels in that complex area. Electron microscopy is not routinely used; adequate diagnostic information can be obtained from sections stained with hematoxylin and eosin and from immunofluorescence studies.

Immunofluorescence. Immunofluorescence is a laboratory technique for demonstrating the presence of tissue-bound and circulating antibodies.[1] Most chronic bullous disorders have specific antibodies that are either fixed to some component of skin or are circulating. Many laboratories around the country provide this testing service and supply transport media and mailing containers for tissue specimens. (Examples are Beutner Laboratories, Buffalo, N.Y., 1-716-838-0549; IMMCO Diagnostics, Buffalo, N.Y., 1-800-537-TEST; and Mayo Medical Laboratories, Rochester, Minn., 1-800-533-1710.) Freezing of specimens is no longer required.

MAJOR BULLOUS DISEASES

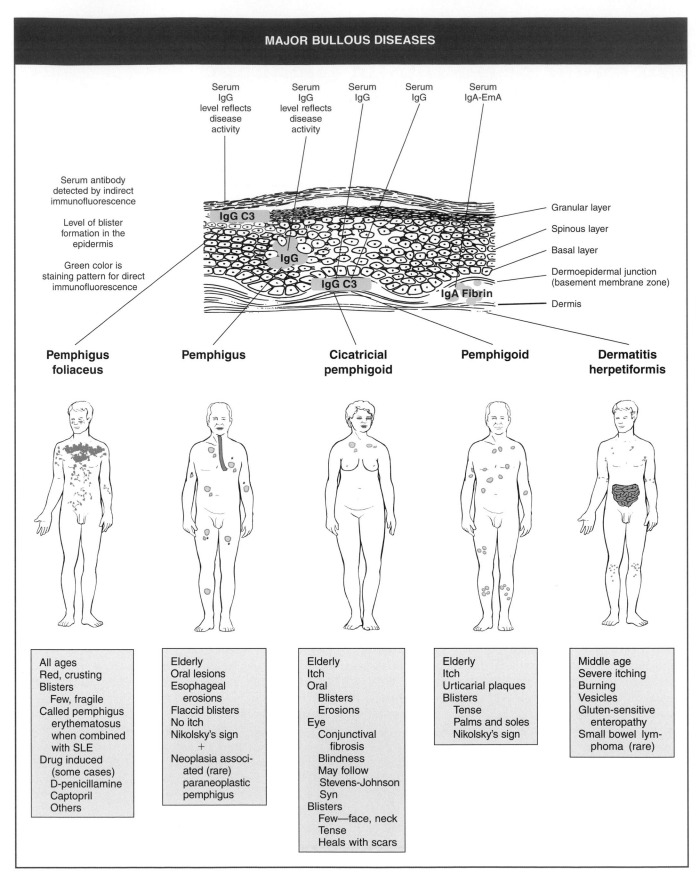

Serum IgG level reflects disease activity

Serum IgG level reflects disease activity

Serum IgG

Serum IgG

Serum IgA-EmA

Serum antibody detected by indirect immunofluorescence

Level of blister formation in the epidermis

Green color is staining pattern for direct immunofluorescence

IgG C3

IgG

IgG C3

IgA Fibrin

Granular layer

Spinous layer

Basal layer

Dermoepidermal junction (basement membrane zone)

Dermis

Pemphigus foliaceus

Pemphigus

Cicatricial pemphigoid

Pemphigoid

Dermatitis herpetiformis

All ages
Red, crusting
Blisters
    Few, fragile
Called pemphigus
    erythematosus
    when combined
    with SLE
Drug induced
    (some cases)
    D-penicillamine
    Captopril
    Others

Elderly
Oral lesions
Esophageal
    erosions
Flaccid blisters
No itch
Nikolsky's sign
    +
Neoplasia associ-
    ated (rare)
    paraneoplastic
    pemphigus

Elderly
Itch
Oral
    Blisters
    Erosions
Eye
    Conjunctival
        fibrosis
    Blindness
    May follow
        Stevens-Johnson
        Syn
Blisters
    Few—face, neck
    Tense
    Heals with scars

Elderly
Itch
Urticarial plaques
Blisters
    Tense
    Palms and soles
    Nikolsky's sign

Middle age
Severe itching
Burning
Vesicles
Gluten-sensitive
    enteropathy
Small bowel lym-
    phoma (rare)

IgA-EmA=IgA antiendomysial antibodies.
Serum antibody—detected by indirect immunofluorescence.

Direct immunofluorescence (skin). Direct immunofluorescence is designed for demonstration of tissue-bound antibody and complement. Sectioned biopsy specimens are treated with fluorescein-conjugated antisera to human immunoglobulins (IgG, IgA, IgM, IgD, and IgE), C3, and fibrin; they are then examined with a microscope equipped with a special light source.

Indirect immunofluorescence (serum). Indirect immunofluorescence is used for demonstration of circulating antibodies directed against certain skin structures. Thin sections of animal squamous epithelium (monkey esophagus, etc.) are first incubated with the patient's serum. Skin-reacting antibodies in the serum attach to specific components of the animal epithelium. Fluorescein-labeled anti–human IgG antiserum is then added for specific identification of the circulating antibody. The circulating antibody responsible for the IgA deposition has not yet been identified, and indirect immunofluorescence is negative.

Figure 16-1
Bullous diseases in the epidermis and dermoepidermal junction.

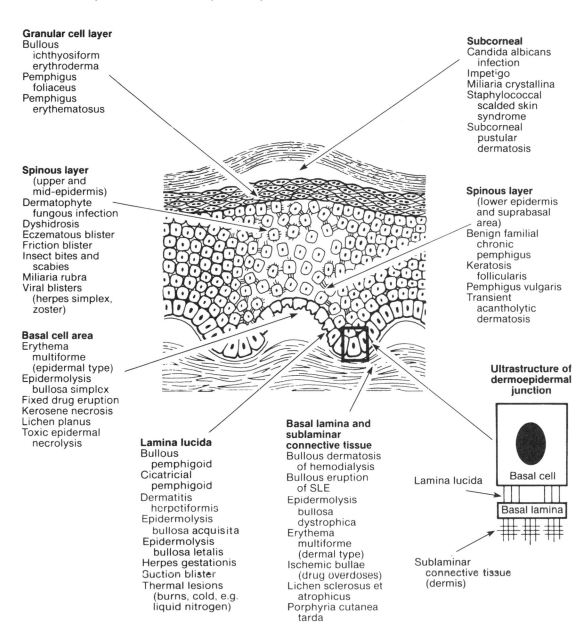

Granular cell layer
Bullous
   ichthyosiform
   erythroderma
Pemphigus
   foliaceus
Pemphigus
   erythematosus

Spinous layer
   (upper and
   mid-epidermis)
Dermatophyte
   fungous infection
Dyshidrosis
Eczematous blister
Friction blister
Insect bites and
   scabies
Miliaria rubra
Viral blisters
   (herpes simplex,
   zoster)

Basal cell area
Erythema
   multiforme
   (epidermal type)
Epidermolysis
   bullosa simplex
Fixed drug eruption
Kerosene necrosis
Lichen planus
Toxic epidermal
   necrolysis

Subcorneal
Candida albicans
   infection
Impetigo
Miliaria crystallina
Staphylococcal
   scalded skin
   syndrome
Subcorneal
   pustular
   dermatosis

Spinous layer
   (lower epidermis
   and suprabasal
   area)
Benign familial
   chronic
   pemphigus
Keratosis
   follicularis
Pemphigus vulgaris
Transient
   acantholytic
   dermatosis

Lamina lucida
Bullous
   pemphigoid
Cicatricial
   pemphigoid
Dermatitis
   herpetiformis
Epidermolysis
   bullosa acquisita
Epidermolysis
   bullosa letalis
Herpes gestationis
Suction blister
Thermal lesions
   (burns, cold, e.g.
   liquid nitrogen)

**Basal lamina and
sublaminar
connective tissue**
Bullous dermatosis
   of hemodialysis
Bullous eruption
   of SLE
Epidermolysis
   bullosa
   dystrophica
Erythema
   multiforme
   (dermal type)
Ischemic bullae
   (drug overdoses)
Lichen sclerosus et
   atrophicus
Porphyria cutanea
   tarda

**Ultrastructure of
dermoepidermal
junction**

Basal cell

Lamina lucida

Basal lamina

Sublaminar
connective tissue
(dermis)

Specimen Selection for Diagnosis of Vesiculo-Bullous Disorders

		Tissue (for direct immunofluorescence)		Serum	Tissue
		Normal tissue (mm from edge of lesion)	Perilesional tissue	Indirect immunofluorescence shows	Lesion—histology shows
SKIN	Pemphigus (all forms)	BX—3mm	BX	Pemphigus and pemphigoid antibodies Can differentiate various forms of pemphigus Levels have prognostic value	Acantholysis
	Pemphigoid (all forms) Epidermolysis bullosa acquisita Linear IgA disease	BX—3mm	BX	Pemphigus and pemphigoid antibodies Levels not of prognostic value	Subepidermal bulla
	Porphyria Pseudo-porphyria Bullous lichen planus Lichen planus	NN	BX	Serum porphyrin (positive only in porphyria)	Subepidermal bulla
	Dermatitis herpetiformis	BX—3-5 mm	NN	Endomysial IgA antibodies Levels have prognostic value	Subepidermal bulla
	Hailey-Hailey Darier's disease	NN	BX		Acantholysis
ORAL (mucosal biopsy)	Cicatricial pemphigoid Erosive lichen planus Pemphigus vulgaris	BX—10 mm	BX	Pemphigus and pemphigoid antibodies (positive in only few cases with conventional techniques)	Same as skin biopsy
OCULAR (conjuctiva biopsy)	Ocular cicatricial pemphigoid	NN	BX	Pemphigus and pemphigoid antibodies (positive in only few cases with conventional techniques)	Same as skin biopsy

Modified from *Immunopathologic studies of the skin*, Buffalo, NY, Beutner Laboratories.
BX = Biopsy.
NN = Not needed.

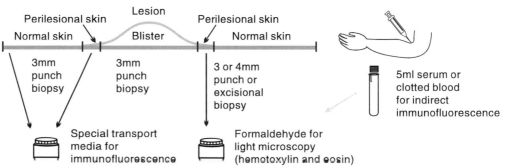

Figure 16-2
Specimen selection for diagnosis of vesiculo-bullous disorders. *(Adapted from* Handbook: Immunopathologic Studies of the Skin, *Beutner Laboratories, Buffalo, NY.)*

TABLE 16-1 Bullous and Vasculitic Disorders—Immunofluorescence Tests

	Selection of biopsy site for direct immunofluorescence*	Biopsy findings: direct immunofluorescence	Serum findings: circulating antibody detected by indirect immunofluorescence
Bullous pemphigoid	Erythematous perilesional skin or mucosa	IgG and/or C3, also other Ig in BMZ; linear—about 50%-80%; deposits disappear as disease subsides. Biopsy normal forearm skin for this study. Biopsy split in 1M NaCl: IgG is in BMZ of roof (and less often in the floor) of split.	IgG class BMZ antibodies—about 70%; level does not correlate with disease activity
Cicatricial pemphigoid	Erythematous perilesional skin or mucosa	IgG and/or C3, also other Ig in BMZ; linear—about 10%-80% Biopsy split in 1M NaCl: IgG is in BMZ of roof (and less often in the floor) of split.	IgG and IgA class BMZ antibodies—10% routine preparation; 82% on salt-split human skin substrate
Epidermolysis bullosa acquisita†	Erythematous perilesional skin or mucosa	Ig and/or C3 in BMZ; linear—almost 100%. Biopsy split in 1M NaCl: IgG is in BMZ of floor of split.	IgG class BMZ antibodies—about 25%
Dermatitis herpetiformis Classic	Perilesional skin or any normal skin	IgA, also F and C in dermal papillae; granular or fibrillar—more than 90% in normal skin	IgA class EMA in about 70% AGA in about 60% ARA in about 36%
Linear IgA disease	Perilesional skin or any normal skin	IgA—100%, also F, rarely C, at BMZ; linear	IgA class BMZ antibodies—about 10% incidence
Henoch-Schönlein purpura	Lesions no older than 24 to 48 hours	Granular IgA in vessels	None
Herpes gestationis	Erythematous perilesional skin	C (100%), Ig (30%-50%) in BMZ; linear	HG factor—about 50%; IgG class BMZ antibodies—about 20%
Pemphigus, all forms except Hailey-Hailey disease	Erythematous perilesional skin	IC deposits of IgG—about 80%; deposits disappear as disease subsides.	IC antibodies—more than 90%; level correlates with disease activity
Erythema multiforme	Edge of involved skin Lesions no older than 24 to 48 hours	Granular IgG and C3 deposits in blood vessels	None
Leukocytoclastic vasculitis	Lesions no older than 24 to 48 hours	Granular Ig (mostly IgM), C3, and F in vessels	None
Lichen planus	Edge of involved skin; avoid old lesions or ulcers	Ig, C and F in cytoid bodies in epidermis, F around rete pegs	None
Porphyria cutanea tarda and other forms of porphyria	Edge of involved skin, sun-exposed	Strong, homogeneous IgG in and around vessel walls, also immunofluorescent band at BMZ	Vascular IgG (IgA and fibrin); IgG in BMZ in lesional skin only
Benign chronic bullous dermatosis of childhood	Erythematous perilesional skin	Same as for dermatitis herpetiformis or pemphigoid	Same as for dermatitis herpetiformis or pemphigoid

Modified from *Handbook of clinical relevance of tests*, IMMCO Diagnostics, Buffalo, NY.
IC, intercellular area of stratum spinosum; *BMZ*, basement membrane zone; *Ig*, immunoglobin; *F*, fibrin or fibrinogen; *C*, complement; *HG*, herpes gestationis factor; *EMA*, endomysial antibodies; *AGA*, antigliadin antibodies; *ARA*, antireticulin antibodies.
*For most bullous diseases two biopsies are recommended: (1) from edge of a fresh lesion and (2) from adjacent normal skin.
†To differentiate epidermolysis bullosa acquisita from bullous pemphigoid, further direct immunofluorescence studies on lesional biopsy specimens and on normal skin split at the lamina lucida by NaCl are required to demonstrate the location of immunoreactants, laminin, and type IV collagen.

Dermatitis Herpetiformis and Linear IgA Bullous Dermatosis

Dermatitis herpetiformis is a rare, chronic, intensely burning, pruritic vesicular skin disease associated in most instances with a subclinical gluten-sensitive enteropathy and IgA deposits in the upper dermis. The reported prevalence in northern Europe is 1.2 to 39.2 per 100,000. The prevalence in Utah in 1987 was 11.2 per 100,000. The mean age of onset of symptoms for male patients was 40.1 years, and that for female patients was 36.2 years.[2] Dermatitis herpetiformis is rare in children. There is a strong association with specific human histocompatibility leukocyte antigens: HLA-B8 (60%), HLA class II antigens HLA-DR3 (95%), and HLA-DQw2 (100%).[3,4]

Linear IgA bullous dermatosis has clinical features similar to those of dermatitis herpetiformis, but has a different histologic and immunofluorescence pattern and there is no associated small bowel disease. Sulfones produce a dramatic response within hours, but without drugs, some patients have chosen suicide as the only means of relief.

Clinical presentation. Dermatitis herpetiformis usually begins in the second to fifth decade, but many cases have been reported in children.[5] The disease is rarely seen in blacks or Asians. Dermatitis herpetiformis presents initially with a few itchy papules or vesicles that are a minor annoyance; they may be attributed to bites, scabies, or neurotic excoriation, and they sometimes respond to topical steroids. In time the disease evolves into its classic presentation of intensely burning urticarial papules, vesicles, and, rarely, bullae, either isolated or in groups such as in herpes simplex or zoster (therefore the term *herpetiformis*).

The vesicles are symmetrically distributed and appear on the elbows, knees, scalp and nuchal area, shoulders, and buttocks (Figures 16-3, 16-4, and 16-5). They are rarely found in the mouth. The distribution may be more generalized. Destruction of the vesicles by scratching provides relief but increases the difficulty of locating a primary lesion for biopsy. Intact lesions for biopsy may be found on the back.

The symptoms vary in intensity, but most people complain of severe itching and burning. One should always think of dermatitis herpetiformis when the symptom of burning is volunteered. The symptoms may precede the onset of lesions by hours, and patients can frequently identify the site of a new lesion by the prodromal symptoms. Treatment does not alter the course of the disease. Most patients have symptoms for years, but approximately one third are in permanent remission.

The vesicular-bullous form is confused with bullous erythema multiforme and bullous pemphigoid. A strong association between dermatitis herpetiformis and diverse thyroid abnormalities has been reported and most likely represents a grouping of immune-mediated disorders. Hypothyroidism was the most common, occurring in 14% of patients. There were clinical or serologic abnormalities in 50% of patients with dermatitis herpetiformis.[6]

Celiac-type dental enamel defects. Celiac-type permanent-tooth enamel defects were found in 53% of patients with dermatitis herpetiformis. The grades of these defects were milder than those described for severe celiac disease. This finding suggests that these patients were already suffering from subclinical gluten-induced enteropathy in early childhood, when the crowns of permanent teeth develop.[7]

Linear IgA bullous dermatosis. Linear IgA bullous dermatosis may present clinically as typical dermatitis herpetiformis, typical bullous pemphigoid, or in an atypical morphologic pattern, and it has histologic features similar to dermatitis herpetiformis. Drugs are responsible for some cases.[8] Immunofluorescence shows IgA along the epidermal basement membrane zone (BMZ). There is no gluten-sensitive enteropathy. Some patients have a circulating-IgA class anti-BMZ antibody on indirect immunofluorescence.

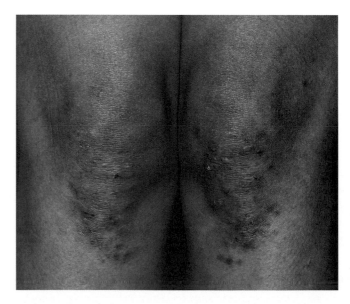

Figure 16-3
Dermatitis herpetiformis. Vesicles are symmetrically distributed on the knees. Most have been excoriated.

Figure 16-4
Dermatitis herpetiformis. Groups of vesicles on an
inflamed base. Lesions are usually not as numerous
as in pemphigus or pemphigoid.

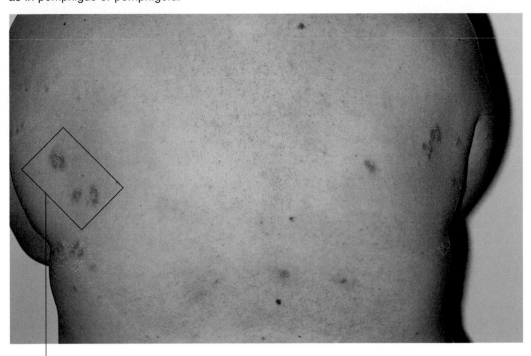

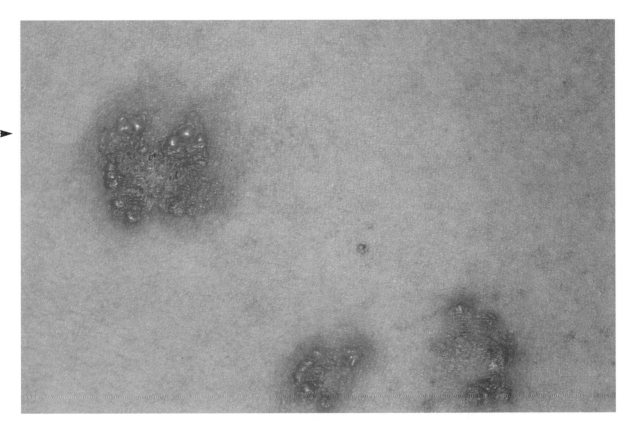

Figure 16-5
Dermatitis herpetiformis. Enlargement of inset of Figure
16-4 shows vesicles that resemble a herpes virus infection;
therefore the designation *herpetiformis.*

GLUTEN-SENSITIVE ENTEROPATHY

A gluten-sensitive enteropathy with patchy areas of villous atrophy and mild intestinal wall inflammation is found in the majority of patients with dermatitis herpetiformis. The changes in the small intestine are similar to but less severe than those found in ordinary gluten-sensitive enteropathy; symptoms of malabsorption are rarely encountered. Fewer than 20% of patients have malabsorption of fat, D-xylose, or iron. A significant correlation was found between IgA antiendomysial antibodies (IgA-EmA) and the severity of gluten-induced jejunum damage. Serum IgA-EmA were present in approximately 70% of patients with dermatitis herpetiformis on a normal diet. IgA-EmA were positive in 86% of dermatitis herpetiformis patients with subtotal villous atrophy, and 11% of dermatitis herpetiformis patients with partial villous atrophy or mild abnormalities. IgA-EmA antibodies disappear after 1 year of a gluten-free diet with the regrowth of jejunal villi. The relationship between IgA-EmA and villous atrophy is a useful diagnostic marker since the enteropathy present in dermatitis herpetiformis is usually without symptoms and therefore difficult to identify.[9]

In patients with dermatitis herpetiformis, ordinary gluten-sensitive enteropathy, and other diseases involving immunologic dysfunction, such as Graves' disease and Sjögren's syndrome, there is a marked increase in the prevalence of the histocompatibility antigens HLA-B8/-DRw3. Patients with linear IgA bullous dermatosis have no evidence of small bowel disease and have a normal prevalence of the above-mentioned histocompatibility antigens.

LYMPHOMA

Small bowel lymphoma and nonintestinal lymphoma have been reported in patients with dermatitis herpetiformis and celiac disease. Typical patients are those who have jejunal villous atrophy and do not adhere rigidly to a gluten-free diet. One author suggests that a gluten-free diet should be started in every patient with dermatitis herpetiformis and villous atrophy, even though gluten-induced abnormalities in the gut have been present for some years before diagnosis, despite the lack of epidemiologic evidence that a gluten-free diet reduces the incidence of lymphoma in dermatitis herpetiformis.[10]

DIAGNOSIS OF DERMATITIS HERPETIFORMIS

Skin biopsy. Figure 16-6 is an example of new red papular lesions that have not blistered. Subepidermal clefts of evolving vesicles, and neutrophils and eosinophils in microabscesses within dermal papillae, are demonstrated. Linear IgA bullous dermatosis histologically resembles dermatitis herpetiformis or bullous pemphigoid.[11]

Immunofluorescence studies. Skin biopsies for immunofluorescence studies are taken from adjacent normal or faintly erythematous skin because the diagnostic Ig deposits are usually destroyed during the blistering process. More than 90% of patients with dermatitis herpetiformis have granular or fibrillar IgA deposits in the dermal papillae; patients with linear IgA bullous dermatosis have linear deposits of IgA in the BMZ.[12] This includes patients treated with sulfones. Multiple specimens may be needed to obtain positive findings because of the focal nature of deposits. Normal skin sites of more than 3 mm from a lesion or sites in areas not commonly involved may test negative for such IgA deposits.

IgA antiendomysial (IgA-EmA), IgA-reticulin, and IgA-gliadin autoantibodies. Circulating antibodies to endomysium, reticulin, and gliadin occur in patients with gluten-sensitive enteropathy (i.e., dermatitis herpetiformis and celiac disease). IgA antiendomysial antibodies to the endomysium (an intermyofibrial substance) on esophageal smooth muscle are found in the serum of patients with dermatitis herpetiformis; they disappear with strict adherence to a gluten-free diet and reappear when gluten is consumed.[13] Serologic studies for the presence of IgA-EmA are highly specific and are found in approximately 70% of all patients with dermatitis herpetiformis[14] who are not on a gluten-free diet, in almost 100% of patients with dermatitis herpetiformis and a grade 3 or 4 flattening of the intestinal mucosa,[15] and in all untreated patients with celiac disease. The antibodies are absent in linear IgA bullous dermatosis. The titers of IgA-EmA parallel the degree of jejunal involvement. The incidence of antibody decreases to 0% when gluten is strictly avoided for 3 months. The test is especially useful for patients in whom the histologic and direct immunofluorescence studies are negative or equivocal.[16] Reticulin antibodies occur in 36% of patients. Antigliadin antibodies are detected in two thirds of dermatitis herpetiformis patients and are not disease specific since increased frequencies of these antibodies are also detected in patients with pemphigus and pemphigoid.[17]

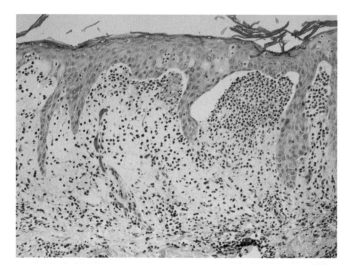

Figure 16-6
Dermatitis herpetiformis. Subepidermal clefts with microabscesses of neutrophils and eosinophils in the dermal papilla.

Trial of sulfones. Patients with a classic history and vesicular eruption may be given a trial of sulfone therapy if they are very uncomfortable. The dramatic relief of symptoms within hours or a few days supports the diagnosis of dermatitis herpetiformis.

Treatment

Dapsone or sulfapyridine. These drugs control but do not cure the disease. Dapsone is more effective than sulfapyridine. The mechanism of action is unknown but possibly is explained by lysosomal enzyme stabilization. For adults, the initial dosage of dapsone is 100 to 150 mg given orally once a day. Itching and burning are controlled in 12 to 48 hours, and new lesions gradually stop appearing. The dosage is adjusted to the lowest level that provides acceptable relief; this is usually in the range of 50 to 200 mg/day. Some patients' symptoms are controlled with 25 mg/day, whereas others may require up to 400 mg/day. Probenecid blocks the renal excretion of dapsone, and rifampin increases the rate of plasma clearance. Dapsone produces dose-related hemolysis, anemia, and methemoglobinemia to some degree in all patients. A leukocyte count and hemoglobin determination should be done weekly when possible for the first month, monthly for 6 months, and semiannually thereafter. Methemoglobinemia, although not usually a significant problem, may cause a blue-gray cyanosis. The coadministration of cimetidine is reported to reduce dapsone-dependent methemoglobinemia in dermatitis herpetiformis patients.[18] Patients with glucose-6-phosphate dehydrogenase (G6PD) deficiency may have a profound hemolysis during sulfone or sulfapyridine therapy, and those at risk of having the deficiency (blacks, Asians, and those of Mediterranean descent) should have a G6PD level ordered before starting therapy.

ADVERSE REACTIONS. Peripheral motor neuropathy may develop during the first few months of dapsone therapy. Generally, high dosages from 200 to 500 mg/day or high cumulative doses in the range of 25 to 600 gm have been implicated.[19] Typically, the distal upper and lower extremities, particularly the hand muscles, are involved. Paresthesia and weakness are the most common complaints, and atrophy of interosseus muscles is often found. Patients complain of difficulty with manual tasks and gait disturbance. Foot-drop is a common manifestation. Rarely, sensory involvement manifested by paresthesia, diminished pain, and numbness accompanies the motor disorder.[20] Symptoms slowly but invariably improve over months to years when the medication is stopped. Sulfapyridine, a short-acting sulfonamide (starting dosage, 500 to 1500 mg/day), can be substituted for dapsone and does not cause neuropathy. Agranulocytosis and aplastic anemia rarely occur but have resulted in death.

The sulfone syndrome,[21] consisting of fever, malaise, exfoliative dermatitis, lymphadenopathy, and hemolytic anemia, is a rare complication. Hypersensitivity hepatitis has been reported as a component of the syndrome.[22] Blood and liver function studies usually become normal within a few months after the patient stops taking dapsone.

Dapsone appears to be safe during pregnancy.[23]

Gluten-free diet. Strict adherence to a gluten-free diet for at least 6 months allows most patients to begin a decrease in or possibly a discontinuation of sulfone therapy. The diet has to be followed for many months (often 2 years) before medications can be discontinued.[24] Although intestinal villous architecture improves, symptoms and lesions recur in 1 to 3 weeks if a normal diet is resumed. Current evidence indicates that a gluten-free diet needs to be continued indefinitely. Patients found to have a linear IgA immunofluorescence pattern do not have villous atrophy and do not respond to a gluten-free diet.

Products must be chosen carefully, since some so-called gluten-free foods contain high levels of gliadin, the enterotoxic agent in gluten.[25] Gluten is in all grains except rice and corn. Gluten-free foods can be ordered from ENER-G Foods, Inc., 6901 Fox Ave. SO, P.O. Box 24723, Seattle, WA 98124-0723, 1-800-331-5222. The Gluten Intolerance Group of North America, P.O. Box 23053, Seattle, WA 98102-0353, 1-206-325-6980, publishes a newsletter and offers other services. Books describing gluten avoidance are available.*

Elemental diet. Dietary factors other than gluten may be important in the pathogenesis of dermatitis herpetiformis. Various substances can act as antigens; if the antigens can be eliminated, no new harmful immune complexes are formed. Most antigens that lead to humoral immune responses are proteins; therefore, a diet without full proteins (elemental diet) is not likely to contain major antigens. In one study, a diet of amino acids, fat, and carbohydrates produced a rapid benefit and allowed a significant reduction in the dosage of dapsone within 2 weeks.[26] A significant improvement in clinical disease activity, independent of gluten administration, and in small bowel morphology are also seen with an elemental diet.[27]

Tetracycline and nicotinamide. Successful treatment of dermatitis herpetiformis and linear IgA bullous dermatosis[28] with tetracycline (500 mg one to three times daily) or minocycline (100 mg twice daily) and nicotinamide (500 mg two or three times daily) is reported. Stopping either nicotinamide or minocycline resulted in a flare of the dermatitis herpetiformis.

---

*For example, Powers M: *Gluten-free and good*, ed 2, St Charles, Mo, 1983, Old Town Press.

Bullae in Diabetic Persons

Crops of bullae may appear abruptly in diabetic persons, usually on the feet and lower legs. They usually develop overnight without preceding trauma. There is little pain or discomfort. Different epidermal split levels and subepidermal separation have been reported.[29] The bullae arise from a noninflamed base, are usually multiple, and vary in size from 1 to several cm.[30] Occasionally they are huge, involving the entire dorsum of the foot or a major portion of the lower leg (Figure 16-7). The bullae are tense and rupture in approximately 1 week, leaving a deep, painless ulcer that forms a firmly adherent crust. Even if not infected, these large ulcers take many weeks to heal. Many patients never have another episode, whereas others have recurrences.

No immunopathologic features are found. The cause is unknown but is possibly ischemic.[31]

Treatment. Ulcers may be compressed several times a day with tepid Burow's solution or silver nitrate. The clean, superficial ulcer base is painted twice a day with 2% merbromin (Mercurochrome), and the surrounding skin is cleaned with hydrogen peroxide. The treatment of deeper erosions and ulcers is described in Chapter Three.

Pemphigus

Pemphigus is a rare, lethal, autoimmune, intraepidermal blistering disease involving the skin and mucous membranes. Circulating IgG autoantibodies directed against the cell surface of keratinocytes destroy the adhesion between epidermal cells, producing blisters.[32] The disease is associated with two kinds of HLA-DR4, DQ8 haplotypes dominantly distributed among Jewish patients, and these plus DR6, DQ5 haplotypes in non-Jewish patients.[33] The mean age of onset is in the sixth decade. Lever[34] classifies pemphigus into two categories: pemphigus vulgaris; with pemphigus vegetans considered to be a variant, and pemphigus foliaceus, with pemphigus erythematosus designating the localized disease. Sixty-one percent have a neoplasm of the immune system.[35] Pemphigus is a disease that is more heard of than seen.

PEMPHIGUS VULGARIS

Pemphigus vulgaris is the most common form of pemphigus.[36] Oral erosions usually precede the onset of skin blisters by weeks or months (Figure 16-8). In one study, the soft palate was involved in 80% of cases at initial presentation.[37] Nonpruritic skin blisters varying in size from 1 to several cm appear gradually and may be localized for a considerable length of time, but they invariably become generalized if left untreated (Figure 16-9). The blisters rupture easily because the vesicle roof, which consists of only a thin portion of the upper epidermis, is very fragile. Application of pressure to small intact bullae causes the fluid to dissect laterally into the midepidermal areas altered by bound IgG (Nikolsky's sign). Exposed erosions last for weeks before healing with brown hyperpigmentation but without scarring. Blisters, erosions, and lines of erythema may appear in the esophageal mucosa.[38] Death formerly occurred in all cases, usually from cutaneous infection, but now occurs in only 10% of cases, usually from complications of steroid therapy. Pemphigus vegetans, a very rare form of pemphigus vulgaris, consists of large verrucous confluent plaques localized to flexural areas.

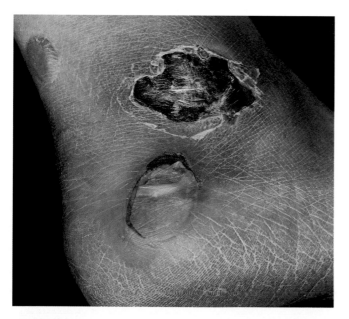

Figure 16-7
Bullae in a person with diabetes. Large bullae may appear spontaneously in diabetics.

PEMPHIGUS VULGARIS

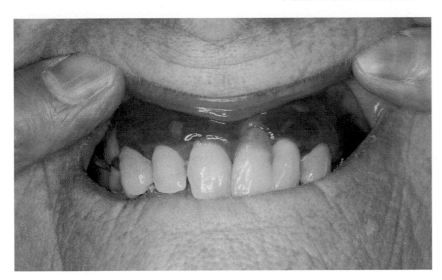

Figure 16-8
Oral erosions commonly occur and may precede the onset of skin blisters by weeks or months.

Figure 16-9
Flaccid blisters rupture easily because the roof, which consists only of a thin portion of the upper epidermis, is very fragile. Healing is with brown hyperpigmentation, but without scarring.

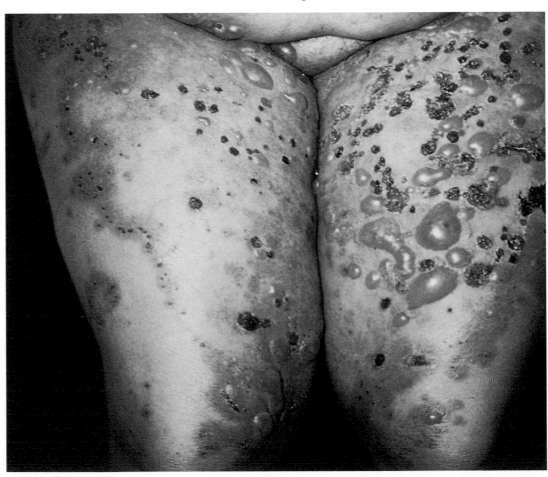

PEMPHIGUS FOLIACEUS, IgA PEMPHIGUS, AND PEMPHIGUS ERYTHEMATOSUS

The age of onset varies more widely in pemphigus foliaceus and pemphigus erythematosus than in pemphigus vulgaris, and there is no racial prevalence. Oral lesions are rarely present. The disease begins gradually on the face (Figure 16-10) in a "butterfly" distribution or first appears on the scalp, chest, or upper back as localized or broad, continuous areas of erythema, scaling, crusting, or, occasionally, bullae (Figure 16-11). Fogo selvagem (Portuguese for "wild fire") is an endemic form of pemphigus foliaceus found in certain rural areas of Brazil and Colombia.[39,40] Chronic exposure to black fly antigens may precipitate IgG4 antibody[41] formation, which may cross-react with epidermal antigens and cause fogo selvagem.[42]

IgG autoantibodies and C3 can be demonstrated high in the epidermis and in the granular layer and presumably are responsible for cleft formation. The vesicle roof is so thin that it ruptures; this is why intact blisters are not usually seen.

Serum leaks out and desiccates, forming the localized or broad areas of crust (Figure 16-12). Intact thin-walled blisters are sometimes seen near the edge of the erosions. The site of blister formation in the horizontal plane of the stratum corneum can be demonstrated in skin biopsy specimens after the upper portion of the epidermis has been dislodged with lateral finger pressure (Nikolsky's sign). IgA pemphigus has clinical and histologic similarity to subcorneal pustular dermatosis and pemphigus foliaceus. IgA antibodies are bound to the epidermal cell surface, and half of the patients have circulating IgA anti–cell surface antibodies.[43,44]

Pemphigus erythematosus, also known as *Senear-Usher syndrome*, may actually be a combination of localized pemphigus foliaceus and systemic lupus erythematosus, because many of these patients have a positive antinuclear antibody and a positive lupus band test result (deposits of Ig or complement, or both, at the dermoepidermal junction).[45] If the eruption becomes more diffuse or generalized, the term *pemphigus foliaceus* is used. The disease may last for years and may be fatal if not treated.

Figure 16-10
Pemphigus erythematosus. Serum and crust with occasional vesicles are present on the face in a butterfly distribution.

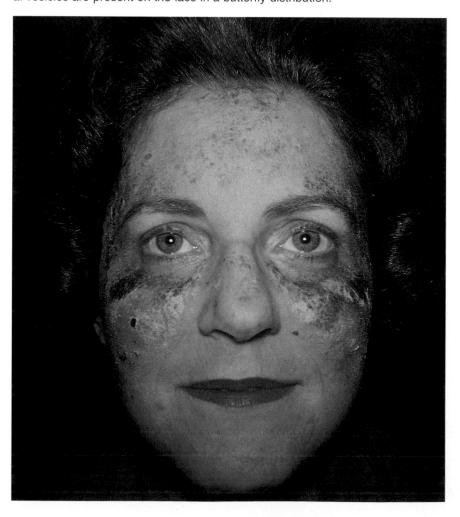

PEMPHIGUS FOLIACEUS

Figure 16-11
The symmetrical distribution of red, eroded, crusted lesions. Occasionally vesicles are seen at the edge of a lesion.

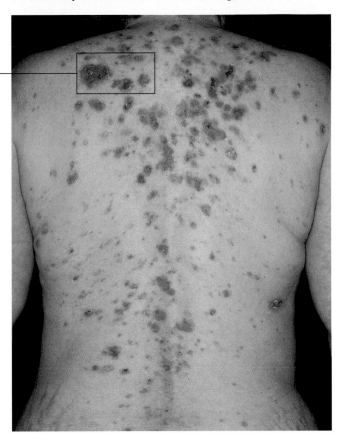

Figure 16-12
Inset of Figure 16-11. The vesicle roof is so thin that it ruptures, leaving erosions with areas of crust.

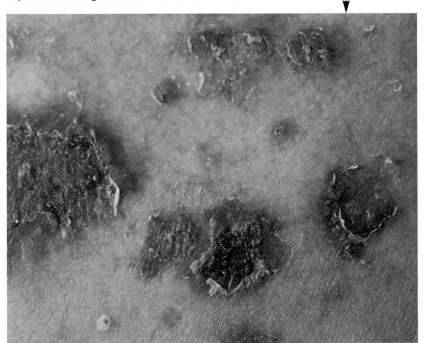

PEMPHIGUS IN ASSOCIATION WITH OTHER DISEASES

Myasthenia gravis and thymoma have been reported on many occasions in association with pemphigus (usually erythematosus and vulgaris).[46,47] The clinical course is variable, but most patients develop myasthenia gravis, followed by the detection of thymus disease, and finally by the appearance of pemphigus. Malignancy, usually of the lymphoid or reticuloendothelial system, occurs more frequently in patients with pemphigus than in normal persons. Paraneoplastic pemphigus is described below.

Drug-induced v. drug-triggered pemphigus. Pemphigus foliaceus has been reported in approximately 5% of patients taking 500 to 2000 mg of D-penicillamine or captopril[47] for any length of time from 2 months to 4 years.[48] Most cases were mild. Patients with pemphigus induced by SH drugs (drugs containing a sulfhydryl radical, e.g., penicillamine or captopril) show spontaneous recovery in 39.4% and 52.6% of cases, respectively, once the drug is discontinued.[49,50]

Pemphigus induced by other drugs shows spontaneous recovery in only 15% of cases. This suggests that penicillamine (SH drugs) induces pemphigus, whereas other drugs only trigger the disease in patients with a predisposition.[51]

The pemphigus-like eruption is not always limited, and the mortality approaches 10%.[52]

Paraneoplastic pemphigus (neoplasia-associated pemphigus). Paraneoplastic pemphigus (PNP) is a newly described, unique autoimmune disease with clinical and histologic features of both Stevens-Johnson syndrome and pemphigus vulgaris, in association with non-Hodgkin's lymphomas and other malignant neoplasms.[53-55] There are painful mucosal ulcerations,[56] conjunctival reactions,[57] and polymorphous skin lesions[58,59] on the trunk and extremities that usually progress to blisters (see box above, right). Antibodies against epithelial proteins are present in desmosomes and hemidesmosomes in the epidermis. The prognosis is poor except for some patients who undergo total resection of their neoplasm.

Neoplasia-associated pemphigus may be a more precise term for this disorder because the course of the blistering eruption does not always parallel the course of the underlying cancer.[60]

Laboratory diagnosis of paraneoplastic pemphigus

Histology. The histologic findings show features of pemphigus and erythema multiforme. There are intraepithelial clefts with epidermal acantholysis. In addition, there are dyskeratotic keratinocytes, vacuolar change of the basilar epidermis, and epidermal exocytosis of inflammatory cells.[61,62]

Direct immunofluorescence. Testing of mucous membrane and skin biopsies shows IgG staining of cell-surface proteins (intercellular substance) and deposition at the BMZ.

Indirect immunofluorescence. Indirect immunofluorescence with rat bladder substrate is used to differentiate PNP from classic pemphigus. Circulating IgG anti–cell-surface

---

CRITERIA FOR THE DIAGNOSIS OF NEOPLASIA-INDUCED PEMPHIGUS

(A patient is considered to have neoplasia-induced pemphigus if all three major or two major and two or more minor criteria are met.)

MAJOR CRITERIA

Polymorphous mucocutaneous eruption
Concurrent internal neoplasia
Characteristic serum immunoprecipitation findings

MINOR CRITERIA

Positive cytoplasmic staining of rat bladder epithelium by indirect immunofluorescence
Intercellular and basement membrane zone immunoreactants on direct immunofluorescence of perilesional tissue
Acantholysis in biopsy specimen from at least one anatomic site of involvement

From Camisa C: *Arch Dermatol* 129:883-886, 1993.

---

and anti-cytoplasmic antibodies occur in a pattern and intensity unique to these patients.[63]

DIAGNOSIS OF PEMPHIGUS

Skin biopsy for light microscopy. A small, early vesicle or skin adjacent to a blister biopsied with a 3- or 4-mm punch shows an intraepidermal bulla, acantholysis (separation of epidermal cells near the blister following dissolution of the intercellular cement substance), and a mild-to-moderate infiltrate of eosinophils (Figures 16-13 and 16-14).

Direct immunofluorescence of skin. Two biopsies are recommended. One biopsy specimen should be taken from the edge of a fresh lesion and the second from an adjacent normal area. Two biopsies are especially helpful in evaluation of oral lesions because lesional sites are frequently denuded. Specimens are deposited in transport media available from specialized laboratories around the country. These are transported unrefrigerated. IgG and, in most instances, C3 are found in the intercellular substance areas of the epidermis. Direct immunofluorescence study on the esophagus was reported positive in all patients.[38]

Indirect immunofluorescence. Patients with pemphigus foliaceus have antibodies to a complex of three polypeptides 260-kd, 160-kd (desmoglein), and 85-kd (plakoglobin) (the foliaceus complex); patients with pemphigus vulgaris have antibodies to a complex of 210-kd, 130-kd, and 85-kd (plakoglobin) polypeptides (the vulgaris complex).[64] Serum IgG antibodies can be demonstrated by indirect immunofluorescent staining and are present in all forms of true pemphigus in approximately 75% of patients with active disease. The antibodies of pemphigus vulgaris and its variants can be distinguished from those of pemphigus foliaceus and its variants in approximately 90% of cases by testing on two tissue substrates. In these cases titers are reported on two substrates. In most cases the level of circulating intercellular substance IgG antibody reflects the activity of disease, rising during periods of activity and falling or disappearing during times of remission.[65] Periodic serum tests to detect changes in titers are helpful in evaluating the clinical course.[66] Serum should be tested every 2 to 3 weeks until remission, and every 1 to 6 months thereafter.

TREATMENT

Corticosteroids and immunosuppressive agents. Both high-dose corticosteroid (more than 120 mg/day)[34,67] therapy and low-dose (60 mg/day)[68] therapy have been advocated. A recent study demonstrated that although a more rapid initial control was achieved with the high-dose regimen, this regimen did not have any long-term benefit over the low-dose regimen with respect to the frequency of relapse or the incidence of complications.

Low-dose regimen. A single daily dose of 1 mg/kg/day of prednisolone or prednisone is given. Patients are treated until remission—a state in which no new blisters develop for at least 1 week. Prednisolone is tapered at 10 mg monthly. When the daily dose of 20 mg prednisolone is reached, adjuvant therapy of 15 mg methotrexate weekly or 100 mg cyclophosphamide[69] daily is added. Prednisolone is then gradually decreased 2.5 mg per month. After 1 year, if the patient is well, the adjuvant therapy is gradually decreased. A major relapse (blisters involving more than 50% of body surface area) is treated with the original starting dosage. All other relapses are treated by doubling the dosage of prednisolone. The value of adjuvant therapy has been questioned for bullous pemphigus by the authors of this regimen[68] and by others.[70]

Adjuvants. Because of the potential toxicity of systemic corticosteroids, another drug may be initiated for the long term. The adjuvant therapy (corticosteroid-sparing medication) is initiated with or after starting corticosteroids. Cyclophosphamide (1.5 to 2.5 mg/kg/day),[69] chlorambucil, azathioprine (1.5 to 2.5 mg/kg/day),[71] dapsone,[72] cyclosporine,[73] and gold,[74,75] plasma exchange,[76] and extracorporeal photopheresis,[77] have been used for adjuvant therapy.[70,78] Hydroxychloroquine 200 mg twice a day was reported to be an effective adjuvant in patients with persistent and widespread pemphigus foliaceus. This was especially true when photosensitivity was present.[79]

Pulse therapy. Conventional long-term, high-dose corticosteroid therapy for pemphigus causes many side effects. Pulse treatment regimens have been reported. On 3 consecutive days, 100 mg dexamethasone is administered intravenously and, on day 1, 500 mg cyclophosphamide is administered intravenously. Between pulses patients receive 50 mg cyclophosphamide orally per day. Initially the pulses are repeated every 2 weeks and later at 10-week intervals. In this report, after 6 months (14 to 48 treatments) 50% to 100% of patients with various forms of pemphigus were clear.[80,81] A similar program using only monthly pulse doses of cyclophosphamide 500 to 1000 mg per treatment also provided control for cases that had failed to respond to oral steroids and other agents.[82]

The combination of nicotinamide (1.5 gm/day) and tetracycline (2 gm/day) or minocycline (100 mg twice a day) was found to be an effective alternative to steroids in superficial pemphigus (pemphigus foliaceus and pemphigus erythematosus) and a steroid-sparing adjuvant, rather than a steroid alternative for pemphigus vulgaris.[83]

Pemphigus in remission. Direct immunofluorescence (DIF) should be performed before therapy is discontinued. A negative DIF finding is a good indicator of remission.[84]

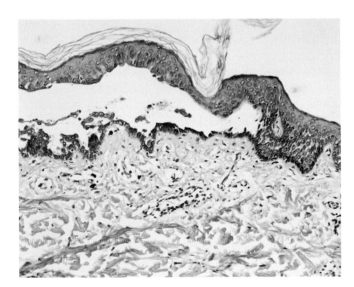

Figure 16-13
Pemphigus vulgaris. The epidermal separation occurs low in the epidermis.

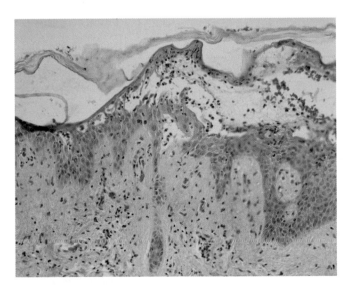

Figure 16-14
Pemphigus foliaceus. The intraepidermal separation appears high in the epidermis.

The Pemphigoid Group of Diseases

Bullous pemphigoid, herpes gestationis, and cicatricial pemphigoid are autoimmune subepidermal blistering diseases with circulating IgG and basement membrane zone–bound IgG antibodies and C3.

BULLOUS PEMPHIGOID

Bullous pemphigoid is a rare, relatively benign subepidermal blistering disease of unknown origin in which IgG autoantibodies are found both circulating and bound in the lamina lucida region of the basement membrane zone (BMZ) of the epidermis. The BMZ-bound autoantibodies result in activation of complement and chemotaxis and degranulation of leukocytes. The leukocytes release proteolytic enzymes that cause basement membrane destruction, resulting in dermal-epidermal separation. The final result is a subepidermal blister.

There is no racial or gender prevalence, and there are no known HLA associations. Pemphigoid is a disease of the elderly, with most cases occurring after age 60, although cases have been reported in children. There have been many reports of the coexistence of bullous pemphigoid with other disorders, but their association is probably coincidental.[85] There is little evidence of an association of bullous pemphigoid with internal malignancy.[86-88] Drugs are often suspected of causing pemphigoid;[89] stopping medication or changing to a different oral medication may help.

Clinical manifestations. Oral blisters, if present, are mild and transient. Pemphigoid begins with a localized area of erythema or with pruritic urticarial plaques that gradually become more edematous and extensive. A diagnosis of hives is frequently made in this preblistering stage. The amount of itching varies but is usually moderate to severe. A group of elderly patients had itching for a mean period of 10 months before the diagnosis was made.[90] In most cases the plaques turn dark red or cyanotic in 1 to 3 weeks, resembling erythema multiforme, as vesicles and bullae rapidly appear on their surface.

The eruption is usually generalized, but the most common sites are the lower part of the abdomen, the groin, and the flexor surfaces of the arms and legs. The palms and soles are affected (Figure 16-15). The 1- to 7-cm bullae appear isolated or in clusters and are tense with good structural integrity, in contrast to the large, flaccid, easily ruptured bullae of pemphigus. Firm pressure on the blister will not result in extension into normal skin as occurs in pemphigus; therefore Nikolsky's sign is negative. Most bullae rupture within a week, leaving an eroded base that, unlike the situation with pemphigus, does not spread and heals rapidly.

The course is variable. Untreated pemphigoid may remain localized and undergo spontaneous remission, or it may become generalized. The disease duration varies from 9 weeks to 17 years (estimated median treatment time 2 years 1 month) with periods of remission followed by recurrences that may be less severe than the initial episode. Throughout this impressive disease, patients remain afebrile, relatively

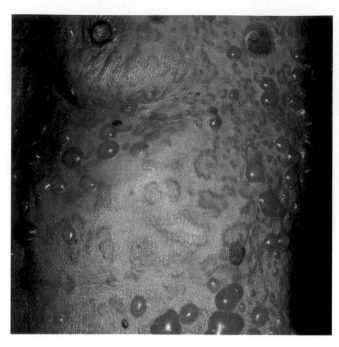

Figure 16-15
Bullous pemphigoid. Generalized eruption with tense blisters arising from an edematous, erythematous annular base.

comfortable, and ambulatory. No clinical, immunologic, or immunogenetic factors are predictive of disease duration.[91]

Many localized clinical variants of bullous pemphigoid have been reported (vesicular, vegetating, hyperkeratotic, erythrodermic) that have the same histologic and immunologic characteristics as generalized bullous pemphigoid. Bullous pemphigoid may occur at sites of trauma and with little spread of the condition outside such areas.[92,93] The diagnosis is confirmed by histology and direct and/or indirect immunofluorescence. See the next section on localized bullous pemphigoid.

Differential diagnosis. The differential diagnosis includes epidermolysis bullosa acquisita, dermatitis herpetiformis, pemphigus, bullous systemic lupus erythematosus, and bullous drug eruptions.

Laboratory. Peripheral blood eosinophilia occurs in 50% of patients, and elevated serum IgE in 70%.

Skin biopsy for light microscopy. There are two important features to demonstrate in biopsy specimens of bullous diseases: the level of cleft formation (i.e., intraepidermal or subepidermal) and the presence or absence of an inflammatory infiltrate, as well as the type of cell present (eosinophils or neutrophils, etc.). Bullae in pemphigoid may arise from inflamed (infiltrate-rich) or noninflamed (infiltrate-poor) skin; the most information is provided through a biopsy on an early bulla on inflamed skin. Histologically, there are subepidermal bullae with eosinophils in the dermis and bullae cavities (Figure 16-16).

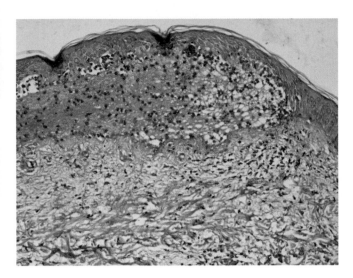

Figure 16-16
Bullous pemphigoid. A subepidermal blister contains numerous eosinophils.

Direct immunofluorescence (DIF) of skin. Another 3- or 4-mm punch biopsy specimen is taken and submitted in special transport media. The highest diagnostic yield for DIF comes from biopsies of inflamed skin next to a blister. DIF is positive in a high percentage of patients even after treatment is initiated. The yield is 62% from oral mucosal biopsies.[94]

DIF shows IgG and/or C3 and, sometimes, IgA, IgM, and fibrin in a linear band at the BMZ. Bullous pemphigoid and epidermolysis bullosa acquisita (EBA) are characterized by linear IgG deposits along the BMZ. Patients with EBA are more likely to have IgG staining without concomitant C3 deposition than are patients with bullous pemphigoid.[95] Biopsy specimens treated with 1 mol/L sodium chloride separate through the lamina lucida. The IgG appears in the dermal side of the split specimens in EBA and predominantly or exclusively in the epidermal side in bullous pemphigoid.[96,97] DIF studies relate to treatment responses. As the disease subsides, complement C3 deposits disappear. Normal skin of the forearm can be used for such studies.

Indirect immunofluorescence. Circulating IgG antibodies are present in approximately 70% of cases, but their level does not correlate with disease activity as it does in pemphigus.[98,99] These antibodies detect the 230-kd major or the 160- to 180-kd minor bullous pemphigoid antigens synthesized by keratinocytes.

Treatment. The clinical course was documented in 82 bullous pemphigoid patients treated with a variety of medications. Considerable heterogeneity in the course was demonstrated. The duration varied from 9 weeks to 17 years. The remission rate was 30% at 2 years and 50% at 3 years. Late relapse was observed after disease-free intervals of more than 5 years. The mortality rate at 1 year was 19%, and treatment was believed to be contributory in seven deaths.[91]

Itching is controlled with hydroxyzine (Atarax) 10 to 50 mg every 4 hours as needed. Systemic steroids combined with immunosuppressive agents such as azathioprine, cyclophosphamide, methotrexate, or chlorambucil have been the mainstay of therapy. The toxicity of these drugs seems disproportionate to the low risk of the disease. Antibiotics, dapsone, and topical steroids may be a safe and effective alternative for some patients. For more information, see the treatment section for cicatricial pemphigoid.

Topical steroids. Topical steroids are an alternative in the treatment of limited bullous pemphigoid.[100] In one series, clobetasol propionate cream was applied twice daily to affected skin until all lesions were healed and for 2 weeks thereafter. Complete epithelialization was achieved in every case within 4 to 17 days of treatment. After discharge, patients received decreasingly less potent corticosteroid creams as maintenance therapy for between 5 weeks and 13 months. Seventy percent of patients remained in remission on this regimen.[101]

Antibiotics. Studies have reported an excellent clinical response when localized or generalized bullous pemphigoid was treated with tetracycline, minocycline, or erythromycin, with or without niacinamide. The recommended schedules are tetracycline or erythromycin 1.0 to 2.5 gm/day, or minocycline 200 mg/day and niacinamide 1.5 to 2.5 gm/day. In a recent study patients with generalized bullous pemphigoid were treated with tetracycline (2 gm daily) without niacinamide.[102] Bulla formation was significantly reduced within 1 week and stopped within 1 to 3 weeks. The 2-gm dosage was maintained for 1 to 2 months, decreased by 500-mg decrements every month, and then stopped. These drugs may suppress the inflammatory response at the BMZ, inhibit neutrophil chemotaxis, and increase cohesion of the dermoepidermal junction.[103,104] The effect may be enhanced by a synergetic effect of niacinamide.

Sulfones. Forty-four percent of patients with bullous pemphigoid respond to treatment with sulfapyridine or dapsone, and their disease can be completely controlled without the use of prednisone.[105] The response occurs within 2 weeks; the maximum dosage is usually 100 mg/day of dapsone.[106] The dosage is regulated according to the patient's response. Dapsone therapy is described in detail in the dermatitis herpetiformis treatment section earlier in this chapter.

Prednisone and immunosuppressive drugs (adjuvant therapy). The mainstay of therapy in past years has been systemic corticosteroids. Noncontrolled trials have reported the use of adjuvant therapies with steroid-sparing effects. These have included azathioprine,[99] cyclophosphamide, chlorambucil, and methotrexate. A large, randomized, multicenter, unblind study was designed to assess the efficacy of azathioprine or plasma exchange when added to conventional dosages of prednisolone. The study demonstrated that neither azathioprine nor plasma exchange is effective enough to be used routinely as an adjuvant to corticosteroids in the management of bullous pemphigoid.[107]

Patients who do not respond to attempts to control their conditions with antibiotics and dapsone and require suppression may be treated with prednisone or prednisolone.

Most authorities recommend an initial dosage of 1 mg/kg per day in two daily doses. Most patients are controlled in 28 days and the dosage can be gradually tapered. The schedule used in one study was to taper to a daily dose of 0.5 mg/kg at 3 months and 0.2 mg/kg at 6 months.[107]

The time required for resolution with prednisone depends on the number of blisters on day 1.[108] The addition of dapsone to the existing regimen of corticosteroids may help to produce a clinical remission, to lower the dosage of prednisone, and to taper off prednisone more easily.[109] Consider adjuvant immunosuppressive therapy with cyclophosphamide or azathioprine if dapsone and prednisone fail (see treatment section for cicatricial pemphigoid).

Ultraviolet light and scratching may induce bullae and should be avoided.[110] One should consider stopping or changing oral medications that are sometimes suspected of causing pemphigoid.

LOCALIZED PEMPHIGOID

Cicatricial pemphigoid (mucosal surfaces), localized childhood vulvar pemphigoid, pretibial pemphigoid[111] (nonscarring bullous lesions predominantly on the legs of women), localized chronic pemphigoid of Brunsting-Perry[112] (crops of grouped blisters on the head and neck that heal with atrophic scars), dyshidrosiform pemphigoid[113] (vesiculobullous hemorrhagic lesions of the palms and soles), and pemphigoid vegetans (erosive and vegetating plaques)[114] are variants of localized pemphigoid. These patients possess the same circulating IgG autoantibodies as patients with generalized bullous pemphigoid.[115] Direct immunofluorescence is, however, a less useful diagnostic test in localized bullous pemphigoid; the intensity of the reaction correlates roughly with extent of disease.[116]

Cicatricial pemphigoid. Seen in the elderly, cicatricial pemphigoid, or benign mucous membrane pemphigoid, is a rare, chronic, subepidermal blistering and scarring disease.[117,118] The oral cavity and the eye are most frequently involved.[119] Unlike bullous pemphigoid, there are few remissions.

Oral disease. The mouth is involved in 85% of cases. Desquamative gingivitis is the most frequent manifestation. The gingiva appears red with diffuse or patchy involvement (Figure 16-17). Oral vesiculobullous lesions form, then rupture, leaving clean, noninflamed erosions that are relatively painless and do not interfere with eating. The vermilion border of the lips is spared, in contrast to the situation with pemphigus. Hoarseness is a sign of laryngeal involvement (8% of cases).

Ocular disease. The eye is involved in 65% of cases. Unilateral conjunctivitis is often the initial presentation; within 2 years the disease is usually bilateral. Fibrosis beneath the conjunctival epithelium is the primary destructive process. Gradual shrinkage of the conjunctiva leads to obliteration of the conjunctival sac (Figure 16-18). Reduced tearing with erosion and neovascularization of the cornea leads to corneal opacification and perforation. Fibrous conjunctival adhesions become more numerous; the disease leads to blindness in approximately 20% of cases. Patients with only ocular lesions are classified as having ocular cicatricial pemphigoid. These patients have lower in vivo deposits of IgG and C3, higher deposits of fibrin, absence of circulating antibodies, and negative serologic reactivity to bullous pemphigoid antigens.[120] Severe ocular mucosal injury, such as that which occurs in Stevens-Johnson syndrome, may be a precipitating factor in the development of ocular cicatricial pemphigoid. The time lag between the

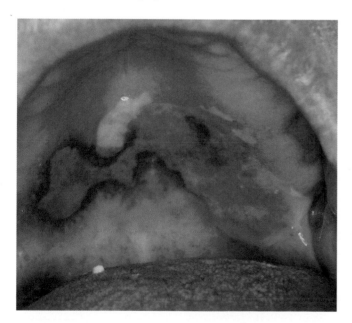

Figure 16-17
Cicatricial pemphigoid. Large, oral-cavity erosions.

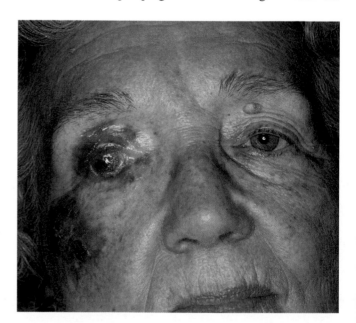

Figure 16-18
Cicatricial pemphigoid involving the conjunctiva and surrounding skin.

onset of Stevens-Johnson syndrome and cicatricial pemphigoid ranged from a few months to 31 years.[121] Prolonged periods of remission after stopping therapy occur in one third of patients. Follow-up must be continued for life, because relapse occurs in 22% of those who were in remission and not undergoing therapy.[122]

Skin disease. Approximately 25% of patients develop cutaneous lesions consisting of scattered tense vesicles or bullae that arise from a red base, usually on the face, neck, and scalp. Vesicles rupture and leave an erosion that eventually heals with or without atrophic scars. Fibrous adhesions and atrophy can occur on the penis, vulva, vagina (17% of cases), and anus. When there is involvement of the head and neck but not the mucous membrane, the disease is known as the *Brunsting-Perry* type of cicatricial pemphigoid.

Diagnosis. The biopsy shows a subepidermal bulla with little inflammation. Direct immunofluorescence of lesional, perilesional, and normal mucous membrane biopsy specimens shows linear deposition of complement and IgG and, less often, IgA. Circulating IgG and IgA antibodies are found in 10% of cases with routine techniques and up to 82% when salt-split human skin is used as a substrate. The autoantibodies bind to the epidermal roof in most cases.[123]

Treatment. A detailed description of topical and systemic therapy appears in a clinical review.[117]

Plan of therapy. Treat localized disease with topical therapy and use intralesional steroids if that fails. Start dapsone if topical therapy is ineffective. Patients not responsive to dapsone after 12 weeks are treated with prednisone with or without dapsone. Immunosuppressive agents and prednisone are used if dapsone fails.[124] Cyclophosphamide is tried first, azathioprine is the alternate choice. The response is slow. The skin and oral lesions respond more quickly and predictably than the eye lesions. Most patients require long-term suppression. Taper and withdraw drugs when a remission is achieved.

Topical therapy

ORAL CAVITY. Debride dead tissue from the oral mucosa. Hydrogen peroxide, elixir of dexamethasone, and elixir of diphenhydramine are each diluted with tap water to a concentration of 1:4 or 1:6, as tolerated. They are not swallowed. Before meals patients rinse with hydrogen peroxide and diphenhydramine (reduces pain, does not suppress taste completely as does viscous lidocaine). After meals patients rinse with hydrogen peroxide to remove food particles and debris, then with dexamethasone for its antiinflammatory effect. Between meals and before bedtime, patients rinse with hydrogen peroxide, then with dexam-

ethasone. This schedule is demanding but effective. Treat oral lesions with fluocinonide gel, which is more adherent and results in better patient compliance than triamcinolone acetonide in Orabase. Food can be puréed in a blender if eating is painful.

EYES. Lubricate frequently with artificial tears and ointments. Infection of the lids is treated with topical or systemic antibiotics. Topical steroids are not effective.

Intralesional therapy. Lesions of the skin, oral cavity, nose, genitalia, and anus respond to intralesional steroids. Inject high in the dermis to avoid atrophy. Use triamcinolone acetonide (dilution of 5 to 10 mg/ml); repeat every 2 to 4 weeks.

Systemic therapy

DAPSONE. Dapsone (75 to 200 mg/day) is the drug of first choice; it controls the inflammation[125] in most patients and achieves a remission in others.[126]

CORTICOSTEROIDS. Prednisone (20 to 80 mg daily) is used. The initial dose depends on the severity of the disease. A twice daily dosage is used during the acute stage and changed to single daily morning dose after new blister formation stops. Taper dosage slowly to avoid a relapse. Pulse therapy has been reported to be effective for bullous pemphigoid (see treatment section on bullous pemphigoid).

IMMUNOSUPPRESSIVE AGENTS (ADJUVANT THERAPY). Immunosuppressive agents have a corticosteroid-sparing effect. They are started when corticosteroids are initiated or shortly afterward. Cyclophosphamide (1.5 to 2.5 mg/kg/day) is superior to azathioprine but is more toxic. Azathioprine (1.5 to 2.5 mg/kg/day) is the alternate choice. A significant response requires 8 to 12 weeks.

ANTIBIOTICS. Infections of the mucous membranes and skin are treated with systemic antibiotics (e.g., doxycycline 200 mg/day).

Surgical therapy Surgery to deal with scarring and to prevent blindness, upper airway stenosis, or esophageal stricture is performed after disease activity has stopped.

Localized vulvar pemphigoid. Childhood localized vulvar pemphigoid is a morphologic variant of bullous pemphigoid.[127,128] Patients present with recurrent vulvar vesicles and ulcers. Scarring may or may not occur. As with generalized pemphigoid, direct immunofluorescence shows linear IgG and C3 at the basement membrane, and indirect immunofluorescence is positive in some cases. Lesions may be treated with a group III through V topical steroid. Oral erythromycin may be effective, as is reported for generalized pemphigoid. Periodic outbreaks have been reported to occur for 3 years. Cases have been misdiagnosed as child abuse.[129,130]

HERPES GESTATIONIS (PEMPHIGOID GESTATIONIS)

Herpes gestationis (HG), an intensely pruritic, blistering disease of pregnancy, occurs in fewer than 1 in 50,000 pregnancies.[131] There is a genetic predisposition; 90% of patients express class II antigens (HLA-DR3 and HLA-DR4) and a class III antigen (C4).[132] HG appears to be mediated by an Ig-G1 specific for a 180-kd component of hemidesmosomes. The disease may appear for the first time during any pregnancy, but once it has occurred, it tends to reappear earlier and be more severe during any subsequent pregnancy. The disorder usually appears during the second or third trimester but may occur from the second week to the early postpartum period. It disappears 1 or 2 months after delivery and recurs with subsequent pregnancies. The newborn fetus has cutaneous involvement 10% of the time. HG is associated with an increase in prematurity.[133]

Clinical presentation. The intensity of disease varies.

HG may be subclinical or mild and nonvesicular during one pregnancy, and explosive and vesiculobullous during another.[134] Edematous plaques occur in crops on the abdomen and extremities and coalesce into bizarre polycyclic rings covering wide areas of the skin (Figure 16-19). As with pemphigoid, within days to weeks the tense blisters evolve from the edematous plaques, rupture to leave slowly healing denuded areas, and heal without scarring; they do cause postinflammatory hyperpigmentation. Spontaneous clearing may be seen during the latter period of the pregnancy, but flares are seen at the time of delivery in 75% to 80% of cases. Mild recurrences may occur with menstruation and the use of oral contraceptives. Mucous membrane involvement is rare.

Diagnosis. Biopsy specimens taken from inflamed skin adjacent to a blister exhibit histologic features similar to those of pemphigoid. A bandlike deposit of C3 in most cases and IgG in 10% of cases can be demonstrated at the BMZ by direct immunofluorescence. Circulating IgG (the so-called herpes gestationis factor) is difficult to find with conventional indirect immunofluorescence techniques. The herpes gestationis factor avidly fixes complement. Therefore a special technique, complement immunofluorescence, which requires a fresh source of complement, is most successful. The herpes gestationis factor can pass through the placenta and may be responsible for the transient pemphigoid-like skin lesions present in some newborns of affected mothers.[135] Peripheral eosinophilia is the only other common laboratory abnormality.

Treatment. Systemic steroids (starting dosage of prednisone 40 mg/day) are most often required for control. As with pemphigoid, the dosage is adjusted to disease response. Topical steroids are useful only for mild activity.

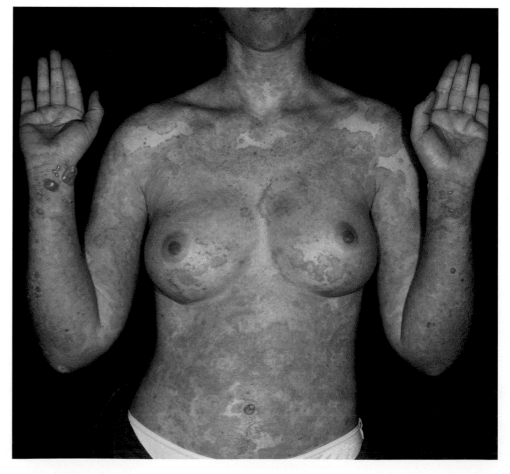

Figure 16-19
Herpes gestationis. Blisters arise from erythematous, edematous polycyclic rings.

BENIGN CHRONIC BULLOUS DERMATOSIS OF CHILDHOOD

Chronic bullous dermatosis of childhood is a rare, non-hereditary, subepidermal blistering disease with clinical features similar to those of bullous pemphigoid and dermatitis herpetiformis except that there is only moderate itching.[136] Large, tense subepidermal bullae appear in clusters on the face (particularly around the mouth), lower trunk, inner thighs, and genitalia. A significant number of patients have linear IgA deposits at the BMZ, circulating IgA anti-BMZ antibodies,[137] and normal jejunal biopsy results.[138,139] The prognosis is good: the disease eventually clears after remissions and exacerbations, and always before puberty. Corticosteroids are used only if dapsone fails.

Pemphigoid-like Disease

EPIDERMOLYSIS BULLOSA ACQUISITA

Epidermolysis bullosa acquisita (EBA) is a rare, subepidermal, blistering disorder associated with autoimmunity to type VII collagen, which is the collagen localized to anchoring fibrils within the dermoepidermal junction of skin. The clinical and histologic picture may mimic bullous or cicatricial pemphigoid and bullous systemic lupus erythematosus (BSLE). It is characterized by a chronic course, poor response to therapy, and occasional remissions. It is seen in children[140] and adults. There are two distinctive clinical presentations that are not mutually exclusive.[141] Diagnosis requires immunofluorescence studies of serum and biopsy specimens. Type VII collagen (the protein component of anchoring fibrils that fortify the attachment of the epidermis to the dermis) is the target molecule in EBA. Type VII collagen contributes to lamina densa-dermal adhesion by cross-linking lamina densa and dermal matrix proteins. Autoantibodies contribute to blisters by interfering with type VII collagen function.[142] Autoantibodies to type VII collagen are also present in BSLE—evidence that EBA and BSLE share an immunogenetic predisposition to C-VII autoimmunity.[143,144]

Classic epidermolysis bullosa acquisita. The classic presentation of EBA is marked by skin fragility characteristic of mechanobullous diseases.[145] Classic EBA presents with tense blisters on a noninflammatory base. They appear in trauma-prone areas of the hands and feet. The lesions heal with scarring and milia formation that resembles porphyria cutanea tarda. Some of these patients may have a scarring alopecia and nail dystrophy. Mucous membrane involvement may occur, and, when this is extensive, the clinical presentation may mimic atypical cicatricial pemphigoid.

Bullous pemphigoid-like epidermolysis bullosa acquisita. Approximately 50% of patients with EBA present this type of clinical picture early in the course of their disease. Tense blisters on an inflammatory base are widely distributed on the trunk and flexural surfaces. There is pruritus, minimal skin fragility, and healing of some of the lesions without scarring and milia.

Diagnosis. Special immunofluorescence tests are required to differentiate EBA from bullous pemphigoid (see Table 16-1). Direct immunofluorescence of perilesional skin shows linear and homogeneous deposits of IgG and C3[146] in the BMZ, bullous pemphigoid shows the same picture. These two diseases can be distinguished by studies of serum tested by indirect immunofluorescence on salt-split normal skin or by obtaining a fresh perilesional skin biopsy, inducing a split at the lamina lucida, and testing for the site of IgG deposition by direct immunofluorescence. Deposition of IgG on the dermal side of the separation differentiates EBA from bullous pemphigoid, which shows IgG on the epidermal side of the separation.[96,97] Indirect immunofluorescence studies of serum with 1 mol/L NaCl-separated human skin shows IgG anti-BMZ autoantibody (antitype VII collagen antibodies) bound to the dermal side of the separation.

Treatment. Most patients respond poorly to topical and systemic therapy. Some patients respond to high-dose prednisone therapy. Cyclosporine (6 mg/kg/day)[147-149] and high-dose intravenous immunoglobulins[150] may be effective.

BENIGN FAMILIAL CHRONIC PEMPHIGUS

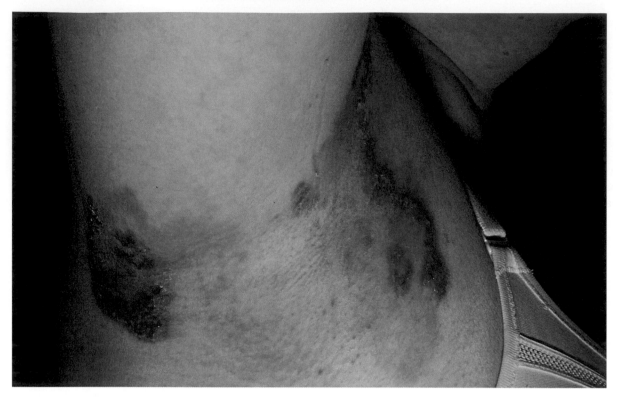

Figure 16-20
Vesicles are grouped in an annular or serpiginous pattern. The vesicles rupture and are replaced by an advancing rim of scale and by crust similar to that seen in impetigo and tinea. The active border extends peripherally, leaving a pale, hypopigmented center.

Figure 16-21
Erythematous annular plaques with vesicles and scale near the advancing border.

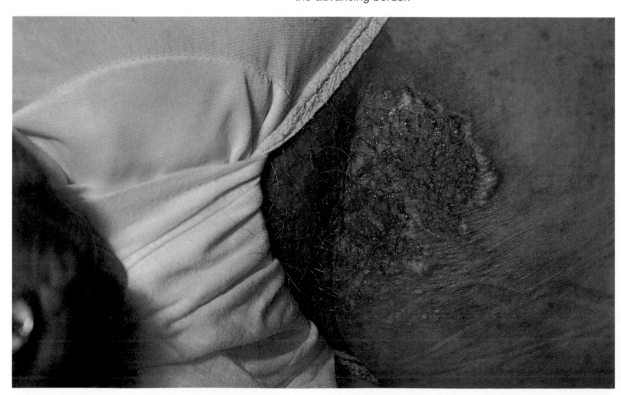

Benign Familial Chronic Pemphigus

Benign familial chronic pemphigus (Hailey-Hailey disease) is a rare, autosomal dominant,[151] intraepidermal, nonscarring bullous disease characterized by erosions, blisters, and warty papules. The disease first appears in adolescence or early adult life, usually during the summer; it is characterized by remissions and exacerbations. Lesions develop on areas exposed to ultraviolet light (nape of the neck and back) and on areas subjected to friction and maceration (axillae and groin) (Figures 16-20 and 16-21). Friction, heat, and sweating exacerbate the lesions, and pain may limit physical activities. Infection with staphylococci, herpes simplex virus,[152] or *Candida* may also precipitate the disease. Longitudinal white bands are present in the fingernails in 71% of patients.[153] Suction tests on clinically normal skin demonstrated a widespread subclinical abnormality in keratinocyte adhesion.[154] An ultraviolet provocation test has been used to identify genetic carriers of Hailey-Hailey disease.[155]

Nonintertriginous lesions. The eruption begins with a group of pruritic vesicles arising from a red or noninflamed base; they are grouped in an annular or serpiginous pattern. The vesicles rupture quickly and are replaced by an advancing rim of scale and crust similar to that seen in impetigo and tinea. The active border extends peripherally, leaving a pale, hypopigmented center. New crops of vesicles appear on the border but rupture so quickly that they may not be appreciated. These moist, indurated plaques ooze serum. Lesions may heal spontaneously in colder weather.

Intertriginous lesions. Vesicles sometimes appear in intertriginous lesions, but most often the patient has broad, moist, red, fissured areas or vegetating warty papules[156] and plaques that do not extend beyond the opposing skin surfaces of the groin or axillae. Intertriginous lesions are chronic and respond slowly to therapy, especially in obese patients.

Treatment

Nonintertriginous lesions. Oral antibiotic therapy (e.g., erythromycin, dicloxacillin, or a cephalosporin) should be started, followed in 3 or 4 days by administration of a group III through V topical steroid. Most lesions of the back and neck respond quickly to this simple program, and treatment is stopped when the lesions have healed. Sunscreens should be worn on exposed surfaces in the summer.

Intertriginous lesions. Groin and axillary lesions may be infected with bacteria and yeast. Therapy with one of the above oral antibiotics is started, and antiyeast creams (e.g., ketoconazole) are applied. Cream is applied to moist lesions and compressed with cool Burow's or silver nitrate solution. Compressing is discontinued once the surfaces are dry, and group V topical steroid creams are applied twice a day until lesions have healed.[153] Chronic and unresponsive lesions have been treated successfully by excision, topical cyclosporine,[157] carbon dioxide laser,[158,159] split-thickness skin grafting,[160] and dermabrasion.[161]

Epidermolysis Bullosa

Epidermolysis bullosa is a term given to three major groups and approximately 16 variants of rare dominant and recessive genetic diseases in which minor trauma causes noninflammatory blistering (mechanobullous diseases).[162] The pathogenesis is unknown. These diseases are classified as scarring or nonscarring and histologically by the level of blister formation.

Clinical classification (scarring vs. nonscarring). The clinical classification is based on the presence or absence of dystrophic changes and scarring. The intraepidermal forms (epidermolysis bullosa simplex) do not scar. Junctional forms (junctional epidermolysis bullosa) manifest as atrophy. Dermal forms (dystrophic epidermolysis) result in atrophy and scarring.

Histologic classification (level of blister formation). Classification is based on light and electron microscopic levels of separation:

Split-through epidermal basal cells—intraepidermal types
Split-through basement membrane area—junctional types
Split-through upper dermis—dermal forms

Epidermolysis bullosa simplex. The disease is autosomal dominant. Sporadic cases may arise by new mutation. Blistering begins in infancy or childhood, especially on the hands and feet or any other point of trauma, and heal without scarring. The major complication is infection.

Junctional epidermolysis bullosa. The disease is autosomal recessive. In most cases severe generalized blistering of the skin with the exception of the palms and soles begins in infancy. There is no scarring. Extensive involvement of the mouth, larynx, eyes, and esophagus is often present. The dentition may become defective. Most patients die in early childhood.

Dystrophic epidermolysis bullosa. The disease may be either autosomal dominant or autosomal recessive. There is great variation in the severity of the several forms of dystrophic epidermolysis bullosa. The severe, recessive form exhibits repeated cycles of blistering and scarring that lead to fusion of the digits, producing the so-called mitten deformity.

Diagnosis. Electron microscopic examination of the skin is the standard for diagnosis. Monoclonal antibodies have recently been used for diagnosis. Immunofluorescence tests for localization of type IV collagen, laminin, and pemphigoid antibodies in the roof or floor of bullae help differentiate the forms of epidermolysis bullosa.

Management. Patients must avoid trauma. Dilantin, a known collagenase inhibitor, is not an effective treatment for recessive dystrophic epidermolysis bullosa. Genetic counseling is essential, and fetal skin biopsy techniques have been developed for prenatal diagnosis. Additional information can be obtained from the Dystrophic Epidermolysis Bullosa Research Foundation, 141 Fifth Avenue, Suite 7-S, New York, NY 10010; 1-212-693-6610.

The Newborn with Blisters, Pustules, Erosions, and Ulcerations

There are more than 30 diseases in the newborn that can present with blisters, pustules, erosions, and ulcerations. For diagnostic purposes they are divided into infectious causes, common transient skin lesions, and uncommon and rare causes (Table 16-2). The most common transient diseases are described below. A complete list is presented in the boxes below and on p. 523. The following laboratory tests may be helpful: bacterial, viral, or fungal cultures; Gram stain; Wright's stain; Tzanck smears; potassium hydroxide (KOH) preparations; and skin biopsies.

Common transient skin lesions

Erythema toxicum neonatorum. Lesions are not present at birth. Erythema toxicum neonatorum (ETN) (toxic erythema of the newborn) occurs in 20% to 50% of term infants—usually second and later deliveries—who are otherwise healthy. It is rare in premature infants and in those weighing less than 2500 gm. Most cases occur between 24 and 48 hours of age.

The rash often begins on the face; the trunk, proximal extremities, and buttocks are commonly involved. Palms and soles are not affected. Lesions may localize at pressure sites. Four types of lesions occur: macules, wheals, papules, and pustules. Tiny papules and pustules are superimposed on macules or wheals. New lesions appear as older lesions resolve. Wright's stain of a pustule shows numerous eosinophils. Peripheral eosinophilia is unusual.

Transient neonatal pustular melanosis. Lesions are present at birth but may be overlooked for 1 or 2 days. Transient neonatal pustular melanosis (TNPM) occurs in 2% to 5% of term blacks and 0.6% of whites who are otherwise healthy. Vesiculopustules, with no underlying erythema, rupture and form a hyperpigmented macule with a collarette of scale. Lesions may be solitary or grouped; most are 2 to 3 mm. They are located on the forehead, behind the ears, under the chin, on the neck and back, and on the hands and feet. The palms and soles may be affected. Lesions are very superficial, located within or just beneath the stratum corneum. Wright's stain shows polymorphonuclear neutrophilic leukocytes (PMNs); eosinophils may predominate. No treatment is necessary. Pustules resolve in a few days; pigmented macules may last for several weeks to months.

A clear-cut differentiation between TNPM and ETN is not always possible. The name *sterile transient neonatal pustulosis* has been proposed to unify these conditions.

Miliaria. Lesions occur approximately 1 week after birth. Miliaria or heat rash occurs in warm climates, while warming in an incubator, during a fever, or from wearing occlusive dressings or warm clothing. Eccrine sweat-duct occlusion is the initial event. The duct ruptures, leaks sweat into the surrounding tissues, and induces an inflammatory

---

CONDITIONS WHERE PUSTULES OR VESICLES PREDOMINATE

COMMON CAUSES

Erythema toxicum neonatorum
Miliaria
Neonatal acne
Neonatal candidiasis
Neonatal pustular melanosis
Staphylococcal pyoderma

UNCOMMON CAUSES

Acropustulosis of infancy
Congenital candidiasis
Herpes simplex
Incontinentia pigmenti
Scabies

RARE CAUSES

Acrodermatitis enteropathica
Congenital self-healing histiocytosis
Cytomegalovirus
Eosinophilic pustular folliculitis
Hyperimmunoglobulin E syndrome
Listeria monocytogenes
Neonatal Behçet's disease
Varicella

From Frieden IJ: *Curr Probl Dermatol* 4:123, 1992.

CONDITIONS WHERE BULLAE MAY PREDOMINATE

COMMON CAUSES

Bullous impetigo
Sucking blisters

UNCOMMON CAUSES

Epidermolysis bullosa
Staphylococcal scalded skin syndrome

RARE CAUSES

Acrodermatitis enteropathica
Aplasia cutis congenita
Chronic bullous dermatosis of childhood
Congenital protein C or S deficiency
Congenital syphilis
Diffuse cutaneous mastocytosis
Ectodermal dysplasias
Epidermolytic hyperkeratosis
Erythropoietic porphyria
Maternal bullous disease
Neonatal varicella
Perinatal gangrene of the buttock
Pseudomonal infection
Toxic epidermal necrolysis

From Frieden IJ: *Curr Probl Dermatol* 4:123, 1992.

response. Occlusion occurs at two different levels to produce two distinct forms of miliaria. In miliaria crystallina, occlusion of the eccrine duct at the skin surface results in accumulation of sweat under the stratum corneum. The lesion appears as a clear dew drop. There is little or no erythema. The vesicles appear individually or in clusters. Miliaria rubra results from occlusion of the intraepidermal section of the eccrine sweat duct. Papules and vesicles surrounded by a red halo or diffuse erythema develop as the inflammatory response develops. A cool water compress and proper ventilation are all that is necessary to treat this self-limited process.

Neonatal acne. Lesions occur 1 to 2 weeks after birth in approximately 20% of newborns. Comedones, papules, and pustules occur in the same distribution as in adolescent acne. Lesions resolve spontaneously.

CONDITIONS WHERE EROSIONS OR ULCERATIONS MAY PREDOMINATE

COMMON CAUSES

Skin changes due to perinatal or neonatal trauma
Sucking blisters

UNCOMMON CAUSES

Aplasia cutis congenita
Epidermolysis bullosa
Herpes simplex, especially congenital
Staphylococcal scalded skin syndrome

RARE CAUSES

Aspergillus infection
Congenital erosive and vesicular dermatosis
Congenital protein C deficiency
Ectodermal dysplasias
Group B streptococcal infection
Hemangiomas and vascular malformations
Intrauterine varicella infection
Neonatal Behçet's disease
Neonatal lupus erythematosus
P. aeruginosa (ecthyma gangrenosum)
Perinatal gangrene of the buttock
Toxic epidermal necrolysis

From Frieden IJ: *Curr Probl Dermatol* 4:123, 1992.

TABLE 16-2 Differential Diagnosis: Blisters and Pustules in the Newborn

Disease	Usual age	Skin: Morphology	Skin: Usual distribution	Clinical: Other	Diagnosis/Findings
INFECTIOUS CAUSES					
Staphylococcal pyoderma	Few days to weeks	Pustules, bullae, occasional vesicles	Mainly diaper area, periumbilical	Boys more than girls; may be in epidemic setting	Gram stain: polymorphonuclear neutrophilic leukocytes, gram+ cocci in clusters. Bacterial culture
Staphylococcal scalded skin syndrome	3 to 7 days; occasionally older	Erythema, cutaneous tenderness, superficial blisters, erosions	Generalized, begins on the face; blistering and erosions in areas of mechanical stress	Irritability, fever	Skin biopsy: separation upper epidermis. Bacterial cultures: blood, urine, etc.
Group A streptococcal disease	Few days to weeks	Isolated pustules, honey-crusted areas	No specific area predisposed	Moist umbilical stump; occasional cellulitis, meningitis, pneumonia	Gram stain: gram + cocci in chains. Bacterial culture
Group B streptococcal disease	At birth or first few days	Vesicles, bullae, erosions, honey-crusted lesions	No specific area predisposed	Pneumonia, bacteremia	Gram stain: gram + cocci chains. Bacterial culture
Listeria monocytogenes	Usually at birth	Hemorrhagic pustules and petechiae	Generalized, especially trunk and extremities	Septic; respiratory distress; maternal	Gram stain: gram + rods. Bacterial culture
Haemophilus influenzae	Birth or first few days	Vesicles and crusted areas	No specific area predisposed	Bacteremia, meningitis may be present	Gram stain: small gram-bacilli. Bacterial culture
Pseudomonas aeruginosa	Days to weeks	Erythema, pustules, hemorrhagic bullae, necrotic ulcerations	Any area; may concentrate in diaper area	Prematurity, history of surgery, GI or pulmonary anomalies are risk factors	Skin or tissue Gram stain: gram-rods. Cultures of skin, blood, etc.
Congenital syphilis	Usually at birth	Blisters or erosions on dusky or hemorrhagic base	Palms, soles, knees, abdomen	Low birth weight, hepatosplenomegaly, metaphyseal dystrophy	Dark field of involved skin. Incompletely treated maternal syphilis
Congenital candidiasis	At birth or first week	Erythema and fine papules evolve into vesicles and pustules	Any part of body; palms and soles often involved	Prematurity, foreign body in cervix or uterus are risk factors	KOH: hyphae, budding yeast
Neonatal candidiasis	Weeks to months	Scaly red patches with satellite papules and pustules	Diaper area or intertriginous areas	Usually none; previous antibiotic prescribed	KOH: hyphae, budding yeast
Aspergillus	5 days +	Morphology: pustules rapidly evolve to other ulcers	Any area	Extreme prematurity/immunocompromised host	Skin biopsy: septate hyphae. Tissue fungal culture
Neonatal herpes simplex	Usual: 5 to 14 days	Vesicles, crusts, erosions may be grouped or not. May follow dermatome	Anywhere; scalp monitor site, torso, oral lesions are most frequent sites	Signs of sepsis; irritability and lethargy; eye, CNS are frequent sites of disease	Tzanck, viral culture

Intrauterine herpes simplex	At birth	Vesicles, widespread bullae, erosions, scars, missing skin	Anywhere on body	Low birth weight; microcephaly, chorioretinitis	Tzanck, viral culture
Fetal varicella infection	At birth	Usually scarring, limb hypoplasia, erosions	Anywhere; usually extremities	Maternal varicella first trimester	Tzanck, viral culture
Neonatal varicella	0 to 14 days	Vesicles on an erythematous base; may be very numerous	Generalized distribution	Maternal varicella 7 days before to 2 days after delivery	Tzanck, viral culture
Scabies	3 to 4 weeks or later	Papules, nodules, crusted area	Generalized, palms, soles	Others in family with itching or rash	Scabies prep: mites (eggs, feces)
TRANSIENT SKIN LESIONS					
Erythema toxicum neonatorum	Usually 24 to 48 hours	Erythematous macules, papules, and pustules	Buttocks, torso, proximal extremities. No palms, soles	Usually term infants over 2500 gm	Wright's stain: eosinophils
Neonatal pustular melanosis	At birth	Pustules without erythema; hyperpigmented macules; some have collarette of scale	Anywhere; most common on forehead, behind ears, neck, back, fingers, toes	Term infants; more common in black infants	Wright's stain: PMNs, occasional eosinophils
Miliaria crystallina	Usually first week of life	Dewdrop-like vesicles, very superficial, no erythema	Forehead, upper trunk, volar forearms most common sites	May be history of warm incubator, occlusive clothing, dressings	Usually clinical; Wright's Gram stain negative
Miliaria rubra	Days to weeks	Erythematous papules with superimposed pustules	Same as miliaria crystallina	Same as miliaria crystallina	Usually clinical; skin biopsy if doubt
Sucking blisters	At birth	Flaccid bulla or bullae on nonerythematous base	Radial forearm, wrist, hand, dorsal, thumb, index finger	Infants sucks vigorously on affected areas	Clinical diagnosis
Neonatal acne	3 to 4 weeks	Comedones, papules, pustules	Mainly cheeks, forehead	Comedones clue to diagnosis	Clinical diagnosis
Skin changes of perinatal/neonatal trauma	Birth to few days	Erosions on scalp, perineal or scalp gangrene (rare)	Scalp, perineum, heels	History fetal monitoring, vacuum extraction, neonatal intensive care	Usually clinical diagnosis
UNCOMMON AND RARE CAUSES					
Perinatal gangrene of the buttock	First few hours to days of life	Erythema or blanching, then localized gangrene, hemorrhagic bulla	Buttock, perineal area; unilateral	Variable history, umbilical artery catheterization	Clinical diagnosis

Continued.

TABLE 16-2, cont'd Differential Diagnosis: Blisters and Pustules in the Newborn

Disease	Usual age	Skin: Morphology	Skin: Usual distribution	Clinical: Other	Diagnosis/Findings
Acropustulosis of infancy	Birth or first days or weeks	Vesicles and pustules	Hands and feet, especially medial	Severe pruritus; lesions come in crops on palms and soles	Clinical. Skin biopsy: intraepidermal pustule
Congenital self-healing histiocytosis	Usually at birth	Erythematous papules, pustules, vesicles, crusting	Generalized distribution	Check lymph nodes, liver, spleen, blood, bones	Skin biopsy: large histiocytes
Diffuse cutaneous mastocytosis	Birth, first weeks of life	Bullae, infiltrated skin, hives, dermographism	Generalized distribution, bleeding, diatheses	Wheezing, diarrhea	Skin biopsy: infiltrate of mast cells
Maternal bullous disease	At birth	Tense or flaccid bullae or erosions	Generalized distribution	Maternal history of blistering disease	Maternal history, direct immuno-fluorescence
Neonatal lupus erythematosus	Birth, first few days	Erosions, other scaly or atrophic plaques	Face, upper torso	Occasional pancytopenia; heart block	Skin biopsy: epidermal atrophy and vascular interface dermatitis; positive maternal neonatal serology (anti-SSA, SSB)
Neonatal Behçet's disease	Congenital or first few days	Mucous membrane erosions, pustules and necrotic ulcers	Oral, genital mucosa; extremities, especially periungual	Maternal history of Behçet's disease	Circulating immune complexes; elevated IgG, decreased total hemolytic complement
Chronic bullous dermatosis of childhood	One congenital case	Tense blisters, often grouped with rosettes, sausage-shaped	Generalized; may concentrate in perineum	Neonatal case: severe eye involvement, milia	Skin biopsy: subepidermal bulla direct immunofluorescence: linear IgA
Toxic epidermal necrolysis	Birth to few weeks of age	Diffuse skin erythema, tenderness, erosions	Generalized distribution	Graft-vs.-host disease *Klebsiella* sepsis, etc	Skin biopsy: full-thickness necrosis
Erosive and vesicular dermatosis	Birth	Vesicles and erosions	Generalized, over 75% of body	? infection or placental infarctions	? Clinical
Hemangiomas and vascular malformations	Birth or first few weeks	Ulcerations overlie macular erythema or obvious vascular anomaly	Ear, lip, perineum, extremities	Contiguous vascular anomaly usually evident	Clinical
Eosinophilic pustular folliculitis	Birth or later	Multiple pustules, crusted area	Scalp, hands, feet	Frequent eosinophilia	Skin biopsy: folliculitis with eosinophils
Acrodermatitis enteropathica	Weeks to months	Sharply demarcated psoriasiform plaques, sometimes vesicles and bullae	Periorificial and acral	Diarrhea, irritability, alopecia, history of hyperalimentation	Serum zinc level less than 50
Epidermolysis bullosa	Birth, rarely later	Bullae or erosions, milia nail dystrophy in dystrophic EB, occasional aplasia cutis	Anywhere, especially extremities, mucosa	Other epithelial tissues, ie,GI, genitourinary, cornea, trachea, may be affected	Skin biopsy for electron micro-scopy or immunofluorescence mapping

	Age of onset	Lesions	Distribution	Associated features	Diagnosis
Epidermolytic hyperkeratosis	Birth	Bullae, erosions, ichthyotic areas of skin	Generalized; blisters more on hands and feet	Family history may be positive	Skin biopsy: big keratohyaline granules
Incontinentia pigmenti	Birth or first weeks	Linear streaks of erythematous papules and vesicles	Generalized following Blaschko's lines	Family history may be positive; eye, CNS, and other abnormalities	Skin biopsy: eosinophilic spongiosis and dyskeratosis
Hyperimmunoglobulin E syndrome	Days to weeks	Multiple vesicles, grouped and individual	Generalized distribution	Recurrent *S. aureus* infection, eosinophilia	? clinical (IgE not high in newborn period)
Aplasia cutis congenita	Birth	One or multiple membrane-covered, depressed areas of skin or raw, ulcerated areas	Usually scalp, may be elsewhere	May be associated with epidermal nevus, placental infarctions, etc.	Clinical or skin biopsy
Ectodermal dysplasias (ED)	Congenital or early infancy	Vesicles or bullae	Depends on specific kind; acral in some; Blaschko's lines in Goltz syndrome	Sweating, limb, oral abnormalities, vary with specific kind of ED	Usually clinical diagnosis
Erythropoietic porphyria	Early infancy	Vesicles or bullae	Photodistribution	Hemolytic anemia, pink urine	High porphyrins in blood, urine
Protein C or S deficiency	Birth or first days of life	Hemorrhagic bullae and cutaneous infarctions	May be focal or generalized	Blood picture consistent with disseminated intravascular coagulation	Absent protein C or S in blood

From Frieden IJ: *Curr Probl Dermatol* 4:123, 1992.

REFERENCES

1. Ullman S: Immunofluorescence and diseases of the skin, *Acta Dermato-Venereologica* (Suppl) 140:1-31, 1988.
2. Smith JB, Tulloch JE, et al: The incidence and prevalence of dermatitis herpetiformis in Utah, *Arch Dermatol* 128:1608-1610, 1992.
3. Cuartero BG, Santamaria MJ, et al: Dermatitis herpetiformis vs. celiac disease, *An Esp Pediatr* 37:307-310, 1992.
4. Hall RP, Otley C: Immunogenetics of dermatitis herpetiformis, *Semin Dermatol* 10:240-245, 1991.
5. Ermacora E et al: Long-term follow-up of dermatitis herpetiformis in children, *J Am Acad Dermatol* 15:24-30, 1986.
6. Cunningham MJ, Zone JJ: Thyroid abnormalities in dermatitis herpetiformis: prevalence of clinical thyroid disease and thyroid autoantibodies, *Ann Intern Med* 102:194-196, 1985.
7. Aine L, Maki M, et al: Coeliac-type dental enamel defects in patients with dermatitis herpetiformis, *Acta Derm Venereol* 72:25-27, 1992.
8. Kuechle MK et al: Drug-induced linear IgA bullous dermatosis: report of six cases and review of the literature, *J Am Acad Dermatol* 30:187-192, 1994.
9. Volta U, Molinaro N, et al: Correlation between IgA antiendomysial antibodies and subtotal villous atrophy in dermatitis herpetiformis, *J Clin Gastroenterol* 14:298-301, 1992.
10. Gawkrodger DJ, Barnetson RSC: Dermatitis herpetiformis and lymphoma, *Lancet* 2:987, 1982.
11. Smith SB et al: Linear IgA bullous dermatosis v dermatitis herpetiformis: quantitative measurements of dermoepidermal alterations, *Arch Dermatol* 120:324-328, 1984.
12. Hall RP: The pathogenesis of dermatitis herpetiformis: recent advances, *J Am Acad Dermatol* 16:1129-1144, 1987.
13. Leonard JN et al: IgA anti-endomysial antibody detection in the serum of patients with dermatitis herpetiformis following gluten challenge, *Arch Dermatol Res* 277:349-351, 1985.
14. Beutner EH et al: Sensitivity and specificity of IgA-class antiendomysial antibodies for dermatitis herpetiformis and findings relevant to their pathogenic significance, *J Am Acad Dermatol* 15:464-473, 1986.
15. Chorzelski TP et al: IgA anti-endomysium antibody: a new immunological marker of dermatitis herpetiformis and coeliac disease, *Br J Dermatol* 111:395-402, 1984.
16. Accetta P et al: Anti-endomysial antibodies, *Arch Dermatol* 122:459-462, 1986.
17. Kumar V, Zane H, et al: Serologic markers of gluten-sensitive enteropathy in bullous diseases, *Arch Dermatol* 128:1474-1478, 1992.
18. Coleman MD, Rhodes LE, et al: The use of cimetidine to reduce dapsone-dependent methaemoglobinaemia in dermatitis herpetiformis patients, *Br J Clin Pharmacol* 34:244-249, 1992.
19. Waldinger TP et al: Dapsone induced peripheral neuropathy, *Arch Dermatol* 120:356-359, 1984.
20. Ahrens EM, Meckler RJ, Callen JP: Dapsone-induced peripheral neuropathy, *Int J Dermatol* 25:314-316, 1986.
21. Millikan LE, Harrell ER: Drug reactions to the sulfones, *Arch Dermatol* 102:220, 1970.
22. Johnson DA et al: Liver involvement in the sulfone syndrome, *Ann Intern Med* 146:875, 1986.
23. Kahn G: Dapsone is safe during pregnancy, *J Am Acad Dermatol* 13:838-839, 1985.
24. Garioch JJ et al: 25 years' experience of a gluten-free diet in the treatment of dermatitis herpetiformis, *Br J Dermatol* 131:541-545, 1994.
25. Ciclitira PJ et al: Evaluation of a gluten free product containing wheat gliadin in patients with coeliac disease, *Br Med J* 289:83, 1984.
26. van der Meer JB: Gluten-free diet and elemental diet in dermatitis herpetiformis, *Int J Dermatol* 29:679-692, 1990.
27. Kadunce DP, McMurry MP, et al: The effect of an elemental diet with and without gluten on disease activity in dermatitis herpetiformis, *J Invest Dermatol* 97:175-182, 1991.
28. Peoples D, Fivenson DP: Linear IgA bullous dermatosis: successful treatment with tetracycline and nicotinamide, *J Am Acad Dermatol* 26:498-499, 1992.
29. Toonstra J: Bullosis diabeticorum: report of a case with a review of the literature, *J Am Acad Dermatol* 13:799-805, 1985.
30. Bernstein JE et al: Bullous eruption of diabetes mellitus, *Arch Dermatol* 115:324-325, 1979.
31. Goodfield MJD et al: Bullosis diabeticorum, *J Am Acad Dermatol* 15:1292-1294, 1986.
32. Korman N: Pemphigus, *J Am Acad Dermatol* 18:1219-1238, 1988.
33. Ahmed AR, Mohimen A, et al: Linkage of pemphigus vulgaris antibody to the major histocompatibility complex in healthy relatives of patients, *J Exp Med* 177:419-424, 1993.
34. Lever WF: Pemphigus and pemphigoid, a review of the advances made since 1964, *J Am Acad Dermatol* 1:1-31, 1979.
35. Younus J, Ahmed AR: The relationship of pemphigus to neoplasia, *J Am Acad Dermatol* 23:498-502, 1990.
36. Becker BA, Gaspari AA: Pemphigus vulgaris and vegetans, *Dermatol Clin* 11:429-452, 1993.
37. Lamey PJ, Rees TD, et al: Oral presentation of pemphigus vulgaris and its response to systemic steroid therapy, *Oral Surg Oral Med Oral Pathol* 74:54-57, 1992.
38. Trattner A, Lurie R, et al: Esophageal involvement in pemphigus vulgaris: A clinical, histologic, and immunopathologic study, *J Am Acad Dermatol* 24:223-226, 1991.
39. Diaz LA, Sampaio SA, et al: Endemic pemphigus foliaceus (fogo selvagem). I. Clinical features and immunopathology, *J Am Acad Dermatol* 20:657-669, 1989.
40. Diaz LA, Sampaio SA, et al: Endemic pemphigus foliaceus (fogo selvagem): II. Current and historic epidemiologic studies, *J Invest Dermatol* 92:4-12, 1989.
41. Rock B, Martins CR, et al: The pathogenic effect of IgG4 autoantibodies in endemic pemphigus foliaceus (fogo selvagem), *N Engl J Med* 320:1463-1469, 1989.
42. Lombardi C, Borges PC, et al: Environmental risk factors in endemic pemphigus foliaceus (fogo selvagem). "The Cooperative Group on Fogo Selvagem Research," *J Invest Dermatol* 98:847-850, 1992.
43. Supapannachart N, Mutasim DF: The distribution of IgA pemphigus antigen in human skin and the role of IgA anti-cell surface antibodies in the induction of intraepidermal acantholysis, *Arch Dermatol* 129:605-608, 1993.
44. Beutner EH, Chorzelski TP, et al: IgA pemphigus foliaceus. Report of two cases and a review of the literature, *J Am Acad Dermatol* 20:89-97, 1989.
45. Amerian ML, Ahmed AR: Pemphigus erythematosus: presentation of four cases and review of the literature, *J Am Acad Dermatol* 10:215-222, 1984.
46. Cruz PD, Coldiron BM, Sontheimer RD: Concurrent features of cutaneous lupus erythematosus and pemphigus erythematosus following myasthenia gravis and thymoma, *J Am Acad Dermatol* 16:472-480, 1987.
47. Kuechle MK et al: Angiotensin-converting enzyme inhibitor-induced pemphigus: three cases and literature review, *Mayo Clin Proc* 69:1166, 1994.
48. Ahmed R: Pemphigus associated with D-penicillamine. In Ahmed AR, moderator: Pemphigus: current concepts, *Ann Intern Med* 92:396-405, 1980.
49. Levy RS, Fisher M, Alter JN: Penicillamine: review and cutaneous manifestations, *J Am Acad Dermatol* 8:548-558, 1983.
50. Mutasim DF, Pelc NJ, et al: Drug-induced pemphigus, *Dermatol Clin* 11:463-471, 1993.
51. Wolf R, Tamir A, et al: Drug-induced versus drug-triggered pemphigus, *Dermatologica* 182:207-210, 1991.
52. Kohn SR: Fatal penicillamine-induced pemphigus foliaceus-like dermatosis, *Arch Dermatol* 122:17, 1986.
53. Anhalt GJ, Kim SC, et al: Paraneoplastic pemphigus. An autoimmune mucocutaneous disease associated with neoplasia, *N Engl J Med* 323:1729-1735, 1990.
54. Mutasim DF, Pelc NJ, et al: Paraneoplastic pemphigus, *Dermatol Clin* 11:473-481, 1993.
55. Camisa C, Helm TN, et al: Paraneoplastic pemphigus: a report of three

cases including one long-term survivor, *J Am Acad Dermatol* 27:547-553, 1992.

56. Helm TN, Camisa C, et al: Paraneoplastic pemphigus. A distinct autoimmune vesiculobullous disorder associated with neoplasia, *Oral Surg Oral Med Oral Pathol* 75:209-213, 1993.

57. Meyers SJ, Varley GA, et al: Conjunctival involvement in paraneoplastic pemphigus, *Am J Ophthalmol* 114:621-624, 1992.

58. Tankel M, Tannenbaum S, et al: Paraneoplastic pemphigus presenting as an unusual bullous eruption, *J Am Acad Dermatol* 29:825-828, 1993.

59. Fried R, Lynfield Y, et al: Paraneoplastic pemphigus appearing as bullous pemphigoid-like eruption after palliative radiation therapy, *J Am Acad Dermatol* 29:815-817, 1993.

60. Camisa C: Paraneoplastic pemphigus is a distinct neoplasia-induced autoimmune disease, *Arch Dermatol* 129:883-886, 1993.

61. Mehregan DR, Oursler JR, et al: Paraneoplastic pemphigus: a subset of patients with pemphigus and neoplasia, *J Cutan Pathol* 20:203-210, 1993.

62. Horn TD, Anhalt GJ: Histologic features of paraneoplastic pemphigus, *Arch Dermatol* 128:1091-1095, 1992.

63. Helou J et al: Accuracy of indirect immunofluorescence testing in the diagnosis of paraneoplastic pemphigus, *J Am Acad Dermatol* 32:441-447, 1995.

64. Korman NJ, Eyre RW, et al: Demonstration of an adhering-junction molecule (plakoglobin) in the autoantigens of pemphigus foliaceus and pemphigus vulgaris, *N Engl J Med* 321:631-635, 1989.

65. Sams WM, Gammon WR: Mechanism of lesion production in pemphigus and pemphigoid, *J Am Acad Dermatol* 6:431-449, 1982.

66. David M et al: The usefulness of immunofluorescent tests in pemphigus patients in clinical remission, *Brit J Derm* 120:391-395, 1989.

67. Lever WF, Schaumburg-Lever G: Treatment of pemphigus vulgaris, *Arch Dermatol* 120:44-47, 1984.

68. Ratnam KV, Phay KL, et al: Pemphigus therapy with oral prednisolone regimens. A 5-year study, *Int J Dermatol* 29:363-367, 1990.

69. Ahmed AR, Hombal S: Use of cyclophosphamide in azathioprine failures in pemphigus, *J Am Acad Dermatol* 17:437-442, 1987.

70. Bystryn JC: Adjuvant therapy of pemphigus, *Arch Dermatol* 120:941-951, 1984.

71. Aberer W et al: Azathioprine in the treatment of pemphigus vulgaris, *J Am Acad Dermatol* 16:527-533, 1987.

72. Basset N et al: Dapsone as initial treatment in superficial pemphigus, *Arch Dermatol* 123:783-785, 1987.

73. Lapidoth M et al: The efficacy of combined treatment with prednisone and cyclosporine in patients with pemphigus: preliminary study, *J Am Acad Dermatol* 30:752-757, 1994.

74. Thomas I: Gold therapy and its indications in dermatology, *J Am Acad Dermatol* 16:845-854, 1987.

75. Poulin Y, Perry HO, Muller SA: Pemphigus vulgaris: results of treatment with gold as a steroid-sparing agent in a series of thirteen patients, *J Am Acad Dermatol* 11:851-857, 1984.

76. Bystryn JC: Plasmapheresis therapy of pemphigus, *Arch Dermatol* 124:1702-1704, 1988.

77. Gollnick HP, Owsianowski M, et al: Unresponsive severe generalized pemphigus vulgaris successfully controlled by extracorporeal photopheresis, *J Am Acad Dermatol* 28:122-124, 1993.

78. Piamphongsant T, Ophaswongse S: Treatment of pemphigus, *Int J Dermatol* 30:139-146, 1991.

79. Hymes SR, Jordon RE: Pemphigus foliaceus. Use of antimalarial agents as adjuvant therapy, *Arch Derm* 128:1462-1464, 1992.

80. Pasricha JS, Das SS: Curative effect of dexamethasone-cyclophosphamide pulse therapy for the treatment of pemphigus vulgaris, *Int J Dermatol* 31:875-877, 1992.

81. Appelhans M, Bonsmann G, et al: Dexamethasone-cyclophosphamide pulse therapy in bullous autoimmune dermatoses, *Hautarzt* 44:143-147, 1993.

82. Pandya AG, Sontheimer RD: Treatment of pemphigus vulgaris with pulse intravenous cyclophosphamide, *Arch Dermatol* 128:1626-1630, 1992.

83. Chaffins ML, Collison D, et al: Treatment of pemphigus and linear IgA dermatosis with nicotinamide and tetracycline: a review of 13 cases, *J Am Acad Dermatol* 28:998-1000, 1993.

84. Ratnam KV, Pang BK: Pemphigus in remission: value of negative direct immunofluorescence in management, *J Am Acad Dermatol* 30:547-550, 1994.

85. Taylor G, Venning V, et al: Bullous pemphigoid and autoimmunity, *J Am Acad Dermatol* 29:181-184, 1993.

86. Venning VA, Wojnarowska F: The association of bullous pemphigoid and malignant disease: a case control study, *Br J Dermatol* 123:439-445, 1990.

87. Ortiz LJ, Vazquez M, et al: Bullous pemphigoid and malignancy, *Bol Asoc Med P R* 82:458-459, 1990.

88. Lindelof B, Islam N, et al: Pemphigoid and cancer, *Arch Dermatol* 126:66-68, 1990.

89. Smith EP, Taylor TB, et al: Antigen identification in drug-induced bullous pemphigoid, *J Am Acad Dermatol* 29:879-882, 1993.

90. Bingham EA et al: Prolonged pruritus and bullous pemphigoid, *Clin Exp Dermatol* 9:564, 1984.

91. Venning VA, Wojnarowska F: Lack of predictive factors for the clinical course of bullous pemphigoid, *J Am Acad Dermatol* 26:585-589, 1992.

92. Macfarlane AW, Verbov JL: Trauma-induced bullous pemphigoid, *Clin Exp Dermatol* 14:245-249, 1989.

93. Liu HH et al: Clinical variants of pemphigoid, *Int J Dermatol* 25:17-27, 1986.

94. Anstey A, Venning V, et al: Determination of the optimum site for diagnostic biopsy for direct immunofluorescence in bullous pemphigoid, *Clin Exp Dermatol* 15:438-441, 1990.

95. Smoller BR, Woodley DT: Differences in direct immunofluorescence staining patterns in epidermolysis bullosa acquisita and bullous pemphigoid, *J Am Acad Dermatol* 27:674-678, 1992.

96. Gammon WR, Kowalewski C, et al: Direct immunofluorescence studies of sodium chloride–separated skin in the differential diagnosis of bullous pemphigoid and epidermolysis bullosa acquisita, *J Am Acad Dermatol* 22:664-670, 1990.

97. Domloge-Hultsch N, Bisalbutra P, et al: Direct immunofluorescence microscopy of 1 mol/L sodium chloride–treated patient skin, *J Am Acad Dermatol* 24:946-951, 1991.

98. Person JR, Rogers RS III: Bullous and cicatricial pemphigoid: clinical, histopathologic, and immunopathologic correlations, *Mayo Clin Proc* 52:54-66, 1977.

99. Ahmed AR, Maize JC, Provost TT: Bullous pemphigoid: clinical and immunologic follow-up after successful therapy, *Arch Dermatol* 113:1043-1046, 1977.

100. Paquet P, Richelle M, et al: Bullous pemphigoid treated by topical corticosteroids, *Acta Derm Venereol* 71:534-535, 1991.

101. Westerhof W: Treatment of bullous pemphigoid with topical clobetasol propionate, *J Am Acad Dermatol* 20:458-461, 1989.

102. Thomas I, Khorenian S, et al: Treatment of generalized bullous pemphigoid with oral tetracycline, *J Am Acad Dermatol* 28:74-77, 1993.

103. Berk MA, Lorincz AL: The treatment of bullous pemphigoid with tetracycline and niacinamide, *Arch Dermatol* 122:670-674, 1986.

104. Thornfeldt CR, Menkes AW: Bullous pemphigoid controlled by tetracycline, *J Am Acad Dermatol* 16:305-310, 1987.

105. Person JR, Rogers RS: Bullous pemphigoid responding to sulfapyridine and the sulfones, *Arch Dermatol* 113:610-615, 1977.

106. Venning VA, Millard PR, et al: Dapsone as first line therapy for bullous pemphigoid, *Br J Dermatol* 120:83-92, 1989.

107. Guillaume JC, Vaillant L, et al: Controlled trial of azathioprine and plasma exchange in addition to prednisolone in the treatment of bullous pemphigoid, *Arch Dermatol* 129:49-53, 1993.

108. Chosidow O, Etienne SD, et al: Pharmacokinetics of prednisone and prednisolone in bullous pemphigoid patients, *Int J Clin Pharmacol Ther Toxicol* 29:376-380, 1991.

109. Jeffes E, Ahmed AR: Adjuvant therapy of bullous pemphigoid with dapsone, *Clin Exp Dermatol* 14:132-136, 1989.

110. Dahl MC, Cook LJ: Lesions induced by trauma in pemphigoid, *Br J Dermatol* 101:469-473, 1979.

111. Borradori L, Prost C, et al: Localized pretibial pemphigoid and pemphigoid nodularis, *J Am Acad Dermatol* 27:863-867, 1992.

112. Leenutaphong V, von Kries R, et al: Localized cicatricial pemphigoid (Brunsting-Perry): electron microscopic study, *J Am Acad Dermatol* 21:1089-1093, 1989.

113. Descamps V, Flageul B, et al: Dyshidrosiform pemphigoid: report of three cases, *J Am Acad Dermatol* 26:651-652, 1992.

114. Chan LS, Dorman MA, et al: Pemphigoid vegetans represents a bullous pemphigoid variant. Patient's IgG autoantibodies identify the major bullous pemphigoid antigen, *J Am Acad Dermatol* 28:331-335, 1993.

115. Domloge-Hultsch N, Utecht L, et al: Autoantibodies from patients with localized and generalized bullous pemphigoid immunoprecipitate the same 230-kd keratinocyte antigen, *Arch Dermatol* 126:1337-1341, 1990.

116. Weigand DA, Clements MK: Direct immunofluorescence in bullous pemphigoid: effects of extent and location of lesions, *J Am Acad Dermatol* 20:437-440, 1989.

117. Ahmed AR, Kurgis BS, et al: Cicatricial pemphigoid, *J Am Acad Dermatol* 24:987-1001, 1991.

118. Mutasim DF, Pelc NJ, et al: Cicatricial pemphigoid, *Dermatol Clin* 11:499-510, 1993.

119. Ahmed AR, Hombal SM: Cicatricial pemphigoid, *Int J Dermatol* 25:90-96, 1986.

120. Chan LS, Yancey KB, et al: Immune-mediated subepithelial blistering diseases of mucous membranes. Pure ocular cicatricial pemphigoid is a unique clinical and immunopathological entity distinct from bullous pemphigoid and other subsets identified by antigenic specificity of autoantibodies, *Arch Dermatol* 129:448-455, 1993.

121. Chan LS, Soong HK, et al: Ocular cicatricial pemphigoid occurring as a sequela of Stevens-Johnson syndrome, *JAMA* 266:1543-1546, 1991.

122. Neumann R, Tauber J, et al: Remission and recurrence after withdrawal of therapy for ocular cicatricial pemphigoid, *Ophthalmology* 98:858-862, 1991.

123. Sarret Y, Hall R, et al: Salt-split human skin substrate for the immunofluorescent screening of serum from patients with cicatricial pemphigoid and a new method of immunoprecipitation with IgA antibodies, *J Am Acad Dermatol* 24:952-958, 1991.

124. Tauber J, Sainz de la Maza M, et al: Systemic chemotherapy for ocular cicatricial pemphigoid, *Cornea* 10:185-195, 1991.

125. Fern AI, Jay JL, et al: Dapsone therapy for the acute inflammatory phase of ocular pemphigoid, *Br J Ophthalmol* 76:332-335, 1992.

126. Rogers RS III, Seehafer JR, Perry HO: Treatment of cicatricial (benign mucous membrane) pemphigoid with dapsone, *J Am Acad Dermatol* 6:215-223, 1982.

127. Saad RW, Domloge-Hultsch N, et al: Childhood localized vulvar pemphigoid is a true variant of bullous pemphigoid, *Arch Dermatol* 128:807-810, 1992.

128. Guenther LC, Shum D: Localized childhood vulvar pemphigoid, *J Am Acad Dermatol* 22:762-764, 1990.

129. Levine V, Sanchez M, et al: Localized vulvar pemphigoid in a child misdiagnosed as sexual abuse, *Arch Dermatol* 128:804-806, 1992.

130. Marren P, Wojnarowska F, et al: Vulvar involvement in autoimmune bullous diseases, *J Reprod Med* 38:101-107, 1993.

131. Shornick JK: Herpes gestationis, *J Am Acad Dermatol* 17:539-556, 1987.

132. Shornick JK, Artlett CM, et al: Complement polymorphism in herpes gestationis: association with C4 null allele, *J Am Acad Dermatol* 29:545-549, 1993.

133. Shornick JK, Black MM: Fetal risks in herpes gestationis, *J Am Acad Dermatol* 26:63-68, 1992.

134. Shornick JK: Herpes gestationis, *Dermatol Clin* 11:527-533, 1993.

135. Shornick JK et al: Herpes gestationis: clinical and histologic features of twenty-eight cases, *J Am Acad Dermatol* 8:214-224, 1983.

136. Marsden RA et al: A study of benign chronic bullous dermatosis of childhood and comparison with dermatitis herpetiformis and bullous pemphigoid occurring in childhood, *Clin Exp Dermatol* 5:159, 1980.

137. Roberts LJ, Sontheimer RD: Chronic bullous dermatosis of childhood: immunopathologic studies, *Pediatr Dermatol* 4:6-10, 1987.

138. Sweren RJ, Burnett JW: Benign chronic bullous dermatosis of childhood: a review, *Cutis* 29:350, 1982.

139. Wojnarowska F et al: Chronic bullous disease of childhood, childhood cicatricial pemphigoid, and linear IgA disease of adults, *J Am Acad Dermatol* 19:792-805, 1988.

140. Arpey CJ, Elewski BE, et al: Childhood epidermolysis bullosa acquisita. Report of three cases and review of literature, *J Am Acad Dermatol* 24:706-714, 1991.

141. Woodley DT: Epidermolysis bullosa acquisita, *Progr Dermatol* 22:1-13, 1988.

142. Karpati S, Stolz W, et al: In situ localization of IgG in epidermolysis bullosa acquisita by immunogold technique, *J Am Acad Dermatol* 26:726-730, 1992.

143. Gammon WR: Epidermolysis bullosa acquisita: a disease of autoimmunity to type VII collagen, *J Autoimmun* 4:59-71, 1991.

144. Boh E, Roberts LJ, et al: Epidermolysis bullosa acquisita preceding the development of systemic lupus erythematosus, *J Am Acad Dermatol* 22:587-593, 1990.

145. Gammon WR et al: Epidermolysis bullosa acquisita—a pemphigoid-like disease, *J Am Acad Dermatol* 11:820-832, 1984.

146. Mooney E, Falk RJ, et al: Studies on complement deposits in epidermolysis bullosa acquisita and bullous pemphigoid, *Arch Dermatol* 128:58-60, 1992.

147. Mallett RB, Holden CA: Clearing of epidermolysis bullosa acquisita with cyclosporine, *J Am Acad Dermatol* 24:1034-1035, 1991.

148. Merle C, Blanc D, et al: Intractable epidermolysis bullosa acquisita: efficacy of cyclosporin A, *Dermatologica* 181:44-47, 1990.

149. Gupta AK, Ellis CN, et al: Oral cyclosporine in the treatment of inflammatory and noninflammatory dermatoses. A clinical and immunopathologic analysis, *Arch Dermatol* 126:339-350, 1990.

150. Meier F, Sonnichsen K, et al: Epidermolysis bullosa acquisita: efficacy of high-dose intravenous immunoglobulins, *J Am Acad Dermatol* 29:334-337, 1993.

151. Richard G, Linse R, et al: Genetics of Hailey-Hailey familial chronic benign pemphigus, *Dermatol Monatsschr* 176:673-681, 1990.

152. Peppiatt T, Keefe M, et al: Hailey-Hailey disease—exacerbation by herpes simplex virus and patch tests, *Clin Exp Dermatol* 17:201-202, 1992.

153. Burge SM: Hailey-Hailey disease: the clinical features, response to treatment and prognosis, *Br J Dermatol* 126:275-282, 1992.

154. Burge SM, Millard PR, et al: Hailey-Hailey disease: a widespread abnormality of cell adhesion, *Br J Dermatol* 124:329-332, 1991.

155. Richard G, Linse R, et al: Hailey-Hailey disease. Early detection of heterozygotes by an ultraviolet provocation tests—clinical relevance of the method, *Hautarzt* 44:376-379, 1993.

156. Langenberg A, Berger TG, et al: Genital benign chronic pemphigus (Hailey-Hailey disease) presenting as condylomas, *J Am Acad Dermatol* 26:951-955, 1992.

157. Jitsukawa K, Ring J, et al: Topical cyclosporine in chronic benign familial pemphigus (Hailey-Hailey disease), *J Am Acad Dermatol* 27:625-626, 1992.

158. Kartamaa M, Reitamo S: Familial benign chronic pemphigus (Hailey-Hailey disease). Treatment with carbon dioxide laser vaporization, *Arch Dermatol* 128:646-648, 1992.

159. McElroy JA, Mehregan DA, et al: Carbon dioxide laser vaporization of recalcitrant symptomatic plaques of Hailey-Hailey disease and Darier's disease, *J Am Acad Dermatol* 23:893-897, 1990.

160. Menz P, Jackson IT, Connolly S: Surgical control of Hailey-Hailey disease, *Br J Plast Surg* 40:557-561, 1987.

161. Kirtschig G, Gieler U, et al: Treatment of Hailey-Hailey disease by dermabrasion, *J Am Acad Dermatol* 28:784-786, 1993.

162. Uitto J, Christiano AM: Inherited epidermolysis bullosa. Clinical features, molecular genetics, and pathoetiologic mechanisms, *Dermatol Clin* 11:549-563, 1993.

CHAPTER SEVENTEEN

Connective Tissue Diseases

Connective tissue diseases (lupus, dermatomyositis, scleroderma, overlap syndromes) are a group of multisystem illnesses of unknown etiology. They have no typical pattern of onset, duration, or organ involvement. This variability makes classification and diagnosis difficult; therefore a list of clinical diagnostic criteria has been established for each entity and is tabulated in the text.

Connective tissue diseases can be more accurately described as autoimmune diseases. Many serum antibodies directed at cellular components (autoantibodies) have been found in each disease and are probably responsible for the clinical manifestations.

Figure 17-1

Clinical and laboratory characteristics of systemic lupus erythematosus (SLE). *(Modified from American Rheumatism Association [ARA] criteria. Copyright 1979, CIBA Pharmaceutical Company, Division of Ciba-Geigy Corporation. Reprinted with permission from* Clinical Symposia, *illustrated by Frank H. Netter, M.D. All rights reserved.)*

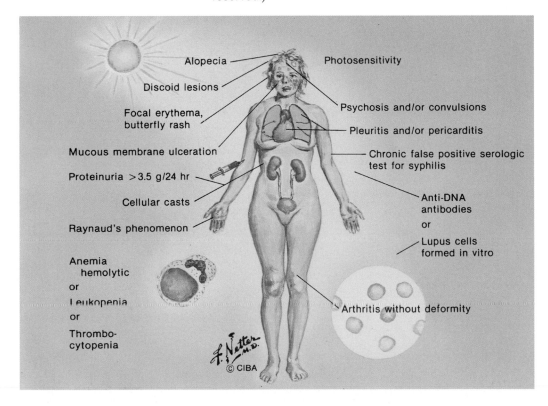

Diagnosis

The diagnosis of connective tissue disease is made by the clinical picture. Antibodies to cell components (typically nuclear antigens) are present in these multisystem disorders. Detecting and defining them helps support the clinical diagnosis and provides information about subsets of disease and prognosis. A large number of antibodies are reported in the literature. The problem is knowing which tests to order and how to interpret them. An approach to the diagnosis of connective tissue diseases is shown in the box on pp. 534 to 535.

Antinuclear antibody (ANA) testing

ANAs are detected by the indirect immunofluorescence test. It is performed by applying test serum to a tissue section (mouse liver or human epithelial cells [HEp-2]). Antibodies to nuclear antigens attach to the various components of the nucleus. Fluorescein-labeled antihuman immunoglobulins are applied to the preparation and react with ANAs that have attached to the nucleus. The preparation is visualized with a fluorescent microscope. Diverse patterns of nuclear fluorescence (homogeneous, peripheral, speckled, or nucleolar) reflect the binding of antibodies to different nuclear components. Nuclear staining patterns were once used as criteria for subsetting,[1] but, with the availability of direct measurements for specific autoantibodies, pattern identification has become less important. The test requires interpretation by visual inspection and consequently lacks a high degree of specificity.

ANA screening. ANA is the first test to order when collagen vascular disease is suspected (Table 17-1). The routine test method used is indirect immunofluorescence on mouse liver substrate. If results of this test are negative, ANA on HEp-2 (human epithelial cell tissue substrate) should be ordered; many ANA-negative patients react with HEp-2 substrate. Many laboratories use HEp-2 routinely.

ANA patterns and titers. If ANA is positive, one of the four patterns (homogeneous, peripheral, speckled, nucleolar) is identified and reported, and the serum is titered. A number of specific antibodies can cause each pattern. The ANA test determines that ANAs of a certain group are present, but it does not identify them.

Specific diagnostic antibody tests. Specific antibody tests should be ordered. The clinical presentation and ANA pattern help to determine which test to order (Tables 17-2 and 17-3). Some laboratories offer tests for groups of antigens (i.e., ANA profiles.)

TABLE 17-1 ANA-Screening Test

ANA (on HEp-2 cells)	Frequency of ANA positivity (%)
Systemic lupus erythematosus	95-100
Drug-induced lupus erythematosus	100
Scleroderma	60-95
Sjögren's syndrome	80
Polymyositis-dermatomyositis	49-74
Rheumatoid arthritis	40-60
Mixed connective tissue disease	100
Normals	<4

Modified from Harmon CE: *Med Clin North Am* 69:547-563, 1985.

TABLE 17-2 Autoantibody Tests for Connective Tissue Diseases

Antibody	Clinical significance
Antinuclear antibodies	Screening for SLE* and PSS
Centromere antibodies	Marker for CREST
nDNA antibodies	Marker for SLE
DNP antibodies	Marker for SLE
Histone antibodies	To exclude drug-induced LE
ENA: Sm antibodies	Marker for SLE
RNP antibodies	SLE, MCTD, scleroderma
SS-A (Ro)/SS-B (La) antibodies	SLE, Sjögren's syndrome, SCLE, and others
Scl-70 antibodies	Marker for scleroderma
Jo-1 antibodies	Marker for polymyositis
PCNA	SLE with high incidence of proliferative glomerulonephritis
Ku (Ki) antibodies	Polymyositis/scleroderma overlap, SLE
Phospholipid antibodies (lupus anticoagulant)	Marker for SLE subset with thrombosis: frequent aborters

Modified from *Handbook: clinical relevance of tests*, Buffalo, NY, 1993, IMMCO Diagnostics.
*SLE, systemic lupus erythematosus; PSS, progressive systemic sclerosis; DNP, deoxyribonuclear protein; LE, lupus erythematosus; ENA, extractable nuclear antigens; MCTD, mixed connective tissue disease; SCLE, subacute cutaneous lupus erythematosus; PCNA, proliferating cell nuclear antigen.

TABLE 17-3 Diagnostic Significance of Immunologic Findings in Serum and Skin Biopsies in Connective Tissue Diseases

Disease	Biopsy findings: direct immunofluorescence	Serum findings	Relevance
Systemic LE	LE* band (granular immune deposits, IgG, and/or IgM) IgA, C3 at DEJ in lesional and/or normal skin: (over 90% in sun-exposed skin)	ANA elevated titers (about 95%-99%); nDNA antibodies about 50%-75%; DNP antibodies <50%: Sm antibodies in about 20%; RNP antibodies in about 25%-30%: SS-A antibodies in about 30%-40%: SS-B antibodies in about 10%-15%; phospholipid antibodies in about 30%-50%: PCNA antibodies in about 2%-10%: Ku (Ki) antibodies in about 10%	DIF, ANA, and ENA usually diagnostic; nDNA and Sm antibodies diagnostic markers
Discoid LE	LE band, mostly IgG and C in lesion ONLY	Essentially negative; ANA titers usually in normal range	LE band highly characteristic
Subacute cutaneous LE	LE band in lesion	ANA positive in 70%; SS-A (Ro) antibodies positive in more than 60%	DIF and anti-SS-A (Ro) highly characteristic
Neonatal LE	LE band in lesion (about 50%)	ANA positive in 30%; antibodies to SS-A (Ro) in 100%; antibodies to SS-B (La) in about 60%	DIF and anti-SS-A (Ro) highly characteristic
Drug-induced LE	LE band in lesion (rare)	ANA positive in more than 90%; histone positive about 90%; other antibodies to nDNA and ENA negative	DIF and histone antibodies in absence of other nuclear antibodies highly characteristic
Mixed connective tissue disease	Nuclear IgG or LE band in normal and/or lesional epidermis	Speckled ANA antibodies in more than 95% and RNP antibodies in more than 90%	Serology and/or DIF of nuclei diagnostic for MCTD, SLE, or PSS
Sjögren's syndrome	Negative	ANA positive in about 55%; antibodies to SS-A (Ro) in 43%-88%; SS-B (La) in 14%-60%; RF positive	Positive serum results support diagnosis
Progressive systemic sclerosis (scleroderma)	Nucleolar IgG in epidermis in few cases; most negative	ANA (about 85%) speckled or nucleolar; centromere antibody in CREST (70% to 90%); Scl-70 antibodies in diffuse sclerosis (45%) and in acrosclerosis (15% to 20%)	DIF limited value; centromere antibodies diagnostic marker in CREST; Scl-70 antibodies diagnostic marker in scleroderma
Polymyositis/dermatomyositis	Negative	ANA usually positive (more than 80%); Jo-1 antibodies in 30% PM, 10% DM; SS-A (Ro) antibodies in 55% PM/scleroderma overlap; Ku (Ki) antibodies in 10% PM/scleroderma overlap	Limited value, but positive serum results support diagnosis
Rheumatoid arthritis	Negative	ANA usually negative or low titer; RF positive in about 90%; RANA positive in about 70% to 90% and 95% of RF-negative cases	Positive serum results support diagnosis

Modified from *Handbook: clinical relevance of tests*, Buffalo, NY, 1993, IMMCO Diagnostics.
*LE, lupus erythematosus; DEJ, dermal-epidermal junction; DNP, deoxyribonuclear protein; PCNA, proliferating cell nuclear antigen; DIF, direct immunofluorescence; ENA, extractable nuclear antigen; MCTD, mixed connective tissue disease; SLE, systemic lupus erythematosus; PSS, progressive systemic sclerosis; RF, rheumatoid factor; PM, polymyositis; DM, dermatomyositis; RANA, antibodies to rheumatoid arthritis associated nuclear antigen.

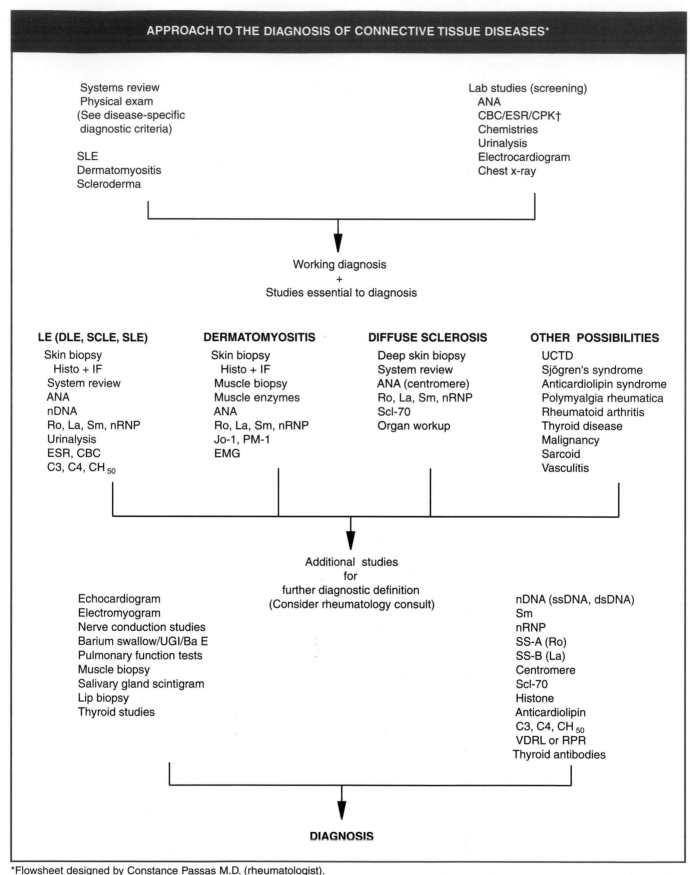

APPROACH TO THE DIAGNOSIS OF CONNECTIVE TISSUE DISEASES*

Systems review
Physical exam
(See disease-specific
  diagnostic criteria)

SLE
Dermatomyositis
Scleroderma

Lab studies (screening)
ANA
CBC/ESR/CPK†
Chemistries
Urinalysis
Electrocardiogram
Chest x-ray

Working diagnosis
+
Studies essential to diagnosis

LE (DLE, SCLE, SLE)
Skin biopsy
  Histo + IF
System review
ANA
nDNA
Ro, La, Sm, nRNP
Urinalysis
ESR, CBC
C3, C4, CH $_{50}$

DERMATOMYOSITIS
Skin biopsy
  Histo + IF
Muscle biopsy
Muscle enzymes
ANA
Ro, La, Sm, nRNP
Jo-1, PM-1
EMG

DIFFUSE SCLEROSIS
Deep skin biopsy
System review
ANA (centromere)
Ro, La, Sm, nRNP
Scl-70
Organ workup

OTHER POSSIBILITIES
UCTD
Sjögren's syndrome
Anticardiolipin syndrome
Polymyalgia rheumatica
Rheumatoid arthritis
Thyroid disease
Malignancy
Sarcoid
Vasculitis

Additional studies
for
further diagnostic definition
(Consider rheumatology consult)

Echocardiogram
Electromyogram
Nerve conduction studies
Barium swallow/UGI/Ba E
Pulmonary function tests
Muscle biopsy
Salivary gland scintigram
Lip biopsy
Thyroid studies

nDNA (ssDNA, dsDNA)
Sm
nRNP
SS-A (Ro)
SS-B (La)
Centromere
Scl-70
Histone
Anticardiolipin
C3, C4, CH $_{50}$
VDRL or RPR
Thyroid antibodies

DIAGNOSIS

*Flowsheet designed by Constance Passas M.D. (rheumatologist).
†CBC, complete blood count; ESR, erythrocyte sedimentation rate; CPK, creatine phosphokinase; IF, immunofluorescence; UCTD, undifferentiated connective tissue disease (formerly mixed CTD); EMG, electromyogram; ENA, extractable nuclear antigens; SLE, systemic lupus erythematosus; PSS, progressive systemic sclerosis; SCLE, subacute cutaneous lupus erythematosus; DLE, discoid lupus erythematosus.

ANA TEST +

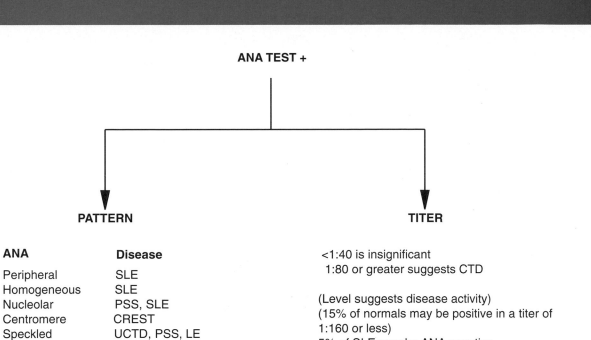

PATTERN

ANA	Disease
Peripheral	SLE
Homogeneous	SLE
Nucleolar	PSS, SLE
Centromere	CREST
Speckled	UCTD, PSS, LE

(patterns indicate disease trends but are not specific)

TITER

<1:40 is insignificant
1:80 or greater suggests CTD

(Level suggests disease activity)
(15% of normals may be positive in a titer of 1:160 or less)
5% of SLE may be ANA negative

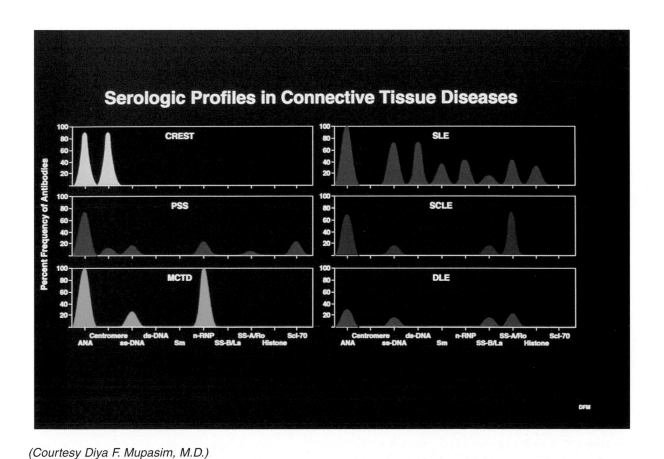

(Courtesy Diya F. Mupasim, M.D.)

Lupus Erythematosus

CLINICAL CLASSIFICATION

Lupus erythematosus (LE) is a multisystem disease of unknown origin characterized by the production of numerous diverse types of autoantibodies that, through immune mechanisms in various tissues, cause several combinations of clinical signs, symptoms (Table 17-4), and laboratory abnormalities (Table 17-5).

The prevalence of LE in North America and northern Europe is about 40 per 100,000 population. There appears to be a higher incidence in black Americans and in Hispanics. Over 80% of cases occur in women during childbearing years.

An attempt to establish criteria for diagnosis resulted in the development by the American Rheumatism Association[2] of a list of 11 clinical and immunologic parameters (Table 17-6). The presence of four or more of the 11 parameters, serially or simultaneously, is believed to be compatible with the diagnosis of LE. Those criteria in a modified form are illustrated in Figure 17-1, p. 531.

Attempts have been made to group patients into subsets to define more homogeneous groups with a predictable course or response to treatment. Recently, subsets of LE have been defined by cutaneous manifestations present in some form in most patients with lupus.[3] The classification proposed in Table 17-7 divides cutaneous LE into three types on the basis of the clinical appearance of the skin lesion: chronic cutaneous LE (scarring, discoid LE [DLE]), subacute cutaneous LE (SCLE), and acute cutaneous LE (ALE). An overview of the lupus syndromes appears in Figure 17-2.

TABLE 17-4 Cumulative Clinical Features in 150 Patients with SLE

Manifestation	Percent
Cutaneous	88
Malar rash	61
Alopecia	45
Photosensitivity	45
Mucosal ulcers	23
Discoid rash	15
Nodules	12
Musculoskeletal	83
Arthritis	76
Ischemic necrosis	24
Myositis	5
Serositis	63
Pleurisy	57
Pericarditis	23
Peritonitis	8
Neuropsychiatric	83
Central nervous system	39
Peripheral neuropathy	21
Organic psychosis	16
Seizures	13
Raynaud's phenomenon	44
Vasculitis	43
Cutaneous	27
Mesenteric	13
Digital ulcers	9
Leg ulcers	6
Nephritis	31
Nephrotic syndrome	13
Chronic renal failure	3
Cardiopulmonary	5

From Hochberg MC et al: *Medicine* 64:285-295, 1985.

TABLE 17-5 Cumulative Laboratory Features in 150 Patients with SLE

Manifestation	Percent
Hematologic	
Anemia	57
Leukopenia	41
Thrombocytopenia	30
Direct Coombs' positive	27
Immunologic	
Hypocomplementemia	59
Rheumatoid factor	34
Hyperglobulinemia	30
Chronic BFP-STS*	26
Antinuclear antibodies	94
Anti-ssDNA	89
LE cells	71
Anti-nRNP	34
Anti-Sm	17
Anti-nDNA	28
Anti-Ro (SSA)	32
Anti-La (SSB)	12

From Hochberg MC et al: *Medicine* 64:285-295, 1985.
*Biologic false-positive test for syphilis.

TABLE 17-6 The 1982 Revised Criteria for Classification of Systemic Lupus Erythematosus*

Criterion	Definition
1. Malar rash	Fixed erythema, flat or raised, over the malar eminences, tending to spare the nasolabial folds
2. Discoid rash	Erythematous raised patches with adherent keratotic scaling and follicular plugging; atrophic scarring may occur in older lesions
3. Photosensitivity	Skin rash as a result of unusual reaction to sunlight, by patient history or physician observation
4. Oral ulcers	Oral or nasopharyngeal ulceration, usually painless, observed by a physician
5. Arthritis	Nonerosive arthritis involving two or more peripheral joints, characterized by tenderness, swelling, or effusion
6. Serositis	Pleuritis: convincing history of pleuritic pain or rub heard by a physician or evidence of pleural effusion OR Pericarditis: documented by ECG or rub or evidence of pericardial effusion
7. Renal disorder	Persistent proteinuria greater than 0.5 gm per day or greater than 3+ if quantification not performed OR Cellular casts: may be red cell, hemoglobin, granular, tubular, or mixed
8. Neurological disorder	Seizures: in the absence of offending drugs or known metabolic derangements (e.g., uremia, ketoacidosis, or electrolyte imbalance) OR Psychosis: in the absence of offending drugs or known metabolic derangements (e.g., uremia, ketoacidosis, or electrolyte imbalance)
9. Hematologic disorder	Hemolytic anemia: with reticulocytosis OR Leukopenia: less than 4000/mm^3 total on two or more occasions OR Lymphopenia: less than 1500/mm^3 on two or more occasions OR Thrombocytopenia: less than 100,000/mm^3 in the absence of offending drugs
10. Immunologic disorder	Positive LE cell preparation OR Anti-DNA: antibody to native DNA in abnormal titer OR Anti-Sm: presence of antibody to Sm nuclear antigen OR False-positive serologic test for syphilis known to be positive for at least 6 months and confirmed by *Treponema pallidum* immobilization or fluorescent treponemal antibody absorption test
11. Antinuclear antibody	An abnormal titer of antinuclear antibody by immunofluorescence or an equivalent assay at any time and in the absence of drugs known to be associated with "drug-induced lupus" syndrome

From Tan EM et al: *Arthritis Rheum* 25:1271, 1982.
*The proposed classification is based on 11 criteria. For the purpose of identifying patients in clinical studies, a person shall be said to have systemic lupus erythematosus if any 4 or more of the 11 criteria are present, serially or simultaneously, during any interval of observation.

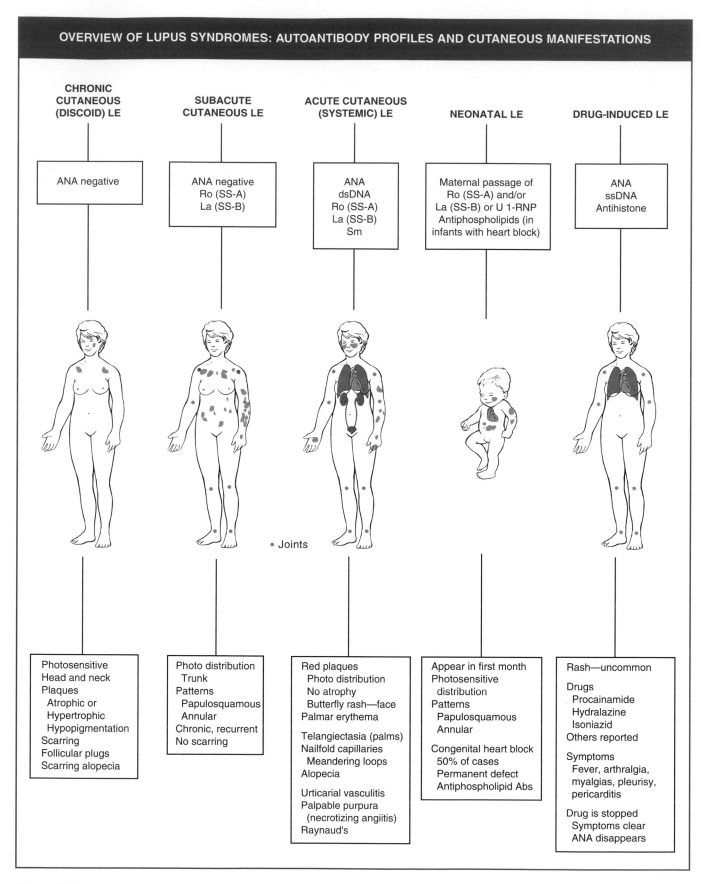

Figure 17-2

TABLE 17-7 Classification of Cutaneous Lupus Erythematosus			
	Clinical forms	**Clinical and laboratory features**	**Histologic features**
DLE, 15%-20%*	Localized Generalized (lesions above and below the neck) Hypertrophic	Usually localized, chronic, scarring lesions of head or neck region or both lasting months to years Usually no extracutaneous disease (5% of patients develop SLE) Antinuclear antibodies occasionally present in low titer; anticytoplasmic antibodies not present Anti-dsDNA† antibodies rarely present Subepidermal immunoglobulin deposits commonly found in lesions (75%), but rarely present in uninvolved skin Simultaneous occurrence of severe systemic lupus erythematosus with nephritis is rare	Hydropic degeneration of the epidermal basal cell layer with focal epidermal atrophy Heavy mononuclear cell infiltrate in upper dermis, periappendageal and perivascular regions, extending into the deep dermis
SCLE, 10%-15%*	Papulosquamous (psoriasiform), 8% Annular-polycyclic, 5%*	Usually widespread, nonscarring lesions with associated scaling, depigmentation, and telangiectasias on face, neck, upper and extensor arms (photosensitive distribution) lasting weeks to months; lesions often exacerbated by exposure to sun Usually associated with extracutaneous disease, but severe renal or central nervous system disease uncommon Antinuclear and anticytoplasmic antibodies frequently present (60% of patients) Anti-dsDNA antibodies present in low serum concentrations in 30% of patients; hypocomplementemia rare HLA-A1, B8, and DR3 significantly increased Subepidermal immunoglobulin deposits present in only 50% of lesions and 30% of uninvolved skin	Marked hydropic changes along epidermal basal cell layer Moderate mononuclear cell infiltrate in superficial dermis only Pilosebaceous atrophy, hyperkeratosis; direct IF staining reveals discrete, speckled IgG deposits in the basal cell cytoplasm associated with Ro/SSA antibodies
Acute cutaneous LE, 30%-50%*	Localized, indurated erythematous lesions (malar areas of face—butterfly rash) Widespread indurated erythema (face, scalp, neck, upper chest, shoulders, extensor arms, backs of hands)	Transient (hours to days) Multisystem disease usually present; renal disease common Antinuclear antibodies usually present Anti-dsDNA antibodies present in 60%-80% of patients, often in high concentration; hypocomplementemia common Subepidermal immunoglobulin deposits commonly found in lesional (>95%) and exposed nonlesional (75%) skin	Hydropic changes along epidermal basal layer Sparse mononuclear cell infiltrate and upper dermal edema

Modified from Gilliam JN, Sontheimer RD: *J Am Acad Dermatol* 4:471, 1981; and Valesk JE et al: *J Am Acad Dermatol* 27:194, 1992.
*Estimated percentage incidence in systemic lupus erythematosus.
†dsDNA, double-stranded DNA.

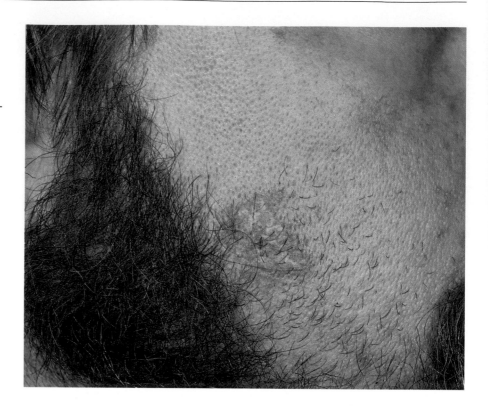

Figure 17-3
Chronic cutaneous LE (discoid LE). An early lesion. Well-defined, elevated, flat-topped plaques with adherent scale.

CHRONIC CUTANEOUS LE (DISCOID LE)

Patients with DLE have a low incidence of systemic disease.[4] The disease is more common in females, and it has a peak incidence in the fourth decade. Less than 2% of patients with DLE develop the disease before 10 years of age.[5] Trauma and ultraviolet light exposure (UVB) may initiate and exacerbate lesions.

The face is the most commonly affected area, but lesions may occur on any body surface. Lesions are usually asymmetrically distributed and begin as asymptomatic, well-defined, elevated, red-to-violaceous, 1- to 2-cm, flat-topped plaques with firmly adherent scale (Figure 17-3). The scale penetrates into the orifices of the hair follicle. Peeling the scale reveals an undersurface that has the appearance of a carpet penetrated by several carpet tacks; it is called *carpet tack scale* (Figure 17-4). Carpet tack scale is most apparent on the face and scalp where the follicular orifices are larger.

Atrophy occurs in both the epidermis and the dermis. Epidermal atrophy occurs early and gives the surface either a smooth white or a wrinkled appearance. Follicular plugs may be prominent (Figure 17-5, *A* and *B*). These lesions endure for months and either resolve spontaneously or progress with further atrophy, ultimately forming smooth white or hyperpigmented depressed scars with telangiectasia and scarring alopecia.[6,7] Occasionally plaques become thick (hypertrophic DLE).[8] DLE can cover wide areas of the face, causing disfigurement (Figure 17-5, *C* and *D*). Hypopigmentation is particularly disfiguring for blacks. The laboratory and histologic features are outlined in Tables 17-7 and 17-8. The presence of anti-ssDNA occurs with widespread active disease.[9]

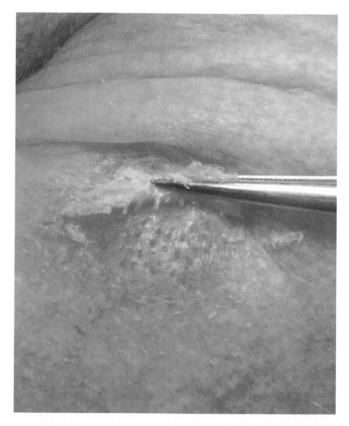

Figure 17-4
Chronic cutaneous LE (discoid LE). Carpet tack scale created by keratin plugs that penetrate deep into the hair follicle.

Figure 17-5 Chronic cutaneous LE (discoid LE).
A, Close-up of a lesion from patient in *D*. The plaque has been present for months. There is hypopigmentation and prominent follicular plugging.
B, Prominent follicular plugging in a plaque of discoid LE located in the scalp.
C, Lesions that are several months old are hypopigmented and atropic.
D, Patient in *C* elected not to be treated and worked outside without sun protection. Eighteen months later significant disease progression has occurred. Plaques have thickened, become more hypopigmented, and developed hyperpigmentation at the borders. Rapid improvement occurred after starting hydroxychloroquine (200 mg) twice a day.

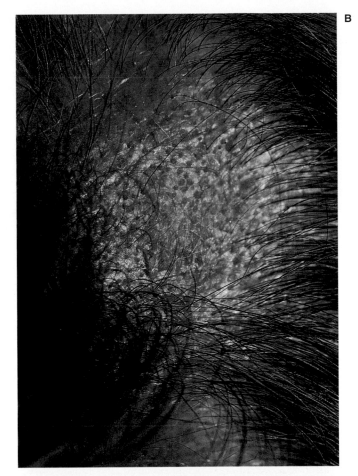

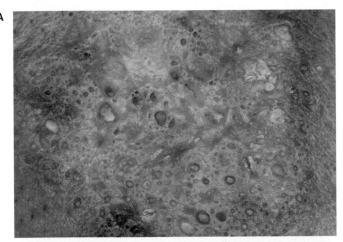

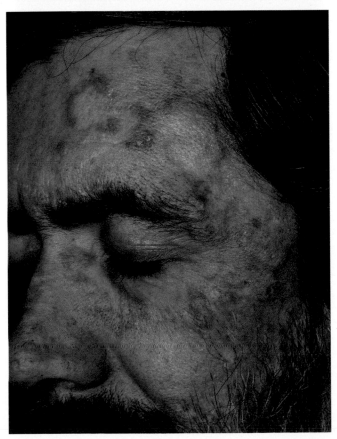

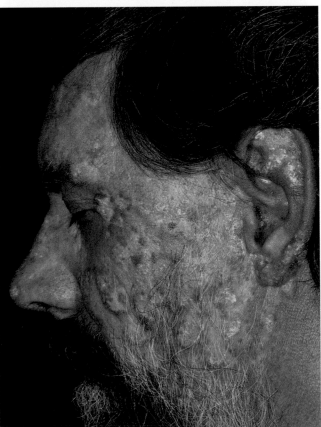

SUBACUTE CUTANEOUS LE

SCLE encompasses the clinical spectrum of cutaneous LE between the chronic destructive DLE and the erythema of acute cutaneous LE. However, SCLE can be associated with the full spectrum of LE-associated phenomena (see Table 17-6). Like DLE, the individual lesions of SCLE may last for months; in contrast to DLE, they heal without scarring. Most patients with SCLE are white females.

Two morphologic varieties are a papulosquamous pattern (Figure 17-6) and an annular-polycyclic pattern (Figure 17-7). Both occur most often on the trunk; one predominates. The lesions spare the knuckles (Figure 17-8), the inner aspects of the arms, the axillae, and the lateral part of the trunk.[10] They are rarely seen below the waist. A subtle gray hypopigmentation and telangiectasia are frequently seen in the center of annular lesions, bordered by erythema and a superficial scale. Follicular plugging, adherent hyperkeratosis, scarring, and dermal atrophy that are characteristic of DLE are not prominent features of SCLE. Hypopigmentation and telangiectasia become more evident as individual lesions resolve. The hypopigmentation fades after several months, but the telangiectasia may persist. The disease tends to be chronic and recurrent, lasting for years. SCLE and antibodies to Ro/SSA have been associated with hydrochlorothiazide therapy.[11]

Other dermatologic manifestations are photosensitivity (85% to 52%), periungual telangiectasia (51% to 22%), discoid LE (35% to 19%), and vasculitis (12%).[10,12] Systemic manifestations (arthritis/arthralgia [74% to 43%], renal disease [19% to 11%], serositis [12%], central nervous system [CNS] symptoms [19% to 6%]) are not severe and follow a benign course.[12]

The laboratory and histologic features of SCLE are outlined in Tables 17-7 and 17-8. Antibodies to Ro/SSA are present in 29% of patients.[12]

Figure 17-6
Subacute cutaneous LE (papulosquamous pattern). Lesions are confined to exposed areas on the upper half of the body. *(Photograph was digitally modified to illustrate the contrast between exposed and nonexposed skin surfaces.)*

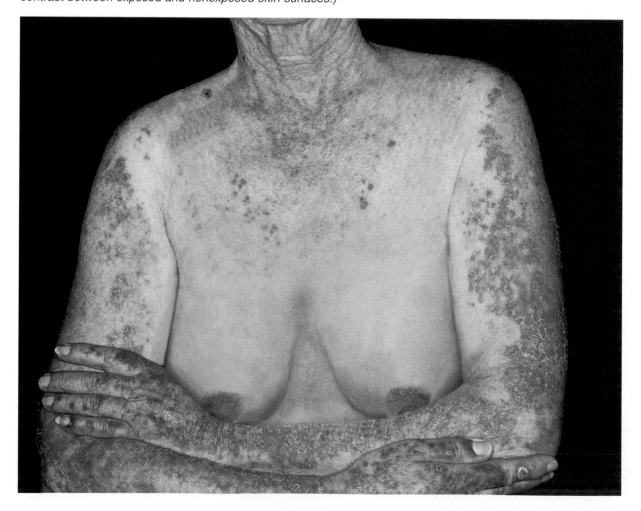

TABLE 17-8 Comparison of Laboratory Findings in the Cutaneous Subsets of LE

Finding	DLE (%)	SCLE (%)	ALE (%)
ANA titer ($\geq$1:160)	4	63	98
Anti-dsDNA	Rare	30	60-80
ESR greater than 30	Few	59	90
LE cell preparation	2	55	80
Low C3 or CH$_{50}$	Rare	Rare	90
WBC less than 4000	7	19	17
Rheumatoid factor latex test positive	15	19	37
Low hemoglobin level	Few	15	50
VDRL biologic false-positive	Few	7	22
Direct immunofluorescence and the lupus band test			
Lesion	90	60	95
Normal sun-exposed	0	46	75
Normal nonexposed	0	26	50

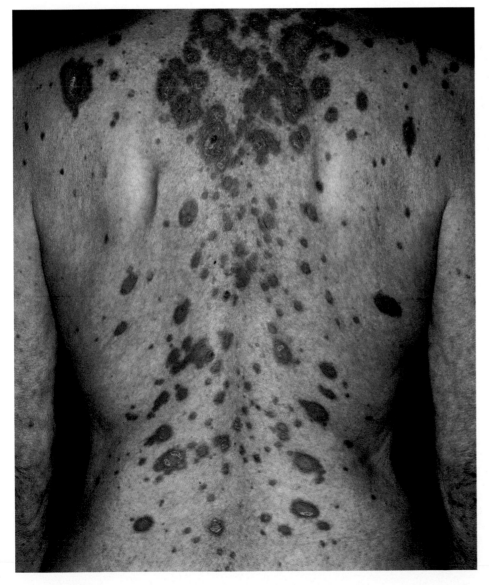

Figure 17-7
Subacute cutaneous LE (annular-polycyclic pattern). The annular plaques have an erythematous scaly border, the central area is hypopigmented, and the eruption is confined to the back and hands.

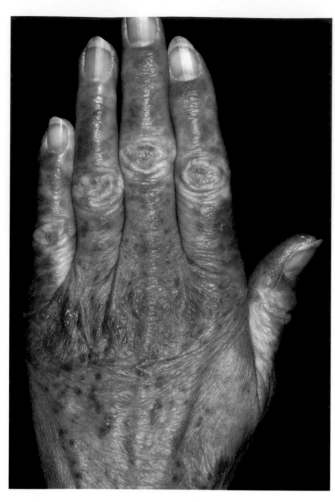

Figure 17-8
Cutaneous LE. In contrast to dermatomyositis, erythema and telangiectasia spare the knuckles.

Figure 17-9
Acute cutaneous LE (systemic LE). The classic butterfly rash occurs in 10% to 50% of patients with acute LE.

ACUTE CUTANEOUS LE

The rash of ALE consists of superficial-to-indurated, non-pruritic, erythematous-to-violaceous plaques; these occur primarily on sun-exposed areas of the face, chest, shoulders, extensor arms, and backs of the hands (Figure 17-8). There may be fine scaling on the surface, but atrophy does not occur. Superficial erythematous plaques may last for a few days, becoming more intense as disease activity increases and fading with improvement in systemic symptoms. The most indurated hivelike plaques remain relatively fixed in shape and may persist for months. The classic butterfly rash (Figure 17-9) over the malar and nasal area occurs in 10% to 50%[13] of patients with ALE, but it is not the most common cutaneous presentation. Erysipelas, rosacea, seborrheic dermatitis, and polymorphous light eruption may occur in the central face area and may easily be confused with acute LE. Flare of lupus during pregnancy is common and occurs significantly more frequently than does flare in nonpregnant SLE patients or in the same patients after pregnancy.[14]

OTHER CUTANEOUS SIGNS OF LE

Telangiectasia. Telangiectasia is a prominent feature of connective tissue disease. Telangiectasia occurs on the palms and fingers in association with palmar erythema; it resembles that observed in liver disease and pregnancy (Figure 17-10). Short, linear telangiectasias are a frequent finding in SLE. Using the ophthalmoscope technique described later in this chapter, nailfold capillary microscopy reveals tortuous, "meandering" capillary loops in 53% of patients with SLE.[15] Usually some disorganization of the capillary pattern is present, but avascular areas are rare, and the capillaries are not widened (see Figure 17-19).

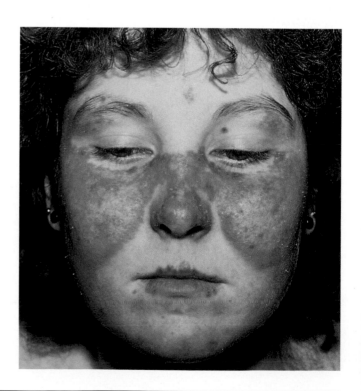

Alopecia. Alopecia is one of the major features of SLE and occurs in more than 20% of cases. Both scarring and nonscarring alopecia occur. Nonscarring hair loss occurs more frequently in SLE, and scarring alopecia is more common in DLE. In nonscarring alopecia the scalp may show focal or diffuse areas of erythema and scale similar to that seen with seborrheic dermatitis. The hair, especially in the frontal areas, becomes coarse and dry. The fragile, poorly formed shafts break, leaving patches of short, unmanageable hair, called *lupus hair*. The scalp and hair eventually become normal as disease activity wanes.

Scarring alopecia of the scalp is a classic sign of DLE (Figure 17-11). The disease begins with scalp erythema, scale, and follicular plugging (keratotic projections from the hair follicles), followed by signs of atrophy and scarring. The skin surface becomes white, smooth, and telangiectatic and is depressed below the normal level. Hair follicles are destroyed during the inflammatory and scarring process, resulting in permanent alopecia. Hair loss is haphazard in distribution, in contrast to the nonscarring hair loss of alopecia areata. At times the scarring is minimal, and the diagnosis of scarring alopecia caused by LE is not confirmed until the biopsy and immunofluorescence studies are obtained.

Urticaria. The reported incidence of urticaria or urticaria-like lesions with LE varies between 7% and 28%.[16] Urticaria is the presenting sign in approximately 5% of cases.[17] Clinically, lesions may be indistinguishable from typical hives; but unlike hives, they are usually nonpruritic, persist for days, and remain relatively fixed in position. This clinical presentation is typical of urticarial vasculitis. In most cases a biopsy reveals necrotizing vasculitis, and the lupus band test is generally positive. Therefore the hivelike lesions are probably a result of immune complex deposition rather than a manifestation of allergy.

Vasculitis. Palpable purpuric lesions identical to those exhibited in necrotizing angiitis occur in SLE. Lesions are most common on the lower legs and may progress to ulceration.[18]

Raynaud's phenomenon. Raynaud's phenomenon is another major diagnostic criterion for SLE. It occurs in 20% or more of SLE patients and may precede other signs and symptoms of SLE by months or years.[19] Progression to digital ulceration is more common in scleroderma.

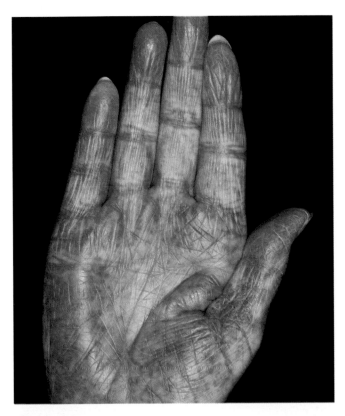

Figure 17-10
Cutaneous LE. Erythema and telangiectasia may appear on the palms.

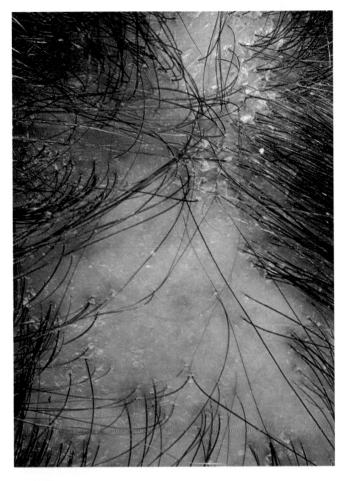

Figure 17-11
Chronic cutaneous LE (discoid LE). Scarring alopecia of the scalp, end-stage disease.

DRUG-INDUCED LE

Hydralazine, procainamide, isoniazid, and, rarely, other drugs can induce a lupuslike syndrome. Patients treated with the usual doses of hydralazine have a relatively low incidence of positivity for ANAs and a very low rate of occurrence of the clinical syndrome.[20] Procainamide is the most common cause of drug-related lupus in the United States. Up to 80% of patients taking procainamide have a positive ANA. Approximately 30% of that group have clinical symptoms.

Induction of autoimmunity by drugs. These structurally different drugs may have functional groups that are oxidized by leukocyte myeloperoxidase in activated phagocytic cells.[21-24] For example, in the presence of activated neutrophils, procainamide is transformed metabolically to procainamide-hydroxylamine, which could then haptenize a protein on the surface of monocytes and induce autoantibodies that are directed against nuclear histone components.

Clinical features. Most commonly the onset of symptoms occurs many months after the drug has been initiated. It is characterized by fever, arthralgia, myalgias, pleurisy, and pericarditis, and it may have an abrupt onset. Rashes are very uncommon.[25,26] Renal involvement and CNS disease are rare. The symptoms generally resolve within days to weeks after the drug is discontinued, and the ANA disappears.

Diagnosis. There are no specific diagnostic criteria for drug-related lupus. Several determinations should be made before the diagnosis is made. There should have been no history suggestive of SLE before drug therapy was started. Antibodies to histones occur in virtually all patients.[27] A positive ANA should be detectable, with at least one clinical feature of SLE during sustained treatment. The ANA consists of anti–single stranded DNA rather than double-stranded native DNA as in classic LE. There should be rapid improvement in the clinical symptoms, a gradual fall in the ANAs and other serologic changes when the drug is withdrawn.[28] Complement levels are normal.

Patient profile. A liver acetyltransferase enzyme inactivates these drugs. Patients can be categorized as either slow or fast acetylators. Slow acetylators develop ANA and clinical symptoms earlier than fast acetylators.[29]

Treatment. Patients with pericarditis, pleural effusions, or pulmonary infiltrates often require prednisone. They respond quickly, and prednisone can be tapered and then discontinued over a few months.[30]

NEONATAL LE

Neonatal LE (NLE) is an immune-mediated disease characterized by subacute cutaneous lupuslike annular and polycyclic lesions, congenital heart block, or both. Individuals who have had NLE may develop connective tissue disease in adulthood. NLE is caused by the transplacental passage of maternal IgG anti-Ro/SSA and/or anti-La/SSB or anti-U1RNP.[31] Most babies of mothers with anti-Ro/SSA, anti-La/SSB, or anti-U1RNP autoantibodies do not develop NLE. There is no way to determine which fetus or infant will be affected. Anti-Ro/SSA are the predominant autoantibodies, and are found in approximately 95% of cases.[31] The skin lesions (present in approximately 50% of affected infants) usually appear within the first month of life, may be initiated by sun exposure, and heal without scarring or atrophy within 6 months.[32] The autoantibodies disappear with the rash. The congenital heart block (present in approximately 50% of affected infants) is a permanent defect that develops in utero during the late second and the third trimesters of pregnancy. Many babies require pacemakers, and approximately 10% die from complications related to cardiac disease. The proposed cause is that the anti-Ro/SSA antibody binds with an autoantigen in the heart and produces an inflammatory process, resulting in fibrotic replacement and destruction of one or more of the following: the sinoatrial bundle, the atrioventricular bundle, or the bundle of His.[33]

Approximately 50% of mothers have clinical features of either Sjögren's syndrome or LE at the time of birth, but more than 85%, with time, demonstrate the onset of sicca symptoms (dry eyes, dry mouth) and/or joint stiffness, arthralgias, or swelling.[34] Of anti-Ro/SSA-positive patients, 90% to 95% possess either the HLA- DR2 or DR3 phenotype.[35] Of lupus patients with abnormal fetal heart rate, 100% have antibodies to phospholipids (lupus anticoagulant).

Management. Two lesional skin biopsies are taken: one for hematoxylin and eosin and the other for immunofluorescence. The finding of anti-Ro/SSA antibody in the infant and mother confirms the diagnosis. Mothers are advised that the risk of a similarly affected infant in subsequent pregnancies is approximately 25%.[34] Patients with heart block may be asymptomatic or require pacemakers.

DIAGNOSIS AND MANAGEMENT OF CUTANEOUS LE

Lupus is an uncommon disease that has been described extensively in the medical literature and in the lay press. Some patients are familiar with the term and fear the worst when informed of their diagnosis. They should be assured that the disease in the majority of patients can be controlled

---

WORKUP FOR SUSPECTED CUTANEOUS LE (DLE, SCLE, SLE)

- Biopsy for histology: lesion
- Biopsy for immunofluorescence: old lesion

If either is consistent with LE:
- System review
- ANA
- nDNA
- Antibodies-SSA (Ro), SSB (La), Sm, nRNP
- Urinalysis
- ESR, CBC
- C3 C4 CH_{50}

with existing therapy, but that periodic clinical and laboratory evaluations are necessary to monitor disease activity.

Management consists of defining the type of cutaneous subset, performing a physical examination to document systemic symptoms, obtaining a battery of relevant blood studies as a baseline for diagnosis and later comparison as disease activity changes (see the box on p. 546), obtaining a biopsy of lesional skin for routine histology and immunofluorescence, and, if appropriate, obtaining a biopsy of nonlesional skin for immunofluorescence and topical and/or systemic treatment. A discussion of systemic symptom management is beyond the scope of this book.

Laboratory studies. A compilation of some of the studies used for the evaluation of LE is listed in the box on p. 546. Patients with chronic cutaneous LE but without evidence of systemic disease should have a similar evaluation for documentation, because a few of these patients may later develop SLE. A comparison of the laboratory findings in the cutaneous subsets of LE is found in Table 17-8. Changes in values of some of these tests may reflect changes in disease activity (Table 17-9).

Antinuclear and anticytoplasmic antibodies. The production of antinuclear and anticytoplasmic antibodies is a fundamental characteristic of LE. Numerous diverse antibodies are produced, and most laboratories have access to facilities that can measure the antibodies listed in Table 17-2. Measurement of these antibodies provides valuable information for diagnosis and prognosis. Quantitative measurement of some of these antibodies, such as anti–double-stranded DNA, can be made, and changes in levels assist in determining disease activity.

Measurement of ANA was the first test available for directly measuring antinuclear antibodies in a qualitative and quantitative manner. The test is positive in the vast majority of patients with LE (see Tables 17-1, 17-3, and 17-5) and is presently an important screening test. The LE cell preparation is no longer a standard screening test.

The ANA test is a nonspecific test that detects many types of antinuclear antibodies. The significance of titers varies with different laboratories, but generally titers below 1:16 are believed to be negative, whereas titers above 1:64 indicate possible SLE. Extremely high titers such as 1:32,000 may be found. Unfortunately the titer level or change of titer has not been a reliable indicator of disease activity.

Skin biopsy, direct immunofluorescence, and the lupus band test. A biopsy of skin lesions in patients with DLE and systemic lupus erythematosus (SLE) provides important diagnostic information. The histologic characteristics are listed in Table 17-7. Direct immunofluorescence of skin (lupus band test) has been used for years for the diagnosis of the various forms of lupus.

Lupus band test. The term *lupus band test* (LBT) refers to direct immunofluorescence examination of normal sun-protected, normal sun-exposed, or lesional skin. Deposits of one or more immunoglobulins (IgG, IgM, IgA, and/or C3) are found at the dermoepidermal junction and in the walls of dermal vessels in patients with DLE, SCLE, and SLE. Although many other diseases can show dermoepidermal junction fluorescence, the lesions of LE characteristically have bright, thick bands composed of more than one immunoglobulin (especially IgG), whereas other diseases have faint or fibrillar bands with a single immunoglobulin (usually IgM).

It is essential that the test be interpreted by experienced laboratories. The frequency of positive tests varies, depending on the type of skin lesion, duration of the lesion, site of biopsy, presence or absence of systemic disease, and duration of treatment.

The practical value of the LBT has been questioned. Recent studies suggest that the test does not aid in predicting which patients with undifferentiated connective tissue disease will develop SLE, and that the LBT is not a useful diagnostic tool in the differential diagnosis of SLE.[36,37]

The test does provide one piece of data that, when used in combination with other studies, may help to characterize this complex disease and differentiate it from others. In the same patients, the band appears as systemic disease activity increases and disappears with spontaneous remission and in those who improved with hydroxychloroquine,[38] prednisone, and/or cytotoxic drugs. A single skin biopsy specimen must be interpreted cautiously in relation to the nature and degree of disease activity; in the same patient the LBT may be positive at one site and negative at another.[39]

Most hospitals do not have the facilities to perform the LBT. Cutaneous immunofluorescence laboratories in various parts of the country provide a liquid transport medium and mailing packages (see p. 499); therefore freezing specimens is unnecessary. A 3- or 4-mm punch biopsy should be submitted.

TABLE 17-9	Laboratory Studies Used to Determine Degree of Systemic Activity of LE	
Laboratory study	**Change of value with increased systemic activity**
Lupus band test	Converts to positive
C3, C4, CH$_{50}$	Concentration decreases
Anti-nDNA antibody	Concentration may increase
LE cell test	Converts to positive
Lymphocyte count	Number decreases
ESR	Value increases

TREATMENT

Sunscreens. Sunlight in the UVA and UVB regions can induce and exacerbate all forms of lupus erythematosus.[40] Patients should avoid direct exposure to sunlight, particularly during the summer and between the hours of 10 A.M. and 3 P.M. Broad-spectrum sunscreens with a sun protection factor of maximum value (greater than 15) that block UVB and UVA light should be applied if sun exposure is anticipated.[41] Patients should be encouraged to apply sunscreens as a routine procedure after morning washing during the summer months.

Topical corticosteroids. Topical corticosteroids are the agents of first choice for all forms of cutaneous LE. Groups I through V topical steroids are required to control DLE. They may be applied three times a day to all active lesions, including those on the face. Patients should be encouraged to restrict application to the active lesion and to avoid normal surrounding skin. Lesions of SCLE and ALE may be treated with groups III through V topical steroid applied three times a day. Those who do not respond should be advanced to group II topical steroids. Discontinue treatment when lesions have cleared.

Intralesional corticosteroids. DLE lesions that are resistant to topical steroids may be managed well with periodic intralesional injections of steroids (e.g., equal parts of 1% xylocaine or saline and triamcinolone acetonide [Kenalog] 10 mg/ml). Lesions frequently become inactive after a single injection and may remain in remission for months. The steroid should be injected with a 27- or 30-gauge needle with sufficient solution to blanch the lesion—approximately 0.1 ml/1.0 cm lesion.

Antimalarials. Antimalarials are effective in the treatment of all forms of cutaneous LE.[42,43] Fear of retinal toxicity resulted in a substantial reduction in the use of these agents; but it was later discovered that excessive daily dosages influenced retinal damage. A review article provides recommendations for use and reassurance that toxicity can be avoided.[44] The recommended safe and effective dosage for an individual weighing 150 pounds is 200 mg of hydroxycholoroquine (Plaquenil) twice a day.[45] Patients can be maintained on this dosage as long as needed, but they should have periodic eye evaluations. By performing serial testing of the foveal reflex and of the reaction of visual fields to red targets,[46] the ophthalmologist can detect a state of "premaculopathy." Testing is done before treatment and every 6 to 12 months during therapy. While the patient is on therapy, premaculopathy is defined as the loss of foveal reflex or the development of paracentral scotomata to red test objects. It is a state of functional loss that is reversible by discontinuation of the drug.

Antimalarials are maintained at the previously recommended dosages until the lesions resolve. They are then reduced to the lowest possible dosage to maintain control. Patients with quiescent SLE who are taking hydroxychloroquine are less likely to have a clinical flare-up if they are maintained on the drug. The discontinuation of treatment in patients with quiescent disease is associated with a 2.5-fold increase in the risk of new clinical manifestations or, in the case of previous manifestations, a recurrence or an increase in severity.[47]

Dapsone. Antimalarials are the drugs of first choice for cutaneous LE when topical steroids have failed. Dapsone (initial dosage 100 mg/day) is an effective alternative for all forms of cutaneous LE.[48-53] The dosage is adjusted after evaluation of clinical response and side effects. Dapsone therapy is described on p. 507.

Oral corticosteroids. Occasionally patients with cutaneous LE do not respond to topical steroids, antimalarials, or dapsone. Such patients should discontinue other forms of therapy and begin prednisone at dosages high enough to control the disease (e.g., 15 mg twice a day), until control is obtained. Oral steroids are then tapered and discontinued; the patient is once more given a trial of conventional therapy.

Other treatments. Azathioprine (100 to 150 mg/ day),[54-56] thalidomide (50 to 300 mg/day),[57-59] and acitretin (50 mg/day)[60] are effective for severe, chloroquine-resistant DLE. Isotretinoin (1 mg/kg/day) is reported to be effective for patients with DLE and SCLE.[61] Treatment with isotretinoin resulted in rapid clinical improvement; recurrences were rapid when the drug was discontinued.[62] Hypertrophic keratotic forms of DLE also respond to isotretinoin.[63,64] Methotrexate may also be effective as a corticosteroid-sparing agent.[65] A recent report shows that a combination of niacinamide and tetracycline or erythromycin are effective for treating discoid lupus erythematosus.[66]

Dermatomyositis and Polymyositis

Dermatomyositis (DM) and polymyositis (PM) are rare inflammatory muscle diseases. There is evidence that DM results from immune-mediated vessel injury in which complement is bound and activated to completion in the intramuscular arterioles and capillaries and results in the destruction of muscle fibers.[67,68] The term *polymyositis* is reserved for cases in which skin inflammation is absent. Although patients of any age may be affected, most patients are either children or adults over age 40. Adult DM can be associated with malignancy and collagen vascular diseases. The clinical picture varies considerably, and the following classification and diagnostic criteria (see the box below) of the idiopathic inflammatory myopathies have been suggested.[69,70]

Classification of idiopathic inflammatory myopathies

Group I	PM
Group II	DM
Group III	PM or DM with malignancy
Group IV	Childhood PM or DM
Group V	PM or DM associated with collagen-vascular disease

DIAGNOSTIC CRITERIA FOR DERMATOMYOSITIS AND POLYMYOSITIS

MAJOR CRITERIA

Proximal symmetric muscle weakness
Compatible muscle biopsy
Myopathy, or inflammatory myositis
Compatible electromyography
Elevated skeletal muscle enzymes (e.g., CPK, aldolase, SGOT)
Compatible dermatologic features

EXCLUSION OF OTHER DISORDERS CAUSING A MYOPATHY

Neurologic disease
Muscular dystrophies
Infections
Toxins
Endocrinopathies

CONFIDENCE LIMITS

Definite PM: three or four criteria (DM + rash)
Probable PM: two criteria (DM + rash)
Possible PM: one criterion (DM + rash)

Modified from Bohan A, Peter JB, Bowman RL, et al: *Medicine* 56:255-286, 1977; and Callen JP: *Dis Mon* 33:237-305, 1987.

POLYMYOSITIS

Symmetric proximal muscular weakness, especially of the hips and thighs, is characteristic of PM. The onset is insidious; patients first note difficulty rising from a chair. Neck muscles are commonly involved, leading to weakness in raising the head ("drooped head"). Dysfunction of the pharyngeal muscles may lead to dysphagia and aspiration pneumonia. Respiratory muscles of the chest wall can be involved. Distal strength is usually preserved. Myalgias can occur, and tenderness is uncommon. Arthralgias are a presenting sign in 41% of patients.[71] Weakness progresses over weeks to months; spontaneous remission may occur. Deep tendon reflexes remain normal and atrophy occurs late in the course of the disease. The muscle changes are indistinguishable from those seen in DM.

DERMATOMYOSITIS

The associated features of PM may precede by months, accompany, or follow the skin signs. Proximal muscle weakness is the most common presenting manifestation; the rash is present in only approximately 40% of patients when they are first evaluated.[72,73] The cutaneous changes sometimes precede the onset of muscle weakness by more than a year.[74] The course of adult DM may be acute, chronic, recurrent, or cyclic. DM tends to be a more severe disease than PM,[74] with a more severe myopathy. DM occurs in all age groups and equally in males and females. The frequency of malignancy is equally increased in DM and PM. There are five dermatologic features of DM: the pathognomonic heliotrope, Gottron's papules, a photosensitive violaceous eruption, periungual telangiectasia, and poikiloderma. The term *amyopathic dermatomyositis* has been applied to three groups of patients: those with cutaneous changes only, those with cutaneous changes only at baseline with subsequent development of myositis, and those with cutaneous changes with normal muscle enzyme serum levels at baseline but with myositis demonstrated by electromyography and/or muscle biopsy specimens.[75-78]

Heliotrope erythema of eyelids. *Heliotrope erythema of the eyelids* (*heliotrope*: violet color) is a term used to describe the violaceous discoloration around the eyes (Figure 17-12). It is a pathognomonic sign of DM. Periorbital edema and violet discoloration may be either the earliest cutaneous sign or a residual finding as diffuse erythema fades.

Gottron's papules. Gottron's papules, a pathognomonic sign of DM, are round, 0.2- to 1-cm, smooth, violaceous-to-red, flat-topped papules that occur over the knuckles, along the sides of the fingers (Figure 17-13), and sometimes over the knees and elbows. Lupus of the back of the hand usually spares the knuckles (see Figure 17-8). Several lesions appear simultaneously any time during the course of the disease; they tend to remain fixed in position. Approximately 60% to 80% of DM patients have Gottron's papules sometime during the course of the disease.

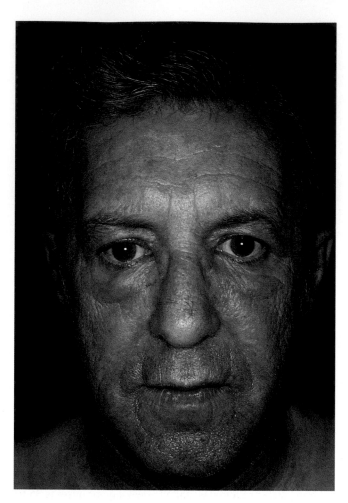

Figure 17-12
Dermatomyositis. Heliotrope (violaceous) discoloration around the eyes and periorbital edema.

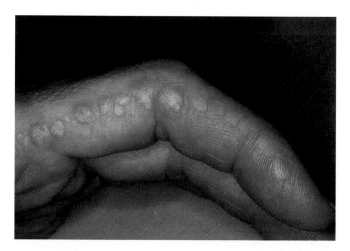

Figure 17-13
Dermatomyositis. Gottron's papules, a pathognomonic sign of dermatomyositis, are round, smooth, violaceous-to-red, flat-topped papules that occur over the knuckles and along the sides of the fingers.

Violaceous scaling patches. A characteristic violet erythema with or without scaling occurs in a localized or diffuse distribution. The localized eruption appears symmetrically over bony prominences such as the knees, elbows, and interphalangeal joints (Figure 17-14). DM typically involves the knuckles and spares the skin over the phalanges. The distribution is reversed in SLE when the skin over the phalanges is involved and the knuckles are spared (see Figure 17-8). The diffuse form begins as a patchy, diffuse, dusky-red or violet erythema of the sun-exposed areas of the face, neck, back, and arms and later may involve the buttocks and legs. Over time the rash becomes confluent, and involved areas become minimally raised and slightly scaly. A diffuse, deep red erythema (malignant erythema) may appear superimposed on the existing eruption in patients with an evolving malignancy. Photosensitivity is common. The rash tends to be confined to sun-exposed areas and is worse after sun exposure.

Periungual erythema and telangiectasia. Clinically these are similar to those seen in other connective tissue diseases. The telangiectasia is most prominent on the proximal nailfold and appears as irregular, red, linear streaks (Figure 17-15). Nailfold capillary microscopy using the ophthalmoscope (see Figure 17-19) reveals a pattern identical to that seen in scleroderma but quite different from that seen in SLE. Therefore this technique may help to distinguish DM from SLE. The cuticles are thick, rough, hyperkeratotic, and irregular (moth-eaten appearance).

Poikiloderma. Late in the course of the disease, as the erythema fades, a highly characteristic pattern may occur in the same sun-exposed areas occupied by the diffuse erythema. *Poikiloderma* is a descriptive term for the pattern that consists of finely mottled white areas and brown pigmentation, telangiectasia, and atrophy. Poikiloderma also occurs as an isolated phenomenon with mycosis fungoides and other rare dermatologic conditions.

Scaly red scalp. Scalp scaling may be a sign of DM. Erythematous, scaly, atrophic scalp lesions initially diagnosed as psoriasis, seborrheic dermatitis, or lupus erythematosus were reported in a series of patients with DM.[79]

Dermatomyositis with malignancy. There is an increased incidence of malignancy in adult DM and PM.[80,81] The association is largely with malignant neoplasms diagnosed at or before the time of diagnosis of PM and DM.[82] Patients over the age of 50 are at greatest risk. It is reported to be as high as 5 to 7 times that of an age-matched population.[83] Tumors may appear at any site, but the most common sites in order of frequency are the breast, lung, ovary, stomach, colon, uterus, and nasopharynx.[84] Myopathy antedated the diagnosis of cancer in approximately 60% of patients by a mean interval of 11 months.[85] In 30% of patients the tumor appeared first, and symptoms of DM subsequently appeared, with a mean interval of 16 months. The rash and symptoms of DM may clear following resection of the tumor. Recurrence of dermatomyositis may indicate the occurrence of a second primary malignancy or recurrent cancer.

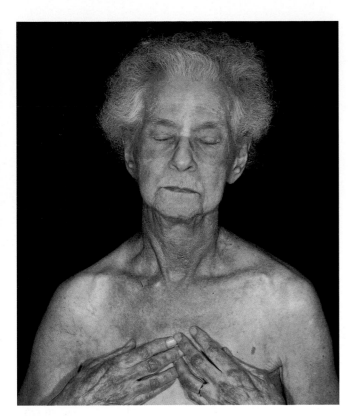

Figure 17-14
Dermatomyositis. Violaceous scaling patches on the face and dorsal interphalangeal joints. The knuckles are involved; they are spared in SLE.

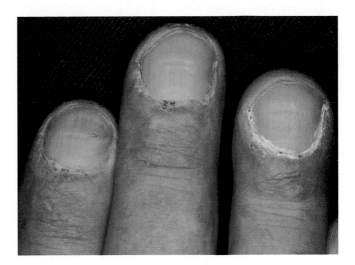

Figure 17-15
Dermatomyositis. Periungual erythema and telangiectasia similar to that seen in other connective tissue diseases.

Childhood dermatomyositis. Juvenile dermatomyositis is characterized by a nonsuppurative myositis that causes symmetric weakness, rash, and vasculitis affecting the GI tract and the myocardium.[86] Calcinosis of subcutaneous tissue (occurs in approximately two thirds of patients and is complicated by recurrent infections),[87] muscle atrophy, residual proximal weakness, contractures, Raynaud's phenomenon, and arthritis are possible late sequelae.[88] Some 50% of children have a very acute, rapidly progressive disease, whereas the remainder present subacutely with rash and a gradually progressive weakness of muscles, joint contractures, and, very infrequently, calcinosis.[89] The course of treated patients is variable: 25% are well in 2 years, 31% experience recurrences when steroids are stopped after remission, and 44% have continuous disease for more than 2 years despite continual corticosteroid therapy.[90] The creatine phosphokinase is elevated when there is acute muscle damage; antinuclear antibodies are usually present. The clinical course and survival improves significantly with intensive early therapy with corticosteroids and physical therapy; as many as 92% survive and as many as 85% are functionally normal after 5 years.[91] The incidence of cancer is low. Death can occur in the acute phase due to myocarditis, progressive unresponsive myositis, perforation of the bowel as a sequel to vasculitis ulceration, or, occasionally, lung involvement.

Overlap syndromes. Myositis may occur during the course of other connective tissue diseases such as scleroderma, rheumatoid arthritis, and LE. The most common association is with scleroderma and is termed *sclerodermatomyositis*. Apparently sclerodermatomyositis is a distinct overlap syndrome, with features of SLE, scleroderma, and PM; it is called *mixed connective tissue disease*. Of these patients, 80% are females, and the peak age of onset is 35 to 40. Clinically, females come to the physician with swollen hands and tapered fingers, Raynaud's phenomenon, abnormal esophageal motility, myositis, and lymphadenopathy. High titers of antibody (anti-RNP) to an extractable nuclear antigen called *ribonucleoprotein* (RNP) occur in all such patients but are not unique to mixed connective tissue disease. ANA is present, but Sm is absent.

Diagnosis. Diagnostic measures include muscle biopsy from weak muscles, skin biopsy of involved skin, and electromyography and measurement of muscle enzymes. (See the box below.) One or more of these parameters may be normal at the time of diagnosis or during the course of the disease, therefore a complete evaluation is needed in all cases.[92]

WORKUP FOR SUSPECTED DERMATOMYOSITIS

- Skin biopsy for histology and immunofluorescence
- Muscle biopsy
- Muscle enzymes
- Electromyography
- ANA
- Antibodies-SSA (Ro), SSB (La), Sm, nRNP, Jo-1, PM-1

Muscle enzymes. Serum muscle enzymes (creatine kinase [CK], aspartate aminotransferase [AST], and alanine aminotransferase [ALT]) are measured both for diagnostic purposes and to monitor disease activity.[93] Although some patients with myositis have normal CKs, most experts use the CK as a guide to clinical response or reactivation of the myositis.[72] Measuring urinary creatine (not creatinine) in a 24-hour collection is an early and sensitive indicator of muscle injury and a better indicator of activity than the serum creatine kinase. The test is especially useful when serum creatine is normal.

Muscle biopsy, electromyography, magnetic resonance imaging (MRI), and phosphorus 31 magnetic resonance spectroscopy (MRS). Muscle biopsies from the same patient may vary. Several specimens may have to be taken to demonstrate an abnormality.[83] A weak muscle should be sampled and will show muscle fiber and capillary damage. Lymphocytes and macrophages partially invade non-necrotic fibers.[96] Electromyographic studies are also indicated to diagnose the disease but not to follow disease activity. MRI may help to establish the diagnosis, to find an appropriate muscle biopsy site, and to monitor the progress of the disease.[94] It is difficult to determine whether immunosuppressive therapy should be stopped when there is discordance between clinical symptoms (weakness) and tests (muscle enzyme levels, strength testing, and MRI).

MRS is a noninvasive test that can be used when decisions are made about changes in therapy. It provides the most reliable data to document flares of disease activity and periods of relative inactivity.[95]

Antibody tests. Specific autoantibody tests (ANA, Jo-1, SSA [Ro], Ku [Ki]) should be ordered (see Tables 17-2 and 17-3). These tests are of limited value in making the diagnosis, but positive serum results help to support it. Serologic studies such as rheumatoid factor, ANA, anti-Ro/SSA, anti-La/SSB, and anti-RNP are performed to rule out associated collagen vascular diseases.

Evaluation for possible malignancy. Patients with DM should be evaluated for internal malignancy. A recent review suggests that the discovery of most internal neoplasms resulted from history, physical examination, and routine laboratory studies.[97] A "blind" or nondirected malignancy search was of no value in any of the cases analyzed. Complete history and physical examination in a search for malignancy should be repeated at certain intervals (e.g., every 6 months, particularly in the older age group of patients). All unusual signs, symptoms, and laboratory values should be pursued.

Treatment

Corticosteroids and immunosuppressive drugs. Oral corticosteroids are the treatment of first choice for most adults who have skin and muscle symptoms.[74] It is important to start at a high enough dosage to control the disease and then to taper slowly. Prednisone (usually 60 mg/day in divided doses) is initiated, gradually tapered, and changed to an alternate-day schedule after disease activity improves, as indicated by improving clinical signs and decreasing levels of muscle enzymes. Most patients begin to improve after the first month. Immunosuppressive drugs such as methotrexate (up to 7.5 to 15 mg/wk or up to 50 mg intravenously once each week),[98,99] azathioprine (2 mg/kg/day orally), or chlorambucil are substituted for or used in addition to prednisone for patients who do not improve after 3 to 6 weeks of prednisone.[100] Methotrexate is effective, but side effects are common. Patients should be monitored for toxic effects on the liver.[101] The cutaneous eruption often resists systemic therapy. Groups IV and V topical steroids reduce the erythema but do not clear the eruption. Exposure to sunlight should be minimized; broad spectrum sunscreens are important.

Antimalarials. Antimalarials are effective in treating the cutaneous lesions of DM.[102,103] Hydroxychloroquine sulfate (200 to 400 mg/day) is prescribed. Chloroquine phosphate (250 to 500 mg/day) is an alternative to hydroxychloroquine failures. Another option is to add oral quinacrine hydrochloride (100 mg/day) to either hydroxychloroquine or chloroquine.[72] Antimalarials have no effect on muscle disease.

Intravenous immune globulin. In several studies with small numbers of patients, high-dose intravenous immune globulin has been shown to be a safe and effective treatment for refractory dermatomyositis.[104,105] Patients are treated with varying schedules (1 gm/kg daily for 2 days each month or 0.4 gm/kg daily for 5 days each month).[106,107] Intravenous immune globulin may be effective as initial therapy and may replace or reduce the need for steroid and immunosuppressive medications.[108]

Cyclosporine. In three recent reports with small numbers of patients, juvenile dermatomyositis patients who had not responded fully to steroids and other immunosuppressants were successfully treated with cyclosporine.[109,110] Cyclosporine-A allowed a decreased dosage of corticosteroids and provided an associated "catch-up" growth in another study.[111] Cyclosporine is associated with significant renal toxicity.

Physical therapy. Bed rest is essential for patients with active muscle disease. Physical therapy is very important in the management of DM. Prednisone and immunosuppressive agents treat inflammation, but they do not make muscles strong. An aggressive-passive physical therapy program should be started, and, as muscle pain decreases, an active exercise program should be begun.

The signs and symptoms of DM often clear shortly after the removal of a malignancy.

Prognosis. There is a poor prognosis when muscle weakness has existed for more than 4 months before diagnosis,[92] with dysphagia, pulmonary disease and malignancy,[70] and for DM patients with a lack of creatine kinase elevation.[112] The cumulative survival rate is as high as 73% after 8 years.[73]

Scleroderma

Scleroderma is a disease characterized by sclerosis of the skin and visceral organs, vasculopathy (Raynaud's phenomenon), and autoantibodies. The spectrum of disease is wide, with systemic and localized forms (see the box below).

CLASSIFICATION OF SCLERODERMA AND SCLERODERMA-LIKE DISORDERS

SYSTEMIC SCLEROSIS

Diffuse scleroderma (10% of cases of systemic sclerosis)
  Skin—bilateral symmetric fibrosis of skin, face, proximal and distal portions of the extremities
  Visceral disease—relatively early appearance
CREST syndrome (90% of cases of systemic sclerosis)
  Skin—relatively limited involvement, often confined to fingers and face
  Visceral disease—delayed appearance
Overlap syndromes
  Sclerodermatomyositis
  Mixed connective tissue diseases

LOCALIZED SCLERODERMA

Morphea
  Plaquelike
  Guttate
  Generalized
  Subcutaneous and keloid morphea
Linear scleroderma
En coup de sabre (with or without facial hemiatrophy)

CHEMICAL-INDUCED SCLERODERMA-LIKE CONDITIONS

Vinyl chloride disease
  Pentazocine-induced fibrosis
  Bleomycin-induced

EOSINOPHILIC FASCIITIS PSEUDOSCLERODERMA

Edematous (scleredema, scleromyxedema)
Indurative (amyloidosis, porphyria cutanea tarda, carcinoid syndrome, phenylketonuria)
Atrophic (progeria, Werner's syndrome, lichen sclerosis et atrophicus)

Adapted from Masi AT et al: *Bull Rheum Dis* 3:1-6, 1981.

SYSTEMIC SCLEROSIS

Systemic sclerosis has a reported incidence of 2 to 12 cases per million people per year. There are two major subsets of the systemic forms: diffuse scleroderma and CREST syndrome. The criteria for the diagnosis of scleroderma are listed in the box below. CREST (calcinosis cutis, Raynaud's phenomenon, esophageal involvement, sclerodactyly, telangiectasia) syndrome is slowly progressive. Diffuse scleroderma can be rapidly progressive and potentially fatal; there is symmetric fibrous thickening and hardening (sclerosis) of the skin and fibrous and degenerative changes in synovium, digital arteries, and certain internal organs, most notably the esophagus, intestinal tract, heart, lungs, and kidneys (Tables 17-10 and 17-11).[113]

Overlap syndromes exist in which typical scleroderma skin changes accompany a variety of other skin and internal diseases.

Localized scleroderma is restricted to the skin in an asymmetric manner. The other forms are rare and are not discussed here. Raynaud's phenomenon precedes or is an early manifestation in the majority of cases. All forms of scleroderma are more common in females.

Chemically induced scleroderma

Scleroderma-like diseases can be induced by a number of chemical compounds, such as plastics, solvents, and drugs. Contaminated rapeseed oil is the cause of toxic oil syndrome, and L-tryptophan induces eosinophilia-myalgia syndrome. Paraffin and silicon can trigger so-called adjuvant disease. Long-term exposure to silica can lead to idiopathic scleroderma.[114,115] This supports the hypothesis that collagen disease may be attributable to the occupations of hypersusceptible persons.

SCLERODERMA CRITERIA

Major criteria
  Proximal sclerosis—single major criterion (91% sensitivity and greater than 99% specificity)*

Minor criteria
  Sclerodactyly
  Digital pitting scars of fingertips or loss of substance of the finger pad
  Pulmonary fibrosis-bibasilar

One major criterion or two or more minor criteria were found in 97% of patients with definite systemic sclerosis, but in only 2% of the comparison patients with SLE, PM/DM, or Raynaud's phenomenon†

*From American Rheumatism Association: *Arthritis Rheum* 23:581-590, 1980.
†Excludes localized scleroderma and pseudoscleroderma.

TABLE 17-10 Organ Involvement in Progressive Systemic Sclerosis

Organ	Involvement (%)
Skin	98
Esophageal atrophy or fibrosis	74
Small intestinal atrophy or fibrosis	48
Large intestinal atrophy or fibrosis	39
Myocardial fibrosis	81
Pericardium*	53
Pericardial effusion	35
Pulmonary interstitial fibrosis	74
Pleural disease	81
Kidneys†	58
Skeletal muscle atrophy	41
Skeletal muscle round cell infiltration	8
Thyroid (fibrosis)	24
Adrenal atrophy	26
Cancer	2

Adapted from D'Angelo WA et al: *Am J Med* 46:428-440, 1969.
*Pericarditis (fibrous or fibrinous) or pericardial adhesions.
†Any of the following: (1) fibrinoid necrosis of afferent arterioles or glomeruli; (2) hyperplasia of interlobular artery; or (3) thickening of basement membrane or wire-loop.

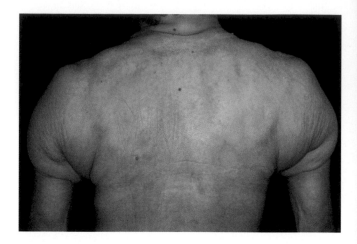

Figure 17-16
Scleroderma. Diffuse systemic sclerosis. Diffuse sclerosis of the limbs.

TABLE 17-11 Signs of Visceral Involvement in Systemic Sclerosis

	Mild	Severe
Raynaud's	Less than five times a day	More than 15 times/day, or digital ulcerations, or both
Esophagus	Dysphagia to solid foods; normal barium swallow	Dysphagia to solid and soft foods and weight loss (>10%); abnormal barium swallow with dilation of the lower two thirds of the esophagus
Lung	No symptoms: vital capacity >70% predicted and CO_2-diffusing capacity between 50% and 75% of predicted, Po_2 >80 mm Hg	Dyspnea + vital capacity <50% of predicted or CO_2-diffusing capacity <33% of predicted, Po_2 <69 mm Hg
Heart	Nonspecific ST-T changes	Angina, definite ischemic changes by ECG*, hypokinesis by MUGA scan or an ejection fraction <30%
Muscle	Mild EMG or CK abnormalities	Definite myositis clinically, biochemically, by EMG, or by muscle biopsy
Kidney	Mild hypertension or a serum creatinine 1.5 times normal, or a creatinine clearance >80%, or a 24-hour protein of <500 mg	Refractory hypertension, or a serum creatinine 4 times normal, or a creatinine clearance <20%, or a 24-hour protein >3 gm

From Casas JA, Subauste CP, Alarcon GS: *Ann Rheum Dis* 46:763-767, 1987.
*ECG, electrocardiogram; EMG, electromyogram; CK, creatine kinase; MUGA, multiunit gated acquisition.

Diffuse scleroderma

Initial signs and symptoms. Presenting signs are skin thickening of the hands and/or Raynaud's phenomenon (64%);[116] rheumatic complaints, including arthralgias and stiffness of the knees (30%); or weakness, weight loss, easy fatigability, stiffness, edema, and diffuse musculoskeletal aching.

Skin. The disease typically remains confined to the fingers, hands, and face for months or years but may progress to involve the forearms, legs, and eventually the entire body (Figure 17-16). In both systemic sclerosis and CREST syndrome there are three stages of skin disease: (1) edematous, (2) indurative or sclerotic, and (3) atrophic.[117]

In the edematous phase the skin is thickened and swollen and appears tense, with nonpitting edema producing the classic early signs of a masklike facies and "sausaging" of the fingers. Hand motion is restricted. The disease progresses to the indurative phase, and skin becomes hard, stiff, and bound down. Hand motion is further restricted. Hair loss and anhydrosis reflect fibrosis and degeneration of appendages. Mottled brown pigmented and hypopigmented areas occur on the forearms, upper thorax, chest, and scalp. Ulcerations, telangiectasia, and atrophy gradually appear. The skin of the fingers and hands becomes thin, shiny, smooth, and tightly bound down with the fingers contracted (sclerodactyly: "claw deformity") (Figure 17-17, *A*). The fingers narrow or taper distally, and the terminal phalanges become shortened as a result of distal bone resorption.

Repeated and increasingly severe attacks of Raynaud's phenomenon lead to fingertip ulcerations that leave pitted or star-shaped scars (Figure 17-17, *B*). Facial skin contracts and appears fixed to bone. The nose becomes beak shaped, and the skin about the mouth is drawn into furrows that radiate from the mouth. The curvature of the mouth becomes smaller, and the lips are thinned. Telangiectatic mats appear on the hands, face, and trunk, and dilated capillary loops are found at the proximal nailfold. Atrophy and softening of the dermis eventually make the skin more pliable.

Figure 17-17 Scleroderma (acrosclerosis).

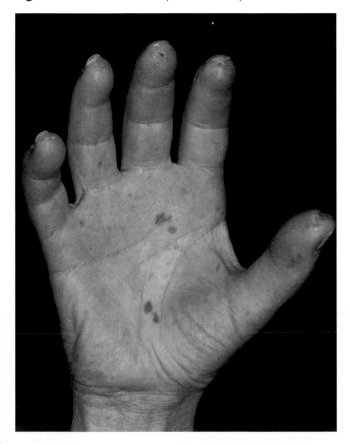

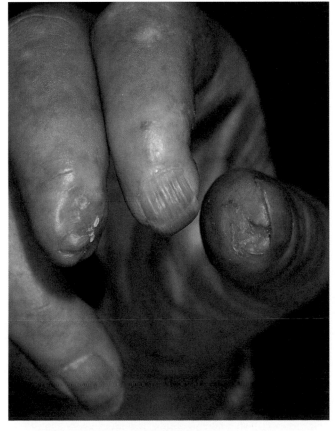

A, The skin is tightly bound down. The fingers are contracted. Telangiectatic mats are evident on the palms. There are fingertip ulcerations.

B, Fingertips are narrowed, and the fingers are shortened as a result of distal bone resorption.

Raynaud's phenomenon. Raynaud's syndrome is a vasospastic disorder precipitated by temperature changes. The term *Raynaud's phenomenon* is used when the changes occur in scleroderma or other connective tissue diseases, and the term *Raynaud's disease* is used when the syndrome occurs in the absence of other conditions. Raynaud's phenomenon is the first symptom of systemic sclerosis in 47% of patients, preceding the onset of sclerodermatous skin changes by several months or years. It occurs during the course of the disease in 90% to 95% of patients.[118] One study showed that 18% of patients with Raynaud's syndrome had systemic sclerosis.[119] The phenomenon does not commonly occur with morphea or other localized forms of scleroderma.

Raynaud's phenomenon represents an episodic vasoconstriction of the digital arteries and arterioles that is precipitated by cold or stress. It is much more common in women. There are three stages during a single episode: pallor (white), in which vasospasm causes the fingers to turn white, cold, numb, and painful; cyanosis (blue), in which relaxation of vasospasm occurs; and hyperemia (red), in which relaxation results in reactive hyperemia and the fingers turn red.

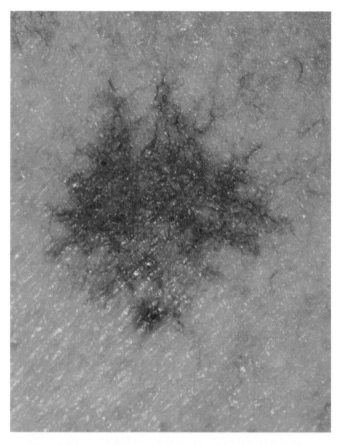

Figure 17-18
Scleroderma. Telangiectatic mats. The telangiectasias of CREST syndrome and scleroderma have a unique morphology. They occur as flat (macular), 0.5-cm, rectangular collections of uniform, tiny vessels.

Nailfold capillary patterns as detected by nailfold capillary microscopy may help distinguish Raynaud's disease (no scleroderma) from Raynaud's phenomenon (associated with scleroderma). A decrease in capillary loops[120,121] occurs in Raynaud's phenomenon. This fact may help to predict which cases of Raynaud's syndrome will evolve into systemic sclerosis.

Telangiectasias. The telangiectasias of CREST syndrome and scleroderma have a unique morphology. They occur as flat (macular), 0.5-cm, rectangular collections of uniform, tiny vessels; these are the so-called telangiectatic mats (Figure 17-18). These mats are most commonly found on the face, lips, palms, and backs of the hands.[122] Telangiectasias may be present around the lips, tongue, and mucous membranes. Involvement of the oral mucosa also suggests Rendu-Osler-Weber disease (hereditary hemorrhagic telangiectasia).

Gastrointestinal tract. Fibrosis and atrophy of smooth muscle can occur in any part of the GI tract. Approximately 10% of patients may have GI symptoms before the appearance of skin changes.[123] Dysphagia is the most common sign of GI involvement.

Esophageal dysfunction with hypomotility, dysphagia, reflux esophagitis, and fibrotic strictures occurs in approximately 90% of patients. Gastroesophageal reflux rather than impaired motility is the major cause of esophageal symptoms.[124] Cinefluoroscopic and manometric studies reveal reduced or absent peristalsis of the lower third of the esophagus. Recently, extremely sensitive, noninvasive scintigraphic procedures have become available for quantitative assessment of esophageal function.[125,126] There is no increased frequency of esophageal carcinoma.[127]

Intestinal dilation and hypoperistalsis are the most common small bowel abnormalities. They lead to a "stagnant loop" syndrome with bacterial overgrowth, malabsorption, and steatorrhea. A characteristic mucosal fold pattern is called the *hide-bound small bowel* of scleroderma.[128] Bleeding gastric telangiectasias located primarily in the upper part of the GI tract can result in severe blood loss.[129] Wide-mouthed sacculations, loss of colonic haustration, and constipation occur with colonic involvement.

Lungs. Lung disease is a frequent cause of death. Abnormal pulmonary function studies with reduced vital and total lung capacity are usually the first signs of lung disease. Dyspnea is the most common symptom; moist basilar rales are the most frequent sign. Interstitial fibrosis and thickening of the alveolar septa are the most common histologic changes. Fibrotic changes typically involve the lower lung fields, and pleural effusions are unusual. A diffuse reticulonodular interstitial pattern in a basilar distribution may be seen in the chest x-ray film. Pulmonary hypertension occurs in 33% of patients.[130]

Kidneys. Renal disease and hypertension are the major causes of death in patients with systemic scleroderma. The appearance of proteinuria, hypertension, or azotemia are poor prognostic signs, and death usually occurs in less than 1 year.[131]

Other organs. Myocardial fibrosis results in arrhythmias, and pulmonary fibrosis leads to pulmonary hypertension and right-sided heart failure. Polyarthralgia or arthritis was among the initial symptoms in 41% of patients.[132,133] Sclerosis of the frenulum may immobilize the tongue. Fibrosis of the minor salivary glands may cause the clinical features of Sjögren's syndrome.

Prognosis. Baseline factors that are most predictive of a poor outcome (rapidly progressive disease and early death) included the presence of abnormal cardiopulmonary signs and abnormal urine sediment (pyuria, hematuria).[134] A subset of patients with scleroderma with antibodies to centromere and histone have severe pulmonary or vascular disease.[135]

CREST syndrome

A more benign, chronic, and localized variant of scleroderma is called *CREST syndrome* (formerly known as *acrosclerosis*). The five clinical features of this disease (calcinosis cutis, Raynaud's phenomenon, esophageal involvement, sclerodactyly, and telangiectasia) are discussed in detail in the section on systemic sclerosis. Calcinosis is a unique feature of CREST.

Calcinosis. Subcutaneous calcinosis occurs most commonly on the palmar aspects of the tips of the fingers. Calcinosis also occurs over the bony prominences of the knees, elbows, spine, and iliac crests. The deposits appear as firm, subcutaneous nodules that may eventually rupture at the surface, discharging fragments of calcium. In response to this foreign material, the skin surrounding the calcium becomes painful, red, and sometimes chronically infected, requiring courses of oral antibiotics.

Although patients with CREST syndrome can progress to more involved systemic disease, those with the clinical and serologic markers of the syndrome have a more benign course than patients with diffuse scleroderma.

The clinical differentiation between CREST syndrome and Osler's disease (telangiectasia hereditaria hemorrhagica) is difficult because telangiectasia may be the most prominent clinical feature in both disorders. However, patients with CREST syndrome usually have anticentromere antibodies in the serum.

Diagnosis of diffuse scleroderma

Specific circulating antibodies are useful in establishing the diagnosis. Most other laboratory studies are nonspecific. (See the box below.)

Autoantibodies. Antinuclear antibodies can be detected in more than 85%-95% of patients with systemic sclerosis. Centromere antibody is found most frequently in patients with limited SSc; they are found in as many as 96% of patients with CREST or acroscleroderma and sclerosis limited to the digits,[136] and in only 21% of patients with diffuse sclerosis[137] (Table 17-12).

The frequency of antibodies in patients with systemic sclerosis is as follows: centromere (21%-32%), Scl-70 (45%), and nucleolar (15%). More than one of the three antibodies is rarely demonstrated in any one serum. One of them is found in two thirds of sera from patients with SSc. Scl-70 antibody is found almost exclusively in sera from patients with extensive SSc (involving the skin of the trunk).[138]

A subset of patients with antibodies to centromere and histone have severe pulmonary or vascular disease.[135]

Other studies. Hypergammaglobulinemia (most often IgG) occurs in approximately 50% of patients. The erythrocyte sedimentation rate (ESR) is elevated (20 to 80) in 60% of cases.[118] There are many other nonspecific findings.

WORKUP FOR DIFFUSE SCLEROSIS

- Deep skin biopsy
- System review
- Office nailfold capillary microscopy
- ANA (centromere)
- Antibodies-SSA (Ro), SSB (La), Sm, nRNP Scl-70
- Organ workup

TABLE 17-12 Immunologic Characteristics of Scleroderma

ANA	Fluorescence	Frequency (%)	Clinical feature
Centromere	Discrete speckles	96	CREST
Scl-70	Fine speckles with or without nucleolar	55	Diffuse scleroderma
Nucleolar	Several nucleolar	60	CREST or diffuse polymyositis, overlap syndromes

Office nailfold capillary microscopy

A technique has been described for characterizing the telangiectasias seen in the proximal nailfold of the various connective tissue diseases. The scleroderma pattern is distinctive and is also seen in dermatomyositis. Familiarity with this technique may help to differentiate patients with lupus and dermatomyositis from patients who have cutaneous eruptions that appear to be similar. The technique used by Minkin and Rabhan[15] is as follows:

A drop of mineral oil is placed on each nailfold. The ophthalmoscope is set at +40, resulting in a ×10 magnification. The instrument is placed close to, but not in touch with, the oil. Generally the capillaries are best seen in the nailfold of the fourth finger. Since the field of observation is smaller

normal

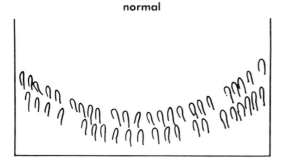

**scleroderma
and dermatomyositis**

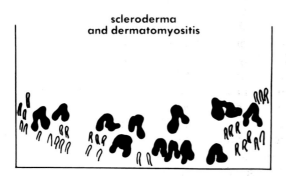

lupus erythematosus

Figure 17-19
Office nailfold capillary microscopy. In normal people the capillaries are seen as fine regular loops. In scleroderma and dermatomyositis the capillary loops are enlarged, deformed, and dilated. Many capillary loops have been lost. In lupus the capillaries are tortuous but there is little dilation of capillary loops. *(From Minkin W, Rabhan NB:* J Am Acad Dermatol *7:190, 1982.)*

Figure 17-20 Nailfold capillary microscopy. Scleroderma, dermatomyositis.

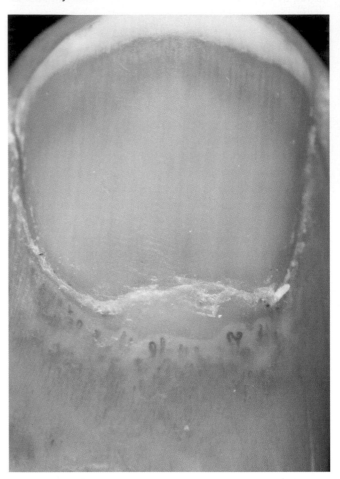

A, The dilated, tortuous capillary loops and avascular areas are obvious.

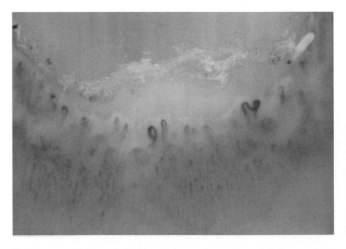

B, Close-up view of *A*. There are enlarged and deformed, dilated capillaries. Loss of capillaries has produced many avascular areas. Normal capillary loops are seen near the bottom of the picture.

than in wide-field microscopy, the ophthalmoscope must be moved over the entire nailfold. A technique for using a television camera to record nailfold capillary characteristics has been described.[139]

Normal. In normal people the capillaries are seen as fine, regular loops with a small, even space between the afferent and efferent limbs, in a row perpendicular to the nail (Figure 17-19).

Overlap syndromes (scleroderma, dermatomyositis). The scleroderma pattern (megacapillaries and/or avascularity) (Figure 17-20) seen in 74% of patients with scleroderma consists of enlarged and deformed capillaries with dilation of both limbs of the loop, which is often engorged with blood ("sausage loop"). There is marked disorganization of the loop arrangement. Loss of capillaries produces many avascular areas and disruption of the orderly appearance of the capillary bed. Patients with Raynaud's phenomenon who present with avascularity and/or a mean of more than two megacapillaries per digit are likely to progress to a scleroderma spectrum disorder.[140-142] The same pattern is seen in 82% of patients with dermatomyositis.

Mixed connective tissue disease. The scleroderma pattern is present in 63%, the lupus pattern in 22%, and 73% have bushy capillary formation. The presence of bushy capillaries suggests mixed connective tissue disease (Figure 17-21).[142]

Lupus. In lupus there are tortuous, "meandering" capillary loops, but there is relatively little dilation of the capillary limbs. At times the loop length is increased and may resemble a renal glomerulus. There is usually some disorganization of the capillary pattern, but only rarely are avascular areas seen.

The changes are distinctive enough that a relatively inexperienced observer can accurately distinguish between patients with scleroderma and those with systemic LE or rheumatoid arthritis.[143] There is a close association between the degree of visible capillary abnormalities and organ involvement.[144]

Treatment

Systemic therapy. Commonly used therapy often hinging on the organ system involved includes colchicine, corticosteroids, calcium channel blockers, angiotensin-inhibiting drugs, and intestinal motility stimulants (cisapride).[145]

Penicillamine (500 to 1500 mg/day) is often the treatment of choice for progressive systemic sclerosis. The clinical response to this agent is variable. It acts by blocking cross-linkages during collagen synthesis.[146] Skin thickness is reduced, and the progression of visceral disease is slowed. An open prospective uncontrolled trial of oral calcitriol (1,25-dihydroxy vitamin D_3) 1.75 μg/day (mean) for 6 to 36 months with systemic sclerosis provided significant clinical improvement.[147] Azathioprine, chlorambucil, cyclosporine, colchicine, corticosteroids, cyclophosphamide, intravenous 5-fluorouracil,[148] potassium *para*-aminobenzoate, and vasodilators are effective in some patients.

Management of cutaneous disease. Cutaneous ulcers are protected with an occlusive dressing such as Duoderm. Ischemic digital-tip ulcers may be protected with a small plastic 'cage.' Infection is signalled by abrupt erythema, swelling, and increased pain and is usually due to staphylococcus. Adequate skin lubrication is difficult to maintain. Patients should bathe less and use moisturizers. Pruritus tends to occur early in the course of diffuse disease, especially over the forearms, and disappears after months or several years. Antipruritic moisturizers such as Sarna lotion may help.

No satisfactory medical approaches to calcinosis have yet been developed. Simple surgical excision may be performed if the overlying skin is intact and is not infiltrated with calcium, which may interfere with wound healing. When skin breakdown and draining fistulous tracts occur from deeper deposits in deeper levels, primary wound closure is not possible. Intense, sterile, inflammatory reactions surrounding hydroxyapatite deposits, along with constitutional symptoms such as low-grade fever, may be dramatically improved by a course of oral colchicine 0.5 mg once or twice daily for 7 to 10 days.

A daily physical therapy program emphasizing full range of motion of all large joints is important.

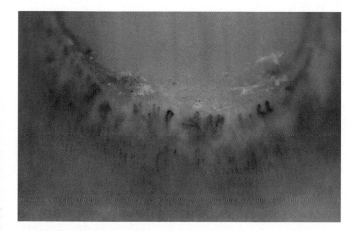

Figure 17-21
Nailfold capillary microscopy. Mixed connective tissue disease. Presence of bushy capillaries is suggestive of mixed connective tissue disease.

LOCALIZED SCLERODERMA

Raynaud's phenomenon, acrosclerosis, or involvement of internal organs does not occur in localized scleroderma. There are three variants: morphea, linear scleroderma, and en coup de sabre.

Morphea

Morphea is more common in females; it can occur at any age but is more common after age 30. Like scleroderma, morphea begins spontaneously and involves thickening or sclerosis of the skin. The two diseases differ in appearance, in the extent of the lesions, and in evolution. Scleroderma appears as a bound-down skin thickening with minor skin color change, progresses to involve large contiguous areas of skin, and does not improve with time. The lesions of morphea begin as one-to-several circumscribed areas of purplish induration (Figure 17-22).

After weeks or months the major portion of the central region of discoloration becomes thickened, firm, hairless, and ivory-colored. The smooth, dull, white, waxy surface is elevated, in contrast to the diffusely bound-down skin of scleroderma. The violaceous or lilac-colored active inflammatory border is a highly characteristic feature of morphea. During the active stage, the round-to-oval plaques slowly extend peripherally but do not increase very much in size. Active lesions persist for 1 to 25 years. Inactive lesions leave their mark. Although much of the induration and skin thickening disappear, previously involved sites may exhibit atrophy and a mottled brown hyperpigmentation at the border and in the previously thickened plaque area (Figure 17-23). The remainder of the lesion becomes hypopigmented.

Multiple small, white plaques (guttate morphea) are a rare form of morphea. Most reported cases are probably cases of lichen sclerosis et atrophicus, and in fact the two diseases may appear simultaneously in the same patient.[149]

Figure 17-22
Morphea. Early lesions with a violaceous or lilac-colored active inflammatory border.

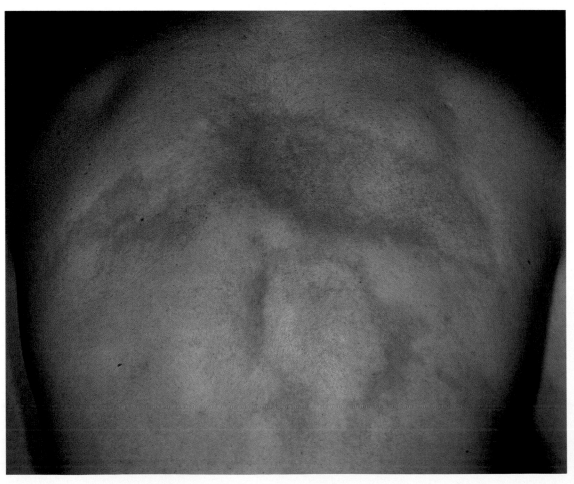

Laboratory diagnosis. Anti-DNA antibodies have been reported in some children. The presence of antihistone antibodies (AHAs) has been demonstrated in localized scleroderma. AHAs were detected in 42% of patients with localized scleroderma and in 87% of patients with generalized morphea.[150,151] The presence of AHAs strongly correlated with the number of morphea lesions, the total number of lesions, and the number of involved areas of the body. ANAs did not correlate with the presence or number of linear lesions. The relationship of morphea to *Borrelia* infection remains undetermined.

Biopsy. The histopathologic features vary with the course of the disease. Early active lesions reveal inflammatory cells in the dermis and subcutaneous tissue. Inflammation is most marked at the violaceous border. The collagen becomes eosinophilic and increases to occupy portions of the subcutaneous fat. Inflammation and sclerosis diminish with time.

Treatment. Asymptomatic plaques should probably be left alone to resolve spontaneously. Topical steroids and occlusion may induce slight improvement.

Inducing atrophy by infiltrating with triamcinolone acetonide (10 mg/ml) may be useful in areas where skin thickening has resulted in discomfort or limitation of motion. Thickened tissue offers great resistance to infiltration, and scattered pitted areas of atrophy rather than a uniform decrease in plaque thickness may result.

Hydroxychloroquine sulfate (200 mg) may be considered for patients who have multiple lesions that on skin biopsy are shown to be in an active inflammatory stage.[152] The adult dosage is 200 mg of hydroxychloroquine twice a day. Induration may be markedly reduced or disappear in 2 to 4 months. The medication should be discontinued after lesions improve. The fundi should be examined by an ophthalmologist before antimalarials are started and should be monitored periodically. Oral calcitriol (1,25 dihydroxy vitamin D_3) 0.50 to 0.75 μg for 3 to 7 months showed a beneficial effect in generalized morphea during an open study.[153] Rapidly deteriorating, generalized morphea has been helped with sulfasalazine (Azulfidine) 1 to 4 gm/day.[154]

Figure 17-23
Morphea. Inactive disease with atrophy and mottled hyperpigmentation.

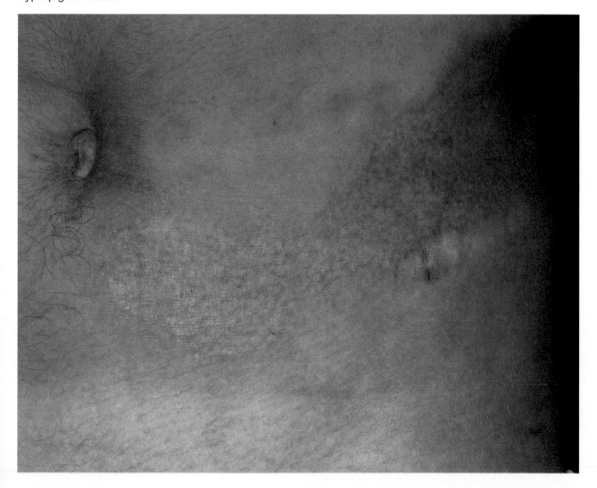

Linear scleroderma

Lesions of linear scleroderma have bands of sclerotic skin that often cross joint lines and lead to mild, but occasionally severe and disabling, joint contractures. Unlike oval plaque morphea, the inflammatory and fibrotic process may involve the underlying subcutaneous tissue and muscle, causing the fibrotic band to be more firmly anchored (Figure 17-24). One large study provides the following data.[155] The female-to-male ratio is 4:1, and 83% of patients are under age 25 when the disease begins. Trauma to the involved site precedes the lesions in 23% of cases. The onset is usually slow and insidious. Most lesions occur on the extremities, and two or more lesions appear simultaneously (61%), often bilaterally (46%). Joint contractures occur in 56% of patients. The typical patient has active disease for 2 to 3 years.

Laboratory. In one study, peripheral blood eosinophilia (200 to 2500 cells/mm^3) occurred in 50% of patients with early active disease and declined with time.[156] The frequency of antinuclear antibodies (HEp-2 cells) was 46%. Antibodies to single-stranded DNA were present in 50% of patients and were more common in those with joint contractures and disease duration of greater than 2 years, but the level of antibody does not correlate with extent of disease.[157] Morphea occurred in 50% of patients.

Treatment. Early and continued physical therapy is crucial to maintain adequate joint motion.

En coup de sabre

The most distinctive form of localized scleroderma is morphea of the frontoparietal face and scalp regions, called *en coup de sabre*, so named because it appears that the blade of a sabre has struck a sharp, deep, vertical line on the face (Figure 17-25). The involved site may show all of the features of morphea. In time, atrophy of one side of the face may occur, giving the impression that a blade was turned to the side to remove a thickness of skin after landing vertically.

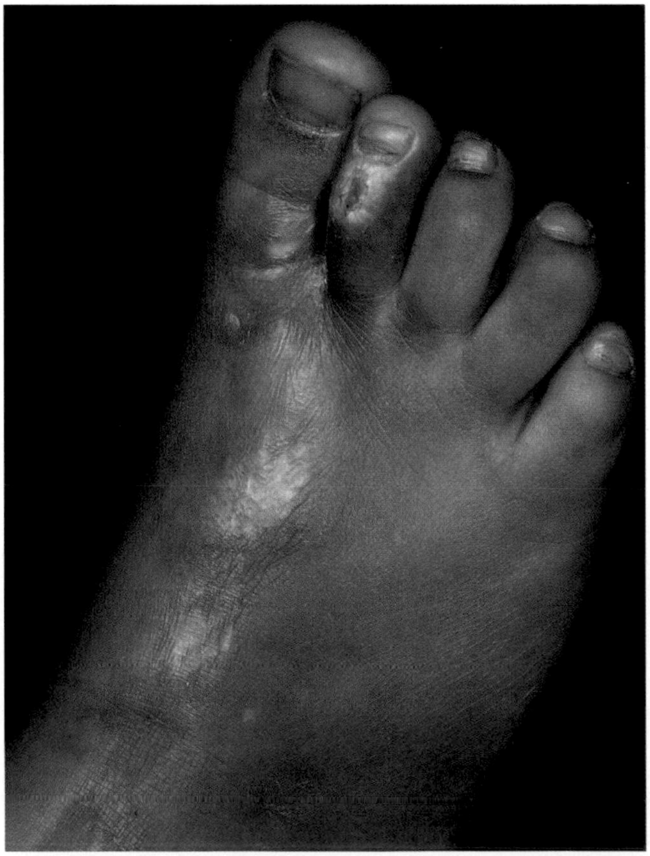

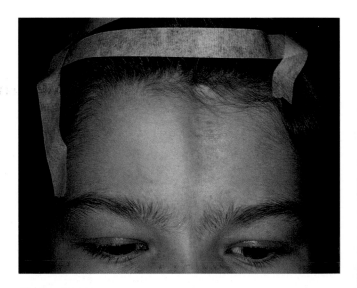

Figure 17-25
Morphea "en coup de sabre."

Figure 17-24
Morphea. Linear pattern.

REFERENCES

1. Provost TT: Subsets in systemic lupus erythematosus: review article, *J Invest Dermatol* 72:110-113, 1979.
2. Tan EM et al: The 1982 revised criteria for the classification of systemic lupus erythematosus, *Arthritis Rheum* 25:1271-1277, 1982.
3. Gilliam JN, Sontheimer RD: Distinctive cutaneous subsets in the spectrum of lupus erythematosus, *J Am Acad Dermatol* 4:471-475, 1981.
4. O'Loughlin S, Schroeter AL, Jordan RE: Study of lupus erythematosus with particular reference to generalized discoid lupus, *Br J Dermatol* 99:1-11, 1978.
5. George PM, Tunnessen W Jr: Childhood discoid lupus erythematosus, *Arch Dermatol* 129:613-617, 1993.
6. de Berker D, Dissaneyeka M, et al: The sequelae of chronic cutaneous lupus erythematosus, *Lupus* 1:181-186, 1992.
7. Wilson CL, Burge SM, et al: Scarring alopecia in discoid lupus erythematosus, *Br J Dermatol* 126:307-314, 1992.
8. Uitto J et al: Verrucous lesions in patients with discoid lupus erythematosus, *Br J Dermatol* 98:507-520, 1978.
9. Callen JP, Fowler JF, Kulick KB: Serologic and clinical features of patients with discoid lupus erythematosus: relationship of antibodies to single-stranded deoxyribonucleic acid and of other antinuclear antibody subsets to clinical manifestations, *J Am Acad Dermatol* 13:748-755, 1985.
10. Sontheimer RD, Thomas JR, Gilliam JN: Subacute cutaneous lupus erythematosus: a cutaneous marker for a distinctive lupus erythematosus subset, *Arch Dermatol* 115:1409-1415, 1979.
11. Reed BR et al: Subacute cutaneous lupus erythematosus associated with hydrochlorothiazide therapy, *Ann Intern Med* 103:49-51, 1985.
12. Callen JP, Kulick KB, Stelzer G, et al: Subacute cutaneous lupus erythematosus: clinical, serologic, and immunogenetic studies of forty-nine patients seen in a nonreferral setting, *J Am Acad Dermatol* 15:1227-1237, 1986.
13. Tuffanelli DL, DuBois EL: Cutaneous manifestations of systemic lupus erythematosus, *Arch Dermatol* 90:377, 1964.
14. Petri M, Howard D, et al: Frequency of lupus flare in pregnancy. The Hopkins Lupus Pregnancy Center experience, *Arthritis Rheum* 34:1538-1545, 1991.
15. Minkin W, Rabhan NB: Office nail fold capillary microscopy using ophthalmoscope, *J Am Acad Dermatol* 7:190-193, 1982.
16. O'Loughlin, Schroeter AL, Jordan RE: Chronic urticaria-like lesions in systemic lupus erythematosus, *Arch Dermatol* 114:879-883, 1978.
17. Sanchez NP et al: The clinical and histopathologic spectrums of urticarial vasculitis: study of forty cases, *J Am Acad Dermatol* 7:599-605, 1982.
18. Christian CL, Sergent JS: Vasculitis syndromes: clinical and experimental models, *Am J Med* 61:385-392, 1976.
19. Kallenberg CGM, Wouda AA: The systemic involvement and immunologic findings in patients presenting with Raynaud's phenomenon, *Am J Med* 69:675-680, 1980.
20. Litwin A, Adams LE, Zimmer H, et al: Immunologic effects of hydralazine in hypertensive patients, *Arthritis Rheum* 24:1074-1078, 1981.
21. Uetrecht JP: The role of leukocyte-generated reactive metabolites in the pathogenesis of idiosyncratic drug reactions, *Drug Metab Rev* 24:299-366, 1992.
22. Rubin RL: Autoantibody specificity in drug-induced lupus and neutrophil-mediated metabolism of lupus-inducing drugs, *Clin Biochem* 25:223-234, 1992.
23. Hofstra AH, Uetrecht JP: Reactive intermediates in the oxidation of hydralazine by HOCl: the major oxidant generated by neutrophils, *Chem Biol Interact* 89:183-196, 1993.
24. Provost TT, Watson R, Gaither KK, et al: The neonatal lupus erythematosus syndrome, *J Rheumatol* 14 (suppl 13):199-205, 1987.
25. Totoritis MC, Rubin RL: Drug-induced lupus: genetic, clinical and laboratory features, *Postgrad Med* 78:149-161, 1985.
26. Cush JJ, Goldings EA: Southwestern internal medicine conference: Drug-induced lupus: clinical spectrum and pathogenesis, *Am J Med Sci* 290:36-45, 1985.
27. Totoritis MC, Tan EM, McNally EM, et al: Association of antibody to histone complex H2A-H2B with symptomatic procainamide-induced lupus, *N Engl J Med* 318:1431-1436, 1988.
28. Hess E: Drug-related lupus (editorial), *N Engl J Med* 31:1460, 1988.
29. Reidenberg MM et al: Acetylator phenotype in idiopathic systemic lupus erythematosus, *Arthritis Rheum* 23:569-573, 1980.
30. Rothfield N: Current approach to SLE and its subsets, *Dis Mon*, October 1982.
31. Lee LA: Neonatal lupus erythematosus, *J Invest Dermatol* 100:9S-13S, 1993.
32. Lee LA: Maternal autoantibodies and pregnancy—II: The neonatal lupus syndrome, *Baillieres Clin Rheumatol* 4:69-84, 1990.
33. Alexander E, Buyon JP, et al: Anti-Ro/SS-A antibodies in the pathophysiology of congenital heart block in neonatal lupus syndrome, an experimental model. In vitro electrophysiologic and immunocytochemical studies, *Arthritis Rheum* 35:176-189, 1992.
34. McCune AB, Weston WL, Lee LA: Maternal and fetal outcome in neonatal lupus erythematosus, *Ann Intern Med* 106:518-523, 1987.
35. Ivarellos A et al: Relationship of HLA-DR and MT antigens to autoantibody expression in systemic lupus erythematosus, *Arthritis Rheum* 26:1533-1535, 1983.
36. Smith CD, Marino C, Rothfield NF: The clinical utility of the lupus band test, *Arthritis Rheum* 27:382-387, 1984.
37. Goldstein R, Thompson FE, McKendry RJR: Diagnostic and predictive value of the lupus band test in undifferentiated connective tissue disease: a followup study, *J Rheumatol* 12:1093-1096, 1985.
38. Chieregato G, Peroni A, et al: Effects of hydroxychloroquine on 'band test' in discoid lupus erythematosus, *Dermatologica* 180:130-132, 1990.
39. Jacobs MI, Schned ES, Bystryn J-C: Variability of the lupus band test, *Arch Dermatol* 119:883-889, 1983.
40. Lehmann P, Holzle E, et al: Experimental reproduction of skin lesions in lupus erythematosus by UVA and UVB radiation, *J Am Acad Dermatol* 22:181-187, 1990.
41. Callen JP, Roth DE, et al: Safety and efficacy of a broad-spectrum sunscreen in patients with discoid or subacute cutaneous lupus erythematosus, *Cutis* 47:130-132, 1991.
42. Dubois EL: Antimalarials in the management of discoid and systemic lupus erythematosus, *Semin Arthritis Rheum* 8:33-51, 1978.
43. Weiss JS: Antimalarial medications in dermatology. A review, *Dermatol Clin* 9:377-385, 1991.
44. Olansky AJ: Antimalarials and ophthalmologic safety, *J Am Acad Dermatol* 6:19-23, 1982.
45. Potter B: Hydroxychloroquine, *Cutis* 52:229-231, 1993.
46. Weiner A, Sandberg MA, et al: Hydroxychloroquine retinopathy, *Am J Ophthalmol* 112:528-534, 1991.
47. The Canadian Hydroxychloroquine Study Group: A randomized study of the effect of withdrawing hydroxychloroquine sulfate in systemic lupus erythematosus, *N Engl J Med* 324:150-154, 1991.
48. Coburn PR, Shuster D: Dapsone and discoid lupus erythematosus, *Br J Dermatol* 106:105-106, 1982.
49. Ruzicka T, Goerz G: Dapsone in the treatment of lupus erythematosus, *Br J Dermatol* 104:53-56, 1981.
50. Hall RP et al: Bullous eruption of systemic lupus erythematosus—dramatic response to dapsone therapy, *Ann Intern Med* 97:167-170, 1982.
51. Matthews CNA, Saihan EM, Warin RP: Urticarial-like lesions associated with systemic lupus erythematosus: response to dapsone, *Br J Dermatol* 99:455-457, 1978.
52. Holtman JH, Neustadt DH, et al: Dapsone is an effective therapy for the skin lesions of subacute cutaneous lupus erythematosus and urticarial vasculitis in a patient with C2 deficiency, *J Rheumatol* 17:1222-1225, 1990.
53. Lindskov R, Reymann F: Dapsone in the treatment of cutaneous lupus erythematosus, *Dermatologica* 172:214-217, 1986.
54. Tsokos GC, Caughman SW, Klippel JH: Successful treatment of generalized discoid skin lesions with azathioprine, *Arch Dermatol* 121:1323-1325, 1985.

55. Shehade S: Successful treatment of generalized discoid skin lesions with azathioprine, *Arch Dermatol* 122:376-377, 1986.

56. Callen JP, Spencer LV, et al: Azathioprine. An effective, corticosteroid-sparing therapy for patients with recalcitrant cutaneous lupus erythematosus or with recalcitrant cutaneous leukocytoclastic vasculitis, *Arch Dermatol* 127:515-522, 1991.

57. Hasper MF: Chronic cutaneous lupus erythematosus, *Arch Dermatol* 119:812-815, 1983.

58. Knop J et al: Thalidomide in the treatment of sixty cases of chronic discoid lupus erythematosus, *Br J Dermatol* 108:461-466, 1983.

59. Atra E, Sato EI: Treatment of the cutaneous lesions of systemic lupus erythematosus with thalidomide, *Clin Exp Rheumatol* 11:487-493, 1993.

60. Ruzicka T, Sommerburg C, et al: Treatment of cutaneous lupus erythematosus with acitretin and hydroxychloroquine, *Br J Dermatol* 127:513-518, 1992.

61. Newton RC et al: Mechanism-oriented assessment of isotretinoin in chronic or subacute cutaneous lupus erythematosus, *Arch Dermatol* 122:170-176, 1986.

62. Shornick JK, Formica N, et al: Isotretinoin for refractory lupus erythematosus, *J Am Acad Dermatol* 24:49-52, 1991.

63. Green SG, Piette WW: Successful treatment of hypertrophic lupus erythematosus with isotretinoin, *J Am Acad Dermatol* 17:364-368, 1987.

64. Rubenstein DJ, Huntley AC: Keratotic lupus erythematosus: treatment with isotretinoin, *J Am Acad Dermatol* 14:910-914, 1986.

65. Wilke WS, Krall PL, et al: Methotrexate for systemic lupus erythematosus: a retrospective analysis of 17 unselected cases, *Clin Exp Rheumatol* 9:581-587, 1991.

66. White SD, Rosychuk RA, et al: Use of tetracycline and niacinamide for treatment of autoimmune skin disease in 31 dogs, *J Am Vet Med Assoc* 200:1497-1500, 1992.

67. Kissel JT, Mendell JR, Rammohan KW: Microvascular deposition of complement membrane attack complex in dermatomyositis, *N Engl J Med* 314:329-334, 1986.

68. Kissel JT, Halterman RK, et al: The relationship of complement-mediated microvasculopathy to the histologic features and clinical duration of disease in dermatomyositis, *Arch Neurol* 48:26-30, 1991.

69. Pearson CM, Bohan A: The spectrum of dermatomyositis. Symposium on rheumatic diseases, *Med Clin North Am* 61:439-457, 1977.

70. Bohan A, Peter JB, Bowman RL, et al: A computer-assisted analysis of 153 patients with polymyositis and dermatomyositis, *Medicine* 56:255-286, 1977.

71. Hoffman GS et al: Presentation, treatment and prognosis of idiopathic inflammatory muscle disease in a rural hospital, *Am J Med* 75:433-438, 1983.

72. Callen JP: Dermatomyositis, *Dis Mon* 33:305-327, 1987.

73. Hochberg MC, Feldman D, Stevens MB: Adult onset polymyositis/dermatomyositis: an analysis of clinical and laboratory features and survival in 76 patients with a review of the literature, *Semin Arthritis Rheu* 15:168-178, 1986.

74. Rockerbie NR et al: Cutaneous changes of dermatomyositis precede muscle weakness, *J Am Acad Dermatol* 20:629-632, 1989.

75. Stonecipher MR, Jorizzo JL, et al: Cutaneous changes of dermatomyositis in patients with normal muscle enzymes: dermatomyositis sine myositis? *J Am Acad Dermatol* 28:951-956, 1993.

76. King L Jr, Park JH, et al: Evaluation of muscles in a patient with suspected amyopathic dermatomyositis by magnetic resonance imaging and phosphorus-31-spectroscopy, *J Am Acad Dermatol* 30:137-138, 1994.

77. Euwer RL, Sontheimer RD: Amyopathic dermatomyositis: a review, *J Invest Dermatol* 100:124S-127S, 1993.

78. Euwer RL, Sontheimer RD: Amyopathic dermatomyositis (dermatomyositis sine myositis). Presentation of six new cases and review of the literature, *J Am Acad Dermatol* 24:959-966, 1991.

79. Kasteler JS, Callen JP: Scalp involvement in dermatomyositis: often overlooked or misdiagnosed, *JAMA* 272:1939, 1994.

80. Sigurgeirsson B, Lindelof B, et al: Risk of cancer in patients with dermatomyositis or polymyositis. A population-based study, *N Engl J Med* 326:363-367, 1992.

81. Bonnetblanc JM, Bernard P, et al: Dermatomyositis and malignancy. A multicenter cooperative study, *Dermatologica* 180:212-216, 1990.

82. Manchul LE et al: The frequency of malignant neoplasms in patients with polymyositis-dermatomyositis: a controlled study, *Arch Intern Med* 145:1835-1839, 1985.

83. Bohan A, Peter JB: Polymyositis and dermatomyositis, *N Engl J Med* 292:344-347, 1975.

84. Barnes BE: Dermatomyositis and malignancy: a review of the literature, *Ann Intern Med* 84:68-76, 1976.

85. Masters R: Case records of the Massachusetts General Hospital. Case 33 1977, *N Engl J Med* 297:378-383, 1977.

86. Pachman LM: Juvenile dermatomyositis: a clinical overview, *Pediatr Rev* 12:117-125, 1990.

87. Moore EC, Cohen F, et al: Staphylococcal infections in childhood dermatomyositis—association with the development of calcinosis, raised IgE concentrations and granulocyte chemotactic defect, *Ann Rheum Dis* 51:378-383, 1992.

88. Hiketa T, Matsumoto Y, et al: Juvenile dermatomyositis: a statistical study of 114 patients with dermatomyositis, *J Dermatol* 19:470-476, 1992.

89. Ansell BM: Juvenile dermatomyositis, *J Rheumatol Suppl* 33:60-62, 1992.

90. Spencer CH et al: Course of treated juvenile dermatomyositis, *J Pediatr* 105:399-408, 1984.

91. Miller LC, Michael AF, Kim Y: Childhood dermatomyositis, *Clin Pediatr* 26:561-566, 1987.

92. Tymms KE, Webb J: Dermatopolymyositis and other connective tissue diseases: a review of 105 cases, *J Rheumatol* 12:1140-1148, 1985.

93. Tymms KE, Beller EM, et al: Correlation between tests of muscle involvement and clinical muscle weakness in polymyositis and dermatomyositis, *Clin Rheumatol* 9:523-529, 1990.

94. Fraser DD, Frank JA, Dalakas M: Magnetic resonance imaging in the idiopathic inflammatory myopathies, *J Rheumatol* 18:1693-1699, 1991.

95. Park JH et al: MRI and P-31 magnetic resonance spectroscopy provide unique quantitative data useful in the longitudinal management of patients with dermatomyositis, *Arthritis Rheum* 37:736-746, 1994.

96. Carpenter S, Karpati G: The pathological diagnosis of specific inflammatory myopathies, *Brain Pathol* 2:13-19, 1992.

97. Callen JP: The value of malignancy evaluation in patients with dermatomyositis, *J Am Acad Dermatol* 6:253-259, 1982.

98. Miller LC, Sisson BA, et al: Methotrexate treatment of recalcitrant childhood dermatomyositis, *Arthritis Rheum* 35:1143-1149, 1992.

99. Sinoway PA, Callen JP: Chlorambucil: an effective corticosteroid-sparing agent for patients with recalcitrant dermatomyositis, *Arthritis Rheum* 36:319-324, 1993.

100. Ramirez G, Asherson RA, et al: Adult-onset polymyositis-dermatomyositis: description of 25 patients with emphasis on treatment, *Semin Arthritis Rheum* 20:114-120, 1990.

101. Zieglschmid-Adams ME et al: Treatment of dermatomyositis with methotrexate, *J Am Acad Dermatol* 32:754-757, 1995.

102. Woo TY et al: Cutaneous lesions of dermatomyositis are improved by hydroxychloroquine, *J Am Acad Dermatol* 10:592-600, 1984.

103. James WD, Dawson N, Rodman OG: The treatment of dermatomyositis with hydroxychloroquine, *J Rheumatol* 12:1214-1216, 1985.

104. Barron KS, Sher MR, et al: Intravenous immunoglobulin therapy: magic or black magic, *J Rheumatol Suppl* 33:94-97, 1992.

105. Lang BA, Laxer RM, et al: Treatment of dermatomyositis with intravenous gammaglobulin, *Am J Med* 91:169-172, 1991.

106. Dalakas MC, Illa I, et al: A controlled trial of high-dose intravenous immune globulin infusions as treatment for dermatomyositis, *N Engl J Med* 329:1993-2000, 1993.

107. Cherin P, Herson S, et al: Efficacy of intravenous gammaglobulin therapy in chronic refractory polymyositis and dermatomyositis: an open study with 20 adult patients, *Am J Med* 91:162-168, 1991.

108. Cherin P et al: Intravenous gammaglobulin as first line therapy in polymyositis and dermatomyositis: an open study of 11 adult patients, *J Rheumatol* 21:1092-1097, 1994.

109. Grau JM et al: Cyclosporine A as first choice therapy for dermatomyositis, *J Rheumatol* 21:381-382, 1994.

110. Pistoia V, Buoncompagni A, et al: Cyclosporin A in the treatment of juvenile chronic arthritis and childhood polymyositis-dermatomyositis. Results of a preliminary study, *Clin Exp Rheumatol* 11:203-208, 1993.

111. Hamill G, Saunders C, et al: "Catch-up" growth in steroid dependent dermatomyositis treated with cyclosporin-A, *Eur J Med* 1:16-18, 1992.

112. Fudman EJ, Schnitzer TJ: Dermatomyositis without creatine kinase elevation: a poor prognostic sign, *Am J Med* 80:329-332, 1986.

113. Rodman GP: When is scleroderma not scleroderma? The differential diagnosis of progressive systemic sclerosis, *Bull Rheum Dis* 31:7-10, 1981.

114. Haustein UF, Ziegler V, et al: Chemically-induced scleroderma, *Hautarzt* 43:469-474, 1992.

115. Pelmear PL, Roos JO, et al: Occupationally induced scleroderma, *J Occup Med* 34:20-25, 1992.

116. Rodman GP: The natural history of progressive systemic sclerosis, (diffuse scleroderma), *Bull Rheum Dis* 13:301-304, 1963.

117. Rocco VK, Hurd ER: Scleroderma and scleroderma-like disorders, *Semin Arthritis Rheum* 16:22-69, 1986.

118. Tuffanelli DL, Winkelmann RK: Systemic scleroderma: a clinical study of 727 cases, *Arch Dermatol* 84:359-371, 1961.

119. Blunt RJ, Porter JM: Raynaud syndrome, *Semin Arthritis Rheum* 10:281-308, 1981.

120. Houtman PM, Kallenberg CGM, Fidler V, et al: Diagnostic significance of nailfold capillary patterns in patients with Raynaud's phenomenon, *J Rheumatol* 13:556-563, 1986.

121. Lee P et al: Digital blood flow and nailfold capillary microscopy in Raynaud's phenomenon, *J Rheumatol* 13:564-569, 1986.

122. Braverman IM: *Skin signs of systemic disease*, ed 2, Philadelphia, 1981, WB Saunders.

123. Kinder RR, Fleischman R: Systemic scleroderma: a review of organ systems, *Int J Dermatol* 13:362-395, 1974.

124. Orringer MB et al: Gastroesophageal reflux in esophageal scleroderma: diagnosis and implications, *Ann Thorac Surg* 21:601-606, 1976.

125. Davidson A, Russell C, Littlejohn GO: Assessment of esophageal abnormalities in progressive systemic sclerosis using radionuclide transit, *J Rheumatol* 12:472-477, 1985.

126. Carette S, Lacourciere Y, Lavoie S, et al: Radionuclide esophageal transit in progressive systemic sclerosis, *J Rheumatol* 12:478-481, 1985.

127. Segel MC, Campbell WL, Medsger TA Jr, et al: Systemic sclerosis (scleroderma) and esophageal adenocarcinoma: Is increased patient screening necessary? *Gastroenterology* 89:485-488, 1985.

128. Horowitz AL, Meyers MA: The "hide-bound" small bowel of scleroderma: characteristic mucosal fold pattern, *Am J Roentgen Rad Ther Nucl Med* 119:332-334, 1973.

129. Allende HD, Ona FV, Noronha AI: Bleeding gastric telangiectasia. Complication of Raynaud's phenomenon, esophageal motor dysfunction, sclerodactyly, and telangiectasia (REST) syndrome, *Am J Gastroenterol* 75:354-356, 1981.

130. Ungerer RG et al: Prevalence and clinical correlates of pulmonary arterial hypertension in progressive systemic sclerosis, *Am J Med* 75:65-74, 1983.

131. Cannon PJ et al: The relationship of hypertension and renal failure in scleroderma (progressive systemic sclerosis) to structural and functional abnormalities of the renal cortical circulation, *Medicine* 53:1-46, 1974.

132. Rodman GP, Medsger TA Jr: The rheumatic manifestations of progressive systemic sclerosis (scleroderma), *Clin Orthop* 57:81-93, 1968.

133. Rodman GP, Medsger TA Jr: Musculoskeletal involvement in progressive systemic sclerosis (scleroderma), *Bull Rheum Dis* 17:419-422, 1966.

134. Bulpitt KJ, Clements PJ, et al: Early undifferentiated connective tissue disease: III. Outcome and prognostic indicators in early scleroderma (systemic sclerosis), *Ann Intern Med* 118:602-609, 1993.

135. Martin L, Pauls JD, et al: Identification of a subset of patients with scleroderma with severe pulmonary and vascular disease by the presence of autoantibodies to centromere and histone, *Ann Rheum Dis* 52:780-784, 1993.

136. Tuffanelli DL et al: Anticentromere and anticentriole antibodies in the scleroderma spectrum, *Arch Dermatol* 119:560-566, 1983.

137. Giordano M et al: Different antibody patterns and different prognosis in patients with scleroderma with various extent of skin sclerosis, *J Rheumatol* 13:911-916, 1986.

138. Ullman S, Halberg P, et al: Serology in patients with scleroderma, *Ugeskr Laeger* 155:472-476, 1993.

139. Studer A, Hunziker T, et al: Quantitative nailfold capillary microscopy in cutaneous and systemic lupus erythematosus and localized and systemic scleroderma, *J Am Acad Dermatol* 24:941-945, 1991.

140. Zufferey P, Depairon M, et al: Prognostic significance of nailfold capillary microscopy in patients with Raynaud's phenomenon and scleroderma-pattern abnormalities. A six-year follow-up study, *Clin Rheumatol* 11:536-541, 1992.

141. Maricq HR: Capillary abnormalities, Raynaud's phenomenon, and systemic sclerosis in patients with localized scleroderma, *Arch Dermatol* 128:630-632, 1992.

142. Granier F, Vayssairat M, Priollet P, et al: Nailfold capillary microscopy in mixed connective tissue disease, *Arthritis Rheum* 29:189-195, 1986.

143. McGill NW, Gow PJ: Nailfold capillaroscopy: A blinded study of its discriminatory value in scleroderma, systemic lupus erythematosus, and rheumatoid arthritis, *Aust NZ J Med* 16:457-460, 1986.

144. Schmidt K-U, Mensing H: Are nailfold capillary changes indicators of organ involvement in progressive systemic sclerosis? *Dermatologica* 176:18-21, 1988.

145. Perez MI, Kohn SR: Systemic sclerosis, *J Am Acad Dermatol* 28:525-547, 1993.

146. Steen VD, Medsger TA Jr, Rodnan GP: D-Penicillamine therapy in progressive systemic sclerosis (scleroderma), *Ann Intern Med* 97:652-659, 1982.

147. Humbert P et al: Treatment of scleroderma with oral 1,25-dihydroxy vitamin D_3: evaluation of skin involvement using noninvasive techniques, *Acta Derm Venerol (Stockh)*, 73:449-451, 1993.

148. Casas JA, Subauste CP, Alarcon GS: A new promising treatment in systemic sclerosis: 5-fluorouracil, *Ann Rheum Dis* 46:763-767, 1987.

149. Uitto J, Santa Cruz DJ, Bauer EA: Morphea and lichen sclerosus et atrophicus, *J Am Acad Dermatol* 3:271-279, 1980.

150. Sato S et al: Clinical characteristics associated with antihistone antibodies in patients with localized scleroderma, *J Am Acad Dermatol* 31:567-571, 1994.

151. Sato S et al: Antigen specificity of antihistone antibodies in localized scleroderma, *Arch Dermatol* 130:1273-1277, 1994.

152. Winkelmann RK: Localized cutaneous scleroderma, *Semin Dermatol* 4:90-103, 1985.

153. Hulshof MM et al: Oral calcitriol as a new therapeutic modality for generalized morphea, *Arch Dermatol* 130:1290-1293, 1994.

154. Czarnecki DB, Taft EH: Generalized morphea successfully treated with salazopyrin, *Acta Derm Venereol* (Stockh) 62:81-82, 1982.

155. Falanga V, Medsger TA Jr, Reichlin M, et al: Linear scleroderma. Clinical spectrum, prognosis, and laboratory abnormalities, *Ann Intern Med* 104:849-857, 1986.

156. Falanga V, Medsger TA Jr: Frequency, levels, and significance of blood eosinophilia in systemic sclerosis, localized scleroderma, and eosinophilic fasciitis, *J Am Acad Dermatol* 17:648-656, 1987.

157. Falanga V, Medsger TA, Reichlin M: High titers of antibodies to single-stranded DNA in linear scleroderma, *Arch Dermatol* 121:345-347, 1985.

CHAPTER EIGHTEEN

Hypersensitivity Syndromes and Vasculitis

An overview of the hypersensitivity and vasculitic syndromes is presented on pp. 568 and 569.

Erythema Multiforme

Erythema multiforme (EM) is a relatively common, acute, often recurrent inflammatory disease.[1] Many factors have been implicated in the etiology of EM, including numerous infectious agents, drugs, connective tissue diseases, physical agents, x-ray therapy, pregnancy, and internal malignancies. In approximately 50% of cases no cause can be found. EM is commonly associated with a preceding herpes simplex or mycoplasma infection, such as primary atypical pneumonia.

Herpes-associated recurrent erythema multiforme. Only a few of the many individuals who experience recurrent herpes simplex virus infection also develop herpes-associated EM. Some adults and children[2] develop EM after each episode of herpes simplex.[3,4] A difference in the HSV-specific immune response does not explain this phenomenon.[5]

Skin biopsies of EM lesions[6] from patients with recurrent disease showed HSV-specific DNA in most cases.[7,8]

Pathogenesis

Recent studies suggest that immune complex formation and subsequent deposition in the cutaneous microvasculature may play a role in the pathogenesis of EM.[9] Circulating complexes and deposition of C3, IgM, and fibrin around the upper dermal blood vessels have been found in the majority of patients with EM.[10] Histologically, a mononuclear cell infiltrate is present about these same upper dermal blood vessels; in the other immune complex–mediated cutaneous vasculitis (leukocytoclastic vasculitis), polymorphonuclear leukocytes are present.

Clinical manifestations

The prodromal symptoms, morphologic configuration of the lesions, and intensity of systemic symptoms vary. Milder forms of the disease may be preceded by malaise, fever, or itching and burning at the site where the eruption will occur. The cutaneous eruptions are most distinctive, and classification is based on their form.

Target lesions and papules. Target lesions and papules are the most characteristic eruptions. Dusky red, round maculopapules appear suddenly in a symmetric pattern on the backs of the hands and feet and the extensor aspect of the forearms and legs. The trunk may be involved in more severe cases. Early lesions itch, burn, or are asymptomatic. The diagnosis may not be suspected until the nonspecific early lesions evolve into target lesions during a 24- to 48-hour period (Figures 18-1 and 18-2). The classic "iris" or target lesion results from centrifugal spread of the red maculopapule to a circumference of 1 to 3 cm as the center becomes cyanotic, purpuric, or vesicular. Partially formed targets with annular borders or target lesions on the palms and soles are less distinctive and clinically resemble urticaria. Individual lesions heal in 1 or 2 weeks without scarring but with hypopigmentation or hyperpigmentation, while new lesions appear in crops. Bullae and erosions may be present in the oral cavity. The entire episode lasts for approximately 1 month.

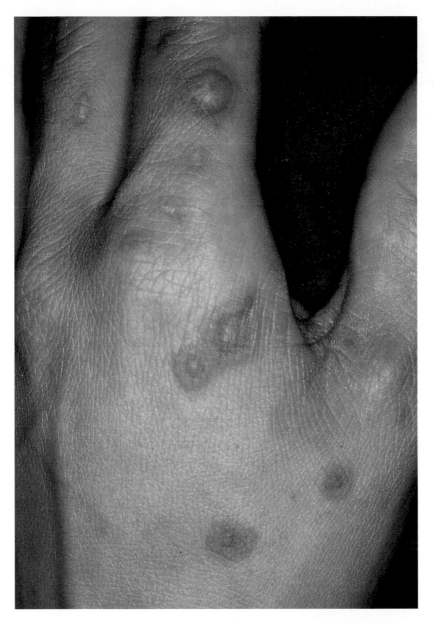

Figure 18-1
Erythema multiforme. Classic iris lesions.

Figure 18-2
Erythema multiforme. An episode may be precipitated by herpes simplex infection.

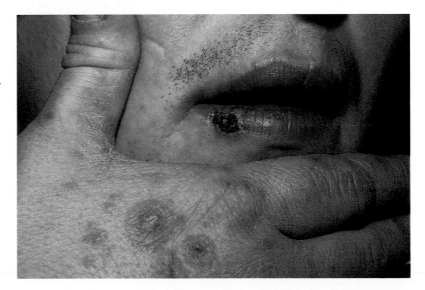

HYPERSENSITIVITY SYNDROMES

Erythema Multiforme	Stevens-Johnson Syndrome	Toxic Epidermal Necrolysis	Erythema Nodosum	Sweet's Syndrome (Acute febrile neutrophilic dermatosis)

Herpes simplex
Mycoplasm pneu-
  moniae
Other infections
Drugs
Malignancies
Others

Drugs
  Phenytoin
  Phenobarbital
  Sulfonamides
  Penicillins
  Others
Infections

Drugs
  Phenytoin
  Phenobarbital
  Sulfonamides
  Ampicillin
  Allopurinol
  Thiacetazone
  Isoniazid
  NSAIDS
Others

Infections
  Streptococci
  Tuberculosis
  *Coccidioido-
    mycosis*
  Others
Drugs
  Sulfonamides
  Oral contracep-
    tives
Systemic illness
  Sarcoidosis
  Ulcerative colitis
  Crohn's disease
  Lymphoma
  Leukemia
Pregnancy

Infections
Autoimmune
  disorders
Lymphoma
Solid tumors

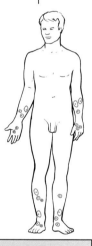
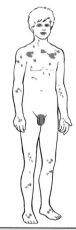
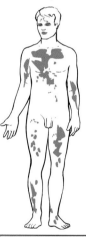
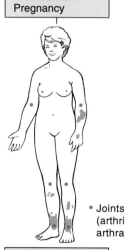
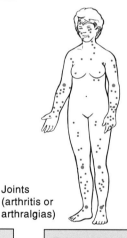

• Joints
  (arthritis or
  arthralgias)

Age 20-40
Prodrome
Few symptoms

Urticarial papules
Target lesions or
  vesicles and
  bullae
  Backs of hands
  Palms
  Soles
  Extensor limbs
  Generalized
Mucous mem-
  branes
  Minimal lesions
Recur in crops for
  2 to 3 weeks
Oral lesions (few)

Children, young
  adults
Prodrome
  URI symptoms
  Fever (high)
  Sore throat
  Cough

Bullae
Crops of lesions
  Skin
  Conjunctivae
  Mouth
  Genitalia
Ulcerative stom-
  atitis
Corneal ulcera-
  tions
Hacking cough
  Pneumonitis

Prodrome
  Fever
  Headache
  Sore throat

SJS-like mucous
  membrane dis-
  ease
Stomatitis
Conjunctivitis
Hot erythema
Painful skin
Blisters and bullae
Detachment of the
  epidermis—
  diffuse
Bronchopneumonia
Septicemia

Female:male 3:1
Age 20-40
Prodrome
  Fever
  Malaise

Skin
  Red swellings
  Shins
  Forearms (lateral
    surfaces)
Arthralgias
Arthritis
Hilar adenopathy

Female:male 3:1
Middle-aged
Influenza-like ill-
  ness or intesti-
  nal infection

Skin lesions
  1-3 weeks later
Nonspecific infec-
  tion
  Respiratory tract
  GI tract
Painful red, round
  plaques
Fever or
Low temperature
Malaise
Arthralgias
Arthritis
Conjunctivitis

Polys >70%
Leukocytosis
  >8000

VASCULITIC SYNDROMES

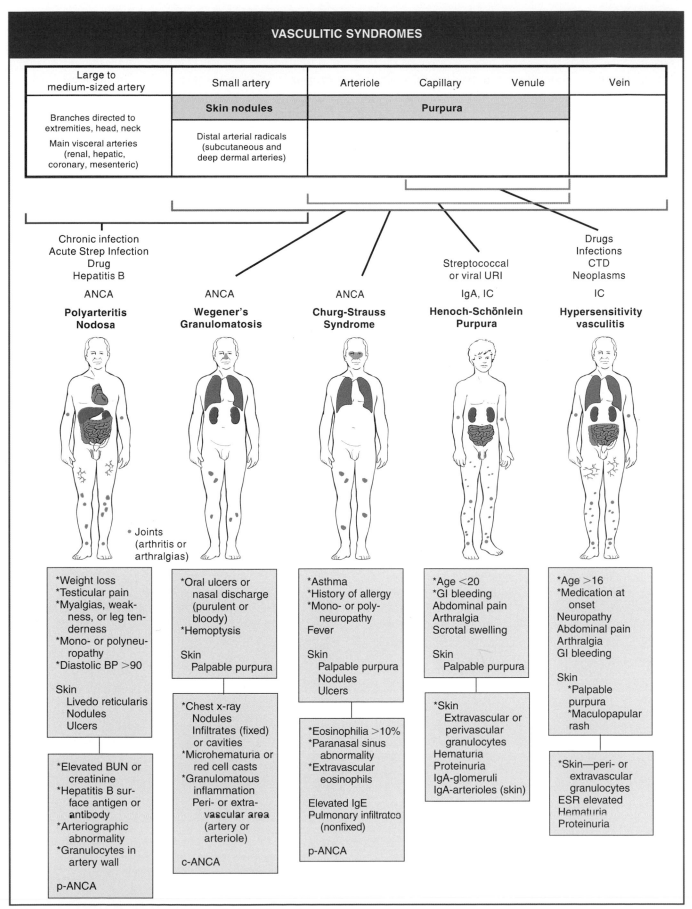

Large to medium-sized artery	Small artery	Arteriole	Capillary	Venule	Vein
	Skin nodules	**Purpura**			
Branches directed to extremities, head, neck Main visceral arteries (renal, hepatic, coronary, mesenteric)	Distal arterial radicals (subcutaneous and deep dermal arteries)				

Chronic infection
Acute Strep Infection
Drug
Hepatitis B

ANCA

Polyarteritis Nodosa

Streptococcal
or viral URI

Drugs
Infections
CTD
Neoplasms

ANCA

Wegener's Granulomatosis

ANCA

Churg-Strauss Syndrome

IgA, IC

Henoch-Schönlein Purpura

IC

Hypersensitivity vasculitis

• Joints (arthritis or arthralgias)

*Weight loss
*Testicular pain
*Myalgias, weakness, or leg tenderness
*Mono- or polyneuropathy
*Diastolic BP >90

Skin
Livedo reticularis
Nodules
Ulcers

*Elevated BUN or creatinine
*Hepatitis B surface antigen or antibody
*Arteriographic abnormality
*Granulocytes in artery wall

p-ANCA

*Oral ulcers or nasal discharge (purulent or bloody)
*Hemoptysis

Skin
Palpable purpura

*Chest x-ray
Nodules
Infiltrates (fixed) or cavities
*Microhematuria or red cell casts
*Granulomatous inflammation
Peri- or extravascular area (artery or arteriole)

c-ANCA

*Asthma
*History of allergy
*Mono- or polyneuropathy
Fever

Skin
Palpable purpura
Nodules
Ulcers

*Eosinophilia >10%
*Paranasal sinus abnormality
*Extravascular eosinophils

Elevated IgE
Pulmonary infiltrates (nonfixed)

p-ANCA

*Age <20
*GI bleeding
Abdominal pain
Arthralgia
Scrotal swelling

Skin
Palpable purpura

*Skin
Extravascular or perivascular granulocytes
Hematuria
Proteinuria
IgA-glomeruli
IgA-arterioles (skin)

*Age >16
*Medication at onset
Neuropathy
Abdominal pain
Arthralgia
GI bleeding

Skin
*Palpable purpura
*Maculopapular rash

*Skin—peri- or extravascular granulocytes
ESR elevated
Hematuria
Proteinuria

*1990 American College of Rheumatology criteria of diagnosis.
ANCA-Antineutrophil cytoplasmic autoantibodies.
IC-Immune complex mediated.

Urticarial plaques. Urticarial plaques may occur without classic target lesions in the same distribution as just described. Unlike hives, all lesions are approximately the same size (1 to 2 cm) and remain unchanged for days.

Vesiculobullous form. The distinctive vesiculobullous form of EM begins with 1- to 5-cm, red, edematous plaques on the extensor surfaces of the extremities; they are found less commonly on the trunk. Lesions may be very extensive or confined to a few areas, such as the elbows and knees. Vesicles or bullae arise from a portion (not the entire surface) of the plaque and may be multiple on a single plaque (Figure 18-3). Lesions are itchy, burning, or painful. They heal in approximately 4 weeks; as with fixed drug eruptions, recurrences may be on exactly the same area. Mucous membrane lesions are more common with this form.

Treatment. Mild cases are not treated. Patients with many target lesions respond rapidly to a 1- to 3-week course of prednisone. Prednisone (40 to 80 mg/day) is continued until control is achieved and is then tapered rapidly in 1 week. Treatment with prednisone can successfully abort a recurrence. Oral acyclovir (200 mg, two or three times a day or 400 mg twice a day) used continually prevents herpes-associated recurrent EM in many cases.[11,12] Herpes-associated EM is not prevented if oral acyclovir is administered after a herpes simplex recurrence is evident, and it is of no value after EM has occurred.[13] Acyclovir has been used by some patients continually for years without any apparent ill effects. One group of patients with recurrent EM and without evidence of herpes infection did not respond to acyclovir. Partial or complete suppression was evident in patients treated with dapsone (100 to 150 mg daily). Azathioprine was used successfully in patients with severe disease for whom all other treatments had failed. The response to treatment was dose-dependent (100 to 150 mg daily).[14] The condition recurred on discontinuation of therapy.

The immunomodulator levamisole, which restores the function of phagocytes and T lymphocytes and activates the inflammatory response, was used successfully to treat patients with chronic or recurring oral lesions of EM. It was given as a single dose of 150 mg/day for 3 consecutive days, alone or in combination with prednisone.[15]

The SJS/TEN Spectrum of Disease

Stevens-Johnson syndrome (SJS), and toxic epidermal necrolysis (TEN) have traditionally been considered the most severe forms of erythema multiforme (EM). It was recently proposed that EM major is distinct from SJS and TEN on the basis of clinical criteria. The proposed concept is to separate an EM spectrum from an SJS/TEN spectrum. The first, characterized by typical target lesions, are postinfectious disorders, often recurrent but with low morbidity. The second, characterized by widespread blisters and purpuric macules, are usually severe drug-induced reactions with high morbidity and poor prognosis. In this concept SJS and TEN might be only types of the same drug-induced process that vary in severity.[16] A three-grade classification has been proposed:

SJS=mucosal erosions and epidermal detachment below 10%

Overlap SJS/TEN=epidermal detachment between 10% and 30%

TEN=epidermal detachment more than 30%

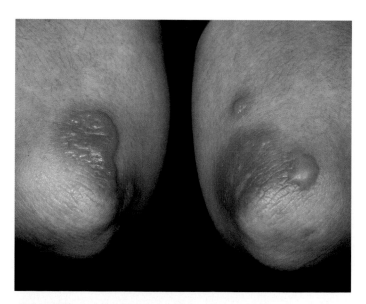

Figure 18-3
Erythema multiforme. Vesiculobullous form. Bullae are arising from a portion of an erythematous plaque.

STEVENS-JOHNSON SYNDROME

Vesiculobullous disease of the skin, mouth, eyes, and genitals is called *Stevens-Johnson syndrome*. The disease occurs most often in children and young adults. The cutaneous eruption is preceded by symptoms of an upper respiratory infection. Bullae occur suddenly 1 to 14 days after the prodromal symptoms, appearing on the conjunctivae, mucous membranes of the nares, mouth (Figure 18-4), anorectal junction, vulvovaginal region, and urethral meatus. Ulcerative stomatitis leading to hemorrhagic crusting is the most characteristic feature. Corneal ulcerations may lead to blindness. A harsh, hacking cough and patchy changes on chest x-ray examination indicate pulmonary involvement.

Skin lesions. Skin lesions in SJS are flat atypical targets or purpuric maculae that are widespread or distributed on the trunk. This is in contrast to the lesions in erythema multiforme, which consist of typical or raised atypical targets or raised edematous papules that are located on the extremities and/or the face.[17]

Patients with limited disease may be weak and lethargic, but the prognosis is good with conservative treatment. Mortality approaches 10% for patients with extensive disease. Fever is high during the active stages. New crops of lesions appear, but the disease is self-limited and resolves in approximately 1 month if there are no complications. Oral lesions may continue for months.

Severe ocular mucosal injury that occurs in Stevens-Johnson syndrome may be a precipitating factor in the development of ocular cicatricial pemphigoid, a chronic, scarring inflammation of the ocular mucosae that can lead to blindness. The time between the onset of Stevens-Johnson syndrome and cicatricial pemphigoid ranges from a few months to 31 years.[18]

Etiology. Drugs are the most common cause (phenytoin, phenobarbital, sulfonamides, penicillins). The disease occurs most often in patients treated for seizure disorders. Upper respiratory tract infection, gastrointestinal (GI) disorders, *Mycoplasma pneumoniae* infection,[19] and herpes simplex virus infection are all implicated. Possible causes should be diligently sought so that recurrences can be avoided.

Diagnosis. A skin biopsy should be performed if the classic lesions are not present. Direct immunofluorescence may be helpful in nontypical cases[9] (see Table 16-1).

Treatment. The use of corticosteroids remains controversial. A study of children suggests that treatment with systemic corticosteroids may be associated with delayed recovery and significant side effects.[20] Other studies conclude that corticosteroids are beneficial and may be lifesaving.[21] Many physicians presented with a sick child who has extensive cutaneous, ocular, and oral lesions elect to treat with oral steroids; most often prednisone (20 to 30 mg twice a day) is given for 1 week until new lesions no longer appear; it is then tapered rapidly.

Itching can be controlled with antihistamines. Cutaneous blisters are treated with cool wet Burow's compresses. Topical steroids should not be applied to eroded areas. Papules and plaques may respond to group II to V topical steroids. Oral symptoms may be relieved by frequent rinsing with lidocaine hydrochloride (Xylocaine Viscous). Patients may tolerate only a liquid or soft diet. Ocular involvement should be monitored by an ophthalmologist. Vitamin A administered topically and systemically was reported to be effective for lacrimal hyposecretion.[22] Secondary infection is treated with oral antibiotics. Stevens-Johnson syndrome associated with herpes simplex virus may be prevented by early use of acyclovir and prednisone.[23]

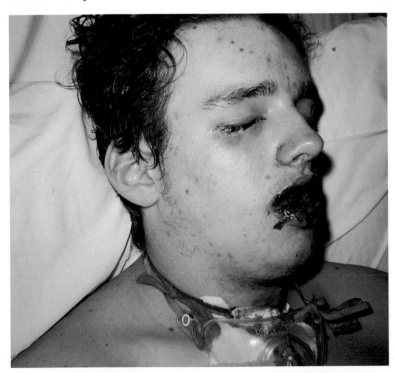

Figure 18-4
Erythema multiforme. Severe bullous form (Stevens-Johnson syndrome). Bullae are present on the conjunctiva and in the mouth.

TOXIC EPIDERMAL NECROLYSIS

Toxic epidermal necrolysis (TEN) is initially seen with Stevens-Johnson–like mucous membrane disease and progresses to diffuse, generalized detachment of the epidermis through the dermoepidermal junction.[24,25] This full-thickness loss of the epidermis results in a mortality of 25% to 100%. Fluid loss is not a major problem; death is usually caused by overwhelming sepsis originating in denuded skin or lungs. TEN is rare, occuring in 1.3 cases per million per year.[26]

The mortality rate is 1% to 5% for Stevens-Johnson syndrome, and 34% to 40% for TEN. Mortality is not affected by the type of drug responsible. In contrast to past series, today there is a high prevalence of human immunodeficiency virus infection among patients with TEN. This high rate of HIV infection is linked to an increased use of sulfonamides—mainly sulfadiazine—in these patients.[27-29] TEN may occur after bone marrow transplantation.[30] It seems to be related to a drug reaction to sulfonamides as often as to acute graft-vs.-host disease.

TEN vs. SSSS. This life-threatening disease is similar in appearance to the staphylococcal scalded skin syndrome (SSSS) (see p. 256), which is induced by a staphylococcal toxin. The split in SSSS, however, is high in the epidermis, just below the stratum corneum, permitting rapid healing of the epidermis without danger of infection. The diagnosis of either TEN or SSSS can be made rapidly by examination of a skin biopsy by frozen section technique.

Pathology and pathogenesis. Histologically there is an early-mild interface dermatitis that evolves into full-thickness necrosis of the epidermis. There is subepidermal blister formation, keratinocyte necrosis, and a sparse lymphohistiocytic infiltrate around superficial dermal blood vessels. Lymphopenia is frequently documented. Cytotoxic T cells (CD8[+] lymphocytes) may contribute to the pathogenesis of blister formation by causing degeneration and necrosis of drug-altered keratinocytes.[31-34]

Etiology. The causes of TEN are the same as those of Stevens-Johnson syndrome, but drugs are most frequently implicated in TEN. The reaction is independent of dosage. In two large series, the culprit drugs included antibiotics (40%), anticonvulsants (11%), and analgesics (5% to 23%). Developing countries have a higher incidence of reactions to antituberculous drugs.[35] The most frequent underlying diseases justifying drug treatment are infections (52.7%) and pain (36%). TEN and other severe cutaneous adverse drug reactions may be linked to an inherited defect in the detoxification of drug metabolites. In a few predisposed patients a drug metabolite may bind to proteins in the epidermis and trigger an immune response, leading to immunoallergic cutaneous adverse drug reaction.[36] The following drugs are most commonly implicated:

Antiepileptic drugs
 Phenytoin
 Phenobarbital
 Carbamazepine
Sulfonamides
Ampicillin
Allopurinol
Antituberculous drugs
 Thiacetazone
 Isoniazid
Nonsteroidal antiinflammatory drugs

Prodromal symptoms. Fever is the most frequent prodromal symptom. Symptoms suggestive of an upper respiratory tract infection, such as headache and sore throat, usually precede the appearance of skin lesions by 1 or 2 weeks. Stomatitis, conjunctivitis, and pruritis occur 1 to 2 days before the onset of the rash.

Skin. TEN begins with diffuse, hot erythema covering wide areas. In hours the skin becomes painful, and with slight thumb pressure the skin wrinkles, slides laterally, and separates from the dermis (Figure 18-5, *A*). This ominous sign (Nikolsky's sign) (Figure 18-5, *B*) heralds the onset of a life-threatening event. Small blisters and large bullae may appear. Nonerythematous skin usually remains intact and the scalp is spared.

Mucous membranes. Inflammation, blistering, and erosion of the mucosal surfaces, especially the oropharynx, are early and characteristic findings. The vaginal tract epithelium frequently blisters and erodes. Pain and erosion of oral mucous membranes interfere with oral intake, and nasogastric or duodenal tube feeding is often required. The rest of the GI tract functions normally if sepsis does not occur.

Eyes. Severe eye involvement is a constant feature. Purulent conjunctivitis leads to swelling, crusting, and ulceration with pain and photophobia. Complications include conjunctival erosions with subsequent revascularization, fibrous adhesions, and corneal ulceration and blindness. Photophobia, mucinous discharge, and decreased visual acuity may last for years.

Respiratory tract. Bronchopneumonia occurs in 30% of reported cases and is the cause of death in many cases. Many patients require intubation or ventilatory support. Respiratory failure can occur, with mucus retention and sloughing of the tracheobronchial mucosa.

Infection. Septicemia and gram-negative pneumonia are the most common causes of death. The lungs and denuded skin are the common portals of entry. The incidence of positive blood culture results is very high when central venous lines are used. Intravenous lines are changed or discontinued if it is probable that they are the source of positive blood culture findings. The urethra is often involved, but the use of Foley catheters can be avoided in many cases.

Fluid and electrolyte loss. Fluid loss in TEN is not as severe as it is in burn patients, but significant losses can occur if xenografts are not applied. Apparently the acute-phase reactants that create massive edema after thermal injury are not released in TEN.

Figure 18-5 Toxic epidermal necrolysis.

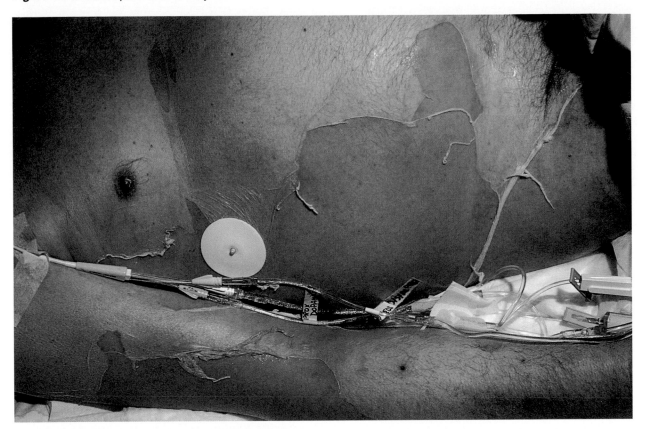

A, Large sheets of full-thickness epidermis are shed.

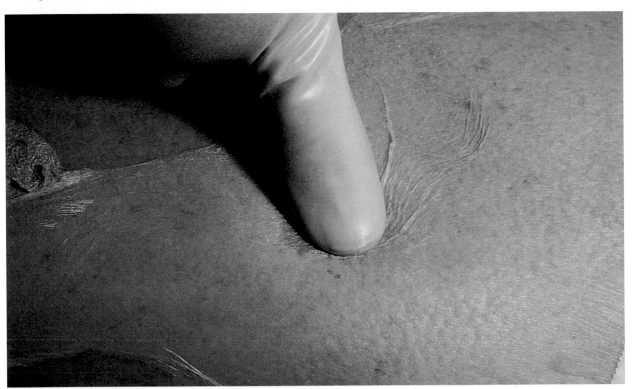

B, Toxic epidermal necrolysis begins with diffuse hot erythema. In hours the skin becomes painful and with slight thumb pressure the skin wrinkles, slides laterally, and separates from the dermis (Nikolsky's sign).

TOXIC EPIDERMAL NECROLYSIS TREATMENT PROTOCOL

1. The patient is taken to the operating room on an urgent basis.
2. All loose skin and blisters are wiped vigorously with a rough washcloth moistened with normal saline solution. No detergents are used.
3. Porcine xenografts are applied to all raw surfaces and stapled in place.
4. The patient is transferred to a warmed, air-fluidized (Clinitron) bed in the burn unit.
5. Initial fluid resuscitation is not required, but careful fluid and electrolyte monitoring is important.
6. The administration of oral steroids is stopped unless medically required; they are tapered if possible.
7. Internal alimentation is established through a nasogastric feeding tube.
8. Systemic antibiotics are used only for specific infections.
9. Intense pulmonary toilet is established.
10. Physical therapy is begun on the day after operation.
11. Dislodged xenografts are replaced.
12. Pain is managed with a "pain cocktail" containing methadone, hydroxyzine, and acetaminophen in cherry syrup. Intravenous narcotics are given as necessary. With the dermis covered, the wounds become essentially pain free.
13. Meticulous eye care is provided hourly. Each day the ophthalmologist removes conjunctival synechiae with a glass rod.
14. Central venous and bladder catheters are avoided.
15. The xenograft becomes brittle and desiccates as the wounds heal beneath it. These areas are trimmed each day.

Modified from Heimbach DM et al: *JAMA* 257:2171-2175, 1987.

Other complications. Leukopenia of uncertain cause may occur. Toxins (e.g., from absorbed silver sulfadiazine) or immune complexes may be the cause.[37-40] In one series, renal involvement consisting of hematuria, proteinuria, and elevated serum creatinine occurred in 50% of patients with Stevens-Johnson syndrome.[41]

Treatment. Separation at the junction of the dermis and epidermis leaves totally viable dermis and intact skin appendages. If the dermis can be protected from toxic detergents, salves, or desiccation, rapid resurfacing by proliferation of epithelium from the skin appendages will occur in approximately 14 days without scarring. Silver sulfadiazine and mafenide acetate (Sulfamylon) delay epithelialization. Silver nitrate wet dressings prevent infection but allow the wounds to dry and cause severe pain during the frequent dressing changes. Synthetic dressings do not adhere well and may become purulent.[42] The conjunctivitis and mucositis also heal without complications if the eyes are meticulously protected.

In one study, cyclophosphamide (100 to 300 mg/day intravenously for 5 days) stopped the blistering, pain, and erythema in a few days. Reepithelialization rapidly occured in 4 to 5 days.[31] Cyclophosphamide inhibits cell-mediated cytotoxicity. Cyclosporine is reported to halt the progression of disease.[43,44] Plasma exchange (1 to 5 sessions) resulted in complete remission in 4 of 5 patients.[45] Good results were also reported with hyperbaric oxygen[46] and plasmapheresis.[47]

Burn center treatment. TEN has pathophysiologic similarities to partial-thickness burn injury and benefits from treatment in a multidisciplinary burn center. The use of a temporary skin substitute is effective for treatment.[48-50] The program used by the University of Washington group,[42] using porcine xenografts, prevents pain and infection, provides the scaffolding for rapid reepithelialization, and avoids the need for steroids (see the box at left). Cryopreserved cadaver allograft skin has also been used successfully as a temporary biologic dressing in the interval before reepithelialization.[51]

Systemic steroids. The use of systemic steroids is still controversial,[52,53] but most authors recommend that steroids not be used.[48]

Steroids cannot prevent the occurrence of TEN, even in high dosages. Patients treated for other diseases with glucocorticosteroids for at least a week prior to the first dermatologic sign of TEN showed no difference in mortality compared with untreated patients.[54] This suggests that steroids do not protect the epidermis from drug-induced keratolysis and that TEN is not an immunologically mediated disease. Improved survival rates have been reported when patients with TEN have been managed without steroids.[55]

Erythema Nodosum

Erythema nodosum (EN) is a nodular erythematous eruption that is usually limited to the extensor aspects of the extremities. EN represents a hypersensitivity reaction to a variety of antigenic stimuli and may be observed in association with several diseases (infections, immunopathies, malignancies) and during drug therapy (with halides, sulfonamides, oral contraceptives). Approximately 50% of cases are idiopathic. The clinical picture is that of a nonspecific systemic illness, with low-grade fever (60%), malaise (67%), arthralgias (64%), and arthritis (31%). Laboratory tests show no specific abnormalities except those related to an underlying disease. Familial EN is reported, with affected family members showing a common haplotype.[56] The incidence has decreased in the antibiotic era. EN is seen more frequently in females.

Clinical manifestations and course. Prodromal symptoms of fatigue and malaise or symptoms of an upper respiratory infection precede the eruption by 1 to 3 weeks.

Arthralgia occurs in more than 50% of patients and begins during the eruptive phase or precedes the eruption by 2 to 8 weeks. Symptoms may disappear in a few weeks or persist for 2 years, but they always resolve without destructive joint changes. The rheumatoid factor is negative. Joint symptoms consist of erythema, swelling, and tenderness over the joint, sometimes with effusions; arthralgia and morning stiffness, most commonly in the knee, but any joint may be affected; and polyarthralgia lasting for days.

The eruptive phase begins with flulike symptoms of fever and generalized aching. The characteristic lesions begin as red, nodelike swellings over the shins; as a rule, both legs are affected. Similar lesions may appear on the extensor aspects of the forearms, thighs, and trunk (Figure 18-6). The border is poorly defined, with size varying from 2 to 6 cm. Lesions are oval, and their long axis corresponds to that of the limb. During the first week the lesions become tense, hard, and painful; during the second week they become fluctuant, as in an abscess, but never suppurate. The color changes in the second week from bright red to bluish or livid; as absorption progresses, it gradually fades to a yellowish hue, resembling a bruise; this disappears in 1 or 2 weeks as the overlying skin desquamates. The individual lesions last approximately 2 weeks, but new lesions sometimes continue to appear for 3 to 6 weeks. Aching of the legs and swelling of the ankles may persist for weeks. The condition may recur for months or years.

Pulmonary hilar adenopathy may develop as part of the hypersensitivity reaction of EN and is seen in cases with diverse causes.[57]

Pathogenesis and etiology. Erythema nodosum is probably a delayed hypersensitivity reaction to a variety of antigens; circulating immune complexes have not been found in idiopathic or uncomplicated cases.[58,59] EN is a reaction pattern elicited by many different diseases (see the box on p. 576). In one large series, 32.5% of cases were idiopathic.[60]

The most common cause today is streptococcal infection and tuberculosis in children and streptococcal infection and sarcoidosis in adults.[61,62]

Coccidioidomycosis (San Joaquin Valley fever) is the most common cause of EN in the west and southwest United States. In approximately 4% of males and 10% of females, the primary fungal infection, which may be asymptomatic or involve symptoms of an upper respiratory infection, is followed by the development of EN. The lesions appear when the skin-test result becomes positive, 3 days to 3 weeks after the end of the fever caused by the fungal infection.

Histoplasmosis, blastomycosis, and lymphogranuloma venereum may cause EN. Leprosy is another possible inciting factor. Clinically, erythema nodosum leprosum resembles EN, but the histologic picture is that of leukocytoclastic vasculitis.

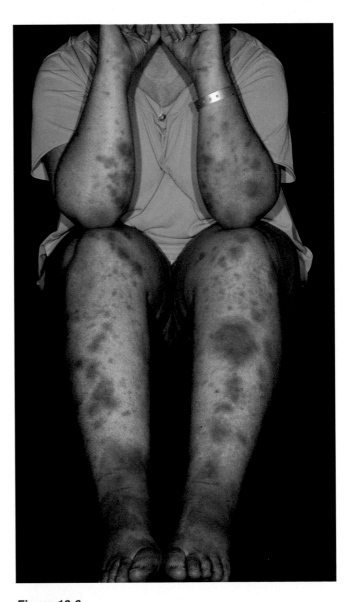

Figure 18-6
Erythema nodosum. Red node-like swelling in the characteristic distribution.

ERYTHEMA NODOSUM—THE MOST COMMON CAUSES

INFECTIONS

Streptococci
Tuberculosis
Psittacosis
Yersiniosis
Lymphogranuloma venereum
Cat-scratch disease
Coccidioidomycosis
Upper respiratory infection

DRUGS

Sulfonamides
Bromides
Oral contraceptives

SYSTEMIC ILLNESSES

Sarcoidosis
Inflammatory bowel disease
Hodgkin's disease

PREGNANCY

Inflammatory bowel diseases such as ulcerative colitis and regional ileitis may trigger EN, usually during active disease with symptoms of abdominal complaints and diarrhea. The mean duration of chronic ulcerative colitis before the onset of EN is 5 years, and the EN is controlled with adequate therapy of the colitis.[63] *Yersinia enterocolitica*, a gram-negative bacillus that causes acute diarrhea and abdominal pain, is a common cause of EN in France and Finland,[64,65] where the initial cases were reported. *Salmonella* and *Campylobacter*[66] have also been implicated.

Sulfonamides, bromides, and oral contraceptives have been reported to cause EN. Several other drugs, such as antibiotics, barbiturates, and salicylates, are often suspected but seldom proved causes of EN.

EN occurs in up to 39%[67] of cases of sarcoidosis and has also been observed in pregnant women.

EN should be considered as a warning signal of impending relapse in a patient with a history of Hodgkin's disease.[68,69]

Dental treatment and the possible presence of infectious dental foci should be considered in the differential diagnosis. EN is reported following dental treatment associated with gingival bleeding or due to infectious dental foci.[70]

Sweet's syndrome (acute febrile neutrophilic dermatosis) and EN are both reactive dermatoses. There are several associated conditions that these disorders have in common. The appearance of both conditions in the same patient has been reported.[71,72]

Many other causes of EN have been reported; most consist of single histories. New etiologies continue to be described.

Diagnosis. Initial evaluation should include throat culture, ASO titer, chest film, PPD skin test, and ESR. The ESR is elevated in all patients with EN.

Patients with GI symptoms should have a stool culture for *Y. enterocolitica*, *Salmonella*, and *Campylobacter*. Bilateral hilar adenopathy on chest x-ray examination does not establish the diagnosis of sarcoidosis, since hilar adenopathy occurs in EN produced by coccidioidomycosis, histoplasmosis, tuberculosis, streptococcal infections, lymphoma, and as a nonspecific reaction in many cases.[73]

The clinical picture is characteristic in most cases and a biopsy is not required. Histologic confirmation is desirable in atypical cases;[74] an excisional rather than a punch biopsy is necessary to sample the subcutaneous fat adequately. Tissue sections show lymphohistiocytic infiltrate, granulomatous inflammation, and fibrosis in the septa of the subcutaneous fat; these are all features of a septal panniculitis.

Differential diagnosis. In Weber-Christian panniculitis, localized areas of subcutaneous inflammation tend to occur on the thighs and trunk rather than on the lower legs. Lesions may suppurate and heal with atrophy and localized depressions. Superficial and deep thrombophlebitis and erysipelas must also be differentiated from EN. Panniculitis secondary to pancreatic disease is associated with evidence of pancreatitis. Erythema induratum is initially seen with dull, red, tender nodules on the calves of women; the nodules often ulcerate and heal with scarring.

Treatment. EN in most instances is a self-limited disease and requires only symptomatic relief with salicylates and bed rest. Cases that are recurrent, unusually painful, or long lasting require a more vigorous approach.

Potassium iodide may be given in doses of 300 mg orally three times each day for 3 to 4 weeks. Different treatment schedules recommend a range of 360 to 900 mg/day.[75,76] Relief of lesional tenderness, arthralgia, and fever may occur in 24 hours. Most lesions completely subside within 10 to 14 days. However, potassium iodide is not effective for all patients with EN. Patients who receive medication shortly after the initial onset of EN respond more satisfactorily than those with chronic EN. Side effects include nasal catarrh and headache.

Corticosteroids are effective but seldom necessary in self-limited diseases. Recurrence following discontinuation of treatment is common, and underlying infectious disease may be worsened.[77]

Indomethacin[78] or naproxen[79] may be more effective than aspirin.

Vasculitis

Cutaneous vasculitis encompasses a highly heterogeneous group of disorders of diverse etiology, pathogenesis, and clinical features (see the box below).

Vasculitis, or angiitis, defined as inflammation of the vessel wall, is probably initiated by immune complex deposition. The cutaneous vasculitic diseases are classified according to the type of inflammatory cell within the vessel walls (neutrophil, lymphocyte, or histiocyte) and the size and type of blood vessel involved (venule, arteriole, artery, or vein). Some vasculitic diseases are limited to the skin; others involve vessels in many different organs.

TYPES OF VASCULITIS CATEGORIZED ON THE BASIS OF PROPOSED PATHOLOGIC MECHANISMS

Immune complex mediated
Henoch-Schönlein purpura
Cryoglobulinemic vasculitis
Lupus vasculitis
Rheumatoid vasculitis
Serum sickness vasculitis
Induced by whole serum
Induced by heterologous proteins
Infection-induced immune complex vasculitis
    Viral (e.g., hepatitis B and C virus)
    Bacterial (e.g., streptococcal)
Paraneoplastic vasculitis
Some drug-induced vasculitis (e.g., sulfonamide)
Behçet's disease
Erythema elevatum diutinum

Antineutrophil cytoplasmic autoantibody (ANCA) associated and possibly ANCA mediated
Wegener's granulomatosis
Microscopic polyarteritis
Churg-Strauss syndrome
Some drug-induced vasculitis (e.g., thiouracil)

Direct antibody attack mediated
Goodpasture's syndrome (mediated by anti-
    basement membrane antibodies)
Kawasaki disease (possibly mediated by anti-
    endothelial antibodies)

Cell mediated
Allograft acute cellular vascular rejection

Unknown
Giant cell (temporal) arteritis
Takayasu arteritis
Polyarteritis nodosa

Adapted from Jennette CJ, Falk RJ: Vasculitis affecting the skin, *Arch Dermatol* 130:899-906, 1994.

The clinical presentation varies with the size of the blood vessel involved and the intensity of the inflammation (Table 18-1; see the comparison of vasculitic syndromes on p. 569). Small-vessel vasculitis—arteriole, capillary, venule—most commonly affects the skin and rarely causes serious internal organ dysfunction, except when the kidney is involved. Muscular arteries acquire focal lesions, leading to aneurysm formation and possibly rupture, or segmental lesions leading to occlusion and distal infarction.

There are numerous cutaneous diseases that histologically show some degree of vessel inflammation. Only those diseases that have inflammation severe enough to cause necrosis of vessel walls are discussed here. *Necrotizing angiitis* is the term given to this group of diseases. These diseases have clinical features that allow one to predict that vessel inflammation and necrosis are taking place and to identify the size of vessel involved[80,81] (Table 18-1). The frequency of the different types of vasculitis is listed in Table 18-2.

Antineutrophil cytoplasmic antibodies. The diagnosis and classification of vasculitis has been revolutionized by the discovery of serum antineutrophil cytoplasmic autoantibodies (ANCAs). ANCAs are a serologic marker for many forms of necrotizing vasculitis and offer insight into its pathogenesis. These autoantibodies against neutrophil granule proteins lead to oxidative injury and extensive tissue damage.[82]

ANCAs have been demonstrated in Wegener's granulomatosis, Churg-Strauss syndrome, pulmonary renal syndrome, microscopic polyarteritis nodosa, leukocytoclastic angiitis, and necrotizing and crescentic glomerulonephritis. The sensitivity of ANCAs for this group of diseases is high when there is renal involvement. The antibodies are moderately sensitive in localized cases (without renal involvement). The titer of ANCAs is not correlated with the severity of vasculitis, but the disappearance of ANCAs is associated with absence of disease activity.[83] Elevated ANCA levels may precede a relapse. Patients have only one or the other of two types of ANCA antibodies.[84]

A theoretic mechanism has been proposed.[85,86] Priming of neutrophils, (e.g., by an infection) causes small amounts of antigens to be released at the cell surface where they can interact with ANCAs. ANCA-activated neutrophils then adhere to endothelial cells via adhesion molecule interactions. These activated and adherent neutrophils then injure endothelial cells (and eventually underlying vessel wall structures) by releasing granule enzymes and toxic oxygen metabolites.

c-ANCA. c-ANCAs ("classic pattern") are directed against the myeloid lysosomal enzyme, proteinase 3, from azurophilic granules. Proteinase 3–specific ANCA (PR3-ANCA) is responsible for most of the cytoplasmic staining pattern on indirect immunofluorescence assay. c-ANCAs are sensitive and specific for active Wegener's granulomatosis and are found in microscopic polyarteritis. Changes in levels of c-ANCAs precede disease activity and may be used as guidelines for treatment.

TABLE 18-1 Clinical Signs of Necrotizing Vasculitis with Respect to Vessel Size Involved

Signs	Diseases
SMALL VESSELS (ARTERIOLE, CAPILLARY, VENULE)	
Urticaria reflects minimal vessel inflammation and necrosis. **Palpable purpura:** exudation and hemorrhage from damaged vessels produce the most characteristic lesion of small-vessel necrotizing vasculitis. The lesion is a red, slightly elevated papule that does not blanch on application of external pressure. **Nodules, bullae, or ulcers** may be present if vessel wall inflammation and necrosis are intense.	Hypersensitivity vasculitis Henoch-Schönlein purpura Essential mixed cryoglobulinemia Vasculitis associated with connective tissue disease Vasculitis associated with malignancies Serum sickness and serum sickness–like reactions Chronic urticaria (urticarial vasculitis) Urticarial prodrome of acute hepatitis type B infection
LARGE VESSELS (SMALL AND MEDIUM-SIZED MUSCULAR ARTERIES)	
Subcutaneous nodules, ulceration, and ecchymoses result from necrosis and thrombosis of larger vessels, which leads to infarction.	Polyarteritis nodosa Churg-Strauss syndrome Wegener's granulomatosis Giant cell (temporal) arteritis

TABLE 18-2 Frequency Distribution of Types of Vasculitis*

Types of vasculitis	No. of cases
Polyarteritis nodosa	118
Churg-Strauss syndrome	20
Wegener's granulomatosis	85
Hypersensitivity vasculitis	93
Henoch-Schönlein purpura	85
Giant-cell (temporal) arteritis	214
Takayasu's arteritis	63
Other vasculitis, type unspecified	129
Vasculitis with a connective tissue disease	141
Kawasaki disease	52
Nonvasculitis	20

*The 48 centers submitted a total of 1020 cases for these studies. The last three groups of patients (n = 213) were excluded from study.

p-ANCA. Antibodies directed against different cytoplasmic constituents of neutrophils (primarily myeloperoxidase [MPO]) produce a perinuclear staining of neutrophils. Patients with p-ANCA (MPO-ANCA) have common features, such as rapidly progressive glomerulonephritic syndrome and pulmonary hemorrhage and purpura. Histologically they have focal segmental necrotizing glomerulonephritis, pulmonary alveolar hemorrhage, and leukocytoclastic vasculitis induced by necrotizing capillaries. p-ANCA occurs in idiopathic crescentic glomerulonephritis, Churg-Strauss syndrome, polyarteritis nodosa with visceral involvement, and vasculitic overlap syndromes. Polyarteritis nodosa limited to the skin and the musculoskeletal system is not associated with ANCA.[87] The specificity for this group of necrotizing vasculitides is high (94% to 99%), although they may occur in patients with hydralazine-induced glomerulonephritis, antiglomerular basement membrane disease, and possibly in some patients with idiopathic systemic lupus erythematosus. p-ANCA of undefined specificity may distinguish ulcerative colitis (sensitivity of 75%) from Crohn's disease (sensitivity of 20%). p-ANCA also occurs in autoimmune liver diseases: in 75% of patients with chronic active hepatitis, in 60% to 85% of those with primary sclerosing cholangitis, and in approximately 30% with primary biliary cirrhosis. p-ANCA is detected in chronic arthritides and in some 5% of healthy controls.[88]

ANCA-laboratory tests. ANCA are detected in serum using normal human neutrophils as the substrate for an indirect immunofluorescence microscopic assay, or by immunochemical tests such as enzyme immunoassay or radioimmunoassay, using specific protein targets. Indirect immunofluorescence microscopy assays demonstrate the two staining patterns (cytoplasmic [c-ANCA] and perinuclear [p-ANCA]) on neutrophils.

Vasculitis of Small Vessels

Most of the diseases characterized by necrotizing inflammation of small blood vessels have a number of features in common. Skin lesions reflect various degrees of small-vessel necrotizing inflammation; the most common is palpable purpura (see Table 18-1). There is hypersensitivity to various antigens (drugs, chemicals, microorganisms, and endogenous antigens) with formation of circulating immune complexes[89] that are deposited in walls of vessels.[90] The vessel-bound immune complexes activate complement that is chemotactic for polymorphonuclear leukocytes. There is an inflammatory response in the walls of small vessels in which leukocytes, by release of lysosomal enzymes, damage vessel walls, causing extravasation of erythrocytes. The term *leukocytoclastic vasculitis* describes the histologic pattern produced when leukocytes fragment (i.e., undergo leukocytoclasis during the inflammatory process, leaving nuclear debris or "dust").

HYPERSENSITIVITY VASCULITIS

Hypersensitivity (leukocytoclastic) vasculitis is the most commonly seen form of small-vessel necrotizing vasculitis. The disease may be limited to the skin or may involve many different organs,[91] in which case it is called *cutaneous-systemic angiitis*.[57] Histologically there is fibrinoid necrosis of small dermal blood vessels, leukocytoclasis, endothelial cell swelling, and extravasation of red blood cells (RBCs).

Diagnosis. Prodromal symptoms include fever, malaise, myalgia, and joint pain. The characteristic lesions are referred to as *palpable purpura*. The lesions begin as asymptomatic, localized areas of cutaneous hemorrhage that acquire substance and become palpable as blood leaks out of damaged vessels. Lesions may coalesce, producing large areas of purpura. Nodules and urticarial lesions may appear. Hemorrhagic blisters and ulcers may arise from these purpuric areas and indicate more severe vessel inflammation and necrosis (Figures 18-7, 18-8, and 18-9). A few-to-numerous discrete, purpuric lesions are most commonly seen on the lower extremities but may occur on any dependent area, including the back if the patient is bedridden, or the arms. Ankle and lower leg edema may occur with lower leg lesions.

Figure 18-7
Hypersensitivity (leukocytoclastic) vasculitis. An intense eruption with several areas of cutaneous necrosis.

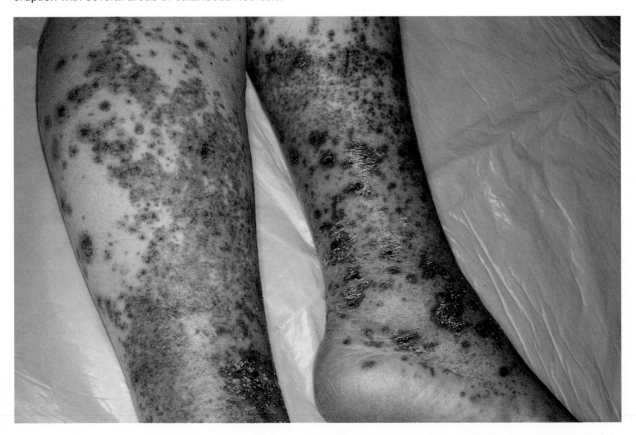

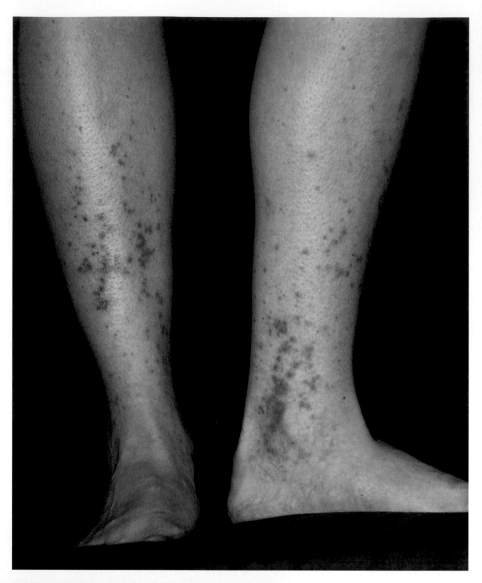

Figure 18-8
Hypersensitivity (leukocytoclastic) vasculitis. Lesions have been present for 4 days and are hemorrhagic.

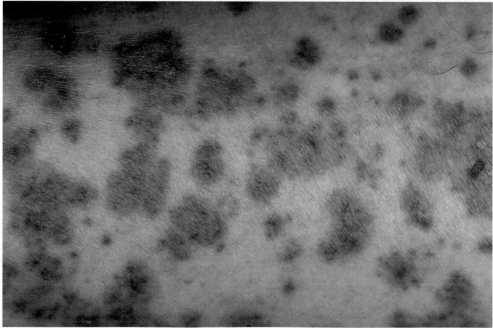

Figure 18-9
Hypersensitivity (leukocytoclastic) vasculitis. Exudation and hemorrhage into the skin make these purpura palpable.

Small lesions itch and are painful; nodules, ulcers, and bullae may be very painful.

Lesions appear in crops, last for 1 to 4 weeks, and heal with residual scarring and hyperpigmentation. Patients may experience one episode if a drug or viral infection is the cause or multiple episodes when the lesions are associated with a systemic disease, such as rheumatoid arthritis or systemic lupus erythematosus. Recurrent crops of new lesions may appear for weeks, months, or years. The disease is usually self-limited and confined to the skin.

Systemic disease. Hypersensitivity vasculitis has many systemic manifestations; the numbers in parentheses in the following discussion indicate the approximate percentage of involvement.[92-94]

An analysis of cutaneous hypersensitivity vasculitis in patients seen by two practicing dermatologists showed that the disease has a better prognosis with less systemic involvement than in those patients seen at medical center clinics.[95,96]

- Kidneys (50%): Kidney disease is the most common systemic manifestation. Mild vasculitis of the kidneys causes microscopic hematuria and proteinuria. Necrotizing glomerulitis or diffuse glomerulonephritis may lead to chronic renal insufficiency and death.
- Nervous system (40%): Peripheral neuropathy with hypoesthesia or paresthesia is more common than central nervous system involvement.
- Gastrointestinal tract (36%): Vasculitis of the bowel causes abdominal pain, nausea, vomiting, diarrhea, and melena.
- Lung (30%): Pulmonary vasculitis may be asymptomatic, detected only as nodular or diffuse infiltrates on chest film; it may be symptomatic, with cough, shortness of breath, and hemoptysis.
- Joints (30%): Symptoms vary from pain to erythema and swelling.
- Heart (50%): Myocardial angiitis produces arrhythmias and congestive heart failure.

Etiology. (1) Drugs—penicillin, thiazides, aspirin, phenothiazines, sulfonamides, iodides, and many others in single case reports; (2) infections—streptococcal upper respiratory tract infections, *Escherichia coli* urinary tract infection, and others; (3) connective tissue disease; (4) malignant neoplasms;[97] and (5) other systemic illnesses. In many cases the cause is not determined. Some of the diseases reported to be associated with hypersensitivity vasculitis are listed in the box below; the incidence of these diseases is listed in the box on p. 582.[97]

SYNDROMES WITHIN THE BROADER GROUP OF HYPERSENSITIVITY VASCULITIS

Henoch-Schönlein purpura
Nonthrombocytopenic purpura, joint, gastrointestinal, renal; postinfection or food allergy; tendency to recur several times and resolve; IgA antibody in immune complexes

Essential mixed cryoglobulinemia
Purpura, arthralgias, anemia, hypergammaglobulinemia, glomerulonephritis; usually IgM rheumatoid factor against IgG; solid evidence for immune complex deposition

Vasculitis associated with connective tissue disease
Usually rheumatoid arthritis and systemic lupus erythematosus; in rheumatoid arthritis, associated with severe erosive and nodular disease; not caused by corticosteroids; combinations of small venule and small- and medium-sized arteries

Vasculitis associated with malignancies
Chronic lymphocytic leukemia, lymphoma, Hodgkin's disease, multiple myeloma

Serum sickness and serum sickness–like reactions
Fever, urticaria, arthralgias, lymphadenopathy 7 to 10 days after primary exposure or 2 to 4 days after secondary exposure (accelerated); heterologous antisera or nonprotein drug (penicillin, sulfa)

Chronic urticaria
Recurrent episodes of urticaria associated with elevated erythrocyte sedimentation rate, normal or low levels of C1q and C4 and episodic arthralgia; biopsy or urticarial plaque shows necrotizing venulitis

Urticarial prodrome of acute hepatitis type B infection
Biopsy shows necrotizing venulitis

Modified from Fauci AS: *Ann Intern Med* 89 (part 1):660-676, 1978.

Evaluation

Clinical studies. Studies to consider are throat culture, antistreptolysin O titer, ESR, platelets, complete blood count (CBC), serum creatinine, urinalysis, antinuclear antibody, serum multiphasic analysis, serum protein electrophoresis, circulating immune complexes, hepatitis B surface antigen, cryoglobulins, CH_{50} (total hemolytic complement), and rheumatoid factor. The ESR is almost always elevated during active vasculitis. A normal ESR in a patient with purpura suggests that immune complex disease is absent. Low complement levels are associated with other features such as renal disease, arthritis, and the presence of immunoreactants deposited along the basement membrane zone of the epidermis.[98]

Skin biopsy. The clinical presentation is so characteristic that a biopsy is generally not necessary. In doubtful cases, a punch biopsy should be taken from an early active lesion. The characteristic mixed infiltrate of mononuclear cells and neutrophils, fibrinoid necrosis of blood vessel walls, and nuclear dust from neutrophil fragmentation (leukocytoclasis) will be obscured if ulcerated lesions are sampled. Patients with deeper levels of vasculitis (down to the lower half of the reticular dermis) have evidence of a more severe clinical disease with systemic involvement.[98]

Immunofluorescent studies. Immunofluorescent studies may be done if the diagnosis cannot be determined from the clinical presentation and skin biopsy. Immune complexes are phagocytized rapidly after deposition in the vessels. Therefore the best time for biopsy of a vessel for immunofluorescence is within the first 24 hours after the lesion forms.

The most common immunoreactants present in and around blood vessels are IgM, C3, and fibrin.[98] The presence of IgA in blood vessels of a child with vasculitis suggests the diagnosis of Henoch-Schönlein purpura (Table 18-3).

Treatment. Identify and remove the offending antigen (i.e., drug, chemical, or infection). No other treatment may be necessary and the disease may clear spontaneously. In other instances the disease persists or becomes recurrent. Short courses of prednisone (40 to 60 mg/day) are effective for most patients. Colchicine, which inhibits neutrophil chemotaxis, is effective in controlling chronic cutaneous hypersensitivity vasculitis.[96,99] The condition is controlled in most patients with 0.6 mg twice daily, effects are seen in 7 to 10 days, and colchicine is tapered and discontinued when lesions resolve. Treatment can be continued for months if necessary, and side effects are minimal. Azathioprine 150 mg/day was used in patients with recalcitrant disease or steroid-induced side effects and produced a good clinical response in 4 to 8 weeks.[96] Dapsone 100 to 150 mg/day controlled three patients in whom disease was confined to the skin.[100] Hydroxychloroquine and nonsteroidal antiinflammatory drugs are not effective. Cyclophosphamide 2 mg/kg/day induced remissions in patients with multiple-organ involvement who were not controlled with prednisone.[101] The drug had no effect on patients with only cutaneous vasculitis.[102]

SPECTRUM AND INCIDENCE OF 101 CASES OF NECROTIZING VASCULITIS

NECROTIZING VASCULITIS ASSOCIATED WITH COEXISTENT DISEASE

Rheumatoid arthritis, 12%
Malignancy, 8%
Polyarteritis nodosa, 7%
Systemic lupus erythematosus, 6%
Sjögren's syndrome, 3%
Wegener's granulomatosis, 3%
Granuloma faciale, 3%
Hypergammaglobulinemic purpura, 2%
Churg-Strauss syndrome, 2%

NECROTIZING VASCULITIS ASSOCIATED WITH PRECIPITATING EVENT

Drug reaction, 13%
Bacterial infection, 8%
Viral infection, 1%

NECROTIZING VASCULITIS OF UNCERTAIN CAUSE

Idiopathic palpable purpura, 13%
Chronic urticaria or angioedema, 10%
Henoch-Schönlein purpura, 4%
Idiopathic vasculitis with nodules, 3%

Data from Sanchez NP, Van Hale HM, Daniel SU WP: *Arch Dermatol* 121:220-224, 1985.

TABLE 18-3 Clinical Features in 25 Patients with Henoch-Schönlein Purpura

Purpura	100%
Arthralgia	84%
Abdominal pain	76%
Nephritis	44%
Gastrointestinal bleeding	40%
Miscellaneous	
Encephalopathy	8%
Orchitis	4%

From Saulsbury FT: *Pediatr Dermatol* 1:195-201, 1984.

HENOCH-SCHÖNLEIN PURPURA

Henoch-Schönlein purpura (HSP), or anaphylactoid purpura, occurs mainly in children between the ages of 2 and 10, although adult cases are reported. It is characterized by palpable purpura over the legs and buttocks, abdominal pain, GI bleeding, arthralgia, hematuria (Table 18-3), and, histologically, by leukocytoclastic vasculitis.[103] All of its features are attributable to the widespread vasculitis believed to be initiated by entrapment of circulating IgA-containing immune complexes in blood vessel walls in the skin, kidney, and GI tract. Leukocytoclastic vasculitis (hypersensitivity vasculitis) and Henoch-Schönlein purpura are similar but separable clinical syndromes.[104]

HSP is usually benign and self-limiting; the degree of renal involvement determines the prognosis. The long-term prognosis is excellent for both adults and children.[105] HSP tends to occur in the springtime; a streptococcal or viral upper respiratory infection may precede the disease by 1 to 3 weeks. A cluster of cases was reported, suggesting that HSP is caused by person-to-person spread of an infectious agent of the respiratory tract to susceptible hosts.[106] A number of infectious agents and drugs have been implicated, but the etiology of HSP remains unknown. In 50% of cases, there are recurrences, typically in the first 3 months; these are milder and more common in patients with nephritis. Prodromal symptoms include anorexia and fever. The clinical features of HSP are as follows.[107]

Skin. Nonthrombocytopenic palpable purpura is most common on the lower extremities and buttocks but can appear on the arms, face, and ears; the trunk is usually spared (Figure 18-10). The lesions evolve from urticarial papules into the classic leukocytoclastic vasculitic lesions within 48 hours. The lesions are 2 to 10 mm in diameter and appear in crops among coalescent ecchymoses and pinpoint petechiae. Lesions fade in several days, more rapidly with bed rest, leaving brown macules. New lesions appear with ambulation.

Abdominal symptoms. GI symptoms occur in 40% to 60% of patients; these include colicky pain, nausea, vomiting, upper GI bleeding, diarrhea, and bloody stool and are potentially the most serious manifestations.[108] Although GI bleeding occurs in 52% of patients, it is self-limiting, and blood transfusions have not been required.[109] Symptoms precede the skin disease by up to 2 weeks and simulate a number of inflammatory or surgically treated bowel diseases. Upper GI endoscopy can be useful in the diagnosis of HSP. Inflammation of the duodenum, especially of the second part, is characteristic of HSP. Upper GI endoscopy shows redness, swelling, petechiae or hemorrhage, or erosions and ulceration of the mucosa. Histology of mucosal biopsy specimens shows nonspecific inflammation with positive staining for IgA in the capillaries.[110] Ultrasound is an important tool in the early diagnosis of intestinal complications.[111,112] It demonstrates edematous hemorrhagic infiltration of the intestinal wall, which can occur in the duodenal, jejunal, and ileal segments, and it detects ileo-ileal

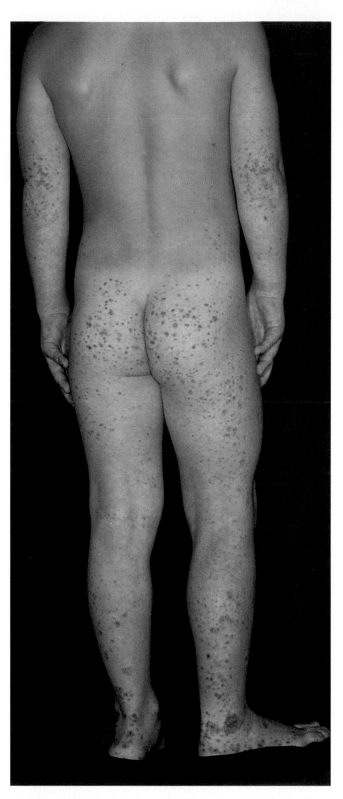

Figure 18-10
Henoch-Schönlein purpura. Palpable purpuric lesions are most common on the lower extremities and buttocks but can appear on the arms, face, and ears; the trunk is usually spared.

intussusception and perforation.[113] Intussusception was confirmed in 1% to 5% of cases.[108]

Joint symptoms. Arthralgia, probably resulting from painful periarticular edema rather than from inflammatory joint disease, involves the ankles, knees, and dorsum of the hands and feet in more than 80% of patients. It is often incapacitating, but it is self-limiting and nondeforming.

Nephritis. Nephritis occurs in 20% to 50% of children. The renal disease is usually milder in children and almost always heals. In 10% to 20% of cases in older children or adults, the nephritis can progress despite the resolution of other disease manifestations. The onset may be acute or delayed. Acute nephritis occurs from 1 to 12 days after the onset of other signs and symptoms. The onset of renal involvement may be delayed for weeks or months in a substantial proportion of patients. Microscopic hematuria is a constant feature, but episodes of gross hematuria occur in 40% of patients with nephritis. Proteinuria and hematuria are found in about 40% of cases. Proteinuria is seen in two thirds of patients with hematuria. IgA nephropathy was found in 8% of children with isolated proteinuria. Urinary abnormalities can persist for 2 to 5 years in patients who develop nephritis in the acute phase of HSP. Progression to nephrotic syndrome and acute and chronic renal failure is possible.[114]

When HSP presents with more than just microhematuria, only 72% of cases proceed to complete recovery.[115] Heavy proteinuria at onset, focal sclerotic and tubulointerstitial changes, and crescents and capsular adhesions are poor prognostic indicators. After a follow-up of at least 8 years, 53% of patients are clinically in remission. Evidence of renal disease may reappear after apparent complete recovery. Childhood HS nephritis requires long-term follow-up, especially during pregnancy. A study of 78 subjects who had HS nephritis during childhood (at a mean of 23.4 years after onset) showed that severity of clinical presentation and initial findings on renal biopsy correlate well with outcome but have poor predictive value in individuals. Forty-four percent of patients who had nephritic or nephrotic syndromes at onset have hypertension or impaired renal function; 82% of those who presented with hematuria (with or without proteinuria) are normal. Sixteen of 44 full-term pregnancies were complicated by proteinuria and/or hypertension, even in the absence of active renal disease.[116]

The renal pathologic findings present a spectrum, from mild focal glomerulitis to necrotizing or proliferative glomerulonephritis with diffuse mesangial proliferation. Diffuse mesangial deposits of IgA are seen on immunofluorescent studies. HS nephritis may be the single most common form of crescentic glomerulonephritis, accounting for 30% of cases.[115] Patients who are HLA-B35 positive may be genetically more susceptible to recurrent episodes of HSP with nephritis, resulting in a protracted illness with significant renal involvement.[117] HS nephritis of the adult carries a high, long-term risk of renal dysfunction.[118]

Acute scrotal swelling. Acute scrotal swelling may be the presenting manifestation. The vasculitis of HSP may involve the scrotum and clinically mimic diseases requiring surgical intervention, such as testicular torsion[119] or an incarcerated inguinal hernia. The ultrasonographic features include marked edema of the scrotal skin and contents with intact vascular flow in the testicles. Nuclear imaging may be used to assess testicular perfusion. These findings help prevent unnecessary surgical exploration.[120]

Pathology. The pathology of HSP is that of an acute vasculitis of arterioles and venules in the superficial dermis and the bowel. Immunofluorescence staining of tissues usually reveals the presence of IgA in the walls of the arterioles and in the renal glomeruli. The serum IgA level is frequently higher than normal.

Diagnosis. There are no diagnostic laboratory tests. CBC, ANA, platelet counts, and coagulation studies are normal. The ESR may be elevated and the serum complement level may be depressed. In one study, serum IgA concentrations were increased in 44% of children.[121] Direct immunofluorescent studies show IgA deposition in blood vessels (75% in affected skin and 67% in uninvolved skin).[122] IgA in vessel walls is a sensitive and specific marker that helps to solidify the diagnosis of HSP. This finding should not be used as the sole criterion for making the diagnosis because it is seen in many other disorders, such as venous stasis and erythema nodosum. One study revealed a significant correlation between plasma levels of anaphylatoxins C3a and C4a and plasma creatinine in patients with nephritis.[123] The role of IgA ANCA has not been defined.[124]

Management. The offending antigen must be identified and removed. The possibilities include infections, malignancies, foods, and drugs. Treatment with corticosteroids[125] or dapsone[126,127] may be useful in early disease before infarction has taken place. In a short-term, double-blind, crossover trial, prednisone had no effect on IgA nephropathy.[115] One study showed that early corticosteroid therapy does not prevent delayed nephritis in children.[128] Another study claims that prednisone given for 2 weeks may prevent nephritis in children who do not already have it when first seen.[115] Plasmapheresis, which removes IgA-immune complexes from the circulation and prevents further vascular damage, was reported to be effective for treating all manifestations of the disease.[129] A 5-year-old girl with severe abdominal pain who did not respond to steroid therapy cleared with intravenous immunoglobulin.[130] A decrease in coagulation factor XIII during the acute phase of the disease correlated with the severity of clinical symptoms, particularly abdominal symptoms, in two reports. Abdominal symptoms and purpura immediately responded to heat-treated, placenta-derived factor XIII concentrate.[131,132]

SCHAMBERG'S DISEASE

Schamberg's disease (progressive pigmented purpuric dermatosis, purpura simplex) is an uncommon eruption characterized by petechiae and patches of brownish pigmentation (hemosiderin deposits), particularly on the lower extremities. Patients are frightened by this vasculitic-appearing eruption, but there is no hematologic disease, venous insufficiency, or associated internal disease. Males are affected more often than females. Children are also affected.[133] Lesions remain for months or years and present only a cosmetic problem. Histologically, there is inflammation and hemorrhage without fibrinoid necrosis of vessels. The cause is unknown, but a cellular immune reaction may play a role.[134,135] In some patients, the eruption was related to medications.[136]

Clinical manifestations. Asymptomatic, irregular, orange-brown patches of varying shapes and sizes appear (Figure 18-11). The most characteristic feature is orange-brown, pinhead-sized "cayenne pepper" spots. Mild erythema and scaling sometimes cause slight itching. Lesions are most common on the lower leg, but they can appear on the upper body. New spots can appear and older ones can fade. In contrast to hypersensitivity vasculitis (palpable purpura), the lesions are macular.

Management. The patient should be assured that there is no systemic disease and informed that pigmentation lasts for years and can be covered with cosmetics, such as Dermablend, if desired. Mild itching and erythema respond quickly to group V topical steroids. Lesions persist, but 67% eventually clear.[137]

Figure 18-11 Schamberg's disease.

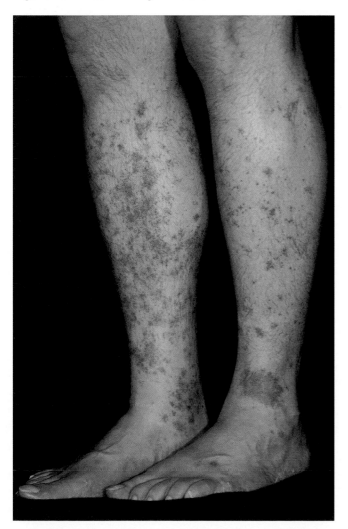

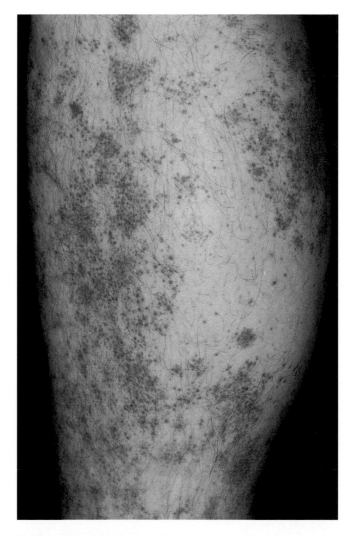

A, Asymptomatic, irregular, orange-brown patches of varying shapes and sizes occur most often on the lower extremities.

B, The most characteristic feature is the orange-brown, pinhead-sized "cayenne pepper" spots.

ESSENTIAL MIXED CRYOGLOBULINEMIA

Cryoglobulinemia may be found in a number of disorders. However, a distinctive syndrome with mixed cryoglobulins has been described for which there is no identifiable underlying disease.[138] Mixed cryoglobulins are immune complexes that cause systemic vasculitis with a variety of symptoms. The features are recurrent palpable purpura of the lower extremities (100%), polyarthralgias without arthritis (72%), and renal disease (55%).[139] The arthralgias are a common presenting symptom and recur throughout the course of the disease. Patients describe a "gelling" of joints on exposure to cold. Clinical signs of renal disease are proteinuria, diastolic hypertension, edema, and renal failure. The prognosis is poor for patients with renal disease.

Cryoprecipitable proteins in serum are greater than 20 mg/100 ml. The serum cryoglobulin concentration does not correlate with disease activity (vasculitis or glomerulonephritis). The cryoglobulins have rheumatoid factor activity and consist of IgM and polyclonal IgG or IgA. Serum protein electrophoresis shows diffuse polyclonal hypergammaglobulinemia without any homogeneous bands in 60% of patients. There is a striking depression of early complement components. The ESR is elevated. Immune complex–mediated renal damage is present in 50% of patients. Many patients have hepatitis B infection,[140] but others do not.[141]

Cutaneous vasculitis and arthralgias require no therapy or are treated with aspirin or other nonsteroidal antiinflammatory agents.

VASCULITIS ASSOCIATED WITH CONNECTIVE TISSUE DISEASE

Typical small-vessel hypersensitivity vasculitis may occur with any of the connective tissue disorders, but most commonly it appears with systemic lupus erythematosus and rheumatoid arthritis. Vessels of all sizes may be involved, with a spectrum of findings ranging from palpable purpura to cutaneous ulcers.

It should not be assumed that leg ulcers in patients with rheumatoid arthritis are vasculitic unless other signs of vasculitis are present.[142] Rheumatoid vasculitis usually develops in patients with long-standing, nodular, severely erosive joint disease who also have hypocomplementemia, very high titers of rheumatoid factor, and often antinuclear antibodies.[143] The vasculitis usually involves the skin and peripheral nerves. Most patients with the early onset of arthritis and vasculitis eventually prove to have rheumatoid vasculitis, systemic vasculitis, or undifferentiated connective tissue syndrome.

Early onset of vasculitis is associated with a poor outcome in patients with undifferentiated connective tissue syndrome and especially with rheumatoid arthritis with rapid progression to vasculitic involvement of the viscera, resulting in death.[144] Patients with rheumatoid arthritis may develop large-vessel vasculitis similar to that seen with polyarteritis nodosa. Morphologically, rheumatoid vasculitis is indistinguishable from polyarteritis nodosa in its distribution and histopathology. Methotrexate may be useful in the treatment of cutaneous vasculitis associated with rheumatoid arthritis.[145]

VASCULITIS ASSOCIATED WITH MALIGNANCY

Small-vessel vasculitis may be seen in association with certain malignancies;[97] these are usually lymphoid or reticuloendothelial neoplasms, such as chronic lymphocytic leukemia, lymphoma, Hodgkin's disease, and multiple myeloma.

URTICARIA

A significant number of patients with chronic urticaria have been shown to have histologic and immunopathologic findings of small-vessel necrotizing vasculitis.[146]

Vasculitis has also been demonstrated in the urticarial plaques of some patients with serum sickness and hepatitis type B infection.[147] These are discussed in Chapter Six.

Churg-Strauss syndrome

Churg-Strauss syndrome (CSS) (allergic granulomatosis) in the past was characterized clinically by the triad of asthma, peripheral eosinophilia (greater than 1500/mm^3) with elevated IgE, and fever. New criteria for classification were established by the American College of Rheumatology in 1990.[148] Asthmatic symptoms develop several months to years before other features of the disease are seen. Vessels are grossly affected, as in polyarteritis nodosa, but histologically these vessels show granulomatous inflammation in addition to leukocyte invasion. Multisystem visceral and cutaneous disease similar to polyarteritis nodosa follows the initial triad of signs and symptoms with hypertension, abdominal pain, neurologic involvement, and pneumonia. The skin is involved in approximately 50% of cases showing palpable purpura, ulcers, infarcts, and deep cutaneous or subcutaneous nodules. Cutaneous involvement generally parallels the systemic course.[149] Antineutrophil cytoplasmic antibodies (p-ANCA) are found in about 60% of cases.[150] Biopsy of an early skin nodule shows vasculitis and eosinophils; older lesions show macrophages and giant cells. Renal involvement is infrequent. The combination of cyclophosphamide, corticosteroids, and plasma exchange is effective.[151]

Vasculitis of Small to Medium Vessels

The consequences of vascular inflammation depend on the size, site, and number of blood vessels affected. Muscular arteries acquire focal lesions (affecting part of the vessel wall), leading to aneurysmal formation and possible rupture, or segmental lesions (affecting the whole circumference), leading to occlusion and distal infarction. The diagnosis depends on a combination of clinical features and characteristic histologic or angiographic appearances.

Kidney disease. In systemic vasculitis the kidney is the organ most commonly involved, and renal biopsy is the single most useful investigation. Renal biopsy should be done if signs of kidney disease appear, because renal failure can develop rapidly. The commonest finding is focal segmental necrotizing glomerulitis; 30% to 50% of specimens show necrotic arteritis. Crescents are common, especially in Wegener's granulomatosis; focal proliferative glomerulonephritis is rare. In contrast to small-vessel disease (Henoch-Schönlein purpura, systemic lupus erythematosus), there is a lack of glomerular immune complex deposition. Renal involvement indicates a poor prognosis, with a 1-year survival in 54% of patients and 5-year survival in 38%,[152] but early aggressive treatment with cyclophosphamide has enhanced the prospects for survival.

Polyarteritis nodosa

The term *nodosa* means a node or swelling. Polyarteritis nodosa (PAN) is a rare disease occurring most commonly in patients older than age 50. Childhood cases are reported.[153,154] There may be a history of chronic infection, drug ingestion, or acute streptococcal infection. Hepatitis (hepatitis B virus) was clinically present in 30% of patients before PAN in one large series.[155] Necrotizing vasculitis occurs in various stages along segments of arteries and at bifurcation points, resulting in clinical signs of ischemia and infarction. Aneurysmal dilation at bifurcation points is detected in visceral organs by angiography and as subcutaneous, sometimes pulsating, nodules in the skin. Multiple organ systems may be involved[156]; the most common are kidney (glomerulosclerosis, cortical infarction), cardiovascular (coronary arteritis [particularly in children], myocardial infarction, hypertension), GI (infarction of bowel segments), and neurologic (asymmetric polyneuritis).

Cutaneous signs. Cutaneous signs are found in approximately 25% of cases. Subcutaneous nodules (less than 2 cm) recur in groups or crops, sometimes along the course of an artery; they are most commonly found on the lower leg. A small, relatively superficial punched-out ulceration occurs in the center of a brownish-tinted area overlying the nodules. Ecchymosis occurs after infarction of vessel walls in a segment or bifurcation.

Laboratory. Childhood cutaneous PAN is frequently associated with antecedent streptococcal infection.[153]

Antineutrophil cytoplasmic antibodies. Antibodies producing a perinuclear staining of ethanol-fixed neutrophils (p-ANCA) occur in PAN with visceral involvement (see earlier section in this chapter on ANCA).[84,150]

Angiography. Angiography can indicate the size and distribution of blood vessels affected but is not diagnostic, since aneurysms are sometimes seen in Wegener's granulomatosis and connective tissue disease arteritis. In up to 70% of cases, celiac axis and bilateral renal angiograms show abnormalities, especially aneurysms.[157] Without treatment, most cases lead to death in less than 2 years.

Treatment. Steroids[158] and cyclophosphamide[159] or azathioprine[160] are effective. In one study, patients with hepatitis B virus–related PAN responded to prednisone, vidarabine, and plasma exchange. The authors claim this regimen is superior to conventional treatment with steroids and cyclophosphamide, which stimulates viral replication.[161]

Cutaneous periarteritis nodosa. A benign, chronically relapsing cutaneous periarteritis nodosa that lacks multisystem involvement but has similar cutaneous lesions has been described.[162,163] The lesions develop a distinctive red, blanchable livedo pattern, usually on the legs. Firm, tender nodules may develop in the red areas. Patients who have a cutaneous disease without clinical or laboratory evidence of systemic disease have a benign course and remain free of systemic disease. A recent study of patients with so-called benign disease revealed signs and symptoms that were indistinguishable from those of classic periarteritis nodosa. The authors suggest that polyarteritis nodosa and benign polyarteritis nodosa are the same disease, with some cases having marked cutaneous involvement and others having relative sparing of the skin and more marked internal organ disease.[164]

Wegener's granulomatosis

Wegener's granulomatosis is a rare, fatal, necrotizing, granulomatous vasculitis that occurs in children and adults[165]; males and females are equally affected. New criteria for classification were established by the American College of Rheumatology in 1990[166] (see the box on p. 569).

Clinical manifestations. The condition is characterized by ulceration and granulomas of the upper and lower respiratory tract, focal and segmental glomerulitis sometimes leading to necrotizing glomerulonephritis, and other multisystem visceral and cutaneous signs similar to the other syndromes of medium-vessel systemic vasculitis. There is nasal, tracheal, bronchial, and laryngeal ulceration, and multiple nodular cavitary infiltrates of the lung parenchyma.[167] Most untreated patients die of renal failure.

Cutaneous signs. Fourteen to forty-seven percent have skin disease with histopathologic findings of necrotizing vasculitis,[168] granulomatous vasculitis, or palisading granuloma.[169] In one study there were palpable purpura (35%), oral ulcers (20%), skin nodules (8%), skin ulcers (7%), and necrotic papules (7%). Dermatologic manifestations were associated with a higher frequency of articular and renal involvement (68% vs. 25% and 80% vs. 47%, respectively).[170]

Antineutrophil cytoplasmic antibodies. ANCAs have been described as sensitive and specific markers for active Wegener's granulomatosis. Wegener's autoantigen, a 29-kD multifunctional protein, is the principal target antigen of autoantibodies associated with Wegener's granulomatosis (see previous section on ANCAs). c-ANCA occurs in more than 90% of patients with extended Wegener's granulomatosis, in 75% of patients with limited Wegener's granulomatosis without renal involvement, and in some 40% to 50% of patients with vasculitic overlap syndromes suggestive of Wegener's granulomatosis, such as microscopic polyarteritis. The presence of c-ANCA is highly specific for those diseases (greater than 98%). Changes in levels of c-ANCA may precede disease activity in some patients who have been in remission or who have low-grade smoldering disease.[88,171]

Treatment. The course of Wegener's granulomatosis has been dramatically improved by treatment with cyclophosphamide and glucocorticoids. Ninety-one percent of patients in one study experienced marked improvement, and 75% achieved complete remission. Fifty percent of remissions were associated with one or more relapses. Disease- and treatment-related morbidity is often profound. Almost all patients have serious morbidity from irreversible features of their disease (86%) or side effects of treatment (42%).[172] Sulfamethoxazole-trimethoprim[173] may be an alternative treatment or may be used with prednisone.[174]

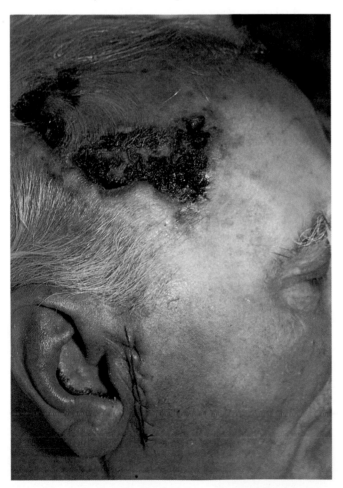

Vasculitis of Large Vessels
Giant-cell (temporal) arteritis

Giant-cell arteritis is a generalized inflammatory disorder involving large and medium-sized arteries. Polymyalgia rheumatica and temporal arteritis may represent different degrees or stages of the same disease.[175] Giant-cell (temporal) arteritis (Figure 18-12) is a necrotizing granulomatous vasculitis of branches of the carotid artery (superficial temporal and occipital and branches of the internal carotid artery); it occurs after age 50. New criteria for classification were established by the American College of Rheumatology in 1990.[176] The syndrome in the prodromal phase produces fever; polymyalgia rheumatica with aching pain and stiffness of the proximal muscles of the neck, shoulders, and hip girdle; and a high erythrocyte sedimentation rate.

In the active phase there is unilateral headache, erythema, and pain over the artery; loss of arterial pulses; tender nodules along the course of the artery; loss of vision; pain while eating; and sometimes massive skin ulceration of the scalp. In the chronic phase symptoms similar to the prodromal phase continue.[177] Management with varying dosages of prednisone has proved effective in resolving symptoms.

Takayasu's arteritis

Takayasu's arteritis is a rare, nonspecific, inflammatory disease of elastic arteries such as the aorta, its larger branches, and the pulmonary artery trunk. The inflammatory lesions are produced in the media and adventitia through the vasa vasorum, and terminate in a diffuse or nodular fibrosis. The male to female sex ratio is 1:4.5. The most frequent age of onset is between 20 and 30 years; the average age of death is between 40 and 50 years. Common clinical symptoms in one study were headache (60%), exertional dyspnea (42%), dizziness (36%), and malaise or weakness (34%). Takayasu's arteritis affected the abdominal aorta (46%) and descending thoracic aorta (37%) more frequently than the ascending aorta (1%) and aortic arch (2%).[178] New active lesions are often observed near the old fibrotic ones. Because the clinical features are determined by the extent and severity of the specific artery involved in the occlusive phase of the disease, total aortography, including coronary angiography, is very important in the initial evaluation of Takayasu's arteritis. The disease is managed surgically with vascular reconstruction[179] or medically with corticosteroids.[180] New criteria for classification were established by the American College of Rheumatology in 1990.

Figure 18-12
Temporal arteritis. There is massive ulceration of the temporal and scalp region. The temporal artery has been biopsied.

NEUTROPHILIC DERMATOSES

Neutrophilic dermatosis represents a continuous spectrum encompassing four entities: subcorneal pustular dermatosis, Sweet's syndrome, erythema elevatum diutinum, and pyoderma gangrenosum. The different neutrophilic dermatoses are manifestations of a potentially multisystemic neutrophilic disease. All may present with pustules, plaques, nodules, and ulcerations. Histologically, a neutrophilic infiltrate appears at variable levels in the epidermis, dermis, and subcutaneous tissue. Systemic manifestations include generalized symptoms and joint, renal, ocular, and lung involvement. There is an overlap in the clinical manifestations of the four entities.[181] Subcorneal pustular dermatosis is very rare and not described here.

Sweet's syndrome (acute febrile neutrophilic dermatosis)

Sweet, in 1964, described a disease with four features: fever; leukocytosis; acute, tender, red plaques; and a papillary dermal infiltrate of neutrophils. This led to the name *acute febrile neutrophilic dermatosis*. Larger series of patients showed that fever and neutrophilia are not consistently present. The diagnosis is based on the two constant features, a typical eruption and the characteristic histologic features; thus the eponym *Sweet's syndrome* (SS) is used. The criteria of the diagnosis of SS are listed in the box at right.

Eighty-six percent of patients are women with a preceding upper respiratory infection. The mean age at presentation is 56 years (range, 22 to 82 years). SS is common in Japan. A genetic predisposition is possible; HLA-Bw54 was found to be a risk factor in a series of Japanese patients with SS.

SS is a reactive phenomenon and should be considered a cutaneous marker of systemic disease. Careful systemic evaluation is indicated, especially when cutaneous lesions are severe or hematologic values are abnormal. Approximately 20% of cases are associated with malignancy. An underlying condition (streptococcal infection, inflammatory bowel disease, myelodysplastic syndrome,[182] non-lymphocytic leukemia and other hematologic malignancies, solid tumors, pregnancy) is found in up to 50% of cases. The association of SS and erythema nodosum and sarcoid[183] has been reported.[71] Attacks of SS may precede the diagnosis of neoplasia by 3 months to 6 years. Patients with associated malignancy are often males with mucosal symptoms, anemia, and frequent recurrence of skin symptoms.[184]

DIAGNOSTIC CRITERIA FOR SWEET'S SYNDROME*

MAJOR CRITERIA

1. Abrupt onset of tender or painful erythematous plaques or nodules occasionally with vesicles, pustules, or bullae
2. Predominantly neutrophilic infiltration in the dermis without leukocytoclastic vasculitis

MINOR CRITERIA

1. Preceded by a nonspecific respiratory or gastrointestinal tract infection or vaccination or associated with:
   - Inflammatory diseases such as chronic autoimmune disorders and infections
   - Hemoproliferative disorders or solid malignant tumors
   - Pregnancy
2. Accompanied by periods of general malaise and fever (>38°C)
3. Laboratory values during onset: ESR >20 mm; C-reactive protein positive; segmented-nuclear neutrophils and stabs >70% in peripheral blood smear; leukocytosis >8000 (three of four of these values necessary)
4. Excellent response to treatment with systemic corticosteroids or potassium iodide

Modified from von den Driesch P: Sweet's syndrome (acute febrile neutrophilic dermatosis), *J Am Acad Dermatol* 31:535-556, 1994.
*Both major and two minor criteria are needed for diagnosis.

Clinical manifestations. Acute, tender, erythematous plaques, nodes, pseudovesicles and, occasionally, blisters with an annular or arciform pattern occur on the head, neck, legs, and arms, particularly the back of the hands and fingers (Figure 18-13). The trunk is rarely involved. Fever (50%); arthralgia or arthritis (62%); eye involvement, most frequently conjunctivitis or iridocyclitis (38%); and oral aphthae (13%) are associated features. Differential diagnosis includes erythema multiforme, erythema nodosum, adverse drug reaction, and urticaria.[185-187] Recurrences are common and affect up to one third of patients.

Laboratory studies. Studies show a moderate neutrophilia (less than 50%), elevated erythrocyte sedimentation rate (greater than 30 mm/hr) (90%), and a slight increase in alkaline phosphatase (83%). ANCAs at a serum dilution of at least 1:20 were demonstrated. The type of ANCA (perinuclear ANCA versus cytoplasmic ANCA) was not subclassified in that report.[188]

Skin biopsy shows a papillary and middermal mixed infiltrate of polymorphonuclear leukocytes with nuclear fragmentation and histiocytic cells. The infiltrate is predominantly perivascular with endothelial-cell swelling in some vessels, but vasculitic changes (thrombosis; deposition of fibrin, complement, or immunoglobulins within the vessel walls; red blood cell extravasation; inflammatory infiltration of vascular walls) are absent.[189,190] A mechanism of disease has been proposed. Histiocyte-derived cytokines secreted either by infiltrating histiocytes in the nonleukemia-associated cases of SS or by tumoral myelomonocytic cells in those associated with leukemia may be responsible for the systemic manifestations and the infiltration with neutrophils in the skin lesions.[191]

Figure 18-13 Sweet's syndrome.

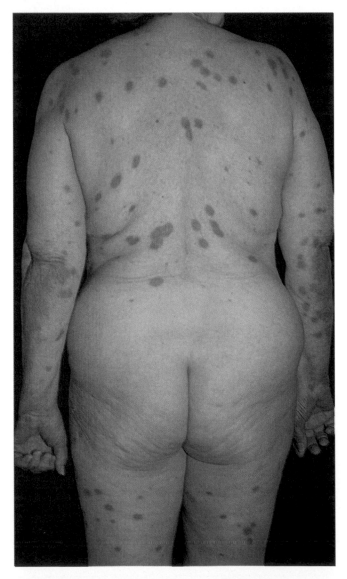

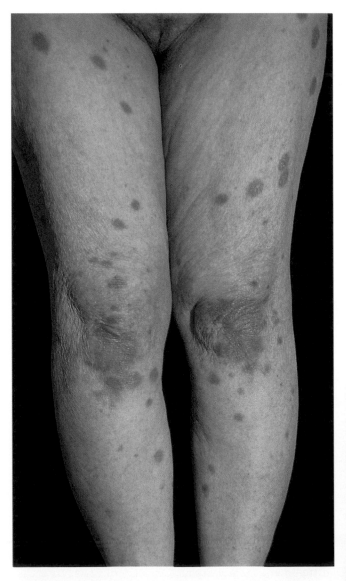

A, Multiple, painful, sharply demarcated, erythematous plaques occur on the neck, upper chest, back, and extremities.

B, Plaques are painful and burning but not itching. The surface is mamillated (papular) or may contain pustules.

Treatment. Systemic corticosteroids (prednisone 0.5 to 1.5 mg/kg of body weight per day) produce rapid improvement. The temperature, WBC count, and eruption improve within 72 hours. The skin lesions clear within 3 to 9 days. Abnormal laboratory values rapidly return to normal. There are, however, frequent recurrences. Corticosteroids are tapered within 2 to 6 weeks to zero. Resolution of the eruption is occasionally followed by milia and scarring. The disease clears spontaneously in some patients. Two patients with SS responded to doxycycline 200 mg daily.[192] Orally administered potassium iodide (15 mg/kg/day) significantly inhibited the neutrophil chemotaxis in peripheral blood[193] and is as effective as corticosteroids. The risk of short-term relapses may be lower. Other alternatives to corticosteroid treatment include colchicine, dapsone, doxycycline, clofazimine, nonsteroidal antiinflammatory agents, and cyclosporine.[194] All of these drugs influence migration and other functions of neutrophils.

Erythema elevatum diutinum

Erythema elevatum diutinum (EED) is a rare skin disease that occurs in men and women (average age, 53 years; range, 32 to 65 years). There are persistent, deep, brown-red–to–purple papules, nodules, and plaques. Blisters and ulcers can develop. Lesions are symmetrically distributed on extensor surfaces on the extremities with a preference for joint regions. Occasionally lesions are found on the buttocks, face, and torso. EED may be a complication of HIV infection.[195]Cutaneous lesions may closely resemble Kaposi's sarcoma.[196]

EED is most likely caused by immune complex deposition (Arthus reaction) in the dermal vessels. Excess exposure to antigens (recurrent infections) or situations in which high levels of antibody occur (e.g., paraproteinemias) are likely to result in immune complexes. Associated medical problems include hypergammaglobulinemia, both monoclonal (IgA clonal gammopathies)[197] and polyclonal;[198] multiple myeloma; and myelodysplasia. EED may precede the myeloproliferative disorders by up to 7.8 years. Chronic infection or recurrent infections (both streptococcal and nonstreptococcal) are also reported.

Histology. Early lesions show leukocytoclastic vasculitis and a massive dermal infiltrate composed mainly of neutrophils, histiocytes/macrophages, and Langerhans' cells. Later lesions contain dense fibrosis and a dermal infiltrate of lymphocytes and histiocytes/macrophages and Langerhans' cells.[199] Lipid material forms in some older lesions. The term *extracellular cholesterosis* is used to describe this process.

Laboratory studies. Laboratory studies to consider for patients with EED include skin biopsy, serum protein electrophoresis, quantitative immunoglobulins, immunoelectrophoresis, cryoglobulins, and complement studies (C3, C4, and CH$_{50}$). Direct immunofluorescence studies are generally nondiagnostic.

Treatment. Dapsone is the treatment of choice. One case of EED that was unresponsive to dapsone was successfully treated with colchicine.[200]

Pyoderma gangrenosum

Pyoderma gangrenosum (PG) is a poorly understood ulcerating skin disease.[201] It often occurs in patients with chronic underlying inflammatory or malignant disease such as ulcerative colitis, rheumatoid arthritis,[202] chronic active hepatitis, Crohn's disease, IgA monoclonal gammopathy,[203] and hematologic and lymphoreticular malignancies; but in 40% to 50% of patients no associated disease is found.[204,205] Trauma may precede PG in a few patients.[206] The disease is recurrent in approximately 30% of patients. In rare instances, PG occurs in children; thus it should be considered in the differential diagnosis of pustular disorders in children with underlying conditions such as ulcerative colitis.[207] A seronegative arthritis affecting large joints is present in approximately 40% of cases.[208]

PG occurs in both ulcerative colitis and in Crohn's disease. Approximately 50% of PG cases occur in association with ulcerative colitis.[63] Approximately 2% of patients with active and extensive ulcerative colitis have PG;[209] and another 4% of patients with active ulcerative colitis have erythema nodosum, which in its early stages can be confused with PG. Males and females are affected equally. The mean duration of chronic ulcerative colitis before the appearance of erythema nodosum and PG is 5 and 10 years, respectively.[63,210] The lesions generally appear during the course of active bowel disease, but they also occur in inactive colitis or less severe disease and may not appear until after colectomy.[211] Pyoderma resolved without intestinal resection in two thirds of patients. Healing after intestinal resection is unpredictable regarding both timing and extent of resection.[212]

Cutaneous manifestations. Lesions are most commonly found on the lower legs, but they may occur on the thighs, buttocks, chest, head, neck,[213] and anywhere on the skin.[214] One study showed that lesions were multiple in 71%, and more than 50% were situated below the knees. The lesion begins as a tender, red macule or papule, pustule, nodule, or bulla. Pustules or vesicles appear on the surface, and the surrounding skin becomes dusky red and indurated. A necrotizing inflammatory process extends peripherally from the primary lesion, resulting in a necrotic ulcer or ulcers with a purulent base with an undetermined purple-to-red margin and a halo of surrounding erythema[215] (Figure 18-14). The fully evolved lesion is generally less than 10 cm, but it may be enormous. The lesions tend to endure, lasting months to years, and heal with cribriform scarring.

Diagnosis. The diagnosis is made by clinical appearance. Histopathologically, PG evolves from folliculitis and abscess formation; it may also show leukocytoclastic vasculitis. The lesions then evolve to suppurative granulomatous dermatitis and finally regress with prominent fibroplasia.[216] These changes are nonspecific, therefore biopsy is of little diagnostic value. No specific abnormal laboratory determination has been found that is useful to diagnosis. Serum protein immunoelectrophoresis may be ordered to test for monoclonal gammopathy.

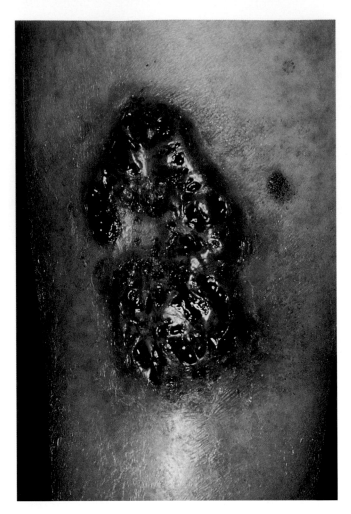

Figure 18-14
Pyoderma gangrenosum. The indurated plaque is ulcerating in several areas.

Treatment. Trauma must be avoided. The small early lesion may be aborted with an intralesional injection of triamcinolone acetonide (Kenalog 10 mg/ml or 40 mg/ml).[217,218] Group II to V topical steroids with or without occlusion may be effective. Systemic corticosteroids are the most consistently reported effective treatment for larger active or fully evolved lesions. Steroids probably do little to alter the natural course of the disease, and in many cases lesions recur after treatment is stopped. Prednisone 40 to 80 mg daily is required for initial control, and the dosage is then tapered and stopped. Dapsone (100 to 400 mg/day) with or without prednisone is effective.[203] The ulcer is treated locally with silver nitrate (1/8%) or Burow's wet compresses applied several times each day. The following drugs have been reported to be effective: minocycline (300 mg/day),[219] cyclosporine,[220-222] clofazimine,[223,224] chlorambucil,[225] methylprednisolone sodium succinate (1 gm infused over 1 hour each day for 5 days),[226,227] potassium iodide,[228] and the topical application of 20% nitrogen mustard.[227,229]

REFERENCES

1. Huff JC, Weston WL, Tonnesen MG: Erythema multiforme: a critical review of characteristics, diagnostic criteria, and causes, *J Am Acad Dermatol* 8:763-775, 1983.
2. Weston WL, Brice SL, et al: Herpes simplex virus in childhood erythema multiforme, *Pediatrics* 89:32-34, 1992.
3. Nesbit SP, Gobetti JP: Multiple recurrence of oral erythema multiforme after secondary herpes simplex: report of case and review of literature, *JAMA* 112:348-352, 1986.
4. Orton PW, Huff JC, Tonnesen MG, et al: Detection of a herpes simplex viral antigen in skin lesions of erythema multiforme, *Ann Intern Med* 101:48-50, 1984.
5. Brice SL, Stockert SS, et al: The herpes-specific immune response of individuals with herpes-associated erythema multiforme compared with that of individuals with recurrent herpes labialis, *Arch Dermatol Res* 285:193-196, 1993.
6. Darragh TM, Egbert BM, et al: Identification of herpes simplex virus DNA in lesions of erythema multiforme by the polymerase chain reaction, *J Am Acad Dermatol* 24:23-26, 1991.
7. Aslanzadeh J, Helm KF, et al: Detection of HSV-specific DNA in biopsy tissue of patients with erythema multiforme by polymerase chain reaction, *Br J Dermatol* 126:19-23, 1992.
8. Miura S, Smith CC, et al: Detection of viral DNA within skin of healed recurrent herpes simplex infection and erythema multiforme lesions, *J Invest Dermatol* 98:68-72, 1992.
9. Buchkell LL, Mackel SE, Jordan RE: Erythema multiforme: direct immunofluorescence studies and detection of circulating immune complexes, *J Invest Dermatol* 74:372, 1980.
10. Finan MC, Schroeter AL: Cutaneous immunofluorescence study of erythema multiforme: correlation with light microscopic patterns and etiologic agents, *J Am Acad Dermatol* 10:497-506, 1984.
11. Lemak MA, Duvic M, Bean SF: Oral acyclovir for the prevention of herpes-associated erythema multiforme, *J Am Acad Dermatol* 15:50-54, 1986.
12. Green JA, Spruance SL, Wenerstrom G, et al: Postherpetic erythema multiforme prevented with prophylactic oral acyclovir, *Ann Intern Med* 102:632-633, 1985.
13. Huff JC: Acyclovir for recurrent erythema multiforme caused by herpes simplex, *J Am Acad Dermatol* 18:197-199, 1988.
14. Schofield JK, Tatnall FM, et al: Recurrent erythema multiforme: clinical features and treatment in a large series of patients, *Br J Dermatol* 128:542-545, 1993.
15. Lozada-Nur F, Cram D, et al: Clinical response to levamisole in thirty-nine patients with erythema multiforme. An open prospective study, *Oral Surg Oral Med Oral Pathol* 74:294-298, 1992.
16. Bastuji-Garin S et al: A clinical classification of cases of toxic epidermal necrolysis, Stevens-Johnson syndrome and erythema multiforme, *Arch Dermatol* 129:92-96, 1993.
17. Haudrey MD et al: Erythema multiforme with mucous membrane involvement and Stevens-Johnson syndrome are clinically different disorders with distinct causes, *Arch Dermatol* 131:539-543, 1995.
18. Chan LS, Soong HK, et al: Ocular cicatricial pemphigoid occurring as a sequela of Stevens-Johnson syndrome, *JAMA* 266:1543-1546, 1991.
19. Levy M, Shear NH: *Mycoplasma pneumoniae* infections and Stevens-Johnson syndrome. Report of eight cases and review of the literature, *Clin Pediatr* 30:42-49, 1991.
20. Rasmussen JE: Erythema multiforme in children: response to treatment with systemic corticosteroids, *Br J Dermatol* 95:181-185, 1976.
21. Patterson R, Grammer LC, et al: Stevens-Johnson syndrome (SJS): effectiveness of corticosteroids in management and recurrent SJS, *Allergy Proc* 13:89-95, 1992.
22. Singer L, Brook U, et al: Vitamin A in Stevens-Johnson syndrome, *Ann Ophthalmol* 21:209-210, 1989.
23. Detjen PF, Patterson R, et al: Herpes simplex virus associated with recurrent Stevens-Johnson syndrome. A management strategy, *Arch Intern Med* 152:1513-1516, 1992.

24. Avakian R, Flowers FP, et al: Toxic epidermal necrolysis: a review, *J Am Acad Dermatol* 25:69-79, 1991.

25. Roujeau JC, Chosidow O, et al: Toxic epidermal necrolysis (Lyell syndrome), *J Am Acad Dermatol* 23:1063-1069, 1990.

26. Roujeau JC, Guillaume JC, et al: Toxic epidermal necrolysis (Lyell syndrome). Incidence and drug etiology in France, 1981-1985, *Arch Dermatol* 126:37-42, 1990.

27. Correia O, Chosidow O, et al: Evolving pattern of drug-induced toxic epidermal necrolysis, *Dermatology* 186:32-37, 1993.

28. Saiag P, Caumes E, et al: Drug-induced toxic epidermal necrolysis (Lyell syndrome) in patients infected with the human immunodeficiency virus, *J Am Acad Dermatol* 26:567-574, 1992.

29. Kimura S, Oka S, et al: Three cases of acquired immunodeficiency syndrome complicated with toxic epidermal necrolysis, *Jpn J Med* 30:553-558, 1991.

30. Villada G, Roujeau JC, et al: Toxic epidermal necrolysis after bone marrow transplantation: study of nine cases, *J Am Acad Dermatol* 23:870-875, 1990.

31. Heng MC, Allen SG: Efficacy of cyclophosphamide in toxic epidermal necrolysis. Clinical and pathophysiologic aspects, *J Am Acad Dermatol* 25:778-786, 1991.

32. Correia O, Delgado L, et al: Cutaneous T-cell recruitment in toxic epidermal necrolysis. Further evidence of CD8+ lymphocyte involvement, *Arch Dermatol* 129:466-468, 1993.

33. Villada G, Roujeau JC, et al: Immunopathology of toxic epidermal necrolysis. Keratinocytes, HLA-DR expression, Langerhans cells, and mononuclear cells: an immunopathologic study of five cases, *Arch Dermatol* 128:50-53, 1992.

34. Miyauchi H, Hosokawa H, et al: T-cell subsets in drug-induced toxic epidermal necrolysis. Possible pathogenic mechanism induced by CD8-positive T cells, *Arch Dermatol* 127:851-855, 1991.

35. Leenutaphong V, Sivayathorn A, et al: Stevens-Johnson syndrome and toxic epidermal necrolysis in Thailand, *Int J Dermatol* 32:428-431, 1993.

36. Wolkenstein P et al: Metabolic predisposition to cutaneous adverse drug reactions, *Arch Dermatol* 131:544-551, 1995.

37. Kim PS et al: Stevens-Johnson syndrome and toxic epidermal necrolysis: a pathophysiologic review with recommendations for a treatment protocol, *J Burn Care Rehabil* 4:91-100, 1983.

38. Goens J et al: Haematological disturbances and immune mechanisms in toxic epidermal necrolysis, *Br J Dermatol* 114:255-259, 1986.

39. Vermeer BJ, Claas FJH: Toxic epidermal necrolysis (letter), *Arch Dermatol* 121:715-716, 1985.

40. Roujeau JC et al: Granulocytes, lymphocytes, and toxic epidermal necrolysis, *Arch Dermatol* 121:305-307, 1985.

41. Ting HC, Adam BA: Stevens-Johnson syndrome: a review of 34 cases, *Int J Dermatol* 24:587-591, 1985.

42. Heimbach DM et al: Toxic epidermal necrolysis: a step forward in treatment, *JAMA* 257:2171-2175, 1987.

43. Hewitt J, Ormerod AD: Toxic epidermal necrolysis treated with cyclosporin, *Clin Exp Dermatol* 17:264-265, 1992.

44. Renfro L, Grant-Kels JM, et al: Drug-induced toxic epidermal necrolysis treated with cyclosporin, *Int J Dermatol* 28:441-444, 1989.

45. Sakellariou G, Koukoudis P, et al: Plasma exchange (PE) treatment in drug-induced toxic epidermal necrolysis (TEN), *Int J Artif Organs* 14:634-638, 1991.

46. Ruocco V, Bimonte D, et al: Hyperbaric oxygen treatment of toxic epidermal necrolysis, *Cutis* 38:267-271, 1986.

47. Kamanabroo D, Schmitz-Landgraf W, Czarnetzki BM: Plasmapheresis in severe drug induced toxic epidermal necrolysis, *Arch Dermatol* 121:1548-1549, 1985.

48. Peters W, Zaidi J, et al: Toxic epidermal necrolysis: a burn-centre challenge, *Can Med Assoc J* 144:1477-1480, 1991.

49. Ward DJ, Krzeminska EC, et al: Treatment of toxic epidermal necrolysis and a review of six cases, *Burns Incl Therm Inj* 16:97-104, 1990.

50. Taylor JA, Grube B, et al: Toxic epidermal necrolysis. A comprehensive approach. Multidisciplinary management in a burn center, *Clin Pediatr* 28:404-407, 1989.

51. Birchall N, Langdon R, Cuono C, et al: Toxic epidermal necrolysis: an approach to management using cryopreserved allograft skin, *J Am Acad Dermatol* 16:368-372, 1987.

52. Tegelberg-Stassen MJ, van Vloten WA, et al: Management of nonstaphylococcal toxic epidermal necrolysis: follow-up study of 16 case histories, *Dermatologica* 180:124-129, 1990.

53. Patterson R, Dykewicz MS, et al: Erythema multiforme and Stevens-Johnson syndrome. Descriptive and therapeutic controversy, *Chest* 98:331-336, 1990.

54. Rzany B, Schmitt H, et al: Toxic epidermal necrolysis in patients receiving glucocorticosteroids, *Acta Derm Venereol* 71:171-172, 1991.

55. Halebian PH et al: Improved burn center survival of patients with toxic epidermal necrolysis managed without corticosteroids, *Ann Surg* 204:503-511, 1986.

56. Elkayam O, Caspi D, et al: Familial erythema nodosum, *Arthritis Rheum* 34:1177-1179, 1991.

57. Braverman IM: Hypersensitivity syndromes. In: *Skin signs of systemic disease*, ed 2, Philadelphia, 1981, WB Saunders.

58. Nunnery E, Persellin RH, Pope RM: Lack of circulating immune complexes in uncomplicated erythema nodosum, *J Rheumatol* 10:991-994, 1983.

59. Fox MD, Schwartz RA: Erythema nodosum, *Am Fam Physician* 46:818-822, 1992.

60. Atanes A, Gomez N, et al: Erythema nodosum: a study of 160 cases, *Med Clin (Barc)* 96:169-172, 1991.

61. Simila S, Pietila J: The changing etiology of erythema nodosum in children, *Acta Tuberculosea et Pneumologica Scandinavica* 46:159, 1965.

62. MacPherson P: A survey of erythema nodosum in a rural community between 1954 and 1968, *Tubercle* 51:324, 1970.

63. Mir-Madjlessi SH, Taylor JS, Farmer RG: Clinical course and evolution of erythema nodosum and pyoderma gangrenosum in chronic ulcerative colitis: a study of 42 patients, *Am J Gastroenterol* 80:615-620, 1985.

64. Debois J et al: *Yersinia entercolitica* as a cause of erythema nodosum, *Dermatologica* 151:65, 1978.

65. Ikeya T, Mizuno E, Takama H: Three cases of erythema nodosum associated with *Yersinia enterocolitica* infection, *J Dermatol (Tokyo)* 13:147-150, 1986.

66. Sanders CJ, Hulsmans RF: Persistent erythema nodosum and asymptomatic *Campylobacter* infection, *J Am Acad Dermatol* 24:285-286, 1991.

67. Atanes A, de Toro J, et al: Study of 94 cases of sarcoidosis with special reference to erythema nodosum, *Rev Clin Esp* 191:65-70, 1992.

68. Simon S, Azevedo SJ, Byrnes JJ: Erythema nodosum heralding recurrent Hodgkin's disease, *Cancer* 56:1470-1472, 1985.

69. Taillan B, Ferrari E, et al: Erythema nodosum and Hodgkin's disease, *Clin Rheumatol* 9:397-398, 1990.

70. Kirch W, Duhrsen U: Erythema nodosum of dental origin, *Clin Invest Med* 70:1073-1078, 1992.

71. Cohen PR, Holder WR, et al: Concurrent Sweet's syndrome and erythema nodosum: a report, world literature review and mechanism of pathogenesis, *J Rheumatol* 19:814-820, 1992.

72. Schlegel Gomez R, Kiesewetter F, et al: Sweet syndrome (acute febrile neutrophilic dermatosis) and erythema nodosum in Crohn disease, *Hautarzt* 41:398-401, 1990.

73. Lofgren S: Erythema nodosum: studies on etiology and pathogenesis in 185 adult cases, *Acta Med Scand* 174 [suppl]:1, 1946.

74. Sanz Vico MD, De Diego V, et al: Erythema nodosum versus nodular vasculitis, *Int J Dermatol* 32:108-112, 1993.

75. Horio T et al: Potassium iodide in the treatment of erythema nodosum and nodular vasculitis, *Arch Dermatol* 117:29-31, 1981.

76. Schultz EJ, Whiting DA: Treatment of erythema nodosum and nodular vasculitis with potassium iodide, *Br J Dermatol* 94:75-78, 1976.

77. Soderstron RM, Krull EA: Erythema nodosum: a review, *Cutis* 21:806-810, 1978.

78. Elizaga FV: Erythema nodosum and indomethacin, *Ann Intern Med* 96:383, 1982.

79. Lehman CW: Control of chronic erythema nodosum with naproxen, *Cutis* 26:66-67, 1980.
80. Bacon PA: Systemic vasculitic syndromes, *Curr Opin Rheumatol* 5:5-10, 1993.
81. Soter NA: Clinical presentations and mechanisms of necrotizing angiitis of the skin, *J Invest Dermatol* 67:354-359, 1976.
82. Charles LA, Caldas ML, et al: Antibodies against granule proteins activate neutrophils in vitro, *J Leukoc Biol* 50:539-546, 1991.
83. Geffriaud-Ricouard C, Noel LH, et al: Clinical spectrum associated with ANCA of defined antigen specificities in 98 selected patients, *Clin Nephrol* 39:125-136, 1993.
84. Niles JL: Value of tests for antineutrophil cytoplasmic autoantibodies in the diagnosis and treatment of vasculitis, *Curr Opin Rheumatol* 5:18-24, 1993.
85. Jennette JC, Ewert BH, et al: Do antineutrophil cytoplasmic autoantibodies cause Wegener's granulomatosis and other forms of necrotizing vasculitis? *Rheum Dis Clin North Am* 19:1-14, 1993.
86. Gross WL, Csernok E, et al: 'Classic' anti-neutrophil cytoplasmic autoantibodies (cANCA), 'Wegener's autoantigen' and their immunopathogenic role in Wegener's granulomatosis, *J Autoimmun* 6:171-184, 1993.
87. Cohen-Tervaert JW, Limburg PC, et al: Detection of autoantibodies against myeloid lysosomal enzymes: a useful adjunct to classification of patients with biopsy-proven necrotizing arteritis, *Am J Med* 91:59-66, 1991.
88. Kallenberg CG, Mulder AH, et al: Antineutrophil cytoplasmic antibodies: a still-growing class of autoantibodies in inflammatory disorders, *Am J Med* 93:675-682, 1992.
89. Mackel SE, Jordon RE: Leukocytoclastic vasculitis: a cutaneous expression of immune complex disease, *Arch Dermatol* 118:296-301, 1982.
90. Gower RG et al: Leukocytoclastic vasculitis: sequential appearance of immunoreactants and cellular changes in serial biopsies, *J Invest Dermatol* 69:477-484, 1977.
91. Sams WM et al: Leukocytoclastic vasculitis (review), *Arch Dermatol* 112:219-226, 1976.
92. Ramsay C, Fry L: Allergic vasculitis: clinical and histological features and incidence of renal involvement, *Br J Dermatol* 81:96, 1969.
93. Winkelman RK, Ditto WB: Cutaneous and visceral syndromes of necrotizing or "allergic" angiitis: a study of thirty-eight cases, *Medicine* 43:59-89, 1964.
94. Lopez LR et al: Gastrointestinal involvement in leukocytoclastic vasculitis and polyarteritis nodosa, *J Rheumatol* 7:677-684, 1980.
95. Ekenstram EA, Callen JP: Cutaneous leukocytoclastic vasculitis, *Arch Dermatol* 120:484-489, 1984.
96. Callen JP, Ekenstam EA: Cutaneous leukocytoclastic vasculitis: clinical experience in 44 patients, *South Med J* 80:848-851, 1987.
97. Greer JM et al: Vasculitis associated with malignancy: experience with 13 patients and literature review, *Medicine (Baltimore)* 67:220, 1988.
98. Sanchez NP, Van Hale HM, Daniel Su WP: Clinical and histopathologic spectrum of necrotizing vasculitis: report of findings in 101 cases, *Arch Dermatol* 121:220-224, 1985.
99. Callen JP: Colchicine is effective in controlling chronic cutaneous leukocytoclastic vasculitis, *J Am Acad Dermatol* 13:193-200, 1985.
100. Fredenberg MF, Malkinson FD: Sulfone therapy in the treatment of leukocytoclastic vasculitis: report of three cases, *J Am Acad Dermatol* 16:772-778, 1987.
101. Fauci AS: Cyclophosphamide, *N Engl J Med* 301:235, 1979.
102. Cupps TR, Springer L, Fauci AS: Cyclophosphamide, *JAMA* 247:1994, 1982.
103. Tapson KM: H-S purpura, *Am Fam Physician* 47:633, 1993.
104. Michel BA, Hunder GG, et al: Hypersensitivity vasculitis and Henoch-Schönlein purpura: a comparison between the 2 disorders. *J Rheumatol* 19:721-728, 1992.
105. Ilan Y, Naparstek Y: Schönlein-Henoch syndrome in adults and children, *Semin Arthritis Rheum* 21:103-109, 1991.
106. Farley TA, Gillespie S, et al: Epidemiology of a cluster of Henoch-Schönlein purpura, *Am J Dis Child* 143:798-803, 1989.
107. Saulsbury FT: Henoch-Schönlein purpura, *Pediatr Dermatol* 1:195-201, 1984.
108. Hu SC, Feeney MS, et al: Ultrasonography to diagnose and exclude intussusception in Henoch-Schönlein purpura, *Arch Dis Child* 66:1065-1067, 1991.
109. Cull DL, Rosario V, et al: Surgical implications of Henoch-Schönlein purpura, *J Pediatr Surg* 25:741-743, 1990.
110. Kato S, Shibuya H, et al: Gastrointestinal endoscopy in Henoch-Schönlein purpura, *Eur J Pediatr* 151:482-484, 1992.
111. Katz S, Borst M, et al: Surgical evaluation of Henoch-Schönlein purpura. Experience with 110 children, *Arch Surg* 126:849-853, 1991.
112. Kagimoto S: Duodenal findings on ultrasound in children with Schönlein-Henoch purpura and gastrointestinal symptoms, *J Pediatr Gastroenterol Nutr* 16:178-182, 1993.
113. Couture A, Veyrac C, et al: Evaluation of abdominal pain in Henoch-Schönlein syndrome by high frequency ultrasound, *Pediatr Radiol* 22:12-17, 1992.
114. Linne T et al: Renal function and biopsy changes during the course of Henoch-Schönlein glomerulonephritis, *Acta Paediatr Scand* 72:97, 1983.
115. Gauthier B: Schönlein-Henoch nephritis and IgA nephropathy in children, *Curr Opin Pediatr* 5:180-185, 1993.
116. Goldstein AR, White RH, et al: Long-term follow-up of childhood Henoch-Schönlein nephritis, *Lancet* 339:280-282, 1992.
117. Nathwani D, Laing RB, et al: Recurrent post-infective Henoch-Schönlein syndrome: a genetic influence related to HLA B35? *J Infect* 25:205-210, 1992.
118. Fogazzi GB, Pasquali S, et al: Long-term outcome of Schönlein-Henoch nephritis in the adult, *Clin Nephrol* 31:60-66, 1989.
119. Chamberlain RS, Greenberg LW: Scrotal involvement in Henoch-Schönlein purpura: a case report and review of the literature, *Pediatr Emerg Care* 8:213-215, 1992.
120. O'Brien WM, O'Connor KP, et al: Acute scrotal swelling in Henoch-Schönlein syndrome: evaluation with testicular scanning, *Urology* 41:366-368, 1993.
121. Petersen S, Taaning E, et al: Immunoglobulin and complement studies in children with Schönlein-Henoch syndrome and other vasculitic diseases, *Acta Paediatr Scand* 80:1037-1043, 1991.
122. Van Hale HM, Gibson LE, Schroeter AL: Henoch-Schönlein vasculitis: direct immunofluorescence study of uninvolved skin, *J Am Acad Dermatol* 15:665-670, 1986.
123. Abou-Ragheb HH, Williams AJ, et al: Plasma levels of the anaphylatoxins C3a and C4a in patients with IgA nephropathy/Henoch-Schönlein nephritis, *Nephron* 62:22-26, 1992.
124. Helander SD et al: Henoch-Schönlein purpura: clinicopathologic correlation of cutaneous vascular IgA deposits and the relationship to leukocytoclastic vasculitis, *Acta Derm Venereol* 75:125, 1995.
125. Wang YJ, Chi CS, et al: Clinical studies of Henoch-Schönlein purpura in Chinese children, *Chung Hua I Hsueh Tsa Chih* 51:345-349, 1993.
126. Ledermann JA, Hoffbrand BI: Dapsone in allergic vasculitis: its use in Henoch-Schönlein disease following vaccination, *J Royal Soc Med* 76:613-614, 1983.
127. Hoffbrand BI: Dapsone in Henoch-Schönlein purpura—worth a trial, *Postgrad Med J* 67:961-962, 1991.
128. Saulsbury FT: Corticosteroid therapy does not prevent nephritis in Henoch-Schönlein purpura, *Pediatr Nephrol* 7:69-71, 1993.
129. Heng MCY: Henoch-Schönlein purpura, *Br J Dermatol* 112:235-240, 1985.
130. Heldrich FJ, Minkin S, et al: Intravenous immunoglobulin in Henoch-Schönlein purpura: a case study, *Md Med J* 42:577-579, 1993.
131. Fukui H, Kamitsuji H, et al: Clinical evaluation of a pasteurized factor XIII concentrate administration in Henoch-Schönlein purpura. Japanese Pediatric Group, *Thromb Res* 56:667-675, 1989.
132. Utani A, Ohta M, et al: Successful treatment of adult Henoch-Schönlein purpura with factor XIII concentrate, *J Am Acad Dermatol* 24:438-442, 1991.

133. Draelos ZK, Hansen RC: Schamberg's purpura in children: case study and literature review, *Clin Pediatr* 26:659-661, 1987.

134. Aiba S, Tagami H: Immunohistologic studies in Schamberg's disease, *Arch Dermatol* 124:1058-1062, 1988.

135. Smoller BR, Kamel OW: Pigmented purpuric eruptions: immunopathologic studies supportive of a common immunophenotype, *J Cutan Pathol* 18:423-427, 1991.

136. Abeck D, Gross GE, et al: Acetaminophen-induced progressive pigmentary purpura (Schamberg's disease), *J Am Acad Dermatol* 27:123-124, 1992.

137. Ratnam KV, Su WP, et al: Purpura simplex (inflammatory purpura without vasculitis): a clinicopathologic study of 174 cases, *J Am Acad Dermatol* 25:642-647, 1991.

138. Meltzer M et al: Cryoglobulinemia: a clinical and laboratory study, *Am J Med* 40:828, 1966.

139. Gorevic PD et al: Mixed cryoglobulinemia: clinical aspects and long-term follow-up of 40 patients, *Amer J Med* 69:287-308, 1980.

140. Levo Y, Gorevic PD, Kassab HJ, et al: Association between hepatitis B virus and essential mixed cryoglobulinemia, *N Engl J Med* 296:1501-1504, 1977.

141. Popp JW Jr, Dienstag JL, Wands JR, et al: Essential mixed cryoglobulinemia without evidence for hepatitis B virus infection, *Ann Intern Med* 92:379-383, 1980.

142. Nishikawa JA: Are leg ulcers in rheumatoid arthritis due to vasculitis? *Eur J Rheumatol Inflamm* 6:288-290, 1983.

143. Gray RG, Poppo MJ: Necrotizing vasculitis as the initial manifestation of rheumatoid arthritis, *J Rheumatol* 10:326-328, 1983.

144. Lakhanpal S, Conn DL, Lie JT: Clinical and prognostic significance of vasculitis as an early manifestation of connective tissue disease syndromes, *Ann Intern Med* 101:743-748, 1984.

145. Upchurch KS, Heller K, Bress NM: Low-dose methotrexate therapy for cutaneous vasculitis of rheumatoid arthritis, *J Am Acad Dermatol* 17:355-359, 1987.

146. Monroe EW et al: Vasculitis in chronic urticaria: an immunopathologic study, *J Invest Dermatol* 76:103-107, 1981.

147. Sergent JS et al: Vasculitis with hepatitis B antigenemia: long term observations in nine patients, *Medicine* 55:1-18, 1976.

148. Masi AT, Hunder GG, et al: The American College of Rheumatology 1990 criteria for the classification of Churg-Strauss syndrome (allergic granulomatosis and angiitis), *Arthritis Rheum* 33:1094-1100, 1990.

149. Gibson LE: Granulomatous vasculitides and the skin, *Dermatol Clin* 8:335-345, 1990.

150. Guillevin L et al: Anticytoplasmic antibodies in systemic polyarteritis nodosa with and without hepatitis B virus infection and Churg-Strauss syndrome: 62 patients, *J Rheumatol (Canada)* 20(3):1345-1349, 1993.

151. Guillevin L, Jarrousse B, et al: Long-term followup after treatment of polyarteritis nodosa and Churg-Strauss angiitis with comparison of steroids, plasma exchange and cyclophosphamide to steroids and plasma exchange. A prospective randomized trial of 71 patients. The Cooperative Study Group for Polyarteritis Nodosa, *J Rheumatol* 18:567-574, 1991.

152. Serra A et al: Vasculitis affecting the kidney: presentation, histopathology and long-term outcome, *Q J Med* 210:181-207, 1984.

153. Siberrg GK et al: Cutaneous polyarteritis nodosa: reports of two cases in children and review of the literature, *Arch Dermatol* 130:884-889, 1994.

154. Seth AP et al: Cutaneous polyarteritis nodosa of childhood, *J Am Acad Dermatol*, 31:561-566, 1994.

155. Guillevin L, Lhote F, et al: Polyarteritis nodosa related to hepatitis B virus. A retrospective study of 66 patients, *Ann Med Interne* 143:63-74, 1992.

156. Cohen RD, Conn DL, Ilstrup DM: Clinical features, prognosis, and response to treatment in polyarteritis, *Mayo Clin Proc* 55:146-155, 1980.

157. Travers RL, Allison DJ, Brettle RP, et al: Polyarteritis nodosa: a clinical and angiographic analysis of 17 cases, *Semin Arthritis Rheum* 8:184-199, 1979.

158. Guillevin L, Fain O, et al: Lack of superiority of steroids plus plasma exchange to steroids alone in the treatment of polyarteritis nodosa and Churg-Strauss syndrome. A prospective, randomized trial in 78 patients, *Arthritis Rheum* 35:208-215, 1992.

159. Guillevin L, Lhote F, et al: Treatment of polyarteritis nodosa and Churg-Strauss syndrome. A meta-analysis of 3 prospective controlled trials including 182 patients over 12 years, *Ann Med Interne* 143:405-416, 1992.

160. Cameron JS: Renal vasculitis: microscopic polyarteritis and Wegener's granuloma, *Contrib Nephrol* 94:38-46, 1991.

161. Guillevin L, Lhote F, et al: Treatment of polyarteritis nodosa related to hepatitis B virus with short-term steroid therapy associated with antiviral agents and plasma exchanges. A prospective trial in 33 patients, *J Rheumatol* 20:289-298, 1993.

162. Diaz-Perez JL, Schroeter AL, Winkelmann RK: Cutaneous periarteritis nodosa, *Arch Dermatol* 116:56-58, 1980.

163. Diaz-Perez JL, Winkelmann RK: Cutaneous periarteritis nodosa, *Arch Dermatol* 110:407-414, 1974.

164. Minkowitz G, Smoller BR, et al: Benign cutaneous polyarteritis nodosa. Relationship to systemic polyarteritis nodosa and to hepatitis B infection, *Arch Dermatol* 127:1520-1523, 1991.

165. Rottem M, Fauci AS, et al: Wegener granulomatosis in children and adolescents: clinical presentation and outcome, *J Pediatr* 122:26-31, 1993.

166. Leavitt, RY, Fauci AS, et al: The American College of Rheumatology 1990 criteria for the classification of Wegener's granulomatosis, *Arthritis Rheum* 33:1101-1107, 1990.

167. Anderson G, Coles ET, et al: Wegener's granuloma. A series of 265 British cases seen between 1975 and 1985. A report by a sub-committee of the British Thoracic Society Research Committee, *Q J Med* 83:427-438, 1992.

168. Mangold MC, Callen JP: Cutaneous leukocytoclastic vasculitis associated with active Wegener's granulomatosis, *J Am Acad Dermatol* 26:579-584, 1992.

169. Patten SF, Tomecki KJ: Wegener's granulomatosis: cutaneous and oral mucosal disease, *J Am Acad Dermatol* 28:710-718, 1993.

170. Francès C et al: Wegener's granulomatosis: dermatologic manifestation in 75 cases with clinicopathologic correlation, *Arch Dermatol* 130:861-867, 1994.

171. Kerr GS, Fleisher TA, et al: Limited prognostic value of changes in antineutrophil cytoplasmic antibody titer in patients with Wegener's granulomatosis, *Arthritis Rheum* 36:365-371, 1993.

172. Hoffman GS, Kerr GS, et al: Wegener granulomatosis: an analysis of 158 patients, *Ann Intern Med* 116:488-498, 1992.

173. McRae D, Buchanan G: Long-term sulfamethoxazole-trimethoprim in Wegener's granulomatosis, *Arch Otolaryngol Head Neck Surg* 119:103-105, 1993.

174. Valeriano-Marcet J, Spiera H: Treatment of Wegener's granulomatosis with sulfamethoxazole-trimethoprim, *Arch Intern Med* 151:1649-1652, 1991.

175. Nordborg E, Nordborg C, et al: Giant cell arteritis, *Curr Opin Rheumatol* 4:23-30, 1992.

176. Hunder GG, Bloch DA, et al: The American College of Rheumatology 1990 criteria for the classification of giant cell arteritis, *Arthritis Rheum* 33:1122-1128, 1990.

177. Hunder GG, Allen GL: Giant cell arteritis: a review, *Bull Rheum Dis* 29:980, 1978.

178. Park YB, Hong SK, et al: Takayasu arteritis in Korea: clinical and angiographic features, *Heart Vessels Suppl* 7:55-59, 1992.

179. Tada Y, Sato O, et al: Surgical treatment of Takayasu arteritis, *Heart Vessels Suppl* 7:159-167, 1992.

180. Hotchi M: Pathological studies on Takayasu arteritis, *Heart Vessels Suppl* 7:11-17, 1992.

181. Vignon-Pennamen MD, Wallach D: Cutaneous manifestations of neutrophilic disease. A study of seven cases, *Dermatologica* 183:255-264, 1991.

182. Soppi E, Nousiainen T, et al: Acute febrile neutrophilic dermatosis (Sweet's syndrome) in association with myelodysplastic syndromes: a report of three cases and a review of the literature, *Br J Haematol* 73:43-47, 1989.

183. Pouchot J et al: Sweet's syndrome and mediastinal lymphadenopathy due to sarcoidosis: three cases of a new association, *Arch Dermatol* 129:1062-1064, 1993.

184. Clemmensen OJ, Menne T, et al: Acute febrile neutrophilic dermatosis—a marker of malignancy? *Acta Derm Venereol* 69:52-58, 1989.

185. Sitjas D, Puig L, et al: Acute febrile neutrophilic dermatosis (Sweet's syndrome), *Int J Dermatol* 32:261-268, 1993.

186. Smolle J, Kresbach H: Acute febrile neutrophilic dermatosis (Sweet syndrome). A retrospective clinical and histological analysis, *Hautarzt* 41:549-556, 1990.

187. Kemmett D, Hunter JA: Sweet's syndrome: a clinicopathologic review of twenty-nine cases, *J Am Acad Dermatol* 23:503-507, 1990.

188. Kemmett D, Harrison DJ, et al: Antibodies to neutrophil cytoplasmic antigens: serologic marker for Sweet's syndrome, *J Am Acad Dermatol* 24:967-969, 1991.

189. Going JJ, Going SM, Myskow MW, et al: Sweet's syndrome: histological and immunohistochemical study of 15 cases, *J Clin Pathol* 40:175-179, 1987.

190. Jordaan HF: Acute febrile neutrophilic dermatosis. A histopathological study of 37 patients and a review of the literature, *Am J Dermatopathol* 11:99-111, 1989.

191. Delabie J, De Wolf-Peeters C, et al: Histiocytes in Sweet's syndrome, *Br J Dermatol* 124:348-353, 1991.

192. Joshi RK, Atukorala DN, et al: Successful treatment of Sweet's syndrome with doxycycline, *Br J Dermatol* 128:584-586, 1993.

193. Honma K, Saga K, et al: Potassium iodide inhibits neutrophil chemotaxis, *Acta Derm Venereol* 70:247-249, 1990.

194. von den Driesch P: Sweet's syndrome (acute febrile neutrophilic dermatosis), *J Am Acad Dermatol* 31:535-556, 1994.

195. Le Boit PE, Cockerell CJ: Nodular lesions of erythema elevatum diutinum in patients infected with the human immunodeficiency virus, *J Am Acad Dermatol* 28:919-922, 1993.

196. Requena L, Sanchez Yus E, et al: Erythema elevatum diutinum in a patient with acquired immunodeficiency syndrome. Another clinical simulator of Kaposi's sarcoma, *Arch Dermatol* 127:1819-1822, 1991.

197. Yiannias JA, el-Azhary RA, et al: Erythema elevatum diutinum: a clinical and histopathologic study of 13 patients, *J Am Acad Dermatol* 26:38-44, 1992.

198. Wilkinson SM, English JS, et al: Erythema elevatum diutinum: a clinicopathological study, *Clin Exp Dermatol* 17:87-93, 1992.

199. Lee AY, Nakagawa H, et al: Erythema elevatum diutinum: an ultrastructural case study, *J Cutan Pathol* 16:211-217, 1989.

200. Henriksson R, Hofer PA, et al: Erythema elevatum diutinum—a case successfully treated with colchicine, *Clin Exp Dermatol* 14:451-453, 1989.

201. Duguid CM, Powell FC: Pyoderma gangrenosum, *Clin Dermatol* 11:129-133, 1993.

202. Ko CB, Walton S, et al: Pyoderma gangrenosum: associations revisited, *Int J Dermatol* 31:574-577, 1992.

203. Powell FC, Schroeter AL, Daniel Su WP, et al: Pyoderma gangrenosum and monoclonal gammopathy, *Arch Dermatol* 119:468-472, 1983.

204. Hickman JG, Lazarus GS: Pyoderma gangrenosum: a reappraisal of associated systemic diseases, *Br J Dermatol* 102:235-237, 1980.

205. Perry HO, Winkelmann RK: Bullous pyoderma gangrenosum and leukemia, *Arch Dermatol* 106:901-905, 1972.

206. Finkel SI, Janowitz HD: Trauma and the pyoderma gangrenosum of inflammatory bowel disease, *Gut* 22:410-412, 1981.

207. Barnes L, Lucky AW, Bucuvalas JC, et al: Pustular pyoderma gangrenosum associated with ulcerative colitis in childhood: report of two cases and review of the literature, *J Am Acad Dermatol* 15:608-614, 1986.

208. Holt PJA et al: Pyoderma gangrenosum: clinical and laboratory findings in 15 patients with special reference to polyarthritis, *Medicine* 59:114-133, 1980.

209. Basler RSW: Ulcerative colitis and the skin, *Med Clin North Am* 64:941-954, 1980.

210. Thornton JR et al: Pyoderma gangrenosum and ulcerative colitis, *Gut* 21:247-248, 1980.

211. Johnson ML, Wilson HT: Skin lesions in ulcerative colitis, *Gut* 10:255-263, 1969.

212. Levitt MD, Ritchie JK, et al: Pyoderma gangrenosum in inflammatory bowel disease, *Br J Surg* 78:676-678, 1991.

213. Synder RA: Pyoderma gangrenosum involving the head and neck, *Arch Dermatol* 122:295-302, 1986.

214. Powell FC et al: Pyoderma gangrenosum: a review of 86 patients, *Q J Med* 55:173-186, 1985.

215. Brunsting LA, Goeckerman WH, O'Leary PA: Pyoderma (ecthyma) gangrenosum: clinical and experimental observations in five cases occurring in adults, *Arch Dermatol Syphilol* 22:655-680, 1930,

216. Hurwitz RM, Haseman JH: The evolution of pyoderma gangrenosum. A clinicopathologic correlation, *Am J Dermatopathol* 15:28-33, 1993.

217. Goldstein F, Krain R, Thornton JL: Intralesional steroid therapy of pyoderma gangrenosum, *J Clin Gastroenterol* 7:499-501, 1985.

218. Jennings JL: Pyoderma gangrenosum: successful treatment with intralesional steroids, *J Am Acad Dermatol* 9:575-580, 1983.

219. Lynch WS, Bergfeld WF: Pyoderma gangrenosum responsive to minocycline hydrochloride, *Cutis* 21:535-538, 1978.

220. Fedi MC, Quercetani R, et al: Recalcitrant pyoderma gangrenosum responsive to cyclosporine, *Int J Dermatol* 32:119, 1993.

221. Magid ML, Gold MH: Treatment of recalcitrant pyoderma gangrenosum with cyclosporine, *J Am Acad Dermatol* 20:293-294, 1989.

222. Elgart G, Stover P, et al: Treatment of pyoderma gangrenosum with cyclosporine: results in seven patients, *J Am Acad Dermatol* 24:83-86, 1991.

223. Kaplan B, Trau H, et al: Treatment of pyoderma gangrenosum with clofazimine, *Int J Dermatol* 31:591-593, 1992.

224. Kark EC, Davis BR: Clofazimine treatment of pyoderma gangrenosum, *J Am Acad Dermatol* 5:346-347, 1981.

225. Callen JP et al: Chlorambucil: an effective corticosteroid-sparing drug for pyoderma gangrenosum, *J Am Acad Dermatol* 21:515-519, 1989.

226. Resnik BI, Rendon M, et al: Successful treatment of aggressive pyoderma gangrenosum with pulse steroids and chlorambucil, *J Am Acad Dermatol* 27:635-636, 1992.

227. Prystowsky JH, Kahn SN, et al: Present status of pyoderma gangrenosum. Review of 21 cases, *Arch Dermatol* 125:57-64, 1989.

228. Richardson JB, Callen JP: Pyoderma gangrenosum treated successfully with potassium iodide, *J Am Acad Dermatol* 28:1005-1007, 1993.

229. Tsele E, Yu RC, et al: Pyoderma gangrenosum—response to topical nitrogen mustard, *Clin Exp Dermatol* 17:437-440, 1992.

CHAPTER NINETEEN

Light-Related Diseases and Disorders of Pigmentation

Photobiology

Sunlight has profound effects on the skin and is associated with a variety of diseases (see the box on p. 598). Ultraviolet light causes most photobiologic skin reactions and diseases. The accepted unit for measuring the wavelength of light is the nanometer (nm). The solar radiation reaching the earth is a continuous spectrum consisting of wavelengths of electromagnetic energy above 290 nm. By convention, ultraviolet light is divided into UVA (320 to 400 nm; long wave, black light), UVB (290 to 320 nm; middle wave, sunburn), and UVC (100 to 290 nm; short wave, germicidal).

UVA causes immediate and delayed tanning and contributes little to erythema and burning. It is constant throughout the day. The longer wavelengths of UVA can penetrate more deeply, reaching the dermis and subcutaneous fat. Chronic exposure to UVA radiation causes the connective tissue degeneration seen in photoaging. UVA augments the carcinogenic effects of UVB. UVA penetrates window glass and interacts with topical and systemic chemicals and medication.

UVB delivers a high amount of energy to the stratum corneum and superficial layers of the epidermis and is primarily responsible for sunburn, suntan, and skin cancers. It produces tanning more efficiently than UVA. It is most intense when the sun is directly overhead between 10 A.M. and 2 P.M. UVB is absorbed by window glass. Prior exposure to UVA enhances the sunburn reaction from UVB.

UVC is almost completely absorbed by the ozone layer and is only transmitted by artificial sources such as germicidal lamps and mercury arc lamps.

CLASSIFICATION OF ABNORMAL REACTIONS TO SOLAR RADIATION

Normal individuals
  Sunburn reaction
  Immediate pigment darkening or tanning reaction
  Delayed tanning (melanogenesis)
Degenerative and neoplastic
  Actinic damage
  Actinic keratosis
  Basal cell carcinoma
  Squamous cell carcinoma
  Malignant melanoma
Idiopathic
  Polymorphous light eruptions
  Hydroa aestivale
  Hydroa vacciniforme
  Solar urticaria
Photosensitivity
  Phototoxicity
  Photoallergy
  Drug eruptions

Photoaggravated diseases
  Acne
  Darier's disease
  Dermatomyositis
  Discoid lupus erythematosus
  Hailey-Hailey disease
  Herpes simplex labialis
  Lichen planus actinicus
  Lymphogranuloma venereum
  Pemphigus foliaceus
  Psoriasis
  Rosacea
Metabolic
  Erythropoietic porphyria
  Erythropoietic protoporphyria
  Porphyria cutanea tarda
  Variegate porphyria

Sun-Damaged Skin

Aging vs. sun damage. Sun exposure is the major cause of the undesirable skin changes often inaccurately perceived as aging. These changes, known as *photoaging*, are caused primarily by repeated sun exposure and not by the passage of time. Many of the clinical signs attributed to aging are actually manifestations of solar damage. The two processes are biologically different.[1,2] The difference can best be demonstrated to patients by comparing the appearance of the skin under the arm near the axillae with the sun-exposed surface of the lower arm.

Normal aging. The skin begins to show signs of aging by ages 30 to 35. Aged skin is thin, fragile, and inelastic. The epidermis becomes thin. There is a gradual loss of blood vessels, dermal collagen, fat, and the number of elastic fibers. There is a reduction in the density of hair follicles, sweat ducts, and sebaceous glands, resulting in a reduction in perspiration and sebum production. Potent steroids should not be used on aged skin with few blood vessels because the steroids are not cleared from the skin as easily as in younger persons.

The skin becomes atrophic and fragile when subcutaneous tissue is lost. Elastic fibers are responsible for the elasticity and resilience of the skin. In normal aging there are loss and fragmentation of elastic fibers, which result in fine wrinkles that resemble crumpled cigarette paper. These shallow wrinkles disappear by stretching. The skin is easily distorted, but it recoils slowly.

Photoaging. Photoaging refers to those skin changes superimposed on intrinsic aging by chronic sun exposure (see the box on p. 599, *top*).[3] Sun-damaged skin is characterized by elastosis (a coarsening and yellow discoloration of the skin), irregular pigmentation, roughness or dryness, telangiectasia, atrophy, deep wrinkling, follicular plugging, and a variety of benign and malignant neoplasms.[4] The epidermis thickens. Although many different cells are affected, it is the elastotic material that accounts for the most striking effects of sun damage.

Solar elastosis is a sign highly characteristic of severe sun damage (Figure 19-1). There is massive deposition in the upper dermis of an abnormal, yellow, amorphous elastotic material that does not form functional elastic fibers. This altered connective tissue does not have the resilient properties of elastic tissue.

Wrinkling becomes coarse and deep rather than fine, and the skin is thickened (Figure 19-2). These wrinkles do not disappear by stretching.[5] Sun-induced wrinkling on the back of the neck shows a series of crisscrossed lines (Figure 19-3) that form a rhomboidal pattern (cutis rhomboidalis nuchae).

Reactive hyperplasia of melanocytes causes persistent pigmentation in the form of freckles, lentigines, and irregular hyperpigmentation and hypopigmentation on the hands, forearms, legs, chest, and back (Figure 19-4).

Blood vessels diminish in number, and the walls of the remaining vessels become thin. Blood vessels need connective tissue for support. Bleeding occurs with the slightest

SUN-INDUCED SKIN CHANGES

TEXTURE CHANGES

Solar elastosis
  Thickened, wrinkled, yellowish skin
Atrophy
  Thinning of the skin; fine wrinkling, prominent blood
    vessels, easy bruising and tearing of the skin, often
    with many linear scars
Wrinkles
  Deep—do not disappear by stretching
    Posterior neck sun damage (cutis rhomboidalis
      nuchae)
    Thickened skin is crisscrossed by deep lines
      creating rhomboidal patterns

VASCULAR CHANGES

Diffuse erythema
  Most apparent in fair-skinned people
Ecchymoses and stellate pseudoscars
  Bleeding into the skin follows minor trauma—only on
    exposed surfaces of the back of the hands and
    arms; associated with atrophy, ease of skin tearing,
    and linear scars
Telangiectasias
  Cheeks, nose, and ears
Venous lake
  Round purple ectatic vessels—lower lips and ears

PIGMENTATION CHANGES

Freckles
  Small, oval, brown macules—primarily on the face
Lentigo
  Large brown macules—face, back of the hands,
    arms, chest, upper back
Guttate hypomelanosis
  Discrete, round, white macules—lower legs and arms
Brown and white pigmentation (irregular)
  Deep brown with areas of hypopigmentation
Poikiloderma of civatte
  Reddish-brown reticulated pigmentation with telang-
    iectasias, atrophy, and prominent hair follicles—
    chest and neck

PAPULAR CHANGES

Nevi
  More numerous on sun-exposed surfaces in predis-
    posed individuals
Yellow papules (solar elastosis)
  Dull-to-bright yellow papules that may coalesce to
    form plaques
Seborrheic keratosis
  Discrete superficial (stuck-on) lesions—more numer-
    ous in sun-exposed areas; flat on extremities, ele-
    vated on the trunk
Comedones and cysts around the eyes (Favre-
  Racouchot syndrome)

---

trauma to the sun-damaged surfaces of the forearms and hands (Figure 19-5) but not to the unexposed surfaces. Making patients aware of this difference convinces them that they do not have a platelet abnormality.

Chronic sun exposure disrupts the maturation of keratinocytes, causing scaling, roughness, seborrheic keratosis (Figure 19-6), actinic keratosis, actinic cheilitis, and squamous cell carcinoma.

Treatment of photoaged skin

Topical tretinoin. Topical application of tretinoin provides some reversal of photodamaged skin (see the box at right).[6] Initially patients experience a subjective tightening of the skin and a pink rosy glow. Objective improvements in wrinkling are seen after 2 to 4 months. The greatest response to therapy occurs during the initial 6 to 9 months.[7,8]

Coarse and fine wrinkles improve. The deepest coarse facial wrinkles are still evident. Most patients experience tretinoin-induced dermatitis when treatment is initiated with the strongest concentration of the cream. The dermatitis can last for weeks to months. A second inflammatory phase occurs in which the erythema is more punctate, and this may represent inflammation of subclinical actinic keratoses.

TOPICAL TRETINOIN— EFFECTS OF TREATMENT

Fine wrinkling—improved
Coarse wrinkling—improved
Tactile roughness—improved
Lentigines—reduction in number
Freckles—reduction in color
Actinic keratoses—decrease in number
Telangiectasia—did not improve
Dermatitis—red, swelling, xerosis, mild scaling
Cutaneous reaction
  Dermatitis—(1 to 10 weeks) xerosis, mild scaling,
    irritation
  Increased pinkness, "rosy glow"
  Inflammation—(3+ months) of presumed subclini-
    cal actinic keratoses

PHOTOAGING

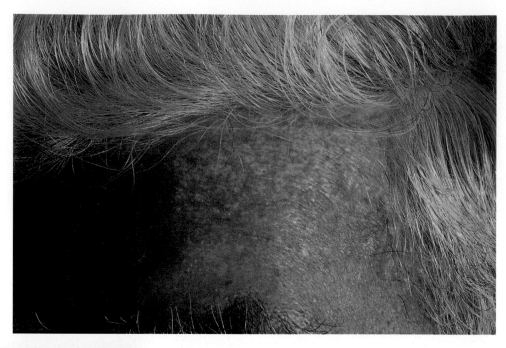

Figure 19-1
Solar elastosis. Numerous yellowish globules in the dermis can be seen through the thin, atrophic epidermis.

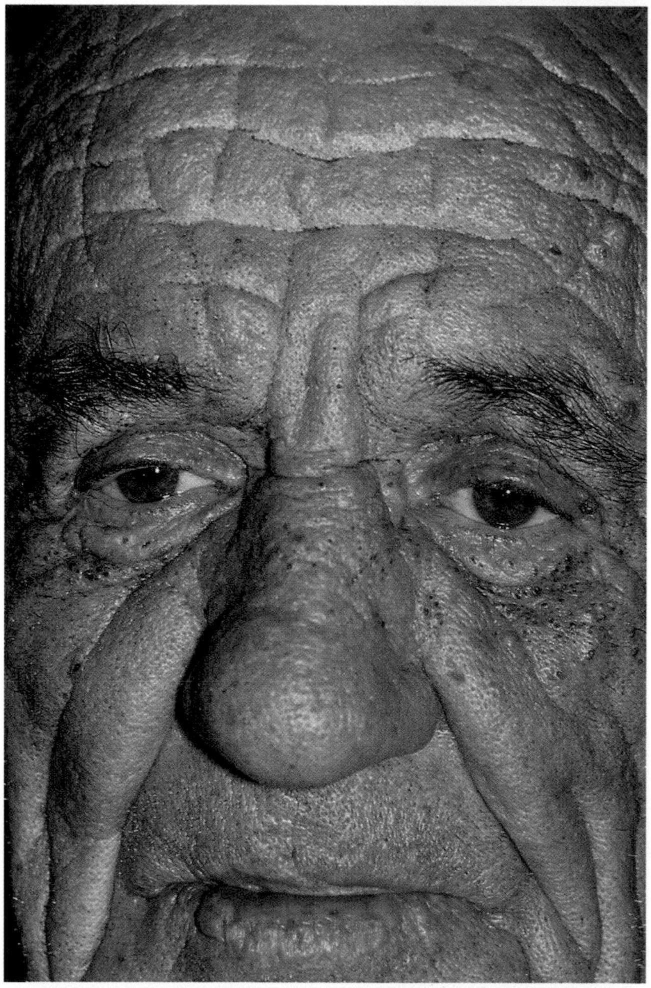

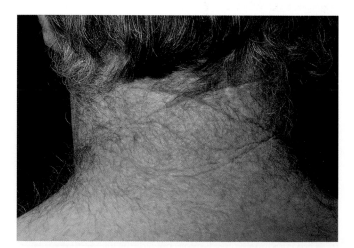

Figure 19-2
Wrinkling becomes coarse and deep rather than fine, and the skin is thickened. Large comedones are present around the eyes.

Figure 19-3
Sun-induced wrinkling on the back of the neck shows a series of crisscrossed lines that form a rhomboidal pattern (cutis rhomboidalis nuchae).

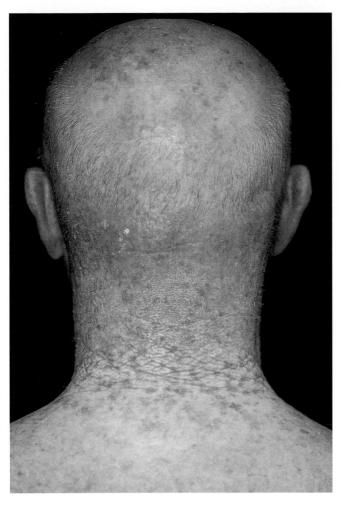

Figure 19-4
Reactive hyperplasia of melanocytes causes lentigines on the upper back. Diffuse persistent erythema is most prominent in fair-skinned people.

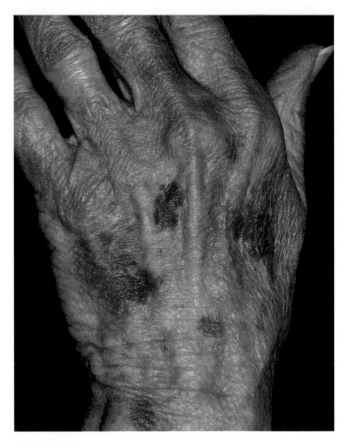

Figure 19-5
Bleeding occurs with the slightest trauma on the sun-damaged surfaces of the forearms and hands but not on the protected, undamaged, unexposed surfaces.

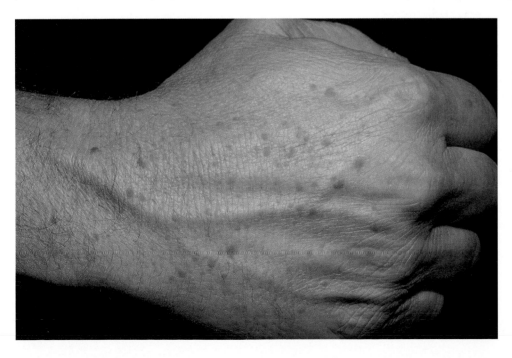

Figure 19-6
Seborrheic keratosis occurs in predisposed individuals.

Hyperpigmented lesions are a predominant component of photoaging in Chinese and Japanese persons; 0.1% tretinoin cream significantly lightens the hyperpigmentation of photoaging in these patients.[9]

Histologically there is increased epidermal hyperplasia, stratum corneum compaction, and increased vascularity in the papillary dermis. The epidermal hyperplasia seen at 24 weeks returns to baseline levels after 48 weeks of therapy despite persistence of clinical benefits in skin roughness and fine wrinkling.[10] In areas of improved hyperpigmentation, there is reduced melanocytic hypertrophy and hyperplasia. The formation of collagen I is significantly decreased in photodamaged human skin, and this process is partly restored by treatment with tretinoin.[11]

TRETINOIN APPLICATION PROCEDURES. The response to tretinoin appears to be dose dependent. Begin with night-time application. Start treatment with cream-based tretinoin (0.025%, 0.05%, 0.1%). A gradual introduction to treatment using every-other-day applications of tretinoin cream (0.025%) is appropriate for patients with sensitive skin (usually type I—see Table 19-1), followed by more frequent applications and higher concentrations when patients accommodate the dermatitis. Patients who complain of greasiness can use tretinoin solution (0.05%) or gel (0.025%, 0.1%) and apply moisturizing cosmetics or lubricating lotions if dryness occurs. Tretinoin can be applied twice a day once patients tolerate daily application.

Different parts of the body vary in the susceptibility to irritation. Frequency of application should be adjusted accordingly. Treatment should not be stopped when inflammation occurs, unless it is severe. The patient's skin never hardens to the effects of tretinoin if treatment is frequently interrupted. Severe inflammatory reactions should be treated with a group V topical steroid. A few days of treatment are sufficient. Sun bathing should be avoided. Daily use of sunscreens should be encouraged. Maximum response occurs after 8 to 12 months of treatment; thereafter application frequency should be reduced to three to four times a week to maintain improvement.[12,13]

Facial chemical peeling and dermabrasion. Phenol and trichloroacetic acid peels and dermabrasion are techniques used to treat photoaged skin.[14] Their use requires special training. The results can be very gratifying.[15]

Alpha-hydroxy acids. Alpha-hydroxy acids have been promoted as improving the appearance of photodamaged skin. One study demonstrated that topical glycolic acid can alleviate the erythema observed after ultraviolet radiation exposure to skin. The antiinflammatory action of glycolic acid may be attributed to its molecular structure, giving it a powerful antioxidant capability, and a subsequent protective effect against free-radically mediated inflammation.[16]

Suntan and Sunburn

Light-induced skin changes depend on the intensity and duration of exposure and genetic factors.

Suntan. A tan protects the body from photoinjury, but ultraviolet-induced injury must occur to produce a tan. Therefore, intentional suntanning is unwise. Repeated brief exposures sufficient to induce tanning add to long-term damage. In general for a given individual, the deeper the tan, the more skin damage suffered in achieving the tan.

Tanning follows moderate and intense sun exposure and occurs in two stages. The first stage, immediate pigment darkening (IPD), is caused primarily by UVA. The skin becomes brown while exposed, but fades rapidly after exposure. IPD is caused by a photochemical change in existing melanin, not by an increase in melanin. A lasting tan requires the synthesis of new melanin; a more lasting tan becomes visible within 72 hours.

Tanning parlors. Evidence shows that tans of comparable degrees acquired from different ultraviolet sources are similar in the amount of photodamage and skin cancer risk that accompanies a tan. Large amounts of radiation are delivered in a short time in commercial tanning parlors. This accelerates photoaging and increases the risk of skin cancer.

Sunburn. The sunburn reaction occurs in stages. With sufficient exposure, erythema appears within minutes (immediate erythema), fades, and then reappears and persists for days (delayed erythema). Vascular permeability of varying degrees results in edema and blisters. Desquamation occurs within a week. Sunburn is best treated with cool wet compresses. Topical anesthetic preparations that contain lidocaine provide some relief. Benzocaine, incorporated into some sunburn preparations, is a sensitizer and should be avoided. A 4- to 6-day course of prednisone (20 mg twice a day for adults) may abort a potentially intense reaction. Protection with sunscreens can, if used properly, prevent burning in even fair-skinned individuals.

Sun Protection

Ultraviolet-induced damage to collagen and elastic fibers and a number of skin cancers[17] can be greatly reduced by high sun protection factor (SPF) sunscreens and other methods to reduce sun exposure. Sun protection may allow for repair of damaged skin. New collagen and elastin may form, and precancerous changes may regress. Substantial lifetime sun exposure occurs with brief incidental exposures such as working outdoors, participating in recreational activities, and walking outside for lunch. Therefore many people need daily protection.

Methods of sun protection. Natural protection is provided by the stratum corneum and the skin pigment, melanin. People vary widely in their natural ability to tan or burn. A sun-reactive skin typing system has been devised to classify individuals as to their ability to tan or burn. These categories (Table 19-1) are useful guides for devising programs for sun protection.

The following are recommended to minimize sun exposure:

1. Avoid sun exposure between 11 A.M. and 3 P.M.
2. Start with short exposures of 15 to 20 minutes in the morning or late afternoon.
3. Wear protective clothing and a hat.
4. Use sunscreens with a high SPF number.

Sunburns are particularly harmful, and great emphasis should be placed on preventing burns. Patients frequently relate that permanent freckling occurred on the upper back after one severe burn. People who take short winter vacations in the south are particularly apt to burn. Total sun exposure during a lifetime is greatest on the face, back of the neck, bald head, upper chest, forearms, backs of the hands, and exposed lower legs. The effects of sunlight can readily be appreciated by comparing the lateral (sun-exposed) surfaces with the medial (sun-protected) surfaces of the forearms of older individuals.

SUNSCREEN APPLICATION

SPF >15

Start use in young children.

Protect all sun-exposed surfaces, including hands, back of neck, ears, lower lips, anterior chest, bald scalp.

Apply routinely each morning after washing or shaving.

There is evidence that skin can repair itself if protected from sun.

Protecting the young. Significant sun exposure occurs during the early years of life when children spend hours playing outside. A study showed that regular use of a sunscreen with an SPF of 15 during the first 18 years of life reduces the lifetime incidence of basal and squamous cell carcinoma by 78%.[18] All children should be protected with high-number SPF sunscreens.

Sunscreens. Sunscreens are topical agents that protect the skin from ultraviolet light (see the Formulary, p. 856). Guidelines for their application are listed in the box above. Sunscreens should not be used as a means of allowing more time in the sun. This negates their beneficial effects.

Sunscreens are topical agents that absorb, scatter, or reflect ultraviolet radiation (UVR) and visible light.[19] UVA agents absorb radiation in the spectral range of 320 to 400 nm. UVB agents absorb radiation in the range of 290 to 320 nm.

Physical sunscreens. Physical sunscreens (referred to as nonchemical sunscreens) are composed of large particles that scatter and reflect light. They are opaque or pigmented and can discolor clothing. The full spectrum of ultraviolet

---

TABLE 19-1 Skin Types and Recommended Sunscreen Protection Factors

Skin type*	Sensitivity to UV light†	Sunburn and tanning history	Recommended sun protection factor‡
I	Very sensitive	Always burns easily; never tans	15 or more
II	Very sensitive	Always burns easily; tans minimally	15 or more
III	Sensitive	Burns moderately; tans gradually and uniformly (light brown)	10 to 15
IV	Moderately sensitive	Burns minimally; always tans well (moderate brown)	8 to 15
V	Minimally sensitive	Rarely burns, tans profusely (dark brown)	8 to 15
VI	Insensitive	Never burns; deeply pigmented (black)	None indicated

Adapted from Pathak MA: *J Dermatol Surg Oncol* 13:739-750, 1987.
*Constitutive color of unexposed buttock skin of individuals of skin types I to III is white and of skin type IV is white or faintly brown. Individuals with skin type V have brown buttock skin, and those with skin type VI have dark brown or black buttock skin.
†Based on first 30 to 45 minutes of sun exposure after winter season or no sun exposure.
‡Based on outdoor field studies.

and visible light (290 to 760 nm) is blocked by these agents. They contain titanium dioxide (5% to 20%), zinc oxide, talc, kaolin, ferric chloride, ichthammol (Ichtyol), or colored clays. These opaque formulations block UVA and are therefore effective for photosensitizing diseases such as polymorphous light eruption, the porphyrias, and lupus erythematosus. Physical sunscreens can be especially useful in areas that burn easily, such as the nose and lips. Products include Covermark, RV Plaque, Dermablend, and many new formulations that contain titanium dioxide.

Chemical sunscreens. Chemical sunscreens absorb radiation. Newer broad-spectrum chemical sunscreens include a combination of chemicals that absorb both UVB and UVA radiation. *Para*-aminobenzoic acid (PABA) was the first chemical sunscreen agent, but its potential to cause allergic reactions has limited its use. Chemical sunscreens include PABA esters, salicylates, cinnamates, and benzophenones.

UVB CHEMICAL BLOCKING AGENTS. PABA esters, including amyl dimethyl (Padimate A or Escolol 506) and octyl dimethyl (Padimate O or Escolol 507), block UVB. Padimate O is the bestselling sunscreen chemical in the United States. Salicylates (octyl salicylate; homomenthyl salicylate, also known as homosalate) are weak and must be used in high concentrations. Cinnamate 2-ethylhexyl *p*-methoxycinnamate (Parsol MCX) is the most commonly used cinnamate.

UVA CHEMICAL BLOCKING AGENTS. Benzophenones mainly block UVA, but their absorbency range extends into the UVB range. Benzophenone derivatives include dioxybenzone (206 to 380 nm), sulisobenzone, oxybenzone (270 to 350 nm), and Parsol 1789 (avobenzone). These sunscreens are most commonly combined with a strong UVB absorber such as Padimate O.

Water-resistant sunscreens. Many new preparations resist removal by bathing. The vehicle is the most important factor in determining water resistance. Some are thick and unpleasant. DuraScreen 30 is highly water resistant.

Sun protection factor. The effectiveness of sunscreens is expressed as the *sun protection factor*, or *SPF*. The SPF is defined as the ratio of the least amount of UVB energy (minimum erythema dose) required to produce a minimum erythema reaction through a sunscreen product film to the amount of energy required to produce the same erythema without any sunscreen application. For an individual who wears a sunscreen with an SPF of 8, eight times longer than usual is required to develop erythema. The SPF for commercially available products is derived from tests with laboratory light sources and therefore is not a true measure of the sunscreen's ability to protect. SPF values were determined for a number of products using natural sunlight, and these were found to be lower than those derived in the laboratory. These values, along with other characteristics of a number of commercially available sunscreen products, are listed in the Formulary on p. 856.

Choice of sunscreen strength. A sunscreen with an SPF of 15 or greater is recommended under most conditions. Sun protection does not increase proportionally with the designated SPF. In the higher range of SPFs, the differences become less meaningful. An SPF of 15 indicates 93% protection; an SPF of 34 indicates 97% protection.

Frequency of use. The majority of lifetime sun exposure occurs during multiple brief exposures that are not intended to produce tanning; therefore daily sun protection should be encouraged. People who sunburn easily or those who have light complexions or sun-sensitivity disorders should use a high SPF sunscreen every day, all year round, particularly if they live in more equatorial latitudes. Sunscreens should be applied once in the morning and reapplied after swimming and heavy exercise. Encourage people to have sunscreens available in the bathroom and to make morning application part of their daily ritual.

Adverse reactions to sunscreens. Contact dermatitis and staining of clothing may occur with sunscreens. Allergic reactions occur more frequently to preservatives or fragrances than to the active ingredients. Irritation to creams is much more common than allergy to a component.

Sunscreens do not promote tanning. Since people vary greatly in their ability to burn, those who want some degree of tan should choose a product with an SPF of 2 to 8 and increase exposure times in a conservative manner.

Unprotected, chronically exposed children can acquire significant actinic damage by the time they reach age 15. The effects of this damage may become apparent after age 20. All sun-exposed surfaces, including the hands, back of the neck, ears, and lower lips, should be protected. As a matter of routine, sunscreen should be applied in the morning after shaving or washing when exposure is anticipated.

Vitamin D levels. Regular use of sunscreens does not result in vitamin D levels outside the normal range.[20]

Sunless or self-tanning lotions. Sunless or self-tanning lotions contain dihydroxyacetone (DHA), which darkens the skin by staining. Staining of skin occurs when DHA combines with free amino groups in skin proteins (keratin) in the stratum corneum to form brown products called *melanoidins*. Little to no sunscreen protection is provided by their use. Some products are formulated with standard sunscreens; the duration of UV protection is more short-lived than that of the skin-color change.

The newer preparations are cosmetically acceptable, as opposed to the orange color that was produced by older formulations. A color change can be seen within an hour of application. The desired tanned appearance can be achieved with two to four applications separated by several hours. The appearance can be maintained by further applications every 2 to 4 days. The face requires fewer but more frequent reapplications than the extremities to achieve the desired appearance. The depth of color directly correlates with thickness and compactness of the stratum corneum. Rougher, hyperkeratotic skin takes up the color more unevenly, as does older skin or mottled or freckled skin. Scars color poorly. The most even color is obtained when the skin is lightly buffed or abraded before application to enhance its smoothness.[21]

Polymorphous Light Eruption

Polymorphous light (PML) eruption is the most common light-induced skin disease seen by the practitioner. Not only does the clinical picture vary, but symptoms may vary over the years. There are several morphologic subtypes,[22] but individual patients tend to develop the same type each year. Lesions usually heal without scarring. The eruption appears first on limited areas, but becomes more extensive during sub-

sequent summers. Most people with PML eruption have exacerbations each summer for many years; a few have temporary remissions. The disease may begin at any age. The amount of light exposure needed to elicit an eruption varies greatly from one patient to another. Patients can tolerate a certain minimum exposure time, such as 30 minutes, after which the eruption appears. Light sensitivity decreases with repeated sun exposure; this phenomenon is referred to as *hardening*. The

POLYMORPHOUS LIGHT ERUPTION

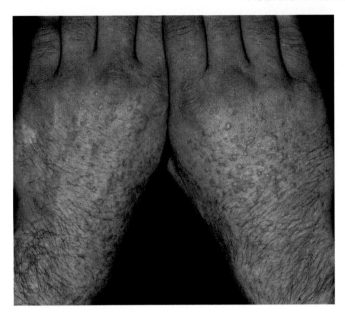

Figure 19-7
Papular type.

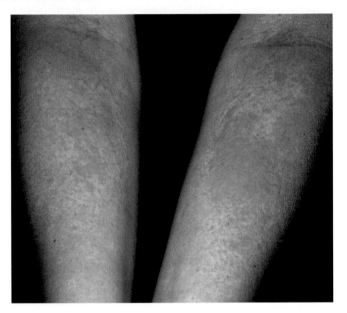

Figure 19-8
Plaque type.

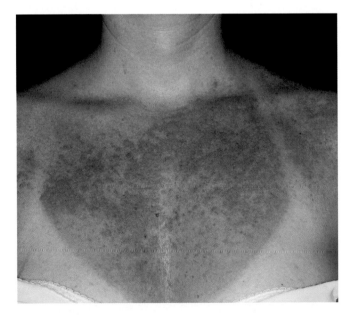

Figure 19-9
Plaque type.

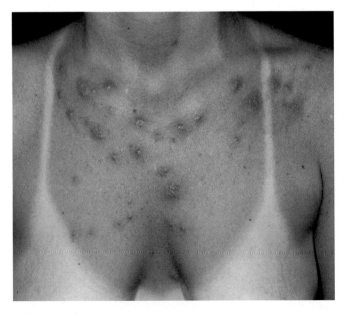

Figure 19-10
Papulovesicular type.

eruption may cease to appear after days or weeks of repeated sun exposure. Those exposed to sunlight year round rarely acquire PML eruption. Most patients have symptoms 2 hours after exposure. In a 7-year follow-up study, 57% of patients reported a decreased sun sensitivity, including 11% in whom the PML eruption totally cleared; none of the patients developed systemic lupus erythematosus.[23]

Hereditary PML eruption (actinic prurigo). Hereditary PML eruption occurs in the Inuit of North America and in Native Americans of North, Central, and South America. Its transmission appears to be autosomal dominant with incomplete penetrance and variable expressivity. In northern latitudes, the eruption appears on sun-exposed areas of the body as early as March and persists through October.[24] The face is the most commonly involved area. The majority of patients are sensitive to UVA light. The younger ages of onset (up to 20 years of age) are associated with cheilitis and more acute eruptions and are more likely to improve over 5 years. Those who develop actinic prurigo as adults (21 years of age and older) tend to have a milder and more persistent dermatosis.[25]

Clinical presentation. The most common initial symptoms are burning, itching, and erythema. The eruption usually lasts for 2 or 3 days, but in some cases it does not clear until the end of summer. Many patients experience malaise, chills, headache, and nausea starting approximately 4 hours after exposure but lasting only 1 or 2 hours. The most commonly involved areas are the vee of the chest (the area exposed by open-necked shirts), the backs of the hands, extensor aspects of the forearms, and the lower legs of women. Women are affected more often than men. Reports vary as to the wavelength of light responsible for inducing lesions. The wavelength of light necessary to elicit the eruption varies with each patient. Many react to UVB, others to UVA,[26] or some to both.[27]

Clinical subtypes. There are a number of clinical types of PML eruption.[22]

PAPULAR TYPE. The papular type is the most common form (Figure 19-7). Small papules are disseminated or densely aggregated on a patchy erythema.

PLAQUE TYPE. The plaque type is the second most common pattern. Plaques may be superficial or urticarial. They may coalesce to form larger plaques and at times are eczematous (Figures 19-8 and 19-9).

PAPULOVESICULAR TYPE. The papulovesicular type is less common. It occurs primarily on the arms, lower limbs, and vee area of the chest and usually begins with urticarial plaques from which groups of vesicles arise (Figure 19-10). Itching is common and is usually moderate or marked.[28]

ERYTHEMA MULTIFORME TYPE. Erythema multiforme–type lesions and distribution are similar to classic erythema multiforme, with lesions most frequent on the backs of the hands and extensor forearms.

HEMORRHAGIC TYPE. The hemorrhagic type may first appear as hemorrhagic papules or purpura. This form is rare.

DIFFERENTIAL DIAGNOSIS. The papular form resembles atopic dermatitis. PML eruption is less pruritic and occurs in a sun-exposed distribution, not in crease areas as does atopic dermatitis.

Systemic and discoid lupus erythematosus plaquelike lesions and histology may be identical to PML eruptions. The characteristic direct and indirect immunofluorescence patterns of lupus erythematosus clarify the diagnosis.

Diagnosis. The histologic features are not diagnostic. Immunofluorescence is negative. Phototesting is not essential but, when performed, must include both UVB and UVA testing.

Treatment

TOPICAL STEROIDS. Short, intermittent 3- to 14-day courses of groups II to V topical steroids are effective.[29]

PROTECTION. Sun exposure during times of maximum intensity (between 11 A.M. and 3 P.M.) should be avoided. Sunscreens with maximum sun-protecting factors should be used. Groups II through V topical steroids reduce pruritis and hasten resolution. Short courses of oral steroids are useful for very itchy, widespread eruptions or for patients who flare during a course of phototherapy or photochemotherapy.

DESENSITIZATION WITH PHOTOTHERAPY. Many patients improve with repeated exposure to sunlight; this is the so-called phenomenon of hardening. This practice is safe; therefore controlled exposure to sunlight or artificial ultraviolet light sources should be the first type of treatment. Patients treated with UVB in the dermatologist's office receive five exposures per week for 3 weeks in the spring, with gradually increasing exposure doses.[30-32] Hardening may also be accomplished with either UVA (340 to 400 nm)[33] or UVA and UVB (300 to 400 nm) (10 exposures to UV light).[34]

Protective clothing should be worn over involved areas.

PSORALEN UVA (PUVA). Trioxsalen (Trisoralen) and natural sunlight[34] treatment is simple and effective for patients who do not improve with the above routine measures and for those who have significant eruptions each summer. A 5-mg dose of trioxsalen should be given for every 20 to 25 pounds of body weight (average dosage, 5 to 6 tablets), followed by sunlight in 2 hours or more. In the early spring the patient should be exposed to 15 minutes of sunlight the first day, and the exposure increased by several minutes each day. Topical steroids should be applied if the disease is activated by treatment. Maximum protection is reached 3 weeks after a 1-week course of treatment, and a single course offers a minimum of 6 weeks of protection. The course is repeated each month during the spring and summer months. Protective glasses such as NoIR should be worn for the remainder of the day after taking psoralens.

The same treatment can be acquired in the dermatologist's office using artificial UVA light and 8-methoxypsoralen. A remission can be obtained for most patients by treating two or three times each week for 4 to 12 weeks in the early spring.[27,31,32,35] See the section on treatment of psoriasis for details.

ANTIMALARIALS. Antimalarials may be effective and should be considered for patients who are not protected by sunscreens and do not respond to UVB or PUVA phototherapy.[36] Antimalarials need to be used only during the summer months; therefore the total necessary dose is small. A 3-month trial (hydroxychloroquine 400 mg/day for the first month and 200 mg/day thereafter) has been effective in reducing rash and irritation.[37] Although the risk of eye damage is slight, ophthalmologic examinations should be obtained periodically to monitor for antimalarial toxicity.

Beta carotene is somewhat effective for prophylactic treatment of PML eruption, but the skin turns yellow-orange. In one study, only 30% of patients responded satisfactorily to a dosage of 3 mg/kg body weight continued throughout the summer.[35]

Hydroa Aestivale and Hydroa Vacciniforme

Hydroa aestivale (summer prurigo of Hutchinson) and hydroa vacciniforme are rare but very distinctive light-induced eruptions. They may represent a type of PML eruption that is peculiar to children. The onset is before puberty, and males are affected more frequently. Moderate itching occurs before and during the eruption. The lesions of hydroa aestivale consist of papules with weeping and crusting. The eruption is most prominent on the face, ears, and backs of the hands, but involvement of non–sun exposed areas, especially the buttocks, is not uncommon. The rash fades but may persist through the winter months. There is evidence of genetic transmission. In many cases UVB light reproduces the lesions.

Hydroa vacciniforme (Figure 19-11) is similar to hydroa aestivale, except that tense, umbilicated vesicles resembling smallpox appear on the face, ears, chest, and backs of the hands; after they break and form a crust, they may heal with scarring. UVA light reproduced the eruption in one case.[38] Both diseases usually clear after puberty. Avoiding the sun and using sunscreens, group V topical steroids, and wet compresses and antimalarials can control these diseases.

Figure 19-11
Hydroa vacciniforme. Umbilicated vesicles resembling smallpox in a sun-exposed distribution on a young boy.

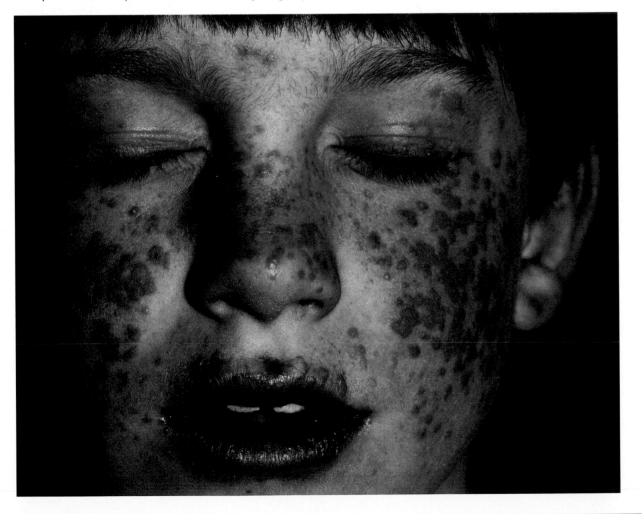

Porphyrias

The porphyrias are a group of diseases caused by inborn enzymatic defects in the heme biosynthetic pathway. (Table 19-2). Each type of porphyria is associated with a specific enzymatic defect that results in an excess of a specific porphyrin (Table 19-3). The porphyrias are classified into two groups, erythropoietic and hepatic, on the basis of the principal site of the specific enzymatic defect. They are differentiated by measuring heme precursors in urine, feces, erythrocytes, and plasma. Most forms are inherited as mendelian autosomal dominants.

Two main types of clinical manifestation occur: life-threatening attacks of acute porphyria and skin photosensitization. Attacks of the acute porphyrias (acute intermittent porphyria, variegate porphyria, and hereditary coproporphyria) are important because they may be life-threatening. The nonacute porphyrias (porphyria cutanea tarda and erythropoietic porphyria) present as skin photosensitization.

TABLE 19-2 Clinical Features of the Porphyrias

Type of porphyria	Heredity	Age of onset	Cutaneous manifestations	Extra-cutaneous manifestations	Laboratory findings			
					Urine	Feces	Erythrocytes	Plasma fluorescence emission peak (nm)
ERYTHROPOIETIC								
Erythropoietic porphyria	AR*	Infancy	Blisters Severe scarring	Red teeth Hemolytic anemia	Uro I Copro I	Copro I	Uro I Stable fluorescence	615
Erythropoietic protoporphyria	AD	Childhood	Burning Edema Thickening Rarely blisters	Rarely occurs Fatal liver disease Gallstones	Negative	Protoporphyrin continuously	Protoporphyrin Transient fluorescence	632
HEPATIC, ERYTHROPOIETIC								
Hepatoerythropoietic porphyria	AR	Infancy	Blisters Severe scarring Thickening	Decreased liver function	Uro I Uro III	Copro I Copro III Isocoproporphyrin	Protoporphyrin	
HEPATIC								
Acute intermittent porphyria	AD	Adolescence	Negative	Abdominal pain Neuropathy Psychosis	ALA and PBG continuously	Negative	Negative	615
Variegate porphyria	AD	Young adulthood	Same as porphyria cutanea tarda	Same as acute intermittent porphyria	ALA and PBG during attacks Copro > Uro	Protoporphyrin continuously Some Copro X-porphyrin	Negative	624-626
Porphyria cutanea tarda	AD	Middle age	Blisters Scarring Thickening Scleroderma-like features	Decreased liver function Siderosis	Uro I > Uro III continuously Continuous fluorescence	Isocoproporphyrin > Copro	Negative	615
Hereditary coproporphyria	AD	Young adulthood	Same as porphyria cutanea tarda	Same as acute intermittent porphyria	Copro, ALA, and PBG during attacks	Copro III continuously	Negative	615

Modified from Sekula SA, Tschen JA, Rosen T: *Am Fam Physician* 219-232, 1986.
*Uro, uroporphyrin; Copro, coproporphyrin; ALA, aminolevulinic acid; PBG, porphobilinogen; AR, autosomal recessive; AD, autosomal dominant.

The skin lesions in porphyria cutanea tarda (the commonest cutaneous porphyria), variegate porphyria, hereditary coproporphyria, and congenital erythropoietic porphyria are similar: mechanical fragility, subepidermal bullae, hypertrichosis, and pigmentation. Erythropoietic protoporphyria is characterized by acute photosensitivity without these lesions.

All types show excess porphyrin metabolites in blood, urine, or feces and in various tissues such as skin and liver. Porphyrins are red-brown pigments. Certain porphyrin metabolites (porphyrinogens) accumulate in the skin and are auto-oxidized to become porphyrins. Porphyrins absorb UVA light in the 400-to-410 nm range (Soret band). These excited porphyrins generate peroxides that cause the blisters seen in porphyria cutanea tarda and variegate porphyria.

PORPHYRIA CUTANEA TARDA

Porphyria cutanea tarda (PCT) is the most common type of porphyria. PCT results from a deficiency of hepatic uroporphyrinogen decarboxylase activity. Both acquired and familial forms exist and are commonly associated in adults with liver disease and hepatic iron overload. The acquired ("sporadic") form is most often precipitated by alcohol.[39] Estrogens, oral contraceptives, certain environmental pollutants, and iron overloading may precipitate PCT. There is also a dominantly inherited form. Most people who consume alcohol or take estrogens do not develop porphyria; therefore it is likely that genetic factors are important in the pathogenesis of nonfamilial cases. This genetic predisposition may explain why some patients on chronic hemodialysis develop PCT.[40] Some of these patients with chronic renal failure have highly increased uroporphyrin concentrations. There is a strong association between hepatitis C virus infection and PCT.[41]

TABLE 19-3 Classification of the Porphyrias

Type of porphyria	Enzyme defect	Recommended tests
ERYTHROPOIETIC		
Erythropoietic porphyria	Uroporphyrinogen III cosynthetase	Urine porphyrins, erythrocyte porphyrins
Erythropoietic protoporphyria	Ferrochelatase (heme synthetase)	Urine, fecal, erythrocyte porphyrins
HEPATIC, ERYTHROPOIETIC		
Hepatoerythropoietic porphyria	Ferrochelatase, uroporphyrinogen decarboxylase	Urine, fecal, erythrocyte porphyrins
HEPATIC		
Acute intermittent porphyria	Uroporphyrinogen 1 synthetase	Urine PBG, porphyrins; erythrocyte uroporphyrinogen I synthetase; erythrocyte δ-aminolevulinate dehydratase
Variegate porphyria	Protoporphyrinogen oxidase	Urine PBG, porphyrins; fecal porphyrins (erythrocyte uroporphyrinogen I synthetase and δ-aminolevulinate dehydratase may be necessary)
Porphyria cutanea tarda	Uroporphyrinogen decarboxylase	Urine porphyrins
Hereditary coproporphyria	Coproporphyrinogen oxidase	Urine PBG, porphyrins; fecal porphyrins (erythrocyte uroporphyrinogen I synthase and δ-aminolevulinate dehydratase may be necessary)
INTOXICATION PORPHYRIA (CHEMICALS)		
	Variable	Erythrocyte porphyrins; urine δ-ALA, PBG, porphyrins; fecal porphyrins*

PBG, porphobilinogen; ALA, δ-aminolevulinate.
*In some cases the quantitation of erythrocyte zinc protoporphyrin is necessary to distinguish intoxication porphyria from protoporphyria.

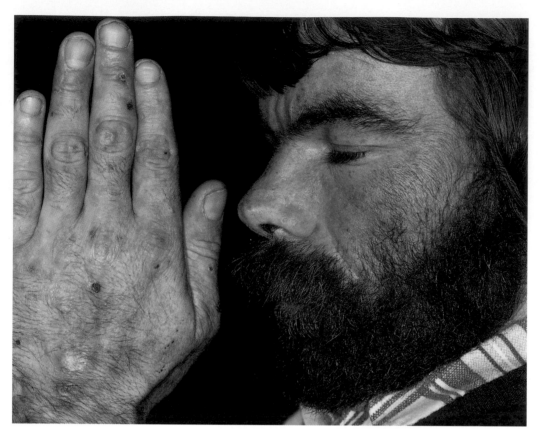

Figure 19-12
Porphyria cutanea tarda. There is increased facial hair around the eyes. Chronic sun exposure has resulted in blistering, erosions, and atrophic scars on the backs of the hands.

Clinical manifestations. The clinical features in order of frequency are blistering in sun-exposed areas, increased skin fragility, facial hypertrichosis, hyperpigmentation, sclerodermoid changes, and dystrophic calcification with ulceration (Figure 19-12).[42] Milia form in previously blistered sites on the hand (Figure 19-13). The classic form of epidermolysis bullosa acquisita has similar features (see Chapter Sixteen).

Diagnosis. The patient's urine may have a red-brown discoloration ("port-wine urine") from high levels of porphyrin pigments. It may show a bright pink fluorescence under a Wood's light. PCT may be confused with other forms of porphyria and other bullous diseases. Assays of fecal, plasma, urinary, and red blood cell porphyrins should be ordered, especially if other forms of porphyria are in the differential diagnosis. The diagnosis is confirmed by demonstrating an elevated urine uroporphyrin level. A 24-hour collection of urine contains different amounts of the various porphyrins in ratios that can be diagnostic. The fraction reported as uroporphyrin dominates the urinary assay in PCT, usually being present in a ratio of 4:1 or more to the coproporphyrin fraction. Quantitative assays of the various porphyrins must be performed to obtain a reliable diagnosis.

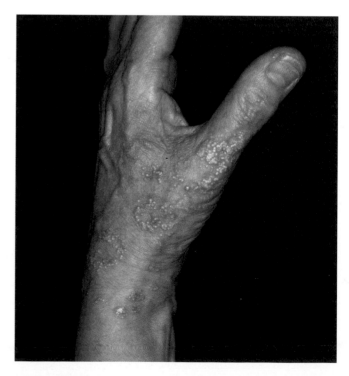

Figure 19-13
Porphyria cutanea tarda. White milia form during the healing process.

Treatment

Phlebotomy. Iron removal by phlebotomy is the treatment of choice. It reduces hepatic iron stores and produces remissions of several years' duration. One unit of blood should be removed every 2 to 4 weeks until the hemoglobin drops to 10 gm/dl or until the serum iron drops to 50 μg/dl. The average number of units required for remission varies between 8 and 14.[43] Measuring plasma uroporphyrin is an effective way to monitor the progress of patients with PCT. Treatment should continue until plasma uroporphyrin drops under 10 mmol/L.[44]

Chloroquine. Chloroquine in very low dosages may also be used. Chloroquine causes the release of hepatic tissue–bound uroporphyrin, and subsequently it is rapidly eliminated by the plasma and excreted by the urine. A too-rapid release of porphyrins might severely affect liver function. Complete clinical and biochemical response has occurred with the use of chloroquine 125 mg twice weekly for 8 to 18 months. Remission in most patients has been for more than 4 years.[45]

Combined treatment with repeated bleeding and chloroquine results in remission in an average of 3.5 months. The time necessary for remission with chloroquine alone is 10.2 months. The time for remission with phlebotomy alone is 12.5 months.[46]

Complete elimination of alcohol and exposure to other hepatotoxins resulted in complete clinical clearing of bullae and skin fragility in 2 months to 2 years in one series of patients.[47]

Sunscreens that block UVA light should be used. Physical sunblockers that contain titanium dioxide are moderately effective.[48]

PSEUDOPORPHYRIA

Pseudoporphyria (a therapy-induced bullous photosensitivity disorder) is a condition that mimics PCT in almost every aspect, except that porphyrin levels in the urine, plasma, and stools are normal. Uroporphyrins are elevated in patients with bullous dermatosis associated with hemodialysis.[49] The condition is precipitated by certain drugs, including tetracyclines, furosemide, nalidixic acid, dapsone, pyridoxine, and naproxen.[50,51] Pseudoporphyria was reported in up to 12% of juvenile rheumatoid arthritis patients treated with naproxen.[52,53] Patients exposed to light in sunbeds have developed pseudoporphyria.[54] There is increased skin fragility, easy bruising, and light-provoked bullae on the dorsum of the hand followed by healing with scarring and milia (Figure 19-14). The onset of bullae may occur 1 week after the drug has been initiated or may not occur for months. An important clue to the diagnosis is that few patients with pseudoporphyria have hypertrichosis, hyperpigmentation, or the sclerodermoid changes found in PCT.[55] The histology (subepidermal bullae with no inflammation, thickened dermal capillary walls with deposition of periodic acid/Schiff-positive material) and immunofluorescent findings (IgG and C deposition at the dermoepidermal junction) are identical to those found in PCT. Stopping the drug is curative in most cases, but remission may not occur for months.

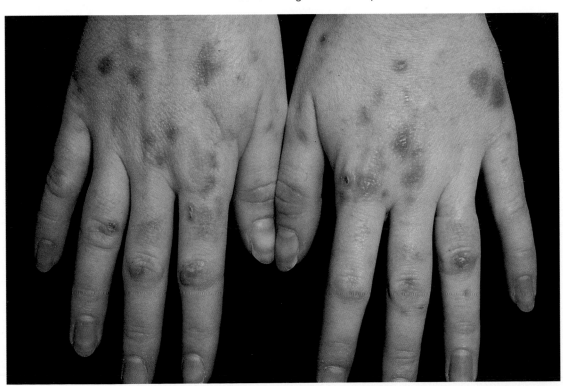

Figure 19-14
Pseudoporphyria. Light-provoked bullae on the back of the hands, followed by healing with scarring, is precipitated by certain drugs such as naproxen.

ERYTHROPOIETIC PROTOPORPHYRIA

Erythropoietic protoporphyria (EPP) differs clinically from PCT. This disease begins in childhood. There are few or no blisters; rather, children complain of burning and redness when exposed to sun or ultraviolet light. There are no porphyrins in the urine. EPP is an autosomal dominant hereditary disorder with irregular penetrance. It is characterized by a deficiency of ferrochelatase, the terminal enzyme in the heme biosynthetic pathway that catalyzes the insertion of ferrous iron into protoporphyrin IX to form heme. The enzyme deficiency causes the accumulation of the photoreactive molecule protoporphyrin in various tissues. Protoporphyrin overproduction occurs mainly in erythroid tissue. Circulating erythrocytes leak protoporphyrin, which accumulates in skin cells. The release of protoporphyrin from erythrocytes is greatly increased if the erythrocytes are exposed to small amounts of light. The cutaneous symptoms are elicited by protoporphyrin-sensitized photodamage of endothelial cells.[56]

Clinical manifestations. The disease is often suspected in infancy or childhood when patients cry or complain of burning of the skin on the face and hands within minutes of sun exposure. Exposure through window glass also elicits symptoms. Hours later, diffuse swelling or erythema appears, and burning persists (Figure 19-15). Purpura may occur, but vesiculation is uncommon. Often, acute changes are not seen. The period of sun exposure required to elicit burning varies from day to day. Several hours of exposure may be tolerated. A "priming phenomenon" has been reported.[57] A certain duration of exposure "primes" the skin so that a short period of additional sun exposure in the same area, even the next day, produces symptoms. It may then take several days after symptoms have developed to regain the usual degree of tolerance. Patients may present with a waxy, cobblestone-like induration of the involved skin. When this change occurs over the knuckles and fingers, the hands look old ("old knuckles"). This is a pathognomonic change in children. Depressed scars form on the nose, cheeks, and dorsum of the hands. Large second-degree phototoxic burns of the abdominal wall have occurred after prolonged exposure to light during surgery.[58]

Most treated patients function well and have a normal life span. Protoporphyrins may accumulate in hepatocytes and cause liver disease.

Liver disease. Excess protoporphyrin affects hepato-biliary structures, and a spectrum of changes, which range from ultrastructural bile canalicular damage to cirrhosis or acute hepatic failure, may occur. The course is unpredictable. Patients may be stable for several years after evidence of liver function abnormalities. Then, within weeks, hepatic failure may develop, requiring urgent orthotopic liver transplantation.[58,59] Gallstones may occur in young children.

Laboratory. Erythrocyte and plasma protoporphyrin and fecal protoporphyrin levels are elevated (see Table 19-2). Fluorescence microscopy is a highly reliable screening test for the detection of increased red cell porphyrins.[60] The urine is normal. Red blood cell protoporphyrins are also increased in iron deficiency anemia and lead poisoning, but photosensitivity is absent. Liver biopsy may show periportal fibrosis.

Treatment. Oral beta carotene (Solatene 30 mg) is helpful in treating the skin photosensitivity.[61,62] Improvement occurs within 1 month of initiating treatment. The children's dosage is 30 mg once, twice, or three times a day. The adult dosage is 60 to 180 mg/day. The skin becomes yellow in 4 to 6 weeks; stools are orange. Therapy is used from early spring through the fall. Pyridoxine was associated with a marked reduction in photosensitivity without evidence of adverse effects in two patients who were only moderately responsive to beta carotene and sunscreens. The reported effective dosage is 25 to 100 mg/hour for 6 to 10 doses during the day; protection was maintained when the dosage was lowered to 100 mg three times a day.[63] Terfenadine (H_1-receptor antagonist) causes a significant inhibition of the immediate flare reaction, but does not alter the erythemal response.[64] Iron therapy may be considered for prophylaxis of hepatic failure.[65] Red blood cell exchange transfusions have been reported to be effective. Cholestyramine 4 gm three times a day is reported to decrease photosensitivity and porphyrin levels. Photoprotection against UVA by chemical sunscreens and physical sunscreens that contain microfine titanium dioxide is helpful. Products containing microfine titanium dioxide offer superior photoprotection for patients who are abnormally sensitive to long wavelength ultraviolet radiation.[48]

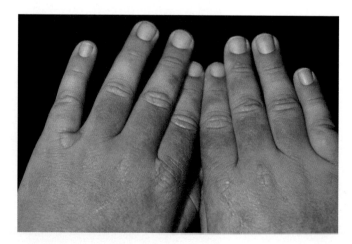

Figure 19-15
Erythropoietic protoporphyria. There are few or no blisters. Burning and redness occur with sun exposure. *(Courtesy Maureen Poh-Fitzpatrick M.D.)*

Phototoxic Reactions

Phototoxic reactions are nonallergic cutaneous responses induced by a variety of topical and systemic agents. The frequency of these eruptions has decreased as informed physicians, aware of the photosensitive potential of certain drugs, have chosen alternatives. Phototoxicity occurs when a photosensitizer is absorbed into the skin either topically or systemically in appropriate concentrations and is exposed to adequate amounts of specific wavelengths of light, usually UVA. Theoretically, if sufficient quantities of chemical and light are delivered, the reaction should occur in all exposed individuals. In fact, the response varies.

Topical exposure. Exposure to plants or chemicals that contain light-sensitizing compounds followed by exposure to certain activating wavelengths of ultraviolet light produces a highly characteristic eruption. A minimum response consists of an almost imperceptible erythema, followed by prolonged hyperpigmentation. A maximum response consists of tingling of the exposed skin and erythema that occur shortly after exposure, followed within hours by burning edema and vesiculation at the end of 24 hours. This is followed by a bullous reaction that lasts for days (Figure 19-16, *A*). Linear streaks (similar to poison ivy) of erythema and vesicles produced by drawing the offending agent across the skin surface are particularly characteristic of topical exposure. Desquamation occurs, and residual hyperpigmentation may persist for 1 year or more (Figure 19-16, *B*).

Figure 19-16 Phototoxic eruption.

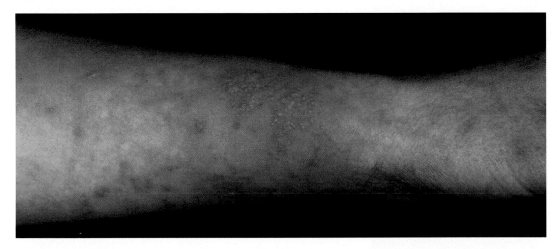

A, Diffuse erythema and vesiculation occurred 24 hours after preparing celery in a commercial processing plant.

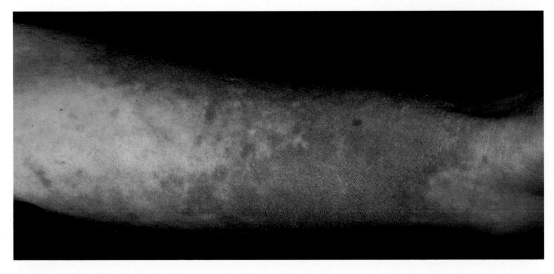

B, The patient pictured in *A* developed diffuse hyperpigmentation in the previously inflamed areas 2 weeks after the acute episode.

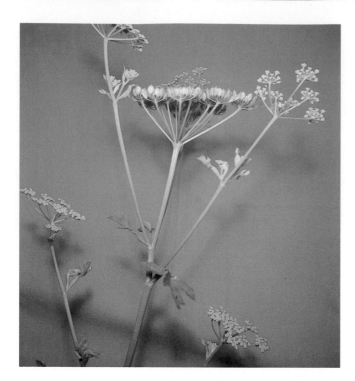

Figure 19-17
Wild parsnip. Cause of phototoxic eruptions.

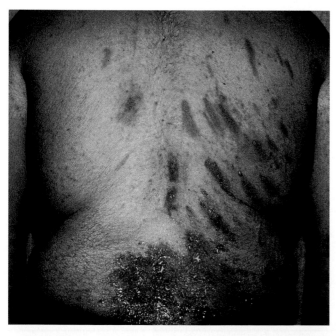

Figure 19-18
Phytophotodermatitis. Streaks of vesicles occurred after the patient lay in a field of wild parsnips and was then exposed to sunlight.

Phytophotodermatitis. Exposure to plants[66] that contain light-sensitizing compounds[67] such as furanocoumarins (psoralens) can cause intense reactions. Examples are exposure to celery by salad makers and grocery workers,[68] wild parsnip (Figures 19-17 and 19-18) in meadows, the rind and pulp of limes,[69-71] berlock dermatitis caused by the psoralen compounds in oil of bergamot (used in some perfumes) (Figure 19-19), and the leaves and young fruits of figs.[72]

The distribution of phototoxic reactions is sharply limited to areas of sun exposure. Topical exposure to solutions or plants produces bizarre patterns of inflammation, such as streaks from brushing against a plant or haphazard lines from celery juice.

Drugs. Exposure to certain drugs[73,74] (see the box on p. 615) may result in a generalized intense erythema in sun-exposed skin. Long lists of drugs reported to cause photosensitivity have been compiled. These are misleading because many are from single case reports. Thiazide diuretics are common offenders.[75] The characteristic areas are the forehead, nose, malar eminences, cheeks, upper ears, lateral and posterior neck, vee of the chest, extensor surfaces of the forearms, backs of the hands, and prominences of the pretibial and calf areas. The upper eyelids, nasolabial folds, and submental areas are typically spared. Photoonycholysis, which is the separation of the nails from the nailbeds, may occur with drugs such as demeclocycline hydrochloride (Declomycin) and tetracycline.

Management. In most instances withdrawal of the drug results in clearance of the clinical reaction. The patient should never take the offending drug again. In rare instances, photosensitivity persists for months or years. These patients may benefit from treatment with PUVA.[76] Topical steroids provide some relief, but oral steroids are often necessary. When simple elimination fails to establish the offending agent, phototesting by physicians experienced with such procedures should be performed.[77]

Photoallergy

Photoallergic reactions are now rare and are primarily of historic interest. Ultraviolet light initiates a reaction between skin protein and a chemical or drug to form an antigen. A delayed hypersensitivity reaction follows, and the clinical presentation is, like poison ivy, eczematous inflammation. Photoallergic contact dermatitis to PABA and structurally related PABA sunscreen has been documented.[78] Musk ambrette in cologne and perfumes is a contemporary cause of photoallergy. Some patients without additional drug exposure continue to flare for years when exposed to sunlight; this is termed a *persistent light reaction.*

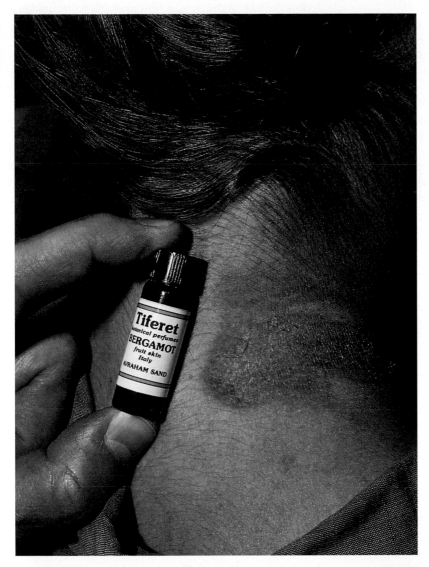

Figure 19-19
Phototoxic reaction (berlock dermatitis).
Oil of bergamot (used in some perfumes)
contains psoralens, which can cause erythema
followed by prolonged hyperpigmentation after
exposure to light.

AGENTS CAUSING PHOTOTOXIC REACTIONS

INTERNAL DRUGS

Chlorpromazine
Chlorothiazides
Tetracyclines
Demeclocycline (Declomycin)
8-methoxypsoralens
Trimethylpsoralen
Nalidixic acid
Amiodarone
Piroxicam (Feldene)
Sulfonamides
Furosemide

TOPICAL AGENTS

Coal tar derivatives
Perfumes

PLANTS CONTAINING PSORALEN COMPOUNDS (PHYTOPHOTODERMATITIS)

Celery
Gas plant (burning bush, dittany)
Meadow grass (agrimony)
Parsnip (wild parsnip)
Persian limes
Wild angelica
Angelica
Cow parsley
Carrot (wild)
Fig (wild)
Sweet orange
False bishop's weed
Hogweed
Rue
Many others reported, but rare

Disorders of Hypopigmentation

Diseases that present with hypopigmentation or hyperpigmentation are listed in Table 19-4. The most common and distinctive are described in the following paragraphs.

VITILIGO

The word *vitiligo* is derived from the Greek *vitelius*, meaning calf. The white spots of vitiligo resemble white patches on a calf. Vitiligo is an acquired loss of pigmentation characterized histologically by absence of epidermal melanocytes. It may be an autoimmune disease associated with antibodies (vitiligo antibodies) to melanocytes.[79] Studies suggest there is some genetic mechanism involved in the etiology of vitiligo and that it is polygenic in nature.[80] There is a positive family history in at least 30% of cases. Both sexes are affected equally. Approximately 1% of the population is affected; 50% of cases begin before age 20. The pigment loss may be localized or generalized.[81] Many patients feel embarrassed. Physicians should be especially alert to the effects of disfigurement.[82]

Clinical manifestations. There are two types (A and B) (Table 19-5). In the more common type A there is a fairly symmetric pattern of white macules with well-defined borders. The borders may have a red halo (inflammatory vitiligo) or a rim of hyperpigmentation. The loss of pigmentation may not be apparent in fair-skinned individuals, but it may be disfiguring in blacks. Initially the disease is limited; it then progresses slowly over years. Commonly involved sites include the backs of the hands, the face, and body folds, including axillae and genitalia (Figures 19-20 to 19-23). White areas are common around body openings such as the eyes, nostrils, mouth, nipples, umbilicus, and anus. Vitiligo occurs at sites of trauma (Köebner's phenomenon), such as around the elbows and in previously sunburned skin. Many patients with vitiligo develop halo nevi.

Childhood vitiligo. Childhood vitiligo is a distinct subset of vitiligo. There is an increased incidence of segmental vitiligo (type B vitiligo), of autoimmune and/or endocrine disease, of premature graying in immediate and extended family members, and of organ-specific antibodies, in addition to a poor response to topical PUVA therapy.[83] Children under age 10 can be treated with topical psoralens and UVA light or topical steroids.[84]

Wood's light examination. Examination with the Wood's light accentuates the hypopigmented areas and is useful for examining patients with light complexions. The axillae, anus, and genitalia should be carefully examined. These areas are frequently involved but often clinically inapparent without the Wood's light.

Associated findings. Most patients with vitiligo have no other associated findings; however, vitiligo has been reported to be associated with alopecia areata, hypothyroidism, Graves' disease, Addison's disease, pernicious anemia, insulin-dependent diabetes mellitus, uveitis, chronic mucocutaneous candidiasis, the polyglandular autoimmune syndromes, and melanoma.[85] Thyroid disorders have been reported in as many as 30% of vitiligo patients.[86] Circulating autoantibodies such as antithyroglobulin and antimicrosomal and antiparietal cell antibodies have been found in more than 50% of patients.[87] Vitiligo is part of the Vogt-Koyanagi syndrome of vitiligo, uveitis, and deafness.

TABLE 19-4 Disorders of Pigmentation

Hypopigmentation	Hyperpigmentation
Acquired	Circumscribed brown
Chemical-induced	Café-au-lait spots
Halo nevus	Diabetic dermopathy
Idiopathic guttate	Erythema ab igne
hypomelanosis	Fixed drug eruption
Leprosy	Freckles
Leukoderma associated	Lentigo in children
with melanoma	Peutz-Jeghers
Pityriasis alba	syndrome
Postinflammatory	Lentigo in adults
hypopigmentation	Melasma
Tinea versicolor	Phytophotodermatitis
Vitiligo	Diffuse brown
Congenital	Addison's disease
Albinism, partial	Biliary cirrhosis
(piebaldism)	Hemochromatosis
Albinism, total	Malignant melanoma
Nevus anemicus	(metastatic)
Nevus depigmentosus	
Piebaldism	
Tuberous sclerosis	

TABLE 19-5 Vitiligo (Types A and B) Clinical Manifestations

	Type A	Type B
Distribution	Nondermatomal	Dermatomal (zosteriform)
Ratio	3	1
Onset	Any age (50% before age 20)	Young
Activity	Lifelong	Rapid spread 1 year
Associated with halo nevus	Yes	No
Köebner's phenomenon	Yes	No
Associated with immunologic diseases	Yes	No

Modified from Koga M, Tango T: *Br J Dermatol* 118:223-228, 1988.

VITILIGO

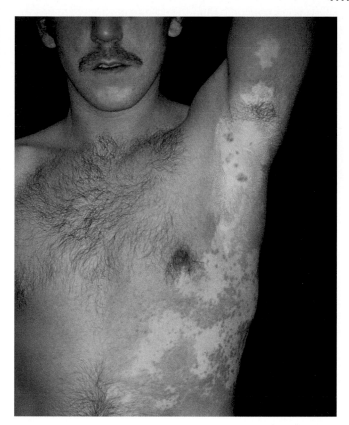

Figure 19-20
Body folds, including the axillae, are commonly involved. Wood's light examination may be necessary to demonstrate this in patients with light skin.

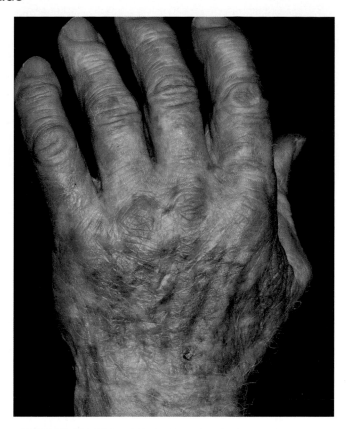

Figure 19-21
The back of the hand is a commonly involved site.

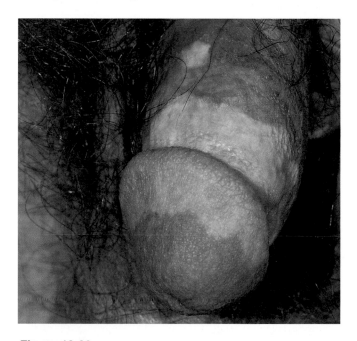

Figure 19-22
The penis is a commonly involved site.

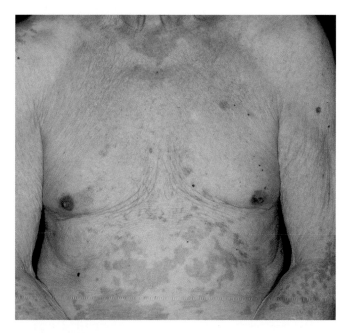

Figure 19-23
There is almost total loss of pigment. Monobenzone (Benoquin), a potent depigmenting agent, could be used for cosmetic purposes to remove the remaining pigment.

Treatment. Depigmented skin is devoid of melanocytes in the epidermis. Repigmentation is caused by activation and migration of melanocytes from a melanocytic reservoir located in the hair follicles.[88] Therefore skin with little or no hair (hands and feet) or with white hair responds poorly to treatment. When a vitiliginous spot repigments, it repigments from the follicle and spreads outward. Melanocytes divide rapidly after any inflammatory process or following UV radiation. PUVA produces inflammation in the skin at the depth of the hair follicle. Cytokines released by the inflammatory process may stimulate melanocytes to proliferate and migrate out. The melanocytes are more susceptible to drug injury from psoralens when they get into the interfollicular space. Some clinicians change to low-dose UVB to encourage melanocyte proliferation and migration.

INDICATIONS. Treatment is necessary only for patients in whom the disease causes considerable emotional and social distress. Vitiligo in individuals with fair complexions is usually not a significant cosmetic problem. The condition becomes more apparent in the summer months when tanning accentuates normal skin. Tanning may be prevented with sunscreens that have an SPF of 15 or higher. Vitiligo is a significant cosmetic problem in people with dark complexions, and repigmentation with psoralens may be worthwhile.

Topical therapy. Topical psoralens and topical steroids have been used with some success in patients with limited areas of pigmentation (see the box below). Some dermatologists who have years of experience with phototherapy will not use topical psoralens. They believe that the potential for

phototoxicity to produce severe burns is too great. The edges where there is residual pigmentation always hyperpigment. This disappears with time.

PUVA. See the box on p. 619 for treatment protocol. Patients should be selected carefully for psoralen photochemotherapy. They should be informed that in approximately 50% of patients there may be some repigmentation following 150 to 200 PUVA treatments over 12 to 24 months.[89] Vitiligo of the backs of the hands almost never responds.[90] Repigmentation may not be complete, and the partially treated areas may appear more bizarre than they did initially. The response is slow. Dark-skinned patients respond better than fair-skinned patients. Children under age 10 are generally not treated with oral phototherapy. Patients with fair skin, types I and II, are unlikely to benefit from PUVA unless there is marked disfigurement.

The new micronized crystalline form of methoxsalen is the preferred drug because it is consistently absorbed. (Trioxsalen is erratically absorbed.) Start with a small dosage and slowly increase until mild erythema is produced, then maintain that dosage. Follicular repigmentation usually begins after 15 or 20 treatments. Significant repigmentation may occur after 50 treatments. Patients may be given a trial off of therapy for a couple of months. They may continue to repigment during this period.

Some patients spontaneously repigment, sometimes after moderate sun exposure. UVB or PUVA can then be used to encourage further repigmentation. Reevaluate patients every 2 or 3 months. Therapy should be stopped if no color returns after this period. Patients who respond usually keep their pigment. Patients who have actively spreading vitiligo should not be treated; treatment does not halt the spread of the disease.

PUVASOL (PSORALENS AND SUNLIGHT). The following program is to be used with natural sunlight. Start with trioxsalen, which is less phototoxic than methoxsalen. The dose should be taken 2 to 4 hours before measured periods of sun exposure. Maximum solar radiation is received between 11 A.M. and 3 P.M. The patient should be treated only twice each week during the first 2 weeks to determine the degree of sun sensitivity. Treatments may be more frequent after this initial period. A persistent, faint erythema is the desired result. The schedule in Table 19-6 is suitable for most patients.

Response to treatment. Improvement begins with perifollicular pigmentation, which then enlarges. Repigmentation occurs at the borders but at a slower rate. Best results are obtained on the face and neck. The face begins to respond after 25 treatments, other areas after 50. Results are poor on the hands and feet and over bony prominences. Focal vitiligo responds better than generalized vitiligo (i.e., it responds to 100 treatments or less, whereas generalized vitiligo requires as many as 200 treatments).[91] Most patients who respond do not develop new areas of pigment loss. The appearance of new or enlarged macules indicates the possible beginning of treatment failure. Maintenance therapy is

---

VITILIGO (LOCALIZED) TREATMENT PROTOCOL

Indications
  Pigment loss less than 20% to 25% of body surface
  Adults and children over age 2
Topical psoralens
  Dilute stock 8-methoxypsoralen solution with Cetaphil or petrolatum to make a 0.1% solution.
    1. Apply the 0.1% solution 90 minutes before UVA exposure
    2. Initial exposure should be 0.12 or 0.25 J/cm^2.
    3. Increase 0.12 or 0.25 J/cm^2/treatment to trace phototoxicity.
Prevention of severe phototoxic reactions after each treatment
    1. Wash after treatment and apply sunscreens.
    2. Avoid sun exposure for 36 hours (sunscreens are not totally effective.)
Topical steroids
  Midpotency steroids (e.g., triamcinolone 0.1%, desonide 0.05%):
    1. Apply cream once each day.
    2. Optimum results require at least 3 to 4 months.

GUIDELINES FOR ORAL PHOTOCHEMOTHERAPY

PATIENT SELECTION

Highly motivated

Detailed information about treatment modalities (length, duration, need for compliance required)

Contraindications (absolute and relative)

History of cutaneous malignant tumors

Prior exposure to carcinogenic agents (arsenic, Grenz-ray or x-ray therapy)

History of photosensitivity or photomediated disorders

Conditions potentially aggravated by PUVA (cataracts, aphakia)

Severe cardiovascular, hepatic, or renal disease

Pregnancy and lactation.

CLINICAL INDICATORS OF RESPONSE

Poor response

Segmental vitiligo

Acrofacial and mucous membrane involvement, white hair on vitiligo macules, dorsal hands and feet, fingers and toes, palms and soles

Good response

Face, neck, trunk, proximal arms and legs

Presence of multiple perifollicular macules

VARIABLES OF TREATMENT

Psoralen

*TMP (0.6 to 0.8 mg/kg), less erythematogenic than 8-MOP, selectively used for outdoor treatment and occasionally for patients with skin types I and II

8-MOP (Oxsoralen Utra) (0.2 to 0.4 mg/kg), used in a controlled therapeutic environment (high-intensity UVA sources) or in patients with skin types III and IV

Ingestion of tablets/capsules in a single dose 1 to 2 hours before anticipated exposure. When available, determinations of serum psoralen levels useful

UV source

Sunlight between 11:00 A.M. and 3:00 P.M. or high-intensity long-wave UV radiation

UV dosimetry

Sunlight: 5 to 10 minutes of summer sunlight, gradually increased by 5 minutes every two treatments, until a maximum of 45 minutes is reached

High-intensity PUVA lights: Initial UVA exposure should be 1.0 J and increments (twice weekly, not on 2 consecutive days) of 0.5 (8-MOP) to 1.0 (TMP) J per treatment until evidence of response or of phototoxicity.

Frequency: at least twice a week. Ideally one treatment every 3rd day. Increased risk of phototoxic side effects without increased response rate with more frequent treatments

Persistent erythema is not required for repigmentation

Duration

12 months or more as continuously as possible for best results

PRECAUTIONS

Avoidance of unnecessary sunlight exposure throughout the remainder of the day after PUVA treatment

Wearing UVA-blocking sunglasses required during the day of treatment. Precise and appropriate advice required for the choice of sunglasses

From Nordlund JJ, Ortonne J-P: *Curr Prob Dermatol* 4(1):21, 1992.
*TMP,4,5',8-trimethylpsoralen; 8-MOP, 8-methoxypsoralen; UVA, UV light type A; 5-MOP, 5-methoxypsoralen; PUVA, psoralen and UVA treatment.

TABLE 19-6 Treatment of Vitiligo with Psoralens: Suggested Sun Exposure Guide

	Basic skin color	
Treatment	Light	Medium
Initial exposure	15 min	20 min
Second exposure	20 min	25 min
Third exposure	25 min	30 min
Fourth exposure	30 min	35 min
Subsequent exposures	Gradually increase exposure on the basis of erythema and tenderness	

not required. Totally repigmented macules should remain filled with 85% certainty; those incompletely filled in are likely to reverse and depigment.

Grafting and transplantation. Several surgical procedures have been developed for treating depigmented skin. These include grafting suction-blistered epidermis, minigrafts, and transplantation of in vitro–cultured epidermis bearing melanocytes.[92]

Systemic steroids. Systemic corticosteroids can arrest the progression of vitiligo and lead to repigmentation in a significant proportion of patients, but may also produce unacceptable side effects. Oral mini-pulse therapy with 5 mg betamethasone/dexamethasone was reported to arrest the progression and induce spontaneous repigmentation in some vitiligo patients. To minimize the side effects, betamethasone as a single oral dose was taken after breakfast on 2 consecutive days per week. The progression of the disease was arrested in 89% with active disease, whereas some patients needed an increase in the dosage to 7.5 mg per day to achieve a complete arrest of lesions. Within 2 to 4 months, 80% of the patients started having spontaneous repigmentation of the existing lesions that progressed with continued treatment.[93]

Cosmetics. For cosmetic purposes, lesions may be temporarily dyed brown with Dy-O-Derm or Vita-dye. Cosmetics that camouflage, (i.e., Dermablend and Covermark; see the Formulary) effectively hide the white patches. Each product comes in several shades.

The sunless or self-tanning lotions that contain dihydroxyacetone (DHA) darken the skin by staining. These preparations work best in vitiligo patients with skin phototypes II and III and are particularly useful if their normal skin is already tanned. The major problem is color blending and matching at the border of vitiliginous and normal skin.[21]

Depigmentation of remaining normal skin. Patients with more than 40% involvement of the skin surface may choose to remove the remaining normal skin pigment with 20% monobenzone (Benoquin cream). Monobenzone destroys melanocytes and can cause contact dermatitis. Therefore, as a test before starting generalized therapy, monobenzone should be applied to a single pigmented spot daily for 1 week. Thereafter larger pigmented areas are treated twice daily for more than 6 to 9 months, not 4 months as is stated in the *Physicians' Desk Reference.* Application for 3 to 4 years may be necessary. Resistant areas such as the hands are treated with monobenzone under Saran Wrap occlusion. Patients may note an inflammatory response within the pigmented skin but not in the white skin. The monobenzone can be diluted to a 10%, 5%, or lower concentration for these patients. A group VI topical steroid may also be used to control inflammation.

Depigmentation is usually done in regions to limit drug absorption. Start with the face and upper extremity areas, then treat lower extremity sites. Truncal areas are last, and many patients choose to leave their trunk its normal color. The rate of depigmentation can vary from weeks to 4 years.

People assisting others with application of monobenzone must wear gloves and use applicators to prevent depigmenting their own skin.

Patients must understand that this is a permanent procedure. They will be sun sensitive for the rest of their lives and must use sunscreen during sun exposure. The results of treatment are usually very gratifying.

Patients who would like some skin color after treatment can use beta carotene (Solatene) 60 mg three times a day for 6 weeks, followed by 30 mg three times a day for maintenance.

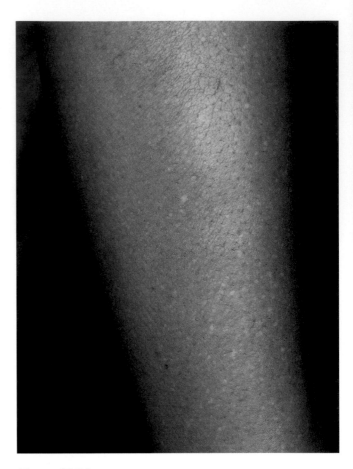

Figure 19-24
Idiopathic guttate hypomelanosis. White spots on the arms and lower legs occur in the middle-aged and the elderly.

IDIOPATHIC GUTTATE HYPOMELANOSIS

Idiopathic guttate hypomelanosis (white spots on the arms and legs) is characterized by 2- to 5-mm white spots with sharply demarcated borders. They are located on the exposed areas of hands, forearms, and lower legs of middle-aged and elderly people (Figure 19-24). Patients have signs of early aging and sun exposure, including seborrheic keratoses, lentigines, and xerosis in the same areas. A subset of these patients have lesions unrelated to sun exposure.[94] The condition is asymptomatic. There is no treatment.

PITYRIASIS ALBA

Pityriasis alba is a common finding that is probably more usual in patients with the atopic diathesis (see Chapter Five). The condition appears in most instances before puberty. The face, neck, and arms are the most common sites. The lesions begin as a nonspecific erythema and gradually become scaly and hypopigmented. The hypopigmentation is transient and caused by mild dermal inflammation and the ultraviolet screening effect of the scaly skin. The condition gradually improves after puberty. Treatment consists of lubrication. Mild inflammation responds to group V topical steroids, but the degree of pigmentation is not affected by any treatment.

The condition is often confused with vitiligo and tinea versicolor. Vitiligo does not scale. The potassium hydroxide preparation is positive in tinea versicolor.

NEVUS ANEMICUS

Nevus anemicus is a rare congenital lesion most frequently observed on the chest or back of females. The lesion usually consists of a well-defined white macule with an irregular border, often surrounded by smaller white macules beyond the border of the major lesion (Figure 19-25). Histologically the skin appears normal; the pale color has been attributed to local blood vessel sensitivity to catecholamines.[95,96] Special stains confirm the presence of melanin and melanocytes. The lesion is most often confused with tinea versicolor or vitiligo. The white macule lacks the scale of tinea and, during Wood's light examination, does not become as prominent as vitiligo.

TUBEROUS SCLEROSIS

Hypopigmented macules (oval, ash leaf–shaped, or stippled) that are concentrated on the arms, legs, and trunk are the earliest signs of tuberous sclerosis[97,98] (Figure 19-26; see also Chapter Twenty-six). They are present in 40% to 90% of patients with the disease, and they number from 1 to 32 in affected individuals.

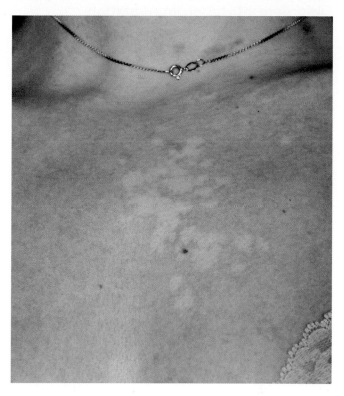

Figure 19-25
Nevus anemicus.

Figure 19-26
Tuberous sclerosis. Ash leaf–shaped hypopigmented macules.

Disorders of Hyperpigmentation

FRECKLES

Freckles, or ephelides, are small, red or light brown macules that are promoted by sun exposure and fade during the winter months. They are usually confined to the face, arms, and back. The number varies from a few spots on the face to hundreds of confluent macules on the face and arms. They occur as an autosomal dominant trait and are most often found in individuals with fair complexions. The use of sunscreens prevents the appearance of new freckles and helps prevent the darkening of existing freckles that typically accompanies sun exposure.

LENTIGO IN CHILDREN

A lentigo is a small (0.5- to 2-cm) tan, brown, or black oval-to-round macule that is darker than a freckle and is not affected by sunlight. Freckles darken with sun exposure. Lentigines may increase in number during childhood and adult life or fade at any time. The Peutz-Jeghers syndrome refers to mucocutaneous pigmentation consisting of many blue-brown lentigines, less than 0.5 cm in diameter, on the buccal mucosa and other areas of the glabrous skin, accompanied by generalized intestinal polyposis.[99,100]

LENTIGO IN ADULTS

Lentigo, or liver spot, occurs in sun-exposed areas of the face, arms, and hands (Figure 19-27). The lesions vary in size from 0.2 to 2 cm and become more numerous with advancing age. A biopsy should be taken from any lentigo that develops a highly irregular border, localized increase in pigmentation, or localized thickening to rule out lentigo maligna melanoma. Cryotherapy is an effective treatment. Topical 0.1% tretinoin significantly improves both clinical and microscopic manifestations of liver spots. After 10 months, 83% of patients with facial lesions who were treated with tretinoin had lightening of these lesions. The lesions do not return for at least 6 months after therapy is discontinued.[101]

Hyperpigmented lesions are a predominant component of photoaging in Chinese and Japanese persons; 0.1% tretinoin cream significantly lightens the hyperpigmentation of photoaging in these patients.[9] Hydroquinone preparations are occasionally useful for bleaching these lesions.

MELASMA

Melasma (chloasma or mask of pregnancy) is an acquired brown hyperpigmentation involving the face and neck in genetically predisposed women. The pigmentation develops slowly without signs of inflammation and may be faint or

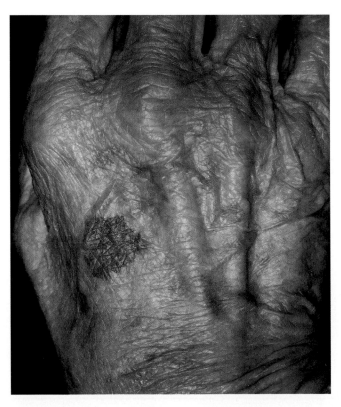

Figure 19-27
Lentigo (liver spots). A brown macule that appears in chronically sun-exposed areas.

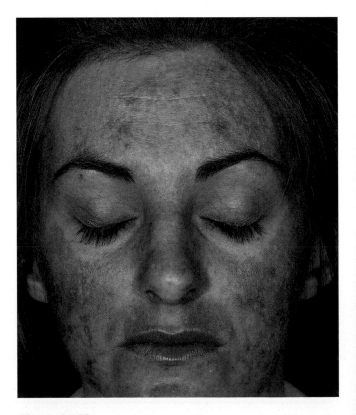

Figure 19-28
Melasma (mask of pregnancy). Diffuse brown hyperpigmentation may occur during pregnancy or while taking oral contraceptives.

dark. There is an increased number and activity of melanocytes in the epidermis and an increased number of melanophages in the dermis. The forehead, malar eminences, upper lip, and chin are most frequently affected (Figure 19-28). Melasma occurs during the second or third trimester of pregnancy, gradually fades after delivery, and darkens with subsequent pregnancies. Melasma occurs in some women taking oral contraceptives.[102] There are four types based on Wood's light examination: (1) an epidermal type that shows enhancement of color contrast, (2) a dermal type that does not, (3) a mixed type that shows no or slight enhancement, and (4) Wood's lamp inapparent, which is seen in dark individuals. The epidermal type responds to depigmenting agents; the dermal pigmentation resists the action of bleaching agents.

Treatment. Sun exposure must be minimized. Sunscreens that block both UVA and UVB light should be used.

DEPIGMENTING AGENTS. Depigmentation may be accomplished with the use of bleaching creams that contain hydroquinone.[103,104] This agent is available in 2% concentrations without prescription (Porcelana) and by prescription in 3% (Melanex) and 4% (Eldoquin-Forte, Eldopaque-Forte, and Solaquin Forte) concentrations (see the Formulary). The medication should be applied twice daily, once in the morning and before bedtime. Hydroquinone is an irritant and a sensitizer, and skin should be tested for sensitivity before use by applying a small amount to the cheek or arm once each day for 2 days (open patch testing). The development of intense erythema or vesiculation indicates an allergic reaction and precludes further use. Products such as Eldopaque have a tinted sunblocking cream base. Patients who object to a tinted preparation may use products that contain benzophenone and PABA ester sunscreens such as Solaquin Forte. These preparations must be used for months and in many cases result in gradual depigmentation. Skin must be protected with broad-spectrum sunscreens both during and after treatment. Tretinoin (Retin-A) enhances the epidermal penetration of hydroquinone and is often prescribed to be used at a different time of day. Start with a low concentration of tretinoin. Increase the concentration until slight irritation occurs. Hydroquinones also bleach freckles and lentigines, but not café-au-lait spots or pigmented nevi.

TRETINOIN. Topical tretinoin used alone produces significant clinical improvement of melasma, mainly due to reduction in epidermal pigment, but improvement occurs slowly over several months.[105] Chemabrasion with 30% to 50% trichloroacetic acid in water is also effective. Darker complected individuals are poor candidates for chemical peels because postinflammatory hyperpigmentation frequently occurs.

CAFÉ-AU-LAIT SPOTS

Café-au-lait spots are uniformly pale brown macules that vary in size from 0.5 to 20 cm and can be found on any cutaneous surface (Figure 19-29). (See also Chapter Twenty-six, p. 793.) They may be present at birth, are estimated to be present in 10% to 20% of normal children, and increase in number and size with age. Six or more spots greater than 1.5 cm in diameter are presumptive evidence of neurofibromatosis (von Recklinghausen's disease) in young children over 5 years of age. In children under 5 years of age, five or more café-au-lait spots greater than 0.5 cm in diameter suggest the diagnosis of neurofibromatosis. Café-au-lait spots are present in 90% to 100% of patients with von Recklinghausen's disease. Smaller spots 1 to 4 cm in diameter in the axillae (axillary freckling or Crowe's sign) are a rare but diagnostic sign of neurofibromatosis. There is no increased incidence of café-au-lait spots in tuberous sclerosis.[106] Lesions that are similar but that have a more irregular border (shaped like "the coast of Maine") are seen in polyostotic fibrous dysplasia (Albright's syndrome). The smooth, regular border of the café-au-lait macules of neurofibromatosis has been compared to "the coast of California."

Macromelanosomes, or larger-than-normal pigment granules, have been detected with the electron microscope in the café-au-lait spots of some patients with neurofibromatosis, but their absence does not rule out the diagnosis. Café-au-lait spots cannot be lightened by hydroquinone bleaching agents.

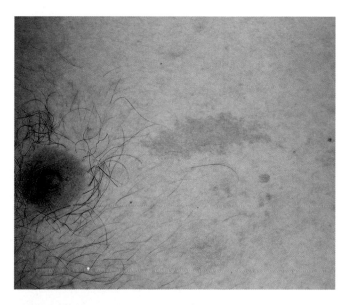

Figure 19-29
Café-au-lait spots. Irregular brown macules that are found in 10% to 20% of normal children. Number and size are increased in neurofibromatosis. (See Figure 26-11.)

DIABETIC DERMOPATHY

Asymptomatic, round, atrophic hyperpigmented areas on the shins (shin spots) are the most common cutaneous manifestation of diabetes. Lesions may also appear on the forearms, the anterior surface of the lower thighs, and the sides of the feet. Men are affected twice as often as women, and the incidence is greatest in patients with diabetic neuropathy. They may be initiated by trauma. Lesions begin as round-to-oval, flat-topped, red, scaly papules that may become eroded. The lesions eventually clear or heal with epidermal atrophy or hyperpigmentation.

ERYTHEMA AB IGNE

Chronic exposure to heat from a wood stove, fireplace, electric blanket, electric heater, hot water bottle, or hot compress may cause a distinctive cutaneous eruption with a reticular pattern. The eruption initially appears as bands of erythema, but brown hyperpigmentation develops with repeated exposure (Figure 19-30).

Erythema ab igne may develop in patients who apply local heat or hot water bottles to painful metastatic and primary tumors.[107]

The pigmentation, caused by melanin,[108] may fade in time or may be permanent. The eruption must be differentiated from livido reticularis, which occurs with diseases such as leukocytoclastic vasculitis. Livido reticularis is a reddish-purple reticular pigmentation, probably caused by restricted blood flow through the horizontal venous plexus. The color persists, but brown hyperpigmentation does not occur.

Figure 19-30
Erythema ab igne. Reticular brown hyperpigmentation that develops in areas chronically exposed to heat. A heating pad used for several months produced the eruption depicted here.

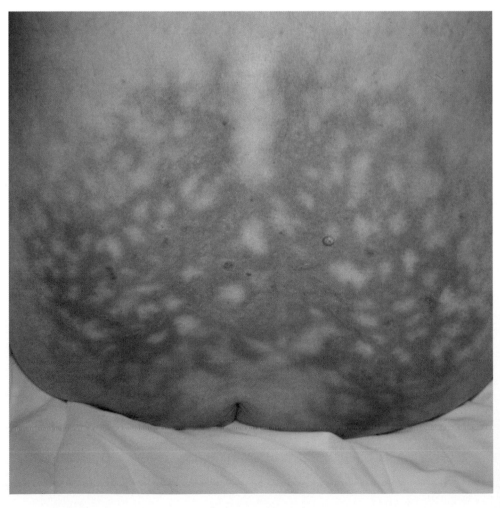

REFERENCES

1. Kligman AM, Lavker RM: Cutaneous aging: the differences between intrinsic aging and photoaging, *J Cutaneous Aging Cosmetic Dermatol* 1:5-12, 1988.
2. Kligman LH, Kligman AM: The nature of photoaging: its prevention and repair, *Photodermatology* 3:215-227, 1986.
3. Taylor CR, Stern RS, et al: Photoaging/photodamage and photoprotection, *J Am Acad Dermatol* 22:1-15, 1990.
4. Gilchrest BA: Overview of skin aging, *J Cutaneous Aging Cosmetic Dermatol* 1:1-3, 1988.
5. Tsuji T, Yorifuji T, Hayashi Y, et al: Two types of wrinkles in aged persons (letter), *Arch Dermatol* 122:22-23, 1986.
6. Weiss JS et al: Topical tretinoin improves photoaged skin, *JAMA* 259:527-532, 1988.
7. Weiss JS, Ellis CN, Headington JT, et al: Topical tretinoin in the treatment of aging skin, *J Am Acad Dermatol* 19:169-175, 1988.
8. Andreano JM, Bergfeld WF, et al: Tretinoin emollient cream 0.01% for the treatment of photoaged skin, *Cleve Clin J Med* 60:49-55, 1993.
9. Griffiths CE, Goldfarb MT, et al: Topical tretinoin (retinoic acid) treatment of hyperpigmented lesions associated with photoaging in Chinese and Japanese patients: a vehicle-controlled trial, *J Am Acad Dermatol* 30:76-84, 1994.
10. Bhawan J et al: Reversible histologic effects of tretinoin on photodamaged skin, *J Geriatr Dermatol* 3(3):62-67, 1995.
11. Griffiths CE, Russman AN, et al: Restoration of collagen formation in photodamaged human skin by tretinoin (retinoic acid), *N Engl J Med* 329:530-535, 1993.
12. Green LJ, McCormick A, et al: Photoaging and the skin. The effects of tretinoin, *Dermatol Clin* 11:97-105, 1993.
13. Ellis CN, Weiss JS, et al: Sustained improvement with prolonged topical tretinoin (retinoic acid) for photoaged skin, *J Am Acad Dermatol* 23:629-637, 1990.
14. Matarasso SL, Salman SM, et al: The role of chemical peeling in the treatment of photodamaged skin, *J Dermatol Surg Oncol* 16:945-954, 1990.
15. Stuzin JM, Baker TJ, et al: Treatment of photoaging. Facial chemical peeling (phenol and trichloroacetic acid) and dermabrasion, *Clin Plast Surg* 20:9-25, 1993.
16. Perricone NV: An alpha hydroxy acid acts as an antioxidant, *J Ger Derm* 1(2):101-104, 1993.
17. Wulf HC, Poulsen T, Brodthagen H, et al: Sunscreens for delay of ultraviolet induction of skin tumors, *J Am Acad Dermatol* 7:194-202, 1982.
18. Stern RS, Weinstein MC, Baker SG: Risk reduction for nonmelanoma skin cancer with childhood sunscreen use, *Arch Dermatol* 122:537-545, 1986.
19. Patel NP, Highton A, Moy RL: Properties of topical sunscreen formulations, *J Dermatol Surg Oncol* 18:316-320, 1992.
20. Marks R et al: The effect of regular sunscreen use on vitamin D levels in an Australian population, *Arch Dermatol* 131:415-421, 1995.
21. Levy SB: Dihydroxyacetone-containing sunless or self-tanning lotions, *J Am Acad Dermatol* 27:989-993, 1992.
22. Holzle E, Plewig G, von Kries R, et al: Polymorphous light eruption, *J Invest Dermatol* 88(suppl):32-38, 1987.
23. Jansen CT, Karvonen J: Polymorphous light eruption, *Arch Dermatol* 120:862-865, 1984.
24. Fusaro RM, Johnson JA: Topical photoprotection for hereditary polymorphic light eruption of American Indians, *J Am Acad Dermatol* 24:744-746, 1991.
25. Lane PR, Hogan DJ, et al: Actinic prurigo: clinical features and prognosis, *J Am Acad Dermatol* 26:683-692, 1992.
26. Holzle E, Plewig G, Hofmann C, et al: Polymorphous light eruption: experimental reproduction of skin lesions, *J Am Acad Dermatol* 7:111-125, 1982.
27. Ortel B, Tanew A, Wolff K, et al: Polymorphous light eruption: action spectrum and photoprotection, *J Am Acad Dermatol* 14:748-753, 1986.
28. Elpern DJ, Morison WL: Papulovesicular light eruption, *Arch Dermatol* 121:1286-1288, 1985.
29. Lane PR, Moreland AA, et al: Treatment of actinic prurigo with intermittent short-course topical 0.05% clobetasol 17-propionate. A preliminary report, *Arch Dermatol* 126:1211-1213, 1990.
30. Morison WL, Momataz K, Mosher DB, et al: UV-B phototherapy and prophylaxis of polymorphous light eruption, *Br J Dermatol* 106:231-233, 1982.
31. Murphy GM, Logan RA, Lovell CR, et al: Prophylactic PUVA and UVB therapy in polymorphic light eruption: a controlled trial, *Br J Dermatol* 116:531-538, 1987.
32. Addo HA, Sharma SC: UVB phototherapy and photochemotherapy (PUVA) in the treatment of polymorphic light eruption and solar urticaria, *Br J Dermatol* 116:539-547, 1987.
33. Berg N et al: Ultraviolet A phototherapy and trimethylpsoralen UVA photochemotherapy in polymorphous light eruption—a controlled study, *Photodermatol Photoimmunol Photomed* 10:139-143, 1994.
34. Rucker BU, Haberle M, et al: Ultraviolet light hardening in polymorphous light eruption—a controlled study comparing different emission spectra, *Photodermatol Photoimmunol Photomed* 8:73-78, 1991.
35. Parrish JA et al: Comparison of PUVA and beta-carotene in the treatment of polymorphous light eruption, *Br J Dermatol* 100:187-198, 1979.
36. Epstein JH: Polymorphous light eruption, *J Am Acad Dermatol* 3:329-343, 1980.
37. Murphy GM, Hawk JLM, Magnus IA: Hydroxychloroquine in polymorphic light eruption: a controlled trial with drug and visual sensitivity monitoring, *Br J Dermatol* 116:379-386, 1987.
38. Eramo LR, Garden JM, Esterly NB: Hydroa vacciniforme, *Arch Dermatol* 122:1310-1313, 1986.
39. Thiers BH: The porphyrias, *J Am Acad Dermatol* 5:621-625, 1981.
40. Poh-Fitzpatrick M et al: Porphyria cutanea tarda in two patients treated with hemodialysis for chronic renal failure, *N Engl J Med* 299:292-294, 1978.
41. Conroy-Cantilena C, Vilamidou L: Porphyria cutanea tarda in hepatitis C virus–infected blood donors, *J Am Acad Dermatol* 32:512-514, 1995.
42. Grossman M et al: Porphyria cutanea tarda: clinical features and laboratory findings in 40 patients, *Am J Med* 67: 277-286, 1979.
43. Cripps DJ: Hospital management of the dermatologic patient: the porphyrias, *Semin Dermatol* 5:55-68, 1986.
44. Adjarov D, Kerimova M: Effective control of patients with porphyria cutanea tarda by measuring plasma uroporphyrin, *Clin Exp Dermatol* 16:254-257, 1991.
45. Kordac V et al: Chloroquine in the treatment of porphyria cutanea tarda. *N Engl J Med* 296:949, 1977.
46. Seubert S, Seubert A, et al: Results of treatment of porphyria cutanea tarda with bloodletting and chloroquine, *Z Hautkr* 65:223-225, 1990.
47. Topi GC, Amantea A, Griso D: Recovery from porphyria cutanea tarda with no specific therapy other than avoidance of hepatic toxins, *Br J Dermatol* 111:75-82, 1984.
48. Diffey BL, Farr PM: Sunscreen protection against UVB, UVA and blue light: an in vivo and in vitro comparison, *Br J Dermatol* 124:258-263, 1991.
49. Poh-Fitzpatrick MB, Sosin AE, Bemis J: Porphyrin levels in plasma and erythrocytes of chronic hemodialysis patients, *J Am Acad Dermatol* 7:100-104, 1982.
50. Judd LE, Henderson DW, Hill DC: Naproxen-induced pseudoporphyria, *Arch Dermatol* 122:451-454, 1986.
51. Suarez SM, Cohen PR, et al: Bullous photosensitivity to naproxen: "pseudoporphyria," *Arthritis Rheum* 33.903-908, 1990.
52. Lang BA, Finlayson LA: Naproxen-induced pseudoporphyria in patients with juvenile rheumatoid arthritis, *J Pediatr* 124:639-642, 1994.
53. Allen R, Rogers M, et al: Naproxen induced pseudoporphyria in juvenile chronic arthritis, *J Rheumatol* 18:893-896, 1991.

54. Stenberg A: Pseudoporphyria and sunbeds, *Acta Derm Venereol* 70:354-356, 1990.

55. Poh-Fitzpatrick MB: Porphyria, pseudoporphyria, pseudopseudoporphyria, *Arch Dermatol* 122:403-404, 1986.

56. Brun A, Sandberg S: Mechanisms of photosensitivity in porphyric patients with special emphasis on erythropoietic protoporphyria, *J Photochem Photobiol B* 10:285-302, 1991.

57. Poh-Fitzpatrick MB: The "priming phenomenon" in the acute phototoxicity of erythropoietic protoporphyria, *J Am Acad Dermatol* 21:311, 1989.

58. Shehade SA, Chalmers RJ, et al: Predictable and unpredictable hazards of erythropoietic protoporphyria, *Clin Exp Dermatol* 16:185-187, 1991.

59. Mercurio MG, Prince G, et al: Terminal hepatic failure in erythropoietic protoporphyria, *J Am Acad Dermatol* 29:829-833, 1993.

60. Todd DJ, Nesbitt GS, et al: Erythropoietic protoporphyria. The problem of a suitable screening test, *Acta Derm Venereol* 70:347-350, 1990.

61. Mathews-Roth MM et al: Beta-carotene as a photoprotective agent in erythropoietic protoporphyria, *N Engl J Med* 282:1231-1234, 1970.

62. Mathews-Roth MM: Erythropoietic protoporphyria—diagnosis and treatment, *N Engl J Med* 297:98, 1977.

63. Ross JB, Moss MA: Relief of the photosensitivity of erythropoietic protoporphyria by pyridoxine, *J Am Acad Dermatol* 22:340-342, 1990.

64. Farr PM, Diffey BL, et al: Inhibition of photosensitivity in erythropoietic protoporphyria with terfenadine, *Br J Dermatol* 122:809-815, 1990.

65. Gordeuk VR et al: Iron therapy for hepatic dysfunction in erythropoietic protoporphyria, *Ann Intern Med* 105:27, 1986.

66. Kavli G, Volden G: Phytophotodermatitis, *Photodermatology* 1:65-75, 1984.

67. Benezra C, Ducombs G: Molecular aspects of allergic contact dermatitis to plants: recent progress in phytodermatochemistry, *Dermatosen* 35:4-11, 1987.

68. Berkley SF et al: Dermatitis in grocery workers associated with high natural concentrations of furanocoumarins in celery, *Ann Intern Med* 105:351-355, 1986.

69. Gross TP et al: An outbreak of phototoxic dermatitis due to limes, *Am J Epidemiol* 125:509-514, 1987.

70. White W: Club Med dermatitis, *N Engl J Med* 314:319-320, 1986.

71. Nigg HN, Nordby HE, et al: Phototoxic coumarins in limes, *Food Chem Toxicol* 31:331-335, 1993.

72. Watemberg N, Urkin Y, et al: Phytophotodermatitis due to figs, *Cutis* 48:151-152, 1991.

73. Ljunggren B, Bjellerup M: Systemic drug photosensitivity, *Photodermatology* 3:26-35, 1986.

74. Epstein JH, Wintroub BU: Photosensitivity due to drugs, *Drugs* 30:42-57, 1985.

75. Addo HA, Ferguson J, Frain-Bell W: Thiazide-induced photosensitivity: a study of 33 subjects, *Br J Dermatol* 116:749-760, 1987.

76. Robinson HN, Morison WL, Hood AF: Thiazide diuretic therapy and chronic photosensitivity, *Arch Dermatol* 121:522-524, 1985.

77. Holzle E, Neumann N, et al: Photopatch testing: the 5-year experience of the German, Austrian, and Swiss Photopatch Test Group, *J Am Acad Dermatol* 25:59-68, 1991.

78. Thune C: Contact and photocontact allergy to sunscreens, *Photodermatology* 1:5-9, 1984.

79. Naughton GK, Reggiardo D, Bystryn J-C: Correlation between vitiligo antibodies and extent of depigmentation in vitiligo, *J Am Acad Dermatol* 15:978-981, 1986.

80. Bhatia PS, Mohan L, et al: Genetic nature of vitiligo, *J Dermatol Sci* 4:180-184, 1992.

81. Lerner AB, Norland JJ: Vitiligo: the loss of pigment in skin, hair, and eyes, *J Dermatol* 5:1, 1978.

82. Porter JR, Beuf AH, et al: The effect of vitiligo on sexual relationships, *J Am Acad Dermatol* 22:221-222, 1990.

83. Halder RM et al: Childhood vitiligo, *J Am Acad Dermatol* 16:948-954, 1987.

84. Esterly NB (ed): Management of vitiligo in children, *Pediatr Dermatol*, 3:498-510, 1986.

85. Bolognia JL, Pawelek JM: Biology of hypopigmentation, *J Am Acad Dermatol* 19:217-255, 1988.

86. Cunliffe WJ, Hall R, Newell DJ, et al: Vitiligo, thyroid disease and autoimmunity, *Br J Dermatol* 80:135-139, 1968.

87. Korkij W et al: Tissue-specific autoantibodies and autoimmune disorders in vitiligo and alopecia areata: a retrospective study, *J Cutan Pathol* 11:522-530, 1984.

88. Cui J, Shen LY, et al: Role of hair follicles in the repigmentation of vitiligo, *J Invest Dermatol* 97:410-416, 1991.

89. Wildfang IL, Jacobsen FK, et al: PUVA treatment of vitiligo: a retrospective study of 59 patients, *Acta Derm Venereol* 72:305-306, 1992.

90. Mosher DB, Fitzpatrick TB, Ortonne JP: Abnormalities of pigmentation. In: *Dermatology in general medicine*, New York, 1987, McGraw-Hill.

91. Lassus A et al: Treatment of vitiligo with oral methoxsalen and UVA, *Photodermatology* 1:170-173, 1984.

92. Falabella R, Escobar C, Borrero I: Transplantation of in vitro-cultured epidermis bearing melanocytes for repigmenting vitiligo, *J Am Acad Dermatol* 21:257-264, 1989.

93. Pasricha JS, Khaitan BK: Oral mini-pulse therapy with betamethasone in vitiligo patients having extensive or fast-spreading disease, *Int J Dermatol* 32:753-757, 1993.

94. Falabella R et al: On the pathogenesis of idiopathic guttate hypomelanosis, *J Am Acad Dermatol* 16:35-44, 1987.

95. Greaves MW, Birkett D, Johnson C: Nevus anemicus: a unique catecholamine-dependent nevus, *Arch Dermatol* 102:172-176, 1970.

96. Mountcastle EA, Diestelmeier MR, Lupton GP: Nevus anemicus, *J Am Acad Dermatol* 14:628-632, 1986.

97. Hurwitz S, Braverman IM: White spots in tuberous sclerosis, *J Pediatr* 77:587-594, 1970.

98. Fitzpatrick TB et al: White leaf-shaped macules, earliest visible sign of tuberous sclerosis, *Arch Dermatol* 98:1-6, 1968.

99. Reid JD: Intestinal carcinoma in the Peutz-Jeghers syndrome, *JAMA* 229:833, 1974.

100. Papaioannon A, Critselis A: Malignant changes in the Peutz-Jeghers syndrome, *N Engl J Med* 289:694, 1973.

101. Rafal ES, Griffiths CE, et al: Topical tretinoin (retinoic acid) treatment for liver spots associated with photodamage, *N Engl J Med* 326:368-374, 1992.

102. Sanchez NP et al: Melasma: a clinical, light microscopic, ultrastructural, immunofluorescence study, *J Am Acad Dermatol* 4:698-710, 1981.

103. Pathak MA et al: Treatment of melasma with hydroquinone, *J Invest Dermatol* 76:324, 1981.

104. Kligman AM, Willis I: A new formula for depigmenting human skin, *Arch Dermatol* 111:40-48, 1975.

105. Griffiths CE, Finkel LJ, et al: Topical tretinoin (retinoic acid) improves melasma. A vehicle-controlled, clinical trial, *Br J Dermatol* 129:415-421, 1993.

106. Bell SD, MacDonald DM: The prevalence of café-au-lait patches in tuberous sclerosis, *Clin Exp Dermatol* 10:562-565, 1985.

107. Ashby M: Erythema ab igne in cancer patients, *J R Soc Med* 78:925-927, 1985.

108. Hurwitz RM, Tisserand ME: Erythema ab igne, *Arch Dermatol* 123:21-22, 1987.

CHAPTER TWENTY

Benign Skin Tumors

Seborrheic Keratoses

Seborrheic keratoses (SKs) and nevi are the most common benign cutaneous neoplasms. They are of unknown origin and have no malignant potential. One must be familiar with all of the characteristics and variants of these lesions to differentiate them from other lesions and to prevent unnecessary destructive procedures.[1] SKs can be easily and quickly removed and, if the procedure is correctly executed, heal with little or no scarring. Most people develop at least one SK at some point in their lives. The number varies from less than 20 in most individuals to numerous lesions on the face or trunk. Patients refer to them as warts, but SKs do not contain human papilloma viruses.[2]

Surface characteristics. The surface of SKs are either smooth with tiny, round, embedded pearls or they are rough, dry, and cracked. They are sharply circumscribed and vary from 0.2 cm to more than 3 cm in diameter. They appear to be stuck to the skin surface and, in fact, occur totally within the epidermis. The surface characteristics vary with the age of the lesion and its location. Those on the extremities are often subtle, flat, or minimally raised and are slightly scaly with accentuated skin lines. Lesions on the face (Figures 20-2 and 20-3) and trunk (Figures 20-4 and 20-5) vary considerably in appearance, but the characteristics common to all lesions are the well-circumscribed border, the stuck-on appearance, and the variable tan-brown-black color. When the border is irregular and notched, the SK resembles a malignant melanoma.

Smooth or rough surfaced. The surface characteristics show considerable variation (Figure 20-1; see the box on pp. 628 to 629). Smooth-surfaced, dome-shaped tumors have white or black pearls of keratin, 1 mm in diameter, embedded in the surface. These *horn pearls* are easily seen with a hand lens. The presence of horn cysts on the surface helps to confirm the diagnosis of an SK. Horn cysts are also found on the surface of some dermal nevi (see bottom photo in the box on p. 629). The rough-surfaced SKs are the most common. They are oval-to-round, flattened domes with a granular or irregular surface that crumbles when picked.

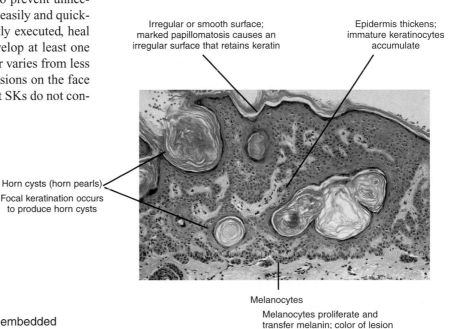

Irregular or smooth surface; marked papillomatosis causes an irregular surface that retains keratin

Epidermis thickens; immature keratinocytes accumulate

Horn cysts (horn pearls)
Focal keratination occurs to produce horn cysts

Melanocytes
Melanocytes proliferate and transfer melanin; color of lesion deepens from brown to black

Figure 20-1
Seborrheic keratosis. Cross-section shows embedded horn cysts.

SEBORRHEIC KERATOSES

ROUGH-SURFACE LESIONS

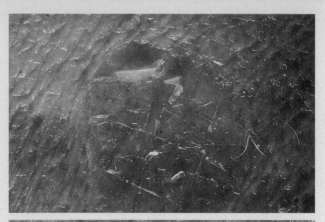

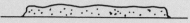

Flat; some scale; light color

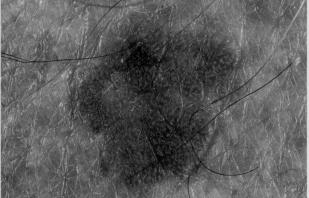

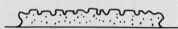

Height increase; lesion appears "stuck on" to surface; color darkens

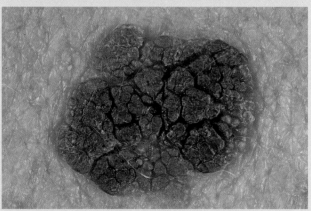

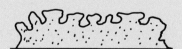

Deep surface cracks appear; keratin can be peeled off; brown or black

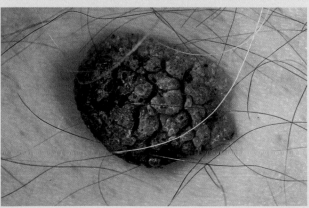

SEBORRHEIC KERATOSES

SMOOTH-SURFACE LESIONS

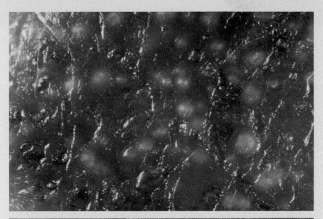

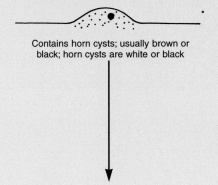

Contains horn cysts; usually brown or black; horn cysts are white or black

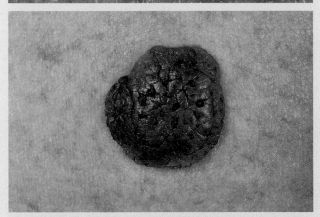

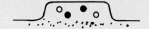

Height increases; horn cysts become more numerous

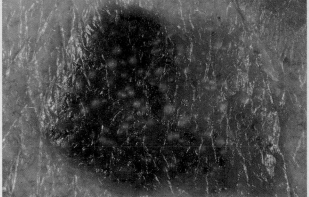

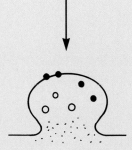

Smooth, dome shaped papule; horn cysts project from surface

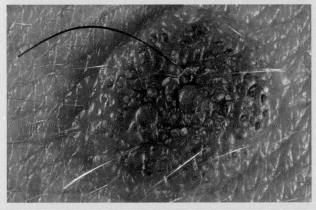

SEBORRHEIC KERATOSIS

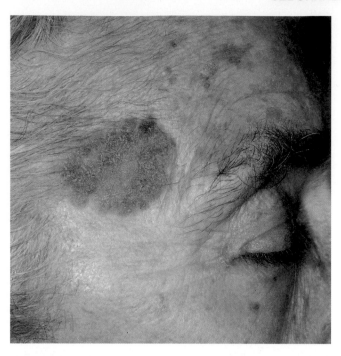

Figure 20-2
Very large lesions may form along the hairline and temple. Flat lesions are usually brown.

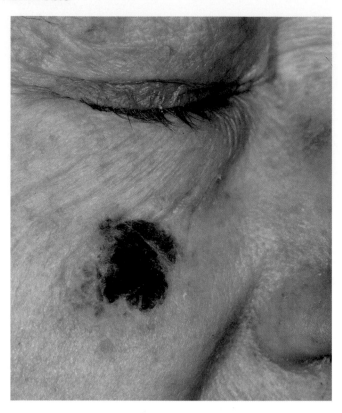

Figure 20-3
Thicker lesions may become dark brown or black.

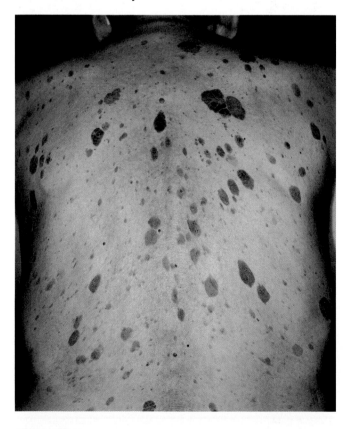

Figure 20-4
Lesions are very common on the back; an individual may have numerous lesions on the sun-exposed back and none on the buttocks.

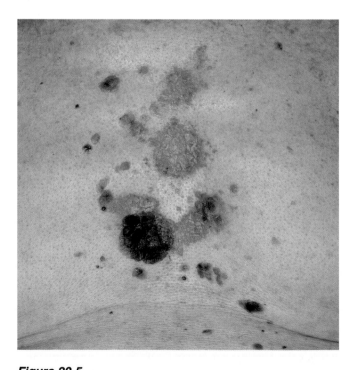

Figure 20-5
The presternal area is a common site. Different levels of keratin retention are depicted here.

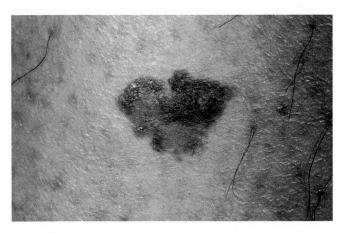

Figure 20-6
Seborrheic keratosis mimicking malignant melanoma. There is variation in pigmentation, and the border is irregular and notched, but the surface is regular with dense keratin.

Seborrheic keratosis vs. malignant melanoma. Many patients present with dark, irregular, sometimes irritated SKs and worry that they are melanomas. SKs can show many of the features of a malignant melanoma, including an irregular border and variable pigmentation (Figures 20-6 to 20-8). The key differential diagnostic features are the surface characteristics. Melanomas have a smooth surface that varies in elevation and in color density and shade. SKs preserve a uniform appearance over their entire surface. Examination with a hand lens is very helpful. Many SKs occur in sun-exposed areas.

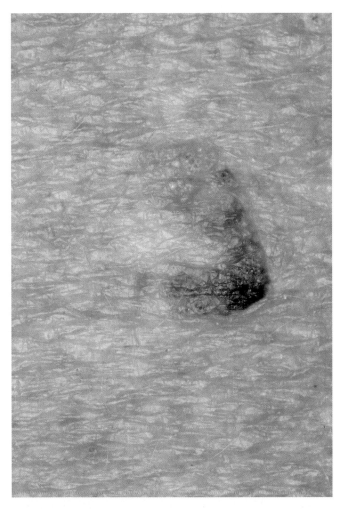

Figure 20-7
Seborrheic keratosis (mimicking melanoma). This flat lesion has many features of a superficial spreading melanoma. The colors are variable and the white area looks like an area of tumor regression.

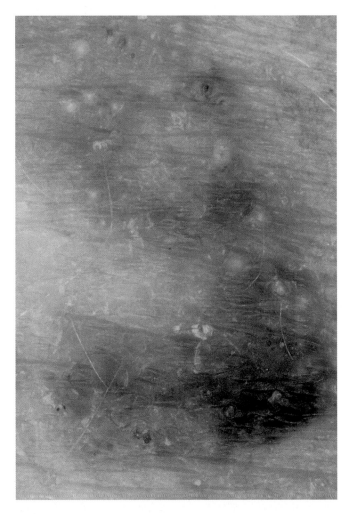

Figure 20-8
Seborrheic keratoses (mimicking melanoma). A magnified view shows several horn cysts that are typically found in seborrheic keratoses and rarely present in melanoma.

Irritated seborrheic keratosis. Although generally asymptomatic, SKs can be a source of itching, especially in the elderly, who have a tendency to unconsciously manipulate these protruding growths. Irritation can be aggravated by chafing from clothing or from maceration in intertriginous areas, such as under the breasts. When inflamed, SKs become slightly swollen and develop an irregular, red flare in the surrounding skin. Itching and erythema can then appear spontaneously in other SKs that have not been manipulated (Figure 20-9) and in areas without SKs. A halo of eczema can appear around SKs; the inflamed border is red, scaly, and may represent a localized form of nummular (coin-shaped) dermatitis.[3,4] The only treatment is to apply topical steroids or to remove all inflamed lesions. With continued inflammation, the SK loses most of its normal characteristics and becomes a bright red, oozing mass with a friable surface that itches intensely (Figure 20-10) and resembles an advanced melanoma or a pyogenic granuloma.

Sign of Leser-Trelat (eruptive SK as a sign of internal malignancy). The sudden appearance of or sudden increase in the number and size of SKs on noninflamed skin has been reported to be a sign of internal malignancy (see Figure 26-2).[5,6] There is a controversy over the sign's validity. Several papers refute its existence,[4,7,8] but single case reports are regularly published. The average age at the time of onset is 61 years. The most common type of associated malignancy is adenocarcinoma (69%); the stomach (40%) is most often involved. In one study, 70% of patients had paraneoplastic disorders such as acanthosis nigricans, acquired ichthyosis, and lanugo hair.[6] Paraneoplastic disorders are cutaneous changes that signal the presence of various internal malignancies. Most patients have metastatic disease when the keratoses appear.[9] The SKs often parallel the course of the malignancy, decreasing in number and size following surgical or chemotherapeutic intervention and returning with recurrence of the cancer, but this is not always the case.

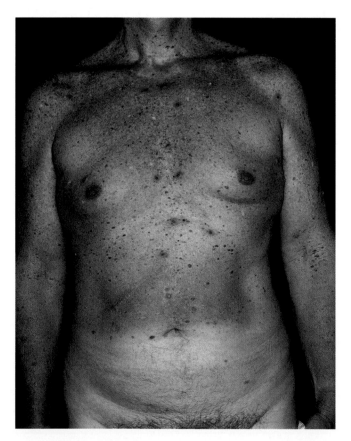

Figure 20-9
Irritated seborrheic keratosis. A single lesion developed an erythematous border; subsequently, inflammation occurred at the base of many other seborrheic keratoses.

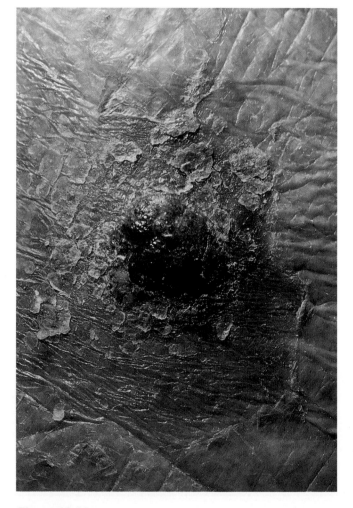

Figure 20-10
Irritated seborrheic keratosis. A bright red, oozing mass simulating a pyogenic granuloma or a melanoma.

Patients with numerous SKs need not be evaluated for malignancy unless the lesions erupt abruptly. Erythrodermatous or eczematous skin[10] can promote the appearance of keratoses, and association with internal malignancy would not be considered in this instance.[11] Keratoses that appear during the course of widespread inflammatory skin disease may regress after the inflammation resolves.[12]

Treatment. Lesions are removed for cosmetic purposes or to eliminate a source of irritation. Since these growths appear entirely within the epidermis, scalpel excision is unnecessary. They are easily removed with cryosurgery or curettage. Lesions to be curetted are first anesthetized with xylocaine introduced with a needle. With multiple strokes, a small curette is smoothly drawn through the lesion (see Chapter Twenty-seven). SKs on the face or on other areas with inappreciable underlying support can be softened before curettage with the electric needle. Monsel's solution controls bleeding, and the site remains exposed to heal. Some lesions are tenaciously fixed to the skin and resist curettage; others are on sites that are difficult to curette, such as the eyelid. These can be dissected with curved, blunt-tipped scissors. Cryosurgery is effective for thin SKs.

Stucco Keratoses

Stucco keratoses, sometimes referred to as *barnacles*, are common, nearly inconspicuous, papular, warty lesions[13] occurring on the lower legs (Figure 20-11), especially around the Achilles tendon area, the dorsum of the foot, and the forearms of the elderly (Figure 20-12). The 1- to 10-mm, round, very dry, stuck-on lesions are considered by most patients to be simply manifestations of dry skin. The dry surface scale is easily picked intact from the skin without bleeding, but it recurs shortly thereafter. The lesions can be removed with curettage or cryosurgery.

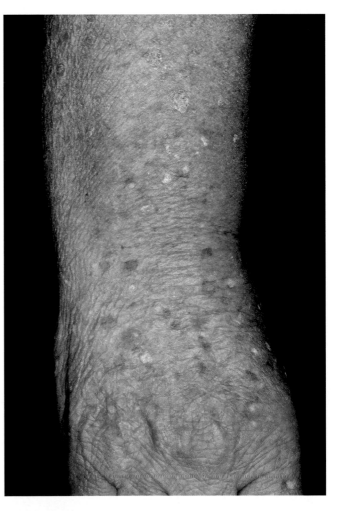

Figure 20-12
Stucco keratosis. Many white, dry, scaly lesions on the forearm and back of the hand. Note also the several brown seborrheic keratoses on the back of the hand.

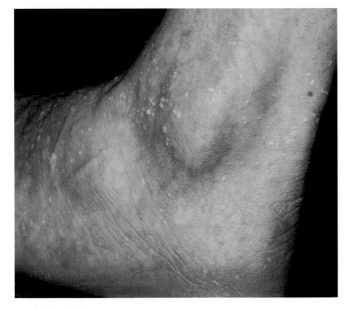

Figure 20-11
Stucco keratosis. Multiple small, scaling lesions in a typical location.

Dermatosis Papulosa Nigra

Young and middle-aged blacks may develop multiple brown-black, 2- to 3-mm, smooth, dome-shaped papules on the face[14] (Figure 20-13). They probably represent a type of SK. Patients who desire removal should be informed that white, hypopigmented scarring may result. The patient's response should be determined by curetting or freezing one or two lesions and permitting them to heal completely.

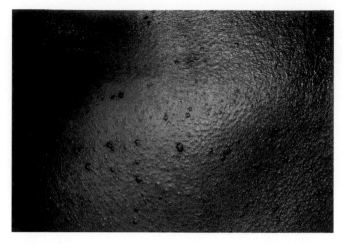

Figure 20-13
Dermatosis papulosa nigra. Seborrheic keratosis–like lesions that appear on the face in blacks.

Cutaneous Horn

Cutaneous horn refers to a hard, conical projection composed of keratin and resembling an animal horn. It occurs on the face, ears, and hands (Figure 20-14) and may become very long. Warts, SKs, actinic keratosis, and squamous cell carcinoma may all retain keratin and produce horns. Treatment is performed by cryosurgery, local scissors excision, or surgical excision.

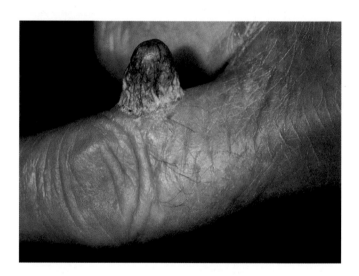

Figure 20-14
Cutaneous horn. A hard conical projection composed of keratin.

Acquired (Digital) Fibrokeratoma

This is a rare lesion of unknown origin that resembles a cutaneous horn or supernumerary digit and occurs around the finger and toes.[15] A short projection of collagen and capillaries is covered by epithelium and, occasionally, by retained keratin[16] (Figure 20-15). It may be surrounded by a collarette of elevated skin. A supernumerary digit, fibroma, and pyogenic granuloma are included in the differential diagnosis. Treatment is performed by simple scissor dissection, and bleeding is terminated by Monsel's solution or electrocautery.

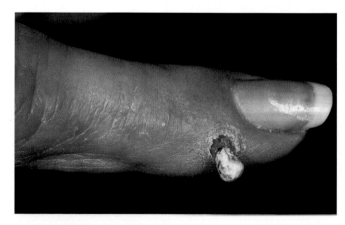

Figure 20-15
Acquired digital fibrokeratoma. A rare lesion resembling a cutaneous horn, the base of which is surrounded by a collarette of elevated skin.

Skin Tags (Achrochordon) and Polyps

Skin tags. Skin tags are common tumors found in approximately 25% of males and females. The most frequent affected area is the axilla (48%), followed by the neck (35%) and inguinal region. The majority of carriers (71%) have no more than three skin tags per location. They can begin in the second decade, with a steady increase in frequency up to the fifth decade; above this age there is no further growth.[17] They begin as a tiny, brown or skin-colored, oval excrescence attached by a short, broad-to-narrow stalk (Figures 20-16 and 20-17). With time, the tumor can increase to 1 cm as the stalk becomes long and narrow (Figure 20-18). Patients complain that when they wear clothing or jewelry, these tumors are annoying. The stalks are easily removed by scissor excision or with a light touch of the electrocautery. Local anesthesia is usually not necessary.

Polyps. Skin polyps have a long, narrow stalk and a broad tip (Figure 20-19). Sometimes they become twisted and compromise the blood supply. Lesions then turn dark brown or black. This sudden change is alarming to patients (Figure 20-20). Polypoid growths may be skin tags, nevi, or melanomas. Polyps occur on the eyelids (Figure 20-17), groin, axilla, or any skin surface except the palms and soles.

Skin tags and colonic polyps. A series of articles claimed that there is an association between skin tags and adenomatous polyps.[18-21] Other studies have claimed that there is no association.[22-24] A prospective study of 98 completely asymptomatic individuals with skin tags was completed. Among these, 33 had polyps: 28 were adenomatous polyps, three were of hyperplastic histology, and two were adenocarcinoma.[25] The authors recommend performing occult blood testing and flexible sigmoidoscopy for an asymptomatic individual whose only marker for colon pathology is the presence of skin tags, reserving colonoscopy for those with a positive family history. A study of 150 consecutive patients who underwent colonoscopy concluded that skin tags as markers of colon neoplasms are insufficient to warrant endoscopic examination.

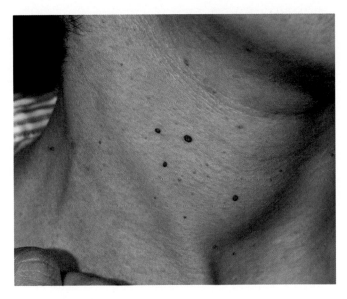

Figure 20-16
Skin tags. Multiple round, black, oval excrescences attached by a short broad-to-narrow stalk.

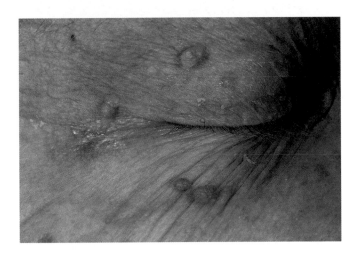

Figure 20-17
Skin tags and polyps are frequently present on the lids.

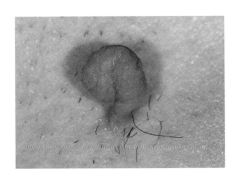

Figure 20-18
Skin tag. A polypoid mass on a long, narrow stalk. Some nevi have an identical appearance.

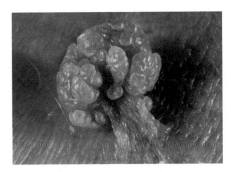

Figure 20-19
Polyp. Polyps contain a long stalk and a broad tip. A biopsy showed this lesion to be a dermal nevus.

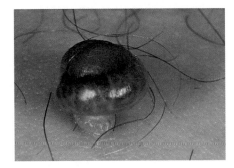

Figure 20-20
Infarcted polyp. Torsion on the stalk can compromise the blood supply. Lesions turn blue-black in hours to days.

Dermatofibroma

Dermatofibromas are common, benign, asymptomatic-to-slightly itchy lesions occurring more frequently in females. They vary in number from 1 to 10 and can be found anywhere on the extremities and trunk, but they are most likely to occur on the anterior surface of the lower legs. Dermatofibromas may not be tumors; rather, they may represent a fibrous reaction to trauma, a viral infection, or an insect bite. They appear as 3- to 10-mm, slightly raised, pink-brown, sometimes scaly, hard growths that retract beneath the skin surface during attempts to compress and elevate them with the thumb and index finger (Figures 20-21 to 20-24). Multiple dermatofibromas (i.e., more than 15) are very rare but have been reported with systemic lupus erythematosus[26] with and without immunosuppressive therapy.

Treatment. Some patients object to the color of the lesion and therefore request excision. These lesions are most commonly found on the lower legs, where elliptic excisions closed with sutures may result in wide, unsightly scars. An alternative is to shave the brown surface with a #15 surgical blade and allow the wound to granulate and reepithelialize. The healed area remains hard because a portion of the fibrous tissue has remained. The brown color may reappear in some lesions. Conservative cryosurgery may also eliminate the color and part of the tumor.[27]

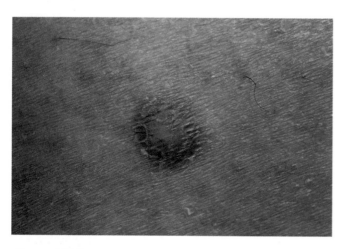

Figure 20-21
Dermatofibroma. A typical lesion on the lower leg that is slightly elevated, round, and hyperpigmented, with a scaling surface.

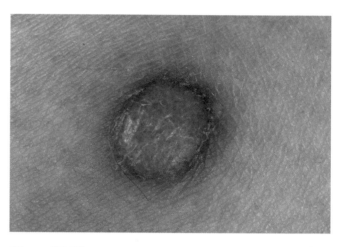

Figure 20-22
Dermatofibroma. Early lesions have a well defined border with an irregular red surface. Brown pigmentation may occur at the periphery after months or years. Pigmentation may extend onto the lesion but almost never reaches the center. Patients often suspect melanoma at this stage.

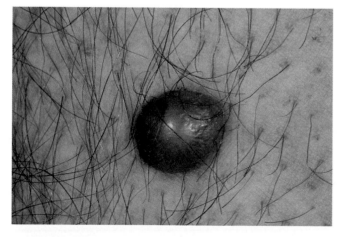

Figure 20-23
Dermatofibroma. This lesion is elevated, very firm, and lacks the typical brown hyperpigmentation of most dermatofibromas.

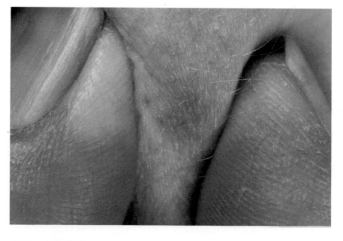

Figure 20-24
Dermatofibroma (retraction sign). Dermatofibromas retract beneath the skin during attempts to compress and elevate them.

Hypertrophic Scars and Keloids

Injury or surgery in a predisposed individual can result in an abnormally large scar. A hypertrophic scar is inappropriately large but remains confined to the wound site and in time regresses; a keloid extends beyond the margins of injury (Figures 20-25, 20-26, and 20-27) and usually is constant and stable without any tendency to subside. There are histologic differences between hypertrophic scars and keloids. Keloids are often symptomatic, and complaints arise because of tenderness, pain, and hyperesthesia, particularly in the early stages of development. Keloids are most common on the shoulders and chest, but they may occur on any skin surface. Blacks are more susceptible and sometimes are victims of facial keloids. Some patients with cystic acne of the back and chest form numerous keloidal scars.

Treatment. There is no routinely effective therapy for all keloids, but a variety of treatment methods exists,[28-30] including intralesional steroid injection, surgical correction, cryotherapy, compression therapy, and irradiation.

Intralesional steroid injections. Fresh, small, and narrow lesions are treated with intralesional injections of corticosteroids at least once every 4 weeks. When the lesion shrinks to near the skin surface, the frequency and concentration of injections should be decreased to avoid overcompensation and telangiectasia. Inducing atrophy with an intralesional injection of triamcinolone acetonide (Kenalog) 10 to 40 mg/ml is adequate for most small lesions; a 27- or 30-gauge needle is used. To distribute the suspension evenly, the triamcinolone should be injected while continuously advancing the needle. Particles of steroid that have not been properly dispersed remain visible as white flecks in the scar tissue. The pressure of the injection should be firm until the lesion blanches. Light cryosurgery prior to the injection facilitates the process. Nitrogen is applied briefly for 2 to 4 seconds until the skin frosts. The keloid is injected 10 to 15 minutes later. This allows better dispersal of the steroid and minimizes deposition into surrounding normal tissue.[31] Early keloids have softer proliferating connective tissue and are more inclined to improve with intralesional injections than are older, inactive lesions.

Surgery and intralesional steroid injections. Surgical removal alone is associated with a 55% to 100% recurrence rate,[28] but better results are realized when intralesional steroids are used following surgery. A typical treatment program involves injecting triamcinolone acetonide 10 to 40 mg/ml into the wound edges after excision. Treatment of the healed site is repeated at 2- to 4-week intervals for 6 months.

Cryotherapy. In one study, cryotherapy with a hand-held liquid nitrogen spray unit resulted in complete flattening in 73% of keloids, most of which were less than 2 years old. At each treatment session, the entire lesion was treated with two or three freeze-thaw cycles. Lesions required 2 to 10 treatment sessions. A topical antibiotic cream and dressing were applied each day during the 1-month healing process. Side effects were limited to hypopigmentation and atrophy.[32]

Silastic gel sheeting. Chronic hypertrophic and keloid scars respond to silicone gel sheeting (e.g., Sil-K, Epi-Derm). These dressings can also prevent keloids from recurring after surgery. In a controlled analysis of fresh surgical incisions, silicone gel sheeting significantly inhibited the formation of hypertrophic scars. Sheeting is used for at least 12 hours daily for 2 months.[33] Beneficial effects are not related to pressure.[34,35]

Compression. Very wide scars or those that can be treated easily with pressure are subjected to compression therapy. Compression devices can be fabricated to treat any area, including the earlobe.

Radiation therapy with surgery. Different protocols are reported. Radiation is usually given within 24 hours after surgery to subdue the second-generation fibroblasts.[36-39] The response rate varies between 92% and 73%. Irradiation at a later time is not helpful.

Figure 20-25
Keloid. A mass of keloids arising in a suture line.

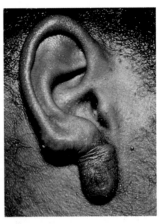

Figure 20-26
Keloid. Huge keloids may form on the ear lobes after any surgical procedure.

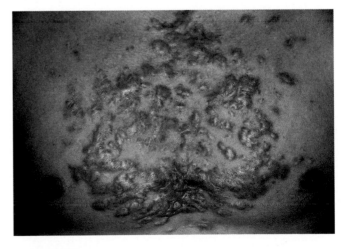

Figure 20-27
Keloid. Numerous confluent keloids arising from a patient with cystic acne.

Keratoacanthoma

Keratoacanthoma (KA) is a relatively common, benign, epithelial tumor, possibly of viral origin,[40] that was previously considered to be a variant of squamous cell carcinoma.[41] It is a disease of the elderly (mean age, 64 years) with an annual incidence rate of 104 per 100,000.[42] It is not associated with internal malignancy.

KA begins as a smooth, dome-shaped, red papule that resembles molluscum contagiosum. In a few weeks the tumor may rapidly expand to 1 or 2 cm and develop a central keratin-filled crater that is frequently filled with crust (Figures 20-28 to 20-31). The growth retains its smooth surface, unlike a squamous cell carcinoma. Untreated, growth stops in approximately 6 weeks, and the tumor remains unchanged for an indefinite period. In the majority of cases it then regresses slowly over 2 to 12 months and frequently heals with scarring. The limbs, particularly the hands and arms, are the most common site; the trunk is the second most common site, but KA may occur on any skin surface. On occasion, multiple KAs appear, or a single lesion extends over several centimeters. These rare variants resist treatment and are unlikely to undergo spontaneous remission.

Treatment. There is no advantage to waiting for spontaneous regression to occur, since most KAs ultimately heal with scarring. KAs are treated surgically or medically. KAs may recur.

Surgery. Electrodesiccation and curettage[43] or blunt dissection[44] (see Chapter Twenty-seven) are efficient and effective for smaller lesions. Excision is effective for large tumors.

5-fluorouracil (topical). In one study, topical 5% fluorouracil cream (Efudex) applied three times a day in the rapid growth phase cured most lesions in 1 to 6 weeks.[45] If possible the central crust should be removed to enhance penetration of medicine. The cream is applied to the lesion and its immediate vicinity, preferably under tape occlusion. Pretreatment with 6% salicylic acid gel (Keralyt) or 20% urea cream (Carmol 20) for lesions on the forearms, hands, or legs enhances penetration of the 5-fluorouracil cream. Lesions on the face and lips may clear in 1 or 2 weeks, but as long as 6 weeks is required for lesions in other areas to respond.

5-fluorouracil (intralesional injection). Excellent results have been reported with 5-fluorouracil injections.[46,47] The tumor is injected with the undiluted solution of 5-fluorouracil 50 mg/ml (available as fluorouracil injection in 500 mg/10 ml ampules). The usual amount is 0.1 to 2 ml, depending on the size of the tumor, injected tangentially into the slopes and then under the tumor. Extravasation of 5-fluorouracil from the central crater causes the amounts absorbed to be less than the amounts injected. Injections are given at 1- to 4-week intervals, depending on the response to treatment. Repeat injections are postponed if a lesion is undergoing necrosis. Patients should be evaluated at weekly intervals. This technique is especially useful for large KAs in difficult locations.[48] Intralesional 5-fluorouracil may be ineffective for older KAs that are not rapidly proliferating. Reported time for healing varies from 1 to 9 weeks.

Podophyllum resin. Podophyllum (20%) in compound tincture of benzoin or alcohol may cure KAs. Remove the central crust and apply podophyllum with a cotton swab. Repeat the treatment every 2 weeks until the lesion disappears.

Methotrexate (intralesional injection). Nine patients with solitary KAs were treated with intralesional methotrexate (MTX).[49] MTX is injected superficially and directly into the lesion at a dose of 12.5 mg/ml. Injections are given at 2-week intervals. Necrosis of the lesion usually begins 5 to 8 days after injection. If complete response is not obtained after two injections, excision is indicated. The mean time to clearing was 3 weeks, with a range of 2 to 4 weeks. All lesions cleared completely, none recurred. Total cumulative dose ranged from 5 to 50 mg. The average amount of MTX per injection was 15 mg. No side effects were noted, and cosmetic results were very good.

Interferon alfa-2a (intralesional injection). Six large KAs were treated with intralesional interferon alfa-2a. Regression occurred in five cases in 3 to 7 weeks, with excellent cosmetic results. The main side effect was pain during injection.[50]

Radiotherapy. KAs that are recurrent after surgical excision or those in which resection would result in cosmetic deformity may benefit from radiotherapy (total doses from 3500 cGy in 15 fractions to 5600 cGy in 28 fractions).[51-53]

Isotretinoin. Patients with multiple KAs have been treated with oral isotretinoin[54] and oral etretinate.[55] Patients with a solitary KA may respond to a short course of isotretinoin. Nine of twelve patients achieved complete resolution of the KA. The average duration of isotretinoin therapy was 6.3 weeks (range, 10 days to 12 weeks) in dosages of 0.5 to 1.0 mg/kg/day.[56]

KERATOACANTHOMA

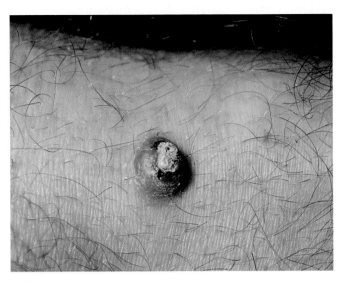

Figure 20-28
An early dome-shaped tumor with a central keratin plug.

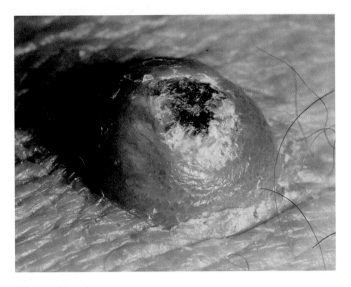

Figure 20-29
Classic presentation of a fully developed tumor.
A round, smooth, dome-shaped mass with a central keratin-filled crater.

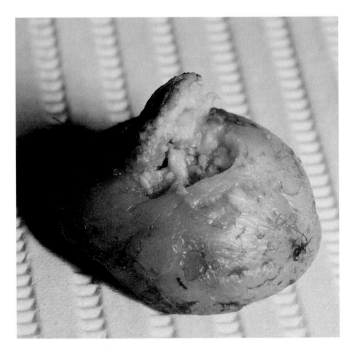

Figure 20-30
The central crust has been elevated from this blunt dissected lesion.

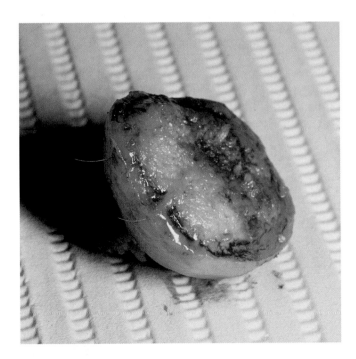

Figure 20-31
The smooth, lobular, intact undersurface of a blunt dissected lesion.

Epidermal Nevus

The term *epidermal nevus* is commonly used to describe a group of cutaneous hamartomas linked by common clinical and histologic features. Linear epidermal nevus or nevus unius lateris (a linear, unilateral, wartlike nevus), nevus verrucosus (a localized, wartlike nevus), and ichthyosis hystrix (an irregular, bilateral, truncal nevus) are some of the names given to variants of epidermal nevus. The term *nevus* means a congenital defect of the skin characterized by the localized excess of one or more types of cells. Histologically the cells are identical to or closely resemble normal cells. *Epidermal nevus* should be used as a general term to designate an excess of one type of epidermally derived cells (e.g., squamous cell or sebocyte). However, the term is commonly reserved for congenital growths in which the predominant cell is the keratinocyte. These nevi arise from the pluripotential germinative cells in the basal layer of the embryonic epidermis. These cells give rise to keratinocytes and skin appendages (hair follicles, sweat glands).

Clinical characteristics. These well-circumscribed growths are present at birth or appear in infancy or childhood. They are round, oval, or oblong; elevated; flat-topped; yellow-tan to dark brown; and have a uniformly warty or velvety surface with sharp borders (Figures 20-32 and 20-33). They appear more commonly on the head and neck; 13% of patients have widespread lesions. Blaschko described a system of lines on the skin that linear nevi follow.[57] These lines represent a developmental growth pattern of the skin (Figure 20-34). Epidermal nevi may spread beyond their original distribution; further progression is unlikely after late adolescence. Nevi present at birth and those on the head are less likely to spread. In spite of their unusual appearance and occasional itching, they are generally inconsequential. Occasionally the growths are very large and disfiguring. Patients with epidermal nevi are at significant risk of having other anomalies in other organ systems.[58] Abnormalities are more likely in patients with widespread nevi. The most common systems involved are skeletal, neurologic, and ocular.

Figure 20-32
Epidermal nevus. A congenital lesion, which is often linear, and has a dark brown, warty, or velvety surface.

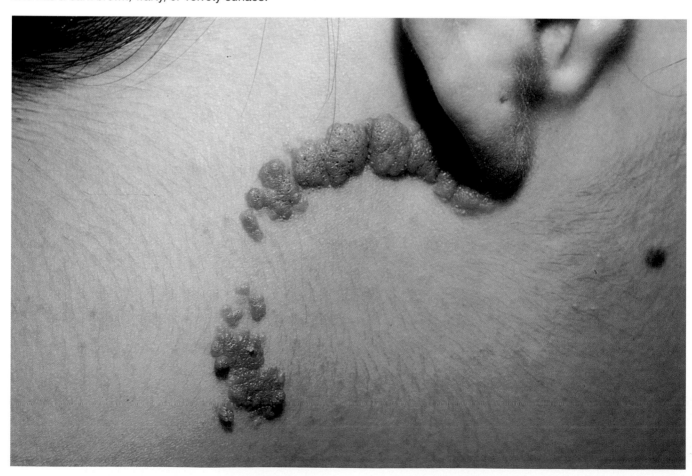

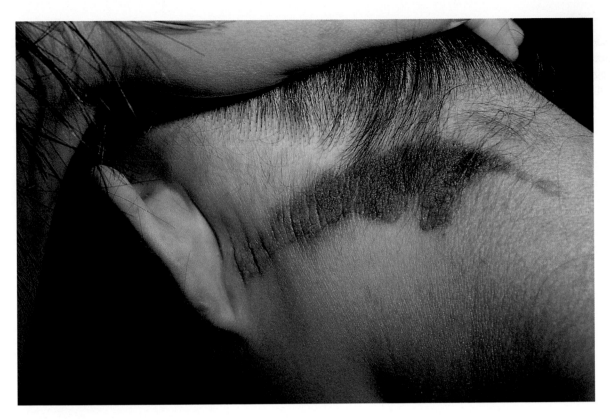

Figure 20-33
Epidermal nevus. A flat, broad lesion that follows Blaschko's lines.

Genetic counseling. The very rare epidermal nevus syndrome consists of extensive epidermal nevi associated with skeletal, ocular, and central nervous system disorders.[59-62] Small lesions are sporadic. Patients do not have a family history of epidermal nevi. Most cases of epidermal nevus syndrome occur sporadically, but there is some suspicion that an autosomal dominant transmission may be present. Inform patients that genetic transmission is possible with large epidermal nevi, but that the data are inadequate to make an accurate determination.

The cause of epidermal nevus syndrome is unknown. Possible explanations are faulty migration and development of embryonic tissue or a developmental error in separation of the ectoderm from the neural tube. Treatment may be attempted with cryosurgery[63] or dermabrasion, but the growths may recur; plastic surgery excision produces the most predictable results.

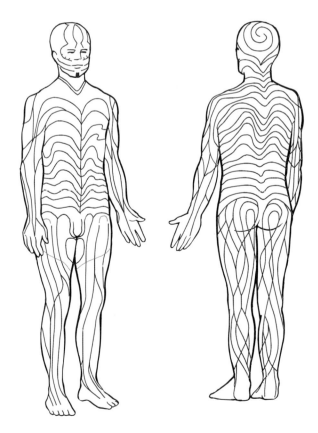

Figure 20-34
Blaschko's lines.

Nevus Sebaceous

Nevus sebaceous is a distinctive growth most commonly found on the scalp (Figure 20-35), followed by the forehead and retroauricular region.[64,65] Involvement of the neck and trunk is exceptional. A nevus of epithelial and nonepithelial skin components, nevus sebaceous sustains age-related modifications in morphology. The nevus occurs singly and is asymptomatic. Two thirds of cases are present at birth; the others develop in infancy or early childhood. Males and females are equally affected. The very rare nevus sebaceous of Jadassohn syndrome consists of the triad of a linear sebaceous nevus, convulsions, and mental retardation. A variety of congenital malformations of the ocular, skeletal, vascular, and urogenital systems have been described in association with nevus sebaceous.[66,67]

Lesions are oval to linear, varying from 0.5 × 1 cm to 7 × 9 cm. The three-stage evolution of the nevoid condition (newborn, puberty, adult) parallels the natural histologic differentiation of normal sebaceous glands. The lesions in infants and younger children are smooth to gently papillat-ed, waxy, hairless thickenings. During puberty there is a massive development of sebaceous glands with epidermal hyperplasia within the lesions (Figure 20-36). At this stage they change clinically by developing a verrucous mulberry irregularity of the surface covered with numerous, closely aggregated, yellow-to-dark brown papules. When this transformation becomes noticeable, parents become worried and seek medical attention.

In approximately 20% of the cases, a third phase of evolution involves the development of secondary neoplasia in the mass of the nevus. A number of benign and malignant "nevoid tumors" may occur, the most common of which is the basal cell epithelioma. The malignant degenerations are relatively low grade; only a few cases of metastasis are reported.[68] Most lesions are sporadic, but cases of inherited nevus sebaceous have been reported.[69]

Treatment. Plastic surgical excision is the treatment of choice. Attempts at local destruction with electrocautery or cryosurgery may lead to recurrence.

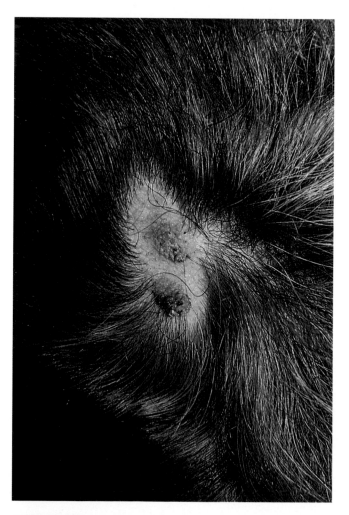

Figure 20-35
Nevus sebaceous. A typical lesion on the scalp of a postpubertal male.

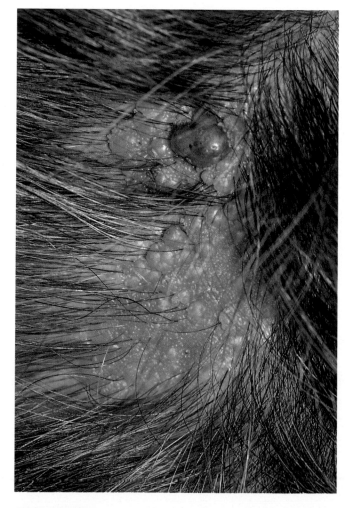

Figure 20-36
Nevus sebaceous. A white globular surface indicative of sebaceous gland hyperplasia that occurs after puberty.

Chondrodermatitis Nodularis Chronica Helicis

This uncommon disorder occurs on the lateral surface of the helix and occasionally on the antihelix, a site rarely occupied by other growths. One (occasionally more) firm, 2- to 6-mm nodule appears spontaneously. It subsequently develops a central scale that lacks the keratinous plug of a keratoacanthoma (Figure 20-37). Removal of the scale reveals a small central erosion. Unlike the full distended margins of a squamous or basal cell carcinoma, the sides of this mass slope down from the center. The small mass is dull red to white and is painful. During the active stage, the base may become red and swollen; pain is constant. Pressure of any type becomes intolerable. As the mass attains its maximum size, it becomes lighter in color but remains symptomatic. The cause of this disorder is unknown, but chronic sun exposure may be a factor. Men over the age of 40 account for 90% of the patients.

Histologically the dermis shows collagen degeneration with granulation tissue, edema, and inflammation.

Treatment

Surgical management. Several techniques have been described. A narrow ellipse is drawn around the nodule, and it is then excised. Vigorously curet the base to remove the soft necrotic cartilage. The end point is reached when the curette is repelled by firm, elastic cartilage. The skin edges are undermined and closed in one layer with 5-0 sutures.[70] Another technique involves making a linear incision over the involved site, dissecting the skin back over the perichondrium, slicing the cartilage horizontally, and then suturing the skin edges.[71] Another method is to excise the nodule with scissors, curet the base, and gently electrodesiccate to eradicate all foci of inflammation. Bleeding is controlled with Monsel's solution. The wound granulates and heals with a defect (see Chapter Twenty-seven). Recurrences are common if all sites of inflammation have not been eradicated. Patients who refuse surgery may be treated with intralesional triamcinolone acetonide (10 to 40 mg/ml) once every 2 to 3 weeks until clear. There is some degree of persistent pain throughout treatment. Surgical intervention is required when this method fails. The CO_2 laser may be used to vaporize the cutaneous nodules and involved cartilage.[72]

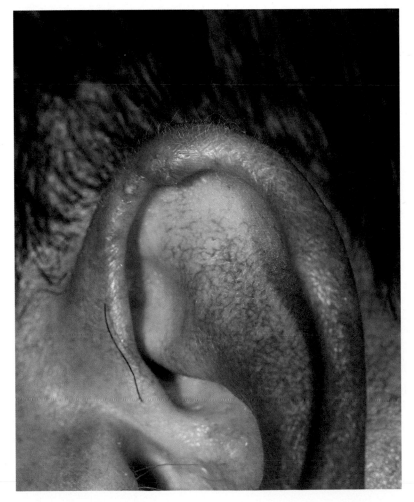

Figure 20-37
Chondrodermatitis nodularis chronica helicis. A painful firm nodule with scaling in the center, occupying a commonly observed site on the lateral surface of the helix.

EPIDERMAL CYSTS

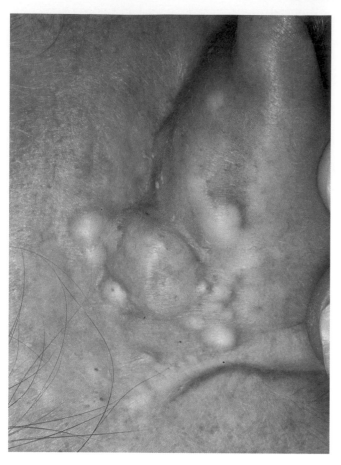

Figure 20-38
The posterior auricular fold is a common place to find one or many epidermal cysts.

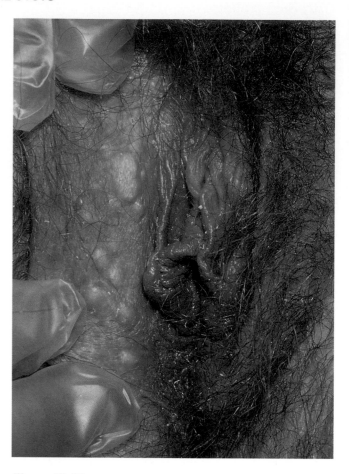

Figure 20-39
Epidermal cysts occur in areas where sebaceous glands are large and numerous, such as on the labia.

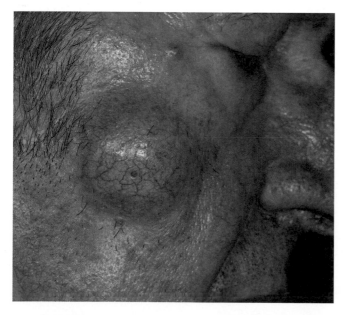

Figure 20-40
The keratin-filled orifice (blackhead) communicating with the surface is not usually as prominent as illustrated here.

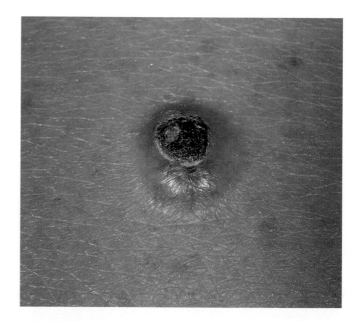

Figure 20-41
Giant comedone. A superficial epidermal cyst commonly found on the back.

Epidermal Cyst

The common epidermal or sebaceous cyst occurs primarily on the face, back or base of the ears, chest, and back or on almost any skin surface (Figures 20-38 and 20-39). Children who are brought to the physician with epidermal cysts or patients with epidermal cysts in unusual areas such as the legs should be suspected of having Gardner's syndrome (see Chapter Twenty-six). The cyst wall is lined with stratified squamous epithelium, which produces keratin. The round, protruding, smooth-surfaced mass is movable and varies in size from a few millimeters to several centimeters. The cyst communicates with the surface through a narrow channel, and the surface opening appears as a small, round, sometimes imperceptible, keratin-filled orifice (i.e., a blackhead) (Figure 20-40). Epidermal cysts may originate from comedones; such lesions are superficial, with a large, black, keratinous plug on the surface. They are referred to as *giant comedones* and are commonly found on the back (Figure 20-41). Cysts may remain small for years or may progressively develop. Spontaneous rupture of the wall results in discharge of the soft, yellow keratin into the dermis. A tremendous inflammatory response ensues, and the sterile purulent material either points and drains through the surface or is slowly reabsorbed. If the wall is destroyed during the inflammatory process, the cyst will not recur.

Treatment. Like boils, fluctuant, inflamed cysts must be drained and evacuated. Small cysts are removed by making a linear incision with a #11 blade over the surface and, if possible, through the orifice. The soft keratinous material is expressed through the incision, and the remaining material is dislodged with a #1 curette. After total evacuation, firm pressure generally forces the cyst wall through the incision, where it can be grasped with the forceps and separated from connective tissue with scissors (this technique is illustrated in Chapter Twenty-seven). To absorb blood and serum, the wound is compressed for several minutes. If necessary, the wound edges may be supported with Steri-strips. Excision is the procedure of choice for large cysts. Cysts may also be excised and sutured or dissected (Figure 20-42).

Pilar Cyst (Wen)

Pilar cysts occur in the scalp and, like epidermal cysts, are freely movable. They are frequently multiple and may become large masses (Figure 20-43). The epithelial-lined wall produces keratin of a different quality than that of the epidermal cyst, but rupture of the wall creates the same intense reaction. The cyst contains concentric layers of dry keratin, which over time may become macerated, soft, and cheesy.

Treatment. Except for the largest structures, pilar cysts can be satisfactorily removed through a linear excision, avoiding suture closure. The following procedure should be used (this procedure is illustrated in Chapter Twenty-seven):

1. Cut the hair over the cyst and make a 3- to 10-mm linear incision.
2. With firm pressure, express the contents and dislodge remaining fragments with a #1 curette.
3. Firmly press the curette against the inner wall of the cyst and move it back and forth to dislodge the cyst from its surroundings. The wall is firm and has a smooth, glazed surface that is easily separated from connective tissue.
4. Hold the cut edge of the cyst with forceps and, while applying continuous pressure to the sides of the wound, separate the cyst from the supporting connective tissue with a blunt dissecting instrument such as a Schamberg or blunt-tipped scissors. The cyst will literally pop out of the wound.
5. To control bleeding, apply firm pressure for 5 minutes. Dressings or bandages are unnecessary.

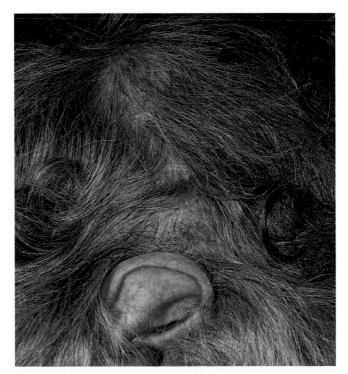

Figure 20-43
Pilar cyst. A freely movable cystic mass found on the scalp. Communication with the surface is rarely observed.

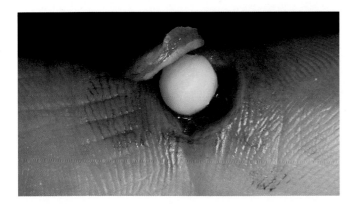

Figure 20-42
Epidermal cyst. The lesion has been dissected intact.

Senile Sebaceous Hyperplasia

Senile sebaceous hyperplasia consists of small tumors composed of enlarged sebaceous glands. They begin as pale yellow, slightly elevated papules; with time they become yellow, dome-shaped, and umbilicated. Senile sebaceous hyperplasia with telangiectasia may be mistaken for a basal cell carcinoma (Figures 20-44 and 20-45). However, close examination of the surface with a hand lens shows a haphazard distribution of vessels on the surface of basal cell carcinoma, whereas the vessels in sebaceous hyperplasia occur only in the valleys between the small yellow lobules. The lesions occur after age 30 in 25% of the population and gradually become more numerous. There is no relationship between the skin type and the occurrence of these lesions. They are commonly found on the forehead, cheeks (Figure 20-46), lower lid, and nose. The etiology remains unclear; chronic solar exposure is not a likely cause.[73]

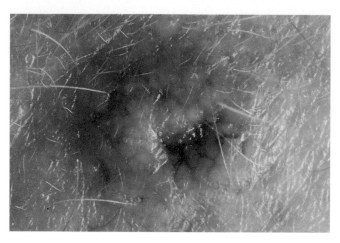

Figure 20-44
Sebaceous hyperplasia. A magnified lesion shows well-defined yellow lobules. Small blood vessels occur between the lobules. Compare this with the position of the blood vessels in a basal cell epithelioma.

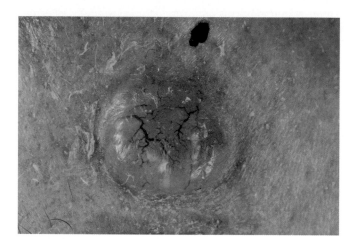

Figure 20-45
Basal cell carcinoma. The blood vessels are haphazardly distributed over the entire surface.

Figure 20-46
Senile sebaceous hyperplasia (cheek). Note central umbilication.

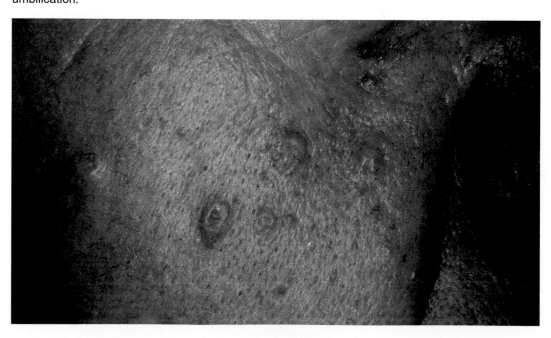

Treatment. Treatment consists of removal of the elevated portion of the papule. A pitted scar results if the entire structure is removed with a curette. The superficial portion of the lesion may be removed by shave excision or destroyed with conservative electrosurgery. Bichloracetic acid can be used for treatment. A tiny amount of acid is carefully applied to the surface with a wooden applicator stick. A stinging sensation occurs and lasts for 24 hours. Polysporin ointment is applied twice a day for 1 week. The treated area forms a crust, heals with residual erythema, and fades over time.[74] Patients with numerous lesions have been reported. Oral isotretinoin (0.5 to 1.0 mg/kg/day) is dramatically effective for these patients. All lesions clear within 2 weeks but recur within 3 weeks after the medication is stopped.[75] It has been speculated that longer treatment (more than 12 weeks) may result in perifollicular fibrosis in the region formerly occupied by the sebaceous gland and may offer a long-term remission. Optimum treatment and dosage schedules have not been established. Long-term isotretinoin therapy may be associated with many side effects.

Syringoma

Syringomas are sweat duct tumors composed of small, firm, flesh-colored dermal papules that occur on the lower lids (Figure 20-47) and, less commonly, on the forehead, chest, and abdomen. Lesions may develop at any age, but they initially appear most frequently during the third and fourth decades; they then slowly become more numerous. The tumors have no malignant potential. They may be removed for cosmetic purposes by electrodesiccation and curettage[76] or excised by gently elevating the small mass with forceps or the curved bevel of a 25-gauge needle and cut out with curved scissors or shaved with a #11 scalpel blade. The oval wound is left to heal by secondary intention.[77,78]

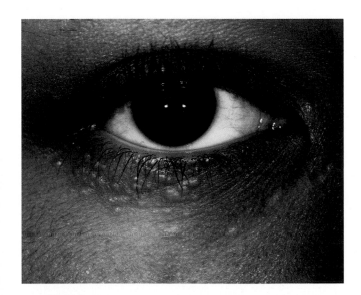

Figure 20-47
Syringoma on the lower lid of a young woman.

REFERENCES

1. Stern RE, Boudreaux C, Arndt KA: Diagnostic accuracy and appropriateness of care for seborrheic keratoses. A pilot study of an approach to quality assurance for cutaneous surgery, *JAMA* 265:74-77, 1991.
2. Zhu WY, Leonardi C, et al: Detection of human papillomavirus DNA in seborrheic keratosis by polymerase chain reaction, *J Dermatol Sci* 4:166-171, 1992.
3. Rosen R, Paver K, et al: Halo eczema surrounding seborrhoeic keratoses: an example of perilesional nummular dermatitis, *Australas J Dermatol* 31:73-76, 1990.
4. Tegner E, Bjornberg A, et al: Halo dermatitis around tumours, *Acta Derm Venereol* 70:31-34, 1990.
5. Venencie PY, Perry HO: Sign of Leser-Trelat: report of two cases and review of the literature, *J Am Acad Dermatol* 10:83, 1984.
6. Holdiness MR: The sign of Leser-Trelat: a review, *Int J Dermatol* 25:564, 1986.
7. Grob JJ, Rava MC, et al: The relation between seborrheic keratoses and malignant solid tumours. A case-control study, *Acta Derm Venereol* 71:166-169, 1991.
8. Lindelof B, Sigurgeirsson B, et al: Seborrheic keratoses and cancer, *J Am Acad Dermatol* 26:947-950, 1992.
9. Czarnecki DB et al: The sign of Leser-Trelat, *Australas J Dermatol* 24:93-99, 1983.
10. Horiuchi Y: Multiple seborrheic verrucae following eczema—a case report, *J Dermatol* 16:505-507, 1989.
11. Brown FC: Sign of Leser-Trelat, *Arch Dermatol* 110:129, 1974.
12. Berman A, Winkelmann RK: Seborrheic keratoses: appearance in course of exfoliative erythroderma and regression associated with histologic mononuclear cell inflammation, *Arch Dermatol* 118:615-618, 1982.
13. Shall L, Marks R: Stucco keratoses. A clinico-pathological study, *Acta Derm Venereol* 71:258-261, 1991.
14. Graham R: What is dermatosis papularis nigra? *Practitioner* 233:635, 1989.
15. Spitalny AD, Lavery LA: Acquired fibrokeratoma of the heel, *J Foot Surg* 31:509-511, 1992.
16. Kint A, Baran R, De Keyser H: Acquired (digital) fibrokeratoma, *J Am Acad Dermatol* 12:816-821, 1985.
17. Banik R, Lubach D: Skin tags: localization and frequencies according to sex and age, *Dermatologica* 174:180-183, 1987.
18. Klein I et al: Colonic polyps in patients with acromegaly, *Ann Intern Med* 97:27-30, 1982.
19. Leavitt J et al: Skin tags: a cutaneous marker for colonic polyps, *Ann Intern Med* 98:928-930, 1983.
20. Chobanian SJ et al: Skin tags as a marker for adenomatous polyps of the colon, *Ann Intern Med* 103:892-893, 1985.
21. Beitler M et al: Association between acrochordons and colonic polyps, *J Am Acad Dermatol* 14:1042-1044, 1986.
22. Dalton AD, Coghill SB: No association between skin tags and colorectal adenomas, *Lancet* 3:1322-1333, 1985.
23. Lubach D, Banik R: Skin tags and colonic polyps, *J Am Acad Dermatol* 16:402, 1987.
24. Luk GD, the Colon Neoplastic Work Group: Colonic polyps and acrochordons (skin tags) do not correlate in familial colonic polyposis kindreds, *Ann Intern Med* 104:209-210, 1986.
25. Chobanian SJ et al: Skin tags as a screening marker for colonic neoplasia, *Gastrointest Endosc* 32:162, 1986.
26. Lu I, Cohen RR, Grossman ME: Multiple dermatofibromas in women with HIV infection and systemic lupus erythematosus, *J Am Acad Dermatol* 32: 901-903, 1995.
27. Lanigan SW, Robinson TWE: Cryotherapy for dermatofibromas, *Clin Exp Dermatol* 12:121-123, 1987.
28. Lawrence WT: In search of the optimal treatment of keloids: report of a series and a review of the literature, *Ann Plast Surg* 27:164-178, 1991.
29. Nemeth AJ: Keloids and hypertrophic scars, *J Dermatol Surg Oncol* 19:738-746, 1993.

30. Datubo-Brown DD: Keloids: a review of the literature, *Br J Plast Surg* 43:70-77, 1990.

31. Ceilley RI, Babin RW: The combined use of cryosurgery and intralesional injections of suspensions of fluorinated adrenocorticosteroids for reducing keloids and hypertrophic scars, *J Dermatol Surg Oncol* 5:54-56, 1979.

32. Rusciani L, Rossi G, et al: Use of cryotherapy in the treatment of keloids, *J Dermatol Surg Oncol* 19:529-534, 1993.

33. Ahn ST, Monafo WW, Mustoe TA: Topical silicone gel for the prevention and treatment of hypertrophic scar, *Arch Surg* 126:499-504, 1991.

34. Quinn KJ et al: Non-pressure treatment of hypertrophic scars, *Burns* 12:102, 1985.

35. Sawada Y, Sone K: Hydration and occlusion treatment for hypertrophic scars and keloids, *Br J Plast Surg* 45:599-603, 1992.

36. Lo TC, Seckel BR, et al: Single-dose electron beam irradiation in treatment and prevention of keloids and hypertrophic scars, *Radiother Oncol* 19:267-272, 1990.

37. Kovalic JJ, Perez CA: Radiation therapy following keloidectomy: a 20-year experience, *Int J Radiat Oncol Biol Phys* 17:77-80, 1989.

38. Sallstrom KO, Larson O, et al: Treatment of keloids with surgical excision and postoperative X-ray radiation, *Scand J Plast Reconstr Surg Hand Surg* 23:211-215, 1989.

39. Darzi MA, Chowdri NA, et al: Evaluation of various methods of treating keloids and hypertrophic scars: a 10-year follow-up study, *Br J Plast Surg* 45:374-379, 1992.

40. Magee KL et al: Human papillomavirus associated with keratoacanthoma, *Arch Dermatol* 125:1587-1589, 1989.

41. Schwartz RA: Keratoacanthoma, *J Am Acad Dermatol* 30:1-19, 1994.

42. Chuang TY, Reizner GT, et al: Keratoacanthoma in Kauai, Hawaii. The first documented incidence in a defined population, *Arch Dermatol* 129:317-319, 1993.

43. Nedwich JA: Evaluation of curettage and electrodesiccation in treatment of keratoacanthoma, *Australas J Dermatol* 32:137-141, 1991.

44. Habif TP: Extirpation of keratoacanthomas by blunt dissection, *J Dermatol Surg Oncol* 6:652-654, 1980.

45. Goette DK: Treatment of keratoacanthoma with topical fluorouracil, *Arch Dermatol* 119:951-953, 1983.

46. Eubanks SW et al: Treatment of multiple keratoacanthomas with intralesional fluorouracil, *J Am Acad Dermatol* 7:126-129, 1982.

47. Goette DK, Odom RB: Successful treatment of keratoacanthoma with intralesional fluorouracil, *J Am Acad Dermatol* 2:212-216, 1980.

48. Parker CM, Hanke W: Large keratoacanthomas in difficult locations treated with intralesional 5-fluorouracil, *J Am Acad Dermatol* 14:770-777, 1986.

49. Melton JL, Nelson BR, et al: Treatment of keratoacanthomas with intralesional methotrexate, *J Am Acad Dermatol* 25:1017-1023, 1991.

50. Grob JJ, Suzini F, et al: Large keratoacanthomas treated with intralesional interferon alfa-2a, *J Am Acad Dermatol* 29:237-241, 1993.

51. Caccialanza M, Sopelana N: Radiation therapy of keratoacanthomas: results in 55 patients, *Int J Radiat Oncol Biol Phys* 16:475-477, 1989.

52. Farina AT et al: Radiotherapy for aggressive and destructive keratoacanthomas, *J Dermatol Surg Oncol* 3:177-178, 1977.

53. Donahue B, Cooper JS, et al: Treatment of aggressive keratoacanthomas by radiotherapy, *J Am Acad Dermatol* 23:489-493, 1990.

54. Levine N, Miller RC, Meyskens FL Jr: Oral isotretinoin therapy: use in a patient with multiple cutaneous squamous cell carcinomas and keratoacanthomas, *Arch Dermatol* 120:1215-1217, 1984.

55. Cristofolini M et al: The role of etretinate (Tigison; Tigason) in the management of keratoacanthoma, *J Am Acad Dermatol* 12:633-638, 1985.

56. Goldberg LH, Rosen T, et al: Treatment of solitary keratoacanthomas with oral isotretinoin, *J Am Acad Dermatol* 23:934-936, 1990.

57. Taieb A, Youbi AE, et al: Lichen striatus: a Blaschko linear acquired inflammatory skin eruption, *J Am Acad Dermatol* 25:637-642, 1991.

58. Rogers M, McCrossin I, Commens C: Epidermal nevi and the epidermal nevus syndrome. A review of 131 cases, *J Am Acad Dermatol* 20:476-488, 1989.

59. Solomon LM, Esterly NB: Epidermal and other congenital organoid nevi, *Curr Probl Pediatr* 6:1-55, 1975.

60. Goldberg LH, Collins SAB, Siegel DM: The epidermal nevus syndrome: case report and review, *Pediatr Dermatol* 4:27-33, 1987.

61. Happle R: How many epidermal nevus syndromes exist? A clinicogenetic classification, *J Am Acad Dermatol* 25:557-560, 1991.

62. Hodge JA, Ray MC, Flynn KJ: The epidermal nevus syndrome, *Int J Dermatol* 30:91-98, 1991.

63. Fox BJ, Lapins NA: Comparison of treatment modalities for epidermal nevus: a case report and review, *J Dermatol Surg Oncol* 11:879-885, 1983.

64. Alessi E, Sala F: Nevus sebaceous: a clinicopathologic study of its evolution, *Am J Dermatopathol* 8:27-31, 1986.

65. Weng CJ, Tsai YC, et al: Jadassohn's nevus sebaceous of the head and face, *Ann Plast Surg* 25:100-102, 1990.

66. Kang WH, Koh YJ, Chun SI: Nevus sebaceous syndrome associated with intracranial arteriovenous malformation, *Int J Dermatol* 26:382-384, 1987.

67. Diven DG et al: Nevus sebaceous associated with major ophthalmologic abnormalities, *Arch Dermatol* 123:383-386, 1987.

68. Tarkhan II, Domingo J: Metastasizing eccrine porocarcinoma developing in sebaceous nevus Jadassohn, *Arch Dermatol* 121:413-415, 1985.

69. Sahl W Jr.: Familial nevus sebaceous of Jadassohn: occurrence in three generations, *J Am Acad Dermatol* 22:853-854, 1990.

70. Coldiron BM: The surgical management of chondrodermatitis nodularis chronica helicis, *J Dermatol Surg Oncol* 17:902-904, 1991.

71. The treatment of chondrodermatitis nodularis with cartilage removal alone, *Arch Dermatol* 127:530-535, 1991.

72. Taylor MB: Chondrodermatitis nodularis chronica helicis. Successful treatment with the carbon dioxide laser, *J Dermatol Surg Oncol* 17:862-864, 1991.

73. Kumar P, Marks R: Sebaceous gland hyperplasia and senile comedones: a prevalence study in elderly hospitalized patients, *Br J Dermatol* 117:231-236, 1987.

74. Rosian R, Goslen JB, et al: The treatment of benign sebaceous hyperplasia with the topical application of bichloracetic acid, *J Dermatol Surg Oncol* 17:876-879, 1991.

75. Burton CS, Sawchuk WS: Premature sebaceous gland hyperplasia: successful treatment with isotretinoin, *J Am Acad Dermatol* 12:182-184, 1985.

76. Stevenson TR, Swanson NA: Syringoma: removal by electrodesiccation and curettage, *Ann Plast Surg* 15:151-154, 1985.

77. Moreno-Gonzalez J, Rios-Arizpe S: A modified technique for excision of syringomas, *J Dermatol Surg Oncol* 15:796-798, 1989.

78. Maloney ME: An easy method for removal of syringoma, *J Dermatol Surg Oncol* 8:973-975, 1982.

CHAPTER TWENTY-ONE

Premalignant and Malignant Nonmelanoma Skin Tumors

Basal Cell Carcinoma

Basal cell carcinoma (BCC) is the most common malignant cutaneous neoplasm found in humans.[1] The most common presenting complaint is a bleeding or scabbing sore that heals and recurs. Unfortunately, in the past there was a tendency to regard BCC as nonmalignant because the tumor rarely metastasizes. BCC advances by direct extension and destroys normal tissue. Left untreated or inadequately treated, the cancer can destroy the whole side of the face or penetrate subcutaneous tissue into the bone and brain.

Risk factors. Fair skin and the degree of sun exposure[2,3] are important risk factors. Outdoor workers and people who live in southern latitudes with higher levels of ambient ultraviolet B radiation are at greater risk. Men have a significantly higher incidence than women.[4] Tanning salons with equipment that emits ultraviolet A or B radiation are also damaging and increase the risk of BCC.

Location. Eighty-five percent of all BCCs appear on the head and neck region; 25% to 30% occur on the nose alone, the most common site. BCC is rarely found on the backs of the hands, although this site receives a significant amount of solar radiation. Tumors also occur in sites protected from the sun, such as the genitals and breasts. BCC in blacks is rare.

Incidence. The tumor may occur at any age, but the incidence of BCC increases markedly after age 40. The incidence in younger people is increasing, possibly as a result of increased sun exposure.[5]

PATHOPHYSIOLOGY

BCCs arise from basal keratinocytes of the epidermis and adnexal structures (hair follicles, eccrine sweat ducts).[6,7] Ultraviolet B (UVB) radiation (sunburn spectrum, 290 to 320 nm) is important for the induction of BCC. UVB radiation damages DNA and its repair system and alters the immune system. Depletion of ozone in the earth's atmosphere results in higher levels of UVB radiation at the earth's surface. Longer wavelength UVA radiation damages DNA and is also carcinogenic.

BCC grows by direct extension and appears to require the surrounding stroma to support its growth. This may explain why the cells are not capable of metastasizing through blood vessels or lymphatics. The course of BCC is unpredictable. BCC can remain small for years with little tendency to grow, particularly in the elderly, or it may grow rapidly or proceed by successive spurts of extension of tumor and partial regression.[8]

BCC occurs at the site of previous trauma, such as scars, thermal burns, and injury. BCC occurs years later at sites treated with ionizing radiation. The tumor appears 3 months to 7 or more years later at the site of a well-remembered injury.[9]

HISTOLOGY

The cells of a BCC resemble those of the basal layer of the epidermis. They are basophilic, have a large nucleus, and appear to form a basal layer by forming an orderly line around the periphery of tumor nests in the dermis, a feature referred to as *palisading* (Figure 21-1).

There are five major histologic patterns.[10]

1. Nodular (21%): a rounded mass of neoplastic cells with well-defined peripheral contours. Peripheral palisading is well developed (Figure 21-1).
2. Superficial (17%): contains buds of atypical basal cells extending from the basal layer of the epidermis (Figure 21-2).
3. Micronodular (15%): small, rounded nodules of tumor about the size of hair bulbs. Tumor islands are rounded, well demarcated, and demonstrate peripheral palisading.
4. Infiltrative (7%): tumor islands vary in size and show a jagged configuration.
5. Morpheaform (1%): numerous small, elongated islands containing a few cells that appear as strands or cords in a fibrous stroma.

A mixed pattern (two or more major histologic patterns) is present in 38.5% of cases.

CLINICAL TYPES

BCC occurs in many different clinical forms, which vary in appearance and malignant potential.

Nodular BCC. Nodular BCC is the most common form. The lesion begins as a pearly white or pink, dome-shaped papule resembling a molluscum contagiosum or dermal nevus (Figure 21-3). The mass extends peripherally. The lesion may remain flat. Traction on the surrounding skin accentuates the pearly border (Figure 21-4). Telangiectatic vessels become prominent and easily recognizable through the thin epidermis as the lesion enlarges (Figure 21-5). The growth pattern is irregular, forming an oval mass whereby the surface may become multilobular. The center frequently ulcerates and bleeds and subsequently accumulates crust and scale (Figures 21-6 to 21-8). Ulcerated BCCs were formerly designated *rodent ulcers*.

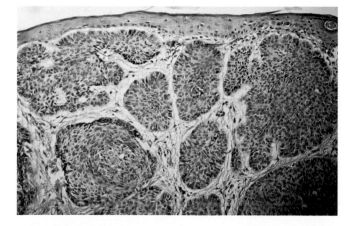

Figure 21-1
Nodular basal cell carcinoma. Nests of atypical basal cells are found in the dermis.

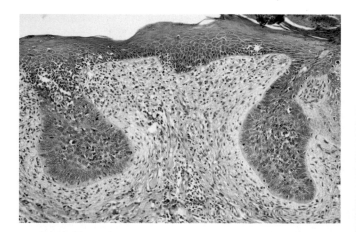

Figure 21-2
Superficial basal cell carcinoma. Buds of atypical basal cells extending from the basal layer of the epidermis.

NODULAR BASAL CELL CARCINOMA

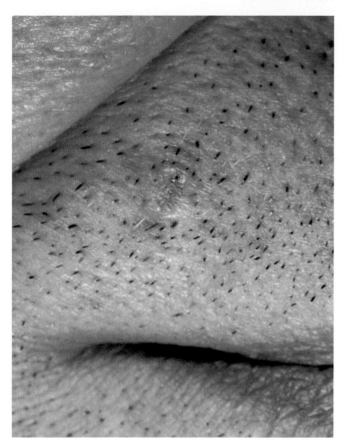

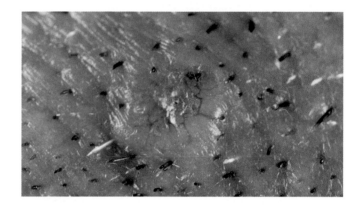

Figure 21-3
A, An early lesion detected only after careful physical examination of the face.

B, Magnification with a hand lens shows a pearly white papule with telangiectatic vessels on the surface.

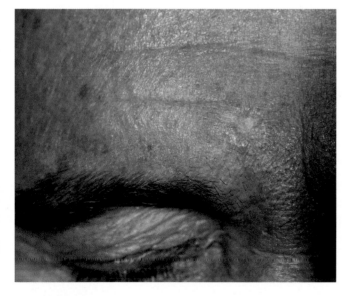

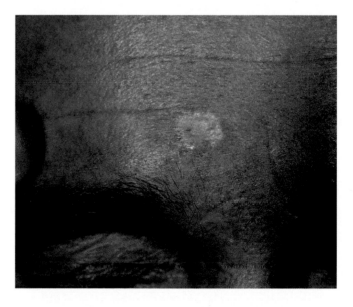

Figure 21-4
A, Early flat lesions are often subtle; telangiectasia and the pearly appearance are not prominent.

B, Traction on the surrounding skin accentuates the firm, pearly border, thus supporting the diagnosis of a nodular BCC.

NODULAR BASAL CELL CARCINOMA

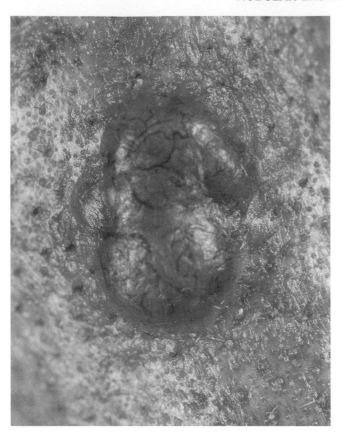

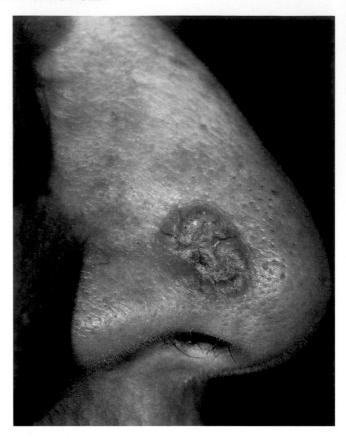

Figure 21-5
Classic presentation. A pink pearly white papule with prominent telangiectatic vessels.

Figure 21-6
The center is ulcerated and is covered with a crust.

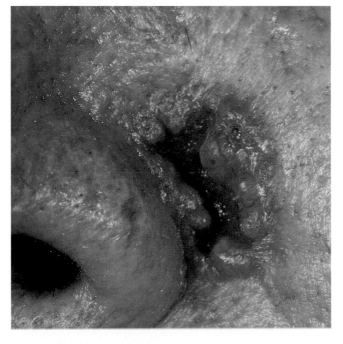

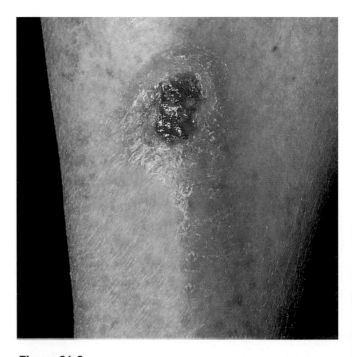

Figure 21-7
 A deep ulcer is surrounded by nodular tumor. In the past this type of lesion was referred to as a *rodent ulcer*.

Figure 21-8
Lesions can appear anywhere on the body. Suspect basal cell carcinoma when a small leg ulcer fails to heal after conventional therapy. Close examination reveals a nodular border.

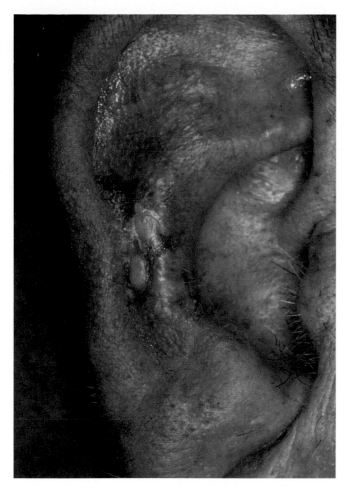

Figure 21-9
Nodular basal cell carcinoma. The lesion appeared to be inflammatory and was treated with topical steroids. After repeated cycles of healing and ulceration, a biopsy proved the diagnosis.

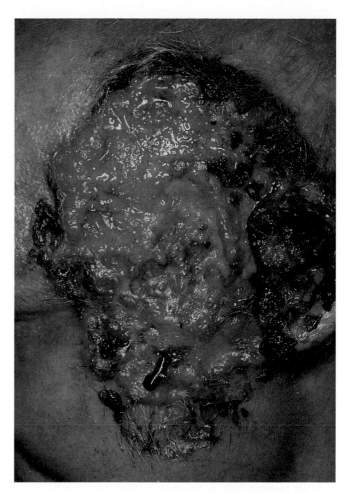

Figure 21-10
Basal cell carcinoma. Recurrence over a broad area after multiple surgical procedures.

Ulcerated areas heal with scarring, and patients often assume their conditions are improving. This cycle of growth, ulceration, and healing continues as the mass extends peripherally and deeper; masses of enormous size may be attained (Figures 21-9 and 21-10). BCCs may present as nonhealing leg ulcers. Biopsy specimens should be taken of leg ulcers that do not respond to treatment.[11] The tissue mass of a nodular BCC has a distinctive consistency that can be appreciated during curettage or biopsy. It has poor cohesive forces and collapses or breaks down when manipulated with a curette. This is an important diagnostic feature that supports the clinical impression during the biopsy procedure.

Pigmented BCC. BCCs may contain melanin that imparts a brown, black, or blue color through all or part of the lesion. Clinically, the lesion resembles a melanoma or pigmented seborrheic keratosis, but close inspection reveals the characteristically elevated, pearly white, translucent border, and the biopsy confirms the diagnosis (Figure 21-11). The histologic pattern most frequently associated with pigment is the nodular pattern.[12]

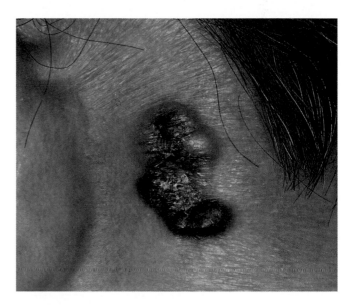

Figure 21-11
Pigmented basal cell carcinoma. A dark mass that resembles a melanoma. The tumor has all of the features of a nodular basal cell carcinoma.

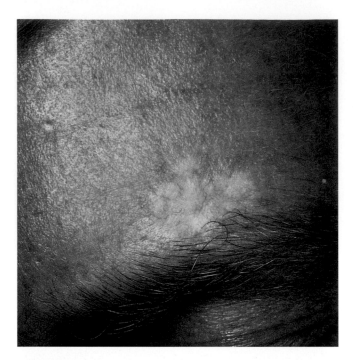

Figure 21-12
Sclerosing basal cell carcinoma. A firm, yellow mass; the surface has a waxy consistency. Borders are ill defined.

Cystic BCC. A variant of nodular BCC appears as a smooth, round, cystic mass. Cystic BCC behaves like nodular BCC.

Sclerosing or morpheaform BCC. Morpheaform BCC is an insidious tumor possessing innocuous surface characteristics that can mask its potential for deep, wide extension. The tumor is waxy, firm, flat-to-slightly raised, either pale white or yellowish, and resembles localized scleroderma, thus the designation *morpheaform* (Figure 21-12). The borders are indistinct and blend with normal skin. Lesions may become depressed and firm, resembling a scar. The tissue is rigid and difficult or impossible to remove with a curette. Localization of this tumor by inspection or biopsy is impossible. The average subclinical extension beyond clinically delineated borders was 7.2 mm in one study.[13] Treatment consists of wide excision or, preferably, Mohs' micrographic surgery.

Superficial BCC. The least aggressive BCC is the superficial BCC. This tumor occurs most frequently on the trunk and extremities, but may occur on the face. There may be one or more lesions. The tumor spreads peripherally, sometimes for several centimeters, and invades after considerable time. Slowly growing lesions may be present for years before patients seek help. The circumscribed, round-to-oval, red, scaling plaque resembles a plaque of eczema, psoriasis, extramammary Paget's disease, or Bowen's disease (Figure 21-13). However, careful inspection of the border reveals its thin, raised, pearly white nature (Figure 21-14). The characteristic features can also be appreciated by eliminating the redness with finger pressure.

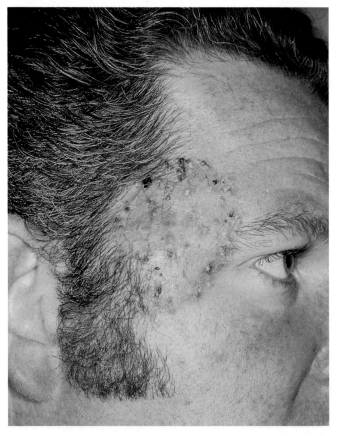

Figure 21-13
Superficial basal cell carcinoma. This large lesion occurred years after trauma. The inflammatory lesion was originally misdiagnosed as psoriasis and tinea.

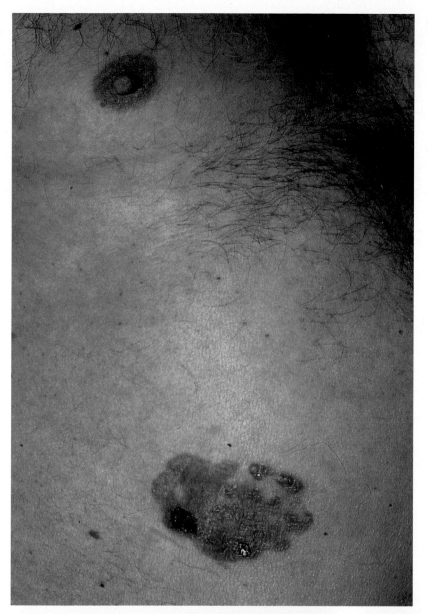

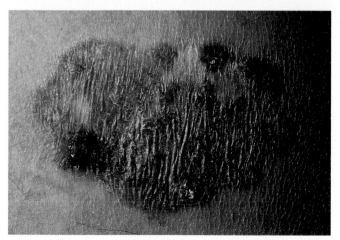

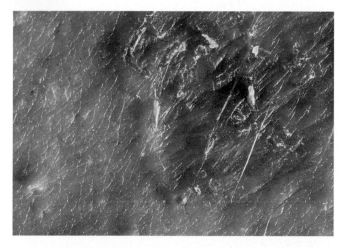

Figure 21-14
Superficial basal cell carcinoma.

A, A large lesion on the trunk that had been slowly growing for 10 years. A diagnosis of eczema had been made, and the lesion was treated with topical steroids.

B, Closer examination of the lesion reveals scale, crusts, and erosions. The border of one section appears elevated even at this magnification.

C, Examination of the border with a hand lens reveals its pearly white characteristics, thus supporting the diagnosis of BCC.

Nevoid BCC syndrome (Gorlin's syndrome). This rare disease is inherited as an autosomal dominant trait with high penetrance and variable expressivity. The gene is located on chromosome 9q22.3-q31.[14,15] It has the following major features: multiple BCCs appear at birth or in early childhood; numerous small pits on the palms and soles (Figure 21-15) (50% to 65%); epithelium-lined jaw cysts, which commonly cause symptoms (65% to 90%); ectopic calcification with lamellar calcification of falx cerebri (80%); and a variety of skeletal abnormalities, especially of the ribs, skull, and spine (70% to 75%).[16] A characteristic facies is present in approximately 70% of patients (Figure 21-16). Numerous associated anomalies may be present (see the box on p. 657).[17,18] There is great variation in the number and behavior of the nevoid BCC. Although many patients have no BCCs or just a few, more than 250 BCCs can be present.[19] Locally destructive tumors are not seen before puberty. Aggressive behavior can occur after puberty, and all patients must be followed closely. Most of the highly invasive tumors involve embryonic cleft areas of the face. Development of multiple BCCs is enhanced by exposure to light and x-ray irradiation,[20] but they also occur on unexposed surfaces.[21] Multiple bilateral jaw cysts are the presenting complaint in approximately 50% of patients; the syndrome was discovered by a dentist, R.J. Gorlin. The cysts appear during the first decade of life and displace the child's teeth, often in the premolar area.[22] They cause pain, drainage, and jaw swelling. The occurrence of multiple skeletal anomalies is highly suggestive and may be the earliest clue to the diagnosis of nevoid BCC syndrome in children. Complete or partial bridging of the sella turcica is present in 75% of patients. Splayed and bifurcated ribs occur in 40% of patients.

The initial evaluation of patients suspected of having BCC syndrome should include the following: (1) detailed family history; (2) dental consultations; and (3) x-rays of jaws, skull, chest, spinal column, and hands.

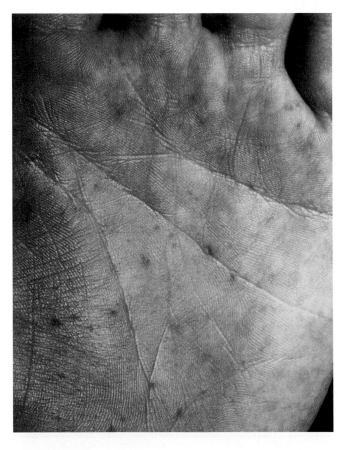

Figure 21-15
Nevoid BCC syndrome. Numerous small pits occur in the palms and soles.

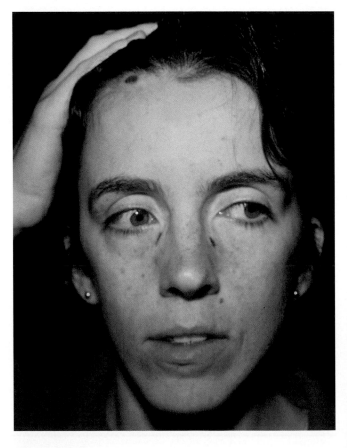

Figure 21-16
Nevoid basal cell carcinoma. Characteristic facies with hypertelorism, prominent suborbital ridges, and a broad nasal root.

NEVOID BASAL CELL CARCINOMA SYNDROME

SKIN

Multiple nevoid basal cell carcinomas
Pits—palms and soles (50% to 65%)
Milia, cysts (epithelial and sebaceous)

FACE AND MOUTH

Multiple jaw cysts (65% to 90%)
    Presenting complaint in 50%
Characteristic facies (70%)
    Mandibular prognathism
    Broadening of the nasal root (25%)
    Frontal/temporoparietal bossing
    Ocular hypertelorism

CENTRAL NERVOUS SYSTEM

Lamellar calcification of falx cerebri (80%)
Bridging of the sella turcica (75%)
Mental retardation
Electroencephalographic abnormalities

SKELETAL SYSTEM ANOMALIES (70% TO 75%)

Rib anomalies (55%): bifurcation and splaying (40%), synostotic, or partial agenesis or rudimentary cervical ribs
Vertebrae (65%): kyphoscoliosis (50%), spina bifida occulta (40%)
Shortened metacarpals (usually 4th, 5th, or both) (28%)
Bone cysts—phalanges and other bones (46%)
Many others

OTHERS

Lymphomesenteric cysts
Ovarian fibromas or cysts

Data from Skully RE, Mark EJ, McNeely BU: *N Engl J Med* 314:700-706, 1986; Gutierrez MM, Mora RG: *J Am Acad Dermatol* 15:1023-1030, 1986; and Gorlin RJ: *Medicine* 66:98-113, 1987.

MANAGEMENT AND RISK OF RECURRENCE

There are several factors to consider before choosing the best treatment modality.[23] The most important are clinical presentation, cell type, tumor size, and location.

Clinical type. Nodular and superficial BCCs are the least aggressive and can be completely removed by electrodesiccation and curettage or by simple surgical excision.

Histologic type. The micronodular, infiltrative, and morpheaform BCCs have a higher incidence of positive tumor margins (18.6%, 26.5%, and 33.3%, respectively) after excision and have the greatest recurrence rate.[10] Clinically, BCCs with these patterns have poorly defined borders and are not apparent during physical examination.[24] They subtly extend into surrounding tissue and are easily missed by blind treatment techniques such as surgical excision. An average of 7.2 mm of subclinical tumor extension was found in mopheaform BCCs in one study, compared with 2.1 mm of extension in well-circumscribed nodular lesions.[13] Routine pathologic examination of surgically excised BCCs may not detect a small nodule or strand of BCC on the other side of the excision margin. These tumors need more aggressive treatment with wide excision or microscopically controlled surgery.

Tumor size. In general, electrodesiccation and curettage afford excellent results for small (less than 2 cm) nodular BCCs located on the forehead and cheeks. Nodular BCCs on the forehead and cheek that are larger and have well-defined margins should be excised and closed; electrosurgery for large tumors may result in large, unsightly scars. The margins of sclerosing BCCs cannot be determined by inspection, and either excision or, preferably, Mohs' micrographic surgery should be performed. Superficial BCCs of any size can be adequately removed by electrosurgery.

Location. Tumors about the nose, eye, and ear require special consideration. BCCs of the medial canthus are particularly dangerous. The skin rests close to bone and cartilage, and tumor cells initially invade and proceed to migrate undetected along periosteum or perichondrium. Healing occurs over inadequately treated tumors, and deep invasion and lateral extension can remain undetected, resulting in a tumor of massive proportions. Extension to the eye and brain is possible.

Relative risk and follow-up. Patients treated for BCC should be followed periodically for 5 or more years.[25] Patients with one BCC often develop another. Of patients with one BCC, 36% to 50% develop a second BCC during the 5 years after treatment.[26,27] In another series, 41% of patients who had two or more previous skin cancers developed another BCC.[28]

Recurrent BCC

Clinical presentation. Inadequately treated BCC may recur. The tumor may be superficial in the scar tissue, on the border, or deep in the dermis or subcutaneous fat (Figure 21-17). The clinical presentation of recurrent BCC sometin.es differs from the original tumor. A tumor that infiltrates scar tissue produces a subtle change in color and consistency that is easily missed. Erosions that appear spontaneously at the border or in the scar are suspicious. The characteristic pearly white border is often absent, but biopsy of the erosion with the curette can reveal the soft, amorphous, gelatinous tissue of BCC extending deep and laterally well beyond the border of the erosion. Deep recurrences show a normal or a brownish erythematous surface and can be confused with epidermal cysts.[29]

Histologic picture, anatomic location, and size are factors in predicting recurrence.

HISTOLOGIC TYPE. Tumors of the morpheaform and basosquamous varieties have the greatest recurrence rate. BCCs that histologically show poor palisading or have a micronodular (islands of tumor) and/or infiltrating strand pattern without sclerotic stroma clinically have poorly defined borders and are not apparent during physical examination.[24] They subtly extend into surrounding tissue and are easily missed by blind treatment techniques such as surgical excision. An average of 7.2 mm of subclinical tumor extension was found in mopheaform BCCs in one study, compared with 2.1 mm of extension in well-circumscribed nodular lesions.[13] As mentioned earlier, routine pathologic examination of surgically excised BCCs may not detect a small nodule or strand of BCC on the other side of the excision margin. These tumors need more aggressive treatment with wide excision or microscopically controlled surgery.

LOCATION. Increasing diameter of the lesion and location of the lesion on various sites of the head, especially the nose and ear, are associated with an increased risk of recurrence, whereas location on the neck, trunk, limbs, or genitalia is associated with a decreased risk of recurrence with curettage-electrodesiccation, radiation therapy, and surgical excision.[30] BCCs on the nose or perinasal area may infiltrate along the perichondrium or penetrate into the embryonic fusion plane of the nasolabial fold, resulting in subclinical extension.

SIZE. The larger the tumor, the greater the chance of recurrence; increased subclinical extension is seen with larger tumors.

Figure 21-17
Recurrent basal cell carcinoma. A haphazard nodular tumor with telangiectasia surrounds and infiltrates under scar tissue.

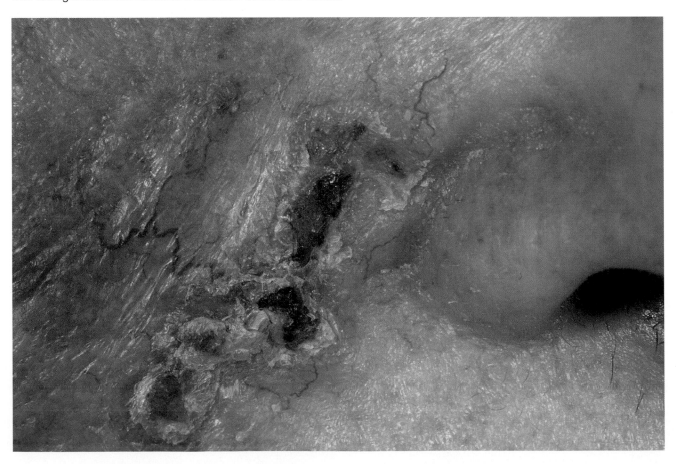

Treatment

The following section outlines various treatment modalities. Specific techniques are described in Chapter Twenty-seven.

Electrodesiccation and curettage. This treatment is most beneficial for nodular BCCs less than 6 mm in diameter, regardless of anatomic site; selected larger BCCs, depending on their anatomic site; and superficial BCCs.[31-36] It is not appropriate for morpheaform BCCs because margins cannot be clinically defined. Lesions on the nose and nasolabial folds may be treated if they are well defined and very small; otherwise these high-risk areas should be treated by Mohs' micrographic surgery. However, the treatment is particularly useful for ear lesions, where mobilization of skin for closure after excision is difficult.

Curettage requires firm dermis on all sides and below the tumor to enable the curette to distinguish between dermis and soft tumor. If the tumor encroaches on the fat, the curette cannot distinguish between fat and soft tumor, and an alternate procedure must be used. Curettage should be avoided for lesions on the back and shoulders, where the dermis is thick, unless the BCCs are superficial and small. Proper technique requires vigorous curettage, usually two to three times; therefore, lesions on the eyelid or lip area are treated by other methods. It is especially useful for lower extremity tumors, where tissue mobilization for excision may be difficult. Wounds created by electrosurgery ooze serum and accumulate crust during a 2- to 6-week healing period. The technique is explained in Chapter Twenty-seven.

Excision surgery. Excision surgery is preferred for large tumors with well-defined borders on the cheeks, forehead, trunk, and legs. The cosmetic result is good and healing time is less than that required for electrosurgery. Excision with primary closure is technically difficult on the ears and nose. The advantage of feeling the tumor with a curette is lost and adequate margins must be taken. A 98% cure rate was achieved in one study when BCCs less than 2 cm were excised with excisional margins of 4 mm around the tumor.[37] One large series revealed 5-year recurrence rates of BCCs excised from various anatomic sites: 0.7% on the neck, trunk, and extremities; 3.2% on the head if lesions were less than 6 mm in diameter; 5.2% on the head if lesions were 6 to 9 mm in diameter; and 9.0% on the head if lesions were 10 mm or more in diameter.[38]

INCOMPLETELY RESECTED BCC. Adequate excision, peripherally and in depth, is the key to surgical control, and the demonstration of tumor cells at the margins of excision is associated with recurrence rates of more than 30%. Data support the policy of immediate re-excision for all patients with incompletely excised basal cell carcinomas rather than a "wait-and-see" policy after incomplete excision.[39] Re-excision may not be necessary if the patient's life span is limited or if treatment of a possible recurrence would not be difficult.

Cryosurgery. Cryosurgery with liquid nitrogen delivered with a spray apparatus or a cryoprobe is appropriate for small-to-large BCCs of the nodular and superficial types with clearly definable margins (laterally and in depth).[40] It is not indicated for tumors deeper than 3 mm unless thermocouples are used to measure depth of freeze. A biopsy is performed as a separate operation before the cryosurgical procedure to determine cell type and extent of the tumor or just before the cryosurgery if there is no doubt about the diagnosis. Postoperative pain is moderate to severe. The appearance of a wound a few days after treatment is sometimes alarming to patients. Cryosurgery techniques are explained in Chapter Twenty-seven.

Mohs' micrographic surgery. Mohs' surgery is a microscopically controlled technique that may be used for all types and sizes of BCCs. The procedure is unnecessarily destructive for smaller lesions or for lesions with well-defined clinical margins, such as nodular or superficial multicentric BCCs.

Mohs' surgery is the treatment of choice for most sclerosing BCCs and other BCCs with poorly defined clinical margins; for tumors in areas of potentially high recurrence, such as the nose or eyelid; for very large primary tumors; and for large recurrent BCCs.[41] The technique is explained in Chapter Twenty-seven.

Radiation. Radiation is useful for elderly patients who cannot tolerate minor surgical procedures. For areas in which preservation of normal surrounding tissue is of prime consideration (e.g., around the eyelids and lips), radiation therapy may produce the best cosmetic result.

The overall 5-year recurrence rate is 7.4%. BCCs less than 10 mm in diameter on the head have a 5-year recurrence rate of 4.4%,[42] whereas those 10 mm or greater in diameter have a rate of 9.5%. The proportion of recurrence-free treatment sites with a good or excellent long-term cosmetic outcome after x-ray therapy (63%) is lower than that of curettage-electrodesiccation (91%) and of surgical excision (84%).[43] Radiation therapy is an effective method of treating recurrent BCCs that are smaller than 1 cm.[44] Therefore, if the long-term cosmetic outcome after treatment is not an overriding concern, x-ray therapy is an effective modality for many primary and recurrent BCCs. The treatment requires a number of outpatient visits that may be difficult for debilitated patients.

5-fluorouracil. 5-fluorouracil (5-FU) should not be used for the treatment of any BCCs, with the exception of some that occur in the rare basal cell nevus syndrome.[45] 5-FU can destroy the surface tumor without affecting deeper cells.

Intralesional interferon alfa[46] and photodynamic therapy. These are new experimental methods of therapy and are not likely to become important therapeutic modalities.

Actinic Keratosis

Actinic keratoses are common, sun-induced, premalignant lesions that increase with age. Light-complected individuals are more susceptible than those with dark complexions. Years of sun exposure are required to induce sufficient damage to cause lesions. Actinic keratoses may undergo spontaneous remission if sunlight exposure is reduced, but new lesions may appear.[47] Patients often present with lesions that were first noticed during the summer, suggesting that the lesions may become more active after sunlight exposure.

Clinical presentation. Actinic keratoses begin as an area of increased vascularity, with the skin surface becoming slightly rough. Texture is the key to diagnosing early lesions. They are better recognized by palpation than by inspection. Very gradually, an adherent yellow crust forms, the removal of which may cause bleeding (Figures 21-18 to 21-21). Individual lesions vary in size from 3 to 6 mm. The extent of disease varies from a single lesion to involvement of the entire forehead, balding scalp, or temples. Induration, inflammation, and oozing suggest degeneration into malignancy. Keratin may accumulate and form a cutaneous horn, particularly on the superior aspects of the pinna (Figure 21-20).

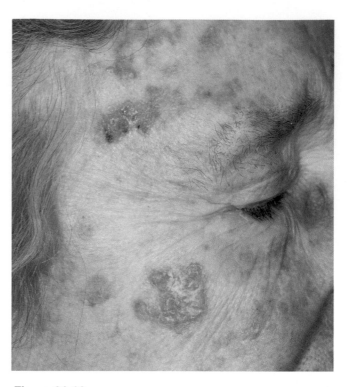

Figure 21-18
Actinic keratosis. Early lesions are present on the forehead. A more advanced lesion with yellow adherent scale is seen on the cheek.

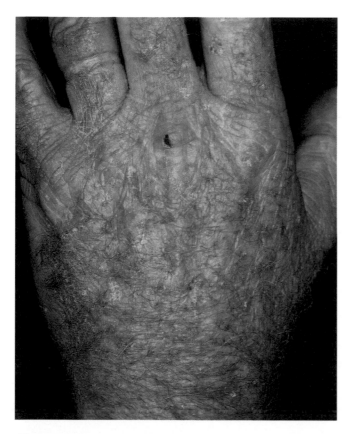

Figure 21-19
Actinic keratosis. Several oval-to-round, red, indurated lesions with adherent scale.

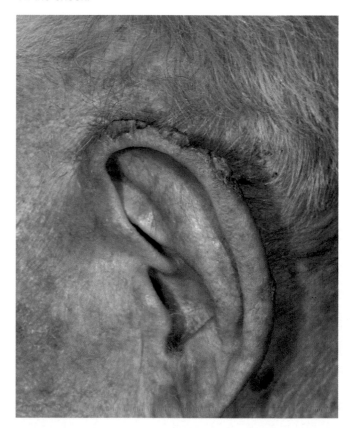

Figure 21-20
Actinic keratosis. Three actinic keratoses are forming cutaneous horns.

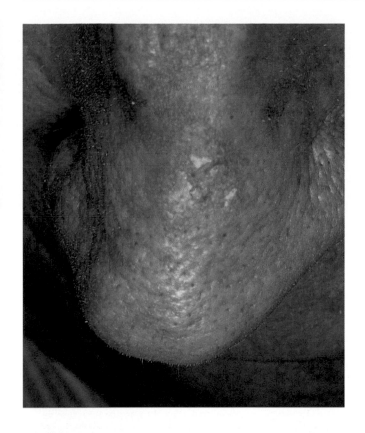

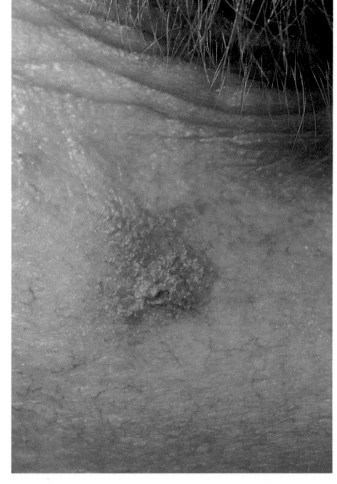

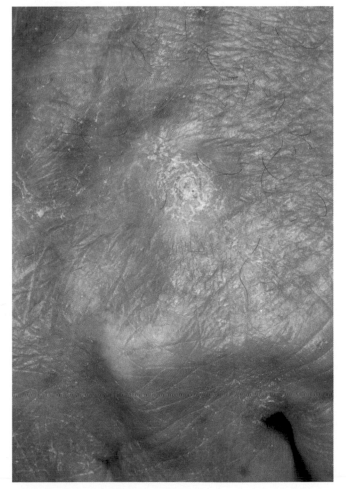

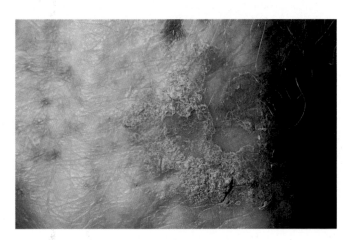

Figure 21-21
Actinic keratosis. These solitary lesions have a red base and the typical dry, adherent, yellow-brown scale.

Histology. Histologically, an actinic keratosis consists of atypical squamous cells confined to the epidermis. The follicles are not involved, so there is no follicular plugging (Figure 21-22). Penetration through the dermoepidermal junction and into the dermis indicates the development of a squamous cell carcinoma.

Transformation into squamous cell carcinoma. After several years, a small percentage of lesions may degenerate into squamous cell carcinomas. A very low yearly transformation rate for single lesions can translate into a substantial lifetime risk of transformation for patients with several actinic keratoses.[48] Up to 60% of squamous cell carcinomas develop from actinic keratosis.[49] Squamous cell carcinomas that evolve from actinic keratosis are not aggressive, but may eventually metastasize.[50] All patients with actinic keratosis should be examined carefully for basal cell carcinomas.

Management

Because actinic keratoses sometimes undergo spontaneous remission, definitive treatment may be delayed for patients with a few superficial lesions. Small lesions should be reexamined at a later date for spontaneous remission. Patients should make every effort to prevent further sun damage. This does not mean that patients must hibernate for a lifetime, but they should understand techniques to reduce sunlight exposure.

Cryotherapy. Cryotherapy is the treatment of choice for most isolated, superficial, actinic keratoses. Actinic keratosis resides in the epithelium. Cryotherapy with liquid nitrogen causes the separation of the epidermis and dermis, resulting in a highly specific, nonscarring method of therapy for superficial lesions. Patients with darker complexions may develop hypopigmented areas after freezing, and treating multiple lesions on the faces of such patients may result in white-spotted faces. 5-FU is the best alternative.

Surgical removal. Individual indurated lesions or those with thick crusts should be removed with minor surgical procedures. It is unnecessary to biopsy lesions less than 0.5 cm. Larger lesions or those occurring about or on the vermilion border of the lips should be examined. Electrodesiccation and curettage easily remove small, thicker lesions. The CO_2 laser may be superior to vermilionectomy for actinic cheilitis too extensive to be treated with topical 5-FU.[51,52]

Figure 21-22
Actinic keratosis. Keratin and crust are present on the surface. Atypical epithelial cells are confined to the epidermis and do not involve the follicular structure.

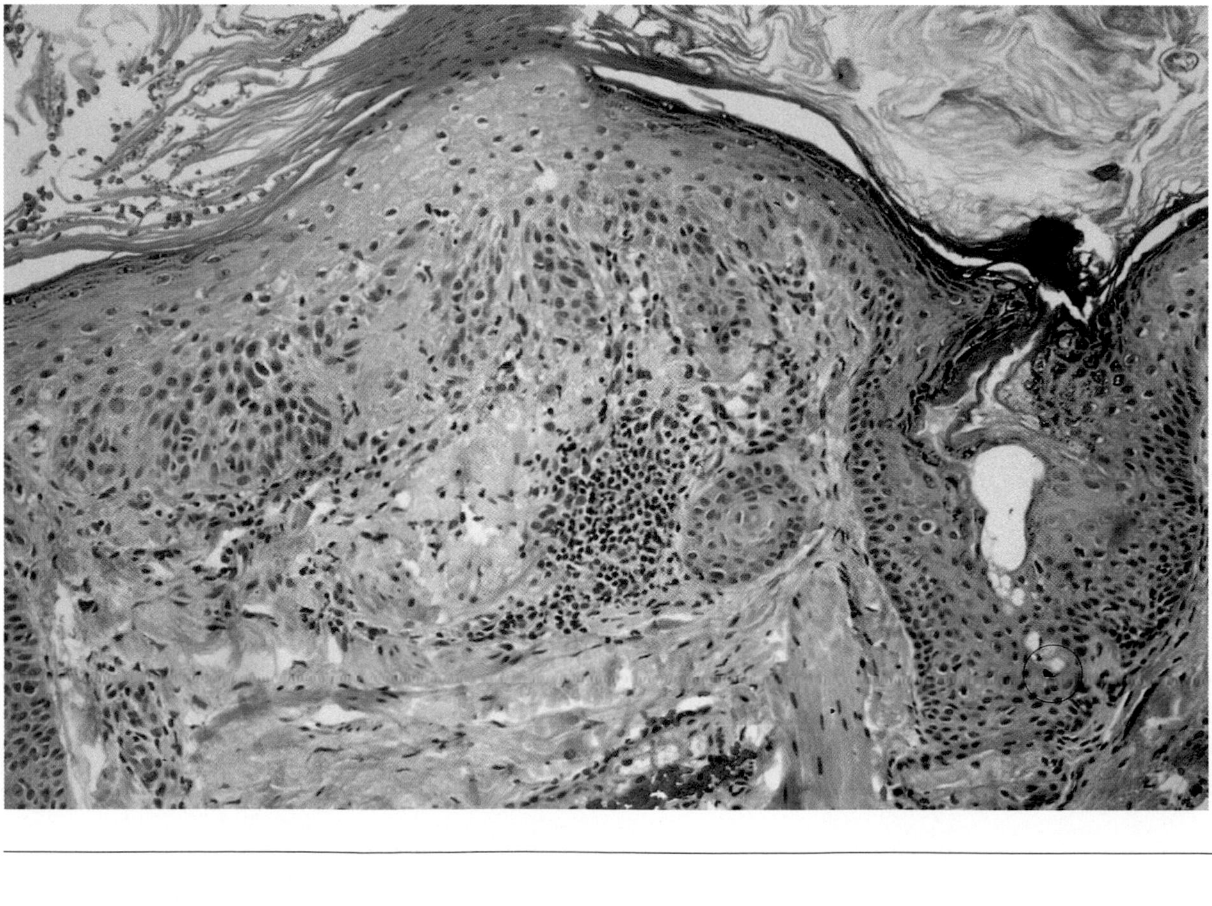

Tretinoin. Experience is accumulating that tretinoin (Retin-A) used alone or in combination with topical 5-FU is an effective treatment for certain actinic keratoses. Patients with mild actinic damage who show only erythema and scaling may be treated with tretinoin 0.05% to 0.1% cream applied once a day.[53] If a few focal areas of scale do not respond after 2 to 4 months, they can be treated with cryotherapy. Tretinoin slightly enhances the effectiveness of 5-FU, thereby shortening treatment time, but intensifying tissue reaction and discomfort. Combination therapy is probably not worth the trouble.

Sunscreens. Regular use of sunscreens prevents the development of solar keratoses.[54] Sunscreens that contain a combination of ingredients to block both the UVA and UVB spectrum of ultraviolet light are most effective. Shade UVA Guard and DuraScreen 30 are examples of commercially available, broad spectrum sunscreens. Sunscreens are best applied in the morning on days when sun exposure is anticipated. Sunscreens should be applied to the face, lower lip, ears, back of the neck, and backs of the hands and forearms. Hats should cover bald heads. The physician should explain that although sunscreens are used, additional lesions may occur, but that many superficial areas of involvement may actually improve.[47]

Acid peels. Glycolic acid is an alpha hydroxy acid that is useful as a chemical peeling agent. Actinic keratoses involve epidermal hyperplasia and retention of stratum corneum. Alpha hydroxy acids applied topically in high concentrations (30% to 70% glycolic acid) cause epidermolysis and elimination of keratosis.[55] Fluorouracil cream may be used for 5 to 7 days prior to the peel to "light up" and identify the lesions. Glycolic acid is applied with a cotton swab to the keratoses, is left on for 5 to 10 minutes, and is then removed with alcohol. Trichloroacetic acid (35%) and Jessner's solution (14 g of resorcinol, 14 g of lactic acid, and 14 g of salicylic acid dissolved in ethanol to make a final solution of 100 ml) induce a medium-depth peel and equal fluorouracil in efficacy.[56]

Topical chemotherapy with 5-fluorouracil. 5-FU is an effective topical treatment for superficial actinic keratosis. Thicker lesions, especially those on the scalp, may evolve into squamous cell carcinomas and should be treated with more aggressive techniques.[57] The agent is incorporated into rapidly dividing cells, resulting in cell death. Normal cells are less affected and clinically appear to be unaffected. Inflammation is induced during this process. Thick, indurated lesions become most inflamed and may best be managed by surgically removing them before instituting topical chemotherapy. The available preparations of 5-FU are listed in Table 21-1 and in the Formulary.

Patients should be cautioned about the various stages of inflammation encountered during treatment. Considerable discomfort may be experienced for 1 week or more during periods of intense inflammation. Pain can be minimized if only small areas are treated at one time; however, many patients wish to treat the full face instead of prolonging the unsightly erythema and crusting for weeks. Lesions on the back of the hands and arms require longer periods of treatment than those on the face. Patients with a small number of lesions may be treated during the summer or winter. Patients with a large number of lesions who work outdoors are best treated in the winter. Pharmaceutical companies that manufacture 5-FU supply patient information sheets with color photographs of the various stages of inflammation.

Topical chemotherapy with masoprocol. Masoprocol (Actinex), a new topical antineoplastic agent, has been approved for treatment of actinic keratoses. A 71.4% reduction in the number of lesions occurs in 1 month when the cream is applied twice a day.[58] Irritation is moderate. Topical 5-FU is more effective.

TABLE 21-1 Guidelines for Choice of 5-FU Concentration and Duration of Therapy According to Site for bid Application

Site	5-FU* (%)	Early signs of inflammation (days)	Duration of treatment (weeks)
Face, lips	1-2	3-5	3
Scalp	5	4-7	4
Neck	5	4-7	4
Arms, hands	5	10-14	6-8
Back	5	10-14	4-6
Chest	5	10-14	4-6

From Goette KD: *J Am Acad Dermatol* 4:633, 1981.
*Topical preparations include Efudex 2% and 5% solutions (10 ml) and 5% cream (25 gm); Fluoroplex 1% solution (30 ml) and 1% cream (30 gm).

Treatment technique (5-FU) and expected results

5-FU is available as a 1% and 5% cream and a 1% and 2% solution. The 1% solution is helpful for the scalp, and the 2% solution is used for individual lesions. There are three schedules for application of topical 5-FU.

Daily bid dosing. Conventional treatment involves application of topical 5-FU twice each day for 3 to 5 weeks. Significant irritation and discomfort is frequently encountered with this schedule (Figure 21-23).

Daily qid dosing (short-term intensive treatment). 5-FU cream or solution is applied four times daily for periods varying between 7 and 21 days, depending on the body location.[59] The same brisk inflammatory reaction and clearing of the majority of actinic keratosis associated with longer courses is realized.

Weekly pulse dosing. A weekly pulse-dosing regimen offers a significant advance in treatment by reducing irritation while producing the same benefit as the daily dosing schedule. Patients apply topical 5-FU in the morning and evening 1 or 2 consecutive days per week. Patients are reexamined in 3 to 4 weeks to assess response and to determine the frequency of application.[60] The average duration of pulse therapy is longer than that of conventional daily therapy (6 to 7 weeks vs. 2 to 4 weeks, respectively). Pulse-treated patients recover more quickly (2 to 4 weeks) than daily-dose treated patients (4 to 8 weeks) because the irritation is much milder.

Some authors suggest using topical steroids during the entire treatment period to suppress inflammation and decrease patient discomfort. This technique, however, may make it difficult to determine when therapy should be stopped. Patients should be evaluated every 2 weeks during the treatment period.

Inflammatory response. In the early inflammatory phase, erythema first appears in treated areas at predictable intervals (see Table 21-1). In the severe inflammatory phase (Figure 21-24, *A*), erythema, edema, burning, stinging, and oozing reach maximum intensity at different intervals, depending on the site treated and the thickness of the lesions. In the lesion disintegration phase (Figure 21-24, *B*), erosion or ulceration, intense inflammation, discomfort, pain, crusting, eschar formation, and evidence of reepithelialization occur. When this phase is reached, treatment stops. Table 21-1 lists the approximate duration of treatment.

Actinic keratosis of the face. Patients with mild damage consisting of erythema and scaling can be treated with tretinoin cream 0.05% alone for several months. Small, superficial lesions that do not respond can then be treated with 5-FU or cryosurgery. Patients with many lesions can be pretreated with tretinoin cream applied once each day for 1 to 3 months. Pretreatment with tretinoin may improve the quality of the dermis and reduce subsequent treatment time with 5-FU. Tretinoin 0.025% cream should be prescribed for patients with sensitive skin. 5-FU may then be applied alone

Figure 21-23 Actinic keratosis—treatment with topical 5-FU.

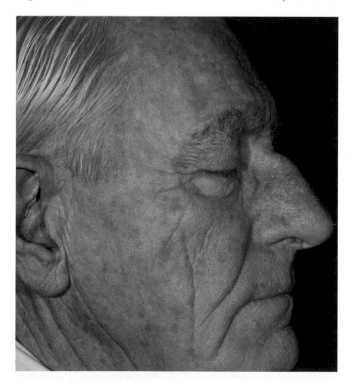

A, Diffuse involvement of the forehead. Lesions are superficial. Lesions on the cheek were not clinically apparent.

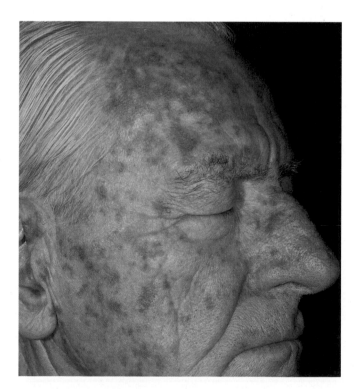

B, Maximum intensity of inflammation was reached 3 weeks after starting treatment. The medication has inflamed the cheek lesions that were not clinically apparent before treatment.

or in combination with tretinoin to complete the treatment program. Combination therapy may shorten the treatment period, but it produces more intense inflammation.

Actinic keratoses of the upper extremity. These lesions are frequently multiple, hyperkeratotic, and distributed over a large area. Hyperkeratosis tends to limit penetration of topical 5-FU. Lesions on the extremities require longer treatment than those on the face. Plastic (Saran Wrap) occlusion is sometimes used to facilitate 5-FU penetration of thicker lesions.

Actinic cheilitis. Actinic cheilitis is treated effectively with 5-FU cream; however, pain and excessive crusting make this a very unpleasant experience for most patients. Some authors suggest using 5% 5-FU cream three times a day for 14 to 18 days to obtain the optimal reaction in the shortest time.[61] The objective is to reduce the morbidity to 2 weeks. Application of 5% lidocaine ointment relieves pain.

Cool compresses are applied several times each day if inflammation is intense. Group V topical steroids may be applied to red areas to suppress inflammation and pruritis.

Appearance of a purulent exudate suggests infection; when this occurs, oral antistaphylococcal antibiotics should be prescribed. In the healing phase (Figure 21-25), residual erythema and hyperpigmentation persist for several weeks.

Contact allergy to 5-FU. Contact allergy to 5-FU should be suspected if intense erythema and vesiculation occur. Patch testing is not reliable because many patients who are allergic to 5-FU do not show a positive patch test reaction.

Prognosis. Patients should remain free of lesions for months and possibly years, but recurrences can be anticipated. Frequently, unsupervised patients inadequately treat their own newly evolving lesions, resulting in surface healing but untreated deeper abnormal cells. For this reason no refills should be indicated on the initial prescription, and patients should be instructed to discard medication when treatment is finished.

Low-fat diet. In patients with a history of nonmelanoma skin cancer, a low-fat diet reduced the incidence of actinic keratosis.[62]

Figure 21-24 Actinic keratosis—treatment with topical 5-FU.

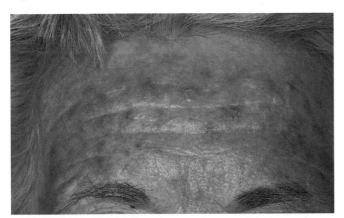

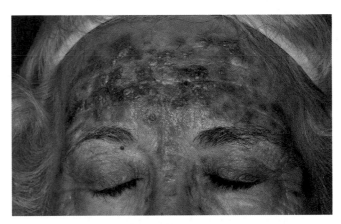

A, Before treatment. Lesions are more advanced than those depicted in Figure 21-23.

B, Three weeks after starting topical 5-FU. Lesion disintegration phase with ulceration and crusting.

Figure 21-25 Actinic cheilitis—treatment with topical 5-FU.

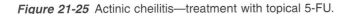

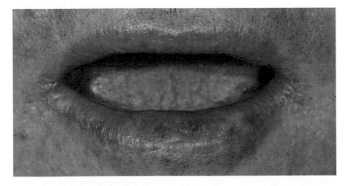

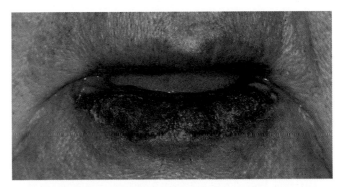

A, Before treatment. The lower lip is pink-white and smooth. The non–sun exposed upper lip is normal.

B, Two weeks after starting topical 5-FU. The entire lower lip is ulcerated.

Squamous Cell Carcinoma

Squamous cell carcinoma (SCC) arises in the epithelium and is common in the middle-aged and elderly population. SCCs are often separated into two major groups based on their malignant potential. Those arising in areas of prior radiation or thermal injury, in chronic draining sinuses, and in chronic ulcers are typically aggressive and have a high frequency of metastasis. SCCs originating in actinically damaged skin are less aggressive and less likely to metastasize.

Risk factors. UVB radiation is important for the induction of SCC. UVB radiation damages DNA (by inducing the formation of pyrimidine dimers) and its repair system and alters the immune system. UVB radiation induces mutation of p53 tumor-suppressor genes. These mutations are found in SCC. Cell-mediated immunity and immune function may be modulated by UVB radiation. Immunosuppression leads to a great increase in the risk of SCC. Renal-transplant recipients have a 253-fold increase in the risk of SCC.[63] Longer wavelength UVA radiation damages DNA and is also carcinogenic. SCC arises in skin that has been damaged by thermal burns or chronic inflammation. It also occurs from epidermal diseases of unknown origin, such as Bowen's disease (see the box below).

Location. Like basal cell carcinoma, SCCs are most common in sun-exposed areas; however, the distribution is different.[64] SCCs are common on the scalp, backs of the hands, and the superior surface of the pinna; BCC is rarely found on these sites.

Incidence. The incidence is highest in lower latitudes such as the southern United States and Australia. The incidence increases rapidly with age and sun exposure and is approximately twice as high in men as in women.

Pathophysiology. Atypical squamous cells originate in the epidermis from keratinocytes and proliferate indefinitely. A flat, scaly lesion becomes an indurated SCC when cells penetrate the epidermal basement membrane and proliferate into the dermis.

Clinical manifestations. SCCs arising from actinic keratosis may have a thick, adherent scale. The tumor is soft and freely movable and may have a red, inflamed base. These lesions are most frequently observed on the bald scalp, forehead (Figure 21-26), and backs of the hands (Figure 21-27). Cutaneous horns may begin as actinic keratosis and degenerate into SCC. SCCs originating on the lip (Figures 21-28 and 21-29) or from apparently normal skin are aggressive and metastasize to the regional lymph nodes and beyond.

Those SCCs beginning in actinically damaged skin, but not from actinic keratosis, appear as firm, movable, elevated masses with a sharply defined border and little surface scale. SCCs that arise in actinically damaged skin were previously thought to have a minimal potential for metastasis; however, such lesions may be aggressive.

Keratoacanthomas vs. SCC. Keratoacanthomas are sometimes difficult to differentiate from SCC. Keratoacanthomas appear suddenly and grow rapidly (see p. 638). They reach a certain size, usually 0.5 cm to 2.0 cm, stop growing, then regress weeks to months later. They begin as red-to-flesh colored, dome-shaped papules with a smooth surface and a central crater filled with a keratinous plug. The pathologist sometimes has difficulty differentiating the benign keratoacanthoma from SCC.

LESIONS FROM WHICH SQUAMOUS CELL CARCINOMA ORIGINATES

Actinic keratosis
   Cutaneous horn
Bowen's disease
   Erythroplasia of Queyrat
Chemical exposure
   Arsenic (internal)
   Tar (external), except therapeutic tars
Leukoplakia
Lichen sclerosis et atrophicus (vulva)
Sites of chronic infection
   Chronic sinus tracts
   Osteomyelitis
Thermal burn scars (Marjolin's ulcer)
   Radiation-damaged skin

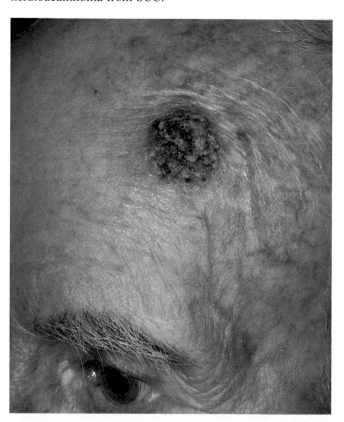

Figure 21-26
Squamous cell carcinoma. Malignant degeneration occurred in an actinic keratosis that had been present for years.

Metastatic potential. The potential for SCCs to metastasize is related to the size, location, degree of differentiation, histologic evidence of perineural involvement, immunologic status, and depth of invasion (Table 21-2).[65,66] SCC first metastasizes to regional lymph nodes in the majority of cases.

TABLE 21-2 Influence of Tumor Variables on Local Recurrence and Metastasis of SCC		
Factor	**Local recurrence**	**Metastasis**
SIZE		
<2 cm	7.4%	9.1%
= or >2 cm	15.2%	30.3%
DEPTH		
<4 mm/Clark I to II	5.3%	6.7%
>4 mm/Clark IV, V	17.2%	45.7%
DIFFERENTIATION		
Well differentiated	13.6%	9.2%
Poorly differentiated	28.6%	32.8%
SITE		
Sun-exposed	7.9%	5.2%
Ear	18.7%	11.0%
Lip	10.5%	13.7%
SCAR CARCINOMA		
(non–sun-exposed)	N/A*	37.9%
PREVIOUS TREATMENT	23.3%	30.3%
PERINEURAL INVOLVEMENT	47.2%	47.3%
IMMUNOSUPPRESSION	N/A	12.9%

From Rowe DE, Carroll RJ, Day CL: *J Am Acad Dermatol* 26:976-990, 1992.
*N/A, Not available

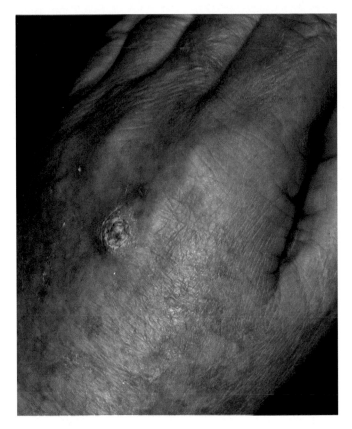

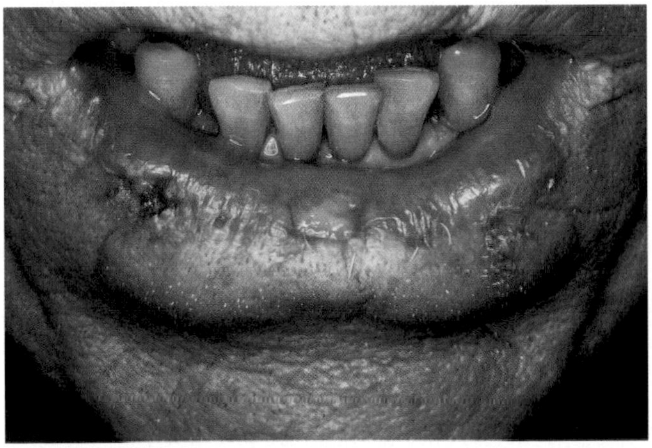

Figure 21-27
Squamous cell carcinoma. Malignant degeneration of an actinic keratosis.

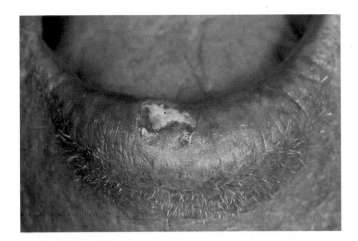

Figure 21-28
Squamous cell carcinoma. Several ulcerated lesions are present on the lower lip of this patient who has spent years working outdoors.

Figure 21-29
Squamous cell carcinoma. The sun-exposed lower lip is a common site. Palpation reveals a deep nodular mass.

Tumor size and depth. In one study, no carcinoma less than 2 mm thick metastasized. Tumors between 2 and 6 mm thick with moderate differentiation and a depth of invasion that does not extend beyond the subcutis can be classified as low-risk carcinomas. The risk of metastasis is high for undifferentiated carcinomas greater than 6 mm thick that have infiltrated the musculature, the perichondrium, or the periosteum.[67] Another study of SCCs on the trunk and extremities showed that, like melanoma, tumor behavior correlated best with the level of dermal invasion and the vertical tumor thickness. Tumors that recurred were at least 4 mm thick and involved the deep half of the dermis or deeper structures. All tumors that proved fatal were at least 10 mm thick.[68] Investigators concluded that patients whose tumors penetrate through the dermis or exceed 8 mm in thickness are at high risk of recurrence or death.

Location. Tumors on the scalp, forehead, ears, nose, and lips are at higher risk.[69] Tumors developing at sites of chronic inflammation, such as ulcers, scar tissue, and previous radiation sites, also have higher rates of metastasis.

Immunologic status. Host immune surveillance plays a role in determining the metastatic potential of SCC.[70] Patients with lymphoproliferative disorders, renal transplants, and those undergoing chronic oral corticosteroid therapy are at high risk. Renal-transplant recipients are at increased risk for skin cancer, most frequently SCC.[71] SCCs are also more aggressive in renal transplant patients, in whom they are associated with a higher risk of metastasis than in the general population. HLA-B mismatching is significantly associated with the risk of SCC in renal-transplant recipients, as is HLA-DR homozygosity.[72]

Mode of spread. Cutaneous SCC may spread by (1) expansion and infiltration, (2) shelving or skating, (3) conduit spread, or (4) metastasis.[73,74] SCC grows locally by expansion and infiltration. When the tumor reaches a hard surface (muscle, cartilage, bone), it may spread laterally (shelves or skates) under normal skin along facial or capsular planes, muscle, perichondrium, and periosteum. Shelving and skating occur in areas with little subcutaneous tissue, such as the scalp, ears, eyelids, nose, and upper lips. The spreading of a tumor along the nerve or vessel in the perineural or perivascular space is called *conduit spread.* This occurs in areas with major nerve trunks on the head and neck. Failure to recognize these three local modes of spread may result in an inadequate surgical procedure. Most SCCs are located on the head and neck. These metastasize, primarily by way of the lymphatics, initially to the superficial (first echelon) draining lymph nodes, then spread to deeper (second echelon) nodes. Distant metastasis occurs by hematogenous dissemination most commonly to the lungs, liver, brain, skin, or bone. SCCs originating on the lip[75,76] (Figures 21-28 and 21-29) and pinna metastasize in 10% to 20% of cases.

TABLE 21-3 Surgical Guidelines for Primary Squamous Cell Carcinoma				
Size	Histologic grade	Anatomic location	Depth of invasion	Surgical margin
<2 cm	1	Low risk*	Dermis	4 mm
> or = 2 cm	2,3,4	High risk†	Subcutaneous tissue	6 mm

From Brodland DG, Zitelli JA: *J Am Acad Dermatol* 27:241-248, 1992.
*Includes tumors less than 1 cm located in "high-risk" areas.
†Scalp, ears, eyelids, nose, and lips.

Treatment. Guidelines of care for cutaneous SCC have been established by the American Academy of Dermatology.[77] Small SCCs evolving from actinic keratosis are treated by electrodesiccation and curettage. Larger tumors or those on or near the vermilion border of the lips are best excised and should include the subcutaneous fat.[64] Histologic microstaging may help to direct therapy. Tumors thinner than 4 mm can be managed by simple local removal. Patients with lesions that are between 4 and 8 mm thick or that exhibit deep dermal invasion should undergo excision. Tumors that penetrate through the dermis are staged by the surgeon and treated with several modalities including excisional and Mohs' surgery,[65] neck dissection, radiation therapy, and chemotherapy.[65,78] Larger tumors or those about the nose and eyes require special consideration (see p. 667). Surgical margins for excision of primary cutaneous SCCs have been proposed (Table 21-3).[69]

Combined systemic therapy with 13-cis-retinoic acid and interferon alpha-2a is highly effective for patients with advanced SCC of the skin.[79]

SQUAMOUS CELL CARCINOMA OF THE EXTREMITIES (MARJOLIN'S ULCER)

Marjolin's ulcer is a term that refers to malignant changes occurring in chronic ulcers of the skin,[80] sinuses, or previous burns.[81] The majority of these lesions are found on the extremities. Different cultures appear to have markedly different susceptibilities to Marjolin's ulcer. Japan, Northern India, and China report high incidences of burn-scar carcinoma. SCCs that occur at sites of chronic inflammation are more aggressive than those that develop from actinic keratosis or Bowen's disease. Their appearance is masked by inflamed hypertrophic tissue.

The overall metastatic rate is greater than 40%. The incidence of regional lymph node involvement from burn-scar carcinoma is approximately 35%. The 5-year survival rate for lower extremity lesions is approximately 30%.[82] Wide local excision has proven unreliable for grade II and grade III disease; amputation and prophylactic node irradiation is recommended.[83] Wide local excision is reserved only for very small lesions that can be radically excised or for grade I lesions.

Bowen's Disease

Bowen's disease, also referred to as *squamous cell carcinoma in situ*, appears mainly on sun-exposed sites. Lesions are found most often on the lower limbs of women and on the scalp and ears of men.[84] Typical lesions are slightly elevated, red, scaly plaques with surface fissures and foci of pigmentation. The borders are well defined (Figures 21-30 and 21-31), and lesions closely resemble psoriasis, chronic eczema, superficial basal cell carcinoma, seborrheic keratosis, and malignant melanoma. The plaque grows very slowly by lateral extension and may eventually, after several months or years, invade the dermis, producing induration and ulceration. When confined to the epidermis the atypical cells, in contrast to actinic keratosis, involve epidermal appendages, particularly the hair follicle (Figure 21-32). Atypical cells are also found at the periphery of lesions in clinically uninvolved skin. Atypical cells in the epidermal lining of the hair follicle, although still confined to the epidermis, are deeper and more difficult to reach by treatment modalities such as topical 5-FU or electrosurgery, which only permit access to superficial areas.

Immunohistochemistry may sometimes be valuable in differentiating Paget's disease, superficial spreading melanoma, and Bowen's disease.[85]

The cause of Bowen's disease is unknown, but several patients with this disease were formerly treated with arsenic. There is no evidence that Bowen's disease is a skin marker for internal malignancy.[86-88]

Treatment. Small lesions may be successfully treated with electrodesiccation and curettage, cryosurgery, or excisional surgery. Larger lesions are treated with excisional surgery[89,90] or 5-FU cream applied twice a day for 4 to 8 weeks. Treatment is discontinued when erosion and superficial necrosis occur. A large area surrounding the lesion should be treated in order to destroy the clinically inapparent disease. Some authors suggest plastic occlusion to enhance penetration to the hair follicle.[91] Acetowhitening is a useful adjunct for surgical management. Acetic acid (vinegar) applied preoperatively more clearly defines clinical margins by disclosing subclinical extension of disease.[92] Photodynamic therapy is an effective alternative for large lesions or those in anatomically difficult areas.[93,94] Photofrin (a tumor-localizing photosensitive substance) is administered intravenously and activated by light from a laser 48 hours later. Cytotoxic substances are released that destroy the malignant tumor and preserve surrounding normal tissues. The most significant side effects are moderate pain and edema. Close follow-up of patients after treatment is required because recurrences are relatively common. Recurrence is related to follicular involvement and ill-defined lateral margins. If left untreated, development of invasive carcinoma is possible but uncommon.

Figure 21-30
Bowen's disease. The red plaque is well defined with scale and some crust on the surface.

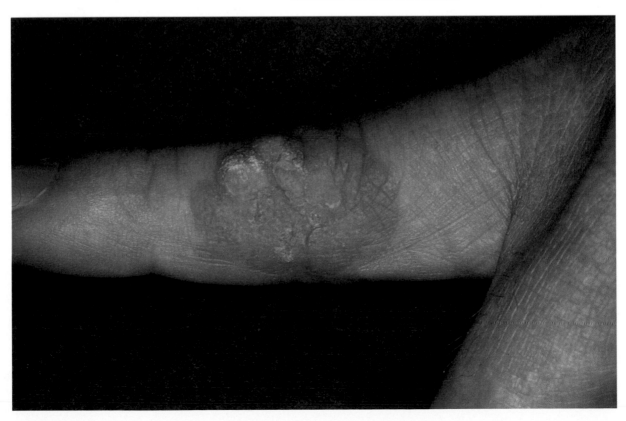

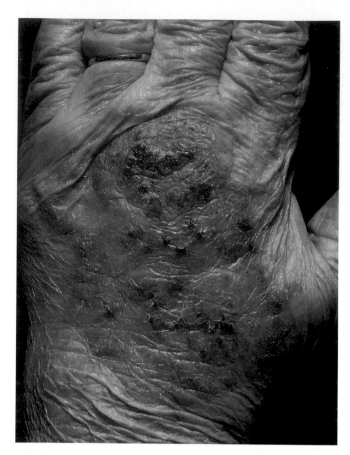

Figure 21-31
Bowen's disease. A large plaque that was misdiagnosed as tinea and psoriasis. Scale and crust form on a surface that intermittently oozes serum.

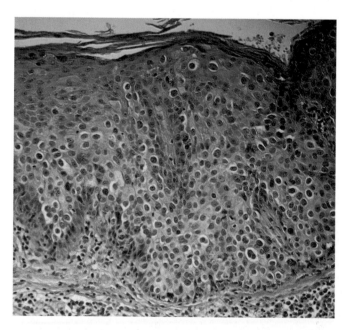

Figure 21-32
Bowen's disease. Atypical cells are present throughout the entire thickness of the epidermis. The dermoepidermal junction remains distinct and intact.

Erythroplasia of Queyrat

Clinically and histologically, erythroplasia of Queyrat of the penis resembles Bowen's disease and is probably the same entity. It appears exclusively under the foreskin of the uncircumcised penis and is a moist, slightly raised, well-defined, red, smooth or velvety plaque (Figure 21-33). Analogous to Bowen's disease of the skin, erythroplasia of Queyrat grows very slowly and has the potential for degeneration into squamous cell carcinoma. Similar lesions may occur on the vulva. 5-FU cream is the treatment of choice. Recurrences are unlikely because the hair follicles that serve as foci for recurrence are absent on the penile mucosa.[95] A 3- to 4-week course is usually required. Use of 5% lidocaine ointment is recommended for pain. CO_2 laser provided good results in one report.[96] Erythroplasia involving the distal glans penis around the urethra and extending into the urethral meatus may require Mohs' microscopically controlled surgery.

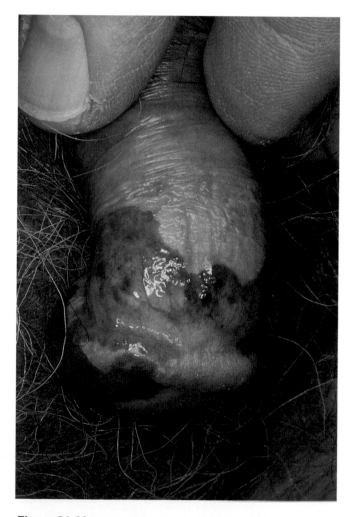

Figure 21-33
Erythroplasia of Queyrat. A moist, glistening, slightly raised plaque. Similar lesions may occur on the vulva.

Leukoplakia

Leukoplakia is a clinical term used to describe a range of nonspecific white lesions, from slightly raised, white, translucent areas to dense, white, opaque lesions, with or without ulceration on the vermilion border of the lips (Figure 21-34), oral mucosa, or vulva. The most common sites of oral leukoplakia are the commissures and the buccal mucosa. Smoking is the most common cause of oral lesions, but chronic irritation from carious teeth or malaligned dentures is also a cause. Histologic changes occur, varying from mild scaling and epidermal thickening with minimal inflammation to varying degrees of dysplasia or carcinoma in situ.[97] Squamous cell carcinoma develops in 17% of all leukoplakia patients.[98,99] In one study of 500 patients with oral leukoplakia, there was squamous cell carcinoma in 9.6% of cases and dysplasia in an additional 24%. Leukoplakia on the floor of the mouth and the ventral surface of the tongue is associated with the highest risk of cancer.[100] Degeneration to carcinoma takes 1 to 20 years. Clinically, the patches are white, slightly elevated, usually well-defined plaques that show little tendency to extend peripherally. The differential diagnosis includes candidiasis, lichen planus, habitual cheek biting, white sponge nevus, and secondary syphilis. A lesion unique to acquired immunodeficiency syndrome (AIDS), termed *hairy leukoplakia*, presents as an asymptomatic, slightly raised, poorly demarcated lesion with a corrugated or "hairy" surface composed of white papillary projections.[101] It occurs principally on the lateral borders of the tongue. *Candida* organisms are frequently observed on the lesion surface. Human papilloma virus and Epstein-Barr virus have been identified in the lesions.[102] Dyskeratosis congenita is a congenital multisystem disorder, characterized by skin pigmentation, dystrophic nails, and leukoplakia.

The clinical appearance of leukoplakia does not generally correlate well with the histopathologic change; therefore, biopsy should be performed for all cases to determine which are precancerous.[103,104] Small lesions may be biopsied and simply followed if the histology is benign. Plaques that histologically exhibit atypical features should be excised, electrodesiccated, destroyed with the laser,[105] or frozen with liquid nitrogen.[106]

Treatment. Leukoplakia of the vulva and the lip can be successfully treated with 5-FU. Lip lesions are treated twice daily with applications of 1% 5-FU solution until erythema and erosions become marked in approximately 10 to 21 days. Discomfort is intense and can be relieved with cool compresses or topical lidocaine gel. Localized dysplastic oral leukoplakia is treated with surgical excision, electrosurgery, or cryosurgery.

Beta-carotene (30 mg/day) produced a major response in 71% of patients with oral leukoplakia in one study. There was no toxicity.[107] However, another study showed isotretinoin is more effective. In that study, isotretinoin (1.5 mg/kg/day) was taken for 3 months, followed by a lower dosage (0.5 mg/kg/day) for 9 months.[108] Many lesions clear spontaneously when cigarette or pipe smoking is stopped.[109] Long-term follow-up is desirable to check for recurrences. Hairy leukoplakia lesions are treated with tretinoin (Retin-A) solution applied with a cotton-tipped applicator once a day. Repeated treatment is necessary as the lesions recur. Lesions contaminated with *Candida* are treated with clotrimazole (Mycelex Troches) dissolved in the mouth five times a day for 5 to 14 days.

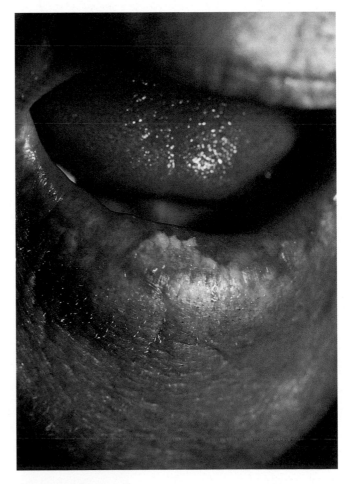

Figure 21-34
Leukoplakia. A thin white plaque had been present on the lip for over 2 years. The patient smoked.

VERRUCOUS CARCINOMA

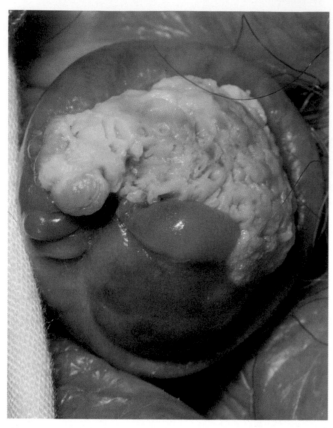

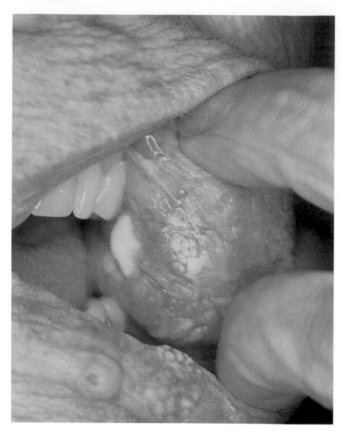

Figure 21-35
The giant condylomata of Buschke-Löwenstein occurs on the male and female genitalia. They initially appear as warts, but grow relentlessly despite multiple attempts at conservative topical and surgical treatment.

Figure 21-36
Oral florid papillomatosis. A white verrucous growth that may extend widely over the oral mucosa.

Figure 21-37
Epithelioma cuniculatum. A lesion was present for months and was suspected of being a plantar wart.

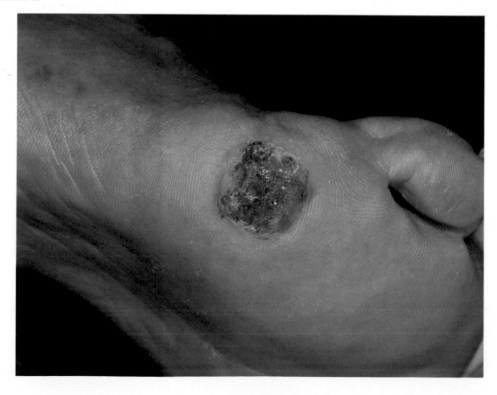

Verrucous Carcinoma

Verrucous carcinoma is a term encompassing three rare entities: epithelioma cuniculatum (plantar surface of the foot), giant condylomata of Buschke-Löwenstein (perineum) (Figure 21-35), and oral florid papillomatosis (Figure 21-36).[110] The term *verrucous carcinoma* was coined to denote a locally aggressive, exophytic, low-grade squamous cell carcinoma with little metastatic potential. Verrucous carcinomas have been reported on many other skin surfaces.[111] Verrucous carcinomas are probably caused by human papilloma viruses (HPV) and are most often associated with HPV-6 and -11.[112,113] They are thought to represent an intermediate lesion in a pathologic continuum from condyloma to squamous cell carcinoma. All three entities have similar biologic potential and show bulky, exophytic, fungating growth, with a high degree of cellular differentiation histologically. A slowly growing tumor extends in surface area and locally compresses and displaces rather than infiltrating contiguous structures and rarely metastasizes. Histologically, the tumor displays massive epidermal thickening with local invasion minus cellular atypia. In their early stages, all tumors may be mistaken for warts (Figure 21-37). However, tumors are unresponsive to locally destructive procedures and slowly, over months or years, increase in size, become indurated, and deeply penetrate the dermis. Conservative local excision,[114] Mohs' microscopically controlled surgery,[115] radiation therapy,[116] CO_2 laser[117] and systemic chemotherapy,[118] etretinate,[119] and interferon[120,121] have all been advocated.

Buschke-Löwenstein tumor. This tumor, a carcinoma-like condylomata acuminata, is verrucous carcinoma of the anogenital mucosal surface. These tumors occur most commonly in uncircumcised men on the glans and prepuce and have the same clinical appearance on the vulva, vagina, cervix,[122] and anorectum. Transformation into invasive carcinoma has been described.[123]

Oral florid papillomatosis. Extensive grey-white, warty tumors with a deeply cleaved surface are found on the gingival mucosa and may extend to the entire oral mucosa and into the larynx and trachea.[124] Local aggression with bone, muscle, and salivary gland invasion occurred in 53% of cases in one study.[125] The tumors are most often reported in the elderly. White sponge nevus is autosomal dominant and is characterized by white lesions that appear from birth to adolescence.

Verrucous carcinoma (epithelioma cuniculatum) plantare. This tumor mimics a variety of other skin lesions with its insidious onset.[126,127] Plantar warts, ischemic ulcers, melanoma, and squamous cell carcinoma must be considered.

Arsenical Keratoses and Other Arsenic-Related Skin Diseases

Pentavalent, inorganic arsenic, dispensed years ago as Fowler's solution (potassium arsenite solution) for psoriasis and other diseases, may cause a number of problems. Arsenical keratoses are discrete, round, wartlike, or pointed keratotic lesions that appear 20 or more years after chronic arsenic ingestion (Figure 21-38). Arsenical keratoses may degenerate into squamous cell carcinoma. Lesions are most common on the palms and soles, but may occur elsewhere. Bowen's disease, multiple basal cell carcinomas, and changes in pigmentation characterized by small, round, white macules ("raindrops on a hyperpigmented background") are additional findings in patients with chronic arsenic ingestion. A significant excess of bladder cancer mortality occurred in patients treated with Fowler's solution.[128] Chronic arsenic toxicity from drinking well water polluted with arsenic occurred in Malaysia[129] from tin-mining soil and in South Calcutta[130] close to a factory that manufactured Paris-green (copper acetoarsenite). Affected persons showed typical skin signs, gastrointestinal symptoms, anemia, signs of liver disease, and peripheral neuropathy. No treatment is necessary for arsenical keratosis unless signs of degeneration occur.

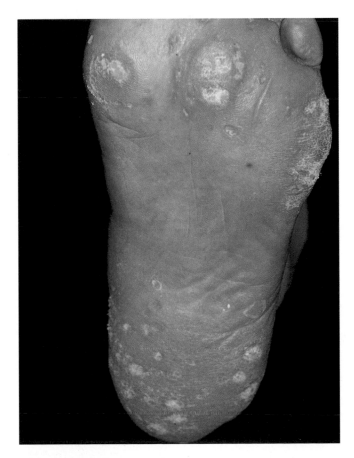

Figure 21-38
Arsenical keratoses. Discrete, wartlike, keratotic lesions occur on the palms and soles.

Cutaneous T-Cell Lymphoma

The term *cutaneous T-cell lymphoma* (CTCL) encompasses a group of distinct lymphomatous neoplasms of helper T cells that present in the skin but later may involve lymph nodes, peripheral blood cells, and the viscera. Mycosis fungoides, Sézary syndrome, and lymphoma cutis are all examples of CTCL. The malignant cells have a marked affinity for the skin, particularly the epidermis, often leading to formation of Pautrier's intraepidermal abscesses. The disease progresses to systemic involvement as the cells lose their affinity for the epidermis. Greater awareness and earlier detection have suggested that CTCL has replaced Hodgkin's disease as the most common adult lymphoma. Unlike other closely related diseases (e.g., adult T-cell leukemic lymphoma), CTCL does not appear to be communicable. Patients with CTCL are heterogeneous with respect to immunocompetence, and this heterogeneity affects their clinical course and response to therapy. The disease was thought to be confined to the elderly, but newer diagnostic techniques show that it starts insidiously in younger adults.[131] A persistent eruption, even in youths and young adults, should be thoroughly evaluated for possible CTCL. Early detection is essential since the disease can be cured in the initial stage when it is confined to the skin. The disease is fatal once systemic spread has occurred. The most common forms of CTCL are mycosis fungoides (MF) and Sézary syndrome (SS), the leukemic phase of MF.

Molecular theory of origin. CTCL is a malignancy of a single clone of CD4-positive T cells that may originate from stimulation by an antigen (possibly from a mutation or a retrovirus). Each patient develops a unique clone of malignant cells with unique surface receptors.[132,133] The disease advances with the development of progressively more aggressive subclones.[134] Initially, Langerhans' cells carry antigens from the skin to peripheral lymph nodes, where they present the antigens to CD4-positive T cells and convert them to cutaneous T-cell lymphoma cells (CTCL cells).[135] The T cells acquire cutaneous lymphoid antigen (CLA) on their surfaces, which acts as a skin-selective homing receptor.[136] CLA permits adherence of the T cell to dermal blood vessels, giving the cells the ability to infiltrate the skin.[137] A unique feature of early-stage CTCL is epidermotropism, in which malignant cells are found in the proximity of the epidermis, where the cellular growth environment is conducive to their proliferation. A second set of antigenic peptides permits immunologic attack against the malignant cells through the use of photopheresis.

Mycosis fungoides

Clinical manifestations. The name *mycosis fungoides* is misleading because the disease is not fungal in origin. MF is a rare T-cell lymphoma that appears to originate in the skin. MF is twice as common in men as in women. Most cases are diagnosed in the fifth and sixth decades, but individuals can develop this disease in childhood and adolescence. Blacks are twice as likely to be affected as whites. The incidence has increased threefold (from 0.19 cases to 0.42 cases per 100,000 population) in the last 20 years. The course is unpredictable, sometimes lasting less than 1 year or lingering for decades. There are four phases in the evolution of the disease: pre-MF, patch, plaque, and tumor. Some patients have only plaques and tumors. Lesions from the last three phases may be present simultaneously. Lymphadenopathy may develop at any stage. Survival time is less than 3 years once the tumor phase begins.[138] Despite the new laboratory diagnostic methods, recognition of the physical signs of the disease by the clinician is still the most sensitive method of detection.

Pre-MF. The pre-MF phase is the first phase in which the diagnosis is suspected, but it cannot be made by clinical or histologic criteria. This premycotic phase persists for months or years and is suspected when inflammation persists and recurs after repeated courses of topical steroids. Spontaneous remissions do occur. Nonspecific pruritic eruptions or pruritus alone may be the only manifestation. A red, scaly, eczematous-like or psoriasis-like eruption and an atrophic, mottled, telangiectatic eruption referred to as *large-patch parapsoriasis* or *poikiloderma vasculare atrophicans* occur. These two latter dermatoses possess characteristic features that allow one to predict with a greater degree of certainty that the evolution of typical MF may occur. These dermatoses can be present for as long as 35 years before the plaques and tumors of MF develop.

ECZEMATOUS FORM. The eczematous form presents with persistent, nonspecific, flat, red, itchy, eczematous areas that resemble asteatotic eczema or atopic dermatitis, except that the lesions tend to remain fixed in location and size, and the margins are sharply delineated (Figure 21-39).

THE POIKILODERMATOUS-PARAPSORIASIS LESION. Lesions of parapsoriasis en plaques are sharply circumscribed and have a faint erythema and sometimes a yellowish cast, a fine scale, and a slightly wrinkled surface. On the trunk and limbs, the lesions are usually 1 to 5 cm and round, oval, or fingerlike (digitate dermatosis). On the buttocks and thighs, where they occur more commonly, lesions present as patches as large as 15 cm. Patients with long-standing parapsoriasis-like lesions that are resistant to conventional treatment require careful monitoring for the possible development of cutaneous lymphoma.[139]

Poikiloderma vasculare atrophicans is a term used to describe lesions that have telangiectasia; "cigarette-paper" skin with fine, wrinkly atrophy; and mottled pigmentation (Figure 21-40). The appearance of poikilodermatous changes is an ominous sign. The terms *parapsoriasis variegata* or

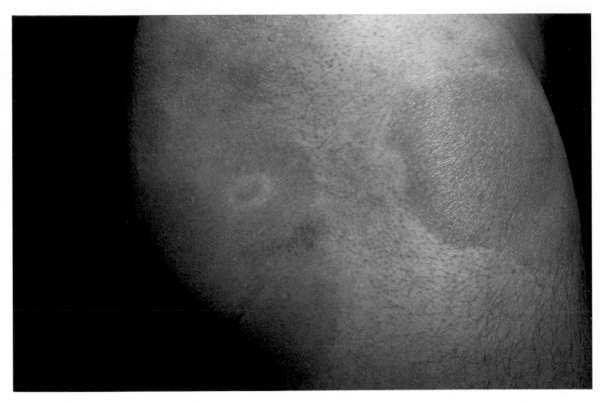

Figure 21-39
Mycosis fungoides. Lesions typical of the eczematous form
or the patch stage. Persistent, flat, red, itchy, well-circumscribed patches can persist for months or years.

Figure 21-40
Mycosis fungoides (poikiloderma vasculare atrophicans).
Red-brown hyperpigmented plaques with an atrophic,
wrinkled surface tend to remain fixed in location.

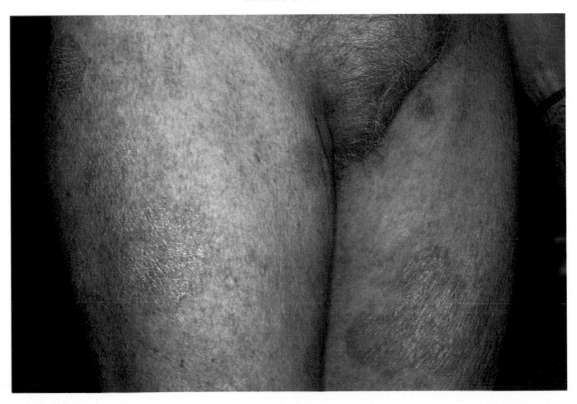

parapsoriasis lichenoides are used to describe variants of these lesions that present with a netlike or reticulated pattern.

Histologic examination shows chronic, nonspecific inflammation in the dermis. The infiltrate may be present as a band in the upper dermis. The inflammatory cells may be polymorphic, and the epidermis may be thickened. A scant number of lymphocytes may be found in the epidermis.

Patch stage. The disease enters the patch stage when histologic changes are characteristic of MF. The morphology of the lesion does not necessarily change (see Figure 21-39).

Plaque stage. The plaque stage is entered gradually when dusky red-to-brown, sometimes scaly areas become elevated above the surrounding uninvolved skin because of acanthosis (thickening of the epidermis). Plaques can arise from uninvolved skin. Itching becomes more persistent and intense and may be intolerable. The plaques vary in shape with round, oval, arciform, or serpiginous patterns, occasionally with central clearing. The extent of involvement varies from a few isolated areas to a major portion of the skin (Figure 21-41). Infiltration of the entire skin produces a thickened red hide with scale (exfoliative dermatitis) or without scale (erythroderma). MF may begin as exfoliative erythroderma. Infiltration and plaques in hairy areas may produce alopecia. Histologically, the plaques exhibit a superficial, deep, perivascular lymphocytic infiltrate with collections of lymphocytes (Pautrier's microabscesses) within a thickened epidermis. The infiltrate becomes mixed (lymphocytes, eosinophils, and plasma cells) as the plaque stage progresses. Some of the lymphocytes are atypical, having a large, hyperconvoluted or cerebriform nucleus ("mycosis cell") (see Figure 21-44). The plaque stage persists for an indefinite period. Plaques regress, remain stationary, or evolve into nodules and tumors.

Tumor stage. Tumors develop from preexisting plaques or erythroderma, or they may originate from red or normal skin (Figure 21-42). Itching may decrease in intensity. Tumors vary in size, some becoming huge or mushroom-shaped (thus the term *mycosis fungoides*, which has been in use for 150 years). Necrosis and ulceration of plaques and tumors are common.

In the early stages, the disease remains confined to the skin. Superficial lymphadenopathy may be detected in the plaque stage, and deep lymphadenopathy with visceral metastasis, such as to the spleen, lungs, or gastrointestinal tract, may occur during the tumor stage.[138]

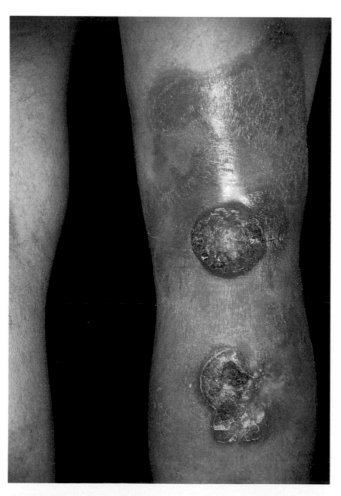

Figure 21-41
Mycosis fungoides. Plaque and tumor stages.

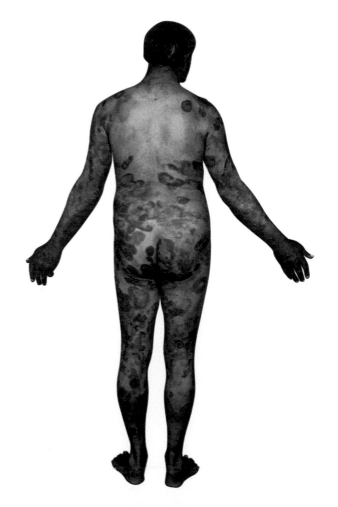

Figure 21-42
Mycosis fungoides. Tumor stage.

Sézary syndrome

Sézary syndrome (SS) is the leukemic form of MF[140] (Figure 21-43). SS consists of the triad of erythroderma, leukemia, and large peripheral lymph nodes. Patients may have generalized pruritus, exfoliative dermatitis and thickening of the skin, ectropion, alopecia, and thickening of the palms and soles. The erythema may wax and wane during the day, or it may disappear and be replaced by plaques and tumors. Erythroderma does not necessarily indicate the presence of SS. Skin biopsy may reveal features resembling those found in the early stages of classic MF.[141] Circulating cells with hyperconvoluted nuclei (Sézary cells) appear to be identical to those found in the skin infiltrates of MF[142] (Figure 21-44).

Diagnosis of CTCL

The diagnosis is made by recognizing the clinical characteristics of the various stages of the disease and is supported by histopathology. It is important to biopsy suspected lesions early enough so that potentially curative treatment can be initiated. Evaluation for systemic involvement includes examination of peripheral blood for Sézary cells and biopsy of palpable lymph nodes. Monoclonal antibody testing and T-cell receptor analysis of peripheral blood and lymph node lymphocytes are new techniques that may help to establish the diagnosis in the earliest stages.[143]

Histology. CTCL presents a difficult diagnostic challenge for the pathologist. The reliability of histopathologic findings is inherently low. Histologic scores do not always correlate with the stages of disease and are not an accurate predictor of clinical outcome. The pathologic diagnosis should be interpreted only in conjunction with the clinical evaluation.[144]

All cells of a clonally derived malignancy, such as CTCL, share a common T-cell receptor. Discovering that many T cells infiltrating a skin lesion have identical T-cell receptor genes suggests that the neoplasm is a malignancy. Examination of the blood and lesions using monoclonal antibodies and T-cell receptor genes may be useful for some patients with erythroderma in which the microscopic appearance is often not diagnostic.[145] At this stage of the disease, the differential diagnosis may include atopic dermatitis, psoriasis, or severe drug reaction. The tests may also be useful in the early nonspecific patch stages of parapsoriasis and eczematous-appearing lesions.

Treatment of CTCL. Some experts feel that the disease can be cured with aggressive treatment when disease is confined to the skin. Stable, localized, nonplaque disease may last for years. Because of the efficacy of topical nitrogen mustard, psoralen activated by UVA light (PUVA), and electron beam therapy in inducing and maintaining remissions, we now rarely see rapid evolution of the disease in patients whose CTCL is diagnosed early.

TOPICAL NITROGEN MUSTARD. Topical nitrogen mustard has been used for more than 20 years and is useful in controlling early-stage disease. An aqueous solution is applied daily to the entire body surface except the groin. Complete responses were achieved in 80%, 68%, and 61% of patients in stages IA, IB, and IIA of the disease, respectively.[146] Topical carmustine (BCNU) is also effective.[147]

PUVA AND UVB. CTCL often begins in sun-shielded regions, such as the buttocks and inferior surface of breasts.

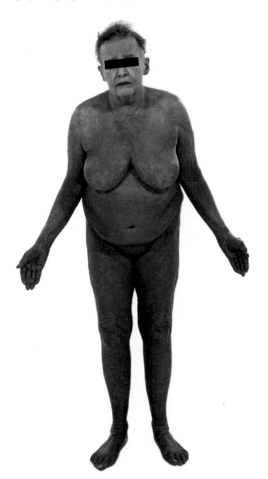

Figure 21-43
Sézary syndrome. Generalized erythroderma with scaling and thickening of the palms and soles.

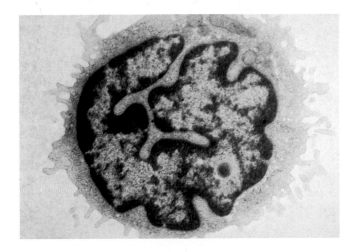

Figure 21-44
Sézary cells. Nuclei are hyperconvoluted.

This suggests that sun exposure to the trunk and extremities alters the environment of certain regions of the skin so that CTCL cells find those sites inhospitable. This may explain why UVB or PUVA therapy can maintain a patient in remission. PUVA is very effective in the limited, "thin," plaque stage of CTCL.[148,149] High rates of remission are induced within 2 to 3 months with a regimen of two or three treatments per week, increasing the dosage of UVA by 0.5 J/cm^2 in alternate treatments, as tolerated. The dosage is held constant, then slowly tapered to once per week, once per 2 weeks, once per month, once every other month for 6 months, and then once every 3 months for an indefinite period. Phototherapy with UVB appears to be effective for patients with early patch-stage CTCL.[150] A combination of interferon and PUVA showed high complete remissions in preliminary studies.[151]

ELECTRON BEAM. Electron beam therapy followed by 6 months of adjuvant chemotherapy (doxorubicin and cyclophosphamide) clearly increased the number and duration of complete remissions and survivals in early-stage patients compared with those treated by electron beam alone. Patients with thick plaques may receive electron beam radiotherapy in 36 doses fractionated to 100 rads each.[152,153]

EXTRACORPOREAL PHOTOPHERESIS. Extracorporeal photopheresis is useful for treating Sézary syndrome and the erythrodermic phase of MF. It is also effective alone or in combination with adjunctive therapy[154] for extensive patch/plaque disease and some tumor-stage disease. Remissions longer than 3 years have been achieved in some patients. Photopheresis involves long-wave radiation (UVA) of leukocytes taken from the patient who has ingested 8-methoxypsoralen, with subsequent reinfusion of the leukocytes to the patient.[155-157] The treatment is given on 2 consecutive days every month for 6 months. Evidence suggests that CTCL cells display small, HLA-associated antigenic peptides on the cell surface that are specific for the malignant clone. Photopheresis alters the peptides. CD8+ cells then recognize the altered peptides and assist in destroying the malignant clone. Patients who have a CD4/CD8 ratio of less than or equal to 5 do better than those with few or no CD8+ cells in their skin.[158]

Individual tumors respond to orthovoltage x-irradiation. Recently published protocols have shown promising results with isotretinoin[159] and acyclovir.[160] All of these treatments for advanced disease may be initially successful in inducing remissions, but none appears to prolong survival.

Lymphomatoid papulosis. Lymphomatoid papulosis is a rare disease in which the skin lesions have a neoplastic-like histology, but the clinical course is benign and chronic.[161] Five percent to 20% of cases evolve into a lymphoma (MF, T-immunoblastic lymphoma, and Hodgkin's disease). Crops of reddish-brown papules undergo central necrosis and spontaneous healing with scar formation. Lesions persist for 2 to 4 weeks before resolving. Papules arise in crops over the trunk and extremities for months to years. The new lesions itch or are painful.

Paget's Disease of the Breast

Paget's disease of the breast results from invasion of the epidermis of the nipple, areola, and surrounding skin by malignant cells originating from an underlying ductal carcinoma.[162] An underlying carcinoma of the breast may be palpated, but in approximately 40% of cases, the cancer is clinically impalpable and radiologically undetectable.[163,164]

Clinical presentation. The disease begins insidiously in one breast with a small area of erythema on the nipple that drains serous fluid and forms a crust (Figure 21-45). The inflammation is usually attributed to trauma, and partial healing comforts the patient. Patients equate lumps rather than inflammatory changes with cancer and, consequently, the disease continues. Malignant cells migrate through the epidermis, and the disease becomes initially apparent on the areola (Figure 21-46) and, at a much later date (a year or more), on the surrounding skin (Figure 21-47). The process appears eczematous, but the plaque is indurated and has sharp margins, which remain relatively fixed for weeks. Ulceration is a late finding. Paget's disease of the male nipple is very rare and is more aggressive than in females.

Diagnosis. Clinically and histologically, the process is very similar to Bowen's disease; however, Bowen's disease of the nipple is very rare. A crucial point to note is that Paget's disease of the breast is a rare, unilateral disease, whereas eczematous inflammation of the nipples is common and almost invariably bilateral. Cytologic diagnosis can be made from nipple scrape smears.[165] A biopsy may be studied with conventional stains and immunohistochemistry. Immunocytochemical techniques are more reliable for distinguishing Paget's disease from superficial spreading malignant melanoma and from primary intraepidermal carcinoma than conventional mucin histochemistry using diastase periodic-acid-Schiff (d-PAS) with and without alcian blue. Positive immunoreactivity occurs with cytokeratin (CAM 5.2), c-erb B-2 oncoprotein (21N), and carcinoembryonic antigen (CEA). CEA is seen in virtually all cases of mammary Paget's disease, with consistent negative immunoreactivity in melanoma and other tumor types.[166,167]

Treatment. After biopsy, treatment is surgical. Cone excision of the nipple-areola complex was described as inadequate in one study.[168] Another study reported success with local radiotherapy when disease was confined to the nipple.[169]

PAGET'S DISEASE OF THE BREAST

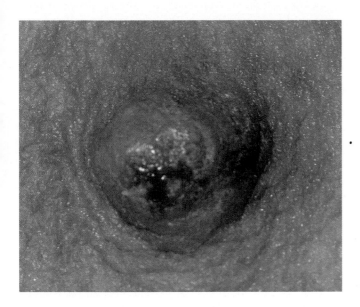

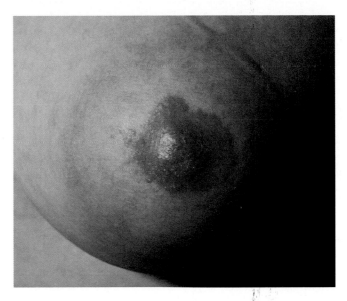

Figure 21-45
Inflammation of both nipples is usually eczema, but inflammation of one nipple is characteristic of Paget's disease. Early Paget's disease appears as little more than a slight irritation, and patients often wait months to inquire about the nonhealing process.

Figure 21-46
The lesion has insidiously spread for 1 year to infiltrate the areola and surrounding skin.

Figure 21-47
A red, scaling plaque drains serous fluid and forms crust. The lesion appears eczematous but, unlike eczema, is unilateral.

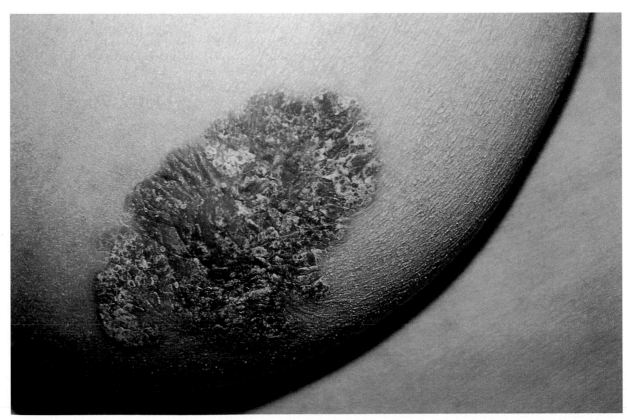

Extramammary Paget's Disease

Extramammary Paget's disease is a rare cutaneous adenocarcinoma that occurs in elderly women more often than in men and is located in the vulva, scrotum, axilla, or the perianal area. Various histochemical studies suggest evidence of sweat gland derivation of the disease.[170,171]

Association with underlying malignancy. The disease may be associated with an underlying adenocarcinoma or carcinoma of the rectum, and 26% of affected patients ultimately die either from the disease itself or from an associated internal malignancy. Twenty-four percent have an associated underlying cutaneous adnexal adenocarcinoma. These patients have a higher mortality rate (46%) than patients with extramammary Paget's disease without underlying cutaneous adnexal adenocarcinoma. Twelve percent of patients with extramammary Paget's disease have an associated concurrent underlying internal malignancy.[172] The location of the underlying internal malignancy is closely related to the location of the cutaneous disease; that is, a perianal location is associated with adenocarcinoma of the digestive system, a penile location is associated with genitourinary malignancy, etc. As with Paget's disease of the breast, the epidermis is infiltrated with malignant cells that migrate laterally. Biopsy often reveals cells that are exterior to the clinically apparent areas, a fact that explains the high rate of recurrence after excision.

Clinical presentation. The disease in males and females appears as a white-to-red, scaling or macerated, infiltrated, eroded, or ulcerated plaque, most frequently observed on the labia majora (Figure 21-48) and scrotum[173] (Figure 21-49). Persistent itching and burning are common. The clinical presentation closely resembles lichen sclerosus et atrophicus, lichen simplex chronicus, leukoplakia, Bowen's disease, or chronic yeast infection.

Histology. Histologically, Paget's disease resembles Bowen's disease and superficial spreading melanoma. Paget's cells are mucin positive, as determined by Hale's colloidal iron stain. The cytoplasm is often PAS-positive and stains with alcian blue at pH 2.5. Immunoperoxidase stains are helpful in establishing the diagnosis and in excluding conditions that resemble Paget's disease. Most cases are CEA positive.[174] CEA is a sweat gland marker. Antikeratin stains Bowen's disease and anti-S-100 protein stain is positive in melanoma.

Management. Conventional surgical excision or Mohs' micrographic surgery,[175] followed optionally by radiation therapy,[176,177] is the treatment for regionally confined disease. A nonradical conservative surgical approach has been advocated. In one study, skinning vulvectomy with split-thickness skin graft, hemivulvectomy, and simple vulvectomy produced excellent results for patients with limited disease without an underlying adenocarcinoma.[178] Fluorescein given intravenously helps to visualize disease margins with the use of an ultraviolet light.[179] Recurrent Paget's disease of the vulva has been treated successfully with topical bleomycin.[180] All patients with extramammary Paget's disease should have a careful physical examination to search for internal malignancy.

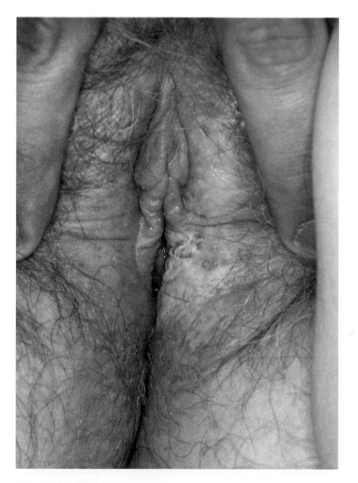

Figure 21-48
Extramammary Paget's disease. A white, eroded plaque with ill-defined borders on the labia.

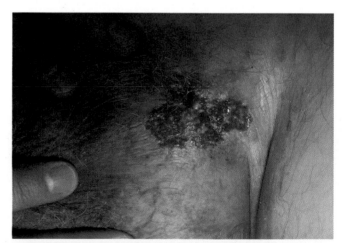

Figure 21-49
Extramammary Paget's disease. Three biopsies were taken before malignant cells were demonstrated at the periphery of this chronic ulcer at the base of the scrotum.

Cutaneous Metastasis

The incidence of cutaneous metastasis in patients with malignancy is approximately 2% to 10%.[181-185] Cutaneous metastases may be the first sign of extranodal metastatic disease, particularly in patients with melanoma, breast cancer, or mucosal cancers of the head and neck.[186] In a series of papers, Brownstein and Helwig[183-185] stated several aspects of cutaneous metastasis. They determined the incidence and relative importance of the sex of the patient, the location of the metastatic growth, the morphology of the metastatic lesion, and the histologic features of the metastatic lesion in identifying the site of the primary tumor. The incidence of some of these features is summarized in Tables 21-4 and 21-5 and is illustrated in Figure 21-50. The most helpful information for localizing the primary tumor is the sex of the patient and the location of the skin tumor.

Morphology of metastatic lesions. The most common representation of cutaneous metastasis is an aggregate of discrete, firm, nontender, skin-colored nodules that appear suddenly, grow rapidly, attain a certain size (often 2 cm), and remain stationary (Figure 21-51). Accurate clinical diagnosis is rare; the lesions are most frequently diagnosed as cysts or benign fibrous tumors. In several instances, the clinical picture is that of a vascular tumor such as a pyogenic granuloma, hemangioma, or Kaposi's sarcoma (Figure 21-52). The periumbilical Sister Mary Joseph's nodule heralds an underlying gastric tumor.

TABLE 21-4 Origins of Skin Metastases

	Men			Women		
Primary site	Cases with skin metastases	%	Primary site	Cases with skin metastases	%
Lung	132	22.4	Breast	380	71.0
Melanoma	103	17.5	Melanoma	49	9.1
Colon and rectum	104	17.7	Colon and rectum	26	4.8
Oral cavity	68	11.6	Ovary	20	3.7
Kidney	35	6.0	Lung	15	2.8
Upper digestive tract	35	6.0	Unknown	9	1.6
Breast	12	2.0	Oral cavity	9	1.6
Stomach	29	4.9	Endometrium	4	0.7
Esophagus	18	3.1	Urinary bladder	6	1.1
Urinary bladder	11	1.9	Uterine cervix	6	1.1
Unknown	11	1.9	Stomach	3	0.6
Pancreas	13	2.2	Bile ducts	3	0.6
Larynx	7	1.2	Pancreas	4	0.6
Liver	4	0.7			
Nasal sinuses	3	0.5			
TOTAL	**587**			**535**	

Adapted from Lookingbill DP, Spangler N, et al: *J Am Acad Dermatol* 29:228-236, 1993; and Brownstein MH, Helwig EB: *Cancer* 29:1298, 1972.

TABLE 21-5 Sites of distant skin metastases

Primary site	Scalp	Face	Neck	Shoulders	Chest	Back	Abdomen	Upper extremities	Lower extremities
Breast	18	2	12	11	4	37	15	16	9
Melanoma	10	7	21	7	28	8	10	21	25
Unknown	4	3	5	0	1	2	5	2	6
Lung	2	1	2	0	9	2	7	1	1
Oral cavity	2	2	4	0	1	1	0	1	0
Colon and rectum	1	1	0	0	2	2	2	0	0

Modified from Lookingbill DP, Spangler N, et al: *J Am Acad Dermatol* 29:228-236, 1993.

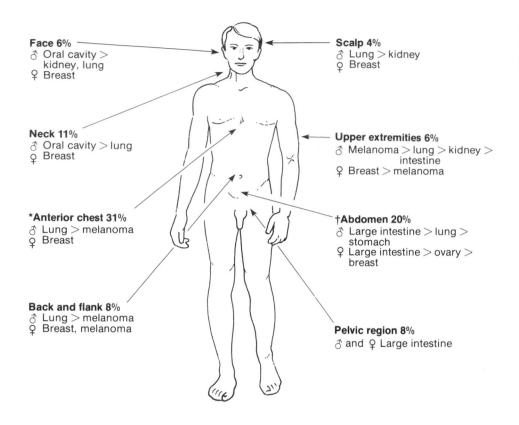

Face 6%
♂ Oral cavity >
kidney, lung
♀ Breast

Scalp 4%
♂ Lung > kidney
♀ Breast

Neck 11%
♂ Oral cavity > lung
♀ Breast

Upper extremities 6%
♂ Melanoma > lung > kidney >
intestine
♀ Breast > melanoma

*Anterior chest 31%
♂ Lung > melanoma
♀ Breast

†Abdomen 20%
♂ Large intestine > lung >
stomach
♀ Large intestine > ovary >
breast

Back and flank 8%
♂ Lung > melanoma
♀ Breast, melanoma

Pelvic region 8%
♂ and ♀ Large intestine

Figure 21-50
Patterns of cutaneous metastasis. 724 patients. Percentages are of the total number of cases. *(Modified from Brownstein MN, Helwig EB: Arch Dermatol 105:862, 1972.)*

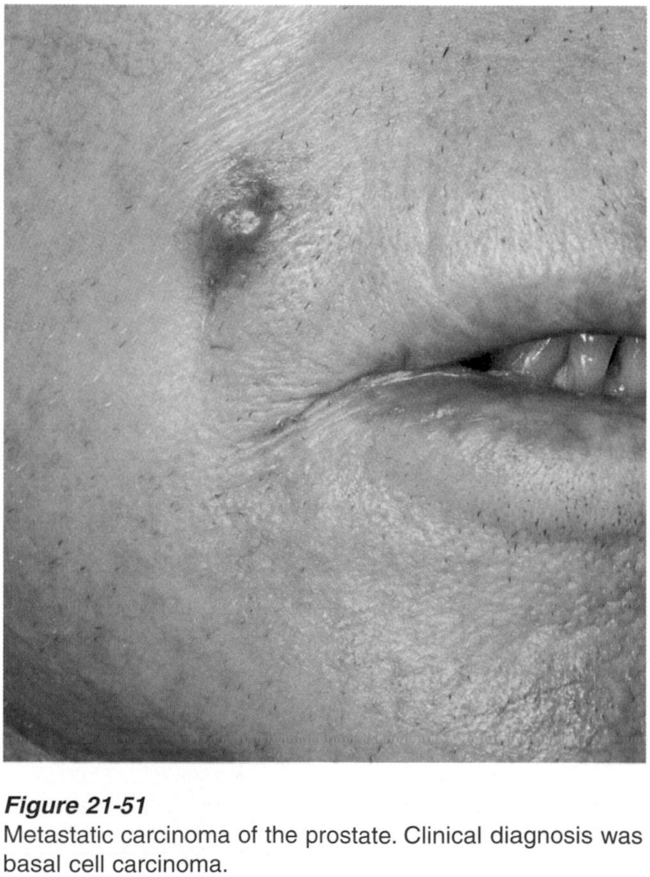

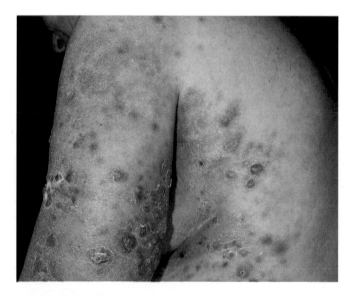

Figure 21-51
Metastatic carcinoma of the prostate. Clinical diagnosis was basal cell carcinoma.

Figure 21-52
Metastatic carcinoma of the breast. Nodules appear vascular and resemble Kaposi's sarcoma.

The second most common pattern of cutaneous metastasis is inflammation with erythema, edema, warmth (Figures 21-53 and 21-54), and tenderness. The primary tumor is usually in the breast, and malignant cells spread to the subepidermal lymphatic vessels, where they create obstruction. The initial diagnosis is frequently a bacterial infection, such as erysipelas or cellulitis. The patient is, however, afebrile and appears to be healthy.

The third and least common pattern simulates a cicatricial condition and resembles discoid lupus erythematosus or morphea. Asymptomatic sclerodermoid plaques, sometimes associated with hair loss (alopecia neoplastica), are most frequently located on the scalp and are caused by metastasis from breast cancer in women and lung or kidney tumors in men. Carcinoma en cuirasse is seen with breast cancer and appears as a hard, infiltrated plaque with a leathery appearance that results from fibrosis and lymph stasis.

Histology of cutaneous metastasis. In general, the histologic features of primary and metastatic tumors are similar, but metastatic tumors are often less differentiated. Frequently, biopsy specimens are not interpreted as originating from a distant site. Adenocarcinoma metastatic to the skin is most often secondary to cancer of the large intestine, lung, or breast. Squamous cell carcinoma metastatic to the skin customarily originates from the oral cavity, lung, or esophagus. Undifferentiated lesions usually originate from the breast or lungs.

Mode of spread. Tumors that invade veins, such as carcinoma of the kidney and lung, frequently present as cutaneous metastasis occurring in diverse skin sites distant from the primary tumor. Cancers that invade lymphatics, such as carcinoma of the breast and squamous cell carcinoma of the oral cavity, appear late in the course of the disease and may invade skin overlying the primary tumor.[74]

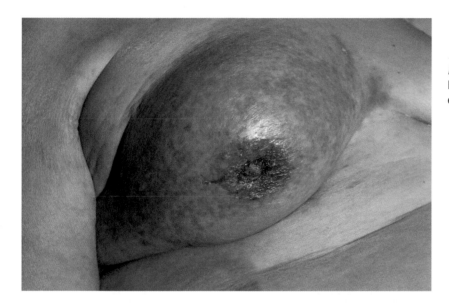

Figure 21-53
Inflammatory cutaneous metastasis with erythema, edema, and crusting.

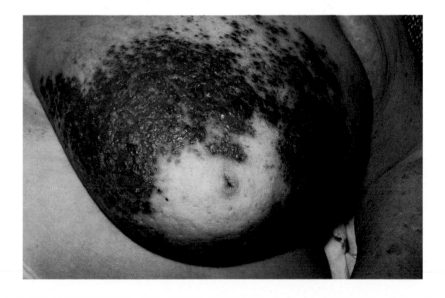

Figure 21-54
Inflammatory cutaneous metastasis. Erosion and crusting resemble infected eczema.

REFERENCES

1. Preston DS, Stern RS: Nonmelanoma cancers of the skin, *N Engl J Med* 327:1649-1662, 1992.
2. Zaynoun S, Ali LA, Shaib J, et al: The relationship of sun exposure and solar elastosis to basal cell carcinoma, *J Am Acad Dermatol* 12:522-525, 1985.
3. Pearl DK, Scott EL: The anatomical distribution of skin cancers, *Int J Epidemiol* 15:502-506, 1986.
4. Reizner GT, Chuang TY, et al: Basal cell carcinoma in Kauai, Hawaii: the highest documented incidence in the United States, *J Am Acad Dermatol* 29:184-189, 1993.
5. Cox NH: Basal cell carcinoma in young adults, *Br J Dermatol* 127:26-29, 1992.
6. Miller SJ: Biology of basal cell carcinoma (part I), *J Am Acad Dermatol* 24:1-13, 1991.
7. Miller SJ: Biology of basal cell carcinoma (part II), *J Am Acad Dermatol* 24:161-175, 1991.
8. Franchimont C et al: Episodic progression and regression of basal cell carcinomas, *Br J Dermatol* 106:305-310, 1982.
9. Rustin MHA, Chambers TJ, Munro DD: Post-traumatic basal cell carcinomas, *Clin Exp Dermatol* 9:379-383, 1984.
10. Sexton M, Jones DB, et al: Histologic pattern analysis of basal cell carcinoma. Study of a series of 1039 consecutive neoplasms, *J Am Acad Dermatol* 23:1118-1126, 1990.
11. Phillips TJ, Salman SM, et al: Nonhealing leg ulcers: a manifestation of basal cell carcinoma, *J Am Acad Dermatol* 25:47-49, 1991.
12. Maloney ME, Jones DB, et al: Pigmented basal cell carcinoma: investigation of 70 cases, *J Am Acad Dermatol* 27:74-78, 1992.
13. Salasche SJ, Amonette RA: Morpheaform basal cell epitheliomas: a study of subclinical extensions in a series of 51 cases, *J Dermatol Surg Oncol* 7:387-393, 1981.
14. Farndon PA, Del Mastro RG, et al: Location of gene for Gorlin syndrome, *Lancet* 339:581-582, 1992.
15. Chenevix-Trench G, Wicking C, et al: Further localization of the gene for nevoid basal cell carcinoma syndrome (NBCCS) in 15 Australasian families: linkage and loss of heterozygosity, *Am J Hum Genet* 53:760-767, 1993.
16. Gorlin RJ: Nevoid basal-cell carcinoma syndrome, *Medicine* 66:98-113, 1987.
17. Gutierrez MM, Mora RG: Nevoid basal carcinoma syndrome. A review and case report of a patient with unilateral basal cell nevus syndrome, *J Am Acad Dermatol* 15:1023-1030, 1986.
18. Evans DG, Ladusans EJ, et al: Complications of the nevoid basal cell carcinoma syndrome: results of a population based study, *J Med Genet* 30:460-464, 1993.
19. Pratt MD, Jackson R: Nevoid basal cell carcinoma syndrome. A 15-year follow-up of cases in Ottawa and the Ottawa valley, *J Am Acad Dermatol* 16:964-970, 1987.
20. Howell JB: Nevoid basal cell carcinoma syndrome, *J Am Acad Dermatol* 11:98-104, 1984.
21. Goldstein AM, Bale SJ, et al: Sun exposure and basal cell carcinomas in the nevoid basal cell carcinoma syndrome, *J Am Acad Dermatol* 29:34-41, 1993.
22. Correl RW: Bilateral cysts of the jaw occurring with multiple skin lesions, *J Am Dent Assoc* 101:978-979, 1980.
23. Drake LA, Ceilley RI, et al: Guidelines of care for basal cell carcinoma. The American Academy of Dermatology Committee on Guidelines of Care, *J Am Acad Dermatol* 26:117-120, 1992.
24. Lang PG, Maize JC: Histologic evolution of recurrent basal cell carcinoma and treatment implications, *J Am Acad Dermatol* 14:186-196, 1986.
25. McDaniel WE: Adequate follow up for treated basal cell carcinoma, *Arch Dermatol* 122:243-244, 1986.
26. Marghoob A, Kopf AW, et al: Risk of another basal cell carcinoma developing after treatment of a basal cell carcinoma, *J Am Acad Dermatol* 28:22-28, 1993.
27. Karagas MR, Stukel TA, et al: Risk of subsequent basal cell carcinoma and squamous cell carcinoma of the skin among patients with prior skin cancer. Skin Cancer Prevention Study Group, *JAMA* 267:3305-3310, 1992.
28. Epstein E: Value of follow-up after treatment of basal cell carcinoma, *Arch Dermatol* 108:798-800, 1973.
29. Leonforte JF: Deep recurrent basal cell epithelioma, *J Am Acad Dermatol* 16:1257-1259, 1987.
30. Dubin N, Kopf AW: Multivariate risk score for recurrence of cutaneous basal cell carcinomas, *Arch Dermatol* 119:373-377, 1983.
31. McDaniel WE: Therapy for basal cell epitheliomas by curettage only, *Arch Dermatol* 119:901-903, 1983.
32. Spiller WF, Spiller RF: Treatment of basal cell epithelioma by curettage and electrodesiccation, *J Am Acad Dermatol* 11:808-814, 1984.
33. Kopf AW et al: Curettage-electrodesiccation treatment of basal cell carcinomas, *Arch Dermatol* 113:439-443, 1977.
34. Whelan CS, Deckers PJ: Electrocoagulation for skin cancer: an old oncologic tool revisited, *Cancer* 47:2280-2287, 1981.
35. Salasche SJ: Curettage and electrodesiccation in the treatment of mid-facial basal cell epithelioma, *J Am Acad Dermatol* 8:496-503, 1983.
36. Silverman MK, Kopf AW, et al: Recurrence rates of treated basal cell carcinomas. Part 2: Curettage-electrodesiccation, *J Dermatol Surg Oncol* 17:720-726, 1991.
37. Wolf DJ, Zitelli JA: Surgical margins for basal cell carcinoma, *Arch Dermatol* 123:340-344, 1987.
38. Silverman MK, Kopf AW, et al: Recurrence rates of treated basal cell carcinomas. Part 3: Surgical excision, *J Dermatol Surg Oncol* 18:471-476, 1992.
39. Richmond JD, Davie RM: The significance of incomplete excision in patients with basal cell carcinoma, *Br J Plast Surg* 40:63-67, 1987.
40. Torre D: Cryosurgery of basal cell carcinoma, *J Am Acad Dermatol* 15:917-929, 1986.
41. Buker JL, Amonette RA: Micrographic surgery, *Clin Dermatol* 10:309-315, 1992.
42. Wilder RB, Kittelson JM, et al: Basal cell carcinoma treated with radiation therapy, *Cancer* 68:2134-2137, 1991.
43. Silverman MK, Kopf AW, et al: Recurrence rates of treated basal cell carcinomas. Part 4: X-ray therapy, *J Dermatol Surg Oncol* 18:549-554, 1992.
44. Wilder RB, Shimm DS, et al: Recurrent basal cell carcinoma treated with radiation therapy, *Arch Dermatol* 127:1668-1672, 1991.
45. Labandter HP, Ryan RF: 5-fluorouracil in management of Gorlin's syndrome, *N Engl J Med* 298:913, 1978.
46. Stenquist B, Wennberg AM, et al: Treatment of aggressive basal cell carcinoma with intralesional interferon: evaluation of efficacy by Mohs surgery, *J Am Acad Dermatol* 27:65-69, 1992.
47. Marks R et al: Spontaneous remission of solar keratoses: the case for conservative management, *Br J Dermatol* 115:649-655, 1986.
48. Dodson JM, De Spain J, et al: Malignant potential of actinic keratoses and the controversy over treatment. A patient-oriented perspective, *Arch Dermatol* 127:1029-1031, 1991.
49. Marks R, Rennie G, Selwood TS: Malignant transformation of solar keratoses to squamous cell carcinoma, *Lancet* 1:795-797, 1988.
50. Moller R, Reymann F, Hou-Jensen K: Metastases in dermatological patients with squamous cell carcinoma, *Arch Dermatol* 115:703-705, 1979.
51. Alamillos-Granados FJ, Naval-Gias L, et al: Carbon dioxide laser vermilionectomy for actinic cheilitis, *J Oral Maxillofac Surg* 51:118-121, 1993.
52. Johnson TM, Sebastien TS, et al: Carbon dioxide laser treatment of actinic cheilitis. Clinicohistopathologic correlation to determine the optimal depth of destruction, *J Am Acad Dermatol* 27:737-740, 1992.
53. Gilchrest BA: Retinoids and photodamage, *Br J Dermatol* 127:14-20, 1992.
54. Thompson SC, Jollcy D, et al: Reduction of solar keratoses by regular sunscreen use , *N Engl J Med* 329:1147-1151, 1993.

55. Moy LS, Murad H, et al: Glycolic acid peels for the treatment of wrinkles and photoaging, *J Dermatol Surg Oncol* 19:243-246, 1993.

56. Lawrence N et al: A comparison of the efficacy and safety of Jessner's solution and 35% trichloroacetic acid vs. 5% fluorouracil in the treatment of widespread facial actinic keratosis, *Arch Dermatol* 131:176-181, 1995.

57. Goette DK: Topical chemotherapy with 5-fluorouracil. A review, *J Am Acad Dermatol* 4:633-649, 1981.

58. Olsen EA, Abernethy ML, et al: A double-blind, vehicle-controlled study evaluating masoprocol cream in the treatment of actinic keratoses on the head and neck, *J Am Acad Dermatol* 24:738-743, 1991.

59. Unis ME: Short-term intensive 5-fluorouracil treatment of actinic keratosis, *Dermatol Surg* 21:162-163, 1995.

60. Pearlman DL: Weekly pulse dosing: effective and comfortable topical 5-fluorouracil treatment of multiple facial actinic keratoses, *J Am Acad Dermatol* 25:665-667, 1991.

61. Bennett R et al: Current management using 5-fluorouracil: 1985, *Cutis*:218, 1985.

62. Black HS et al: Effect of a low fat diet on the incidence of actinic keratosis, *N Engl J Med* 330:1272-1275, 1994.

63. Hartevelt MM, Bavinck JN, et al: Incidence of skin cancer after renal transplantation in the Netherlands, *Transplantation* 49:506-509, 1990.

64. Kwa RE, Campana K, Moy RL: Biology of cutaneous squamous cell carcinoma, *J Am Acad Dermatol* 26:1-26, 1992.

65. Rowe DE, Carroll RJ, et al: Prognostic factors for local recurrence, metastasis, and survival rates in squamous cell carcinoma of the skin, ear, and lip. Implications for treatment modality selection, *J Am Acad Dermatol* 26:976-990, 1992.

66. Dinehart SM, Pollack SV: Metastases from squamous cell carcinoma of the skin and lip, *J Am Acad Dermatol* 21:241-248, 1989.

67. Breuninger H, Black B, et al: Microstaging of squamous cell carcinomas, *Am J Clin Pathol* 94:624-627, 1990.

68. Friedman HI, Cooper PH, Wanebo HJ: Prognostic and therapeutic use of microstaging of cutaneous squamous cell carcinoma of the trunk and extremities, *Cancer* 56:1099-1105, 1985.

69. Brodland DG, Zitelli JA: Surgical margins for excision of primary cutaneous squamous cell carcinoma, *J Am Acad Dermatol* 27:241-248, 1992.

70. Dinehart SM, Chu DZ, et al: Immunosuppression in patients with metastatic squamous cell carcinoma from the skin, *J Dermatol Surg Oncol* 16:271-274, 1990.

71. Boyle J, MacKie RM, et al: Cancer, warts, and sunshine in renal transplant patients: a case-control study, *Lancet* 1:702-705, 1984.

72. Bavinck JN et al: Relation between skin cancer and HLA antigens in renal-transplant recipients, *N Engl J Med* 325:843-848, 1991.

73. Johnson TM, Rowe DE, et al: Squamous cell carcinoma of the skin (excluding lip and oral mucosa), *J Am Acad Dermatol* 26:467-484, 1992.

74. Brodland DG, Zitelli JA: Mechanisms of metastasis, *J Am Acad Dermatol* 27:1-8, 1992.

75. Hosal IN, Onerci M, et al: Squamous cell carcinoma of the lower lip, *Am J Otolaryngol* 13:363-365, 1992.

76. McGregor GI, Davis NL, et al: Impact of cervical lymph node metastases from squamous cell cancer of the lip, *Am J Surg* 163:469-471, 1992.

77. Task Force on Cutaneous Squamous Cell Carcinoma: Guidelines of care for cutaneous squamous cell carcinoma. Committee on Guidelines of Care, *J Am Acad Dermatol* 28:628-631, 1993.

78. Sadek H, Azli N, et al: Treatment of advanced squamous cell carcinoma of the skin with cisplatin, 5-fluorouracil, and bleomycin, *Cancer* 66:1692-1696, 1990.

79. Lippman SM, Parkinson DR, et al: 13-cis-retinoic acid and interferon alpha-2a: effective combination therapy for advanced squamous cell carcinoma of the skin, *J Natl Cancer Inst* 84:235-241, 1992.

80. Stankard CE, Cruse CW, et al: Chronic pressure ulcer carcinomas, *Ann Plast Surg* 30:274-277, 1993.

81. Fleming MD, Hunt JL, et al: Marjolin's ulcer: a review and reevaluation of a difficult problem, *J Burn Care Rehabil* 11:460-469, 1990.

82. Novick M et al: Burn scar carcinoma: a review and analysis of 46 cases, *J Trauma* 17:808-817, 1977.

83. Lifeso RM, Bull CA: Squamous cell carcinoma of the extremities, *Cancer* 55:2862-2867, 1985.

84. Kossard S, Rosen R: Cutaneous Bowen's disease. An analysis of 1001 cases according to age, sex, and site, *J Am Acad Dermatol* 27:406-410, 1992.

85. Reed W, Oppedal BR, et al: Immunohistology is valuable in distinguishing between Paget's disease, Bowen's disease and superficial spreading malignant melanoma, *Histopathology* 16:583-585, 1990.

86. Chuang TY, Tse J, et al: Bowen's disease (squamous cell carcinoma in situ) as a skin marker for internal malignancy: a case-control study, *Am J Prev Med* 6:238-243, 1990.

87. Chute CG, Chuang TY, et al: The subsequent risk of internal cancer with Bowen's disease, *JAMA* 266:816-819, 1991.

88. Lycka BA: Bowen's disease and internal malignancy. A meta-analysis, *Int J Dermatol* 28:531-533, 1989.

89. Rasmussen OO, Christiansen J: Conservative management of Bowen's disease of the anus, *Int J Colorectal Dis* 4:164-166, 1989.

90. Beck DE, Fazio VW: Premalignant lesions of the anal margin, *South Med J* 82:470-474, 1989.

91. Sturm HM: Bowen's disease and 5-fluorouracil, *J Am Acad Dermatol* 1:513-522, 1979.

92. Baker EJ, Hobbs ER: Enhancement of the clinical margins of Bowen's disease by acetowhitening, *J Dermatol Surg Oncol* 16:846-850, 1990.

93. Jones CM, Mang T, et al: Photodynamic therapy in the treatment of Bowen's disease, *J Am Acad Dermatol* 27:979-982, 1992.

94. Buchanan RB, Carruth JA, et al: Photodynamic therapy in the treatment of malignant tumours of the skin and head and neck, *Eur J Surg Oncol* 15:400-406, 1989.

95. Goette DK et al: Erythroplasia of Queyrat: treatment with topically applied 5-fluorouracil, *JAMA* 232:934, 1975.

96. Greenbaum SS, Glogau R, et al: Carbon dioxide laser treatment of erythroplasia of Queyrat, *J Dermatol Surg Oncol* 15:747-750, 1989.

97. Crissman JD, Visscher DW, et al: Premalignant lesions of the upper aerodigestive tract: pathologic classification, *J Cell Biochem Suppl* 1:49-56, 1993.

98. Silverman S Jr, Gorsky M, Lozada F: Oral leukoplakia and malignant transformation: a follow-up study of 257 patients, *Cancer* 53:563, 1984.

99. Dorey JL, Blasberg B, Conklin RJ, et al: Oral leukoplakia: current concepts in diagnosis, management, and malignant potential, *Int J Dermatol* 23:638-642, 1984.

100. Kramer IRH: Oral leukoplakia, *J R Soc Med* 73:765-767, 1980.

101. Lupton GP et al: Oral hairy leukoplakia, a distinctive marker of human T-cell lymphotropic virus type III (HTLV-III) infection, *Arch Dermatol* 123:624-628, 1987.

102. Greenspan D et al: Oral "hairy" leukoplakia in male homosexuals: evidence of association with both papillomavirus and a herpes-group virus, *Lancet* 2:831-834, 1984.

103. Shklar G: Oral leukoplakia, *N Engl J Med* 315:1544-1545, 1986.

104. Banoczy J, Csiba A: Comparative study of the clinical picture and histopathologic structure of oral leukoplakia, *Cancer* 29:1230-1234, 1972.

105. Horch HH, Gerlach KL: CO_2 laser treatment of oral dysplastic precancerous lesions: a preliminary report, *Lasers Surg Med* 2:179-185, 1982.

106. Al-Drouby HAL: Oral leukoplakia and cryotherapy, *Br Dent J* 155:124-125, 1983.

107. Garewal HS, Meyskens F Jr, et al: Response of oral leukoplakia to beta-carotene, *J Clin Oncol* 8:1715-1720, 1990.

108. Lippman SM, Batsakis JG, et al: Comparison of low-dose isotretinoin with beta carotene to prevent oral carcinogenesis, *N Engl J Med* 328:15-20, 1993.

109. Roed-Petersen B: Effect on oral leukoplakia of reducing or ceasing tobacco smoking, *Acta Derm Venereol* 62:164-167, 1982.

110. Schwartz RA: Verrucous carcinoma of the skin and mucosa, *J Am Acad Dermatol* 32:1-21, 1995.

111. Kao GF, Graham JH, Helwig EB: Carcinoma cuniculatum (verrucous carcinoma of the skin): a clinicopathologic study of 46 cases with ultrastructural observations, *Cancer* 49:2395-2403, 1982.

112. Rubben A, Beaudenon S, et al: Rearrangements of the upstream regulatory region of human papillomavirus type 6 can be found in both Buschke-Lowenstein tumours and in condylomata acuminata, *J Gen Virol* 73:3147-3153, 1992.

113. Noel JC, Vandenbossche M, et al: Verrucous carcinoma of the penis: importance of human papillomavirus typing for diagnosis and therapeutic decision, *Eur Urol* 22:83-85, 1992.

114. Frankel AH, Warren AM: Verrucous squamous cell carcinoma, *J Foot Surg* 25:307-310, 1986.

115. Mora RG: Microscopically controlled surgery (Mohs' chemosurgery) for treatment of verrucous squamous cell carcinoma of the foot (epithelioma cuniculatum), *J Am Acad Dermatol* 8:354-362, 1983.

116. Reinecke L, Thornley AL: Case report: radiotherapy—an effective treatment for vaginal verrucous carcinoma, *Br J Radiol* 66:375-378, 1993.

117. Persky M: Carbon dioxide laser treatment of oral florid papillomatosis, *J Dermatol Surg Oncol* 10:64-66, 1984.

118. Ilkay AK, Chodak GW, et al: Buschke-Lowenstein tumor: therapeutic options including systemic chemotherapy, *Urology* 42:599-602, 1993.

119. Burg G, Sobetzko R: Florid oral papillomatosis: an indication for etretinate? *Hautarzt* 41:314-316, 1990.

120. Gilbert P, Beckert R: Combination therapy for penile giant Buschke-Lowenstein condyloma, *Urol Int* 45:122-124, 1990.

121. Gross G, Roussaki A, et al: Recurrent vulvar Buschke-Lowenstein's tumor-like condylomata acuminata and Hodgkin's disease effectively treated with recombinant interferon-alpha 2c gel as adjuvant to electrosurgery, *Curr Probl Dermatol* 18:178-184, 1989.

122. Schwartz RA: Buschke-Lowenstein tumor: verrucous carcinoma of the penis, *J Am Acad Dermatol* 23:723-727, 1990.

123. Creasman C, Haas PA, et al: Malignant transformation of anorectal giant condyloma acuminatum (Buschke-Loewenstein tumor), *Dis Colon Rectum* 32:481-487, 1989.

124. Cannon CR, Hayne ST: Concurrent verrucous carcinomas of the lip and buccal mucosa, *South Med J* 86:691-693, 1993.

125. Rajendran R, Sugathan CK, et al: Ackerman's tumour (verrucous carcinoma) of the oral cavity: a histopathologic study of 426 cases, *Singapore Dent J* 14:48-53, 1989.

126. Smith P Jr, Hylinski JH, et al: Verrucous carcinoma: epithelioma cuniculatum plantare, *J Foot Surg* 31:324-328, 1992.

127. Fugate DS, Romash MM: Carcinoma cuniculatum (verrucous carcinoma) of the foot, *Foot Ankle* 9:257-259, 1989.

128. Cuzick J, Sasieni P, et al: Ingested arsenic, keratoses, and bladder cancer, *Am J Epidemiol* 136:417-421, 1992.

129. Jaafar R, Omar I, et al: Skin cancer caused by chronic arsenical poisoning—a report of three cases, *Med J Malaysia* 48:86-92, 1993.

130. Mazumder DN, Das Gupta J, et al: Environmental pollution and chronic arsenicosis in south Calcutta, *Bull World Health Organ* 70:481-485, 1992.

131. Burns MK, Ellis CN, et al: Mycosis fungoides–type cutaneous T-cell lymphoma arising before 30 years of age. Immunophenotypic, immunogenotypic and clinicopathologic analysis of nine cases, *J Am Acad Dermatol* 27:974-978, 1992.

132. Bertness V et al: T-cell receptor gene rearrangements are clinical markers of human T-cell lymphomas, *N Engl J Med* 313:534-538, 1985.

133. Weiss LM et al: Clonal rearrangements of T-cell receptor genes in mycosis fungoides and dermatopathic lymphadenopathy, *N Engl J Med* 313:539-544, 1985.

134. Heald PW, Edelson RL: New therapies for cutaneous T-cell lymphoma, *Arch Dermatol* 123:189-191, 1986.

135. Broder S et al: The Sézary syndrome: a malignant proliferation of helper T cells, *J Clin Invest* 58:1297-1306, 1976.

136. Borowitz MJ, Weidner A, et al: Abnormalities of circulating T-cell subpopulations in patients with cutaneous T-cell lymphoma: cutaneous lymphocyte-associated antigen expression on T cells correlates with extent of disease, *Leukemia* 7:859-863, 1993.

137. Berg EL, Yoshino T, Rott LS, et al: The cutaneous lymphocyte antigen is a skin lymphocyte homing receptor for the vascular lectin endothelial cell-leukocyte adhesion molecule-1, *J Exp Med* 174:1461-1466, 1991.

138. Epstein EH et al: Mycosis fungoides: survival, prognostic features, response to therapy, and autopsy findings, *Medicine* 15:61-72, 1972.

139. Kikuchi A, Naka W, et al: Parapsoriasis en plaques: its potential for progression to malignant lymphoma, *J Am Acad Dermatol* 29:419-422, 1993.

140. Miller RA et al: Sézary syndrome: a model for migration of T lymphocytes to skin, *N Engl J Med* 303:89-92, 1980.

141. Buechner SA, Winkelmann RK: Sézary syndrome. A clinicopathologic study of 39 cases, *Arch Dermatol* 119:979-986, 1983.

142. Vonderheid EC, Sobel EL, Nowell PC: Diagnostic and prognostic significance of Sézary cells in peripheral blood smears from patients with cutaneous T cell lymphoma, *Blood* 66:358-366, 1985.

143. Lamberg SI et al: Clinical staging for cutaneous T-cell lymphoma, *Ann Intern Med* 100:187-192, 1984.

144. Olerud JE, Kulin PA, et al: Cutaneous T-cell lymphoma. Evaluation of pretreatment skin biopsy specimens by a panel of pathologists, *Arch Dermatol* 128:501-507, 1992.

145. Abel EA et al: Benign and malignant forms of erythroderma: cutaneous immunophenotypic characteristics, *J Am Acad Dermatol* 19:1089-1095, 1988.

146. Vonderheid EC et al: Long-term efficacy, curative potential, and carcinogenicity of topical mechlorethamine chemotherapy in cutaneous T cell lymphoma, *J Am Acad Dermatol* 20:416-428, 1989.

147. Zackheim HS et al: Topical carmustine (BCNU) for mycosis fungoides and related disorders: a 10-year experience, *J Am Acad Dermatol* 9:363-374, 1983.

148. Rosenbaum MM, Roenigk Jr HH, Caro WA, et al: Photochemotherapy in cutaneous T cell lymphoma and parapsoriasis en plaques: long-term follow-up in forty-three patients, *J Am Acad Dermatol* 13:613-622, 1985.

149. Honigsmann H et al: Photochemotherapy for cutaneous T cell lymphoma: a follow-up study, *J Am Acad Dermatol* 10:238-245, 1984.

150. Ramsey DL, Lish KM, et al: Ultraviolet-B phototherapy for early-stage cutaneous T-cell lymphoma, *Arch Dermatol* 128:931-933, 1992.

151. Mostow EN et al: Complete remission in psoralen and UV-A (PUVA)–refractory mycosis fungoides–type cutaneous T-cell lymphoma with combined interferon alfa and PUVA, *Arch Dermatol* 129:747-752, 1993.

152. Braverman IM et al: Combined total body electron beam irradiation and chemotherapy for mycosis fungoides, *J Am Acad Dermatol* 16:45-60, 1987.

153. Hamminga B, Noorkijk EM, van Vloten WA: Treatment of mycosis fungoides: total-skin electron-beam irradiation vs topical mechlorethamine therapy, *Arch Dermatol* 118:150-153, 1982.

154. Bunn PA Jr et al: Systemic therapy of cutaneous T-cell lymphomas (mycosis fungoides and Sézary syndrome), *Ann Intern Med* 121:592-602, 1994.

155. Edelson R et al: Treatment of cutaneous T-cell lymphoma by extracorporeal photochemotherapy. Preliminary results, *N Engl J Med* 316:297-303, 1987.

156. Zic J, Arzubiaga C, Salhany KE, et al: Extracorporeal photopheresis for treatment of cutaneous T-cell lymphoma, *J Am Acad Dermatol* 27:729-736, 1992.

157. Heald P, Rook A, Perez M, et al: Treatment of erythrodermic cutaneous T-cell lymphoma with extracorporeal photochemotherapy, *J Am Acad Dermatol* 27:427-433, 1992.

158. Armus S, Keyes B, et al: Photopheresis for the treatment of cutaneous T cell lymphoma, *J Am Acad Dermatol* 23:898-902, 1990.

159. Kessler JF et al: Isotretinoin and cutaneous helper T-cell lymphoma (mycosis fungoides), *Arch Dermatol* 123:201-204, 1987.

160. Scheman AJ, Steinberg I, Taddeini L: Abatement of Sézary syndrome lesions following treatment with acyclovir, *Am J Med* 80:1199-1202, 1986.

161. Karp DL, Horn TD: Lymphomatoid papulosis, *J Am Acad Dermatol* 30:379-395, 1994.

162. Paone JF, Baker RR: Pathogenesis and treatment of Paget's disease of the breast, *Cancer* 48:825-829, 1981.

163. Vielh P, Validire P, et al: Paget's disease of the nipple without clinically and radiologically detectable breast tumor. Histochemical and immunohistochemical study of 44 cases, *Pathol Res Pract* 189:150-155, 1993.

164. Ikeda DM, Helvie MA, et al: Paget disease of the nipple: radiologic-pathologic correlation, *Radiology* 189:89-94, 1993.

165. Samarasinghe D, Frost F, et al: Cytological diagnosis of Paget's disease of the nipple by scrape smears: a report of five cases, *Diagn Cytopathol* 9:291-295, 1993.

166. Hitchcock A, Topham S, et al: Routine diagnosis of mammary Paget's disease. A modern approach, *Am J Surg Pathol* 16:58-61, 1992.

167. Haerslev T, Krag Jacobsen G: Expression of cytokeratin and erbB-2 oncoprotein in Paget's disease of the nipple. An immunohistochemical study, *APMIS* 100:1041-1047, 1992.

168. Dixon AR, Galea MH, et al: Paget's disease of the nipple, *Br J Surg* 78:722-723, 1991.

169. el-Sharkawi A, Waters JS: The place for conservative treatment in the management of Paget's disease of the nipple, *Eur J Surg Oncol* 18:301-303, 1992.

170. Merot Y et al: Extramammary Paget's disease of the perianal and perineal regions, *Arch Dermatol* 121:750-752, 1985.

171. Hamm H, Vroom TM, Czarnetzki BM: Extramammary Paget's cells: further evidence of sweat gland derivation, *J Am Acad Dermatol* 15:1275-1281, 1986.

172. Chanda JJ: Extramammary Paget's disease: prognosis and relationship to internal malignancy, *J Am Acad Dermatol* 13:1009-1014, 1985.

173. Reedy MB, Morales CA, et al: Paget's disease of the scrotum: a case report and review of current literature, *Tex Med* 87:77-79, 1991.

174. Helm KF, Goellner JR, et al: Immunohistochemical stains in extramammary Paget's disease, *Am J Dermatopathol* 14:402-407, 1992.

175. Coldiron BM, Goldsmith BA, et al: Surgical treatment of extramammary Paget's disease. A report of six cases and a reexamination of Mohs micrographic surgery compared with conventional surgical excision, *Cancer* 67:933-938, 1991.

176. Besa P, Rich TA, et al: Extramammary Paget's disease of the perineal skin: role of radiotherapy, *Int J Radiat Oncol Biol Phys* 24:73-78, 1992.

177. Brierley JD, Stockdale AD: Radiotherapy: an effective treatment for extramammary Paget's disease, *Clin Oncol* 3:3-5, 1991.

178. Bergen S, Di Saia PJ, et al: Conservative management of extramammary Paget's disease of the vulva, *Gynecol Oncol* 33:151-156, 1989.

179. Misas JE, Cold CJ, et al: Vulvar Paget disease: fluorescein-aided visualization of margins, *Obstet Gynecol* 77:156-159, 1991.

180. Watring WG et al: Treatment of recurrent Paget's disease of the vulva with topical bleomycin, *Cancer* 41:10-11, 1978.

181. Lookingbill DP, Spangler N, et al: Cutaneous metastases in patients with metastatic carcinoma: a retrospective study of 4020 patients, *J Am Acad Dermatol* 29:228-236, 1993.

182. Lookingbill DP, Spangler N, et al: Skin involvement as the presenting sign of internal carcinoma. A retrospective study of 7316 cancer patients, *J Am Acad Dermatol* 22:19-26, 1990.

183. Brownstein MH, Helwig EB: Metastatic tumors of the skin, *Cancer* 29:1298-1307, 1972.

184. Brownstein MH, Helwig EB: Patterns of cutaneous metastasis, *Arch Dermatol* 105:862-868, 1972.

185. Brownstein MH, Helwig EB: Spread of tumors to the skin, *Arch Dermatol* 107:80-86, 1973.

186. Poole S, Fenske NA: Cutaneous markers of internal malignancy. I. Malignant involvement of the skin and the genodermatoses, *J Am Acad Dermatol* 28:1-13, 1993.

Nevi and Malignant Melanoma

Melanocytic Nevi

Nevi, or moles, are benign tumors composed of nevus cells that are derived from melanocytes. The well-publicized increase in the incidence of melanoma has stimulated the layperson's interest and concern about pigmented lesions.

Many myths surround moles; for example, that hairs should not be plucked from moles or that moles should not be removed or disturbed. These myths should be clarified.

Nevus cells. The nevus cell differs from melanocytes in a number of ways. The nevus cell is larger, lacks dendrites, has more abundant cytoplasm, and contains coarse granules. Nevus cells aggregate in groups (nests) or proliferate in a nonnested pattern in the basal region at the dermoepidermal junction. Nevus cells in the dermis are classified into types A (epithelioid), B (lymphocytoid), and C (neuroid). Through a process of maturation and downward migration, type A epidermal nevus cells develop into type B cells and then into type C dermal nevus cells.[1]

Incidence and evolution. Moles are so common that they appear on virtually every person. They are present in 1% of newborns and increase in incidence throughout infancy and childhood, reaching a peak at puberty. Size and pigmentation may increase at puberty and during pregnancy. A few may continue to appear throughout life. Nevi may occur anywhere on the cutaneous surface. There is a strong correlation between sun exposure and the number of nevi. Acquired nevi on the buttock or female breast are unusual.

Nevi vs. melanoma. Nevi exist in a variety of characteristic forms that must be readily recognized to distinguish them from malignant melanoma. Except for certain types, such as large congenital nevi and atypical moles, most nevi have a very low malignant potential.

Nevi vary in size, shape, surface characteristics, and color. The important fact to remember is that each individual nevus tends to remain uniform in color and shape. Although various shades of brown and black may be present in a single lesion, the colors are distributed over the surface in a uniform pattern.

Melanomas consist of malignant pigment cells that grow and extend with little constraint through the epidermis and into the dermis. Such unrestricted growth produces a lesion with a haphazard or disorganized appearance, which varies in shape, color, and surface characteristics. Nevertheless, the characteristics of uniformity cannot always be relied on to differentiate benign from malignant lesions because very early melanomas may appear quite uniform, having a round or oval shape with a uniform brown color.

Examination with a hand lens. Careful inspection of suspicious lesions with a powerful hand lens may reveal irregularities in the border or minute areas of regression that suggest malignancy.[2] Dome-shaped, pigmented lesions with uniform speckling over the surface are usually benign dermal nevi (Figure 22-1). A flat, dark macule with a uniform, netlike pattern is usually a lentigo (Figures 22-2 and 22-3).[3] Lentigines with netlike patterns are most often found on the trunk.

COMMON MOLES

Nevi may be classified as acquired or congenital, but a clinical classification based on appearance and conventional nomenclature is used here.[4]

Classification. Common moles are subdivided into three types—junction, compound, and dermal—based on the location of the nevus cells in the skin (see the box on p. 690). The three types represent sequential developmental stages in the life history of a mole. During childhood, nevi begin as flat junction nevi in which the nevus cells are located at the dermoepidermal junction. They evolve into compound nevi when some of the cells migrate into the dermis. Migration of all of the nevus cells into the dermis results in a dermal nevus. Dermal nevi usually form only in adults, but this evolution does not consistently occur.[4] Nevi with cells confined to the dermoepidermal junction area tend to be flat, whereas those with cells confined to the dermis are usually elevated.

SURFACE CHARACTERISTICS OF BENIGN PIGMENTED LESIONS

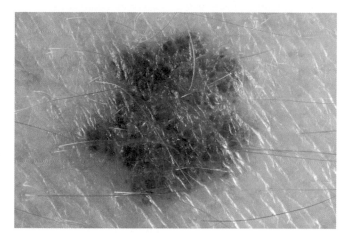

Figure 22-1
Surface speckling (dermal nevus). Examination of the surface of this pigmented lesion with a hand lens reveals uniform speckling over the surface, a characteristic of a benign pigmented nevus.

Figure 22-2

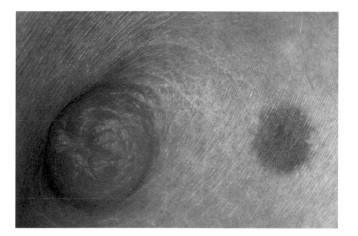

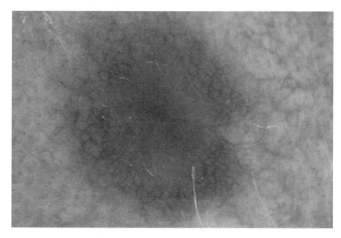

A, A pigmented macule adjacent to the nipple.

B, Examination of the surface of the pigmented macule in *A* reveals a highly uniform, netlike pattern. A biopsy proved that the macule was a lentigo.

Figure 22-3

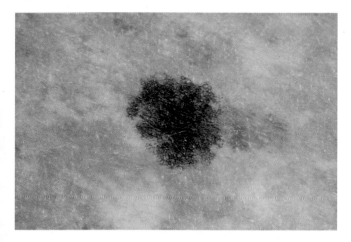

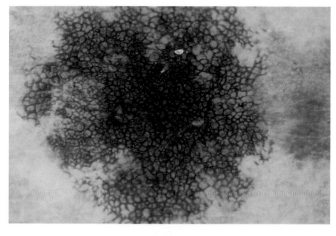

A, A pigmented macule on the sun-exposed upper back. The lesion has an irregular border suggestive of a melanoma.

B, Examination of the surface of the pigmented macule in *A* reveals a highly uniform, netlike pattern. A biopsy proved that the macule was a lentigo.

Junction nevi. Junction nevi are flat (macular) or slightly elevated, and they are light brown to brown-black with uniform pigmentation that may be slightly irregular (Figure 22-4). The surface is smooth and flat to slightly elevated, and the border is round or oval and symmetric. Most lesions are hairless. Junction nevi vary in size from 0.1 to 0.6 cm; some are larger. Junction nevi may change into compound nevi after childhood, but they remain as junction nevi on palms, soles, and genitalia. Junction nevi are rare at birth and generally develop after the age of 2 years. Degeneration into melanoma is very rare.

Compound nevi. Compound nevi are slightly elevated and flesh colored or brown. They are elevated and smooth or warty and become more elevated with increasing age (Figure 22-5). They are uniformly round, oval, and symmetric. Hair may be present. If a white halo appears at the periphery of the lesion, it is referred to as a *halo nevus.*

Dermal nevi. Dermal nevi are brown or black, but may become lighter or flesh-colored with age. Lesions vary in size from a few millimeters to a centimeter. The variety of shapes reflects the evolutionary process in which moles extend downward with age and nevus cells degenerate and become replaced by fat and fibrous tissue.

Dome-shaped lesions are the most common (Figures 22-6 through 22-8). They generally appear on the face and are symmetric, with a smooth surface. They may be white or translucent, with telangiectatic vessels on the surface mimicking basal cell carcinoma. The structure may be warty (Figure 22-9) or polypoid (Figure 22-10). Pedunculated lesions with a narrow stalk are located on the trunk, neck, axilla, and groin. They may appear as a soft, flabby, wrinkled sack (Figure 22-11).

Elevated nevi are exposed and are prone to trauma from clothing and other stimuli, often causing them to bleed and inflame, influencing some patients to suspect malignancy. White borders may appear, creating a halo nevus. Degeneration to melanoma is very rare, but dermal nevi may resemble nodular melanoma; therefore, knowledge of duration is important.

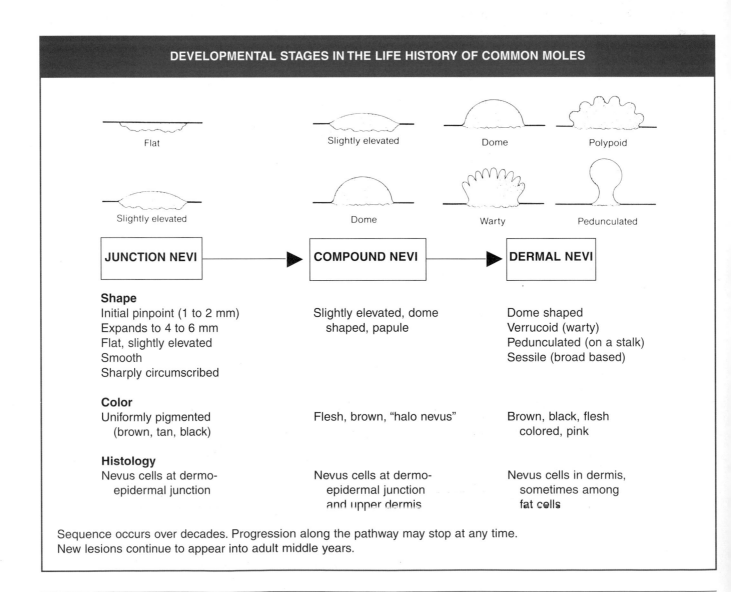

DEVELOPMENTAL STAGES IN THE LIFE HISTORY OF COMMON MOLES

Flat

Slightly elevated

Dome

Polypoid

Slightly elevated

Dome

Warty

Pedunculated

JUNCTION NEVI	COMPOUND NEVI	DERMAL NEVI
Shape Initial pinpoint (1 to 2 mm) Expands to 4 to 6 mm Flat, slightly elevated Smooth Sharply circumscribed	Slightly elevated, dome shaped, papule	Dome shaped Verrucoid (warty) Pedunculated (on a stalk) Sessile (broad based)

Color
Uniformly pigmented
  (brown, tan, black)
	Flesh, brown, "halo nevus"	Brown, black, flesh
		  colored, pink

Histology
Nevus cells at dermo-
  epidermal junction
	Nevus cells at dermo-
	  epidermal junction
	  and upper dermis
		Nevus cells in dermis,
		  sometimes among
		  fat cells

Sequence occurs over decades. Progression along the pathway may stop at any time.
New lesions continue to appear into adult middle years.

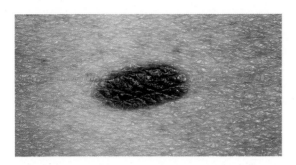

Figure 22-4
Junction nevus. Flat, black, and uniform.

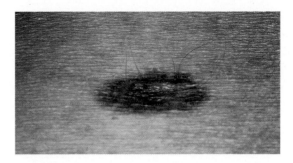

Figure 22-5
Compound nevus. Center is elevated.

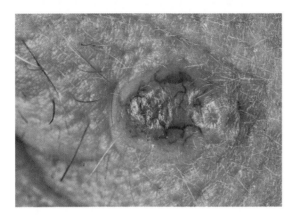

Figure 22-6
Dermal nevus. Flesh colored with surface vessels; resembles basal cell carcinoma.

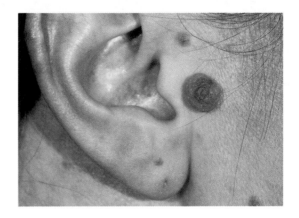

Figure 22-7
Dermal nevus. Dome shaped.

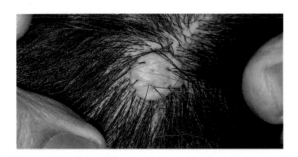

Figure 22-8
Dermal nevus. Flesh colored and dome shaped.

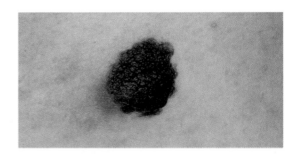

Figure 22-9
Dermal nevus. Warty (verrucous) surface.

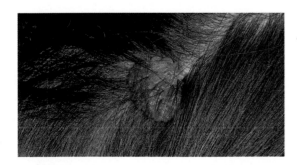

Figure 22-10
Dermal nevus. Polypoid.

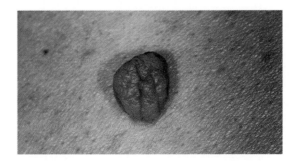

Figure 22-11
Dermal nevus. Pedunculated with a soft, flabby, wrinkled surface.

Management of common moles

Suspicious lesions. Any pigmented lesion suspected of being malignant should be biopsied or referred for a second opinion. Suspicious lesions should be completely removed by excisional biopsy down to and including subcutaneous tissue.

Nevi. Patients frequently request removal of nevi for cosmetic purposes. It is good practice to biopsy all pigmented lesions; therefore, total removal by electrocautery should be avoided. Nevi are removed either by shave excision or by simple excision and closure with sutures. Most common nevi are small and consequently shave excision is adequate.

Recurrent previously excised nevi (pseudomelanoma). Weeks to months after incomplete removal of a nevus, brown macular pigmentation may appear in the scar (Figure 22-12). Some nevus cells remain with shave excision and partial repigmentation is possible. Residual pigmentation may be removed with electrocautery or cryosurgery. An unusual histologic picture resembling melanoma (pseudomelanoma) may follow partial removal of nevi.[5-7] If the repigmented area is excised, the pathologist should always be notified that the submitted tissue was acquired from a previously treated area. Histologically, the melanocytes appear atypical but are confined to the epidermis, and there is no lateral spread of individual melanocytes.

Nevi with small dark spots. A small percentage of small dark dots within melanocytic nevi is due to melanoma. These roundish areas of brown or black hyperpigmentation measure 3 mm or less in diameter and are located peripherally.[8] Biopsy specimens of nevi with small dark dots should be sectioned to ensure histologic examination of this focus of hyperpigmentation.

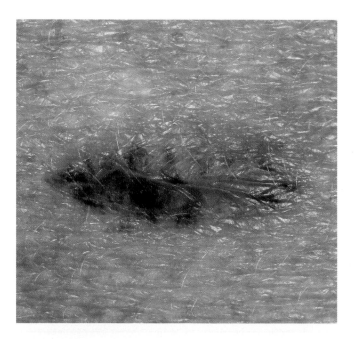

Figure 22-12
Recurrent, previously excised nevi (pseudomelanoma). Brown, macular pigmentation may appear in the scar of an incompletely removed nevus.

SPECIAL FORMS

Special forms of pigmented lesions include congenital nevus, halo nevus, nevus spilus, Becker's nevus, benign juvenile melanoma (Spitz nevus), blue nevus, and labial melanotic macules.

Congenital nevi. Congenital nevi (birthmarks) are present at birth and vary in size from a few millimeters to several centimeters, covering wide areas of the trunk, an extremity, or the face. Not all pigmented lesions present at birth are congenital nevi; café-au-lait spots may also be present at birth. The largest lesions are referred to as *giant hairy nevi.* Giant congenital nevi on the trunk are referred to as *bathing trunk nevi* (Figure 22-13).

Congenital nevi may contain hair; if present, it is usually coarse. Such nevi are uniformly pigmented, with various shades of brown or black predominating (Figure 22-14), but red or pink may be a minor or sometimes predominant color (Figure 22-15). Most are flat at birth, but become thicker during childhood, and the surface becomes verrucous and sometimes nodular.

The risk of developing melanoma in very large lesions is significant.[9] Malignant transformation may occur early in childhood; therefore, large, thick lesions should be removed as soon as possible.[10] The risk of developing malignancy may be related to the number of melanocytes and consequently to the size and thickness; however, melanomas have also developed in small congenital nevi. There is a large risk of melanoma in patients with nevi covering more than 5% of the body surface area.[10] The risk of malignant degeneration for smaller congenital nevi is unknown. A report showed histologic features of congenital nevi in 8.1% of the melanoma specimens studied.[11]

Management. The incidence of melanomas in small congenital nevi is unknown. Persons with large congenital nevi (bathing trunk nevi) are at definite risk for the development of melanoma in childhood, and these nevi are managed by a plastic surgeon. Because of the possibility of malignant degeneration of congenital nevi, some experts recommend that all congenital nevi be considered for prophylactic excision.[12] All congenital moles should be checked by a dermatologist. If a congenital mole is not surgically removed, it should be examined on a regular basis.

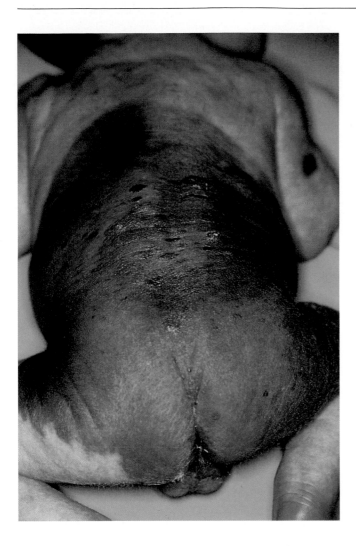

Figure 22-13
Giant congenital nevus (bathing trunk nevus).

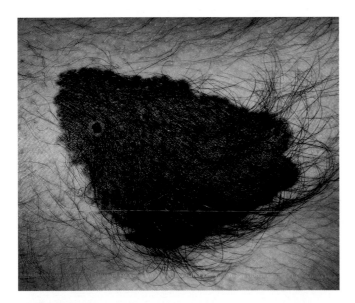

Figure 22-14
Congenital hairy nevus. The border is irregular and appears notched, but that characteristic is maintained in a uniform manner around the entire border.

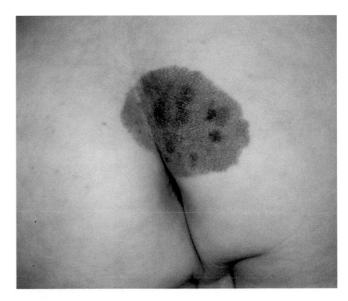

Figure 22-15
Congenital nevus. Pigmentation is variable and nonuniform, but a biopsy showed all such areas were benign.

Figure 22-16 Nevus spilus.

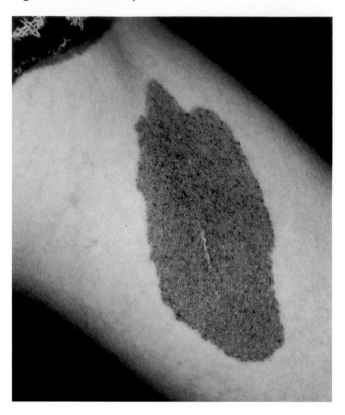

A, A large, brown, macular lesion resembling a café-au-lait spot. Tiny, black papules are uniformly distributed over the surface.

Nevus spilus. Nevus spilus is a hairless, oval or irregularly shaped, brown lesion that is dotted with darker brown-to-black spots.[13,14] The brown area is usually flat, and the black dots may be slightly elevated and contain typical nevus cells (Figure 22-16). There is considerable variation in size, ranging from 1 to 20 cm; they may appear at any age. The anatomic position or time of onset is not related to sun exposure.

Nevus spilus is flat and necessitates excision and closure if the patient desires removal.

Becker's nevus. Becker's nevus is not a nevocellular nevus because it lacks nevus cells. The lesion is a developmental anomaly consisting of either a brown macule (Figure 22-17), a patch of hair, or both (Figure 22-18). Nonhairy lesions may later develop hair. The lesions appear in adolescent men on the shoulder, submammary area, and upper and lower back.[15] Becker's nevus varies in size and may enlarge to cover the entire upper arm or shoulder. The border is irregular and sharply demarcated. Malignancy has never been reported.

Becker's nevus is usually too large to remove and is best left untouched. The hair may be shaved or permanently removed.

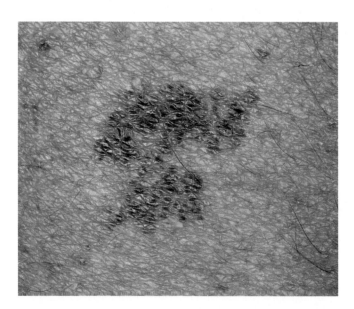

B, The macular pigmentation is less prominent than in the lesion illustrated in *A.*

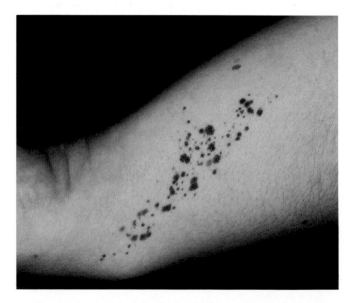

C, The macular pigmentation is almost entirely absent. The multiple papules containing nevus cells predominate. Compare this with *A.*

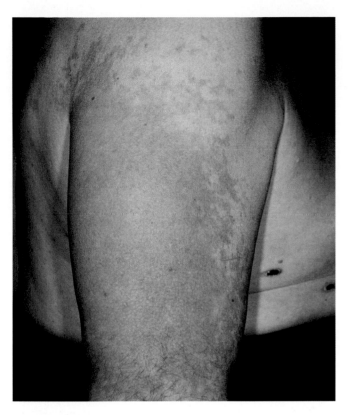

Figure 22-17
Becker's nevus. A huge, brown macule. Only a small area
of this lesion contains hair.

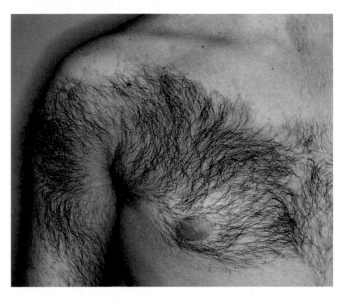

Figure 22-18
Becker's nevus. A typical lesion with macular pigmentation
and hair.

Halo nevi. A compound or dermal nevus that develops a
white border is called a *halo nevus*. The depigmented halo is
symmetric and round or oval with a sharply demarcated border (Figure 22-19). There are no melanocytes in the halo area.
Histologically, chronic inflammatory cells may be present.
Most halo nevi are located on the trunk; they never occur on
palms and soles. Halo nevi develop spontaneously, most
commonly during adolescence. They may occur as an isolated phenomenon or several nevi may spontaneously develop
halos. Halos may repigment with time or the nevus may disappear. Repigmentation does not follow removal of the
nevus. The incidence of vitiligo may be increased in patients
with halo nevi.[16] A halo may rarely develop around malignant
melanoma, but in such instances it is usually not symmetric.

Removal of a halo nevus is unnecessary unless the nevus
has atypical features. Parental concern over this impressive
change is often reason for a conservative excision. In such
cases, the mole part of a halo nevus may be removed by
shave or excision.

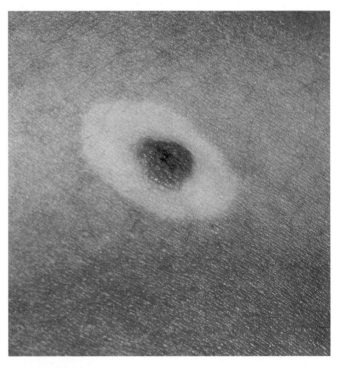

Figure 22-19
Halo nevus. A sharply defined, white halo surrounds this
compound nevus.

Spitz nevus. Spitz nevus, or benign juvenile melanoma,[17] is most common in children, but does appear in adults. The term *melanoma* is used because the clinical and histologic appearance is similar to melanoma. They are hairless, red or reddish-brown, dome-shaped papules or nodules with a smooth (Figure 22-20) or warty surface; they vary in size from 0.3 to 1.5 cm. The color is caused by increased vascularity, and bleeding sometimes follows trauma. Spitz nevi are usually solitary but may be multiple. They appear suddenly and, contrary to slowly evolving common moles, patients can sometimes date their onset. The benign juvenile melanoma should be removed for microscopic examination. Histologic differentiation from melanoma is sometimes difficult.[18]

Blue nevus. The blue nevus is a slightly elevated, round, regular nevus, usually less than 0.5 cm, and contains large amounts of pigment located in the dermis (Figure 22-21). The brown pigment absorbs the longer wavelengths of light and scatters blue light (Tyndall effect). The blue nevus appears in childhood and is most common on the extremities and dorsum of the hands. A rare variant, the cellular blue nevus, is larger (usually greater than 1 cm) and nodular and is frequently located on the buttock. There are reported cases of malignant degeneration of these larger blue nevi into melanomas.[19]

Labial melanotic macule. Brown macules on the lower lip are relatively common, especially in young adult women. Histologically, they resemble freckles and not lentigo, but unlike freckles, they do not darken with sun exposure.[20]

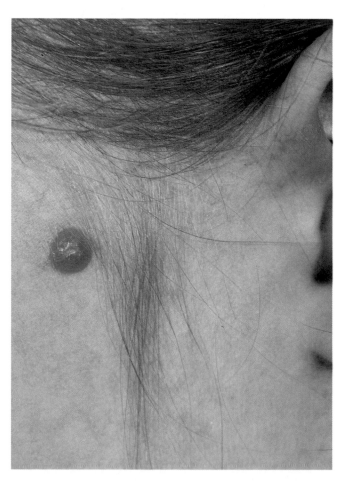

Figure 22-20
Benign juvenile melanoma (Spitz nevus). A reddish, dome-shaped nodule that generally appears in children.

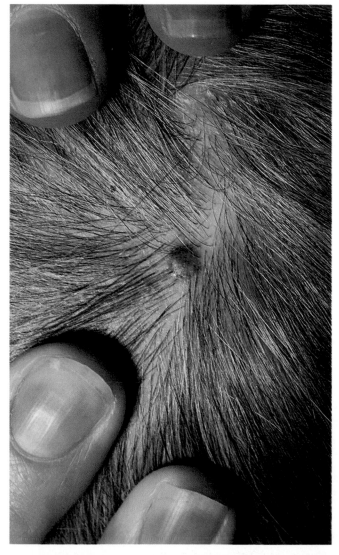

Figure 22-21
Blue nevus. Most lesions are small and round.

ATYPICAL-MOLE SYNDROME

Familial melanoma and melanoma precursors. Cutaneous melanoma may occur as isolated, so-called sporadic cases; in association with multiple atypical nevi; or in familial clusters, in which case it is referred to as the *atypical-mole syndrome* (AMS), formerly known as *dysplastic nevus syndrome*. In the late 1970s, the dysplastic nevus (DN) or atypical mole (AM) was identified in melanoma-prone families. It was then determined that AMs are cutaneous markers that identify specific family members who are at increased risk for melanoma. The AM (Figure 22-22) may also be the single most important precursor lesion of melanoma. These nevi may occur in persons from melanoma-prone families and in persons who lack both a family history and a personal history of melanoma.[21]

Atypical-mole syndrome and familial melanoma. Numerous families with multiple melanoma patients have been reported. These patients usually develop melanoma at a young age, have a predisposition to multiple primary melanomas, and have the tendency to develop thin, superficial-spreading melanomas. Large, unusual-looking moles were initially recognized as a precursor to melanoma in patients with familial cutaneous melanoma. This syndrome was named *B-K mole syndrome* from two of the probands, and the precursor nevi were designated as *B-K moles* and later referred to as *dysplastic nevi.*[22] The syndrome is now called the *atypical-mole syndrome.* Recent estimates suggest that approximately 32,000 persons in the United States have familial atypical-mole syndrome with familial melanoma, accounting for approximately 5.5% of all melanomas diagnosed in this country.[23] Hereditary malignant melanoma and atypical moles represent pleiotropic effects of a mendelian autosomal dominant gene with high penetrance.[24]

One study showed that the hereditary cutaneous malignant melanoma/atypical-mole syndrome does not predispose to other cancers.[25]

Definition. The National Institutes of Health (NIH) Consensus Conference on Diagnosis and Treatment of Early Melanoma has defined the familial atypical mole and melanoma syndrome as (1) the occurrence of malignant melanoma in one or more first- or second-degree relatives; (2) a large number of melanocytic nevi (MN), often more than 50, some of which are atypical and often variable in size; and (3) melanocytic nevi that demonstrate certain histologic features. AMS probably represents a spectrum. At one end all members of a kindred have AMs and some have malignant melanoma (MM). At the other end are persons with one AM without a personal and/or family history of MM.

Association with melanoma. Patients with AMS, familial or sporadic, are at significant risk for developing melanoma.[26,27] Atypical moles have been observed in 8% of patients with nonfamilial (sporadic) melanoma, and the transformation into superficial-spreading melanoma has been photographically documented. Family members without atypical moles do not show any apparent increase in melanoma risk. The frequency of sporadic AMs in the general population is unknown.

Atypical moles are found on the skin of 90% of patients with hereditary melanomas, and more than 50% of melanomas in this group are associated histologically with and probably evolve from atypical moles.[28-31] The lifetime risk of developing cutaneous melanoma among the white population in the United States is approximately 0.8%, or 1 in 125. Persons who have AMs and no family members with the disease have a 6% risk of developing melanoma.[32] Persons who have AMs and a history of melanoma have a 10% risk of getting a second melanoma; persons who have AMs and have a family member with melanoma have a 15% risk. The lifetime risk of melanoma approaches 100% for those people with AMs from families with two or more first-degree relatives who have cutaneous melanoma.[33,34]

Among atypical-mole–bearing family members, those patients with melanoma have very large numbers of nevi more frequently than patients with AMs without melanoma. Family members with AMs have more nevi than do patients who have only common acquired nevi.

Clinical features of atypical moles

Morphology. These unusual nevi differ in a number of important ways from typical acquired pigmented nevi or moles[35] (Table 22-1). Atypical moles are larger than common moles. They have a mixture of colors, including tan, brown, pink, and black. The border is irregular and indistinct

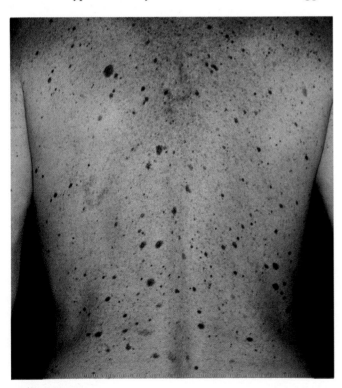

Figure 22-22
Atypical nevi. There are numerous large nevi present. Superficial spreading melanomas have been removed from the upper back and the midline on the right side (note scars). Nevi are larger than 1 cm and irregularly pigmented.

and often fades into the surrounding skin. The surface is complex and variable, with both macular and papular components. A characteristic presentation is a pigmented papule surrounded by a macular collar of pigmentation ("fried-egg lesion"). In one study, the total number of nevi and macular components were the only useful features to predict histologic melanocytic dysplasia. However, "fried-egg lesions" often do not display histologic melanocytic dysplasia. In contrast, the absence of a macular component in melanocytic nevi in a person with fewer than 13 total body nevi accurately predicts the absence of melanocytic dysplasia on histologic examination.[36]

Development and distribution. Atypical moles are not present at birth, but begin to appear in the mid-childhood years as typical common moles. The appearance changes at puberty, and newer lesions continue to appear well after the age of 40.[37] Common moles occur most often on sun-exposed areas. AMs occur in those locations and at unusual sites such as the scalp, buttocks, and breast. The predilection sites for melanoma in familial AMS patients of both sexes correspond with the distribution of nevi; in males nevi and melanoma counts are higher on the back, in females both the back and the lower extremities are affected. These findings strongly suggest an association between nevus distribution and melanoma occurrence and site in familial AMS.[38]

Histology. The NIH Consensus Conference listed the histologic criteria as follows: architectural disorder with asymmetry, subepidermal (concentric eosinophilic and/or lamellar) fibroplasia, and lentiginous melanocytic hyperplasia with spindle or epithelioid melanocytes aggregating in nests of variable size and forming bridges between adjacent rete ridges. Melanocytic atypia may be present to a variable degree. In addition, there may be dermal infiltration with lymphocytes, as well as the "shoulder" phenomenon (intraepidermal melanocytes extending singly or in nests beyond the main dermal component).

Management

Recommendations for management of patients with AMs have been given in the National Institutes of Health Consensus Development Conference statement, October 24-26, 1983.[35] These, along with other recent recommendations, are given in the box above.

RECOMMENDATIONS FOR THE MANAGEMENT OF AMS

- Examine total cutaneous surface every 3 to 12 mo,* beginning around puberty
- Use hair-blower for scalp examination
- Consider total cutaneous photographs as baseline
- Excise lesions suspected to be melanoma
- Educate patient on self-examination of skin
- Recommend sun avoidance and/or protection
- Suggest screening of blood relatives for AM and MM
- Suggest regular ophthalmologic examinations for ocular nevi and ocular melanoma

Modified from Slade J et al: Atypical mole syndrome: risk factors for cutaneous malignant melanoma and implications for management, *J Am Acad Dermatol* 32:479-494, 1995.
*The frequency of follow-up is a function of estimated risk for MM.

TABLE 22-1 Differences Between Atypical Moles and Common Nevi

Characteristics	Atypical moles	Common nevi
Distribution	Back most common, upper and lower limbs, sun-protected areas, female breasts, scalp, buttock, groin	Usually sun-exposed areas; most above the waist
Number	Less than 10 to greater than 100	10 to 40
Age at onset	Appear as normal nevi at age 2 to 6; increase in number and size at puberty; new nevi appear throughout life	Absent at birth; appear at age 2 to 6; grow vertically in uniform manner throughout life; several may appear at puberty
Size	Usually greater than 5 mm and commonly greater than 10 mm	Usually less than 6 mm
Shape and contour	Irregular border; flap (macular) areas; margin fades into surrounding skin, always has a macular component	Round, symmetric, uniformly macular or papular smooth border
Color	Variable within a single lesion; brown, black, red, pink	Uniform tan, brown, black; darken during pregnancy or at adolescence; become lighter with age
Histology	Persistent lentiginous melanocytic hyperplasia Melanocytic nuclear atypia* Lamellar fibroplasia Concentric eosinophilic fibroplasia Sparse, patchy lymphocytic infiltration	Nevus cells at the dermoepidermal junction and/or in the dermis

Modified from Greene MH et al: *N Engl J Med* 312:91, 1985.
*May not be essential to make diagnosis.

Malignant Melanoma

One of the most dangerous tumors, malignant melanoma arises from cells of the melanocytic system. Melanoma has the ability to metastasize to any organ, including the brain and heart. Therefore, it is imperative that all physicians be familiar with the features of early preinvasive melanoma and include a complete skin examination as part of routine physical examinations (Figure 22-23). Referral or excisional biopsy is indicated for suspicious lesions. The previous practice of waiting and watching for a change may result in death. Criteria for the early diagnosis of malignant melanoma have been established and can be appreciated by all physicians and disseminated to patients.

Risk for melanoma. The incidence of melanoma is increasing and may be reaching epidemic proportions. The lifetime risk of cutaneous melanoma for white Americans in 1987 was 1 in 123. It is projected to be 1 in 90 by the year 2000. Many deaths due to melanoma may be prevented by screening those individuals at greatest risk[39,40] (Table 22-2).

Prevention and sun exposure. Increased recreational sun exposure and alterations of the upper atmosphere by pollutants resulting in increased radiation may be the two most important factors in the disproportionate rise in the incidence of melanoma. People who suntan poorly or sunburn easily or who have had multiple or severe sunburns have a twofold to threefold increased risk for developing cutaneous melanoma. Individuals with recreational and vacation sun exposure who experience acute episodic exposures to sunlight may be at greater risk than those with constant occupational sun exposure. [41] It is postulated that sunlight causes cutaneous immunosuppression.

Prevention of melanoma is accomplished by sun protection (especially in childhood) and avoidance of excessive sun exposure. Morbidity and mortality can be reduced by early detection, diagnosis, and treatment.

Sunscreen effectiveness. Chemical sunscreens block UVB but are less effective at blocking UVA, which makes up 90% to 95% of ultraviolet energy in the solar spectrum. Sunscreens prevent erythema and sunburn, but inhibit accommodation of the skin to sunlight, therefore their use may permit excessive exposure of the skin to UVA. Laboratory data suggest that melanoma is promoted by UVA, therefore UVB sunscreens might not be effective in preventing melanoma. Sunscreen use may give people a

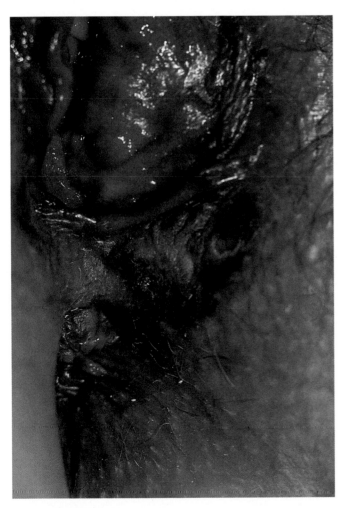

Figure 22-23
Superficial spreading melanoma. Modesty prevented the patient from asking the physician about this lesion, which had been present for 2 years. Fortunately, it was discovered during a complete examination of the skin.

TABLE 22-2 Summary of Risk Factors for the Development of Cutaneous Melanoma	
Risk factor	**Relative risk***
Persistently changed or changing mole Adulthood (≥15 yr vs. <15 yr)	Very high
One or more large or irregularly pigmented lesions	88
Atypical mole(s) and familial melanoma	148
Atypical mole(s) but no familial melanoma	27
Lentigo maligna	10
Congenital mole	21
White race (vs. black)	12
Previous cutaneous melonoma	9
Cutaneous melanoma in parents, children, or siblings	8
Immunosuppression	4
Sun sensitivity	3
Excessive sun exposure	3

From Rhodes AR et al: *JAMA* 258:3147, 1987; copyright 1987, American Medical Association.
*Degree of increased risk for persons with the risk factor compared with persons without the risk factor. Relative risk of 1.0 implies no increased risk.

false sense of security and encourage excessive exposure. Hats, protective clothing, and avoiding sunbathing are more protective than chemical sunscreens.

ABCDs of malignant melanoma recognition. The goal is to recognize melanomas at the earliest stage. Compared to common acquired melanocytic nevi, malignant melanomas tend to have *A*symmetry, *B*order irregularity, *C*olor variegation, and *D*iameter enlargement.[42] Changes in shape and color are important early signs and should always arouse suspicion. Ulceration and bleeding are late signs; hope of cure diminishes greatly if the diagnosis has not been made before such changes occur. The specific signs that appear during the evolution of each type of melanoma are listed and illustrated on the following pages. A list of all possible changes at all stages of development is given in Table 22-3.

Characteristics of benign moles. Benign moles have a more uniform tan, brown, or black color. The border is regular and the lesion is roughly symmetric; if the lesion could be folded in half, the two halves would superimpose. Most acquired benign moles are 6 mm or less in diameter and appeared early in life. The only notable change is a slight uniform elevation during pregnancy or with age.

Clinical classification

Melanoma either begins de novo or develops from a pre-existing lesion, such as a congenital or atypical mole. A classification into several different types was devised after observing that the microscopic anatomy of the tumor at the periphery of the elevated tumor mass was variable and possessed characteristic patterns that could be correlated with distinctive clinical presentations.[43-45] The proposed types are superficial spreading melanoma (SSM), lentigo maligna melanoma (LMM), nodular melanoma (NM), and acral-lentiginous melanoma (ALM).

Many, but not all,[46] pathologists recognize these various clinicopathologic types of melanoma. Some melanomas do not conform to this clinicopathologic classification and may be labeled exclusively malignant melanoma. Malignant melanoma may be a single entity that has various clinical and histologic forms varying with the degree of differentiation of the tumor cell. The potential for a melanocyte to degenerate and become neoplastic is probably influenced by a number of factors, including degree of skin pigmentation, heredity, immunologic status, quantity of solar radiation, sex of the individual, and anatomic position on the body.

TABLE 22-3 Signs Suggesting Malignancy in Pigmented Lesions

Sign	Implication
CHANGE IN COLOR	
Sudden darkening; brown, black	Increased number of tumor cells, the density of which varies within the lesion, creating irregular pigmentation
Spread of color into previously normal skin	Tumor cells migrating through epidermis at various speeds and in different directions (horizontal growth phase)
Red	Vasodilation and inflammation
White	Areas of regression or inflammation
Blue	Pigment deep in dermis, sign of increasing depth of tumor
CHANGE IN CHARACTERISTICS OF BORDER	
Irregular outline	Malignant cells migrating horizontally at different rates
Satellite pigmentation	Cells migrating beyond confines of primary tumor
Development of depigmented halo	Destruction of melanocytes by possible immunologic reaction and inflammation

CHANGES IN SURFACE CHARACTERISTICS

Scaliness
Erosion
Oozing
Crusting
Bleeding
Ulceration
Elevation
Loss of normal skin lines

DEVELOPMENT OF SYMPTOMS

Pruritus
Tenderness
Pain

Growth characteristics. Once a melanocyte becomes neoplastic, constraints on its localization are removed, and it may leave its assigned position at the basal layer of the epidermis. A well-differentiated malignant melanocyte retains its affinity for the epidermis and may grow slowly horizontally, only to be restrained or eliminated in some areas by a still-competent immunologic system. Years of slow growth and regression by a number of such cells on the face produces the LMM.

A more immature group of cells would be more aggressive and extend and regress at a faster rate, stimulating new vessel formation and inflammation. Such biologic behavior could be expected to produce the SSM. Melanomas in which the cells are extending laterally are considered to be in the horizontal (radial) growth phase.[47] This phase may endure for months or years.

A poorly differentiated cell knows no bounds, has no affinity for the epidermis, and grows both horizontally and vertically, producing a mass or NM. Melanomas in which cells have begun to grow vertically into the dermis and form a mass are considered to be in the vertical growth phase. The validity of the type classification has yet to be settled; however, it does enable one to understand the growth and evolution of malignant melanoma and, therefore, is an aid to making an early diagnosis. The various types of melanomas have specific characteristics.[48,49]

Figure 22-24
Distribution of superficial spreading malignant melanoma of the skin in men and women. *(From* Causes and effects of changes in stratospheric ozone: update 1984, *Washington, DC, National Academy Press. Courtesy New York University Melanoma Cooperative Group and the National Academy Press.)*

Superficial spreading melanoma. SSM (Figure 22-25) is most common in middle age, from the fourth to fifth decade. It develops anywhere on the body, but most frequently on the upper back of both sexes and on the legs of women (Figure 22-24). SSM begins in a nonspecific manner and then changes shape by radial spread and regression. The random migration of cells, along with the process of regression, results in lesions with an endless variety of shapes and sizes. The shape is bizarre if left untreated for years. The hallmark of SSM is the haphazard combination of many colors, but it may be uniformly brown or black. Colors may become more diverse as time proceeds. A dull red color is frequently observed, which may occupy a small area or may dominate the lesion. The precursor radial growth phase may last for months or for more than 10 years. Nodules appear when the lesion is approximately 2.5 cm in diameter.[50]

Nodular melanoma. NM (Figure 22-26) occurs most often in the fifth or sixth decade. It is more frequent in males than females, with a ratio of 2:1. It is found anywhere on the body.

NM is most commonly dark brown, red-brown, or red-black and is dome-shaped, polypoid, or pedunculated. It is occasionally amelanotic (flesh colored) and resembles flesh-colored dermal nevi. NM is the type of melanoma most frequently misdiagnosed because it resembles a blood blister, hemangioma, dermal nevus, or polyp (see p. 709).

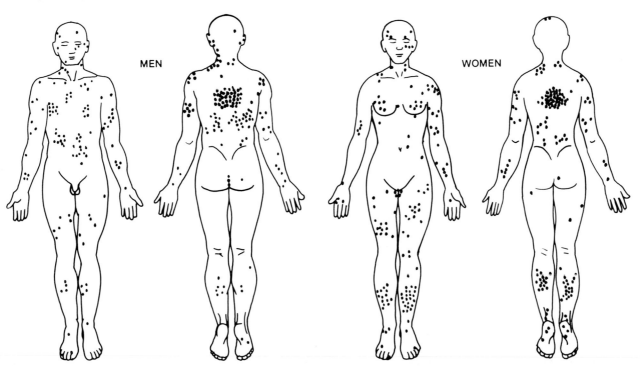

MEN   WOMEN

SUPERFICIAL SPREADING MELANOMA

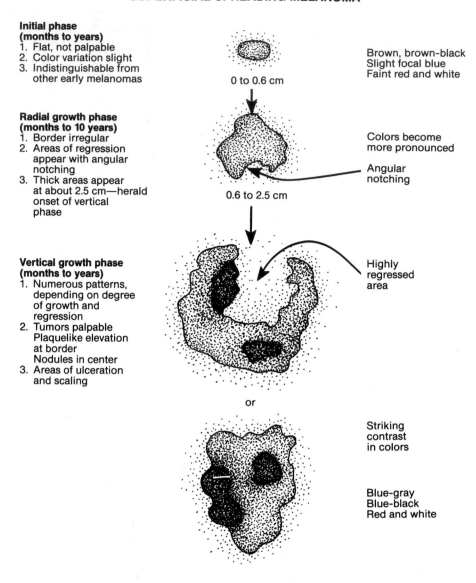

**Initial phase
(months to years)**
1. Flat, not palpable
2. Color variation slight
3. Indistinguishable from other early melanomas

0 to 0.6 cm

Brown, brown-black
Slight focal blue
Faint red and white

**Radial growth phase
(months to 10 years)**
1. Border irregular
2. Areas of regression appear with angular notching
3. Thick areas appear at about 2.5 cm—herald onset of vertical phase

0.6 to 2.5 cm

Colors become more pronounced

Angular notching

**Vertical growth phase
(months to years)**
1. Numerous patterns, depending on degree of growth and regression
2. Tumors palpable
   Plaquelike elevation at border
   Nodules in center
3. Areas of ulceration and scaling

Highly regressed area

or

Striking contrast in colors

Blue-gray
Blue-black
Red and white

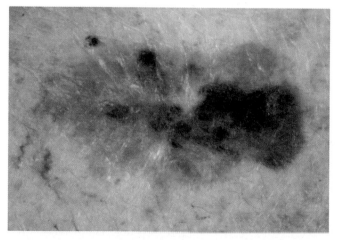

Figure 22-25
Superficial spreading melanomas in all stages of development. The small early lesions have irregular borders, irregular pigmentation, and small white areas indicating regression. The largest tumors show an accentuation of all of these features.

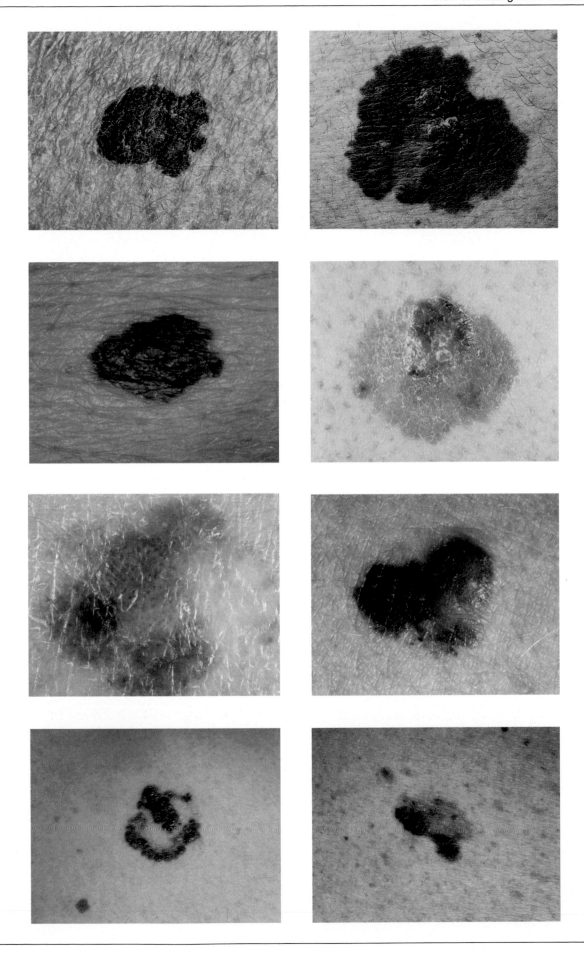

NODULAR MELANOMAS

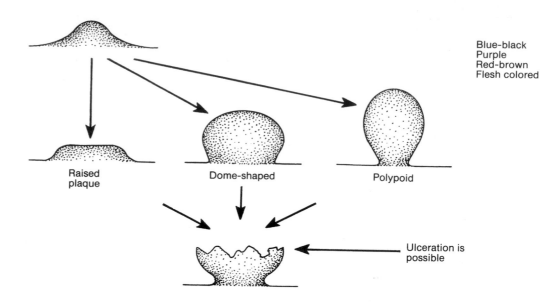

**Initial phase
(weeks or months)**
No radial
growth phase

Vertical growth phase
1. Raised above skin
   with variety of
   shapes
2. Ulceration and
   crust and
   bleeding frequent
3. May resemble
   angioma

Raised plaque

Dome-shaped

Polypoid

Blue-black
Purple
Red-brown
Flesh colored

Ulceration is possible

Pressure test

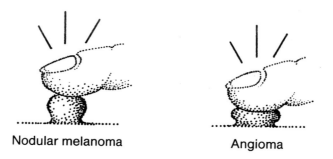

Nodular melanoma

Angioma

Press suspected nodule firmly for 30 seconds;
near-total involution is characteristic of
hemangioma, not melanoma.

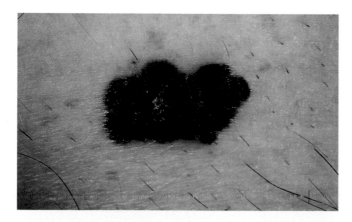
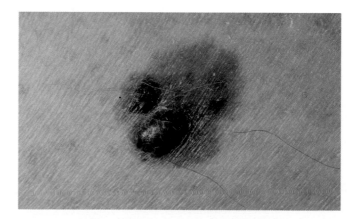

Figure 22-26
There are raised plaque, dome-shaped, and polypoid lesions. Some appear to be
originating from nevi. A halo has developed around one of the plaque-shaped melanomas.

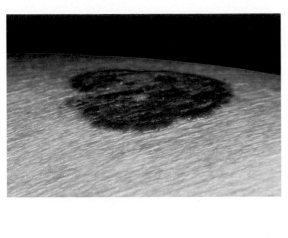

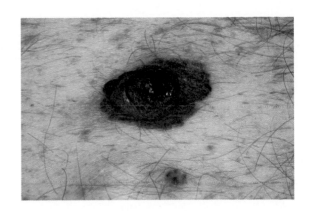

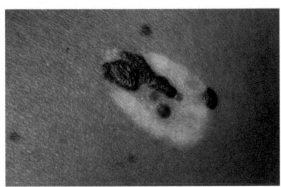

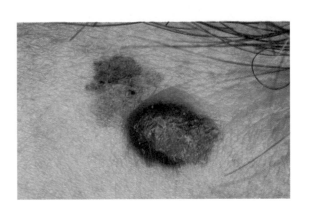

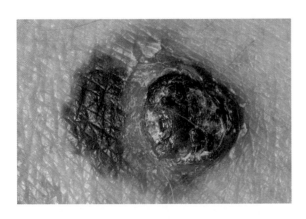

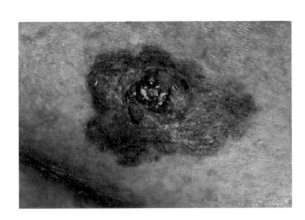

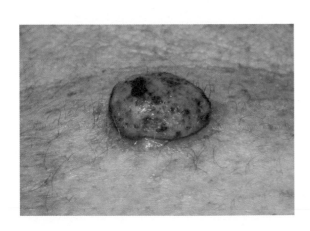

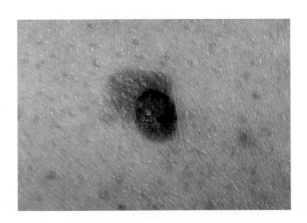

LENTIGO MALIGNA-MELANOMA

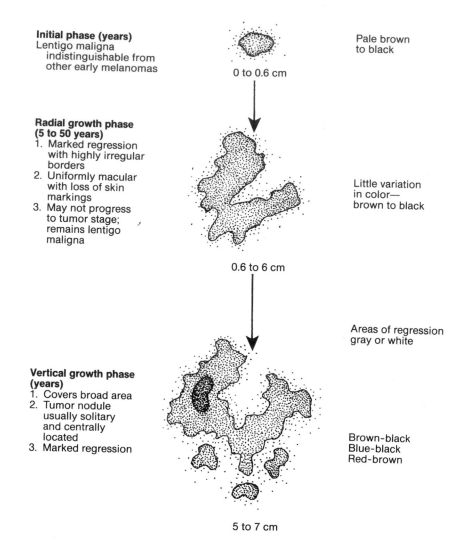

Initial phase (years)
Lentigo maligna
  indistinguishable from
  other early melanomas

0 to 0.6 cm

Pale brown
to black

**Radial growth phase
(5 to 50 years)**
1. Marked regression
   with highly irregular
   borders
2. Uniformly macular
   with loss of skin
   markings
3. May not progress
   to tumor stage;
   remains lentigo
   maligna

0.6 to 6 cm

Little variation
in color—
brown to black

Areas of regression
gray or white

**Vertical growth phase
(years)**
1. Covers broad area
2. Tumor nodule
   usually solitary
   and centrally
   located
3. Marked regression

5 to 7 cm

Brown-black
Blue-black
Red-brown

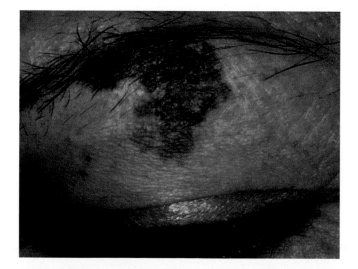

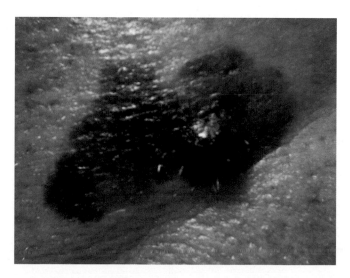

Figure 22-27
The lesions grow slowly and regress for several years, forming highly irregular borders.
The color remains brown or black until the tumor stage is reached. The lesions on p. 707 have been present for years.

Lentigo maligna and lentigo maligna melanoma. LMM (Figure 22-27) usually presents in the sixth or seventh decade. Most are located on the face, but 10% are on other exposed sites, such as arms and legs.

The radial growth phase is called *lentigo maligna* (LM) or *Hutchinson's freckle*. The radial growth phase may last for years and never develop a vertical growth phase. The risk of progression of LM to LMM varies with age, but is lower than commonly believed. For a patient aged 45 years with LM, the estimated risk of developing LMM by age 75 is 3.3%. Estimated lifetime risk of transformation to melanoma is 4.7%. For a patient aged 65 years with LM, the risk of developing LMM is 1.2%, and the lifetime risk of transformation to melanoma is 2.2%. These risk estimates apply to patients in whom LM is discovered incidentally.[51]

LMM may have a complex patten. Years of migration and regression can produce lesions with a shape more varied and bizarre than that of SSM. The color is more uniform than SSM, but red and white may later occur. Tumors are generally in the center of the lesion, away from the border. LMM may ulcerate or undergo changes similar to other lesions when they enter the tumor stage. Nodules are usually single and generally appear when the lesion has assumed a size of 5 to 7 cm, but may occur in much smaller lesions. LMM does not have a better prognosis than other forms of melanoma; as with other types of melanoma, the prognosis depends on tumor thickness.[52]

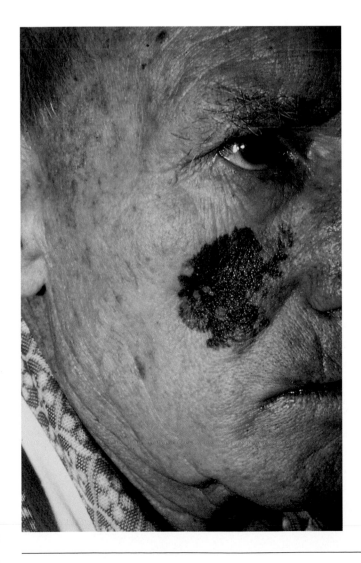

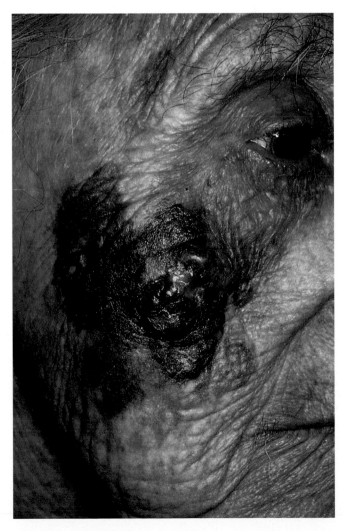

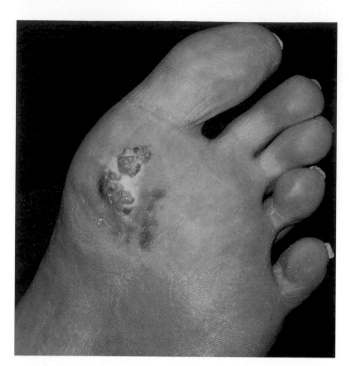

Figure 22-28
Acral-lentiginous melanoma.

Acral-lentiginous melanoma. ALM (Figures 22-28 and 22-29) appears on the palms,[53] soles, terminal phalanges, and mucous membranes.[54] Similar in clinical presentation to LM and LMM, ALM has the same colors and tendency to remain flat. Like LM, plantar melanomas may remain latent for a number of years, making patients with these lesions good candidates for therapeutic cures if detected early.[55] ALM is most frequent in blacks and Asians. The sole of the foot is the most prevalent site of malignant melanoma in non-Caucasians. Small areas of elevation may be associated with deep invasion; the tumor is very aggressive and metastasizes early. The sudden appearance of a pigmented band originating at the proximal nail fold (Hutchinson's sign) is suggestive of acral-lentiginous melanoma (Figure 22-30). Acquired melanocytic lesions on the sole larger than 7 mm in maximum diameter should be examined histologically.

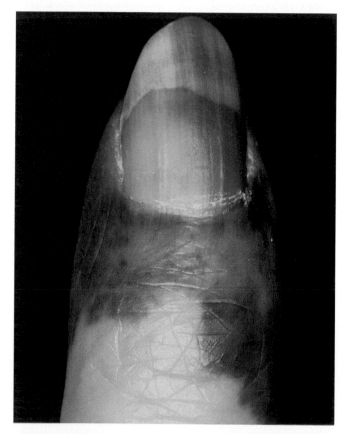

Figure 22-29
Acral-lentiginous melanoma. Macular pigmentation had progressed slowly for over 3 years before the patient consulted a physician.

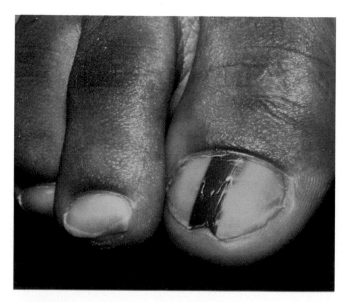

Figure 22-30
Acral-lentiginous melanoma. The sudden appearance of a pigmented band originating at the proximal nail fold (Hutchinson's sign) is suggestive of acral-lentiginous melanoma.

BENIGN LESIONS THAT RESEMBLE MELANOMA

Typical nevi or other lesions, such as those of seborrheic keratosis, may have features that suggest melanoma. These lesions should be biopsied (Figures 22-31 to 22-34).

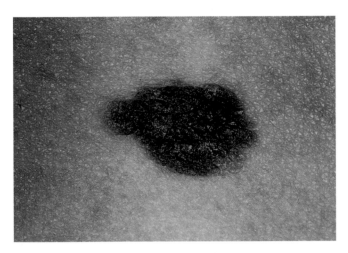

Figure 22-31
Nevus with an irregular border and a variety of colors resembling superficial spreading melanoma.

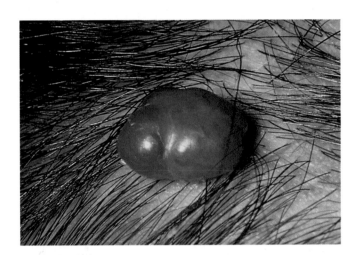

Figure 22-32
Hemangioma (nodular shaped) resembling nodular melanoma.

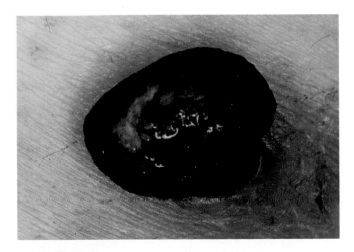

Figure 22-33
Traumatized hemangioma suggesting malignant degeneration.

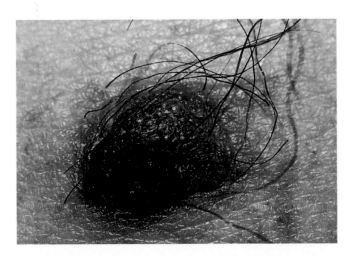

Figure 22-34
Traumatized nevus suggesting malignant degeneration.

DERMOSCOPY

Most pigmented lesions can be diagnosed on the basis of clinical criteria. However, there are many small lesions in which the distinction between a benign and malignant process cannot be made by examination with the naked eye.

Dermoscopy (epiluminescence microscopy) is a technique used to see a variety of structures in pigmented lesions that are not discernible to the naked eye.[56,57] Lotion or mineral oil is applied to the surface of the lesion to make the epidermis more transparent. Then examination with a 10× ocular scope, a microscope ocular eyepiece (held upside down), or a dermatoscope (available from surgical supply houses) reveals several features that are helpful in differentiating between benign and malignant pigmented lesions. This technique provides additional criteria for the diagnosis of melanoma (see boxes on pp. 710 to 713).

Patterns seen by dermoscopy

Reticulated pattern or brown pigment "network." A network of brownish lines over a tan background is seen. It represents pigment in the epidermal basal cells.[58] It is regular or irregular, narrow or wide.

Diffuse pigmentation or blotches. These are irregularly shaped, dark brown or black areas of pigmentation of various sizes. Some resemble "ink spots." They correspond to areas where there is melanin in all levels of the epidermis and/or upper dermis.

Brown globules. These are circular to oval pigmented structures. They represent nests of melanocytes or melanophages at the dermoepidermal junction or in the upper dermis.

Black dots. Black dots are sharply circumscribed and round. They can be various sizes but are often very small. This represents a focal collection of melanin in the stratum corneum.

Depigmented or hypopigmented areas. Zones of relatively lighter pigmentation represent patchy areas of the epidermis that contain less melanin or a relatively thinned epidermis where telangiectasias are often noticeable.

White areas. These areas have no pigment. They correspond to zones with no melanin in the epidermis and dermis. They may have fibroplasia and telangiectasias such as those seen in areas of "regression" of malignant melanomas.

Grey-blue areas. Melanin in the deeper dermis causes the blue hue.

Radial streaming and pseudopods. Linear brown to black streaks radiate from the border of a pigmented lesion into surrounding skin. This feature is also seen in the central areas of lightly pigmented melanomas. Pseudopods are curved extensions. These features are morphologic expressions of the radial growth phase of melanoma.[59]

DERMOSCOPY (EPILUMINESCENCE MICROSCOPY)* OF PIGMENTED LESIONS

BENIGN
Nevi
Lentigo

MALIGNANT
Melanoma

| Regular netlike pattern | **Pigment network** | Irregular, wide Abruptly ends at periphery |

| Regular, homogeneous Gradually thins at periphery | **Diffuse pigmentation** | Heavy, irregular Abruptly ends at periphery |

*Apply lotion or mineral oil to the surface and examine with a hand lens (10× magnification).

DERMOSCOPY (EPILUMINESCENCE MICROSCOPY)* OF PIGMENTED LESIONS

BENIGN
Nevi
Lentigo

MALIGNANT
Melanoma

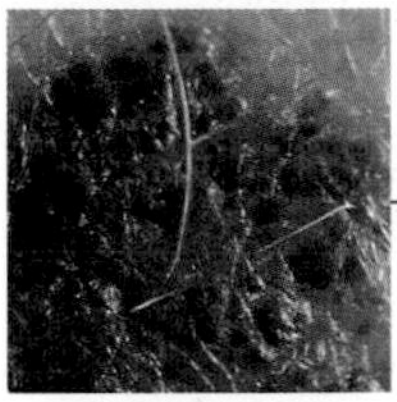

Uniform in size
and shape
Regularly
distributed
——— **Brown globules** ———
Varied in size
and shape
Irregularly
distributed

Uniform in size
and shape
Regularly
distributed
——— **Black dots** ———
Varied in size
and shape
Irregularly
distributed

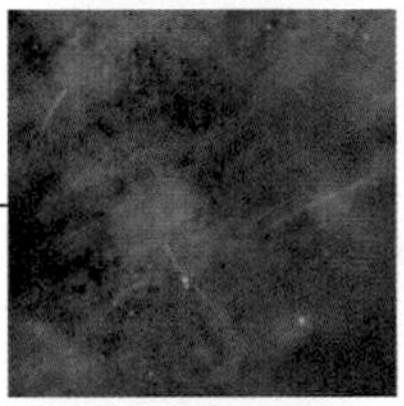

Uniform and
homogeneous
——— **Hypopigmented and depigmented areas** ———
Irregularly
distributed

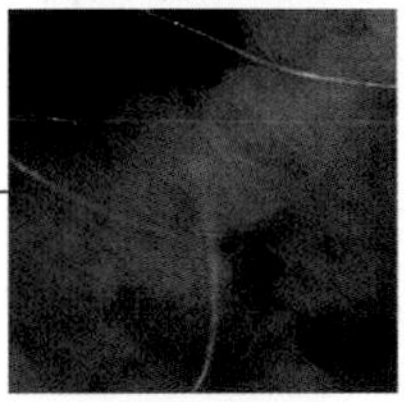

Pseudopods Radial streaming ———
Brown projections
radiating into
normal skin
Called *pseudopods*
when fingerlike
or branched

White areas ——————— No pigment ———

Grey-blue areas ———
Dense ill-
defined areas

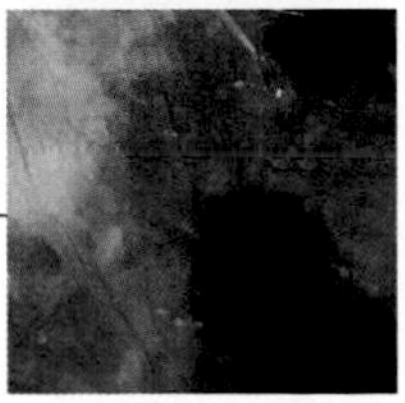

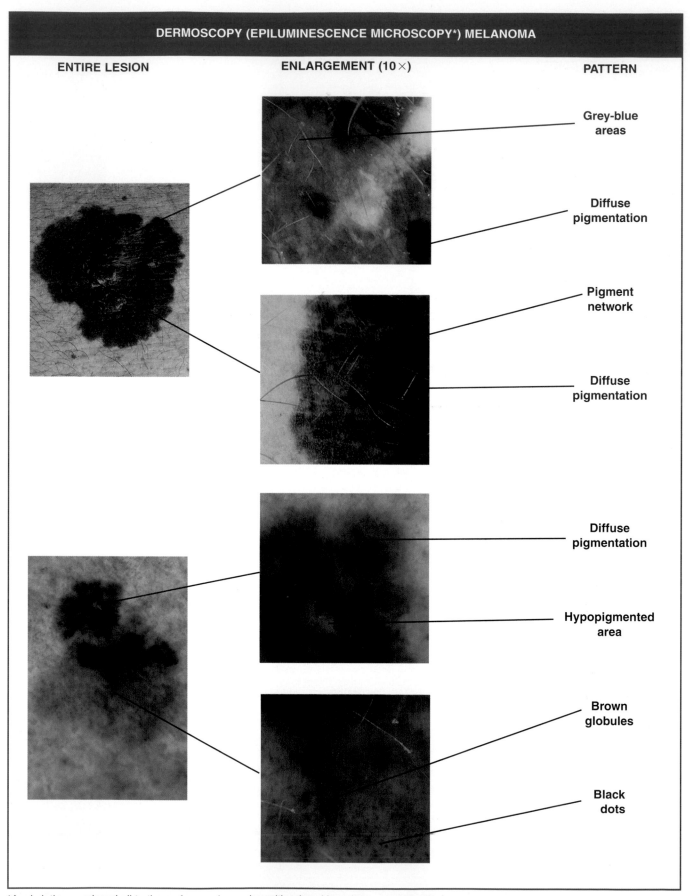

DERMOSCOPY (EPILUMINESCENCE MICROSCOPY*) MELANOMA

ENTIRE LESION   **ENLARGEMENT (10×)**   **PATTERN**

Grey-blue areas

Diffuse pigmentation

Pigment network

Diffuse pigmentation

Diffuse pigmentation

Hypopigmented area

Brown globules

Black dots

*Apply lotion or mineral oil to the surface and examine with a hand lens (10 × magnification).

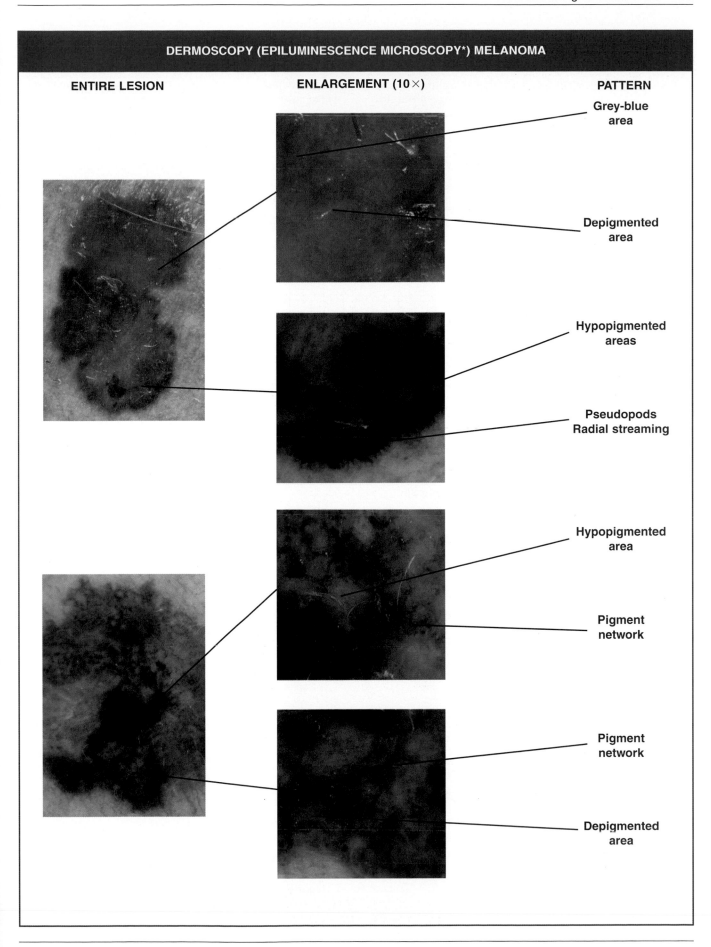

DERMOSCOPY (EPILUMINESCENCE MICROSCOPY*) MELANOMA

ENTIRE LESION   ENLARGEMENT (10×)   PATTERN

Grey-blue area

Depigmented area

Hypopigmented areas

Pseudopods Radial streaming

Hypopigmented area

Pigment network

Pigment network

Depigmented area

BIOPSY

Excisonal biopsy. The prognosis and extent of surgery are based on tumor type, thickness, and level of invasion. The pathologist is capable of reporting this information if provided with an excisional biopsy of the entire lesion that is deep enough to include subcutaneous fat. Whenever possible, a margin of 1 cm should be used, as this is an adequate and definitive treatment in melanomas up to 1 mm in Breslow thickness.

Incisional or punch biopsy. Incisional or punch biopsies are sometimes necessary in surgically sensitive areas, such as the nose and periorbital or digital regions. If total excision is impractical, an incisional biopsy should be taken from what is considered to be the deepest part of the tumor; that

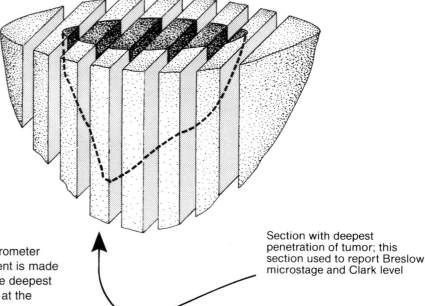

Biopsy specimen   Sections cut by pathologist

Section with deepest penetration of tumor; this section used to report Breslow microstage and Clark level

Figure 22-35
To obtain the Breslow microstage, an ocular micrometer mounted on the microscope is used. Measurement is made from the granular cell layer to the section with the deepest penetration of tumor. When ulceration is present at the surface, measurements starts at the ulcer base.

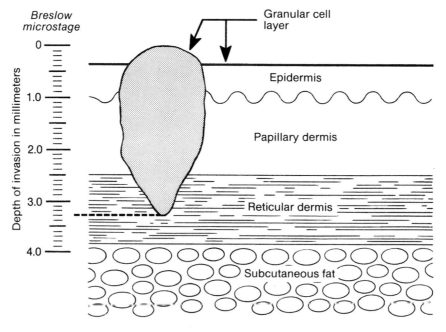

Tumor pictured—reported by pathologist as:
1. Depth of invasion 3.3 mm
2. Clark level 4

is, the area with the highest surface elevation. The darkest area should be sampled in flat lesions. Punch biopsy may not be sufficient because it yields such a small piece of tissue that the problem may go undetected. Studies suggest that cutting into a melanoma by incisional or punch biopsy before definitive surgery does not dislodge malignant cells that could result in systemic metastases.[60,61]

PATHOLOGY REPORT

The pathologist determines the following in the pathology report (Figure 22-35):

Tumor thickness (Breslow microstage). The tumor is step sectioned. The section with the deepest level of penetration of tumor is used to measure thickness. An ocular micrometer is placed on the microscope. The pathologist measures the thickness of the tumor in millimeters from the granular cell layer to the deepest part of the tumor. The report is given as Breslow level, followed by the depth reported in millimeters.[62,63]

Tumor thickness (Clark level). The tumor depth is reported by anatomic site (i.e., epidermis, depth in dermis, etc.) and assigned a Clark level of invasion (Figure 22-35).[64]

Radial growth phase vs. vertical growth phase. The growth phase of the tumor is determined by histologic criteria (see Table 22-7).

Mitotic rate. The mitotic rate per mm^2 is reported.

Tumor-infiltrating lymphocytes. The degree to which lymphocytes infiltrate and disrupt the tumor cell is reported.

Histologic regression. Areas of epidermis that have no recognizable tumor and are flanked by areas of melanoma indicate regression.

CLINICAL STAGING, INITIAL INVESTIGATIONS, AND FOLLOW-UP

Clinical staging. Clinical staging refers to the extent of disease as determined by physical examination. Stage I con-sists of local disease. Stage II is enlarged regional lymph nodes, as determined by palpation. In stage III, there is clinical evidence of disseminated disease through, for instance, positive liver scan or chest x-ray.

Initial investigations. Studies show that the initial staging investigations can be limited to history and physical examinations with baseline chest x-ray. Other examinations have failed to detect metastatic melanoma.[65,66]

Follow-up investigations. Follow-up should include only history, physical examinations, and chest x-rays. Other routine studies have failed to detect metastatic disease.[65]

Follow-up examinations. For those patients who have recurrence of their melanomas, the period of disease-free survival correlates inversely with tumor thickness: the thicker the primary tumor, the shorter the disease-free interval for that group.[67] Table 22-4 shows the observed rate of recurrence by year for patients in each of four tumor thickness groups. Table 22-5 shows suggested schedules of follow-up visits after diagnosis with clinical stage I melanoma. Patients with thicker tumors have elevated risk of recurrence in the early years after diagnosis and need to be followed more frequently.

Patients may develop recurrence after 10 years or more of being disease free. Late recurrence may be local, and survival subsequent to treatment of these metastases is often protracted. Therefore, patients with cutaneous melanoma should be followed for life.[68,69]

One study showed that patients with three or more clinically atypical nevi and patients with atypical nevi plus a history of melanoma had a significantly increased risk for melanoma. No second melanoma developed among patients with previous melanoma who had a normal nevus pattern. The highest risk of melanoma was among patients with atypical nevi and a family history of melanoma. This study showed the value of clinical follow-up of high-risk patients to detect early thin melanomas.[70]

TABLE 22-4 Probability of Recurrence of Melanoma (Based on 1324 Stage I Patients)

Year following diagnosis	Tumor thickness			
	<0.76 mm (381 patients)	0.76-0.149 mm (405 patients)	1.50-4.0 mm (410 patients)	>4.0 mm (128 patients)
1	1.0(%)	5.7(%)	18.8(%)	33.6(%)
2	0.8	3.2	12.5	12.3
3	1.8	4.4	8.3	15.9
4	0.6	5.3	6.3	12.5
5	0.7	3.1	4.7	5.0
6	0.9	5.9	4.8	0
7	0	4.2	3.2	0
8	0	4.4	7.3	0
9	0.4	0	7.7	0
10	0	0	4.1	0

From Kelly JW, Blois MS, Jagebiel RW: *J Am Acad Dermatol* 13:756, 1985.

TABLE 22-5 Follow-up Intervals After Diagnosis of Melanoma

Year following diagnosis	Tumor thickness			
	<0.76 mm	0.76-1.49 mm	1.50-4.0 mm	>4.0 mm
1	6 mos	6 mos	3 mos	2-3 mos
2	12	6	4	3
3	12	6	4	3
4	12	6	4	3
5	12	6	6	6
6	12	6	6	6
7	12	8	6	6
8	12	10	8	8
9	12	10	10	10
10	12	12	10	10

From Kelly JW, Blois MS, Jagebiel RW: *J Am Acad Dermatol* 13:756, 1985.

PROGNOSIS

Clinical stage I

Prognosis in perspective. The following paragraphs list clinical and histologic features of melanoma used to predict prognosis. Tumor thickness has been used as the most important variable in predicting prognosis[71] (Figure 22-36). Vertical growth phase, high mitotic index, marked cytologic atypia, minimal tumor inflammatory infiltrate, presence of regression, presence of plasma cells, male sex, age more than 45 years, and axial anatomic location are all features associated with a poor prognosis.[72] A model has been developed based on these criteria and was found by one group to be 76% accurate in predicting outcome over 10 years. There is, however, a significant population of long-term survivors in whom prognosis cannot be accurately predicted using these features. Some patients with multiple features that suggest a poor prognosis survive for years, whereas others with few such features die rapidly. The following may be used to provide a general sense of prognosis. Individual patients with unique genetic and immunologic characteristics may not fit this model.[73]

Clark et al. developed a model for predicting 8-year survival in individual stage I melanoma patients. The model is based on the following histologic and clinical data (see Figure 22-8).

1. Tumor thickness (Breslow microstage).
2. Tumor thickness (Clark level).
3. Growth phase—radial growth phase or vertical growth phase. Transformed melanocytes first proliferate above the epidermal basement membrane, then invade the papillary dermis (Clark level 2). These are the in situ and microinvasive radial growth phases of melanoma. Tumors larger than 0.76 mm are, with rare exceptions, in the vertical growth phase. Levels 3 and 4 tumors are usually in the vertical growth phase.
4. Mitotic rate.

5. Degree of tumor lymphocyte infiltration.
6. Presence or absence of histologic regression.
7. Record the anatomic site of the primary and the sex of the patient.[74]

Radial growth phase tumors. Melanomas with malignant cells confined above the epidermal basement membrane (in situ) or in the papillary dermis (microinvasive) are called *radial growth phase melanomas.* These are almost always less than .76 mm thick. Projected survival probability is 100%.[75]

Vertical growth phase tumors. Tumors that have invaded the reticular dermis have entered the vertical growth phase. Projected survival probability is determined from the probability tables, using the data collected from the pathologist's report. The prognostic model of Clark et al. (Tables 22-6 through 22-8), based upon the concept of tumor progression and the evaluation of six readily assessible clinical and histologic attributes, has been validated by another study.[76]

Pregnancy, oral contraceptives, prognosis, and risk. On the basis of a limited number of controlled studies, it does not appear that pregnancy before, after, or at the time of diagnosis of stage I MM influences the 5-year survival rate.[77,78]

Oral contraceptive use does not seem to increase the risk of malignant melanoma,[79] except possibly for women aged 30 to 40 years who used oral contraception for 10 years or more or who started to use oral contraception 15 years or more before the diagnosis.[80]

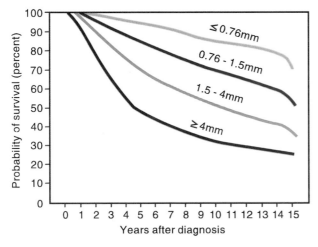

Figure 22-36
Survival of stage I melanoma patients based on tumor thickness. (Data from Slingluff CL Jr, Dodge RK, Stanley WE, et al: *Cancer* 70:1924, 1992.)

TABLE 22-6	Single Variable 8-Year Survival Results for Clinical Stage I Vertical Growth Phase Melanoma	
Variable	**Characteristic**	**% Survival***
Mitotic rate	0.0/mm²	95.1
	0.1-6.0/mm²	79.4
	>6.0/mm²	38.2
Tumor infiltrating lymphocytes	Brisk	88.5
	Nonbrisk	75.0
	Absent	59.3
Thickness	<0.76 mm	93.2
	0.76 mm-1.69 mm	85.6
	1.70 mm-3.60 mm	59.8
	>3.60 mm	33.3
Site	Extremities	87.3
	Head, neck, and trunk	62.4
	Volar or subungual	46.2
Sex	Female	83.8
	Male	56.6
Regression	Absent or incomplete	77.0
	Present	60.0

Modified from Clark WH Jr et al: *J Natl Cancer Inst* 81:1893-1904, 1989.
*8-year survival rate—all other attributes being held constant.

TABLE 22-7 Comparison of Invasive Radial Growth Phase With Vertical Growth Phase

Invasive radial growth phase	Vertical growth phase
Isolated foci of melanoma cells are present in the papillary dermis; they are arrayed as single cells or as small clusters of cells no more than 5 to 10 cells wide	The melanoma cells in the dermis are seen as a contiguous spheric or plaquelike aggregate larger than any nest of radial growth phase cells Such aggregates are easily recognized when thickness is >0.76 mm

Modified from Clark WH Jr et al: *J Natl Cancer Inst* 81:1893-1904, 1989.

TABLE 22-8 Probabilities of 8-Year Survival Given a Thickness of <1.70 mm* or Thickness of ≥1.70 mm*

Mitotic rate/mm²	Til†	Regression	Female				Male			
			Extremities		Head and trunk‡		Extremities		Head and trunk‡	
			<	≥	<	≥	<	≥	<	≥
0.0/mm²	Brisk	Absent	1.0	.99	1.0	.98	1.0	.98	.99	.95
		Present	1.0	.99	.99	.95	.99	.96	.96	.86
	Nonbrisk	Absent	1.0	.98	.98	.94	.99	.95	.96	.84
		Present	.99	.95	.96	.85	.97	.88	.89	.66
	Absent	Absent	.99	.94	.95	.82	.96	.85	.86	.60
		Present	.96	.86	.87	.61	.89	.67	.69	.35
0.1–6.0/mm²	Brisk	Absent	1.0	.98	.98	.94	.99	.95	.95	.84
		Present	.99	.95	.96	.84	.97	.87	.88	.65
	Nonbrisk	Absent	.99	.95	.95	.82	.96	.86	.87	.61
		Present	.96	.86	.87	.62	.90	.68	.70	.36
	Absent	Absent	.95	.83	.84	.57	.87	.63	.65	.31
		Present	.88	.64	.66	.32	.71	.38	.40	.14
>6.0/mm²	Brisk	Absent	.99	.94	.95	.81	.96	.85	.86	.60
		Present	.96	.85	.86	.61	.89	.67	.68	.35
	Nonbrisk	Absent	.95	.84	.84	.57	.88	.63	.65	.31
		Present	.88	.64	.66	.32	.72	.38	.40	.14
	Absent	Absent	.85	.59	.61	.28	.67	.33	.34	.12
		Present	.68	.34	.35	.12	.42	.15	.16	.04

Modified from Clark WH Jr et al: *J Natl Cancer Inst* 81:1893-1904, 1989. All numbers derived from a point-survival probability.
*Vertical growth phase; clinical stage I cases.
†Tumor infiltrating lymphocytes.
‡Also including neck, volar, and subungual primary site location.

SURGICAL MANAGEMENT OF CLINICAL STAGE I MELANOMA

Clinical stage I melanoma is managed surgically. The surgeon must determine the resection margins and decide whether or not to perform a regional node dissection.

Resection margins. Recent data show that a surgical margin of 1 cm is appropriate treatment for most thin melanomas (1 mm or less in Breslow thickness)[81-83] (see Table 22-8 and Figure 22-37). A multiinstitutional study demonstrated that lesions 1 to 4 mm thick can be excised with a 2-cm margin.[84] Compromises are necessary for lesions on the digits and face.

Management of lymph nodes

Therapeutic lymph node dissection. The surgical excision of lymph nodes clinically positive for tumor is referred to as a *therapeutic lymph node dissection*. Surgical excision of metastases to regional lymph nodes can result in a cure. Patients with a primary melanoma who have an enlarged lymph node are treated with radical dissection of all the nodes in the region of the primary cancer.

Elective lymph node dissection. Excision of clinically normal-appearing regional lymph nodes when the primary melanoma is initially diagnosed is known as an *elective lymph node dissection* (ELND). It is performed because of the risk of occult or microscopic metastases. Whether surgery should be performed when there is no indication that the cancer has metastasized is still uncertain.[85,86,87] The consensus at this time is that node dissection can be delayed until regional node metastases becomes evident. Opponents of this "wait-and-see policy" claim that postponing dissection could allow the cancer to spread.

Patients with clinically negative nodes who are likely to benefit from elective lymph node dissection are those with a primary melanoma that is between 1.5 and 4 mm thick. The decision to perform an elective lymph node dissection in this group is at the discretion of the surgeon. If ELND is not performed, careful follow-up and education regarding lymph node self-examination is critical.

Sentinel node mapping and biopsy. Sentinel node biopsy offers an alternative to either elective removal of all nodes in the drainage basin or the "watch and wait" strategy.[88] The technique helps identify occult, microscopic nodal disease. The procedure is performed at the time of wide excision of a primary melanoma to determine whether lymphadenectomy is indicated. A blue dye (patent blue-V or isosulfan blue) is injected intradermally at the site of the melanoma. The dye is rapidly taken up by the lymphatic vessels and carried to the first lymph node ("sentinel node") in the basin to which the melanoma site drains. A small incision is made over the site of the expected lymphatic drainage; the "sentinel node" is identified by its blue staining and is sent for frozen section examination and rapid immunoperoxidase staining. Studies show that the histology of the sentinel lymph node is characteristic of the entire lymph node basin. Skip metastases to nonsentinel nodes are found in fewer than 1% of patients.

Lymphoscintigraphy. The lymphadenectomy site can be determined more accurately by lymphoscintigraphy than by anatomic guidelines and leads to minimum surgical intervention.[89,90] Intradermal lymphoscintigraphy is especially useful for determining the direction of lymphatic drainage in patients who have melanoma on the trunk, where multidirectional lymphatic drainage is likely. Most patients show

Figure 22-37
Melanoma surgical guidelines.

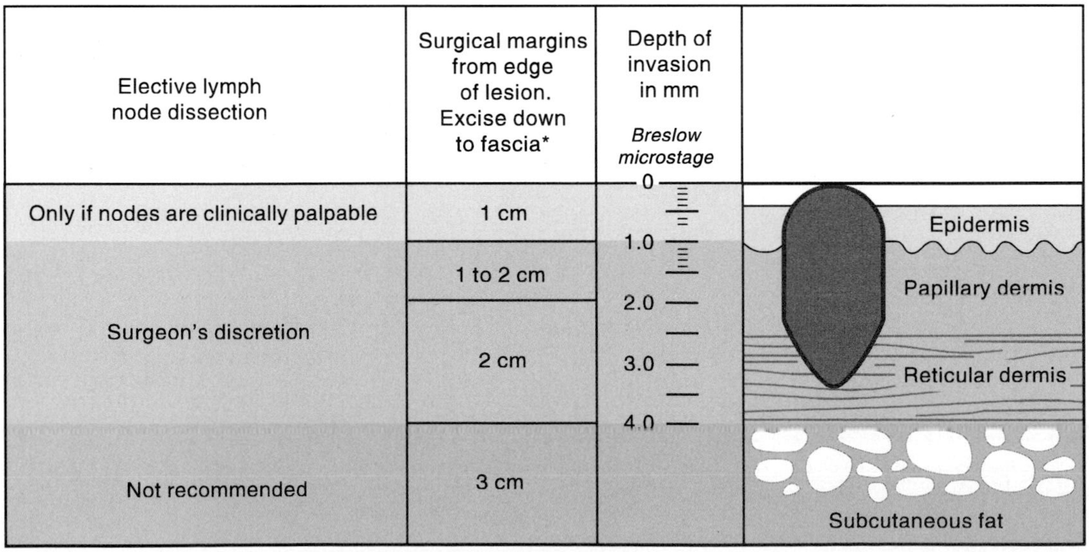

Elective lymph node dissection	Surgical margins from edge of lesion. Excise down to fascia*	Depth of invasion in mm *Breslow microstage*	
Only if nodes are clinically palpable	1 cm	0 — 1.0	Epidermis
Surgeon's discretion	1 to 2 cm	2.0	Papillary dermis
	2 cm	3.0	Reticular dermis
		4.0	
Not recommended	3 cm		Subcutaneous fat

lymph drainage to one or two node groups. Technetium radio-labeled sulfur colloid is injected intracutaneously around the primary site and traced to its lymph node destination.[91] The number and location of interval nodes can be determined and marked on the skin. These and the major lymph channels can be excised at the time of surgery.

Cryosurgery of lentigo maligna. Lentigo maligna is found predominantly in areas of actinic damage where cosmetically unsatisfactory scars may result from conventional surgery. Cryosurgery is an efficient alternative to conventional surgery provided that patients are selected properly and extension of cryonecrosis is monitored.[92]

REFERENCES

1. Elder DE, Greene MH, Bondi EE, et al: Acquired melanocytic nevi and melanoma—the dysplastic nevus syndrome. In Ackerman AB, editor: *Pathology of malignant melanoma,* New York, 1981, Masson.
2. Steiner A, Pehamberger H, Wolff K: In vivo epiluminescence microscopy of pigmented skin lesions. II. Diagnosis of small pigmented skin lesions and early detection of malignant melanoma, *J Am Acad Dermatol* 17:584-591, 1987.
3. Pehamberger H, Steiner A, Wolff K: In vivo epiluminescence microscopy of pigmented skin lesions. I. Pattern analysis of pigmented skin lesions, *J Am Acad Dermatol* 17:571-583, 1987.
4. Cochran AJ, Bailly C, et al: Nevi, other than dysplastic and Spitz nevi, *Semin Diagn Pathol* 10:3-17, 1993.
5. Connors RC, Ackerman AB: Histologic pseudomalignancies of the skin, *Arch Dermatol* 112:1767-1780, 1976.
6. Ronnen M et al: Pseudomelanoma following treatment with surgical excision and intralesional triamcinolone acetonide to prevent keloid formation, *Int J Dermatol* 25:533-534, 1987.
7. Park HK, Leonard DD, Arrington JH, et al: Recurrent melanocytic nevi: clinical and histologic review of 175 cases, *J Am Acad Dermatol* 17:285-292, 1987.
8. Bolognia JL et al: The significance of eccentric foci of hyperpigmentation ("small dark dots") within melanocytic nevi, *Arch Dermatol* 130:1013-1017, 1994.
9. Kopf AW, Bart RS, Hennessey P: Congenital nevocytic nevi and malignant melanomas, *J Am Acad Dermatol* 1:123-130, 1979.
10. Swerdlow AJ et al: The risk of melanoma in patients with congenital nevi: a cohort study, *J Am Acad Dermatol* 32:595-599, 1995.
11. Rhodes AR et al: The malignant potential of small congenital nevocellular nevi. An estimate of association based on a histologic study of 234 primary melanomas, *J Am Acad Dermatol* 6:230-241, 1982.
12. Rhodes AR: Small congenital nevi (reply), *J Am Acad Dermatol* 7:687, 1982.
13. Stewart DM, Altman J, Mehregan AH: Speckled lentiginous nevus, *Arch Dermatol* 114:895-896, 1978.
14. Cohen HJ, Minkin W, Frank SB: Nevus spilus, *Arch Dermatol* 102:433-437, 1970.
15. Bart RS, Kopf A: Extensive melanosis and hypertrichosis (Becker's nevus), *J Dermatol Surg Oncol* 3:379, 1977.
16. Bleehen SS, Ebling FJ: Disorders of skin color. In Rook A, Wilkinson DS, Ebling FJ, et al, editors: *Textbook of dermatology,* ed 2, Oxford, 1979, Scientific Publications.
17. Casso EM et al: Spitz nevi, *J Am Acad Dermatol* 27:901-913, 1992.
18. Binder SW, Asnong C, et al: The histology and differential diagnosis of Spitz nevus, *Semin Diagn Pathol* 10:36-46, 1993.
19. Merkow LP: A cellular and malignant blue nevus, *Cancer* 24:886-896, 1969.
20. Spann CR, Owen LG, Hodge SJ: The labial melanotic macule, *Arch Dermatol* 123:1029-1031, 1987.
21. Newton JA: Familial melanoma, *Clin Exp Dermatol* 18:5-11, 1993.
22. Pellegrini AE: The dysplastic nevus syndrome, What is it? *Am J Dermatopathol* 4:453-454, 1982.
23. Kraemer KH et al: Dysplastic nevi and cutaneous melanoma risk (letter), *Lancet* 2:1076-1077, 1983.
24. Goldstein AM, Tucker MA, et al: The inheritance pattern of dysplastic naevi in families of dysplastic naevus patients, *Melanoma Res* 3:15-22, 1993.
25. Greene MH et al: Hereditary melanoma and the dysplastic nevus syndrome: the risk of cancers other than melanoma, *J Am Acad Dermatol* 16:792-797, 1987.
26. Marghoob AA et al: Risk of cutaneous malignant melanoma in patients with "classic" atypical mole syndrome, *Arch Dermatol* 130:993-998, 1994.
27. Kang S et al: Melanoma risk in individuals with clinically atypical nevi, *Arch Dermatol* 130:999-1001, 1994.
28. Reimer RR et al: Precursor lesions in familial melanoma, a new genetic preneoplastic syndrome, *JAMA* 239:744-746, 1978.
29. Elder DE et al: Dysplastic nevus syndrome: a phenotypic association of sporadic cutaneous melanoma, *Cancer* 46:1787-1794, 1980.
30. Happle R et al: Arguments in favor of a polygenic inheritance of precursor nevi, *J Am Acad Dermatol* 6:540-543, 1982.
31. Greene MH et al: Precursor naevi in cutaneous malignant melanoma: a proposed nomenclature, *Lancet* 2:1024-1027, 1980.
32. Kousseff BG: The genetics of malignant melanomas, *Ann Plast Surg* 28:11-13, 1992.
33. Kraemer KN et al: Risk of cutaneous melanoma in dysplastic nevus syndrome types A and B, *N Engl J Med* 315:1615-1616, 1986.
34. Greene MH et al: Melanoma risk in familial dysplastic nevus syndrome (abstract), *J Invest Dermatol* 82:424, 1984.
35. Precursors to malignant melanoma, National Institutes of Health Consensus Development Conference Statement, Oct 24-26, 1983, *J Am Acad Dermatol* 10:683-688, 1984.
36. Roush GC, Dubin N, et al: Prediction of histologic melanocytic dysplasia from clinical observation, *J Am Acad Dermatol* 29:555-562, 1993.
37. Halpern AC, Guerry D, et al: Natural history of dysplastic nevi, *J Am Acad Dermatol* 29:51-57, 1993.
38. Crijns MB, Bergman W, et al: On naevi and melanomas in dysplastic naevus syndrome patients, *Clin Exp Dermatol* 18:248-252, 1993.
39. Rhodes AR et al: Risk factors for cutaneous melanoma, *JAMA* 258:3146-3154, 1987.
40. Evans RD et al: Risk factors for the development of malignant melanoma-I: review of case-control studies, *J Dermatol Surg Oncol* 14:393-408, 1988.
41. Holman CDJ, Armstrong BK, Heenan PJ: Relationship of cutaneous malignant melanoma to individual sunlight-exposure habits, *J Natl Cancer Inst* 76:403-414, 1986.
42. Nachbar F et al: The ABCD rule of dermatoscopy, *J Am Acad Dermatol* 30:551-559, 1994.
43. Mihm MC et al: Early detection of primary cutaneous malignant melanoma, a color atlas, *N Engl J Med* 289:989-996, 1973.
44. Mihm MC, Clark WH, Reed RJ: The clinical diagnosis of malignant melanoma, *Semin Oncol* 2:105-118, 1975.
45. Kopf AW et al: Clinical diagnosis of cutaneous malignant melanoma. In *Malignant melanoma,* New York, 1979, Masson.
46. Ackerman AB, David KM: A unifying concept of malignant melanoma: biologic aspects, *Hum Pathol* 17:438-440, 1986.
47. Clark WH, Ainsworth AM, Bernardino EA: The developmental biology of primary human malignant melanomas, *Semin Oncol* 2:83-103, 1975.
48. Sober AJ, Fitzpatrick TB, Mihm MC: Primary melanoma of the skin: recognition and management, *J Am Acad Dermatol* 2:179-197, 1980.
49. Sober AJ, Fitzpatrick TB, Mihm MC, et al: Malignant melanoma. In *Dermatology in general medicine,* New York, 1987, McGraw-Hill.
50. McGovern VJ et al: The classification of malignant melanoma and its histologic reporting, *Cancer* 32:1446-1457, 1973.
51. Weinstock MA, Sober AJ: The risk of progression of lentigo maligna to lentigo maligna melanoma, *Br J Dermatol* 116:303-310, 1987.

52. Koh HK et al: Lentigo maligna melanoma has no better prognosis than other types of melanoma, *J Clin Oncol* 2:994-1001, 1984.

53. Dwyer PK, Mackie RM, et al: Plantar malignant melanoma in a white Caucasian population, *Br J Dermatol* 128:115-120, 1993.

54. Sutherland CM, Mather FJ, et al: Acral lentiginous melanoma, *Am J Surg* 166:64-67, 1993.

55. Scrivner D, Oxenhandler RW, Lopez M, et al: Plantar lentiginous melanoma, *Cancer* 60:2502-2509, 1987.

56. Pehamberger H et al: In vivo epiluminescence microscopy: improvement of early diagnosis of melanoma, *J Invest Dermatol* 100:356S-362S, 1993.

57. Kenet RO et al: Clinical diagnosis of pigmented lesions using digital epiluminescence microscopy, *Arch Dermatol* 129:157-174, 1993.

58. Yadau S et al: Histopathologic correlates of structures seen on dermoscopy (epiluminescence microscopy), *Am J Dermatopath* 15(4):297-305, 1993.

59. Menzies SW et al: The morphologic criteria of the pseudopod in surface microscopy, *Arch Dermatol* 131:436-440, 1995.

60. Lederman JS, Sober AJ: Does biopsy type influence survival in clinical stage I cutaneous melanoma? *J Am Acad Dermatol* 13:983, 1985. Letter to the editor questioning results with a reply, *J Am Acad Dermatol* 15:293-294, 1986.

61. Penneys NS: Excision of melanoma after initial biopsy, an immunohistochemical study, *J Am Acad Dermatol* 13:995-998, 1985.

62. Breslow A: Prognosis in stage I cutaneous melanoma: tumor thickness as a guide to treatment. In *Pathology of malignant melanoma*, New York, 1981, Masson.

63. Breslow A et al: Stage I melanoma of the limbs: assessment of prognosis by levels of invasion and maximum thickness, *Tumori* 64:373-384, 1978.

64. Suffin SC, Waisman J, Clark WH, et al: Comparison of the classification by microscopic level (stage) of malignant melanoma by three independent groups of pathologists, *Cancer* 40:3112-3114, 1977.

65. Kersey PA et al: The value of staging and serial follow-up investigations in patients with completely resected, primary, cutaneous malignant melanoma, *Br J Surg* 72:614-617, 1985.

66. Ardizzoni A et al: Stage I-II melanoma: the value of metastatic work-up, *Oncology* 44:87-89, 1987.

67. Kelly JW, Blois M, Sagebiel RW: Frequency and duration of patient follow-up after treatment of a primary malignant melanoma, *J Am Acad Dermatol* 13:756-760, 1985.

68. Shaw HM, Beattie CW, McCarthy WH, et al: Late relapse from cutaneous stage I malignant melanoma, *Arch Surg* 120:1155-1159, 1985.

69. Rogers GS et al: Hazard-rate analysis in stage I malignant melanoma, *Arch Dermatol* 122:999-1002, 1986.

70. MacKie RM, McHenry P, et al: Accelerated detection with prospective surveillance for cutaneous malignant melanoma in high-risk groups, *Lancet* 341:1618-1620, 1993.

71. Morton DL, Davtyan DG, et al: Multivariate analysis of the relationship between survival and the microstage of primary melanoma by Clark level and Breslow thickness, *Cancer* 71:3737-3743, 1993.

72. Wanek LA, Elashoff RM, et al: Application of multistage Markov modeling to malignant melanoma progression, *Cancer* 73:336-343, 1994.

73. Rowley MJ, Cockerell CJ: Reliability of prognostic models in malignant melanoma. A 10-year followup study,. *Am J Dermatopathol* 13:431-437, 1991.

74. Bernengo MG, Reali UM, et al: BANS: a discussion of the problem, *Melanoma Res* 2:157-162, 1992.

75. Guerry D, Synnestvedt M, et al: Lessons from tumor progression: the invasive radial growth phase of melanoma is common, incapable of metastasis, and indolent, *J Invest Dermatol* 100:342S-345S, 1993.

76. Szymik B, Woosley JT: Further validation of the prognostic model for stage I malignant melanoma based on tumor progression, *J Cutan Pathol* 20:50-53, 1993.

77. Driscoll MS, Grin-Jorgensen CM, et al: Does pregnancy influence the prognosis of malignant melanoma? *J Am Acad Dermatol* 29:619-630, 1993.

78. Kjems E, Krag C: Melanoma and pregnancy. A review, *Acta Oncol* 32:371-378, 1993.

79. Palmer JR, Rosenberg L, et al: Oral contraceptive use and risk of cutaneous malignant melanoma, *Cancer Causes Control* 3:547-554, 1992.

80. Le MG, Cabanes PA, et al: Oral contraceptive use and risk of cutaneous malignant melanoma in a case-control study of French women, *Cancer Causes Control* 3:199-205, 1992.

81. Rivers JK: Management of precursors and primary lesions of melanoma, *Curr Opin Oncol* 5:377-382, 1993.

82. NIH Consensus conference. Diagnosis and treatment of early melanoma, *JAMA* 268:1314-1319, 1992.

83. Veronesi U, Cascinelli N: Narrow excision (1-cm margin). A safe procedure for thin cutaneous melanoma, *Arch Surg* 126:438-441, 1991.

84. Balch CM, Urist MM, et al: Efficacy of 2-cm surgical margins for intermediate-thickness melanomas (1 to 4 mm). Results of a multi-institutional randomized surgical trial, *Ann Surg* 218:262-267, 1993.

85. Drepper H, Kohler CO, et al: Benefit of elective lymph node dissection in subgroups of melanoma patients. Results of a multicenter study of 3616 patients, *Cancer* 72:741-749, 1993.

86. Hein DW, Moy RL: Elective lymph node dissection in stage I malignant melanoma: a meta-analysis, *Melanoma Res* 2:273-277, 1992.

87. Lyons JH, Cockerel CJ: Elective lymph node dissection for melanoma, *J Am Acad Dermatol* 30:467-480, 1994.

88. Morton DL, Wen DR, et al: Intraoperative lymphatic mapping and selective cervical lymphadenectomy for early-stage melanomas of the head and neck, *J Clin Oncol* 11:1751-1756, 1993.

89. Uren RF, Howman-Giles RB, et al: Lymphoscintigraphy in high-risk melanoma of the trunk: predicting draining node groups, defining lymphatic channels and locating the sentinel node, *J Nucl Med* 34:1435-1440, 1993.

90. Fisher EB, Lewis V Jr, et al: The role of cutaneous lymphoscintigraphy in determining regional lymph node drainage of truncal melanomas, *Ann Plast Surg* 28:506-510, 1992.

91. Farciano D et al: Lymphoscintigraphy in melanoma patients using Tc-99m dextran, *J Nucl Med* 25:40-41, 1984.

92. Bohler-Sommeregger K, Schuller-Petrovic S, et al: Cryosurgery of lentigo maligna, *Plast Reconstr Surg* 90:436-440, 1992.

CHAPTER TWENTY-THREE

Vascular Tumors and Malformations

Congenital Vascular Lesions

A number of different congenital vascular lesions occur in the skin. Most represent developmental malformations and do not appear to be genetically determined. Vascular structures may be abnormal in size, abnormal in numbers, or both. These varied lesions have been referred to by many terms that have since been abandoned in favor of a simple classification, consisting of two groups, that is based on history and physical examination. The two major categories are hemangiomas and vascular malformations (Table 23-1).[1]

CONGENITAL VASCULAR LESIONS

Hemangiomas
  Strawberry
  Cavernous
  Mixed
Malformations
  Salmon patch
  Port-wine stains
  Syndromes
    Sturge-Weber
    Cobb
    Klippel-Trenaunay-Weber
  Maffuci's
Other arteriovenous malformations

TABLE 23-1 Congenital Vascular Lesions		
	Hemangiomas	**Malformations**
Occurence	40% present at birth Most occur in first year of life	99% present at birth
Location	Common on face, any area	Common on limbs, any area
Appearance	Well delineated	Poorly circumscribed
Course	Rapid neonatal growth	No change in size
	Slow involution	Grows in proportion to child No involution
Vessel type	Predominantly arterial	Predominately venous, but any combination of capillary, venous, arterial, and lymphatic components can occur

Histology	Proliferative phase
	  Endothelial hyperplasia
	Involuting phase
	  Fibrosis, fatty infiltration
	  Diminished cellularity, increased number of
	    mast cells
		Normal endothelial turnover
		Normal number of mast cells

HEMANGIOMAS

Strawberry hemangiomas

Strawberry hemangiomas occur at birth or during the first year of life in 1% to 3% of infants; the female-to-male ratio is 3:1. Many children have one, but several may be present. Most are small, harmless birthmarks that proliferate for 8 to 18 months and then slowly regress over the next 5 to 8 years, leaving normal or slightly blemished skin. They consist of a collection of dilated vessels in the dermis surrounded by masses of proliferating endothelial cells. These cells are responsible for the unique growth characteristics. The lesions begin as nodular masses or as flat, ill-defined, telangiectatic macules that are mistaken for bruises. Strawberry hemangiomas grow rapidly for weeks or months, forming nodular, protuberant, compressible masses of a few millimeters to several centimeters. In rare instances the lesions may almost cover an entire limb. They are bright red, with well-defined borders (Figure 23-1). Vital structures can be compressed (Figure 23-2), and rapidly growing areas may ulcerate; however, most have a benign course. An inactive phase lasting several months is followed by fibrosis and involution. When patients reach age 7, approximately 70% of strawberry hemangiomas have regressed, and more than 90% eventually regress.[2] The mass shrinks and fades in color during the scarring process. Involution begins in most cases by age 3; those present after ages 7 to 9 infrequently undergo further regression. Regression is characterized by normal-appearing skin (approximately 70% of cases) or by atrophy, scarring, telangiectasia, pigmentation changes, and deformity.

Management. Lesions that are relatively small and indolent should remain untouched if they are to involute spontaneously. In most cases, the result is very satisfactory. Patients should be seen regularly to reassure their parents and to monitor growth. Small areas of bleeding and ulceration are treated with cool, wet compresses. Lesions with functional impairment, deep ulceration, or infection are treated. Facial lesions that pose a cosmetic problem are also considered for treatment.

CORTICOSTEROIDS. Rapidly growing lesions or those that have the potential to interfere with vital structures such as the eyes, auditory canals, and airways should be treated with prednisone (2 to 4 mg/kg/day) given in divided doses twice a day.[3,4,5,6] The proliferative phase is inhibited and the hemangioma shrinks in approximately half the cases. Most lesions stabilize and markedly regress in 2 to 4 weeks. Prednisone may then be given in a single, early-morning dose tapered on an alternate-day schedule for a few weeks and then discontinued. Occasionally higher doses may be required. A second course of treatment is given for recurrences. Lesions that do not regress by late childhood may be evaluated for surgical excision.

INTRALESIONAL STEROIDS. Periorbital hemangiomas have been associated with ophthalmic complications in 40% to 80% of cases.[7,8] Strabismus and amblyopia are the most common. Intralesional steroids are frequently used by the ophthalmologist to treat lesions that do not respond to oral steroids (see the box on p. 723).[9,10] In most cases, clinical response is noticed within 1 to 3 days. The first change is a

Figure 23-1
Strawberry hemangioma. A nodular protuberant mass consisting of dilated vessels in the dermis that undergoes spontaneous involution in more than 90% of the cases.

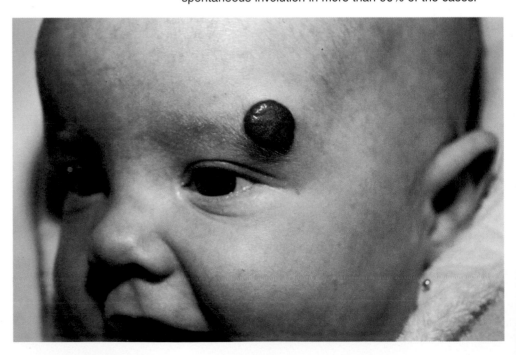

blanching of the vascular pattern, followed by a rapid regression in the size of the mass. Involution is most rapid in the first or second week after treatment. Retinal occlusion is a potential risk. Surgery is used for lesions that do not respond to corticosteroids.

INTERFERON ALFA-2a. In one study, infants with life-threatening or vision-threatening hemangiomas that did not respond to corticosteroid therapy were treated with daily subcutaneous injections of interferon alfa-2a (up to 3 million U per square meter of body-surface area). In 90% of the patients, the hemangiomas regressed by 50% or more after an average of 7.8 months of treatment (range, 2 to 13 months). Transient side effects of treatment with interferon alfa-2a included fever, neutropenia (one patient), and skin necrosis (one patient). No long-term toxicity was observed after a mean follow-up of 16 months.[11]

LASERS. Pulsed dye lasers (yellow laser light) are used to treat some hemangiomas, but the deeper portions are beyond the reach of yellow laser light.[12,13] Some recommend pulsed dye laser treatment of all superficial hemangiomas that appear during the first weeks of life, before they begin to proliferate. Ulcerated, painful hemangiomas respond well. Consider treatment of facial hemangiomas that do not regress by the school-age years to relieve the social burden on young patients. Pulsed dye lasers are also effective for removing residual telangiectasias associated with regression. Superficial coagulation with argon lasers and deeper coagulation with Nd:YAG lasers are associated with significant scarring and generally are not used.

GUIDELINES FOR THE USE OF INTRALESIONAL STEROIDS IN PERIORBITAL HEMANGIOMAS

EVALUATION

History and physical examination
Computed tomography scan
Avoidance of immunization with live virus vaccines
Short-acting, light, general anesthetics

PHARMACOLOGIC AGENTS

40 mg/ml triamcinolone acetonide (Kenalog 40) (1 ml)
    plus
6 mg/ml betamethasone sodium phosphate (Celestone) (1 ml)*
    OR
6 mg equal parts of betamethasone sodium phosphate and betamethasone acetate (Celestone Soluspan)
    OR
4 mg dexamethasone sodium phosphate (Decadron)

PROCEDURE

Anterior approach to the eyelid is preferred.
Multiple injection sites: 0.1 cc aliquot
Aspirate before injecting (27- or 30-gauge needle)
Digital pressure is then applied to avoid hematomas

Repeat up to three times at 8-week intervals or until regression has ceased

Adapted from Reyes BA: *J Dermatol Surg Oncol* 15:828-832, 1989.
*Combines the rapid action of betamethasone with the prolonged action of triamcinolone.

Figure 23-2
Strawberry hemangioma. A rapidly growing mass that is encroaching on the orbit.

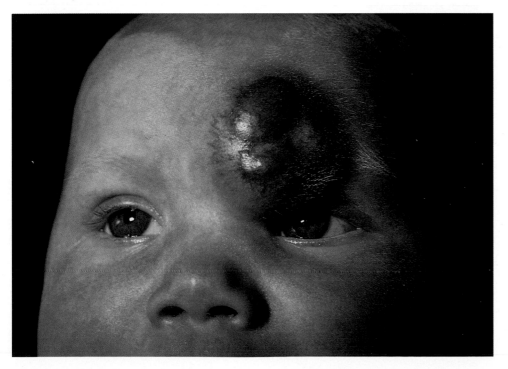

Cavernous hemangiomas

Cavernous hemangiomas are collections of dilated vessels deep in the dermis and subcutaneous tissue that are present at birth. Clinically they appear as pale, skin-colored, red, or blue masses that are ill defined and rounded (Figure 23-3). Like strawberry hemangiomas, the lesions enlarge for several months, become stationary for an indefinite period, and undergo spontaneous resolution. They are managed like strawberry hemangiomas.

Kasabach-Merritt syndrome. Kasabach-Merritt syndrome is a variant of disseminated intravascular coagulation (DIC) in which platelets and clotting factors are locally consumed within a giant hemangioma. There is thrombocytopenia, microangiopathic hemolytic anemia, and an acute or chronic consumption coagulopathy in association with a rapidly enlarging hemangioma (Figure 23-4).[14] The cause of DIC is not known, but blood is static in the venous sinusoids, and both platelets and contact factors may be activated by the abnormal endothelium. Kasabach-Merritt syndrome occurs most often in young infants during the first few weeks of life, but it may occur in adults. The majority of hemangiomas are very large and occur on the limbs or trunk. Prednisone 2 to 4 mg/kg/day is indicated when the hemangioma rapidly enlarges and the platelet count drops precipitously. Other treatments have been reported, including prednisone and epsilon-aminocaproic acid,[15] cryoprecipitate plus intraarterial thrombin and aminocaproic acid,[16] and intermittent pneumatic compression of the affected limb.[17] Pentoxifylline administered orally was successful in one case when other treatments failed.[18]

Three patients with large lesions that were unresponsive to conventional therapies stabilized after 7 days of treatment with interferon alfa-2a alone. (See strawberry hemangioma treatment section on p. 723.)[11]

The condition remits when the hemangioma begins to involute.

Hemangiomas associated with congenital abnormalities. The association of hemangiomas with congenital abnormalities is rare. Most of the vascular lesions associated with congenital malformations and syndromes are malformations, such as the port-wine stain, or other true vascular malformations and not hemangiomas. A few malformation syndromes have an association with cutaneous hemangiomas. These include coarctation of the aortic arch in association with multiple hemangiomas; midline abdominal and sternal defects in conjunction with facial hemangiomas; and spinal cord and vertebral abnormalities with sacral hemangiomas. Large facial hemangiomas (occupying at least one quarter to one half of the facial surface) may be linked to the Dandy-Walker malformation (cystic expansion of the fourth ventricle into the posterior cranial fossa) or other posterior fossa brain abnormalities (e.g., hypoplastic cerebellum, posterior fossa arachnoid cyst).[19] Ophthalmologic disorders (choroidal hemangioma, microphthalmos, and strabismus) may also be present. Brain-imaging studies should be performed on all asymptomatic infants with extensive facial hemangiomas to assess for hydrocephalus and fourth-ventricle anomalies.

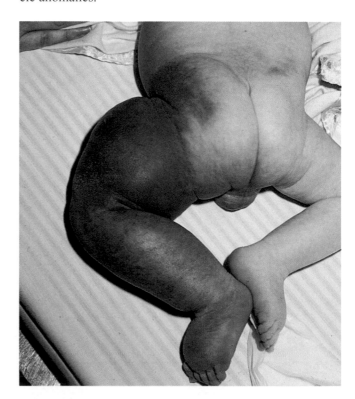

Figure 23-4
Kasabach-Merritt syndrome. Thrombocytopenia, microangiopathic hemolytic anemia, and an acute or chronic consumption coagulopathy occur in association with a rapidly enlarging hemangioma. *(Courtesy Nancy B. Esterly M.D.)*

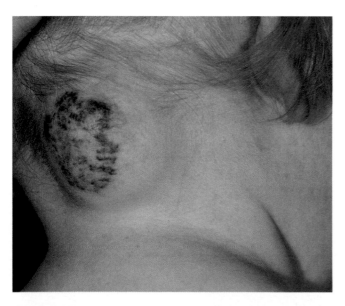

Figuro 23-3
Cavernous hemangioma. Cavernous hemangioma is a collection of dilated vessels deep in the dermis and subcutaneous tissue that presents as a pale, skin-colored, red, or blue mass.

MALFORMATIONS
Port-wine stains (nevus flammeus)

In most cases these distinctive lesions are developmental anomalies that are not genetically transmitted. They are present at birth in 0.1% to 0.3% of infants. Port-wine stains are a significant cosmetic problem that does not fade with age. These nevi are usually unilateral; they frequently occur on the face, but they also appear elsewhere (Figure 23-5). They may be a few millimeters in diameter or may cover an entire limb (Figure 23-6). Size remains stable throughout life. Nevus flammeus appears at birth as flat, irregular, red-to-purple patches. Initially the lesions are smooth, but later they may become papular, simulating a cobblestone surface. Two thirds of all patients develop nodularity or hypertrophy by the fifth decade of life. Unlike the salmon patch, nevus flammeus tends to darken with age. The entire depth of the dermis contains numerous dilated capillaries.

Systemic syndromes. Nevus flammeus may be a component of neurocutaneous syndromes (Table 23-2), such as Sturge-Weber syndrome (nevus flammeus of the trigeminal area) (Figure 23-7) or Klippel-Trenaunay-Weber syndrome. When it occurs over the midline of the back, nevus flammeus may be associated with an underlying spinal cord arteriovenous malformation.

Patients who do not have port-wine stains on the areas served by branches V^1 and V^2 of the trigeminal nerve have no signs or symptoms of eye and/or central nervous system (CNS) involvement (Figure 23-7). Port-wine stains of the eyelids, bilateral distribution of the birthmark, and unilateral port-wine stains involving all three branches of the trigeminal nerve are associated with a significantly higher likelihood of having eye and/or CNS complications. Twenty-four percent of those with bilateral trigeminal nerve port-wine stains have eye and/or CNS involvement, compared with 6% of those with unilateral lesions. All those who have eye and/or CNS complications have port-wine stain involvement of the eyelids; in 91% both upper and lower eyelids are involved, whereas in 9% only the lower eyelid is involved. None of those with upper eyelid port-wine stains alone have eye and/or CNS complications.[21] In summary, patients with port-wine stains of the eyelids, bilateral lesions, and unilateral lesions involving all three divisions of the trigeminal nerve should be studied for glaucoma or for CNS lesions.[21]

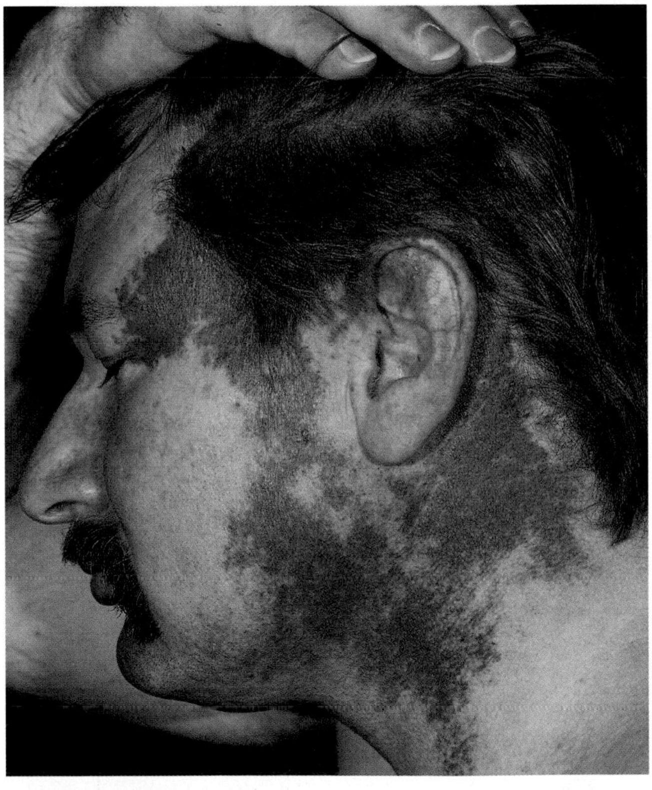

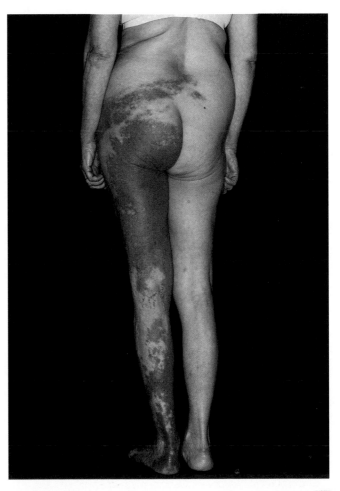

Figure 23-5
Nevus flammeus, An extensive lesion with a relatively smooth surface.

Figure 23-6
Nevus flammeus covering the entire lower limb. The affected limb is 2 inches longer than the normal side.

TABLE 23-2 Neurocutaneous Syndromes with Vascular Abnormalities*

	Cobb syndrome	Sturge-Weber syndrome	Rendu-Osler-Weber syndrome
Synonym	Cutaneomeningo-spinal angiomatosis	Encephalotrigeminal angiomatosis	Hereditary hemorrhagic telangiectasia
Inheritance	Not familial	Dominant partial trisomy or not familial	Autosomal-dominant
Sex distribution	More in males	Equal	Equal
Age of onset	Childhood or adolescence	Two thirds with hemangioma at birth	Childhood
Skin lesion	Port-wine stain or angiokeratomas in dermatomal distribution corresponding within segment or two of area of spinal cord involvement†	Ipsilateral capillary angioma or port-wine stain in distribution of superior and middle branches of the trigeminal nerve†; associated cavernous changes may occur No consistent relationship between extent of skin lesion and degree of meningeal involvement	Telangiectasia (skin and mucous membranes)†
CNS findings	Arteriovenous or venous angioma of the spinal cord† Neurologic signs of cord compression or anoxia	Angioma of meninges† Intracranial gyriform calcifications Mental retardation (60%)† Epilepsy (usually focal)† Hemiparesis contralateral to skin lesions† Visual impairment (50% have one or more of various eye abnormalities)†	Angiomas in the brain or spinal cord with signs of localized tumor
Associated findings	Angioma of vertebrae Renal angioma Kyphoscoliosis	Renal angioma Coarctation of aorta High, arched palate Abnormally developed ears	Pulmonary arteriovenous anastomoses Hemorrhage from lesions in mouth, GI tract, and GU tract and associated anemia
Diagnostic aids	Lateral spine x-ray film Myelography Selective spinal angiography	EEG Skull x-ray film Cerebral angiography	None
Treatment	Surgical removal of spinal cord angioma if possible	Anticonvulsants Surgical removal of intracranial lesion if possible Cosmetic procedures for skin lesions	Cautery of bleeding lesions

From Jessen T, Thompson S, Smith EB: *Arch Dermatol* 113:1582, 1977. Copyright 1977, American Medical Association.
*CNS, central nervous system; GI, gastrointestinal; GU, genitourinary; EEG, electroencephalogram.
†Major component of this syndrome.

Fabry-Anderson syndrome	Ataxia telangiectasia	von Hippel-Lindau disease
Angiokeratoma corporis diffusum	Cephalo-oculocutaneous telangiectasia	Angiomatosis retinae et cerebelli syndrome
Recessive trait (X chromosome)	Autosomal recessive	Autosomal dominant

Males tend to full syndrome:
   Angiokeratomas
   Extremity pain
   High blood pressure
   Cardiomegaly
   Albuminuria
   Hypohidrosis
	Equal	Equal

Childhood	Childhood	Adult
Small clustered angiokeratomas (symmetric, mucosal, increased over bony prominences) Palmar mottling	Telangiectasia (increased in sun-exposed areas)[†] Inelasticity	Port-wine stains in some; most with no cutaneous lesions Café-au-lait spots
Cerebral vascular accidents Neuronal glycolipid deposition (peripheral neuritis)	Progressive cerebellar ataxia (voluntary movements)[†] Ocular telangiectasia (spread from canthal fold)[†] Peculiar eye movements (nystagmus, poor control)[†] Retarded Slow dysarthric speech Decreased tendon reflexes	Cerebellar hemangioblastoma and cyst[†] Spinal hemangioblastoma (rarely) Retinal hemangiomas (tangle of vessels away from disc)[†]
Stooped posture Slender limbs; thin, weak muscles Dilated, tortuous conjunctival and retinal vessels Varicose veins and stasis edema Scant facial hair Hypogonadism	Sinopulmonary infections[†] Hypoplastic or absent thymus Small spleen Retarded growth Malignancies (reticulum cell sarcoma, Hodgkin's disease, lymphosarcoma, gastric carcinoma)	Pheochromocytoma Pancreatic cysts Hepatic angiomas Renal hypernephromas (20%) Polycythema (erythropoietic substance from tumor)
Urinary glycolipids (ceramide trihexoside) Slit lamp Biopsy—renal or marrow (lipid deposits)	Diminished or absent IgA Increased serum alpha-fetoprotein	Hemogram (polycythemia) Urinalysis, excretory urograms Skull x-ray films, angiogram Myelogram
Symptomatic	Control infections Plasma infusions (IgA) Thymus transplant Transfer factor	Supportive

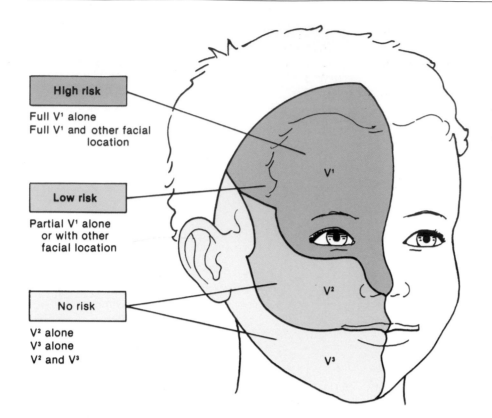

High risk

Full V¹ alone
Full V¹ and other facial
location

Low risk

Partial V¹ alone
or with other
facial location

No risk

V² alone
V³ alone
V² and V³

V¹

V²

V³

Figure 23-7
Facial port-wine stains and risk of
Sturge-Weber syndrome. *(Adapted
from Enjolvas O, Riche MC, Merland
JJ: Pediatrics 76:48, 1985.)*

Figure 23-8

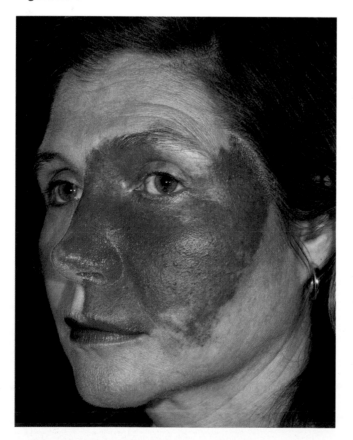

A, Nevus flammeus with a papular surface.

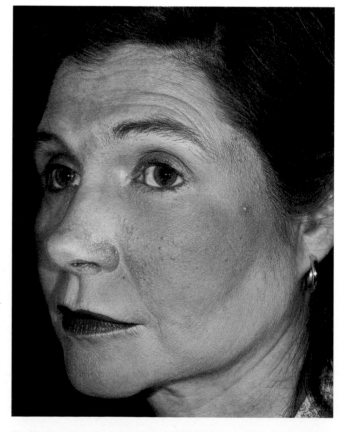

B, Same patient as in *A* after applying Covermark makeup.

Treatment. Port-wine stains have the potential to cause lasting detrimental psychologic effects. The pulsed tunable dye laser is a highly effective method of treatment and should be considered for all affected infants.

LASERS. The pulsed dye laser (yellow light) is selective and limits thermal damage to the cutaneous vasculature.[13,23] Yellow laser light is very effective for nearly all vascular disorders. There is no postlaser-treatment scar formation. Argon lasers (blue-green light) are used to treat melanocytic and selected vascular disorders; they produce some scarring. The CO_2 laser produces the same effect as an electric needle, heating the epidermis and dermis and producing hypertrophic scars.[24]

Individuals are treated as outpatients; patients under 12 years of age usually require some form of sedation or anesthesia, since the procedure is painful and cooperation during the procedure is necessary.

COSMETICS. The cosmetic appearance of some patients with port-wine stains can be significantly improved by using the tinted waterproof makeup, Covermark, manufactured by Lydia O'Leary, Moonachie, NJ (Figure 23-8). Covermark is sold in some drug stores, department stores, and beauty salons. A list of stores carrying Covermark can be obtained directly from the company. Dermablend is a similar product that is generally available in department stores. Both products are available in many shades.

Salmon patches

Salmon patches (stork bite, angel's kiss) are actually variants of nevus flammeus; they are present in approximately 40% to 70% of newborns. They are red, irregular, macular patches resulting from dilation of dermal capillaries. The most common site is on the nape of the neck (Figure 23-9), where the lesion is referred to as a *stork bite*. They are often inconspicuous and covered by hair. Patches that occur on the glabella and upper eyelids are sometimes mistaken for pressure or forceps clamp marks. Salmon patches on the face fade within a year, but those on the nape may persist for life.

Figure 23-9
Salmon patch (stork bite). A variant of nevus flammeus found in many individuals on the nape of the neck.

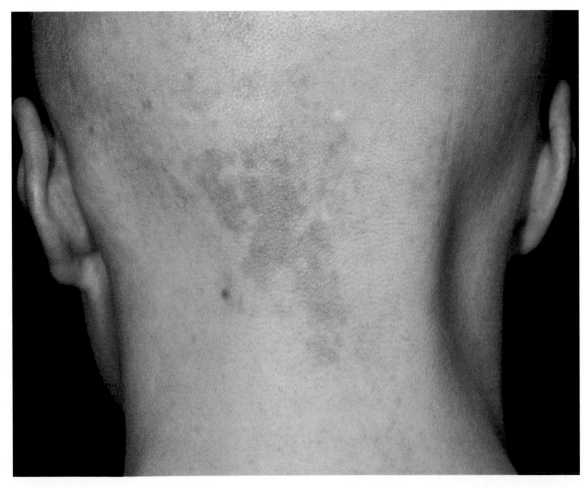

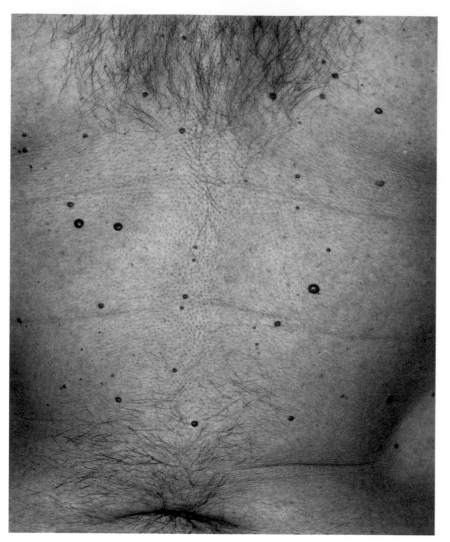

Figure 23-10
Cherry angioma. Multiple small, red papules commonly occur on the trunk.

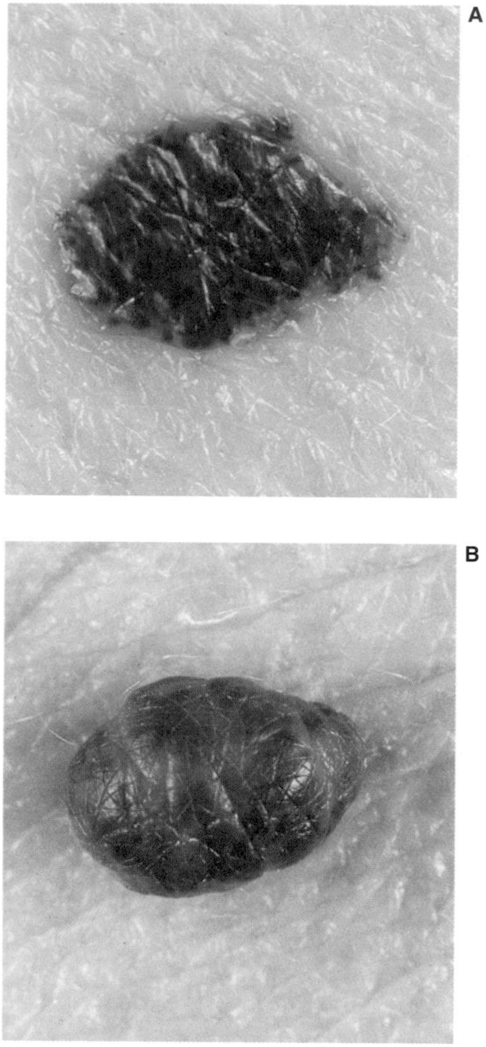

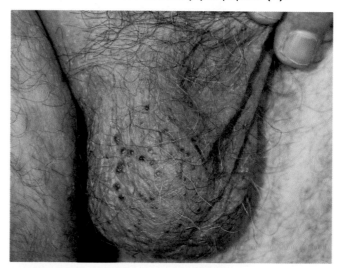

Figure 23-11
Cherry angioma. Lesions may be slightly raised and flat **(A)** or papular **(B)**.

Acquired Vascular Lesions
CHERRY ANGIOMA

The most common vascular malformation is the benign cherry or senile angioma. These 0.5- to 5-mm, smooth, firm, deep red papules (Figures 23-10 and 23-11) occur in virtually everyone after age 30 and numerically increase with age. Patients recognize them as new growths, prompting concerns about malignancy. They are most common on the trunk and vary in number from a few to hundreds. Trauma produces slight bleeding. The papules are easily removed by scissor excision or electrodesiccation and curettage.

ANGIOKERATOMAS

Angiokeratomas are lesions characterized by dilation of the superficial dermal blood vessels and hyperkeratosis of the overlying epidermis. The term is applied to six different vascular malformations. The most common are angiokeratomas of the scrotum (Fordyce) (Figure 23-12) or vulva,[25]

Figure 23-12
Angiokeratomas (Fordyce). Multiple red-to-purple papules consisting of multiple small blood vessels.

characterized by multiple 2- to 3-mm, red-to-purple papules that occasionally bleed with trauma. The onset is between the ages of 20 and 50 years. Increased venous pressure may be implicated, such as occurs with pregnancy and hemorrhoids. If desired, removal is performed by simple scissor excision or electrodesiccation and curettage. The other forms of angiokeratomas are rare. They consist of red-brown-black, hyperkeratotic plaques varying in size and distribution. Numerous cutaneous angiokeratomas are part of the Fabry-Anderson syndrome (see Table 23-2).

VENOUS LAKE

Venous lakes are dark blue, slightly elevated, 0.2- to 1-cm, dome-shaped lesions composed of a dilated, blood-filled vascular channel. They are common on sun-exposed surfaces of the vermilion border of the lip (Figure 23-13) and the ears.[26] They occasionally bleed following trauma and can be removed by electrodesiccation or with the argon[27] or pulsed dye[28] laser.

LYMPHANGIOMA CIRCUMSCRIPTUM

These uncommon but distinctive hamartomatous malformations consist of dilated lymph channels, which may be filled with serosanguineous fluid, that communicate with deeper lymph channels. The appearance of the lesions has been compared to a mass of frog's eggs ("frog spawn"). They consist of tiny to 5-mm, grouped, translucent or hemorrhagic vesicles on a dull red or brown base (Figure 23-14). Some lesions contain a mixture of vascular and lymph channels. Lesions may appear in the setting of postmastectomy lymphedema as a result of lymphatic damage following surgery and radiation.[29] This is referred to as *secondary lymphangioma* (lymphangiectasis).

The malformations consist of a collection of subcutaneous lymphatic cisterns with a thick muscle coat that communicates through dilated channels lined with lymphatic endothelium with the superficial vesicles. There is no communication between the cysts and the adjacent normal lymphatics.[30] The contraction of the muscle coat may force fluid to the surface and create the vesicles. The depth and extent of involvement cannot be adequately estimated from the cutaneous examination. Magnetic resonance imaging has been used to demonstrate accurately the true extent of involvement.[31]

Treatment. Treatment is indicated for cosmetic reasons and to prevent leakage of fluid and recurrent infection. The lesions recur unless the deep communicating cisterns are removed or destroyed. Small groups of surface vessels can be destroyed by electrosurgery. Surgical removal of the subcutaneous cisterns, leaving sufficient skin for primary closure, results in acceptable cure rates. Residual skin vesicles separated from their underlying cysts regress.[32] Surface lymphatic vessels are vaporized, and communicating channels to deeper cisterns are sealed with the CO_2 laser,[33] which, unlike the argon laser, is not color dependent for vaporization.

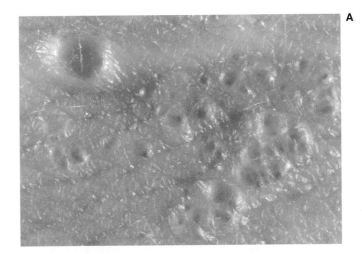

A

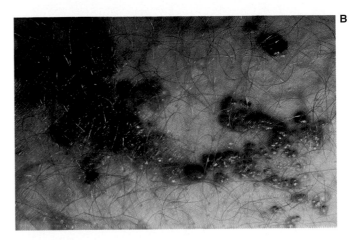

B

Figure 23-14
Lymphangioma circumscriptum. Dilated lymph channels. Appearance has been compared to a mass of frog's eggs ("frog spawn"). Lesions are filled with **(A)** clear or **(B)** blood-tinged fluid.

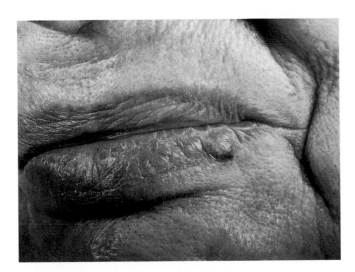

Figure 23-13
Venous lake. A dilated, blood-filled channel typically seen on the lower lip.

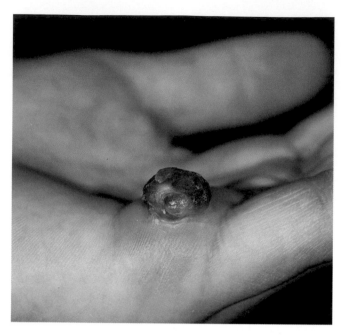

Figure 23-15
Pyogenic granuloma. A dome-shaped tumor with a moist, fragile surface. The lesion may bleed profusely with the slightest trauma.

PYOGENIC GRANULOMA (LOBULAR CAPILLARY HEMANGIOMA)

Pyogenic granuloma is a benign acquired vascular lesion of the skin and mucous membranes that is common in children and young adults. They are small (less than 1 cm), rapidly growing, yellow-to-bright red, dome-shaped (Figures 23-15 and 23-16), fragile protrusions that have a glistening, moist-to-scaly surface.[34] The base of the lesion is often surrounded by a collarette of scale (Figure 23-17). They are most commonly seen on the head and neck region and on the extremities, especially the fingers. Pyogenic granuloma occurs in pregnant women (pregnancy epulis) and is found primarily in the gingiva.[35] The word *epulis* is used to describe a localized growth on the gingiva.

The slightest trauma causes bleeding that is difficult to control. The dermis is composed of a mass of capillaries. *Pyogenic* suggests an infectious origin, but the lesion is a lobular capillary hemangioma that is probably caused by trauma. Pyogenic granuloma-like lesions occur in patients with acquired immunodeficiency syndrome (AIDS) who develop cat-scratch disease.

Treatment consists of firm and thorough curettage of the base and border. Electrodesiccation is often necessary to eradicate the lesions completely and to control bleeding. Pyogenic granuloma recurs if the most minute piece of abnormal tissue remains.[36] Multiple lesions may occur after the excision of a solitary lesion. This is a well-recognized but rare event.[37] Spontaneous resolution usually occurs within 6 months. Pregnancy epulis usually regresses following childbirth.

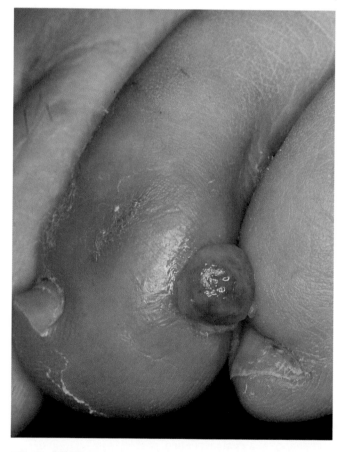

Figure 23-16
Pyogenic granuloma. A large bulbous mass with a glistening surface.

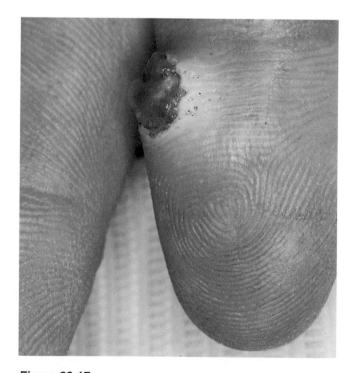

Figure 23-17
Side view of a pyogenic granuloma demonstrating the white collarette of scale often observed at the base.

KAPOSI'S SARCOMA

Kaposi's sarcoma or multiple idiopathic hemorrhagic sarcomas are vascular neoplasms that were rarely seen before the AIDS era. The incidence of HLA-DR5 antigen was reported to be higher in classic and AIDS-associated Kaposi's sarcoma.[38] A recent study demonstrated no association.[39] Kaposi's sarcoma can be divided into five subsets on the basis of clinical and epidemiologic criteria (Table 23-3).[40] The incidence of second malignancies (especially lymphoreticular neoplasms) is increased in classic Kaposi's sarcoma and in Kaposi's sarcoma patients with AIDS. Classic and AIDS-associated Kaposi's sarcoma may be caused by a new herpes virus.[41]

Classic Kaposi's sarcoma. The rare classic form generally appears on the feet or lower legs. It begins as violaceous macules and papules (Figure 23-18) and very slowly progresses to form plaques with multiple red-purple nodules (Figure 23-19). It occurs almost exclusively in elderly males of Jewish, Greek, or Italian descent. Progression of this disease in the elderly is slow and, although lymph node and visceral involvement can occur, most of these patients die of unrelated causes.

Epidemic or AIDS-related Kaposi's syndrome. Overall, 37.4% of AIDS cases are diagnosed with Kaposi's sarcoma prior to death.[42] Epidemiologic features suggest a sexually transmitted cofactor in the pathogenesis of AIDS-associated Kaposi's sarcoma.[41,43] Homosexual men have greater than a 30% incidence of Kaposi's sarcoma, but the incidence is less than 1% in men with hemophilia. Homosexual men living in San Francisco, Los Angeles, and New York City and sexually active, homosexual Canadian men traveling to these cities are far more likely to develop Kaposi's sarcoma than are homosexual men who do not live in or travel to these areas. Kaposi's syndrome probably occurs as a multicentric rather than a metastatic disease in AIDS. Unlike the classic form, lesions are often multifocal and widespread when first detected. They are most commonly found on the trunk and the head and neck areas. Mucous membranes are involved.[44] They initially form slightly raised, oval or elongated, poorly demarcated, rust-colored infiltrates. Rapid progression to red or purple nodules and plaques follows. They may look like granulation tissue, stasis dermatitis, pyogenic granuloma, or capillary hemangiomas.[45] More than half of the patients have generalized lymphadenopathy at the time of first examination. Eventually most patients develop systemic lesions (see Chapter Eleven). It is important to treat cutaneous lesions for cosmetic purposes, because their presence is a constant reminder of a fatal disease.

Endemic African Kaposi's sarcoma. Endemic African Kaposi's sarcoma is a common neoplastic disorder in the sub-Saharan region of Africa. There are two forms: the cutaneous and the lymphatic. Both are rare in patients between 10 and 20 years of age. The cutaneous form typically occurs in men as nodules on the lower legs. Lymph node or systemic involvement is uncommon. The lymphadenopathic form is seen in children younger than 10 years of age. Cutaneous lesions may surface; the prognosis is poor.[46]

Endemic Kaposi's sarcoma responds to local radiation therapy or chemotherapy.[47] Complete (32%) and partial (54%) regression of cutaneous lesions was achieved with radiation therapy, which is the treatment of choice for this disease.[48]

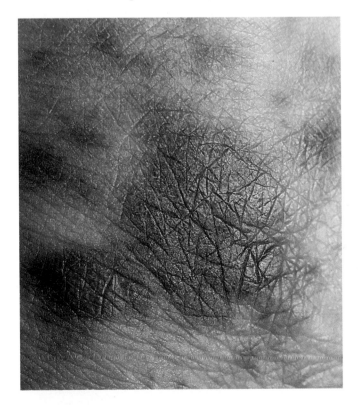

Figure 23-18
Kaposi's sarcoma. Early lesion consisting of violaceous macules and plaques.

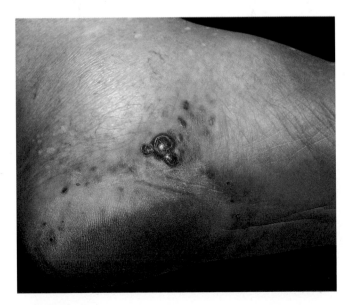

Figure 23-19
Kaposi's sarcoma. Purple nodules are most commonly seen on the lower legs.

Kaposi's sarcoma associated with immunosuppressive states. Azathioprine, cyclophosphamide, cyclosporine, and prednisone, singly or in combination, have been implicated in sporadic cases of Kaposi's sarcoma. Many were renal-transplant patients. Some tumors regressed after therapy was withdrawn,[49] and others responded to radiation.

Treatment. The primary goal of treatment is to improve the cosmetic appearance, to shrink symptomatic oral lesions, and to relieve pain. Most patients can be managed with local therapy.

LIQUID NITROGEN CRYOTHERAPY. Liquid nitrogen cryotherapy is easily applied as a primary therapy and is the treatment of choice for most lesions. A complete response is observed in 80% of treated Kaposi's sarcoma lesions. There is often persistent Kaposi's sarcoma in the deeper dermis under the treated site, but the cosmetic effect is excellent. Patients receive an average of three treatments per lesion. Treatment is repeated at 3 week intervals, allowing adequate healing time. One treatment consisted of two freeze-thaw cycles, with thaw times ranging from 11 to 60 seconds per cycle (range, 10 to 20 seconds for macular lesions; 30 to 60 seconds for papular lesions).[50] Treatment is well tolerated. Blistering occurs frequently, but pain is limited. Secondary infection does not occur. Keep treated lesions covered until they heal because blister fluid may contain HIV.

INTRALESIONAL CHEMOTHERAPY. Intralesional chemotherapy is more effective than cryotherapy for nodular lesions greater than 1 cm in diameter. It is also useful for the treatment of symptomatic oral lesions. Postinflammatory hyperpigmentation may respond to cryotherapy or may be camouflaged with cosmetics. Vinblastine is prepared from stock solutions to the desired concentration. Vinblastine-containing syringes can be stored under refrigeration after preparation. Vinblastine 0.1 mg (0.5 ml of a 0.2 mg/ml solution) is injected per square centimeter of lesion. For lesions that do not respond to 0.1 mg/cm^2, incremental doses to a maximum of 0.2 mg/cm^2 of lesion may be used. Oral lesions and larger cutaneous lesions respond best to 0.2 mg/cm^2. In this setting, increasing the concentration of vinblastine to 0.4 to 0.6 mg/ml is recommended to reduce the volume injected per square centimeter of lesion to 0.5 ml. A maximum total dose of 2 mg during clinic visits is recommended. After a healing interval of 3 weeks, each treated lesion may require an additional 1 to 2 injections for maximal response.[51] Pain lasts for 1 to 2 days. Local anesthesia does not reduce the efficacy of treatment or the pain experienced by the patient.

RADIATION THERAPY. Radiation therapy was the primary form of local therapy for Kaposi's sarcoma before the AIDS epidemic. Response rates of greater than 80% were achieved. Radiation therapy is indicated for large tumor masses, especially those that interfere with normal function. Treated lesions show a 50% reduction in size. A large retrospective study of patients with AIDS-related Kaposi's sarcoma supports the use of a single 8-Gy fraction for all Kaposi's sarcoma lesions of the skin.[52] Another study demonstrated that fractionated radiotherapy to higher total doses results in improved response and control.[53]

Intralesional interferon alfa was demonstrated to be effective in a limited number of studies.[54-56] Systemic interferon or systemic chemotherapy are used to treat extensive visceral disease and widespread cutaneous disease.

TABLE 23-3 Clinical Features of Kaposi's Sarcoma

	Classic	African cutaneous	African lymphadenopathic	AIDS	Immunosuppressive
Epidemiology	Sporadic (endemic)	Endemic	Endemic	Endemic	Sporadic
Age (years)	50-70	<10, >20	<10	25-42	20-80
Mean age	68	35	<10	35	—
M:F ratio	3:1	10-15:1	1-2:1	Male, homosexual	10-1.7:1
Incidence	0.02	—	0.1-0.85*†	40%-70%, up to 90%	—
% Cancers diagnosed	0.06	—	9%	—	—
Sites	Legs, feet	Extremities	Nodes	Head, neck, upper aspect of trunk	Variable
Lesion type	Nodular	Nodular, florid, infiltrating	Lymphadenopathic	Macules, plaques, nodules	Nodules
Node involvement	Rare	Uncommon indolent	Expected	Common	Variable
Course	Indolent	Locally aggressive	Aggressive	Fulminant	Variable
Treatment response	Good	Good	Good initially	Poor	Variable

From Piette WW: *J Am Acad Dermatol* 16:855-861, 1987.
*Cases/100,000 population
†Representative incidence figures from Tanzania.

Telangiectasias

Telangiectasias are permanently dilated, small blood vessels consisting of either venules, capillaries, or arterioles. The maximum diameter is 1 mm. Vessels appear as single strands, in groups as small macules, or with a central punctum. They accompany a variety of diseases and sometimes are clues to the underlying diagnosis (see the box below). Telangiectasias are usually only a cosmetic problem; they rarely bleed.

CLASSIFICATION OF TELANGIECTASIA

PRIMARY (CAUSE UNKNOWN)

Ataxia telangiectasia
Generalized essential telangiectasia
Hemorrhagic hereditary telangiectasia (Rendu-Osler-Weber syndrome)
Spider angiomas
Unilateral nevoid telangiectasia syndrome

SECONDARY (PART OF KNOWN ENTITY)

Actinically damaged skin
After laser or electrosurgery
After cryosurgery
Basal cell carcinoma
Collagen vascular disease
    Dermatomyositis
    Lupus erythematosus
    Scleroderma
Cushing's syndrome
Estrogen excess
    Cirrhosis
    Oral contraceptives
    Pregnancy
Metastatic carcinoma
Necrobiosis lipoidica diabeticorum
Poikilodermas
Pseudoxanthoma elasticum
Radiation therapy injury
Rosacea
Telangiectasia macularis eruptiva perstans (generalized cutaneous mastocytosis)
Topical steroid induced
Xeroderma pigmentosa

SPIDER ANGIOMA

Spider angiomas (nevus araneus) form as arterioles (spider bodies), become more prominent near the surface of the skin, and radiate capillaries (spider legs) (Figure 23-20). They occur in many normal individuals and frequently appear in children. Once formed, they tend to be permanent. Bleeding rarely occurs. Spider angiomas are most common on the exposed surfaces of the face and arms. They increase in number with liver disease and during pregnancy and are probably stimulated by higher-than-normal estrogen concentrations. Spider angiomas should be distinguished from the flat patches of tiny vessels of uniform size (telangiectatic mats) seen in scleroderma.

Treatment. Local anesthesia is optional in the following procedure for treatment. The blood is forced out of the spider by pressing firmly on the lesion; with continuous pressure, the finger is moved slightly to one side to expose the central arteriole, and the central arteriole is gently electrodesiccated. If the arteriole has been destroyed, the radiating capillaries may not fill. Incompletely destroyed lesions may recur. Vigorous desiccation may cause a pitted scar. Lasers are also effective.

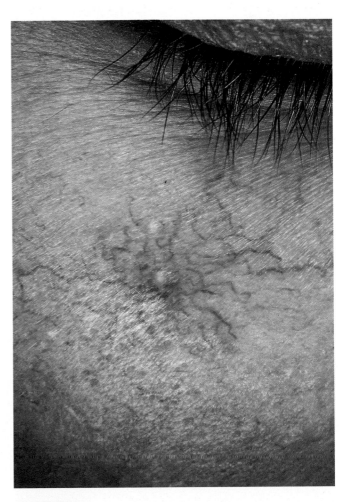

Figure 23-20
Spider angioma. Well-defined, dilated vessels radiate from a central point.

HEREDITARY HEMORRHAGIC TELANGIECTASIA

Hereditary hemorrhagic telangiectasia (HHT) (Rendu-Osler-Weber disease) is an autosomal dominant, inherited malformation of blood vessels. The characteristic lesions begin as tiny, flat telangiectasias, with a few vessels radiating from a single point. In rare instances, there is a large central arteriole as seen in spider angioma. Engorged lesions are fragile and bleed easily with the slightest trauma. Few to numerous lesions occur primarily on the lips, tongue (Figure 23-21), nasal mucosa, forearms, hands, fingers, and throughout the gastrointestinal tract, but any skin area or internal organ may be involved. Hereditary hemorrhagic telangiectasia is the most common cause of pulmonary arteriovenous fistula.[57] Although lesions may be prominent during childhood, they are most often so small and subtle that stretching the lip is required to accentuate them. By the third or fourth decade, telangiectasias become more apparent, and the diagnosis is easily made. Recurrent bleeding from nasal or gastrointestinal telangiectasia can be fatal in a small number of cases. Bleeding points are treated by electrocautery. Two patients with severe epistaxis were treated with low-dose oral aminocaproic acid. Aminocaproic acid at a dosage of 1 to 1.5 gm twice per day with 325 mg of ferrous sulfate per day reduced the number and severity of epistaxis episodes to insignificant levels; epistaxis remained clinically insignificant even when the dosage was reduced to 1.5 to 2 gm per day.[58] Aminocaproic acid most likely inhibits fibrinolysis in the telangiectatic vessel wall, enabling fibrin deposits to seal the bleeding sites effectively. Most patients have a normal life expectancy.

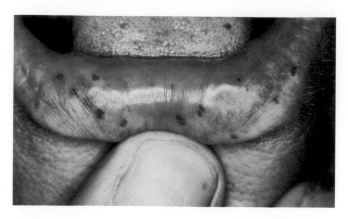

Figure 23-21
Hereditary hemorrhagic telangiectasia. Several lesions are present on the lip and tongue.

UNILATERAL NEVOID TELANGIECTASIA SYNDROME

Telangiectasias that appear in a segmental distribution are called *unilateral superficial telangiectasias*. There are acquired and congenital forms. The acquired form begins with states of increasing estrogen blood levels: (1) at puberty in females, (2) during pregnancy (Figure 23-22), or (3) with alcoholic cirrhosis. In subsequent pregnancies the syndrome recurs once it has appeared, although it may appear for the first time during a second pregnancy.[59,60] Most cases involve the trigeminal, C3, C4, or adjacent dermatomes. The distribution suggests an estrogen-sensitive nevoid anomaly.[61]

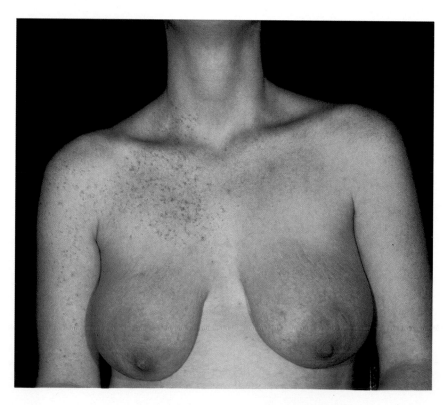

Figure 23-22
Unilateral nevoid telangiectasia syndrome. Telangiectasia appeared on the right chest and arm during pregnancy.

GENERALIZED ESSENTIAL TELANGIECTASIA

Generalized essential telangiectasia is seen primarily in women and is sometimes familial; the average age at onset is 38 years. The telangiectasias slowly progress over years or decades and are not accompanied by associated systemic problems. Lesions appear predominantly on the legs but may appear anywhere (Figure 23-23). Its onset is not related to hormonal stimulation.[62] Autosomal dominant transmission has been suggested. Lesions have been reported to resolve with tetracycline.[63]

SCLERODERMA

The telangiectasias of CREST syndrome and scleroderma have a unique morphology. They occur as flat (macular), 0.5-cm, rectangular collections of uniform tiny vessels; these are the so-called telangiectatic mats (see Figure 17-18). These mats are most commonly found on the face, lips, palms, and backs of the hands.[64] Telangiectasias may be present around the lips, tongue, and mucous membranes. Involvement of the oral mucosa also suggests Rendu-Osler-Weber disease.

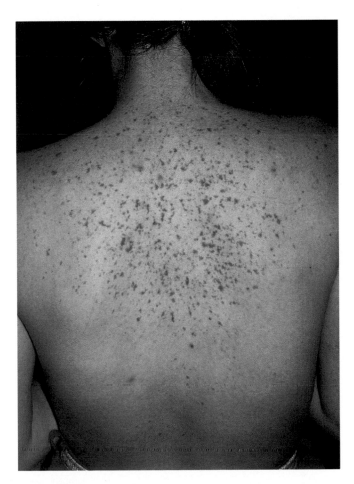

Figure 23-23
Generalized essential telangiectasia. Telangiectasias are seen primarily in women. Lesions appear predominantly on the legs but may appear anywhere.

REFERENCES

1. Mulliken JB, Glowacki J: Hemangiomas and vascular malformations in infants and children: a classification based on endothelial characteristics, *Plast Reconstr Surg* 69:412-422, 1982.
2. Illingworth RS: Thoughts on the treatment of vascular nevi, *Arch Dis Child* 51:138-140, 1976.
3. Edgerton MT: The treatment of hemangiomas: with special reference to the role of steroid therapy, *Ann Surg* 183:517-532, 1976.
4. Brown SH, Neerhout RC, Ronkalsrud GW: Prednisone therapy in the management of large hemangiomas in infants and children, *Surgery* 71:168-173, 1972.
5. Bartoshesky LE, Bull M, Geingold M: Corticosteroid treatment of cutaneous hemangiomas: how effective? *Clin Pediatr* 17:629-638, 1978.
6. Zaren HA, Edgerton MT: Cavernous hemangiomas and prednisolone therapy, *Plast Reconstr Surg* 39:76, 1976.
7. Haik BG, Jakobiec FA, Ellsworth RM, et al: Capillary hemangioma of the lids and orbit: an analysis of the clinical features and therapeutic results in 101 cases, *Ophthalmology* 86:760-792, 1979.
8. Stigmar G, Crawford JS, Ward CM, et al: Ophthalmic sequelae of infantile hemangiomas of the eyelids and orbit, *Am J Ophthalmol* 85:806-813, 1978.
9. Kushner BJ: The treatment of periorbital infantile hemangioma with intralesional corticosteroid, *Plast Reconst Surg* 76:517-524, 1985 and discussion by Edgerton MT: 525-526.
10. Reyes BA: Intralesional steroids in cutaneous hemangioma, *J Dermatol Surg Oncol* 15:828-832, 1989.
11. Ezekowitz RA, Mulliken JB, et al: Interferon alfa-2a therapy for life-threatening hemangiomas of infancy, *N Engl J Med* 326:1456-1463, 1992.
12. Garden JM, Bakus AD, et al: Treatment of cutaneous hemangiomas by the flashlamp-pumped pulsed dye laser: prospective analysis, *J Pediatr* 120:555-560, 1992.
13. Garden JM, Bakus AD: Clinical efficacy of the pulsed dye laser in the treatment of vascular lesions, *J Dermatol Surg Oncol* 19:321-326, 1993.
14. Esterly NB: Kasabach-Merritt syndrome in infants, *J Am Acad Dermatol* 8:504-513, 1983.
15. Dresse MF, David M, et al: Successful treatment of Kasabach-Merritt syndrome with prednisone and epsilon-aminocaproic acid, *Pediatr Hematol Oncol* 8:329-334, 1991.
16. Stahl RL, Henderson JM, et al: Therapy of the Kasabach-Merritt syndrome with cryoprecipitate plus intra-arterial thrombin and aminocaproic acid, *Am J Hematol* 36:272-274, 1991.
17. Aylett SE, Williams AF, et al: The Kasabach-Merritt syndrome: treatment with intermittent pneumatic compression, *Arch Dis Child* 65:790-791, 1990.
18. de Prost et al: Successful treatment of Kasabach-Merritt syndrome with pentoxifylline, *J Am Acad Dermatol* 25: 854-855, 1991.
19. Burns AJ, Kaplan LC, Mulliken JB: Is there an association between hemangioma and syndromes with dysmorphic features? *Pediatrics* 88:1257, 1991.
20. Jessen T, Thompson S, Smith EB: Cobb syndrome, *Arch Dermatol* 113:1587-1590, 1977.
21. Tallman B, Tan OT, et al: Location of port-wine stains and the likelihood of ophthalmic and/or central nervous system complications, *Pediatrics* 87:323-327, 1991.
22. Reference deleted in proofs.
23. Goldman MP, Fitzpatrick RE, et al: Treatment of port-wine stains (capillary malformation) with the flashlamp-pumped pulsed dye laser, *J Pediatr* 122:71-77, 1993.
24. Van Gemert MJC, Welch AJ, Tan OT, et al: Limitations of carbon dioxide lasers for treatment of port-wine stains, *Arch Dermatol* 123:71-73, 1987.
25. Novick NL: Angiokeratoma vulvae, *J Am Acad Dermatol* 12:561, 1985.
26. Goldberg LH, Altman AR: Venous lakes of the ears, *Cutis* Dec:472-473, 1985.

27. Neumann RA, Knobler RM: Venous lakes (Bean-Walsh) of the lips—treatment experience with the argon laser and 18 months follow-up, *Clin Exp Dermatol* 15:115-118, 1990.

28. Gonzalez E, Gange RW, et al: Treatment of telangiectases and other benign vascular lesions with the 577 nm pulsed dye laser, *J Am Acad Dermatol* 27:220-226, 1992.

29. Leshin B, Whitaker DC, Foucar E: Lymphangioma circumscriptum following mastectomy and radiation therapy, *J Am Acad Dermatol* 15:1117-1119, 1986.

30. Whimster IW: The pathology of lymphangioma circumscriptum, *Br J Dermatol* 94:473-486, 1976.

31. McAlvany JP, Jorizzo JL, et al: Magnetic resonance imaging in the evaluation of lymphangioma circumscriptum, *Arch Dermatol* 129:194-197, 1993.

32. Browse NL et al: Surgical management of lymphangioma circumscriptum, *Br J Surg* 73:585-588, 1986.

33. Bailin PL, Kantor GR, Wheeland RG: Carbon dioxide laser vaporization of lymphangioma circumscriptum, *J Am Acad Dermatol* 14:257-262, 1986.

34. Ro BI: Granuloma pyogenicum, *Int J Dermatol* 25:634-635, 1986.

35. Daley TD, Nartey NO, et al: Pregnancy tumor: an analysis, *Oral Surg Oral Med Oral Pathol* 72:196-199, 1991.

36. Patrice SJ, Wiss K, et al: Pyogenic granuloma (lobular capillary hemangioma): a clinicopathologic study of 178 cases, *Pediatr Dermatol* 8:267-276, 1991.

37. Taira JW, Hill TL, et al: Lobular capillary hemangioma (pyogenic granuloma) with satellitosis, *J Am Acad Dermatol* 27:297-300, 1992.

38. Prince HE et al: HLA studies in acquired immune deficiency syndrome patients with Kaposi's sarcoma, *J Clin Immunol* 4:242-245, 1984.

39. Tzfon EE et al: No HLA antigen is significant in classic Kaposi's sarcoma, *J Am Acad Dermatol* 28:118-119, 1993.

40. Tappero JW, Conant MA, et al: Kaposi's sarcoma. Epidemiology, pathogenesis, histology, clinical spectrum, staging criteria and therapy, *J Am Acad Dermatol* 28:371-395, 1993.

41. Moore P, Chang Y: Detection of Herpes virus–like sequences in Kaposi's sarcoma patients with and those without HIV infection, *N Engl J Med* 332:1181-1185, 1995.

42. Hoover DR, Black C, et al: Epidemiologic analysis of Kaposi's sarcoma as an early and later AIDS outcome in homosexual men, *Am J Epidemiol* 138:266-278, 1993.

43. Archibald CP, Schechter MT, et al: Evidence for a sexually transmitted cofactor for AIDS-related Kaposi's sarcoma in a cohort of homosexual men (see comments), *Epidemiology* 3:203-209, 1992.

44. Mitsuyasu RT: Clinical aspects of AIDS-related Kaposi's sarcoma, *Curr Opin Oncol* 5:835-844, 1993.

45. Safai B et al: The natural history of Kaposi's sarcoma in the acquired immunodeficiency syndrome, *Ann Intern Med* 103:747-750, 1985.

46. Ziegler JL: Endemic Kaposi's sarcoma in Africa and local volcanic soils, *Lancet* 342:1348-1351, 1993.

47. Stein ME, Spencer D, et al: Endemic African Kaposi's sarcoma: clinical and therapeutic implications. 10-year experience in the Johannesburg Hospital (1980-1990), *Oncology* 51:63-69, 1994.

48. Stein ME, Lakier R, et al: Radiation therapy in endemic (African) Kaposi's sarcoma, *Int J Radiat Oncol Biol Phys* 27:1181-1184, 1993.

49. Trattner A, Hodak E, et al: The appearance of Kaposi sarcoma during corticosteroid therapy, *Cancer* 72:1779-1783, 1993.

50. Tappero JW, Berger TG, et al: Cryotherapy for cutaneous Kaposi's sarcoma (KS) associated with acquired immune deficiency syndrome (AIDS): a phase II trial, *J Acquir Immune Defic Syndr* 4:839-846, 1991.

51. Boudreaux AA, Smith LL, et al: Intralesional vinblastine for cutaneous Kaposi's sarcoma associated with acquired immunodeficiency syndrome. A clinical trial to evaluate efficacy and discomfort associated with infection, *J Am Acad Dermatol* 28:61-65, 1993.

52. Berson AM, Quivey JM, et al: Radiation therapy for AIDS-related Kaposi's sarcoma, *Int J Radiat Oncol Biol Phys* 19:569-575, 1990.

53. Stelzer KJ, Griffin TW: A randomized prospective trial of radiation therapy for AIDS-associated Kaposi's sarcoma, *Int J Radiat Oncol Biol Phys* 27:1057-1061, 1993.

54. Ghyka G, Alecu M, et al: Intralesional human leukocyte interferon treatment alone or associated with IL-2 in non–AIDS related Kaposi's sarcoma, *J Dermatol* 19:35-39, 1992.

55. Trattner A, Reizis Z, et al: The therapeutic effect of intralesional interferon in classical Kaposi's sarcoma, *Br J Dermatol* 129:590-593, 1993.

56. Tur E, Brenner S, et al: Low-dose recombinant interferon alfa treatment for classic Kaposi's sarcoma, *Arch Dermatol* 129:1297-1300, 1993.

57. Hodgson CH et al: Hereditary hemorrhagic telangiectasia and pulmonary arteriovenous fistula, *N Engl J Med* 261:625-636, 1959.

58. Saba HI et al: Brief report: treatment of bleeding in hereditary hemorrhagic telangiectasia with aminocaproic acid, *N Engl J Med* 330:1789-1790, 1994.

59. Wilkin JK et al: Unilateral dermatomal superficial telangiectasia, *J Am Acad Dermatol* 8:468-477, 1983.

60. Tok J, Berberian BJ, et al: Unilateral nevoid telangiectasia syndrome, *Cutis* 53:53-54, 1994.

61. Uhlin SR, McCarty KS Jr: Unilateral nevoid telangiectatic syndrome: the role of estrogen and progesterone receptors, *Arch Dermatol* 119:226-228, 1983.

62. Person JR, Longcope C: Estrogen and progesterone receptors are not increased in generalized essential telangiectasia, *Arch Dermatol* 121:836-837, 1985.

63. Shelley WB: Essential progressive telangiectasia, *JAMA* 210:1343-1344, 1971.

64. Braverman IM: *Skin signs of systemic disease*, ed 2, Philadelphia, 1981, WB Saunders.

Hair Diseases

Physicians are frequently confronted with hair-related problems. Most complaints are from patients with early-onset pattern baldness. The physician must be able to recognize this normal, inherited hair loss pattern so that detailed and expensive evaluations can be avoided. Other patients have complaints about abnormal hair growth; these diseases must be recognized and not dismissed as balding. The signs of hair loss or excess growth are at times subtle. The signs usually seen with cutaneous disease, such as inflammation, may be absent. A systematic approach to evaluation is essential.

Anatomy and Physiology

Hair follicle. The hair follicle is formed in the embryo by a club-shaped epidermal, down growth, the primary epithelial germ that is invaginated from below by a flame-shaped, capillary-containing dermal structure called the *papilla* of the hair follicle. The central cells of the down growth form the hair matrix, the cells of which form the hair shaft and its surrounding structures. The matrix lies deep within the subcutaneous fat. The mature follicle contains a hair shaft, two surrounding sheaths, and a germinative bulb (Figure 24-1). The follicle is divided into three sections. The infundibulum extends from the surface to the sebaceous gland duct. The isthmus extends from the duct down to the insertion of the erector muscle. The inferior segment, which exists only during the growing (anagen) phase, extends from the muscle insertion to the base of the matrix. The matrix contains the cells that proliferate to form the hair shaft (Figure 24-2). The mitotic rate of the hair matrix is greater than that of any other organ. The cells begin to differentiate at the top of the bulb. The inner and outer root sheaths protect and mold the growing hair. The inner root sheath disintegrates at the duct of the sebaceous gland. Hair growth is greatly influenced by any stress or disease process that can alter mitotic activity.

Hair structure. The hair shaft is dead protein. It is formed by compact cells that are covered by a delicate cuticle composed of platelike scales. The living cells in the matrix multiply more rapidly than those in any other normal human tissue. They push up into the follicular canal, undergo dehydration, and form the hair shaft, which consists of a dense, hard mass of keratinized cells. Normal hairs have a pointed tip. The hair in the follicular canal forms a cylinder of uniform diameter. Short hairs with tapered tips have either short growth cycles or have experienced the recent onset of anagen.

The growing shaft is surrounded by several concentric layers (see Figure 24-2). The outermost glycogen-rich layer is called the *outer root sheath*. It is static and continuous with the epidermis. The inner root sheath (Henle's layer, Huxley's layer, and cuticle) is visible as a gelatinous mass when the hair is plucked. It protects and molds the growing hair but disintegrates before reaching the surface at the infundibulum.

The hair shaft that emerges has three layers—an outer cuticle, a cortex, and sometimes an inner medulla—all of which are composed of dead protein. The cuticle protects and holds the cortex cells together. Split ends result if the cuticle is damaged by brushing or chemical cosmetic treatments. The cortex cells in the growing hair shaft rapidly synthesize and accumulate proteins while in the lower regions of the hair follicle. Systemic diseases and drugs may interfere with the metabolism of these cells and reduce the hair shaft diameter. Pigment-containing melanosomes are acquired deep in the bulb matrix and are deposited in the cortical and medullary cells.

Figure 24-1
Hair follicle. Longitudinal section showing the three sections: the infundibulum, the isthmus, and the inferior segment. *(Courtesy* Hospital Practice.*)*

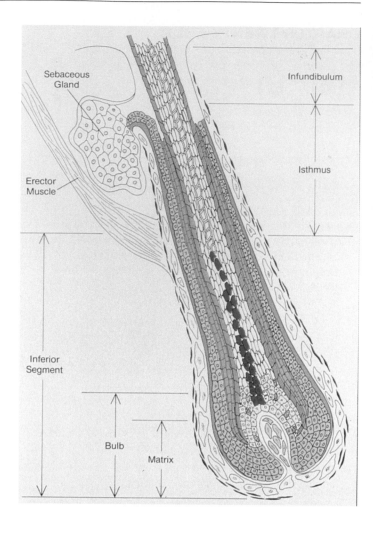

Figure 24-2
Hair bulb. The outer and inner root sheaths mold and protect the growing hair shaft. The hair shaft consists of the medulla, hair cortex, and cuticle. *(Courtesy* Hospital Practice.*)*

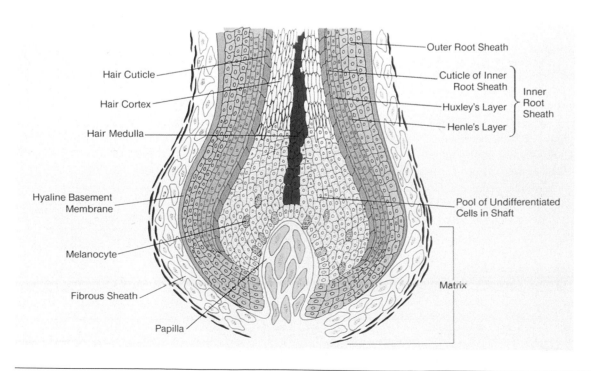

Growth cycle. The average scalp has more than 100,000 hairs. The growth phase of scalp hair is approximately 1000 days (range, 2 to 6 years). Hair in other areas, such as the eyebrows and eyelashes, has a shorter growth phase (1 to 6 months). Scalp hair grows 0.3 to 0.4 mm/day, or approximately 6 inches a year.

Humans have a mosaic growth pattern; hair growth and loss are not cyclic or seasonal, as in some mammals, but occur at random, so that hair loss is continuous (Figure 24-3). There are three stages in the hair growth cycle: catagen (transitional phase), telogen (resting phase), and anagen (growing phase). Approximately 85% to 90% of hairs are in the anagen phase, and 10% to 15% are in the telogen phase; 50 to 100 hairs are lost each day.

Anagen. The anagen or growth phase begins with resumption of mitotic activity in the hair bulb and dermal papilla. The follicle grows down and meets the dermal papilla, recapitulating the embryonic events of development of the hair follicle. A new hair shaft forms and forces the tightly held club hair out. During anagen, hair grows at an average rate of 0.35 mm/day, or 1 cm in 28 days[1]; this rate diminishes with age. Scalp hair remains in an active growing phase for an average of 2 to 6 years. The active growing phase is much shorter and the resting stage is longer for hair on the arms, legs, eyelashes, and eyebrows (30 to 45 days), which explains why these hairs remain short. Approximately 85%

of scalp hairs are in an active growing phase at any one time. Continuous anagen occurs in some dogs (e.g., poodles) and in merino sheep; these animals do not lose or shed hair.

Catagen. Catagen is the phase of acute follicular regression that signals the end of anagen. Approximately 3% of scalp hairs are in this 2- to 3-week transitional phase at any one time. Cell division in the hair matrix stops, and the resting, or catagen, stage begins. The outer root sheath degenerates and retracts around the widened lower portion of the hair shaft to become a club hair. The lower follicle shrinks away from the connective tissue papilla and ascends to the level of the insertion of the erector muscle. The completion of catagen is marked by formation of the normal club hair.

Telogen. All activity ceases and the structure rests during the telogen phase. The telogen phase in the scalp lasts for approximately 100 days.[2] Approximately 10% to 15% of scalp hairs are in the telogen phase at any one time, and these follicles are randomly distributed. The telogen phase is much longer in eyebrow, eyelash, arm, and leg hair. The inactive dead hair, or club hair, has a solid, hard, dry, white node at its proximal end; the white color is due to a lack of pigment. The club hair is firmly held in place and then ejected. A new anagen hair grows and replaces the shed telogen hair. Approximately 25 to 100 telogen hairs are shed each day; possibly twice this number are lost on the days the hair is shampooed. Seasonal shedding occurs in other animals but is random in humans.

Types of hair. There are three types of hair. Lanugo hairs are the fine hairs found on the fetus; similar fine hairs (peach fuzz) found on the adult are called *vellus hairs*. Thick, pigmented hairs are called *terminal hairs*. Those on the top of the head and in the beard, axillary, and pubic areas are influenced by androgens. Hair on the rest of the body is independent of androgens.

Figure 24-3
Growth cycle of hair. **A**, Conclusion of the growth phase. **B**, Transition phase: the inferior segment separates from the papilla. **C**, The club hair ascends to the level of the erector muscle. **D**, The growing cycle resumes. **E**, A new hair forms. **F**, The growing hair forces the club hair out. *(Courtesy Hospital Practice.)*

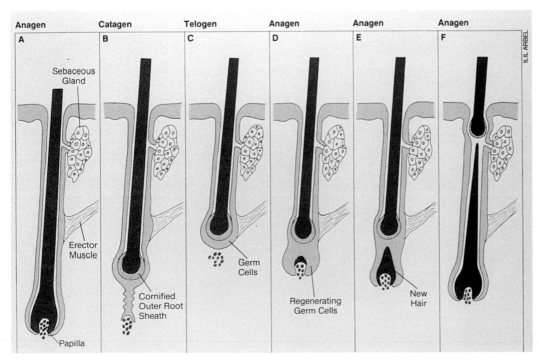

Evaluation of Hair Loss

The causes of hair loss (alopecia) are numerous. A classification is used here that is based primarily on distribution (i.e., localized vs. generalized). A systematic approach for evaluation of hair loss is outlined in the box below. Traditionally, the alopecias have been divided into scarring or nonscarring, but the presence of scarring is sometimes difficult to appreciate, and some diseases cause scarring at one time but not at another. Scarring, when present, is a helpful sign; it should always be sought.

Generalized Hair Loss

Diffuse hair loss (Table 24-1) usually occurs without inflammation or scarring. The loss affects hairs throughout the scalp in a more or less uniform pattern. The hair pluck test is important for differential diagnosis.

Telogen effluvium (loss of resting hair). A number of events have been documented that prematurely terminate anagen and cause an abnormally high number of normal hairs to enter the resting, or telogen, phase (Table 24-2).[3] The follicle is not diseased, but has had its biologic clock reset and undergoes a normal involutional process. Usually no more than 50% of the patient's hair is affected. Scarring and inflammation are absent. Resting hairs on the scalp are retained for approximately 100 days before they are lost; therefore, telogen hair loss should occur approximately 3 months after the event that terminated normal hair growth.

Kligman[4] explained this process and identified the various precipitating events (see Table 24-2). The most common causes are briefly discussed here. High fever from any cause may result in a sudden diffuse loss of club hairs 2 to 3 months later. Hair loss begins abruptly and lasts for approximately 4 weeks. Hair pluck tests show telogen counts that vary from 30% to 60%. Full recovery can be expected.

TABLE 24-1 Hair Loss

Generalized*	Localized†
Telogen effluvium	Androgenic alopecia
Acute blood loss	Male pattern
Childbirth	Female pattern
Crash diets (inadequate protein)	Hirsutism
	Alopecia areata
Drugs	Trichotillomania
Coumarins	Traction alopecia
Heparin	Scarring alopecia
Propanolol	Developmental defects: aplasia cutis
Vitamin A	
High fever	Physical injury: burns, pressure
Hypothyroidism and hyperthyroidism	Infection
Physical stress (e.g., surgery)	Fungal: kerion
	Bacterial: folliculitis, furuncle
Physiologic (e.g., neonate)	Viral: herpes zoster
Psychologic stress	Neoplasms
Severe illness (e.g., systemic lupus erythematosus)	Metastatic carcinoma
	Sclerosing basal cell carcinoma
Anagen effluvium	Others
Cancer chemotherapeutic agents	Lupus erythematosus
	Lichen planus
Poisoning	Cicatricial pemphigoid
Thallium (rat poison)	Scleroderma
Arsenic	
Radiation therapy	
Generalized patchy	
Secondary syphilis: "moth eaten" alopecia	

*Diffuse uniform loss, but many hairs left randomly distributed in area of loss
†Most or all hair missing from involved area.

SYSTEMATIC APPROACH TO EVALUATION OF HAIR LOSS

History
 Sudden vs. gradual loss
 Presence of systemic disease or high fever
 Recent psychologic or physical stress
 Medication or chemical exposure
Examination
 Localized vs. generalized
 Scarring vs. nonscarring
 Inflammatory vs. noninflammatory
 Density: normal or decreased
 Presence of follicular plugging
Skin disease in other areas

Diagnostic procedures
 Hair pluck
  Telogen effluvium vs. anagen effluvium
  Possible trichotillomania
  Potassium hydroxide examination for fungi
  Scalp biopsy
  Scarring alopecia
  Trichotillomania
 Hormone studies

Severe emotional and physical traumas have been documented to cause diffuse hair loss. Hair loss has been reported to occur 2 weeks after severe psychologic or physical trauma, but since that is too short a time for the induction of the telogen phase, the loss must have occurred by another mechanism. Some individuals may experience increased shedding due to idiopathic shortening of anagen (a short anagen syndrome). They have increased shedding and decreased hair length. For every 50% reduction in the duration of anagen, there is a corresponding doubling of follicles in telogen.

Postpartum hair loss. The percentage of follicles in telogen progressively decreases during pregnancy, particularly during the last trimester. Diffuse but primarily frontotemporal hair loss occurs in a significant number of women 1 to 4 months after childbirth. The loss can be quite significant, but recovery occurs in less than 1 year. Hair growth usually returns to the prepregnancy state.

Drugs. Cytotoxic drugs that directly affect hair matrix cell proliferation cause profound hair loss, inducing an anagen effluvium. A large number of drugs probably cause telogen effluvia. These are listed in the box below.

Anagen effluvium. Anagen effluvium (see Tables 24-1 and 24-2) is the abrupt loss of hair from follicles that are in their growing phase. An abrupt insult to the metabolic and follicular reproductive apparatus must be delivered to create such an event. Cancer chemotherapeutic agents and radiation therapy are capable of such an insult.[5,6] The rapidly dividing cells of the matrix and cortex are affected. The insult causes a change in the rate of hair growth but does not convert the follicle to a different growth phase, as occurs in telogen effluvium. High concentrations of antimetabolites or radiation bring the entire metabolic process to an abrupt halt, and the entire hair and hair root are shed intact. The only hairs left are those in the telogen phase. These are dead, wedged into the hair canal, and unaffected by any acute event.

Insults of less intensity slow the mitotic rate of the bulb and cortex cells, causing bulb deformity and narrowing of the lower hair shaft. Narrow, weakened hair shafts are easily broken and shed without bulbs. Since 90% of scalp hairs are in the anagen phase, a large number of hairs can be affected. Patients with 10% to 20% of their hair remaining after an insult almost certainly have had an anagen effluvium. Minoxidil 2% topical has no benefit in the prevention of chemotherapy-induced alopecia.[7]

TABLE 24-2 Features Differentiating Telogen Effluvium and Anagen Effluvium		
Clinical presentation	**Telogen**	**Anagen**
Onset of shedding after insult	2-4 months	1-4 weeks
Percent hair lost	20-50	80-90
Type of hair lost	Normal club (white bulb)	Anagen hair (pigmented bulb)
Hair shaft	Normal	Narrowed or fractured

DRUGS PROBABLY ASSOCIATED WITH TELOGEN EFFLUVIUM

Aminosalicylic acid
Amphetamines
Bromocriptine
Captopril
Carbamazepine
Cimetidine
Coumadin
Danazol
Enalapril
Etretinate
Levodopa
Lithium
Metoprolol
Propanolol
Pyridostigmine
Trimethadione

OFFICE TECHNIQUES OF DIAGNOSING HAIR DISEASE

TELOGEN EFFLUVIUM

Hair shaft examination	Tapered tips, normal shaft
Hair pull	More than six hairs per site
Hair pluck	More than 20% hairs in telogen
Daily counts	Greater than 100, all telogen bulbs
Growth window	Normal growth rate
Part width	Normal to slightly widened
Scalp biopsy	Increased telogen hair bulbs

ANAGEN EFFLUVIUM

Hair shaft examination	Normal shafts
Hair pull	Bulb end tapered, more than six hairs per site
Daily counts	Greater than 100
Part width	Widened

ANDROGENETIC ALOPECIA

Hair shaft examination	Miniaturized hairs
Hair pull	Normal
Daily counts	Usually normal
Part width	Wide in androgen-dependent areas
Scalp biopsy	Classic pathology

ABNORMAL SHAFT FRAGILITY (TRICHORRHEXIS NODOSA)

Hair shaft examination	Structural abnormality present
Hair pull	Abnormal or broken hairs
Daily collections	Broken hairs
Hair growth window	Normal growth rate

TRICHOTILLOMANIA

Hair shaft examination	Broken tips, normal shaft
Hair pull	Normal
Daily counts	Normal
Growth window	Normal growth rate
Scalp biopsy	Classic pathology

From a symposium given by Rebecca J. Caserio, M.D., clinical assistant professor, University of Pittsburgh.

Diagnosing hair disease (see the box at left)

History. Inquire about drugs, severe diet restriction, vitamin A supplementation, and thyroid symptoms. Determine the time of onset and the duration of hair loss. Abrupt-onset telogen effluvium is most often related to a specific event. Gradual or imperceptible onsets are more complicated and involve possible shortened anagen as well as a differential diagnosis that includes alopecia areata, androgenetic alopecia, and diffuse primary scarring alopecias.

Physical examination. Examine the scalp surface and hair shafts. Microscopically examine hair ends and hair shaft diameters.

Observation. Hair density may be reduced by 50% before hair thinning becomes clinically apparent; therefore, observation is an inaccurate method of evaluating density and loss.

Hair shaft examination (clip tests). Grasp 25 to 30 hairs between the thumb and forefinger just at the scalp surface. Cut the hair between the fingers and the scalp. Hair just above the fingers is cut and discarded. Float the hairs onto a wet microscope slide and cover with another slide. Evaluate hair shaft diameters.

Hair pull. Sample 3 cm above the auricle. Tightly grasp 60 hairs firmly between the thumb and forefinger. Exert a slow, constant traction to slightly tent the scalp and slide the fingers up the hair shafts. There should be fewer than six club hairs extracted. Repeat the count on the opposite side of the head and in two other areas. Examine the hair bulbs.

Daily counts. The patient collects hair lost in the first morning combing and includes those lost during washing for 14 days, saving them in clear plastic bags. The patient counts the hairs and records the number on the bags. Examine the hairs under the microscope to determine if the bulbs are anagen or telogen. Daily hair shed counts are not necessary if the pull test is positive. It is normal to lose up to 100 hairs daily and 200 to 250 hairs on the day of shampooing. If the hair is shampooed daily, the counts should be less than 100.

Part width. Make a coronal part with a comb over the vertex. Note the part width. Make a series of parallel parts over the vertex and visually compare the part diameter. Do the same over the occipital and temporal scalp. Visually compare the part diameters in the different anatomic scalp areas. Hair density is greatest in childhood and decreases progressively with age. The hair is less dense in the vertex in both sexes, and thinning increases with age.

Hair growth window. Select an area where the hair fails to grow and an area that can be covered by the remaining hair. Cut the hair short, then shave a 2 × 2 cm square area. Occlude the area with an occlusive dressing and remove it in 1 week if trichotillomania is suspected. Normal growth is 2.5 mm in 1 week and 1 cm in 1 month. This test proves to the patient that the hair is growing.

Hair pluck—trichogram. This is a painful technique but is still used by some clinicians. Abruptly extract hairs from the scalp with a rubber-tipped needle holder.[8] This can be made by placing rubber-tubing needle protectors from prepackaged injectable drugs over the jaws of a small needle holder. The process is as follows. Firmly grasp approximately 50 hairs at the same height and rotate the needle holder one turn to ensure a firm hold on the hairs. Apply slight tension on the hairs; then with a quick, positive, upward motion, extract the hairs. The pain is intense but of short duration. Cut the excess hair 1 cm from the roots, float the hairs onto a wet microscope slide or Petri dish, and examine with a 10× lens (Figure 24-4). A simple technique for staining plucked anagen hairs allows them to be distinguished easily from plucked telogen hairs. Anagen hair dye (4-dimethylaminocinnamaldehyde [DACA]*) reacts with citrulline, an amino acid found only in the internal root sheath. The stain is dropped on the root ends of a hair pluck preparation, and the hairs are moved gently from side to side for 15 to 20 seconds to allow penetration of the dye.

Telogen hairs have small, unpigmented, ovoid bulbs and do not contain an internal root sheath. Anagen hairs have larger, elongated, pigmented (if hair is pigmented) bulbs shaped like the end of a broom, surrounded by a gelatinous internal root sheath.

There are diseases in which hair fragments with absent bulbs are obtained during a hair pull. Processes that interfere with cell division cause the shaft to be poorly formed and therefore apt to break under tension. Alopecia areata, antimetabolite therapy, and small doses of ionizing radiation interrupt the mitotic activity in the cells that normally contribute cells to the growing hair.

---

*Dermatologic Lab and Supply, Inc., Council Bluffs, Iowa, (800) 831-6273.

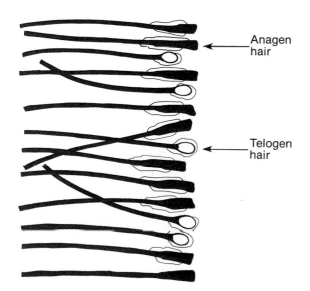

Figure 24-4
Hair pluck preparation showing anagen and telogen hairs.

Localized Hair Loss (see Table 24-1)
ANDROGENIC ALOPECIA IN MEN (MALE-PATTERN BALDNESS)

Baldness in men is not a disease, but rather a physiologic reaction induced by androgens in genetically predisposed men. The pattern of inheritance is probably polygenic.[9] Some young men with rapidly progressive male-pattern baldness have elevated dehydroepiandrosterone sulfate levels, suggesting that adrenal hyperactivity may initiate alopecia in young men who are genetically susceptible.[10] There are two populations of scalp follicles: androgen-sensitive follicles on the top and androgen-independent follicles on the sides and back of the scalp. In genetically predisposed individuals and under the influence of androgens, terminal hair follicles are transformed into velluslike follicles and the terminal hair is shed and replaced by fine light vellus hair. The progression and various patterns of hair loss are classified by Hamilton (Figure 24-5). Triangular frontotemporal recession occurs normally in most young men (type I) and women after puberty. The first signs of balding are increased frontotemporal recession accompanied by midfrontal recession (type II). Hair loss in a round area on the vertex follows, and the density of hair decreases, sometimes rapidly, over the top of the scalp (types III through VII).

Patients who begin balding at an early age are most distressed and are tempted to consult nonphysician "experts" at hair clinics. These clinics offer a variety of topical preparations, none of which has any value whatsoever. Patients who seek advice for hair loss should be warned not to become involved in these long-term and expensive programs. Selected patients may be referred for hair transplants, plastic surgical rotation flaps, or even wigs.

Treatment. The desire for treatment varies. Some men accept the inevitable; others find baldness intolerable. Minoxidil (topical) and several surgical procedures are available.

Minoxidil. Minoxidil (topical)[11] (Rogaine) was approved for the treatment of male-pattern baldness in 1988. A month's supply of the 2% or 5% solution comes with a dropper applicator. The applicator is designed to deliver 1 ml. The medication is applied to a dry scalp twice a day. The hair should not be wet for at least an hour afterward.

Ideal candidates are men under 30 who have been losing hair for less than 5 years. About one third of these patients grow hair that is long enough to be cut or combed.[12] Minoxidil works best in men with small areas of partial hair loss on the vertex. Minoxidil's effect on hair in the frontal and temple areas is not yet known. Hair growth is evident in 8 to 12 months. The solution must be used continually to preserve growth.[13,14] Minoxidil may stop or retard the progression of male-pattern baldness. Adverse effects are limited to local intolerance in a few patients and allergic reactions to minoxidil and the vehicle used.

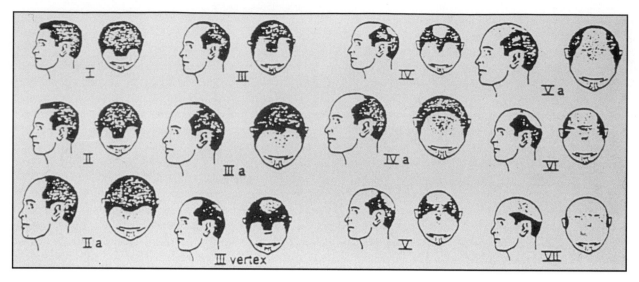

Figure 24-5
Norwood/Hamilton classification of male-pattern baldness.
(From Norwood OT: South Med J *68:1359-1365, 1975.)*

Hair transplants. Hair transplants have been used successfully for years to permanently restore hair. Age is not a determining factor. The new power punch produces a superior graft. Androgen-independent hairs from the lateral and posterior areas of the scalp are used. Some surgeons suture the donor sites after removal of the round graft. The standard graft is a 4-mm cylinder of skin that contains between 8 and 15 hairs. Cylinders of skin 3.5 mm in diameter are removed from the recipient sites, discarded, and replaced with the 4 mm grafts.

The surgeon must have a sense of aesthetics to properly design the anterior hairline. Grafts are first implanted anteriorly to establish a frontal hairline. Subsequent grafts are placed posteriorly in a fan pattern. Grafts are placed at an acute angle of 20 to 30 degrees. An innovation using smaller grafts produces a more natural hairline with a transitional zone. These micrografts and minigrafts soften the frontal hairline. They are prepared by sectioning standard grafts into halves and quarters. The halved and quartered hair grafts are inserted into a slash wound created with a #15 blade.[15]

Many sessions, each approximately 1 month apart, are required. The cost of each punch graft is approximately $40 to $50. More than 300 grafts may be necessary to complete the project.

Scalp reduction and flaps. An anterior-posterior elliptic excision of bald vertex scalp with primary closure can provide an instant hair effect. The procedure can be repeated every 4 weeks until hair margins converge or scalp tissue becomes too thin. Grafts or flaps may be used later to fill any remaining void. Alternately, several types of flaps can be designed by the creative surgeon to fill voids.

Hair weaves. Hair weaves have been refined by the HAIR CLUB FOR MEN (1-800-677-7700) in the United States. They developed a process whereby strands of human hair are applied to a thin nylon filament that is anchored to the scalp with the individual's own hair. The person returns approximately every 6 weeks for a haircut and tightening of the growing anchor hairs. Clients are generally very satisfied with the process and prefer it to a wig.

ADRENAL ANDROGENETIC FEMALE-PATTERN ALOPECIA

Chronic, progressive, diffuse hair loss in women in their 20s and 30s is a frequently encountered complaint. These women, who usually have a normal menstrual cycle and lack any abnormalities on physical examination, have been classified as having "male-pattern baldness," a genetic trait, and have been dismissed without further evaluation. Recent studies have shown that some of these women have increased levels of the serum adrenal androgen dehydroepiandrosterone sulfate (DHEA-S) and a distinct pattern of central scalp alopecia, which has been called *adrenal androgenetic female-pattern alopecia*.

Male-pattern baldness results in a gradual regression of the hair on the central scalp and gradual frontotemporal recession, as well as a gradual decrease in hair shaft diameter in the areas of hair loss. In contrast, most women with diffuse alopecia experience a gradual loss of hair on the central scalp, with retention of the normal hairline without frontotemporal recession. There is a variety of anagen hair diameters. With advancing age, the central thinning becomes more pronounced; in contrast to male-pattern baldness,

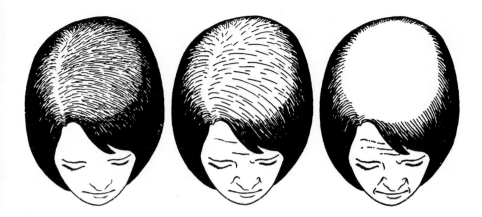

Figure 24-6
Evolution of the female type of androgenic alopecia. *(From Ludwig E:* Br J Dermatol *97:247, 1977.)*

a fringe of hair along the frontal hairline persists (Figure 24-6).[16] In exceptional cases a course similar to that in men is seen, with deep frontotemporal recession.

Laboratory findings. The laboratory investigation of female patients with diffuse alopecia with both female and male patterns is outlined in Table 24-3. Laboratory evaluation for some androgenetic alopecia should initially include determination of the serum DHEA-S and total serum testosterone (T) levels, testosterone-estradiol–binding globulin (TeBG) for the T/TeBG ratio, and serum prolactin levels.[10]

Treatment. A 2% topical minoxidil solution (Rogaine/Regaine) was significantly more effective than placebo in the treatment of female androgenetic alopecia.[17,18] A 5% solution is now available.

See treatment for hirsutism and androgenetic alopecia in men.

TABLE 24-3 Laboratory Values for Evaluation of Diffuse Female Alopecia			
	Female-pattern alopecia	Female-pattern alopecia with hirsutism	Male-pattern alopecia (frontotemporal recession)
DHEA-S*	Normal or elevated	Normal or elevated	Elevated
T	Normal	Normal or elevated	Elevated
TeBG	Normal	Decreased or normal	Decreased or normal
T/TeBG Prolactin†	Normal	Elevated	Elevated

Modified from Kasick JM et al: *Cleve Clin Q* 50:111, 1983.
DHEA-S, dehydroepiandrosterone sulfate; *T*, total serum testosterone; *TeBG*, testosterone-estradiol—binding globulin; *T/TeBG*, androgenic index.
†If elevated, suspect pituitary disease (e.g., pituitary prolactin-secreting adenoma).

HIRSUTISM

Hirsutism is defined as the appearance of excessive coarse (terminal) hair in a pattern not normal in females. Hirsutism by itself or associated with other signs of virilization (see the box at right) may be a sign of an endocrine disorder. Most cases are androgen mediated. In women, androgens originate from the adrenal glands or the ovary. The investigation of cause therefore involves the study of these two organs. Non-androgen–mediated causes are listed in the box on p. 748. Many patients do not have any abnormal studies or any cause for the excess hair growth and are classified as having idiopathic hirsutism.

SIGNS OF VIRILIZATION
Acne and increased sebum production
Clitoral hypertrophy
Decrease in breast size
Deepening of the voice
Frontotemporal balding
Increased muscle mass
Infrequent or absent menses
Heightened libido
Hirsutism
Malodorous perspiration

CAUSES OF HIRSUTISM

HIRSUTISM WITHOUT VIRILIZATION (NON-ANDROGEN–DEPENDENT HIRSUTISM)

Genetic
- Racial
- Familial

Physiologic
- Puberty
- Pregnancy
- Menopause

Endocrine
- Hypothyroidism
- Acromegaly

Congenital lesions
- Hurler's syndrome
- Trisomy E
- De Lange's syndrome

Porphyria

Hamartomas

Drugs
- Androgens
- Diazoxide
- Glucocorticoids
- Minoxidil
- Oral contraceptives (progestational components)
- Phenytoin

CNS lesions
- Multiple sclerosis
- Encephalitis
- Hyperostosis frontalis interna

Achard-Thiers syndrome

HIRSUTISM WITH VIRILIZATION (ANDROGEN-DEPENDENT HIRSUTISM)

Ovarian
- Polycystic ovary syndrome
- Hyperthecosis
- HAIR-AN syndrome (hyperandrogenism, insulin resistance, acanthosis nigricans)
- Tumors

Adrenal
- Congenital adrenal hyperplasias (classic and attenuated forms)
  - 21-hydroxylase deficiency
  - 11-hydroxylase deficiency (rare)
  - 3B-hydroxysteroid dehydrogenase deficiency (rare)
- Tumors
- ACTH-dependent Cushing's syndrome

Excessive body hair. Most women have some terminal hair in the so-called male sexual pattern. Normal variations are great, and women of certain ethnic groups, such as women of eastern Mediterranean descent, may have dense facial and body hair, as well as terminal hair around the areolae and extending from the pubis in the midline of the abdomen. Such individuals would be recognized as normal in their countries of origin and can be reassured. Women who develop hirsutism well after puberty, especially if accompanied by signs of virilization such as infrequent or absent menses, have an abnormal condition and require further evaluation.

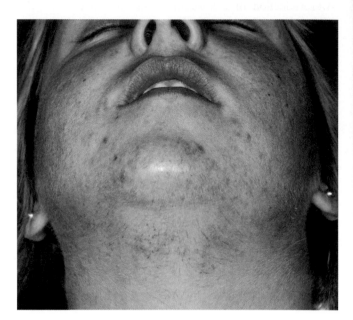

Figure 24-7
Hirsutism (grades II and III). Growth of terminal hair on the chin and neck of a young woman.

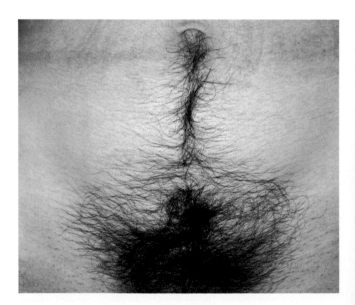

Figure 24-8
Hirsutism. A prominent escutcheon in a woman.

The amount and distribution of hair is an indication of the androgen effect. Vellus hair (narrow, nonpigmented hair) covers most of the body before puberty. Androgen-dependent follicles are located in the beard area, upper back, shoulders, sternum, axillae, and pubis (Figures 24-7 and 24-8). Axillary and pubic follicles are very sensitive to low levels of androgens, whereas follicles on the face and trunk respond only to high levels of androgens. Excess androgens can transform vellus hair in these regions to terminal hair (thick, pigmented hair) and produce hirsutism. Frontotemporal scalp hair recession often is seen with hirsutism.

Androgens. Virilization in women is usually caused by an overproduction of testosterone and other androgens. The higher the production of androgens, the greater the degree of virilization. The four primary circulating androgenic steroids in women are dehydroepiandrosterone (DHEA) and its sulfate (DHEA-S), androstenedione, and testosterone (Figure 24-9). Approximately 50% of the testosterone is secreted from the ovaries and adrenal glands. The remainder is produced from metabolism in the liver, fat, and skin of the prehormones androstenedione, DHEA, and DHEA-S. Androstenedione is produced by both the ovaries and the adrenal glands. DHEA-S originates from the adrenal glands. The liver is the major site of testosterone metabolism. Testosterone overproduction overwhelms the liver's clearance capabilities, and excessive testosterone appears in the circulation. The hair follicle then becomes a site to metabolize the excess testosterone. Metabolism of excess testosterone by the hair follicle leads to excessive coarse hair production.[19]

Testosterone binds to androgen receptors in the hair follicle. The follicular enzyme 5a-reductase is activated and transforms receptor-bound testosterone to 5a-dihydrotestosterone (DHT), which is metabolized to androstanediol. The activated hormones stimulate follicular proliferation, resulting in the growth of thick (terminal) hair.

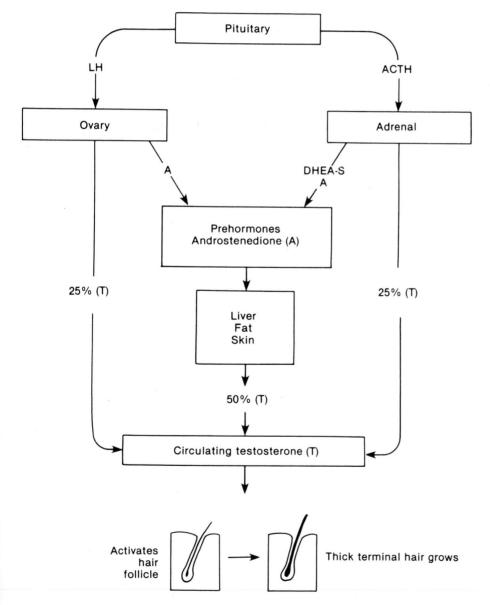

Figure 24-9
Androgen-dependent hirsutism.
T = testosterone; DHEA = dehydroepiandrosterone; DHEA-S = dehydroepiandrosterone sulfate; A = androstenedione.

EVALUATION OF HIRSUTISM

DETERMINE THAT HIRSUTISM ACTUALLY EXISTS

Document degree and distribution. Drug-induced hirsutism (other than androgens) consists of increase in fine hairs (lanugo-like) that is not restricted to androgen-dependent areas

CLASSIFY DEGREE OF FACIAL HIRSUTISM*
(based on distribution and number of terminal hairs)

Grade I	Scattered, chin
Grade II	Clusters, chin
Grade III	Entire chin and anterior neck
Grade IV	Full male beard

HISTORY

Serious disease is suggested by onset of hirsutism well after puberty, rapid progression of hair growth, balding, deepening of the voice, and increased libido.

Idiopathic hirsutism, polycystic ovary disease, and late-onset attenuated congenital adrenal hyperplasia (21-hydroxylase deficiency) usually start at puberty with slowly progressive hair growth. Weight gain and menstrual irregularity are often seen.

Polycystic ovary disease is the most common cause of hyperandrogenism in women. These women show no signs of virilization and minor degrees of hirsutism.

PHYSICAL EXAMINATION

Look for signs of virilization

Determine "clitoral index": the product of the vertical and horizontal dimensions of the glans—normal range 9-35 mm^2. Unequivocal clitoral enlargement (>100 mm^2) suggests severe hyperandrogenicity and is not usually seen in polycystic ovary disease, idiopathic hirsutism, or congenital adrenal hyperplasia.

Pelvic examination: 50% of ovarian tumors are palpable.

Palpate abdomen for adrenal masses.

Acanthosis nigricans suggests insulin resistance.

Examine for signs of Cushing's disease.

PERFORM INITIAL LABORATORY STUDIES (SEE BOX AT RIGHT)

PERFORM FOLLOW-UP STUDIES OR REFER TO ENDOCRINOLOGIST

Adapted from Rittmaster RS, Loriaux DL: *Ann Intern Med* 106:95-107, 1987.
*Data from Birnbaum MD, Rose LI: *Fertil Steril* 32:536, 1979; Rittmaster RS, Loriaux DL: *Ann Intern Med* 106:95-107, 1987; and Braunstein GD: Female reproductive disorders. In Hershman JM, editor: *Management of endocrine disorders*, Philadelphia, 1980, Lea & Febiger.

LABORATORY EVALUATION OF HIRSUTISM

INITIAL VISIT

Virilization (determine degree of severity)

Serum testosterone* and free testosterone (Determine level of circulating testosterone whatever its origin.)

Testosterone-estradiol–binding globulin (To assess the influence of any excess androgenic hormone, whatever its origin. Androgens depress liver synthesis of this binding protein.)

Serum 17-hydroxyprogesterone (between 7:00 and 9:00 A.M.) (if history suggestive of congenital adrenal hyperplasia)

Serum dehydroepiandrosterone sulfate (DHEA-S)[†]

Serum androstenedione[‡]

Serum LH and FSH

Serum thyroxine

Ovarian sonography (ultrasound)

With these tests, the diagnosis can be established in more than 95% of patients at the first visit.

SUBSEQUENT VISITS

Testosterone: normal or slightly elevated
  No further investigation

Testosterone: markedly elevated
  Repeat testosterone test
  Computed tomography (adrenal glands)
  ACTH stimulation test for confirmation—if 17-hydroxyprogesterone elevated
  Surgical exploration
  Urinary free cortisol + overnight dexamethasone suppression test (if Cushing's syndrome suspected)
  Ovarian/adrenal vein catheterization
  Prolactin levels rule out prolactin-secreting tumor

Data from Morris DV: *Clin Obstet Gynecol* 12:649-675, 1985; Hammond MG, Talbert LM, Groff TR: *Postgrad Med* 79:107-113, 1986.
*Serum testosterone levels fluctuate with the menstrual cycle, peaking at midcycle.
†Serum DHEA-S is used as a marker of adrenal androgen production because serum concentrations do not vary with the menstrual cycle and there is little diurnal fluctuation.
‡Serum A concentrations vary as much as 50% over a 24-hour period. There is an increase in mean plasma A levels during midcycle.

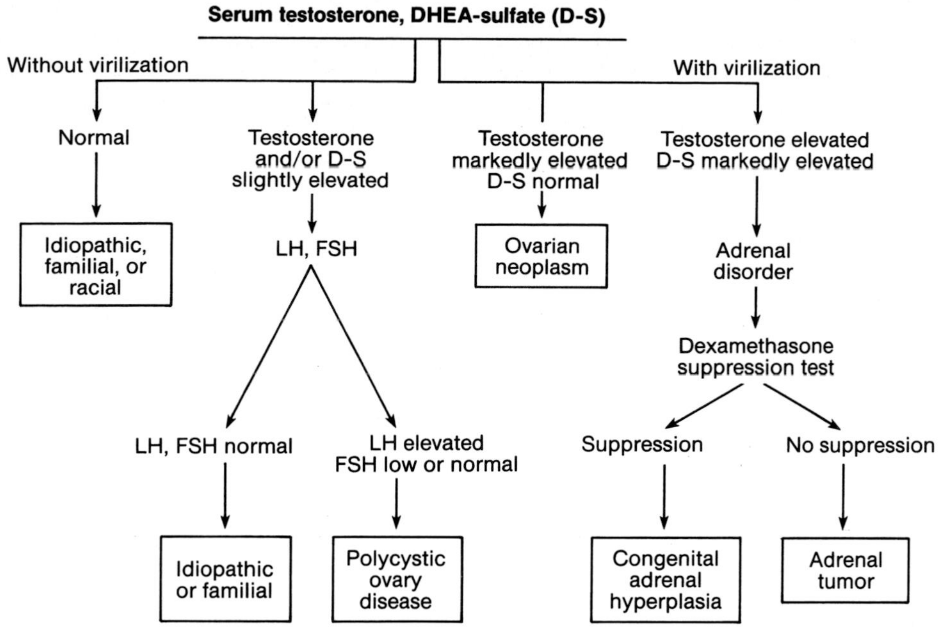

Serum testosterone, DHEA-sulfate (D-S)

Without virilization → Normal → Idiopathic, familial, or racial

Without virilization → Testosterone and/or D-S slightly elevated → LH, FSH

LH, FSH → LH, FSH normal → Idiopathic or familial

LH, FSH → LH elevated FSH low or normal → Polycystic ovary disease

With virilization → Testosterone markedly elevated D-S normal → Ovarian neoplasm

With virilization → Testosterone elevated D-S markedly elevated → Adrenal disorder → Dexamethasone suppression test

Dexamethasone suppression test → Suppression → Congenital adrenal hyperplasia

Dexamethasone suppression test → No suppression → Adrenal tumor

Figure 24-10
Flow sheet for the evaluation of a patient with hirsutism with or without associated virilization. *DHEA-sulfate (D-S)*, dehydroepiandrosterone sulfate; *LH*, luteinizing hormone; *FSH*, follicle-stimulating hormone. *(From Braunstein GD: Female reproductive disorders. In Hershman JM, editor:* Management of endocrine disorders, *Philadelphia, 1980, Lea & Febiger.)*

Androgen production in hirsutism. Mean plasma androgen levels are elevated in women with hirsutism, but there is considerable overlap in values among normal women and women with idiopathic hirsutism and polycystic ovary syndrome. Between 25% and 60% of hirsute women have a normal total plasma testosterone level. A normal plasma testosterone level is found in 80% of women with normal menses. Testosterone production rates are almost always elevated in hirsute women. A normal random plasma testosterone level in a hirsute woman frequently does not accurately reflect the testosterone production rate. The free plasma testosterone level is a more sensitive index of increased testosterone production in women with hirsutism than is the total testosterone level.[20]

Evaluation. A systematic approach for the evaluation of hirsutism is outlined in the boxes on p. 750 and in Figure 24-10.

Treatment. Hirsutism cannot be cured, only suppressed. The problem is cosmetic, and the decision to treat must be made after consideration of the potential side effects of medication. Many women find excess hair intolerable and choose to tolerate side effects.

Treatment begins after ovarian and adrenal disease has been investigated and, if present, is dealt with appropriately (Table 24-4). Oral contraceptives reduce free testosterone. Low-dose glucocorticoids (dexamethasone, prednisone) suppress adrenal gland production and lower DHEA-S levels. Spironolactone, cyproterone acetate, and cimetidine are androgen receptor competitive inhibitors. Spironolactone is used extensively in the United States to treat hirsutism. Cyproterone acetate is available in other countries.

Patients are treated and observed during a 3-month suppression period. Hair growth neither lessens nor worsens during this period. Improvement is observed within 6 to 12 months.

Certain drugs decrease the rate of growth and the size of the hair shaft and lighten hair color, but they do not affect established hairs. These must be removed for best results.

TABLE 24-4 Treatment of Hirsutism

Classification of facial hirsutism*	Adrenal†	Ovarian or‡ idiopathic
I	No treatment needed	Spironolactone, 50 mg/day
II	Dexamethasone, 0.25 mg qhs	Spironolactone, 50-75 mg/day
III	Dexamethasone, 0.5 mg qhs	Spironolactone, 75 mg/day
IV	Dexamethasone, 0.25 mg qhs PLUS Spironolactone, 50 mg/day	Spironolactone, 50-75 mg/day PLUS Norethindrone-mestranol (oral contraceptive)

Modified from Tremblay RR: *Clin Endocrinol Metab* 15:363-371, 1986.
*See the box on p. 750.
†Elevated DHEA-S and/or 17-hydroxyprogesterone and testosterone levels and reduced TeBG.
‡Normal or elevated testosterone levels and reduced TeBG.

Cosmetic approach. Excess facial hair may be plucked, shaved, bleached, wax stripped, or removed by chemical depilatories or electrolysis.[21] Shaving does not increase the thickness or rate of growth, but women are reluctant to use this technique.

Glucocorticoids. Glucocorticoids are most effective for patients whose hirsutism is of short duration. Glucocorticoids suppress adrenocorticotropic hormone (ACTH) and thereby diminish adrenal androgen production. They are used to treat women with congenital adrenal hyperplasia (classic and attenuated forms) and other conditions with increased levels of DHEA-S. Low dosages of glucocorticoids suppress androgen but not adrenal glucocorticoid production. Dexamethasone (0.25 to 1 mg) or prednisone (5 to 7.5 mg) is administered at bedtime. Nighttime administration reduces the early-morning peak of ACTH secretion and generally does not cause the typical side effects of glucocorticoid excess or prolonged adrenal suppression. Dosage adjustments must be made because the dosage required for adrenal suppression, particularly with dexamethasone, varies widely among patients. DHEA-S and morning cortisol levels should be monitored. DHEA-S levels should fall to near-normal range, and cortisol levels should be maintained at normal levels. Treatment is stopped after 1 year, and the patient is observed. Decreased hair growth occurs in approximately 30% to 50% of patients.

Oral contraceptives. Oral contraceptives reduce hair growth in 50% to 75% of women with idiopathic hirsutism and polycystic ovary disease. The estrogen component of oral contraceptives decreases the ovarian and adrenal androgen production and stimulates the liver to produce increased quantities of testosterone-estradiol–binding globulin. The circulating globulin binds and decreases the concentration of active serum androgens. The criteria for choosing an oral contraceptive are the same for hirsutism and acne. Effective preparations are those with high concentrations of estrogen and a progestin with low androgen activity. Agents containing 100 μg of mestranol and 2 mg of norethindrone (Ortho-Novum 2 mg; Norinyl 2 mg) meet this criteria. If the high dosage of estrogen is not tolerated, preparations containing 80 μg of mestranol and 1 mg of norethindrone (Norinyl 1 + 80—21 or 28 days; Ortho-Novum 1/80—21 or 28) may be substituted. Approximately 50% of patients treated with oral contraceptives for 6 months or more show improvement.

Spironolactone. Spironolactone is an antiandrogen that acts at the hair follicle as an androgen receptor competitive inhibitor, resulting in decreased production of dihydrotestosterone, and suppresses androgen production by the gonad and adrenal glands.[22] Antiandrogens do not induce hair loss, but the hair shaft diameter decreases in size, and color lightens. Pregnancy is contraindicated during spironolactone use. Spironolactone is not useful for women with a slight degree of hirsutism. Various studies have used spironolactone in the range of 50 to 200 mg/day. The lower dosage regimens are usually effective and minimize side effects.

The most common side effect is metrorrhagia.[23] This side effect, which for many women is intolerable, increases at higher dosages. Metrorrhagia is minimized by taking spironolactone on days 4 through 21 of the menstrual cycle or adding cyclic estrogen/progesterone therapy to continuous spironolactone therapy.[24] Other, less common, side effects include transient polyuria, fatigue, headache, gastric distress, and breast tenderness. It has been claimed that long-term administration of spironolactone may be associated with an increased incidence of breast cancer.[25]

Cimetidine. Cimetidine blocks androgen action at the hair follicle and would be expected to be effective whether the source of the excess androgen were ovarian or adrenal. However, this drug is less effective than other drugs and is generally not used to treat hirsutism.

Cyproterone acetate (available outside the United States). Cyproterone acetate is a progestogen that suppresses gonadotropin secretion and also acts by blocking androgen receptors.[26] It is used in Europe and in other countries to treat hirsutism. Dosages ranging from 2 to 200 mg/day, generally in combination with ethynyl estradiol, are used. Cyproterone acetate is taken up in adipose tissue and then slowly released, thus rendering the patient susceptible to menstrual irregularity. A reversed sequential regimen was developed to avoid this side effect. It consists of giving cyproterone acetate on days 5 through 15 of the cycle in dosages initially of 50 to 100 mg per day. Ethynyl estradiol is given in a dosage of 50 μg daily from days 5 through 26 of the cycle. Dosage reduction is possible once effective remission of hirsutism occurs. A combination oral contraceptive (Diane) containing cyproterone acetate (2 mg) and estrogen ethynyl estradiol (50 μg) is sometimes used for maintenance. Side effects include nausea, weight gain, breast tenderness, breakthrough bleeding, headache, decreased libido, and depression.

ALOPECIA AREATA

Alopecia areata is a common asymptomatic disease characterized by the rapid onset of total hair loss in a sharply defined, usually round, area. The diagnosis is made by observation. Most patients are under 40 and have no other associated findings. A wide spectrum of involvement is seen. The majority of patients report the sudden occurrence of one or several 1- to 4-cm areas of hair loss on the scalp that can be easily concealed by covering with adjacent hair. The skin is smooth and white or may have short stubs of hair. The hair shaft in alopecia areata is poorly formed and breaks on reaching the surface (Figure 24-11, *A*).

Regrowth begins in 1 to 3 months and may be followed by loss in the same or other areas. The prognosis for total permanent regrowth in cases with limited involvement is excellent. The new hair is usually of the same color and texture, but it may be fine and white (Figure 24-11, *B*). Occasionally the white color remains. The eyelashes, beard, and, rarely, other parts of the body may be involved. Total hair loss of the scalp (alopecia totalis) (Figure 24-11, *C*), seen most frequently in young people, may be accompanied by cycles of growth and loss, but the prognosis for long-term regrowth is poor. Total body hair loss (alopecia universalis) is very rare. The "moth-eaten" or diffuse alopecia of secondary syphilis may be confused with alopecia areata.[27]

Nail changes. Nail pitting and longitudinal striations may be seen in one to all of the nails of some patients with alopecia areata (Figure 24-11, *D*).[28]

Etiology. The etiology is unknown. Stress is frequently cited, but a recent study concludes that there is little evidence that emotional stress plays a significant role in the pathogenesis of alopecia areata.[29] Alopecia areata appears to progress as a wave of follicles prematurely enter telogen.[30] The event weakens or narrows the hair shaft, which continues to grow before the telogen phase is complete. Most weakened hairs fracture when they reach the surface. The affected hairs that are often found retained at the periphery of a lesion have a normal upper shaft and a narrowed base— "exclamation point" hair. There is a peribulbar lymphocytic infiltrate.

Figure 24-11 Alopecia areata.

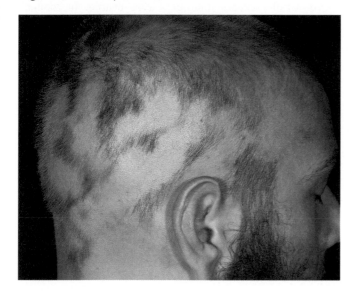

A, Multiple round and oval patches of hair loss.

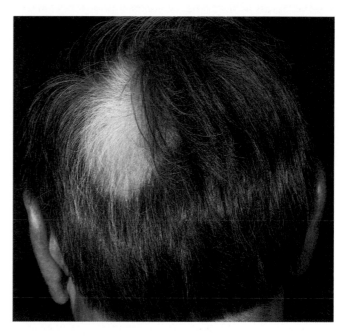

B, The regrown hair is white.

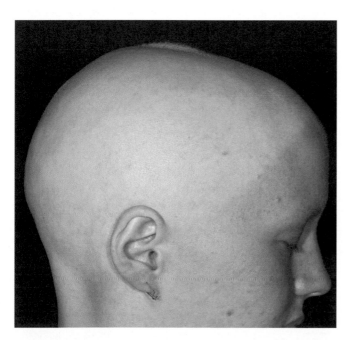

C, Alopecia totalis. The hair has regrown for short periods. The prognosis for normal regrowth is poor.

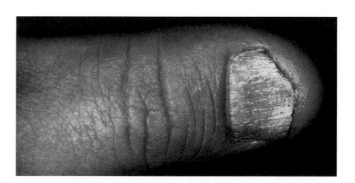

D, Shallow pitting occurs in some patients with alopecia areata.

Alopecia areata may be associated with thyroid disease, pernicious anemia,[31] Addison's disease, vitiligo,[32] lupus erythematosus, ulcerative colitis,[33] and Down's syndrome. Circulating autoantibodies and follicular deposits of C3 and IgG have been reported.[34] The significance of these findings is unknown.

Psychologic implications. Hair plays an important role in one's appearance and self-image and sudden hair loss in a bizarre pattern is psychologically painful.[35] It affects the quality of life and limits social freedom. Those affected equate partial hair loss with balding and fear total hair loss. The appearance is striking, and people stare. Alopecia areata is devastating for image-conscious teenagers. Patients make attempts to hide bald spots by covering them with adjacent long hairs. Those with extensive loss who cannot adequately camouflage the spots may go into hiding or obtain a wig. A network of support groups across the country is available to help people cope with fears, loneliness, and concerns. Patients can contact the Alopecia Areata Foundation* for information about support groups and newsletters. The physician can provide continuing support for this difficult problem.

Treatment

Observation. The majority of patients with a few small areas of hair loss can be assured that the prognosis for regrowth is excellent. If there is great anxiety or if bald areas cannot be concealed, then intralesional injections should be considered.

Intralesional injection. Hair growth can be stimulated in the majority of cases with an intradermal injection of triamcinolone acetonide (Kenalog), 2.5 to 10 mg/ml.[36,37] The suspension is delivered uniformly throughout the bald area by simultaneously injecting and advancing the needle. Just enough of the suspension should be injected to momentarily blanch the skin. Injections may be repeated at 4-week intervals. Atrophy, especially with the 10 mg/ml dosage, is the major side effect. The results in most cases are gratifying, but there is no evidence that intralesional steroid injections alter the course of the disease, and the hair may once again be shed. This treatment should be reserved for patients with a few small areas of hair loss.

Systemic steroids

PULSE CORTICOTHERAPY. Nine patients with recent-onset alopecia areata (1 year) and a bald surface of greater than 30% of the scalp were given 250 mg intravenously of methylprednisolone twice a day on 3 successive days. The course of the ongoing episode of alopecia areata was stopped in eight patients. At the 6-month follow-up, a regrowth on 80% to 100% of the bald surfaces was observed in six patients.[38]

Lower dosages of oral and intramuscular steroids restore hair growth, but the hair is lost when treatment is stopped.[39] In one study, a 6-week taper of prednisone resulted in 25% regrowth in 30% to 47% of patients with mild to extensive alopecia areata, alopecia totalis, or alopecia universalis, with predictable and transient side effects. Two percent topical minoxidil three times daily appeared to help limit post-steroid hair loss.[40]

Anthralin. Anthralin (Drithocreme 1%, 0.5%, 0.25%, or 0.1%) applied once daily in concentrations high enough to induce a visible dermatitis with erythema and mild itching has been reported to induce hair growth.[41] Low dosages of anthralin cause only minimal irritation and are of no benefit.[42] The mechanism of action is unknown, but the treatment is safe and may be considered for refractory cases. Combination therapy with 5% minoxidil plus 0.5% anthralin is more effective than when either drug is used as a single agent.[43]

Photochemotherapy (PUVA). Both topical[44] and oral[45] methoxsalen in combination with long-wave ultraviolet light (UVA) is reported to be successful for some patients, but the relapse rate is high when treatment is stopped. A recent study of 102 patients concluded that PUVA is not an effective treatment for alopecia areata.[46]

Topical allergens. Hair growth may be stimulated by inducing a contact allergy at the sites of hair loss. Diphenylcyclopropenone,[47,48] dinitrochlorobenzene (DNCB),[49] and squaric acid dibutylester[50] induce sensitivity in most individuals and have been used as therapeutic agents in clinical trials.[51] The most frequent side effects are eczematous reactions with blistering, spreading of the induced contact eczema, and sleep disturbances. These agents are moderately effective but are not used in routine practice. The use of DNCB has been curtailed because of its potential carcinogenicity.

Minoxidil (topical solution). Rogaine (topical minoxidil, 2% and 5% solution) is approved for the treatment of male-pattern baldness. The response is variable. Some studies show that the currently available concentration is of limited benefit,[52] whereas others show cosmetically acceptable results in approximately 30% of cases with twice-a-day application.[53] The response is slow and requires months of treatment. Minoxidil does not change the course of the disease, and continual use is required to sustain growth.[54] Maximum results have been obtained when the bedtime minoxidil application was covered with a thin layer of white petrolatum for occlusion.[55]

Other treatments. Topical cyclosporine,[56] oral cyclosporine,[57] oral inosiplex (a synthetic immunomodulator),[58] and topical nitrogen mustard[59] have all been used with some success to treat alopecia areata.[60,61]

Hair weaves and wigs. See treatment section under androgenic alopecia in men. High quality wigs are available.

---

*National Alopecia Areata Foundation, 714 C St., Suite 202, San Rafael, CA 94901, 415 456 4644; Alopecia Areata Association of Canada, 55 McCaul St., Suite 123, Toronto, Ontario, Canada M5T 2W7.

TRICHOTILLOMANIA

Trichotillomania is the act of manually removing hair by manipulation. It is defined in the *Diagnostic and Statistical Manual of Mental Disorders* as an irresistible urge to pull the hair and a sense of relief after the hair has been plucked. This conscious or subconscious habit or tic is most commonly performed by young children, adolescents, and women. The female/male ratio is 2.5:1. Hair is twisted about the finger and pulled or rubbed until extracted or broken. The favorite site is the easily reached frontoparietal region of the scalp, but any scalp area or the eyebrows and eyelashes may be attacked. The affected area has an irregular angulated border, and the density of hair is greatly reduced; but the site is never bald, as in alopecia areata. Several short, broken hairs of varying lengths are randomly distributed in the involved site. Hair that grows beyond 0.5 to 1 cm can be grasped by small fingers and extracted (Figure 24-12).

The symptom may first manifest during inactive periods in the classroom, while watching television, or in bed while waiting to fall asleep. Parents seldom notice the behavior. In many children trichotillomania is triggered by hospitalizations or medical interventions, problems at home, or difficulties at school. Cases also occur with severe sibling rivalry, a disturbed parent-child relationship, and mental retardation.[62] Comorbidity with severe, overt psychopathology increases in incidence, with trichotillomania arising in adolescence and adulthood.[63] Some psychiatrists classify it as an obsessive-compulsive disorder in adults.[64] Increased prevalence has been documented in adults with anxiety and with affective disorders.

Diagnosis. First, the patient should be asked if he or she manipulates the hair. Parents or teachers may be aware of the habit. A potassium hydroxide and Wood's light examination rules out noninflammatory tinea capitis. Areas of alopecia areata are completely devoid of hair. In questionable cases a hair pluck can be performed from the diseased areas; in trichotillomania, it shows no telogen hair roots. Nearly 100% of the hairs are in the active-growing, anagen phase. The absence of telogen hairs is the reason no hair is released on gentle hair traction. Skin biopsy specimens (4- or 5-mm punch extending into the subcutaneous tissue) show normal hairs, absence of hairs in follicles, and no infiltration of leukocytes. Catagen hairs are present in 74%, pigment casts in 61%, and traumatized hair bulbs in 21%; these findings are most evident in areas affected for less than 8 weeks.[65]

Treatment. Many patients are psychologically stable[66] and require only a discussion of the problem with an understanding physician or parent. Many of these cases resolve spontaneously. Advise parents to divert the child's attention when hair is being pulled and to be accepting and supportive rather than judgmental or punitive. Patients with extensive involvement or those who persist in the habit should have a psychiatric evaluation.[67] The relative effectiveness and long-term benefits of behavioral and drug treatments are not established. Clomipramine (Anafranil), a tricyclic antidepressant, appears to be effective in the short-term treatment of trichotillomania,[68] but some patients in one study relapsed at 3-month follow-up while still taking previously effective levels of the drug.[64] Patients treated with fluoxetine (Prozac) in an open 16-week trial improved significantly.[69]

Figure 24-12 Trichotillomania.

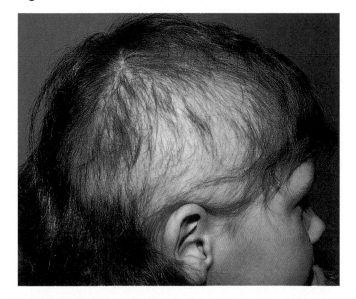

A, Hair has been manually extracted from a wide area of the scalp. There is no inflammation or scarring.

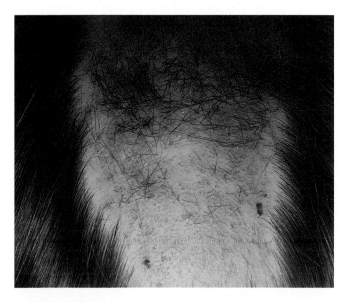

B, Several short hairs are randomly distributed in the involved site.

TRACTION (COSMETIC) ALOPECIA

Prolonged tension created by certain hairstyles, such as braids or pony tails, hair rollers, and hot hair-straightening combs, may result in temporary or, rarely, permanent hair loss in an area corresponding exactly to the stressed hair. The scalp may appear normal or may show evidence of inflammation or scarring. Temporary or permanent occipital alopecia secondary to pressure ischemia may occur on the scalp of patients left on their backs in the same position during surgery.

SCARRING ALOPECIA

A number of diseases cause scarring, and, if they happen to occur in the scalp, hair follicles may be destroyed, resulting in scarring or cicatricial alopecia. Many of these diseases can be recognized by their characteristic presentation.

Discoid lupus erythematosus. Discoid lupus erythematosus presents in the scalp with discrete bald patches showing follicular plugging (see Chapter Seventeen).

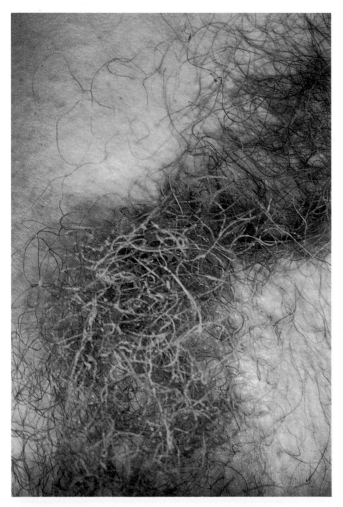

Figure 24-13
Trichomycosis axillaris. Yellow concretions are adherent to the axillary hair. These concretions are composed of a mass of diphtheroid organisms and not fungi.

Erythema and scaling may or may not be present. With time, plugged follicles disappear, and the skin becomes smooth, atrophic, and scarred. Biopsy and immunofluorescence help to establish the diagnosis.

Lichen planus. Lichen planus presents in the scalp with violaceous papules or as an area of alopecia with follicular plugging (see Chapter Eight). If scarring occurs, the follicular plugs are lost, and the diagnosis with biopsy cannot be made with certainty at this stage. This type of scarring alopecia without evidence of lichen planus in other areas has been called *pseudopelade*.

Aplasia cutis congenita. A small blister or eroded area, usually in the midline of the scalp, may be present at birth. It represents a congenital absence of a portion or a full thickness of skin. In most cases the area heals spontaneously. Larger areas of aplasia may be associated with other developmental defects.

Trichomycosis

Trichomycosis is an asymptomatic infection of axillary or pubic hair caused by a corynebacterium. The hair shaft becomes coated with adherent yellow (occasionally red or black), firm concretions[70] (Figure 24-13). Hyperhidrosis is often present. The hair is shaved, and hyperhidrosis is controlled with antiperspirants. Naftifine hydrochloride 1% cream (Naftin) is effective for superficial fungal infections and also has antibacterial properties. It is reportedly effective for trichomycosis.[71]

REFERENCES

1. Munro DD: Hair growth measurement using intradermal sulphur 35 L-cystine, *Arch Dermatol* 93:119, 1966.
2. Rook A, Dawber R: *Diseases of the hair and scalp*, Oxford, 1982, Blackwell Scientific Publications.
3. Headington JT: Telogen effluvium, *Arch Dermatol* 129:356-363, 1993.
4. Kligman AM: Pathologic dynamics of human hair loss. I. Telogen effluvium, *Arch Dermatol* 83:175-198, 1961.
5. Webster JR, Huff S, Gecht MC: Thallotoxicosis, *Arch Dermatol* 78:278, 1958.
6. Levantine A, Almeyda J: Drug induced alopecia, *Br J Dermatol* 89:549, 1973.
7. Granai CO, Frederickson H, et al: The use of minoxidil to attempt to prevent alopecia during chemotherapy for gynecologic malignancies, *Eur J Gynaecol Oncol* 12:129-132, 1991.
8. Maguire HC Jr, Kligman AM: Hair plucking as a diagnostic test, *J Invest Dermatol* 43:77, 1964.
9. Kuster W, Happle R: The inheritance of common baldness: two B or not two B? *J Am Acad Dermatol* 11:921-926, 1984.
10. Pitts RL: Serum elevation of dehydroepiandrosterone sulfate associated with male pattern baldness in young men, *J Am Acad Dermatol* 16:571-573, 1987.
11. Price VH, editor: Rogaine (topical minoxidil, 2%) in the management of male pattern baldness and alopecia areata: proceedings of a symposium; sixteen papers covering all aspects of minoxidil, *J Am Acad Dermatol* 16:647-750, 1987.
12. Rietschel RL, Duncan SH: Safety and efficacy of topical minoxidil in the management of androgenetic alopecia, *J Am Acad Dermatol* 16:677-685, 1987.
13. Olsen EA, Weiner MS: Topical minoxidil in male pattern baldness: effects of discontinuation of treatment, *J Am Acad Dermatol* 17:97-101, 1987.

14. Olsen EA, DeLong ER, Weiner M: Long-term follow-up of men with male pattern baldness treated with topical minoxidil, *J Am Acad Dermatol* 16:688-695, 1987.

15. Pinski JB: Hair transplantation, *Semin Dermatol* 6:249-263, 1987.

16. Ludwig E: Classification of the types of androgenic alopecia (common baldness) occurring in the female sex, *Br J Dermatol* 97:247-254, 1977.

17. De Villez RL, Jacobs JP, et al: Androgenetic alopecia in the female. Treatment with 2% topical minoxidil solution, *Arch Dermatol* 130:303-307, 1994.

18. Jacobs JP, Szpunar CA, et al: Use of topical minoxidil therapy for androgenetic alopecia in women, *Int J Dermatol* 32:758-762, 1993.

19. Kirschner MA: Special topics in endocrinology and metabolism, 6:55-93, 1984.

20. Leshin M: Southwestern internal medicine conference: hirsutism, *Am J Med Sci* 294:369-383, 1987.

21. Richards RN, McKenzie MA, Meharg GE: Electroepilation (electrolysis) in hirsutism, *J Am Acad Dermatol* 15:693-697, 1986.

22. Young RL, Goldzieher JW, Elkind-Hirsch K: The endocrine effects of spironolactone used as an antiandrogen, *Fertil Steril* 48:223-228, 1987.

23. Helfer EL, Miller JL, Rose LI: Side-effects of spironolactone therapy in the hirsute woman, *J Clin Endocrinol Metab* 66:208-211, 1988.

24. Board JA, Rosenberg SM, Smeltzer JS: Spironolactone and estrogen-progestin therapy for hirsutism, *South Med J* 80:483-486, 1987; erratum 80:1067, 1987.

25. Hammerstein J, Moltx L, Schwartz U: Antiandrogens in the treatment of acne and hirsutism, *J Steroid Biochem* 19:591, 1983.

26. Holdaway IM et al: Cyproterone acetate as initial treatment and maintenance therapy for hirsutism, *Acta Endocrinol* 109:522-529, 1985.

27. Lee JY, Hsu ML: Alopecia syphilitica, a simulator of alopecia areata: histopathology and differential diagnosis, *J Cutan Pathol* 18:87-92, 1991.

28. Dotz WI, Lieber CD, Vogt PJ: Leukonychia punctata and pitted nails in alopecia areata, *Arch Dermatol* 121:1452-1454, 1985.

29. van der Steen P, Boezeman J, et al: Can alopecia areata be triggered by emotional stress? An uncontrolled evaluation of 178 patients with extensive hair loss, *Acta Derm Venereol* 72:279-280, 1992.

30. Messenger AG, Slater DN, Bleehen SS: Alopecia areata: alterations in the hair growth cycle and correlation with the follicular pathology, *Br J Dermatol* 114:337-347, 1986.

31. Muller SA, Winkelman RK: Alopecia areata, *Arch Dermatol* 88:290, 1963.

32. Anderson I: Alopecia areata: a clinical study, *Br Med J* 2:1250, 1950.

33. Allen HB, Moschella SL: Ulcerative colitis associated with skin and hair changes, *Cutis* 14:85, 1974.

34. Bystryn J, Orentreich N, Stengel F: Direct immunofluorescence studies in alopecia areata and male pattern alopecia, *J Invest Dermatol* 73:317-320, 1979.

35. Beard HO: Social and psychological implications of alopecia areata, *J Am Acad Dermatol* 14:697-700, 1986.

36. Abell E, Munroe DD: Intralesional treatment of alopecia areata with triamcinolone acetonide by jet injector, *Br J Dermatol* 88:55-59, 1973.

37. Porter D, Burton JL: A comparison of intralesional triamcinolone hexacetonide and triamcinolone acetonide in alopecia areata, *Br J Dermatol* 85:272-273, 1971.

38. Perriard-Wolfensberger J, Pasche-Koo F, et al: Pulse of methylprednisolone in alopecia areata, *Dermatology* 187:282-285, 1993.

39. Winter RJ, Kern F, Blizzard RM: Prednisone therapy for alopecia areata: a follow-up report, *Arch Dermatol* 112:1549-1552, 1976.

40. Olsen EA, Carson SC, et al: Systemic steroids with or without 2% topical minoxidil in the treatment of alopecia areata, *Arch Dermatol* 128:1467-1473, 1992.

41. Schmoeckel C et al: Treatment of alopecia areata by anthralin-induced dermatitis, *Arch Dermatol* 115:1254-1255, 1979.

42. Nelson DA, Spielvogel RL: Anthralin therapy for alopecia areata, *Int J Dermatol* 24(9):606-607, 1985.

43. Fiedler VC, Wendrow A, et al: Treatment-resistant alopecia areata. Response to combination therapy with minoxidil plus anthralin, *Arch Dermatol* 126:756-759, 1990.

44. Mitchell AJ, Douglass MC: Topical photochemotherapy for alopecia areata, *J Am Acad Dermatol* 12:644-649, 1985.

45. Claudy AL, Gagnaire D: PUVA treatment of alopecia areata, *Arch Dermatol* 119:975-978, 1983.

46. Healy E, Rogers S: PUVA treatment for alopecia areata—does it work? A retrospective review of 102 cases, *Br J Dermatol* 129:42-44, 1993.

47. van der Steen PH, Boezeman JB, et al: Topical immunotherapy for alopecia areata: re-evaluation of 139 cases after an additional follow-up period of 19 months, *Dermatology* 184:198-201, 1992.

48. van der Steen PH, van Baar HM, et al: Treatment of alopecia areata with diphenylcyclopropenone, *J Am Acad Dermatol* 24:253-257, 1991.

49. Comments and opinions: Several letters involving the hazards of dinitrochlorobenzene, *Arch Dermatol* 122:11-15, 1986.

50. Caserio RJ: Treatment of alopecia areata with squaric acid dibutyl-ester, *Arch Dermatol* 123:1036-1041, 1987.

51. van der Steen PH, van Baar HM, et al: Prognostic factors in the treatment of alopecia areata with diphenylcyclopropenone, *J Am Acad Dermatol* 24:227-230, 1991.

52. White SI, Friedmann PS: Topical minoxidil lacks efficacy in alopecia areata, *Arch Dermatol* 121:591, 1985.

53. Price VH: Double-blind, placebo-controlled evaluation of topical minoxidil in extensive alopecia areata, *J Am Acad Dermatol* 16:730-736, 1987.

54. Price VH: Topical minoxidil (3%) in extensive alopecia areata, including long-term efficacy, *J Am Acad Dermatol* 16:737-744, 1987.

55. Fiedler-Weiss VC: Topical minoxidil solution (1% and 5%) in the treatment of alopecia areata, *J Am Acad Dermatol* 16:745-748, 1987.

56. De Prost Y et al: Placebo-controlled trial of topical cyclosporin in severe alopecia areata, *Lancet* Oct:803, 1986.

57. Gupta AK, Ellis CN, et al: Oral cyclosporine for the treatment of alopecia areata. A clinical and immunohistochemical analysis, *J Am Acad Dermatol* 22:242-250, 1990.

58. Galbraith GMP, Thiers BH, Jensen J, et al: A randomized double-blind study of inosiplex (Isoprinosine) therapy in patients with alopecia areata, *J Am Acad Dermatol* 16:977-983, 1987.

59. Arrazola JM, Sendagorta E, Harto A, et al: Treatment of alopecia areata with topical nitrogen mustard, *Int J Dermatol* 24:608-610, 1985.

60. Shapiro J: Alopecia areata. Update on therapy, *Dermatol Clin* 11:35-46, 1993.

61. Fiedler VC: Alopecia areata. A review of therapy, efficacy, safety, and mechanism, *Arch Dermatol* 128:1519-1529, 1992.

62. Oranje AP, Peereboom-Wynia JDR, De Raeymaecker DMJ: Trichotillomania in childhood, *J Am Acad Dermatol* 15:614-619, 1986.

63. Swedo SE, Rapoport JL: Annotation: trichotillomania, *J Child Psychol Psychiatry* 32:401-409, 1991.

64. Christenson GA, Mackenzie TB, et al: Characteristics of 60 adult chronic hair pullers, *Am J Psychiatry* 148:365-370, 1991.

65. Muller SA: Trichotillomania: a histopathologic study in sixty-six patients, *J Am Acad Dermatol* 23:56-62, 1990.

66. Christenson GA, Chernoff-Clementz E, et al: Personality and clinical characteristics in patients with trichotillomania, *J Clin Psychiatry* 53:407-413, 1992.

67. Swedo SE et al: A double-blind comparison of clomipramine and desipramine in the treatment of trichotillomania (hair pulling), *N Engl J Med* 321:497-501, 1989.

68. Pollard CA, Ibe IO, et al: Clomipramine treatment of trichotillomania: a follow-up report on four cases, *J Clin Psychiatry* 52:128-130, 1991.

69. Winchel RM, Jones JS, et al: Clinical characteristics of trichotillomania and its response to fluoxetine, *J Clin Psychiatry* 53:304-308, 1992.

70. Levit F: Trichomycosis axillaris: a different view, *J Am Acad Dermatol* 18:778-779, 1988.

71. Rosen T, Krawczynska AM, et al: Naftifine treatment of trichomycosis pubis, *Int J Dermatol* 30:667-669, 1991.

CHAPTER TWENTY-FIVE

Nail Diseases

Anatomy and Physiology

Anatomy. The nail unit consists of several components (Figure 25-1). The nail plate is hard, translucent, dead keratin. The nailfold includes the skin surrounding the lateral and proximal aspects of the nail plate. The proximal nailfold overlies the matrix. Its keratin layer extends onto the proximal nail plate to form the cuticle. Capillary loops at the tip of the proximal nailfold are normally small and inapparent, but they become distinct in diseases such as systemic lupus erythematosus and scleroderma. The proximal nailfold epithelium covers the proximal nail plate for a few millimeters and then makes a 180-degree turn and curves back into direct contact with the nail plate. It makes another 180-degree turn and becomes continuous with the nail matrix.

The matrix epithelium synthesizes 90% of the nail plate. The lunula (white half-moon), which is visible through the nail plate, is the distal aspect of the nail matrix. It is continuous with the nail bed. The nail bed extends from the distal nail matrix to the hyponychium. As the nail streams distally, material is added to the undersurface of the nail, thickening it and making it densely adherent to the nail bed.[1] The nail bed consists of parallel longitudinal ridges with small blood vessels at their base (Figure 25-2). Bleeding induced by trauma or vessel disease, such as lupus, occurs in the depths of these grooves, producing the splinter hemorrhage pattern viewed through the nail plate. The hyponychium is a short segment of skin lacking nail cover; it begins at the distal nail bed and terminates at the distal groove.

Nail biopsy. Ungual biopsies are used to diagnosis tumors, inflammatory disease, and infections. The ideal ungual biopsy is performed after avulsion of the plate. This allows clear visualization of the matrix and bed. A punch or excisional biopsy technique is chosen, which provides a sufficient amount of tissue and produces a minimal amount of scarring.

Nail plate avulsion. One or two percent lidocaine without epinephrine is injected with a 30-gauge needle into the lateral and proximal nailfolds, or a digital block may be used. Carbocaine may be used and is longer acting. Wait at least 3 to 5 minutes after injection until the nail apparatus is fully anesthetized. A wide penrose drain is used as a tourniquet for no more than 10 minutes. The nailfolds are loosened from the nail plate with a 2- to 3-mm nail elevator, 2- to 3-mm dental spatula, or mosquito forceps. The same instrument is then placed under the distal edge of the nail plate and gently pushed distally to proximally to separate the nail plate from the underlying nail bed. Rock the instrument back and forth to ensure full nail-plate/nail-bed separation. Grasp the nail plate with a Kelly hemostat or nail-grasping forceps and gently remove it. After the procedure, the wound is dressed with polysporin ointment, telfa, tube gauze, and then tape.[2]

Paronychial biopsy. Paronychial (proximal and lateral nailfold) lesions can be biopsied by a shave biopsy, a punch biopsy, or removed en bloc by blunt dissection. Elliptic excisional biopsies of the proximal nailfold are performed with the long axis oriented horizontally. Be aware of the insertion of the extensor tendon. Ellipitic excisions of the lateral nailfold are oriented longitudinally.

Nail-matrix biopsy. Nail-matrix biopsy may cause permanent nail dystrophy. The most common reason to biopsy the nail matrix is to exclude the diagnosis of melanoma in a patient with a longitudinal, pigmented band. Care must be taken in nail-matrix biopsy to minimize the risk of permanent nail dystrophy.[3] For longitudinal bands that are 3 mm or narrower, a simple punch biopsy to excise the focus of pigmentation in the matrix is sufficient. More complicated excisional techniques to sample wider lesions are best performed by dermatologic surgeons.[4]

Growth rates. Nails grow continuously, but their growth rate decreases both with age and poor circulation. Fingernails, which grow faster than toenails, grow at a rate of 0.5 to 1.29 mm per week. It takes approximately 5.5 months for a fingernail to grow from the matrix to the free edge and approximately 12 to 18 months for a toenail to be replaced. A reduction in the rate of matrix-cell division occurs during systemic diseases such as scarlet fever, causing thinning of the nail plate (Beau's lines).

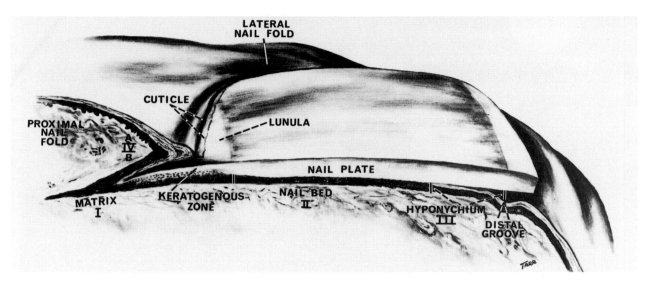

Figure 25-1
Diagrammatic drawing of an adult fingertip, showing nail structures through a longitudinal midline plane. *(From Zaias N, Ackerman BA:* Arch Dermatol *107:193, 1973. Copyright 1973, American Medical Association.)*

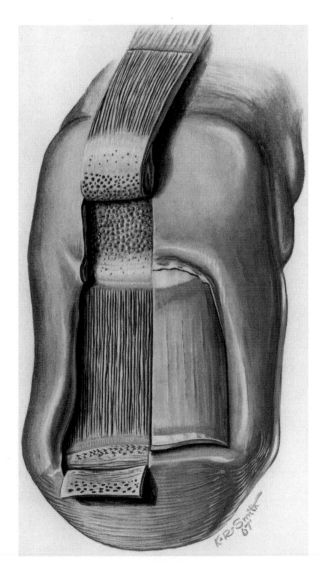

Figure 25-2
Dermal topography underlying nail unit. The nail bed consists of parallel longitudinal ridges with small blood vessels at their base. Anatomic pathology of splinter hemorrhages is obvious. *(From Zaias N, Ackerman BA:* Arch Dermatol *107:193, 1973. Copyright 1973, American Medical Association.)*

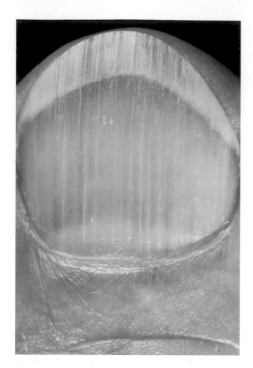

Figure 25-3
Longitudinal ridging. Parallel elevated nail ridges are a common aging change. This change does not indicate any deficiency.

Normal Variations

The shape and opacity of the nail varies considerably among individuals. Aging may increase or decrease nail thickness. Longitudinal ridging (Figure 25-3) is common in aging, but this variant is occasionally observed among the young. Beading occurs at all ages but is more common in the elderly (Figure 25-4). The beads cover part or most of the plate surface and are arranged longitudinally. A pigmented band or bands occur in more than 90% of blacks (Figure 25-5). The sudden appearance of such a band in whites necessitates further investigation.

Nail structure can be altered by primary skin diseases, infections, trauma, internal diseases, congenital syndromes, and tumors. A more detailed discussion with illustrations of the most commonly encountered entities is presented in the following sections.

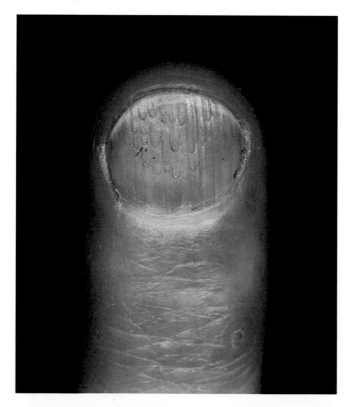

Figure 25-4
Longitudinal ridging and beading. A variant of normal most commonly seen in the elderly.

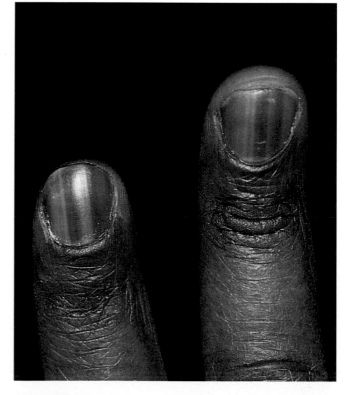

Figure 25-5
Pigmented bands occur as a normal finding in more than 90% of blacks.

Nail Disorders Associated with Skin Disease

Psoriasis. The incidence of nail involvement in psoriasis varies from 10% to 50%. Nail involvement usually occurs simultaneously with skin disease but may occur as an isolated finding. Pitting, onycholysis, discoloration, subungual thickening, and nail-plate alterations take place.[5] Pitting, or sharply defined ice pick–like depressions in the nail plate, is the most common finding (Figure 25-6). The number, distribution, pattern, and depth vary. Pitting is observed in normal nails and with alopecia areata, but, in general, psoriatic pits are deeper. Pits form as the nail substance is shed, which is a process analogous to the shedding of psoriatic skin scale.

Separation of the nail from the nail bed, or onycholysis, is common. Onycholysis is frequently accompanied by yellow discoloration. Separation begins at the distal groove or under the nail plate and may involve several nails. Psoriasis of the hyponychium results in the accumulation of yellow, scaly debris that elevates the nail plate. The debris is commonly mistaken for nail fungus infection. Severe psoriasis of the matrix and nail bed results in grossly malformed nails, and nail-bed splinter hemorrhages are common (Figure 25-7). Treatment is unsatisfactory. Intralesional injections into the matrix with triamcinolone acetonide (Kenalog) (2.5 to 5 mg/ml) delivered with a 30-gauge needle produces the most satisfactory results.[6] This painful procedure is repeated every 3 or 4 weeks. There is little merit in treating psoriatic nails with photochemotherapy (PUVA) or topical 5-fluorouracil (5-FU).

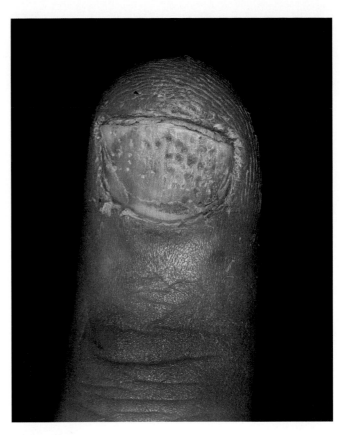

Figure 25-6
Psoriasis. Pitting is the most common nail change found in psoriasis.

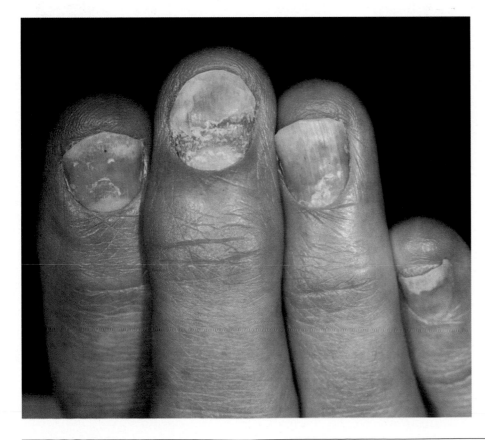

Figure 25-7
Psoriasis. Onycholysis, subungual debris, and nail plate distortion are shown. These changes are often misinterpreted as being fungal in origin.

Lichen planus. Approximately 25% of patients with nail lichen planus (LP) have LP in other sites before or after the onset of nail lesions. Nail LP usually appears during the fifth or sixth decade of life. The matrix, nail bed, and nailfolds may be involved in producing a variety of changes, few of which are characteristic. Minimal inflammation of the matrix induces longitudinal grooving and ridging, which are the most common findings of LP of the nail. The development of severe and early destruction of the nail matrix with scarring characterizes a small subset of patients with nail LP.[7] A pterygium, caused by adhesion of a depressed proximal nailfold to the scarred matrix, may occur after intense matrix inflammation (Figure 25-8). The nail plate distal to this focus is either absent or thinned out. In most cases, nail LP is self-limiting or promptly regresses with treatment.

Permanent damage to the nail is uncommon, even in patients with diffuse involvement of the matrix. Matrix lesions may respond to intralesional triamcinolone acetonide (2.5 to 5 mg/ml) delivered with a 30-gauge needle every 3 or 4 weeks. Severe cases respond to prednisone (20 to 40 mg/day). This may require a long course of treatment in which the possible risks may outnumber the advantages.

Alopecia areata. Many patients with alopecia areata have shallow pitting or surface stippling in a uniform or gridlike pattern (Figure 25-9).

Darier's disease. A number of nail changes are reported with Darier's disease,[8] but white, longitudinal streaks are the most common and the most characteristic.

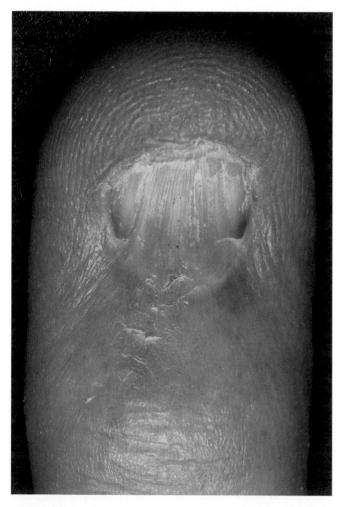

Figure 25-8
Lichen planus. Inflammation of the matrix results in adhesion of the proximal nailfold to the scarred matrix, a pterygium.

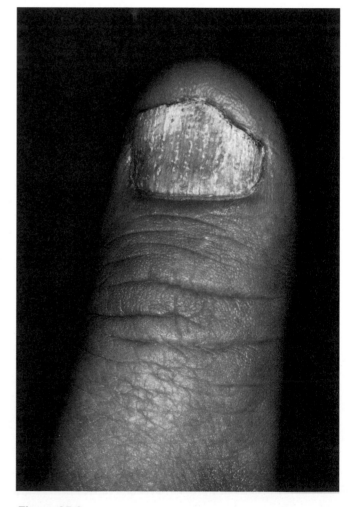

Figure 25-9
Alopecia areata. Shallow pitting occurs in some patients with alopecia areata.

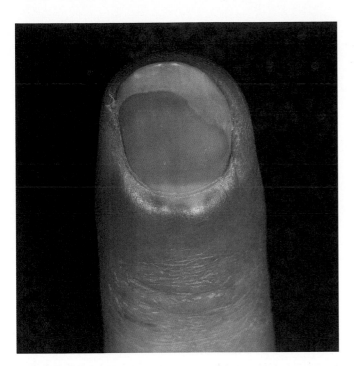

Figure 25-10
Acute paronychia. Erythema and purulent material occur at the proximal nailfold.

Acquired Disorders
BACTERIAL AND VIRAL INFECTIONS

Acute paronychia. The rapid onset of painful, bright red swelling of the proximal and lateral nailfold may occur spontaneously or may follow trauma or manipulation. Superficial infections present with an accumulation of purulent material behind the cuticle (Figure 25-10). The small abscess is drained by inserting the pointed end of a comedone extractor or similar instrument between the proximal nailfold and the nail plate. Pain is abruptly relieved. A diffuse, painful swelling suggests deeper infection, and cases that do not respond to antistaphylococcal antibiotics may require deep incision. Acute paronychia rarely evolves into chronic paronychia.

Chronic paronychia. Chronic paronychia evolves slowly and presents initially with tenderness and mild swelling about the proximal and lateral nailfolds (Figure 25-11). Individuals whose hands are repeatedly exposed to moisture (e.g., bakers, dishwashers, and dentists) are at greatest risk. Manipulation of the cuticle accelerates the process. Typically, many or all fingers are involved simultaneously.

Figure 25-11
Chronic paronychia. Erythema and swelling of the nailfolds. The cuticle is absent. Chronic inflammation has caused horizontal ridging of the nails.

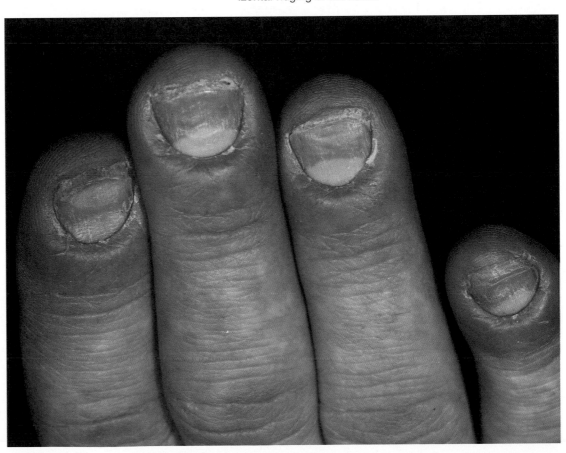

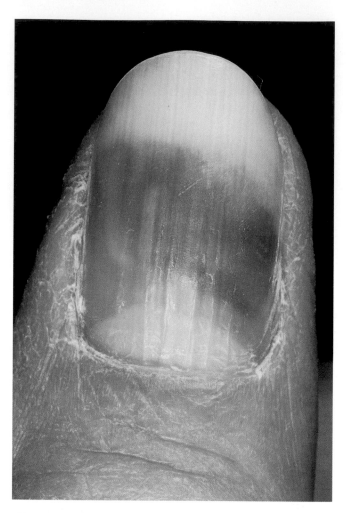

Figure 25-12
Pseudomonas colonized the space between the nail and the nail plate after onycholysis occurred, imparting a green color to the nail plate.

The cuticle separates from the nail plate, leaving the space between the proximal nailfold and the nail plate exposed to infection. Many organisms, both pathogens and contaminants, thrive in this warm, moist intertriginous space. The skin about the nail becomes pale red, tender or painful, and swollen. Occasionally a small quantity of pus can be expressed from under the proximal nailfold. A culture of this material may grow *Candida* or gram-positive and gram-negative organisms. The nail plate is not infected and maintains its integrity, although its surface becomes brown and rippled. There is no subungual thickening such as that present in some fungal infections. The process is chronic and responds very slowly to treatment. Psoriasis of the fingers may present in a similar form.

Treatment. Every attempt must be made to keep the hands dry. One should avoid using medicines with an ointment base, because they are too occlusive and interfere with the necessary drying process. Patients should refrain from washing dishes and from washing their own hair. Rubber or plastic gloves are of some value, but moisture accumulates in them with prolonged use.

Oral antibiotics do not penetrate this distal site in sufficient concentration. Furthermore, the variety of organisms is too numerous to respond to a single oral agent. The most effective treatment is to place one or two drops of 3% thymol in 70% ethanol, which must be compounded by a pharmacist, at the proximal nailfold and to wait for this liquid to flow by capillary action into the space created by the absent cuticle. Slight elevation of the proximal nailfold with a flat toothpick facilitates penetration. This should be repeated two or three times a day for weeks, until the cuticle is re-formed. The cuticle may never re-form in patients with long-standing inflammation. Fluconazole (200 mg/day) for 2 to 4 weeks may control chronic inflammation. Short courses of fluconazole may have to be repeated as the infection recurs.

***Pseudomonas* infection.** Repeated exposure to soap and water causes maceration of the hyponychium and softening of the nail plate. Separation of the nail plate (onycholysis) exposes a damp, macerated space between the nail plate and the nail bed, which is a fertile site for the growth of *Pseudomonas*. The nail plate assumes a green-black color[9] (Figure 25-12). There is little discomfort or inflammation. This presentation may be confused with subungual hematoma (see Figure 25-24), but the absence of pain with *Pseudomonas* infection establishes the diagnosis. Zaias[10] recommends applying a few drops of a one part chlorine bleach/four parts water mixture under the nail three times a day.

Herpetic whitlow. Dentists and nurses used to be at risk of acquiring herpes simplex infection of the fingertip. The risk has greatly diminished with the use of gloves. The appearance and course of the disease resembles that at other body sites, except that there is extreme pain from the swollen fingertips (see Figure 12-29).

FUNGAL NAIL INFECTIONS

Tinea of the nails is also called *tinea unguium*. Dermatophytes *T. rubrum* and *T. mentagrophytes* are responsible for most fingernail and toenail infections, but the so-called nonpathogenic fungi (contaminants), and *Candida* can also infect the nail plate.[11] Multiple pathogens may be present in a single nail. Nail infection may occur simultaneously with hand or foot tinea or may occur as an isolated phenomenon. Toenail infections occur in 15% to 20% of the population between 40 and 60 years of age. The disease may also occur in children.

Trauma predisposes to infection. There is a tendency to label any process involving the nail plate as a fungal infection, but many other cutaneous diseases can change the structure of the nail. Fifty percent of thick nails are not infected with fungus. Differential diagnosis is discussed at the end of this section.

Laboratory diagnosis. The diagnosis of fungal nail infection should be established with both a potassium hydroxide (KOH) examination and a culture. Physicians without the facilities to perform a KOH or culture may obtain these services from specialty laboratories, such as the University Center for Medical Mycology, Department of Dermatology, 11100 Euclid Avenue, Cleveland, Ohio, 44106-5028; 216-844-8580, 216-844-1076 (fax). They provide convienient Derma Pak containers for specimen collection. These small, flat containers can be returned in a regular envelope.

Nail collection techniques for KOH. Confirm the species of fungus before starting oral antifungal treatment. When performing cultures, obtain crumbling debris from under several nails and at different parts (proximal and distal areas of infection) of the infected nail. Collect subungual debris from under the distal edge of the nail with a curet. Sample the nail surface with a curet or scrape it with a #15 scalpel blade. Fungi are found in the nail plate and in the cornified cells of the nail bed. Hyphae that are present in the nail plate may not be viable; therefore, sample the cornified cells of the nail bed if possible.

The nail plate and hard debris can be adequately softened for direct examination by leaving the fragments, along with several drops of potassium hydroxide, in a watch glass covered with a Petri dish for 24 hours. (See Chapter Thirteen on fungal infections for details of the KOH examination.)

Nail collection techniques for culture. First swab the nail plate with alcohol to remove bacteria. Fragments of nail-plate and nail-bed scrapings are inoculated onto Sabouraud's medium with and without antibiotics to identify the fungal species. Use fresh Sabouraud's with antibiotics. Antibiotics degrade in old media and do not effectively suppress bacterial contaminants. The dermatophyte test medium contains the antibiotic cycloheximide and phenol red as a pH indicator. Dermatophytes release alkaline metabolites that turn the medium from yellow to red in 7 to 14 days. Some nondermatophytes, such as *Scopulariopsis, Aspergillus, Penicillium*, black molds, and yeast, may cause a color change and give a false positive reaction.[12]

Patterns of infection. There are four distinct patterns of nail infection described by Zaias.[13] Several patterns of infection may occur simultaneously in the nail plate. *Trichophyton rubrum* and *T. mentagrophytes* invade the nail plate more frequently than *T. violaceum* or *T. tonsurans. Aspergillus, Cephalosporium, Fusarium*, and *Scopulariopsis*, generally considered contaminants or nonpathogens, have been isolated from infected nails. They may be found in any pattern of nail infection, especially distal subungual onychomycosis and white superficial onychomycosis. The contaminants do not respond to griseofulvin or the newer oral antifungal agents. The four patterns of nail infection are illustrated in Figures 25-13, 25-14, and 25-15.

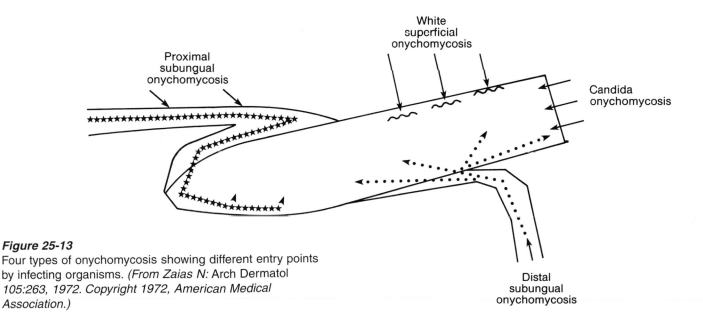

Figure 25-13
Four types of onychomycosis showing different entry points by infecting organisms. *(From Zaias N: Arch Dermatol 105:263, 1972. Copyright 1972, American Medical Association.)*

Distal subungual onychomycosis. Distal subungual onychomycosis (Figure 25-14) is the most common pattern of nail invasion. Fungi invade the hyponychium, the distal area of the nail bed. The distal nail plate turns yellow or white as an accumulation of hyperkeratotic debris causes the nail to rise and separate from the underlying bed. Fungus grows in the substance of the plate, causing it to crumble and fragment. A large mass composed of thick nail plate and underlying debris may cause discomfort with footwear.

White superficial onychomycosis. This is caused by surface invasion of the nail plate, most often by *T. mentagrophytes.* The surface of the nail is soft, dry, and powdery and can easily be scraped away (Figure 25-15). The nail plate is not thickened and remains adherent to the nail bed.

Proximal subungual onychomycosis. Microorganisms enter the posterior nailfold-cuticle area, migrate to the underlying matrix, and finally invade the nail plate from below. Infection occurs within the substance of the nail plate, but the surface remains intact. Hyperkeratotic debris accumulates and causes the nail to separate. Transverse white bands begin at the proximal nail plate and are carried distally with outward growth of the nail plate (see Figure 25-14, *B*). *T. rubrum* is the most common cause. This is the most common pattern seen in patients with AIDS.

Candida *onychomycosis.* Nail-plate infection caused by *C. albicans* is seen almost exclusively in chronic mucocutaneous candidiasis. It generally involves all of the fingernails (Figure 25-16). The nail plate thickens and turns yellow-brown.

Figure 25-14 Distal subungual onychomycosis.

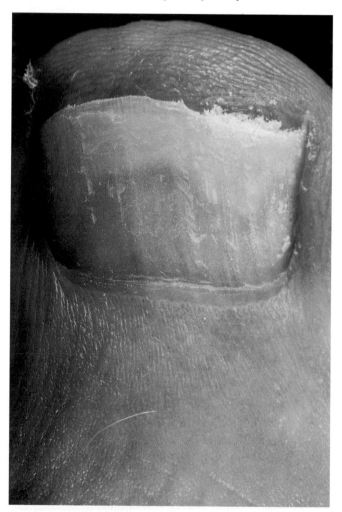

A, Early changes showing subungual debris at the distal end of the nail plate.

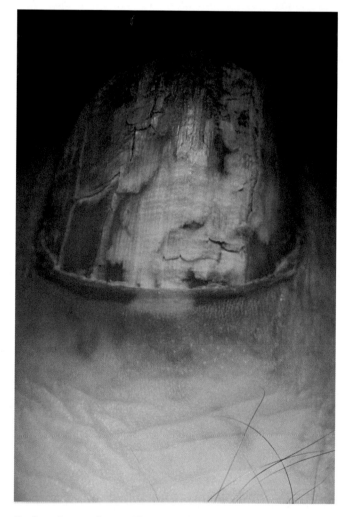

B, An advanced case. The infection has progressed from the distal end to involve the entire nail plate. The nail plate often separates from the nail bed.

There are many other patterns of infection. Linear, yellow or dark brown streaks appear at the distal end and grow proximally in some patterns. In others, some or all of the nail plate may appear yellow; in these areas the nail can be separated from the underlying bed.

Differential diagnosis. Psoriasis is most commonly confused with onychomycosis, and the two diseases may coexist. More confusion exists, since psoriatic nail disease may present as an isolated phenomenon without other cutaneous signs. The single distinguishing feature of psoriasis, pitting of the nail-plate surface, is not a feature of fungal infection. Leukonychia, the occurrence of white spots or bands that appear proximally and proceed out with the nail, is probably caused by minor trauma and may be confused with proximal subungual onychomycosis. Eczema or habitual picking of the proximal nailfold induces the nail plate to be wavy and ridged, but its substance remains intact and hard. Numerous, less common nail diseases may be confused with tinea unguium.

Treatment. Treating tinea of the nails can be discouraging.[19] Topical creams and lotions do not penetrate the nail plate and are of little value except in controlling inflammation at the nailfolds. Expensive, long-term oral therapy, if effective, is often followed by reinfection when the oral medication is discontinued.[20] Oral therapy has the highest success rate with fingernail and nail infections in young individuals. The optimum duration and dosage of these drugs have yet to be determined. (See the box below.) There is evidence that prolonged use of a topical antifungal agent, after clinical response of onychomycosis to an oral agent, may prevent nail reinfection.[21] Use of a topical antifungal cream for 1 year after clinical cure of onychomycosis has prevented reinfection in the 12-month follow-up period.

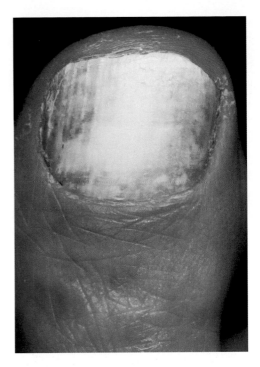

Figure 25-15
White superficial onychomycosis. The surface is soft, dry, and powdery and can easily be scraped away. The nail plate is not thickened and does not separate from the nailbed.

ORAL ANTIFUNGAL AGENTS FOR TREATING TINEA OF THE NAILS	
Drug	**Dosage**
Fluconazole (Diflucan)	One 150-mg dose each week[14]
Itraconazole (Sporanox)	200 mg/day[15] "Pulse dosing": 400 mg/day for first week of each month (16 weeks)
Terbinafine	250 mg/day (12 weeks)[16,17]
Griseofulvin	990 mg/day[18]

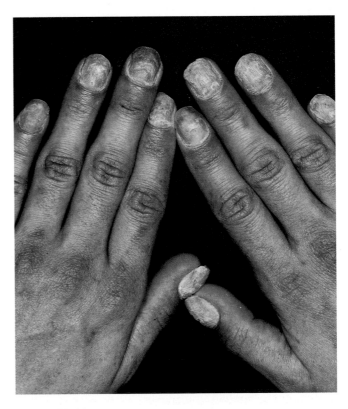

Figure 25-16
Candida onychomycosis in a patient with chronic mucocutaneous candidiasis. All of the fingernails are infected.

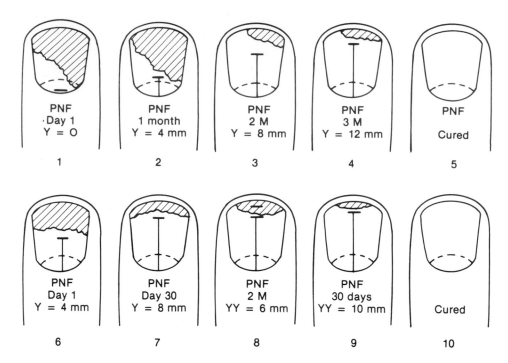

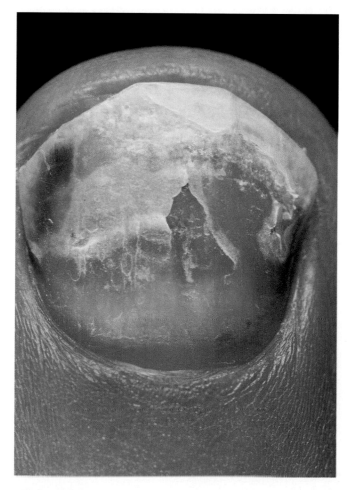

Figure 25-17
Determination of drug effectiveness in onychomycosis. Diagrammatic drawing of the objective method for determining drug effectiveness with antifungal agents in onychomycosis. Chronologic sequence of events in a patient cured with the minimum effective daily dose. The cross-hatched areas are clinical onychomycosis. *X* is a superficial cut made on the normal nail plate adjacent to the onychomycotic border. *Y* is the distance from the proximal nailfold to the onychomycotic border *(X)* and reflects normal nail present. An effective dosage acts as a barrier as in nails 2 through 5. The initial drug dosage became ineffective (nail 8) and required an increase in the drug dose to achieve a cure (nails 9 and 10). *(From Zaias N, Drachman D: J Am Acad Dermatol 9:912-919, 1983.)*

Assessing drug effectiveness.[21] The method described here is used to assess patients with distal subungual onychomycosis (Figure 25-17). When an effective dosage of an oral antifungal agent is given, it acts as a barrier to further proximal nail invasion by the fungus (Figure 25-18). A superficial horizontal cut is made with a scalpel in the midline on the normal nail plate, adjacent to the onychomycotic border. The groove is filled with ink or dye, and a measurement is taken from this point to the proximal nailfold's edge. If an effective dosage is given, the onychomycotic area does not invade proximal to the mark; then the amount of new plate should reflect the normal nail-plate production. The patient returns in 1 month. In most normal, healthy subjects, 1.5 to 2 mm of nail plate grows per month from the large toenails and 3 to 4 mm of nail plate grows per month from the fingernails. If the fungus invades proximal to the horizontal scalpel groove, then the dosage of medication is increased and the measuring process starts anew.

Figure 25-18
Distal subungual onychomycosis treated for 8 weeks. A distinct border separates the normal nail from the infected distal nail plate.

Mechanical reduction of infected nail plate. A nail clipper with plier handles may be used to remove substantial amounts of hard, thick debris. One should insert the pointed tip of the instrument as far down as possible between the diseased nail and the nail bed. Adherent thick nail plate can be reduced by sanding or cutting the surface layers with the clippers. Removal of the infected nail may accelerate resolution of the infection.

Surgical removal. Painful or extremely infected nails (usually the nail of the first toe) can be removed by a simple surgical procedure (see p. 758).

Nonsurgical avulsion of nail dystrophies.[22] Symptomatic dystrophic nails may be painlessly removed with a urea compound (Figure 25-19). The technique has its greatest application in removing hypertrophic mycotic nails and can be used to treat other hypertrophic nail conditions of the nail plate, such as psoriatic nails. The procedure also facilitates subsequent treatment with topical antifungal agents. The technique removes only grossly diseased or dystrophic nails, not normal nails. Urea ointment (Ureacin-40) is commercially available or can be compounded by a pharmacist.

The urea formulation found to be most effective is as follows: urea powder 40%, 120 gm; white beeswax or soft paraffin, 5%, 15 gm; anhydrous lanolin, 20%, 60 gm; white petrolatum, 25%, 75 gm; and silica gel, type H, 10%, 30 gm. Urea powder and silica gel are blended in after the other ingredients have been combined and melted at 85° C. The mixture has a 4-month shelf life.

Cloth adhesive tape is used to cover the normal skin surrounding the affected nail plate, which has been pretreated with tincture of benzoin. The urea compound is generously applied directly to the nail surface and covered with a piece of plastic wrap. This in turn is covered with a finger that is cut from a plastic glove and held in place with adhesive tape. Patients are instructed to keep the area completely dry with the aid of plastic gloves or booties.

An alternate technique uses adhesive felt (mole skin) and waterproof, stretchable tape (Blenderm). A nail-shaped hole is cut in a piece of mole skin, and the mole skin is applied, sticky surface down, on the dorsal aspect of the toe so that just the nail is exposed through the hole. The well is filled with the urea compound and covered with Blenderm tape.[23] The patient returns to the physician in 7 to 10 days. At that time the treated nails are removed, when possible, by either lifting the entire nail plate from the nail bed or by cutting the abnormal portions with a nail cutter. This is followed by light curettage until a clinically normal nail is reached at all margins.

Figure 25-19 Nonsurgical avulsion of nail dystrophies.

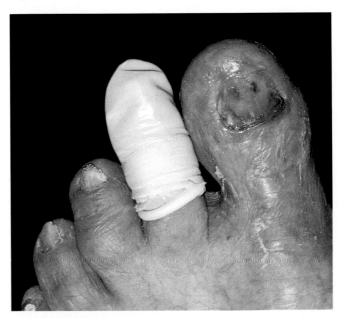

A, Infected nail before application of urea formulation.

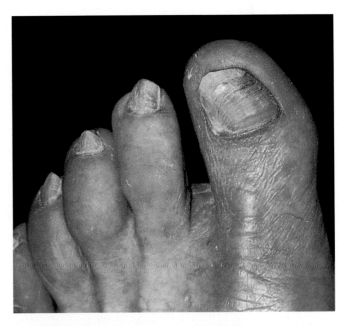

B, Infected nail of the large toe depicted in *A* has been dissolved by the urea formulation.

TRAUMA

Onycholysis. Onycholysis, the painless separation of the nail from the nail bed, is common. Separation usually begins at the distal groove and progresses irregularly and proximally, causing part or most of the plate to become separated (Figure 25-20). The nonadherent portion of the nail is opaque with a white, yellow, or green tinge. The causes of onycholysis include psoriasis, trauma, *Candida* or *Pseudomonas* infections, internal drugs,[24] PUVA photochemotherapy,[25] contact with chemicals, maceration from prolonged immersion, and allergic contact dermatitis (e.g., to nail hardener).[26,27]

When other signs of skin disease are absent, onycholysis is most frequently seen in women with long fingernails. With normal activity, the extended nail inadvertently strikes objects and acts as a lever to pry the nail from the nail bed. Forcing a stylus between the nail plate and bed while manicuring can cause separation. Photoonycholysis may occur with the use of tetracycline antibiotics. Treatment is simple. All of the separated nail is removed, and the fingers are kept dry. Removing the separated nail eliminates the lever, and dryness discourages infection. One should not cover the cut nails; occlusion promotes maceration. Any form of manipulation should be discouraged.

Nail and cuticle biting. Nail biting is a nervous habit that usually begins in childhood and lasts for years. One or all nails may be chewed as far as the lunula. The nail plate is chiseled and bitten from the nail bed by the teeth. Nail growth occurs during periods of physical activity, but periods of physical inactivity seem to promote zealous nail biting. Thin strips of skin on the lateral and proximal nailfold may also be stripped (Figure 25-21). Patients are aware of their habit but seem powerless to control it. Painting the nail plate with a distasteful preparation such as Nail Cure (Purepac) or Sally Hansen Nail Biter may help discourage the habit.

Figure 25-20
Onycholysis. Separation of the nail plate starts at the distal groove. Minor trauma to long fingernails is the most common cause.

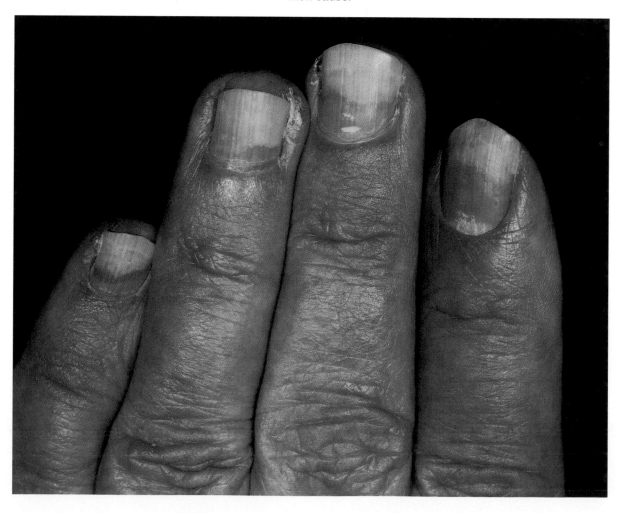

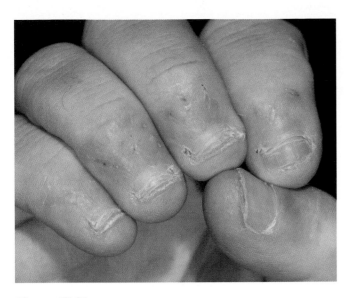

Figure 25-21
Nail and cuticle biting.

Nail plate excoriation. Digging or excoriating the nail plate is much less common than biting. This destructive practice may result in gross deformity of the nail plate.

Hangnail. Triangular strips of skin may separate from the lateral nailfolds, particularly during the winter months. Attempts at removal may cause pain and extension of the tear into the dermis. Separated skin should be cut before extension occurs. Constant lubrication of the fingertips with skin creams and avoidance of repeated hand immersion in water is beneficial.

Ingrown toenail. Ingrown toenails are common; the large toe is most frequently affected. The nail pierces the lateral nailfold and enters the dermis, where it acts as a foreign body. The first signs are pain and swelling. The area of penetration becomes purulent and edematous as exuberant granulation tissue grows alongside the penetrating nail (Figure 25-22). Ingrown nails are caused by lateral pressure of poorly fitting shoes, improper or excessive trimming of the lateral nail plate, or trauma.

Figure 25-22 Ingrown toenail.

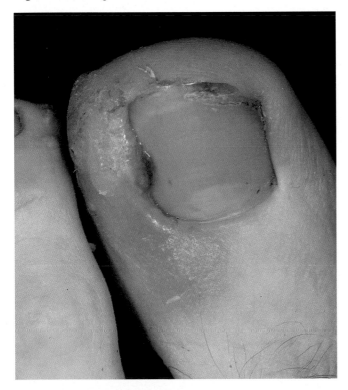

A, Swelling and inflammation occur at the lateral nailfold.

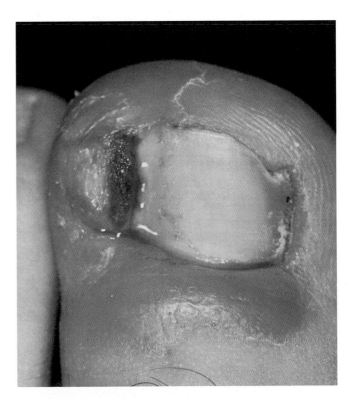

B, Exuberant granulation tissue has appeared alongside the penetrating nail in this long-established case.

Figure 25-23 Phenol matricectomy.

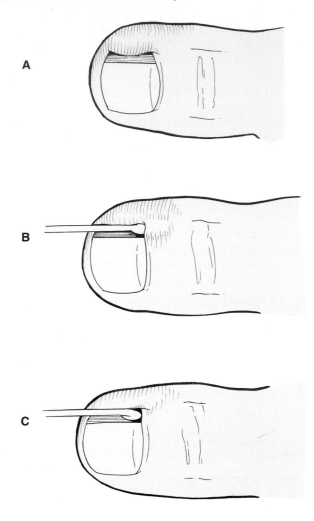

Perform digital block anesthesia with 1% plain lidocaine.

A, A 2- to 3-mm strip of the nail plate is removed. A tourniquet is applied to the digit because the phenol must be applied to a bloodless field.

B, A protective ointment such as vaseline is applied to the surrounding periungual tissues to prevent contact with the phenol solution. Phenol (88% liquified phenol) is applied with a partially stripped cotton applicator (saturated but not dripping). Three 30-second applications are performed during which the matrix is vigorously massaged.

C, A small dermal curette is used to scrape the matrix epithelium. The entire field is then lavaged with 70% isopropyl alcohol.

Treatment

INGROWN NAIL WITHOUT INFLAMMATION. Separate the distal anterior tip and lateral edges of an ingrown toenail from the adjacent soft tissue with a wisp of absorbent cotton coated with collodion. This gives immediate relief of pain and provides a firm runway for further growth of the nail. The collodion fixes the cotton in place, waterproofs the area, and permits bathing. The cotton insert may need reinsertion in 3 to 6 weeks. Cotton without collodion may be used, but it may have to be replaced frequently. This method is not applicable to patients with infected acute inflammation of the lateral nailfold.[28]

INGROWN NAIL WITH INFLAMMMATION. The lateral nailfold is infiltrated with 1% or 2% lidocaine (Xylocaine). Nail-splitting scissors are inserted under the ingrown nail parallel to the lateral nailfold. The tip is inserted toward the matrix until resistance is met, and the wedge-shaped nail is then cut and removed. Granulation tissue is reduced with a silver nitrate application or removed with a curet. For a few days, the inflamed site is treated with a Burow's cool, wet compress until the swelling and inflammation have subsided. Shoes should be worn that allow the toes to fall naturally, without compression. The new nail is forced up and over the lateral nailfold by inserting cotton under the lateral nail margin and allowing it to remain in place for days or weeks.

RECURRENT INGROWN NAIL. Patients with recurrent ingrown nails may require the use of liquid phenol for permanent destruction of the lateral portions of the nail matrix (Figure 25-23).[29-31]

Subungual hematoma. Subungual hematoma (Figure 25-24) may be caused by trauma to the nail plate, which causes immediate bleeding and pain. The quantity of blood may be sufficient to cause separation and loss of the nail plate. The traditional method of puncturing the nail with a red-hot paperclip tip remains the quickest and most effective method of draining the blood. Trauma to the proximal nailfold causes hemorrhage that may not be apparent for days. The nail plate may emerge from the nailfold with blood stains that remain until the nail grows out.

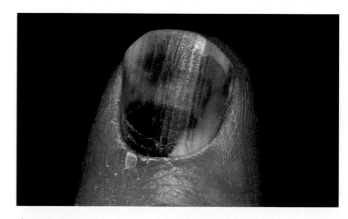

Figure 25-24
Subungual hematoma. A *Proteus* or *Pseudomonas* infection might be suspected if there were no history of trauma.

Nail hypertrophy. Gross thickening of the nail plate may occur with tight-fitting shoes or other forms of chronic trauma. The nail plate is brown, very thick, and points to one side (Figure 25-25). Shoes compress the nail plate against the toe and cause pain. The substance of the nail plate may be reduced with sandpaper or a file, or the nail can be removed and the nail matrix permanently destroyed with phenol so that the nail will not regrow.[29]

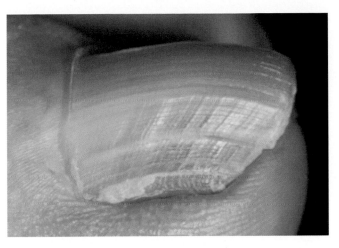

Figure 25-25
Nail hypertrophy. The nail plate becomes thick and distorted, often causing discomfort when shoes are worn.

White spots or bands. White spots (leukonychia punctata) in the nail plate, a very common finding, possibly result from cuticle manipulation or other mild forms of trauma (Figure 25-26). The spots or bands may appear at the lunula or may appear spontaneously in the nail plate and subsequently disappear or grow with the nail.[32]

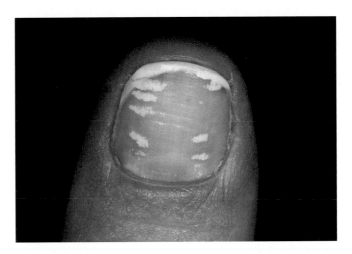

Figure 25-26
White spots (leukonychia punctata). A common finding often mistaken for a fungal infection.

Distal plate splitting (brittle nails). The splitting into layers or peeling of the distal nail plate may resemble or be analogous to the scaling of dry skin (Figure 25-27). This nail change is found in approximately 20% of the adult population.[33] Repeated water immersion increases the incidence of brittle nails, particularly in women.[34] Protection with rubber-over-cotton gloves and application of heavy lubricants directly to the nail plate provide improvement. Local measures to rehydrate the nail plate should be initiated. After the nails have been soaked in water at bedtime, a moisturizer (e.g., an alpha-hydroxy acid or a lactic acid such as Lac-Hydrin) should be applied. The moisturizing agent may be applied under occlusion with a white cotton glove or sock.[35] Nail enamel may slow the evaporation of water from the nail plate. It should be removed and reapplied no more than once a week. Patients with brittle nails who receive the B-complex vitamin, biotin, (2.5 mg/day) may improve and have up to a 25% increase in nail-plate thickness.[36,37]

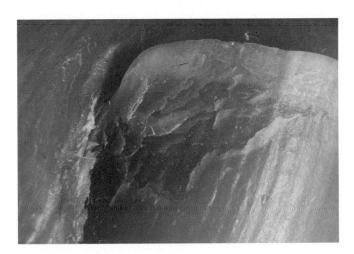

Figure 25-27
Distal nail splitting. The nail splits into layers or the distal nail plate peels, a change analogous to the scaling of dry skin.

Habit-tic deformity. Habit-tic deformity is a common finding and is caused by biting or picking a section of the proximal nailfold of the thumb with the index fingernail. The resulting defect consists of a longitudinal band of horizontal grooves that often have a yellow discoloration. The band extends from the proximal nailfold to the tip of the nail (Figure 25-28). This should not be confused with the nail rippling that occurs with chronic paronychia or chronic eczematous inflammation of the proximal nailfold. The ripples of chronic inflammation appear as rounded waves (Figure 25-29), in contrast to the closely spaced, sharp grooves produced by continual manipulation.

The method of formation is demonstrated for the patient. Some patients are not aware of their habit, and others who admit to nail picking may not realize that they have created the defect. Patients who discontinue manipulation are able to grow relatively normal nails; there are those, however, who find it impossible to stop.

Median nail dystrophy. Median nail dystrophy is a distinctive nail-plate change of unknown origin. A longitudinal split appears in the center of the nail plate. Several fine cracks project from the line laterally, giving the appearance of a fir tree. The thumb is most often affected (Figure 25-30). There is no treatment, and after a few months or years the nail can be expected to return to normal. Recurrences are possible.

Pincer nails (curvature). Inward folding of the lateral edges of the nail results in a tube- or pincer-shaped nail (Figure 25-31). The nail bed is drawn up into the tube and may become painful. The toenails are more commonly involved than the fingernails. Shoe compression is thought to cause pincer nails, but the etiology is uncertain. If pain is significant, surgical removal of the nail or reconstruction of the nail unit is required.

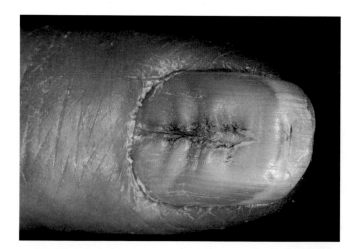

Figure 25-28
Habit-tic deformity. A common finding on the thumbs caused by picking the proximal nailfold with the index finger.

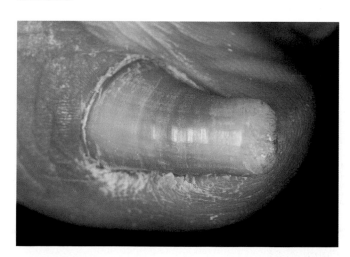

Figure 25-29
Nail rippling caused by chronic inflammation of the proximal nailfold. A normal nail grows once the eczema has been controlled.

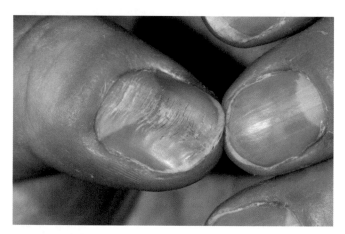

Figure 25-30
Median nail dystrophy.

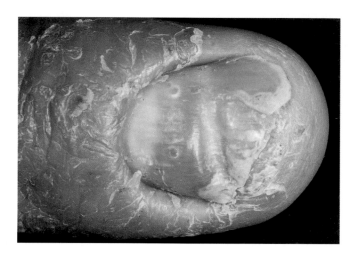

Figure 25-31
Pincer nails (overcurvature). Inward folding of the lateral edges of the nail results in a tube- or pincer-shaped nail.

The Nail and Internal Disease

Beau's lines. Beau's lines are transverse depressions of all of the nails that appear at the base of the lunula weeks after a stressful event has temporarily interrupted nail formation (Figure 25-32). The lines progress distally with normal nail growth and eventually disappear at the free edge. They develop in response to many diseases, such as syphilis, uncontrolled diabetes mellitus, myocarditis, peripheral vascular disease, and zinc deficiency, and to illness accompanied by high fevers, such as scarlet fever, measles, mumps, and pneumonia.[38]

Yellow nail syndrome. The spontaneous appearance of yellow nails occurs before, during, or after certain respiratory diseases and in diseases associated with lymphedema. Patients note that nail growth slows and appears to stop. The nail plate may become excessively curved, and it turns dark yellow. The surface remains smooth or acquires transverse ridges, indicating variations in the growth rate; nails grow at less than half the normal rate. Partial or total separation of the nail plate may occur. The nails show an increased curvature about the long axis, the cuticles and lunulae are lost, and usually all the nails are involved. The nails grow very slowly, at a rate of 0.1 to 0.25 mm/week, compared with 0.5 to 2 mm/week for normal adult fingernails. The diseases reported to be associated with yellow nail syndrome are edema of the lower extremities, facial edema, pleural effusion, bronchiectasis, sinusitis, bronchitis, and chronic respiratory infections.[39] Yellowish nail pigmentation has been reported in patients with AIDS.[40] The nails may spontaneously improve, even when the associated disease does not improve.[41,42] Oral vitamin E in dosages of up to 800 IU/day for up to 18 months may help. Yellow nails that were treated with a 5% vitamin E solution (containing DL-alpha-tocopherol in dimethyl sulfoxide), two drops twice a day to the nail plate, showed marked clinical improvement and an increase in nail-growth rate.[43]

Spoon nails. Lateral elevation and central depression of the nail plate cause the nail to be spoon shaped; this is called

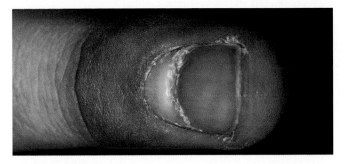

Figure 25-32
Beau's lines. A transverse depression of the nail plate that occurs several weeks after certain illnesses.

koilonychia. Spoon nails are seen in normal children and may persist a lifetime without any associated abnormalities. The spontaneous onset of spoon nails has been reported to occur with iron-deficiency anemia and in 50% of patients with idiopathic hemochromatosis.[44] The nail reverts to normal when the anemia is corrected.

Finger clubbing. Finger clubbing (Hippocratic nails) is a distinct feature associated with a number of diseases, but it may occur as a normal variant. The distal phalanges of the fingers and toes are enlarged to a rounded, bulbous shape. The nail enlarges and becomes curved, hard, and thickened (Figure 25-33). The angle made by the proximal nailfold and nail plate (Lovibond's angle) increases and approaches or exceeds 180 degrees. The proximal nailfold feels as though it is floating on the underlying tissue. Clubbing is associated with a variety of lung diseases, cardiovascular disease, cirrhosis, colitis, and thyroid disease. The changes are permanent.

Terry's nails. Terry's nails are white or light pink but retain a 0.5- to 3-mm normal, pink, distal band (Figure 25-34). The findings are associated with cirrhosis, chronic congestive heart failure, adult-onset diabetes mellitus, and age.[45] It has been speculated that Terry's nails are a part of aging and that associated diseases "age" the nail. These changes are not associated with hypoalbuminemia or anemia.

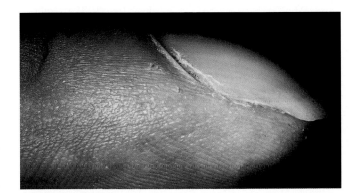

Figure 25-33
Finger clubbing. The distal phalanges are enlarged to a rounded, bulbous shape. The nail enlarges and becomes curved, hard, and thickened.

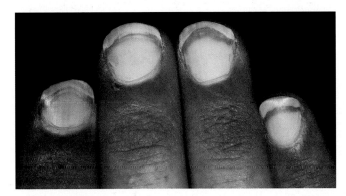

Figure 25-34
Terry's nails. The nail bed is white with only a narrow zone of pink at the distal end.

Congenital Anomalies

Numerous congenital syndromes involve nail changes. The most widely understood syndromes all have autosomal dominant inheritance patterns.

Among other signs of pachyonychia congenita, there are yellow, very thick nail beds with elevated nails, palmar and plantar hyperkeratosis, and white keratotic thickening of the tongue. Some patients have erupted teeth at birth. In nail-patella syndrome, there are defective short nails and small or absent patella, in addition to other signs.

Color and Drug-Induced Changes

Changes in nail color may result from a color change in the nail plate or in the nail bed. Several articles[24,46,47] list changes associated with nail pigmentation. Some of these changes are listed in Tables 25-1 and 25-2. Cancer chemotherapeutic drugs have been associated with a variety of changes in the nail unit (Table 25-3).

TABLE 25-1 Color Changes of Nails

Etiology	Pattern of color change
BROWN NAILS	
Antimalarial drugs	Diffuse blue, brown
Cancer chemotherapeutic agents (Table 25-3)	Transverse black bands
Hyperbilirubinemia	Diffuse brown
Junctional nevi	Longitudinal brown bands
Malnutrition	Diffuse brown or black bands
Melanocyte stimulating hormone oversecretion Addison's disease Cushing's disease (after adrenalectomy) Pituitary tumor	Longitudinal brown bands
Melanoma	Longitudinal bands, may increase with width (Hutchinson's sign)
Normal finding in more than 90% of blacks	Longitudinal brown bands
Photographic developer	Diffuse brown
GREEN NAILS	
Pseudomonas	Green streaks and patches
YELLOW NAILS	
Yellow-nail syndrome	Diffuse yellow
Onycholysis	Distal nail separation
BLUE NAILS (BLACKS)	
Zidovudine treatment for AIDS	Diffuse blue
Antimalarial drugs	Diffuse blue
Minocycline	Diffuse blue
Wilson's disease	Diffuse blue
Hemorrhage	Irregular

TABLE 25-2 White Nail or Nail-bed Changes

Disease	Clinical appearance
Anemia	Diffuse white
Arsenic	Mee's lines: transverse white lines
Cirrhosis	Terry's nails: most of nail, zone of pink at distal end (Figure 25-34)
Congenital leukonychia (autosomal dominant; variety of patterns)	Syndrome of leukonychia, knuckle pads, deafness; isolated finding; partial white
Darier's disease	Longitudinal white streaks
Half-and-half nail	Proximal white, distal pink; azotemia
High fevers (some diseases)	Transverse white lines
Hypoalbuminemia	Muehrcke's lines: stationary paired transverse bands
Hypocalcemia	Variable white
Malnutrition	Diffuse white
Pellagra	Diffuse milky white
Punctate leukonychia	Common white spots
Tinea and yeast	Variable patterns
Thallium toxicity (rat poison)	Variable white
Trauma	Repeated manicure: transverse striations
Zinc deficiency	Diffuse white

TABLE 25-3 Nail Changes Induced by Cancer Chemotherapeutic Drugs

Drug	Apparent change	Site of action/mechanism/comments
Adriamycin (doxorubicin)	Onycholysis; hyperpigmentation; transverse pigmented bands; longitudinal gray, brown, and black pigmented bands; bluish nails	Nail-bed and matrix toxicity
Bleomycin (patient also taking vinblastine)	Onycholysis; "dystrophy"; longitudinal pigmented bands; shedding; thickening nail bed; darkening of nail cuticle	Nail-bed or matrix toxicity
Cancer chemotherapeutic drugs in general	Slow growth; sometimes Beau's lines	Matrix toxicity
	White transverse lines (Mee's lines)	Combination chemotherapy (doxorubicin, cyclophosphamide, vincristine)—nail plate
Cyclophosphamide (Cytoxan)	Hyperpigmentation; transverse pigmented bands; longitudinal pigmented band	Nail-bed and nail-plate color change matrix and bed toxicity
Dacarbazine (DTIC)	Hyperpigmentation	Matrix toxicity
Daunorubicin	Transverse brown-black bands	Probable matrix toxicity
5-fluorouracil (topical and systemic)	Diffuse blue superficial pigment; hyperpigmentation; onycholysis "Dystrophy"; paronychial inflammation; pain and thickening of nail bed; transverse striations, half and half–like nail changes	Superficial blue pigment may be scraped off
Genetic tendency for nail pigmentation postchemotherapy	Brownish	Probable matrix toxicity
Hydroxyurea	Atrophic, brittle nails	Nail-matrix toxicity
Melphalan (Alkeran)	Longitudinal pigmented bands	Nail bed—increase in melanin in basal melanocytes, matrix toxicity
Mercaptopurine	Nail shedding	Probable cytotoxic and photosensitivity effect on bed and matrix
Methotrexate	Hyperpigmentation, acute paronychia	Probable matrix toxicity
Nitrogen mustard	Hyperpigmentation	Probable matrix toxicity
Nitrosoureas	Hyperpigmentation	Probable matrix toxicity

From Daniell CR III, Scher RK: *J Am Acad Dermatol* 10:250-258, 1984.

Tumors

A limited number of tumors have been reported to occur about and under the nails (Table 25-4).

Warts. The most common periungual growth is the periungual wart. It is discussed in Chapter Twelve. Warts are most common in children who bite their nails. Warts on the lateral nailfold and on the fingertip may extend deeply under the nail (Figure 25-35). A longitudinal nail groove may result from warts situated over the nail matrix. Warts are epidermal growths, but, if massive, they can erode the underlying bony matrix by displacement.

Digital mucous cysts. Digital mucous cysts (focal mucinosis) are not true cysts but rather a focal collection of mucin lacking a cystic lining. These soft, dome-shaped, translucent, pink-white structures occur on the dorsal surface of the distal phalanx of the middle-aged and the elderly (Figure 25-36). These structures contain a clear, viscous, jellylike substance that exudes if the cyst is incised. There are two types. The cysts on the proximal nailfold are not connected to the joint space or tendon sheath. They result from localized fibroblast proliferation. Compression of the nail-matrix cells induces a longitudinal nail groove. The cysts located on the dorsal-lateral finger at the distal interphalangeal (DIP) joint are probably caused by herniation of tendon sheaths or joint linings and are related to ganglion and synovial cysts.[48]

Simple surgical excision, intralesional steroid injections, and unroofing of the cyst followed by electrodesiccation and curettage have a high recurrence rate.[49]

Excision of the lesion with its pedicle and associated portions of the joint capsule affords a high cure rate but may result in subsequent partial loss of motion.[50]

TABLE 25-4 Nail-unit Tumors	
Diagnosis	**Clinical findings**
MALIGNANT	
Squamous cell carcinoma	Verrucous lesion, onycholysis or subungual growth; nail-plate destruction
Bowen's disease	Hyperkeratosis and onycholysis
Melanoma	Longitudinal brown subungual band; pigmented macule extending onto the periungual skin (Hutchinson's sign); mass below the nail, loss of nail plate, ulceration.
BENIGN	
Myxoid cyst	Dome-shaped, translucent, proximal nailfold
Acquired digital fibrokeratoma	Looks like a garlic clove with the outer skin stripped off; usually projects from proximal nail groove
Glomas tumor	Red or blue suffusion beneath the nail plate; pressure blanches capillaries and causes pain
Giant cell tumor of tendon sheath	Arises from synovial lining cells associated with the distal interphalangeal joint synovia and tendons; firm and deeply fixed to the underlying fibrous tissue; does not arise on the nail unit
Exostosis	A painful, bony growth; x-ray film confirms diagnosis
Warts	May occur on any surface about the nail; spread by nail biting
Keratoacanthoma	Rapidly growing mass, central crust
Pyogenic granuloma	Red, vascular excrescence often devoid of an epithelial cover; profuse bleeding with slight trauma

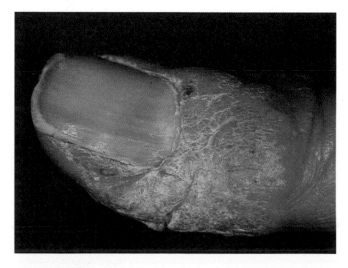

Figure 25-35
Periungual wart.

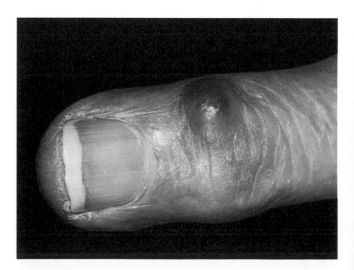

Figure 25-36
Digital mucous cyst.

CRYOSURGERY. Cryosurgery using either the open-spray or the cryoprobe technique yields a cure rate of up to 75%.[51] A local anesthetic is injected prior to treatment. The roof of the cyst is removed with scissors and the gelantinous material is expelled to facilitate freezing of the base of the lesion. Either a flat cryoprobe of approximately the same size as the cyst or a direct intermittent open spray to the center of the lesion is applied. The freeze time is 30 to 40 seconds when the cryoprobe technique is used and 20 to 30 seconds when the open-spray technique is used. The treated site becomes edematous and exudative, and a bulla develops in most cases. Healing is complete in 4 to 6 weeks. Lesions can be re-treated if necessary.

MULTIPLE PUNCTURES. A high cure rate was reported with the simple technique of repeated punctures and expression of the cyst contents (Figure 25-37). Cysts that resisted multiple needlings were usually reduced to small, asymptomatic nodules. Without anesthesia, the cyst is punctured with a medium-sized hypodermic needle (26 gauge) to a depth of 3 to 5 mm. The clear contents, sometimes tinged with blood, are squeezed out by fingertip pressure. The patient is given a supply of needles to repeat the procedure at home if the cyst recurs. From 1 to 10 or more needlings resulted in a cure or in an asymptomatic lesion in 95% of patients.

Pyogenic granuloma. Pyogenic granuloma occasionally occurs in the lateral nailfold. This benign mass of vascular tissue is removed with thorough desiccation and curettage (Figure 25-38). Recurrences are common if any residual tissue is left. Periungual malignant melanoma can mimic pyogenic granuloma.

Nevi and melanoma. Junctional nevi can appear in the nail matrix and produce a brown pigmented band. Brown longitudinal bands are common in blacks (see Figure 25-5) but rare in whites. Melanoma of the nail region, or melanotic whitlow, although rare, is a distinctive lesion (see Figure 22-30). Most are classified as acral lentiginous melanomas. The growth is usually painless and slow, and it can occur anywhere around or under the nail.[52] The lesion may present as a pigmented band that increases in width. There has not been enough experience to make specific recommendations concerning the management of pigmented bands in whites. The spontaneous appearance of such a band is noteworthy to most physicians, who promptly require a biopsy. Benign subungual nevi are rare in whites, so subungual nevoid lesions should be regarded as malignant until proved otherwise.[53]

Figure 25-37 Digital mucous cyst.

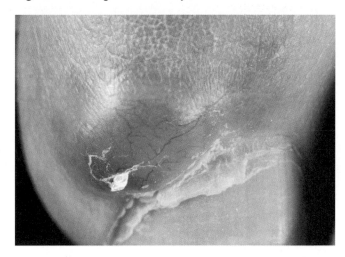

A, Intact cyst.

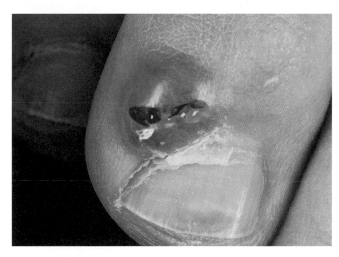

B, Incision with a #11 surgical blade. A clear, sometimes blood-tinged, viscous, jellylike substance exudes when the cyst is incised.

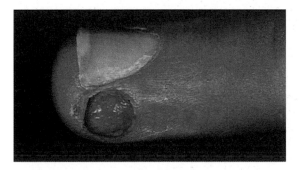

Figure 25-38
Pyogenic granuloma. A pedunculated nodule with a smooth, glistening surface. The surface frequently becomes crusted, eroded, or ulcerated. Minor trauma may produce considerable bleeding.

REFERENCES

1. Johnson M, Comaish JS, Shuster S: Nail is produced by the normal nail bed: a controversy resolved, *Brit J Dermatol* 125:27-29, 1991.
2. Daniel CR: Basic nail plate avulsion, *J Dermatol Surg Oncol* 18:685-688, 1992.
3. Fleegler EJ: A surgical approach to melanonychia striata, *J Dermatol Surg Oncol* 18:708-714, 1992.
4. Rich P: Nail biopsy. Indications and methods, *J Dermatol Surg Oncol* 18:673-682, 1992.
5. Farber EM, Nall L: Nail psoriasis, *Cutis* 50:174-178, 1992.
6. Peachey RDG, Pye RJ, Harman RRM: Treatment of psoriatic nail dystrophy with intradermal steroid injections, *Br J Dermatol* 95:75, 1976.
7. Tosti A, Peluso AM, et al: Nail lichen planus: clinical and pathologic study of twenty-four patients, *J Am Acad Dermatol* 28:724-730, 1993.
8. Zaias N, Ackerman BA: The nail in Darier-White disease, *Arch Dermatol* 107:193-199, 1973.
9. Chapel TA, Adcock M: *Pseudomonas* chromonychia, *Cutis* 27:601-602, 1981.
10. Zaias N: *The nail in health and disease*, New York, 1980, Spectrum Publication.
11. Haneke E: Fungal infections of the nail, *Semin Dermatol* 10:41-53, 1991.
12. Cooper A: The diagnosis of nail fungal infections, *Arch Dermatol* 127:1566-1567, 1991.
13. Zaias N: Onychomycosis, *Arch Dermatol* 105:273, 1972.
14. Nahass GT, Sisto M: Onychomycosis: successful treatment with once-weekly fluconazole, *Dermatology* 186:59-61, 1993.
15. Willemsen M, De Doncker P, et al: Posttreatment itraconazole levels in the nail. New implications for treatment in onychomycosis, *J Am Acad Dermatol* 26:731-735, 1992.
16. van der Schroeff JG, Cirkel PK, et al: A randomized treatment duration-finding study of terbinafine in onychomycosis, *Br J Dermatol* 39:36-39, 1992.
17. Goodfield MJ, Andrew L, et al: Short-term treatment of dermatophyte onychomycosis with terbinafine, *Br Med J* 304:1151-1154, 1992.
18. Korting HC, Schafer-Korting M, et al: Treatment of tinea unguium with medium and high doses of ultramicrosize griseofulvin compared with that with itraconazole, *Antimicrob Agents Chemother* 37:2064-2068, 1993.
19. Davies RR, Everall JD, Hamilton E: Mycological and clinical evaluation of griseofulvin for chronic onychomycosis, *Br Med J* 3:464-468, 1967.
20. Hagermark O, Berlin A, Wallin I, et al: Plasma concentration of griseofulvin in healthy volunteers and outpatients treated for onychomycosis, *Acta Derm Venereol* 56:289-296, 1976.
21. Zaias N, Drachman D: A method for the determination of drug effectiveness in onychomycosis: trials with ketoconazole and griseofulvin ultramicrosize, *J Am Acad Dermatol* 9:912-919, 1983.
22. South DA, Farber EM: Urea ointment in the nonsurgical avulsion of nail dystrophies: a reappraisal, *Cutis* 25:609-612, 1982.
23. Averill RW, Scher RK: Simplified nail taping with urea ointment for nonsurgical nail avulsion, *Cutis* Oct:231-233, 1986.
24. Daniel CR III, Scher RK: Nail changes secondary to systemic drugs or ingestants, *J Am Acad Dermatol* 10:250-258, 1984.
25. Morgan JM, Weller R, et al: Onycholysis in a case of atopic eczema treated with PUVA photochemotherapy, *Clin Exp Dermatol* 17:65-66, 1992.
26. Kechijian P: Onycholysis of the fingernails: evaluation and management, *J Am Acad Dermatol* 12:522-560, 1985.
27. Daniel CR: Onycholysis: an overview, *Semin Dermatol* 10:34-40, 1991.
28. Ilfeld FW: Ingrown toenail treated with cotton collodion insert, *Foot Ankle* 11:312-313, 1991.
29. Siegle RJ, Harkness J, Swanson NA: Phenol alcohol technique for permanent matricectomy, *Arch Dermatol* 120:348-350, 1984.
30. Siegle RJ, Stewart R: Recalcitrant ingrowing nails. Surgical approaches, *J Dermatol Surg Oncol* 18:744-752, 1992.
31. Ceilley RI, Collison DW: Matricectomy, *J Dermatol Surg Oncol* 18:728-734, 1992.
32. Zaun H: Leukonychias, *Semin Dermatol* 10:17-20, 1991.
33. Lubach D et al: Incidence of brittle nails, *Dermatologica* 172:144, 1986.
34. Lubach D, Beckers P: Wet working conditions increase brittleness of nails, but do not cause it, *Dermatology* 185:120-122, 1992.
35. Cohen PR, Scher RK: Geriatric nail disorders: diagnosis and treatment, *J Am Acad Dermatol* 26:521-531, 1992.
36. Hochman LG, Scher RK, et al: Brittle nails: response to daily biotin supplementation, *Cutis* 51:303-305, 1993.
37. Colombo VE, Gerber F, et al: Treatment of brittle fingernails and onychoschizia with biotin: scanning electron microscopy, *J Am Acad Dermatol* 23:1127-1132, 1990.
38. Sweren RJ, Burnett JW: Multiple Beau's lines, *Cutis* 29:41-42, 1982.
39. Venincie PY, Dicken CH: Yellow nail syndrome: report of five cases, *J Am Acad Dermatol* 10:187-192, 1984.
40. Scher RK: Acquired immunodeficiency syndrome and yellow nails, *J Am Acad Dermatol* 18:758-759, 1988 (letter).
41. De Coste SD, Imber MJ, et al: Yellow nail syndrome, *J Am Acad Dermatol* 22:608-611, 1990.
42. Pavlidakey GP, Hashimoto K, Blum D: Yellow nail syndrome, *J Am Acad Dermatol* 11:509-512, 1984.
43. Williams HC, Buffham R, et al: Successful use of topical vitamin E solution in the treatment of nail changes in yellow nail syndrome, *Arch Dermatol* 127:1023-1028, 1991.
44. Chevrant-Breton J et al: Cutaneous manifestations of idiopathic hemochromatosis, *Arch Dermatol* 113:161-165, 1977.
45. Holzberg M, Walker HK: Terry's nails: revised definition and new correlations, *Lancet* April:896-899, 1984.
46. Daniel CR III, Osment LS: Nail pigmentation abnormalities: their importance and proper examination, *Cutis* 30:348, 1982.
47. Unamuno P, Fernandez-Lopez E, et al: Leukonychia due to cytostatic agents, *Clin Exp Dermatol* 17:273-274, 1992.
48. Newmeyer, WL, Kilgore ES Jr, Graham WP: Mucous cysts: the dorsal digital interphalangeal joint ganglion, *Plast Reconstr Surg* 53:313-315, 1974.
49. Sonnex TS: Digital myxoid cysts: a review, *Cutis* Feb:89-94, 1986.
50. Miller PK, Roenigk RK, et al: Focal mucinosis (myxoid cyst). Surgical therapy, *J Dermatol Surg Oncol* 18:716-719, 1992.
51. Kuflik EG: Specific indications for cryosurgery of the nail unit. Myxoid cysts and periungual verrucae, *J Dermatol Surg Oncol* 18:702-706, 1992.
52. Mikhail GR: Subungual epidermoid carcinoma, *J Am Acad Dermatol* 11:291-298, 1984.
53. Shukla VK, Hughes LE: How common are benign subungual naevi? *Eur J Surg Oncol* 18:249-250, 1992.

CHAPTER TWENTY-SIX

Cutaneous Manifestations of Internal Disease

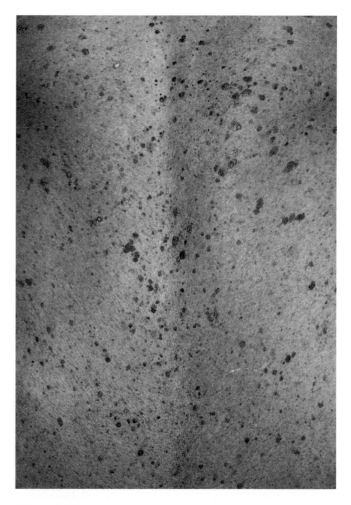

Figure 26-1
A paraneoplastic syndrome; the Leser-Trelat sign. The rapid onset of numerous seborrheic keratoses can be associated with an internal malignancy.

Certain cutaneous diseases are frequently associated with internal disease. The skin disease itself may be inconsequential, but its presence should prompt investigation of possible related internal disorders. A selected group of such diseases is discussed in this chapter. Pigmentary skin changes associated with internal diseases are also discussed in Chapter Nineteen.

Internal Cancer and Skin Disease

The skin can be associated with internal malignancy in a variety of ways. The skin lesions may be a marker for an inherited syndrome (i.e., the genodermatoses), may represent a reaction to the tumor (the paraneoplastic syndromes) (Figure 26-1), may be caused by a carcinogen, may occur as a result of treatment, or may represent direct tumor extension or metastasis to the skin.[1,2,3,4] These disease associations are listed in Table 26-1 and in the boxes on p. 783. Syndromes in which genodermatosis is associated with cancer are discussed later in this chapter.

TABLE 26-1 Cutaneous Lesions and Internal Malignancy

Syndrome	Clinical presentation	Malignancy
Ataxia telangiectasia	Cerebellar ataxia, telangiectasia (e.g., pinna, bulbar conjunctiva)	Reticulum cell sarcoma, Hodgkin's, gastric
Alopecia mucinosa	Patch of follicular papules and boggy infiltrate, face, trunk, scalp	Mycosis fungoides
Amyloidosis	Macroglossia; smooth tongue; shiny, translucent, waxy papules on eyelids, nasolabial folds, lips, and intertriginous areas; "pinch purpura"—skin bleeds with trauma	Multiple myeloma
Acanthosis nigricans	Adult onset in absence of obesity, endocrinopathy, and family history; hyperkeratotic, hyperpigmented skin folds in flexural areas (neck, axillae, antecubital fossa, breast, groin)	Abdominal cancer, other adenocarcinomas
Bazex's syndrome (acrokeratosis para neoplastica)	Three stages: (1) psoriasiform lesions, tips of fingers and toes; (2) keratoderma, hands and feet; (3) lesions extend locally and new lesions appear on knees, legs, thighs, arms	Carcinoma of esophagus, tongue, lower lip, upper lobes of the lungs
Bloom's syndrome	Erythema face ("butterfly area"), stunted growth	Acute leukemia
Carcinoid syndrome	Episodes of flushing (face, neck, chest), dyspnea, asthma, diarrhea, murmur of pulmonary stenosis and insufficiency	Serotonin-containing tumor of body parts such as appendix, small intestine, bronchus
Cowden's syndrome (multiple hamartoma syndrome)	Warty papules on face, hands, mouth	Breast, thyroid
Dermatomyositis (adult)	Heliotrope erythema eyelids, bluish-red plaques on knuckles	Breast, gastrointestinal, genitourinary, lung, ovary
Erythema gyratum repens	Rapidly moving waxy bands of erythema with serpiginous outline and "wood grain" pattern	Breast, lung, stomach, bladder, prostate
Gardner's syndrome	Epidermal cysts, cutaneous osteomas and fibromas, polyps in small and large intestine	Adenocarcinoma of colon
Glucagonoma syndrome	Migratory necrolytic erythema in intertriginous and dependent areas, elevated serum glucagon levels	Glucagon-secreting alpha cell tumor of the pancreas
Hypertrichosis lanuginosa (acquired)	Long hair on face and trunk	Bronchus, gallbladder, rectum
Ichthyosis (acquired)	Generalized scaling, prominent on extremities, spares the flexural area	Hodgkin's disease; other lymphoproliferative malignancies; cancer of lung, breast, cervix
Kaposi's sarcoma	Red papular and nodular neoplasms most common on lower legs	Internal organ Kaposi's sarcoma, high incidence of other cancers
Leser-Trélat sign	Sudden appearance (3-6 months) and rapid increase in size and number of seborrheic keratoses	Colon, breast
Melanosis (generalized)	Generalized cutaneous melanosis	Metastatic melanoma
Metastases to the skin	Metastasis to any cutaneous site	Variety of tumors
Muir-Torre syndrome	Multiple sebaceous adenomas	Visceral carcinomas
Paget's disease (breast)	Eczematous crusted lesion of nipple, areola	Breast
Paget's disease (extramammary)	Eroded scaling plaques of vulva, scrotum, axilla, perianal, groin	Cervical cancer and adenocarcinoma of anus and rectum
Palmoplantar keratoderma (tylosis)	Skin thickening of palms and soles	Gastrointestinal carcinomas
Paraneoplastic pemphigus	Blisters, erosive stomatitis	Lymphoid malignancies, thymomas, sarcomas
Peutz-Jeghers syndrome	Pigmented macules on lips and oral mucosa; polyposis of small intestine	Adenocarcinoma of stomach, duodenum, colon
Sipple's syndrome	Multiple mucosal neuromas	Medullary carcinoma of thyroid, C cell neoplasia, pheochromocytoma
Sweet's syndrome	Fever, painful cutaneous plaques	Hematologic malignancies
Urticaria pigmentosa (disseminated maculopapular form)	Brown-red macules and papules that contain mast cells and urticate when traumatized	Hematologic malignancies
von Hippel-Lindau disease	Angiomas of skin, angiomatosis of cerebellum or medulla	Hypernephroma, pheochromocytoma
von Recklinghausen's neurofibromatosis	Café-au-lait spots, white macules, multiple cutaneous neuromas, internal neuromas	Malignant neurilemnoma, astrocytoma, pheochromocytoma
Wiskott-Aldrich syndrome	Eczematous lesions in atopic dermatitis distribution	Reticuloendothelial malignancy

CANCER SYNDROMES ASSOCIATED WITH CUTANEOUS DISEASE

INHERITED SYNDROMES WITH CUTANEOUS SIGNS—THE GENODERMATOSES (THOSE ASSOCIATED WITH INTERNAL MALIGNANCIES)

(Dermatosis associated with, but not caused by, the tumor)
Ataxia telangiectasia
Basal cell nevus syndrome (Gorlin's syndrome)
Cowden's disease (multiple hamartoma syndrome)
Cronkhite-Canada syndrome
Gardner's syndrome
Howel-Evans syndrome (palmoplantar keratoderma)
Immunodeficiency syndromes
Multiple mucosal neuroma syndrome
Peutz-Jeghers syndrome
Torre-Muir syndrome
von Hippel-Lindau syndrome
von Recklinghausen's syndrome
Werner's syndrome
Wiskott-Aldrich syndrome

PARANEOPLASTIC SYNDROMES (CUTANEOUS REACTIONS TO INTERNAL MALIGNANCIES)

Acanthosis nigricans	Herpes zoster
Acquired hypertrichosis lanuginosa	Keratoacanthomas
	Leser-Trélat sign
Acquired ichthyosis	Migratory thrombophlebitis
Bazek's syndrome	Multiple eruptive angiomas
Carcinoid-flushing	Pruritus
Dermatomyositis	Pyoderma gangrenosum
Erythema gyratum repens	Raynaud's syndrome— atypical
Erythroderma	Urticaria
Glucagonoma syndrome	

HORMONE-SECRETING TUMORS

APUDoma
Ectopic ACTH syndrome
Carcinoid syndrome
Glucagonoma syndrome

CARCINOGEN-INDUCED SKIN CANCERS

Arsenical keratosis
Bowen's disease of covered skin

DISEASES WITH RAPID ONSET OF CUTANEOUS DISEASE

Acanthosis nigricans
Acquired ichthyosis
Eczematous reactions
Eruptive seborrheic keratosis—Leser-Trélat sign
Eruptive lanugo hair—hypertrichosis lanuginosa (acquisita)
Erythema gyratum repens
Figurate erythemas
Multiple eruptive angiomata

SKIN CHANGES ASSOCIATED WITH TREATMENT OF INTERNAL CANCER

STOMATITIS

Acridinyl anisidide
Dactinomycin
Daunorubicin
Doxorubicin
Fluorouracil
Methotrexate
Others—less often

ALOPECIA

Cyclophosphamide
Doxorubicin
Nitrosoureas

HYPERPIGMENTATION (SKIN AND/OR NAIL)

Bisulfan
Bleomycin 30%
Cyclophosphamide >20%
Doxorubicin
Fluorouracil 2% to 5% in sun-exposed areas
Hydroxyurea
Mithramycin—follows intense red eruption 35%

HYPERSENSITIVITY REACTIONS

Asparaginase 22% to 65%—hives
Cisplatin 5%—hives

UNIQUE CUTANEOUS REACTIONS

Acral erythema—cytarabine, combined toxic effects of drugs and radiation
Flushing 35%—mithramycin
Inflammation of preexisting actinic keratoses— fluorouracil
Localized nodules, hands—bleomycin
Papules evolve into pustules, face and trunk— dactinomycin

Modified from Bronner AK, Hood AF: *J Am Acad Dermatol* 9:645-663, 1983.

CUTANEOUS PARANEOPLASTIC SYNDROMES

Paraneoplastic syndromes (PNSs) are diseases that appear before or concurrently with an internal malignancy. They represent a remote or systemic effect of a neoplasm (see the box at left). There is a wide range of categories of PNSs, including endocrine, neurologic, hematologic, rheumatic, renal, and cutaneous. They may be the initial clue to the presence of an underlying neoplasm. The activity of a PNS can parallel the course of the tumor and thus be used as a marker of remission or recurrence. PNSs are estimated to occur in 7% to 15% of patients with cancer.

The cutaneous changes are thought to result from the production of biologically active hormones, growth factors, or antigen-antibody interactions induced by or produced by the tumor.[5,6] Many of these syndromes, such as acanthosis nigricans, are proliferative skin disorders. Products secreted by the tumor, such as transforming growth factor alpha, may stimulate keratinocytes to proliferate.[7]

Cutaneous Manifestations of Diabetes Mellitus

Approximately 30% of patients with diabetes mellitus develop a skin disorder sometime during the course of disease. A list of these disorders follows[8]:

Candida infections (mouth, genital)
Carotenodermia (yellow skin)
Diabetic bullae
Diabetic dermopathy (shin spots)
Diabetic thick skin
Erythema (face, lower legs, feet)
External otitis
Finger pebbles
Foot ulcers
Acanthosis nigricans (insulin resistance syndromes)
Gas gangrene (nonclostridial)
Granuloma annulare (localized or generalized)
Insulin lipodystrophy
Necrobiosis lipoidica
Yellow nails
Perforating disorders
Eruptive xanthomas

Diabetic bullae are described in Chapter Sixteen.

NECROBIOSIS LIPOIDICA

Necrobiosis lipoidica (NL) is a disease of unknown origin, but more than 50% of the patients with NL are generally insulin dependent. The previous term *necrobiosis lipoidica diabeticorum* was changed because a significant minority of patients do not have diabetes. The skin lesions may appear years before the onset of diabetes, and most patients with diabetes do not develop NL. The disease may occur at any age, but it most commonly appears in the third and fourth decades. Most of the patients are females, and in most cases the lesions are confined to the anterior surfaces of the lower legs[9] (Figure 26-2).

The eruption begins as an oval, violaceous patch and expands slowly. The advancing border is red, and the central area turns yellow-brown. The central area atrophies and has a waxy surface; telangiectasias become prominent (Figure 26-3). Ulceration occurs, particularly following trauma, in 13% of cases.[10] In many instances the clinical presentation is so characteristic that biopsy is not required.

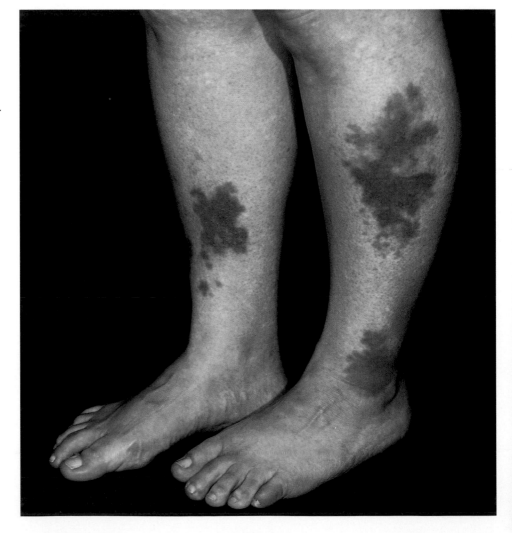

Figure 26-2
Necrobiosis lipoidica. Erythematous violaceous plaques on the anterior surfaces of the lower legs.

Treatment

Topical and intralesional steroids. Topical and intralesional steroids arrest inflammation but promote further atrophy. One large plaque completely involuted after 6 weeks of clobetasol propionate under occlusion.[11] Intralesional injections effectively control small areas of NL, but the concentration of triamcinolone acetonide (10 mg/ml) should be diluted with saline or xylocaine to 2.5 mg/ml to avoid atrophy.

Systemic corticosteroids. A 5-week course of systemic corticosteroids resulted in complete cessation of disease activity and no recurrence in a mean follow-up period of 7 months in 6 patients; however, restitution of atrophic skin lesions was not achieved.[12] Ulceration of NL was successfully treated with oral prednisolone.[10]

Pentoxifylline. Pentoxifylline (Trental) 400 mg three times a day resulted in significant improvement after 1 month of treatment in one patient. Ulcerating NL, resistant to acetylsalicylic acid, healed completely within 8 weeks of administration of 400 mg pentoxifylline twice a day.[13] Pentoxifylline is thought to decrease blood viscosity by increasing fibrinolysis and red blood cell deformability and also to inhibit platelet aggregation.

Aspirin and dipyridamole. A number of changes in the microvasculature occur in the dermis of plaques of NL. The proposed cause is either an immune complex–mediated vasculitis with vascular occlusion in the small vessels or a delayed hypersensitivity reaction. The increased tendency to show spontaneous platelet aggregation may also play a role in vascular occlusion. Treatment has been used to inhibit these changes. Low-dose aspirin and dipyridamole are thought to inhibit platelet aggregation, but reports concerning their efficacy in healing ulcers in plaques of NL are conflicting.[14-16] The recommended treatment is aspirin (3.5 mg/kg every 48 hours),[17] which for the average patient is 325 gm (one tablet), or dipyridamole (Persantine) (25-, 50-, or 75-mg tablets) (2 to 3 mg/kg/day), which for the average patient is 150 to 200 mg daily in divided doses.[18] For effective control of ulceration, platelet-inhibition therapy must be used for a minimum of 3 to 7 months. Recommended treatment schedules should be followed because there is evidence that higher dosages can decrease treatment effectiveness.

Skin grafting. Skin grafting is effective for extensive disease.[19]

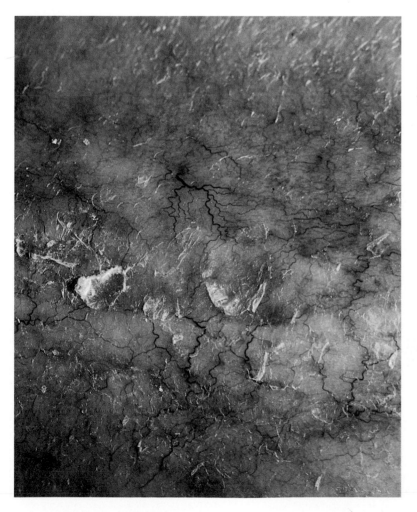

Figure 26-3
Necrobiosis lipoidica. The central area is waxy yellow with prominent telangiectasia.

GRANULOMA ANNULARE

There are conflicting reports about the association of granuloma annulare with diabetes mellitus.[20-22] Most patients with the localized form of granuloma annulare do not have clinical or laboratory evidence of diabetes. The association between disseminated granuloma annulare and diabetes has been established, but the frequency is unknown.[23]

Granuloma annulare is characterized by a ring of small, firm, flesh-colored or red papules (Figure 26-4). The localized form, most common in young adult females, is most frequently found on the lateral or dorsal surfaces of the hands and feet (Figure 26-5). The disease begins with an asymptomatic, flesh-colored papule that undergoes central involution. Over months, a ring of papules slowly increases in diameter to 0.5 to 5 cm (Figure 26-6). The duration of the disease is highly variable. Many lesions undergo spontaneous involution without scarring, whereas others last for years. The familial occurrence of granuloma annulare is uncommon but has been noted in siblings, twins, and successive generations.[24]

Disseminated granuloma annulare occurs in adults and appears with numerous flesh-colored or erythematous papules, some of which form annular rings. The papules may be accentuated in sun-exposed areas. The course is variable; many lesions persist for years.

Generalized perforating granuloma annulare is characterized by 1- to 4-mm, umbilicated papules on the extremities and is most commonly seen in children and young adults. Biopsy shows transepithelial elimination of degenerating collagen fibers. A high incidence of perforating granuloma annulare has been reported in the Hawaiian Islands.[25]

Subcutaneous granuloma annulare occurs in children. The presenting symptom is a rapidly growing, painless, soft-tissue mass of the extremities (most commonly the elbows and knees) or scalp. The mean age at presentation is 3.9 years. Diagnosis requires an excisional biopsy. Lesions may recur after excision. Lesions may resolve spontaneously and recur after excision. No record of progression to systemic illness is reported.[26]

Diagnosis. The clinical presentation is characteristic, and biopsy may not be required. The histology shows collagen degeneration, a feature similar to that seen in necrobiosis lipoidica.

Treatment. Localized lesions are asymptomatic and are best left untreated. Those patients troubled by appearance may be treated with intralesional injections of triamcinolone acetonide (2.5 to 5 mg/ml). The solution should be injected only into the elevated border. Topical steroids have little effect. Disseminated granuloma annulare has been reported to respond to dapsone,[27-30] isotretinoin,[30] etretinate,[31] hydroxychloroquine,[32,33] and niacinamide (1.5 gm/day).

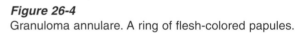

Figure 26-4
Granuloma annulare. A ring of flesh-colored papules.

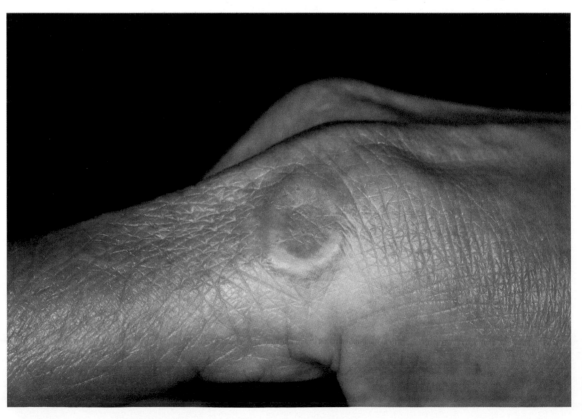

Figure 26-5 Granuloma annulare.

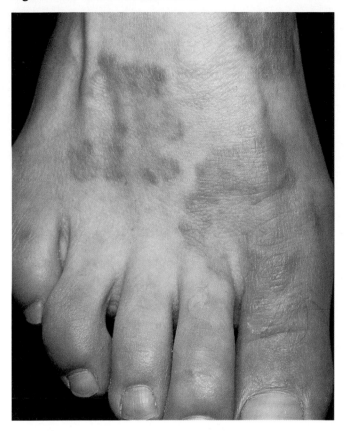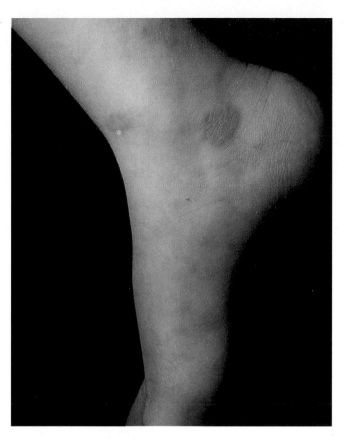

Rings of small flesh-colored or red papules are frequently found on the lateral and dorsal sufaces of the feet.

Figure 26-6
Granuloma annulare is often symmetrically distributed.

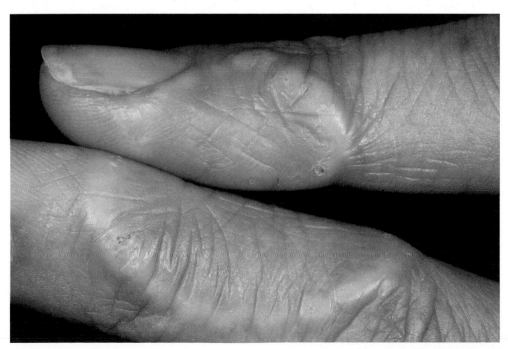

Acanthosis Nigricans

Acanthosis nigricans is a nonspecific reaction pattern that may accompany obesity; diabetes; excess corticosteroids; pineal tumors; other endocrine disorders; multiple genetic variants; drugs such as nicotinic acid, estrogens, and corticosteroids; and adenocarcinoma (see the box at right). In all cases the disease presents with symmetric, brown thickening of the skin. In time the skin may become quite thickened as the lesion develops a leathery, warty, or papillomatous surface (Figure 26-7). The lesions range in severity from slight discoloration of a small area to extensive involvement of wide areas. The most common site of involvement is the axillae, but the changes may be observed in the flexural areas of the neck and groin, the belt line, over the dorsal surfaces of the fingers, in the mouth, and around the areolae of the breasts and umbilicus. During the process there is papillary hypertrophy, hyperkeratosis, and an increased number of melanocytes in the epidermis.

TYPES OF ACANTHOSIS NIGRICANS
Benign
Obesity-associated
Part of a syndrome (many)
Malignant
Acral acanthotic anomaly
Unilateral
Medication-induced

Modified from Schwartz RA: Continuing medical education: acanthosis nigricans, *J Am Acad Dermatol* 31(1):1, 1994.

Figure 26-7
Acanthosis nigricans. The skin is brown and thickened and has a papillomatous surface.

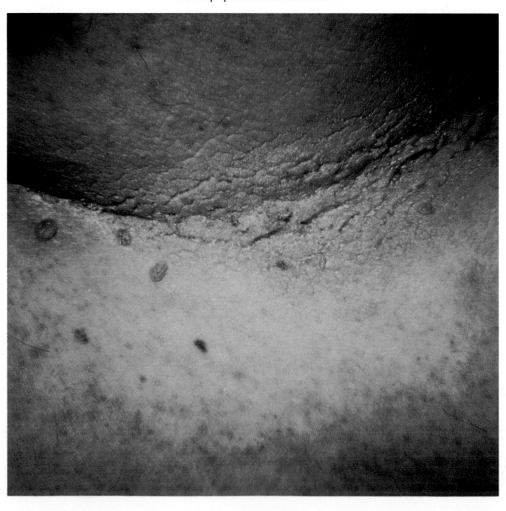

Benign acanthosis nigricans. The majority of cases are idiopathic and are associated with obesity; this process is referred to as *pseudoacanthosis nigricans*. It is postulated that heat, friction, and maceration in the flexural folds are the cause, but in one study of obese patients, those with acanthosis nigricans had fasting plasma insulin levels that were markedly higher than those without acanthosis nigricans. Therefore, acanthosis nigricans may be a cutaneous marker of hyperinsulinemia in obese individuals.[34,35]

The interaction between excessive amounts of circulating insulin with insulin-like growth factor receptors on keratinocytes may lead to the development of acanthosis nigricans.[36]

In rare instances acanthosis nigricans may occur as an autosomal dominant trait with no obesity, associated endocrinopathies, or congenital abnormalities; it may appear at birth or during childhood and is accentuated at puberty.[37] Drug-induced acanthosis nigricans has occurred with the use of nicotinic acid[38] and, rarely, with other agents.[39]

Malignant acanthosis nigricans. The cases of greatest concern are those originating in nonobese adult patients. These cases may result from secretion of tumor products with insulin-like activity or transforming growth factor alpha, which stimulates keratinocytes to proliferate.[7] These patients must be evaluated for internal malignancy. The stomach is the most common site,[40] but cancer in several other areas has been reported.[41] In approximately one third of patients, the skin lesions precede the clinical manifestations of cancer, and in several cases they have disappeared with successful removal of the tumor.[42] A recurrence of acanthosis nigricans may mark the recurrence or metastasis of the previously treated cancer.

Insulin-resistant syndromes. In a large and heterogeneous group of conditions, insulin action at the cellular level is markedly reduced[43] (see the box at right). Acanthosis nigricans appears to represent a cutaneous marker of tissue insulin resistance, irrespective of its cause (antibodies to the insulin receptor or congenital or acquired defects of receptor or postreceptor function).[44-48] These patients may not require insulin therapy, and many do not have diabetes. For patients without diabetes, insulin resistance is established by the documentation of high levels of circulating insulin or by the observation of an impaired response to exogenous insulin. Prolonged hypersecretion of insulin may lead to pancreatic exhaustion, glucose intolerance, and type II diabetes. Hyperandrogenism, insulin resistance, and acanthosis nigricans is called the *HAIR-AN syndrome*. The vulva is the most likely place to find acanthosis nigricans in obese, hirsute, hyperandrogenic, insulin-resistant women.[49]

Treatment. Lesions are usually asymptomatic and do not require treatment. Reducing thicker lesions in areas of maceration may decrease odor and promote comfort. Lac-Hydrin, a 12% lactic acid cream, applied as needed may soften lesions. Retinoic acid (Retin-A cream or gel) applied each day, or less often if irritation occurs, is effective.[50] Oral isotretinoin (Accutane) is useful, but acanthosis nigricans recurs when the drug is discontinued.[51]

ACANTHOSIS NIGRICANS WITH ENDOCRINE DISORDERS ASSOCIATED WITH INSULIN RESISTANCE

TYPE A SYNDROME (HAIR-AN SYNDROME)

HA=Hyperandrogenemia
IR=Insulin resistance
AN=Acanthosis nigricans
Familial
Young women (usually black)
Virilization or accelerated growth
Presentations
  Hirsutism, polycystic ovaries
  Acral hypertrophy, clitoral hypertrophy, muscle cramps
Acanthosis nigricans
  Onset in infancy or childhood
  Rapid progression during puberty
  Generalized
Plasma testosterone levels high

TYPE B SYNDROME

Women (average age 39)
Uncontrolled diabetes
Ovarian hyperandrogenism (premenopausal women)
Autoimmune disease associated
  Systemic lupus erythematosus
  Scleroderma
  Sjogren's syndrome
  Hashimoto's thyroiditis
  Most have only
    Leukopenia and
    Anti-DNA antibodies (high titers)
Acanthosis nigricans
  Varying severity

Xanthomas and Dyslipoproteinemia

The plasma lipids and lipoprotein levels are under the control of a number of genetic and environmental influences. Abnormalities in a number of these lipids or subfractions result in dyslipoproteinemias and xanthomas. Xanthomas are lipid deposits in the skin and tendons that occur secondary to a lipid abnormality. These localized deposits are yellow and are frequently very firm. Although certain types of xanthomas are characteristic of certain lipid abnormalities, none is absolutely specific because the same form of xanthomas occurs in many different diseases[52]; further investigation is always required. The molecular defect of various lipid disorders is now known; however, the classification and diagnosis are still based on history and clinical presentation (Table 26-2).

Pathophysiology. The liver secretes lipoproteins, which are particles composed of various combinations of cholesterol and triglycerides. These particles are made water soluble to facilitate transport to peripheral tissues by polar phospholipids and 12 different specific proteins termed *apolipoproteins*. The apolipoproteins also serve as cofactors for plasma enzymes and interact with cell surface receptors. Lipoproteins are divided into five major classes: chylomicrons, very low-density lipoproteins (VLDL), intermediate-density lipoproteins (IDL), low-density lipoproteins (LDL), and high-density lipoproteins (HDL). LDL and HDL have each been divided into two subfractions.

Classification: primary vs. secondary hyperlipoproteinemia. Dyslipoproteinemias are categorized as primary or secondary. Primary conditions (Table 26-3) are genetically determined and were grouped by Fredrickson into five or six types on the basis of specific lipoprotein elevations.[53] This classification is the major frame of reference for these diseases, but modifications were made as new information became available.[54,55] Secondary hyperlipoproteinemias occur as a result of another disease process that can induce symptoms, lipoprotein changes, and xanthomas that mimic the primary syndromes. Diagnosis should be made as follows:

TABLE 26-2 Xanthomas

Type	Clinical characteristics	Associated lipid abnormality
Xanthelasma	Inner or outer canthus; plane or papular	No lipid abnormality; increased frequency of apo E-ND phenotype and hyperapobetalipoproteinemia; type II*
Eruptive	Crops of discrete yellow papules on an erythematous base on buttocks, extensor aspects of elbows and knees; lesions clear when triglycerides return to normal	Indicative of hypertriglyceridemia and seen with types I, II, IV, and rarely III and diabetes mellitus
Plane	Palms and palmar creases, eyelids, face, neck, chest	Biliary cirrhosis, type III; reported in types II, IV
Tuberous	Lipid deposits in dermis and subcutaneous tissue; plaquelike or nodular; frequently found on the elbows or knees	Hypertriglyceridemia (familial or acquired); types II and III; biliary cirrhosis
Tendinous	Nodules involving the elbows, knees, Achilles tendon, and dorsum of hands and feet	Indicates hypercholesterolemia; type II, occasionally III

*There are five types of familial hyperlipidemia.

TABLE 26-3 Primary Dyslipidemia (the Genetic Dyslipidemias)

Phenotype	Lipoprotein at increased concentration	Cholesterol concentration	Triglyceride concentration	Dermatologic lesion(s)
I	Chylomicrons	+	+ + + +	Eruptive xanthomas
IIa	LDL	+ + + +	+	Tendon, tuberous, and intertriginous xanthomas; xanthelasma
IIb	VLDL and LDL	+ + + +	+ +	Tendon, tuberous, and intertriginous xanthomas, xanthelasma
III	IDL	+ + +	+ + +	Palmar xanthomas
IV	VLDL	+	+ + +	Eruptive xanthomas
V	Chylomicrons and VLDL	+ +	+ + + +	Eruptive xanthomas

1. Determine the type of xanthoma.
2. Measure fasting blood levels of cholesterol, triglycerides, and HDL, then calculate VLDL and LDL.
3. Rule out secondary diseases—see the box at right. The diagnosis of primary hyperlipoproteinemia is one of exclusion.
   a. Thyroid, liver, renal function tests
   b. Glucose tolerance tests
   c. Complete blood count (CBC), serum, and urine immunoelectrophoresis
   d. Chest x-ray film, bone marrow
   e. Antinuclear antibodies (ANA)

Laboratory diagnosis. Measure cholesterol, triglyceride, and HDL levels after a 12- hour fast. If the triglyceride levels are below 400 mg/dl and dysbetalipoproteinemia-type III is not present, the following formulas can be used to calculate VLDL and LDL concentrations. Lipoprotein electrophoresis is not useful as a screening tool, since it is only semiquantitative. A complete quantification of lipoproteins by ultracentrifugation is available at some centers.

VLDL cholesterol = Triglycerides ÷ 5
(Triglycerides in excess of 700 is ÷ 10)
LDL cholesterol = Total cholesterol − (VLDL + HDL)

Xanthelasma and plane xanthomas. Plane xanthomas occur in several areas of the body and are flat or slightly elevated (Figure 26-8). Xanthelasma is the most common form. Xanthelasma can be associated with familial hypercholesterolemia, phenotype IIa or IIb, but 50% of the patients have normal cholesterol levels. Longevity studies have shown that xanthelasma with or without hypercholesterolemia is one of the main risk factors for death from atherosclerotic disease.

SECONDARY DYSLIPIDEMIA

HYPERCHOLESTEROLEMIA

Diet
Hypothyroidism
Obstructive liver disease
Nephrosis
Porphyria
Paraproteinemias (myeloma, lymphoma, cryoglobulinemia, macroglobulinemia)

HYPERTRIGLYCERIDEMIA

Obesity
Diabetes mellitus—uncontrolled
Alcohol ingestion
Renal failure
Systemic lupus erythematosus
Lipodystrophy
Glycogen storage disease
Medications (e.g., estrogens, oral contraceptives, beta-blockers, hydrochlorothiazide, isotretinoin)

Further study of these patients with normal cholesterol and triglycerides often reveals an elevated LDL and VLDL and decreased HDL.[56] This profile is found for patients who have a high risk of atherosclerotic cardiovascular disease. Studies show that numerous people with xanthelasma have an elevated apolipoprotein B[57] and other fractions that are known to be atherogenic. It may be that all patients with xanthelasma have an increased risk for atherosclerosis.

Figure 26-8
Plane xanthomas in a patient with biliary cirrhosis.

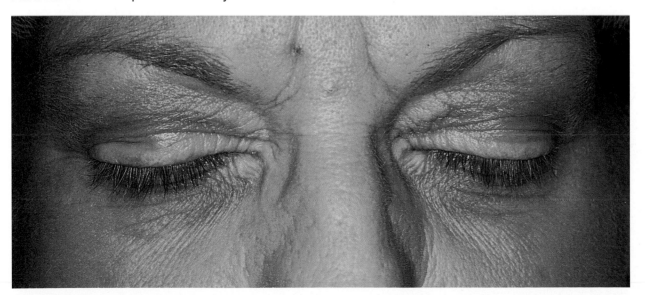

Figure 26-9 Eruptive xanthomas.

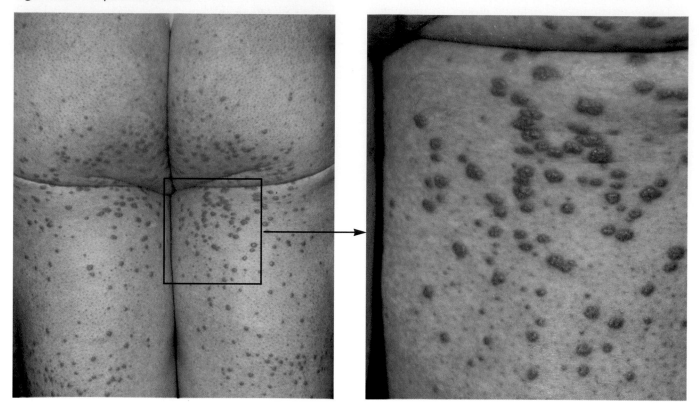

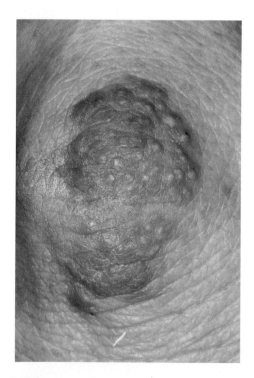

Figure 26-10
Tuberous xanthomas. Groups of yellow papules on the elbows.

Eruptive xanthomas. These are yellow, 1- to 4-mm papules with a red halo around the base. They appear suddenly in crops on extensor surfaces of the arms, legs, and buttocks and over pressure points (Figure 26-9). Lesions clear rapidly when serum lipid levels are lowered.

Tuberous xanthomas. These are slowly evolving yellow papules, nodules, or tumors that occur on the knees, elbows, and extensor surfaces of the body and the palms (Figure 26-10).

Tendinous xanthomas. These smooth, deeply situated nodules are attached to tendons, ligaments, and fascia. They are most often found on the Achilles tendons and the dorsal aspects of the fingers.

Regression of xanthomas. Certain xanthomas disappear with treatment. The eruptive and palmar xanthomas can regress rapidly. The eruptive type of tuberous xanthomas can disappear. Tendinous xanthomatous lesions tend to persist.

Neurofibromatosis

The neurofibromatoses comprise at least two autosomal dominant disorders affecting an estimated 100,000 Americans. These diseases have tumors surrounding nerves. Neurofibromatosis 1 (NF1) is the most common and is characterized by congenital lesions of the skin, central nervous system, bone, and endocrine glands. Neurofibromatosis 2 (NF2) is characterized by bilateral acoustic neuromas and other nerve tumors. Skin and other systemic manifestations are minimal or absent.[58] Café-au-lait macules, freckling, and neurofibromas localized to a segment of the body are called *segmental neurofibromatosis* (NF5). The NF1 gene is located on chromosome 17 and the NF2 gene is found on chromosome 22.

Neurofibromatosis 1. NF1 is a disorder of neural crest–derived cells characterized by the presence of café-au-lait spots, multiple neurofibromas, and Lisch nodules (pigmented iris hamartomas); there are several other less common features. There is considerable variation of manifestations within the same family. It occurs in approximately one of every 3500 births and affects both sexes with equal frequency and severity. Neurofibromatosis is one of the most common mutations in humans; at least half of the cases represent new mutations.

Clinical manifestations

Café-au-lait spots. Café-au-lait spots are light-colored-to-brown macules (see Chapter Nineteen). The criteria for establishing the diagnosis with reference to the number and size of café-au-lait spots[59] are listed below and on p. 796. The spots are present in virtually every patient with neurofibromatosis, usually at birth, but they may not appear for months. Their size and number increase with age (Figure 26-11). Intertriginous freckling, a pathognomonic sign, may occur in the axillae, inframammary region, and groin (Figure 26-12). Café-au-lait macules alone are not absolutely diagnostic of NF1, regardless of their size and number.

Presumptive evidence of neurofibromatosis

- Six or more café-au-lait macules over 5 mm in greatest diameter if prepubertal
- Six or more café-au-lait macules over 15 mm in greatest diameter if postpubertal

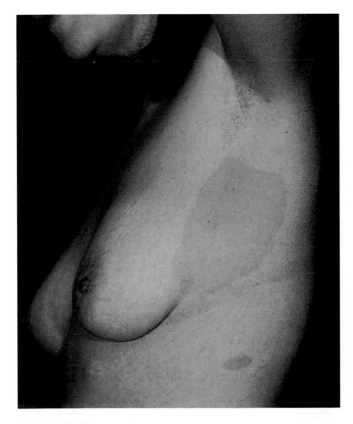

Figure 26-11
von Recklinghausen's neurofibromatosis. Café-au-lait spots vary in size and have a smooth border.

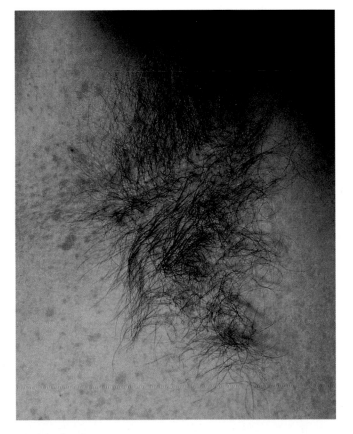

Figure 26-12
von Recklinghausen's neurofibromatosis. Axillary freckling (Crowe's sign)—an almost pathognomonic sign.

Neurofibromas. Tumors are usually not present in childhood, but they begin to appear at puberty. Tumors increase in both number and size as the patient ages. Some patients have only a few small tumors, whereas others develop hundreds over the entire body surface, including the palms and soles (Figure 26-13).

There are three different types of cutaneous tumors. The most common is sessile or pedunculated. Early tumors are soft, dome-shaped papules or nodules that have a distinctive violaceous hue. Digital pressure on the soft tumor causes invagination or "button-holing." When the soft tumors attain a certain size, they bend and hang or become pendulous. The plexiform neuroma is an elongated tumor that occurs along the course of peripheral nerves. *Elephantiasis neuromatosa* is a term used to describe a diffuse tumor of nerve trunks that extends into surrounding tissues, causing gross deformity. This form of neuroma produced the facial deformity in Joseph Merrick of London, England, the man who was described in the play and movie, *The Elephant Man*. Most tumors are benign, but malignant degeneration to a neurofibrosarcoma or malignant schwannoma has been reported in approximately 2% of cases[60]; it rarely occurs before age 40.

Lisch nodules. Lisch nodules (LNs) are pigmented, melanocytic,[61] iris hamartomas (Figure 26-14).[62] They increase in number with age and are asymptomatic. The prevalence of LNs and neurofibromas according to age is shown in Figure 26-15. All adults with neurofibromatosis who are 21 years of age or older have LNs. LNs have never been seen in the absence of neurofibromatosis. They are never the only clinical sign of NF1. They are more likely to be present in younger patients than are neurofibromas (see Figure 26-15) and therefore help to make the diagnosis in younger patients.[63] No association has been found between LNs and overall clinical severity. They are markers for the von Recklinghausen's neurofibromatosis gene; they may be present in immediate relatives who have no cutaneous or other specific signs of the disease.[64] LNs may be seen without the aid of instruments, but slit-lamp examination is essential for differentiation from iris freckles or nevi. Iris freckles are flat and have a lacework structure, whereas LNs are raised, round, dome-shaped, brown papules that are present in both eyes.

Systemic manifestations. Neurofibromatosis has a broad spectrum of systemic manifestations; the most important are listed in the box on p. 795.

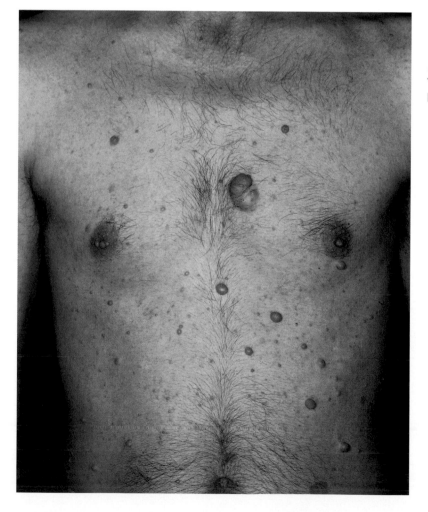

Figure 26-13
von Recklinghausen's neurofibromatosis. Adult patient with hundreds of neurofibromas.

Figure 26-14 von Recklinghausen's neurofibromatosis—Lisch nodules.

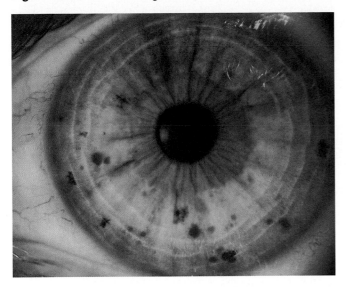

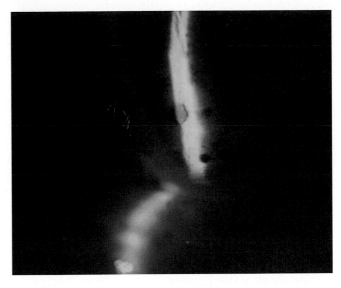

A, Lisch nodules—pigmented iris hamartomas are present in more than 60% of patients with neurofibromatosis who are 7 years of age or older.

B, Slit-lamp examination is essential for differentiation from iris freckles. Iris freckles are flat and have a lace-work structure; Lisch nodules are raised, round, fluffy, and light brown. *(Courtesy Lucian Szmyd M.D.)*

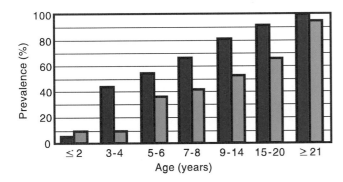

Figure 26-15
Prevalence of Lisch nodules (red bars) and neurofibromas (blue bars) in 167 patients with neurofibromatosis 1, according to age. *(Modified from Lubs ML et al:* N Engl J Med *324:1264, 1991.)*

SYSTEMIC MANIFESTATIONS OF NEUROFIBROMATOSIS

Central nervous system tumors
  Optic gliomas
  Astrocytomas, acoustic neuromas, meningiomas, neurilemomas
Constipation
Headache
Intellectual handicap
Kyphoscoliosis
Macrocephaly
Malignant disease
  Neurofibrosarcoma
  Malignant schwannoma
  Neuroblastoma
  Wilm's tumors
  Rhabdomyosarcoma
  Leukemia
Pheochromocytomas
Premature or delayed puberty
Pseudarthrosis (tibia, radius)
Seizures
Speech impediment
Short stature

From Riccardi VM: *N Engl J Med* 305:1617, 1981.

Natural history. Survival rates are significantly impaired for relatives with neurofibromatosis, are worse in probands, and are worst in female probands. Malignant neoplasms or benign central nervous system tumors occur in 45% of probands. Compared with the general population, male relatives with neurofibromatosis have the same rate of neoplasms, whereas female relatives have a nearly twofold higher rate. Nervous system tumors are disproportionately represented.[65]

Diagnosis. NF1 is considered to be present in an individual with two of the following criteria, provided no other disease accounts for the findings[66]:

- Café-au-lait macules
  Six or more café-au-lait macules over 5 mm in greatest diameter if prepubertal
  Six or more café-au-lait macules over 15 mm in greatest diameter if postpubertal
- Neurofibromas
  Two or more of any type or
  One plexiform neurofibroma
- Axillary or inguinal freckles
- A distinctive osseous lesion, such as sphenoid wing dysplasia or bowing, or thinning of long-bone cortex with or without pseudarthrosis
- Bilateral optic nerve gliomas
- Lisch nodules
  Two or more on slit-lamp examination
- A first-degree relative (parent, sibling, or offspring) with NF1 determined by the above criteria

NF1 should be suspected in children with a large head circumference (above the 97th percentile for age) and one of the following: a mild cognitive impairment, a learning disability, or a selective visual-spatial impairment.

Segmental neurofibromatosis (NF5). In some patients, café-au-lait spots, freckles, and/or neurofibromas are limited to a single dermatomal segment. A postzygotic somatic mutation in a primitive neural crest cell is the most likely causative mechanism for this cutaneous hamartoma.[67,68] The lesions are strictly unilateral and noninherited in most cases; however, in a few patients, the disease becomes generalized.[69] These patients should be examined for LNs and other signs of neurofibromatosis.

Genetic counseling. The patient's offspring, both male and female, have a 50% chance of inheriting this autosomal dominant disease. The penetrance is virtually 100%, but the expressivity is extremely variable. The severity of the disease is highest in those born to an affected mother.[70] Fifty percent of cases are new mutations in which the parents are unaffected. All family members and relatives should be examined for the triad of Lisch iris nodules, solitary neurofibromas, and café-au-lait spots.[64]

The LN is a reliable indicator of NF1; slit-lamp examination is important to establish the diagnosis. All people above the age of 20 who have NF1 also have LNs.[63] Therefore, minimally affected and unaffected parents and adult siblings can be identified. If the diagnosis is in doubt and a child has no LNs, the examination should be repeated periodically. LNs often appear before neurofibromas. Adult siblings and adult children of affected persons can be counseled that their risk of having affected children is the same (approximately 1 in 3500) as that of the parents of patients with sporadic cases if all three elements of the triad are absent.[71] Patients who have a segmental pattern of neurofibromatosis should be counseled that genetic transmission of their trait, though rare, is possible.[72]

Management. There are more than 60 neurofibromatosis clinics in the United States. These clinics are usually based at teaching centers where a group of specialists provides a team approach to management. The National Neurofibromatosis Foundation has a list of clinics and can be reached by calling (800) 323-7938. A genetic counselor is available to speak to the physician or the patient.

Cutaneous tumors may be excised. The patient must be followed closely to detect malignant degeneration of neurofibromas. Genetic counseling is of utmost importance. Periodic complete evaluations are required to detect the numerous possible internal manifestations. Magnetic resonance imaging with gadolinium enhancement is the primary neuroimaging modality used for diagnosis, management, and screening of family members.[73,74]

Tuberous Sclerosis

Tuberous sclerosis (epiloia) is an autosomal dominant disease of variable penetrance that is characterized by multiple hamartomas of the skin, central nervous system, kidneys, heart, retina, and other organs. The skin lesions (adenoma sebaceum, shagreen patch, white macules, or periungual fibromas) are reliable markers of the disease. Tuberous sclerosis affects at least 1 in 10,000 people; two thirds of cases occur sporadically, one third are familial. Mildly affected individuals may be undiagnosed. The triad of epilepsy, angiofibromas (adenoma sebaceum), and mental retardation that is typically associated with tuberous sclerosis is present in only 25% of patients. Mental retardation may be present in less than 50%. The 1992 consensus report of the diagnostic criteria committee of the National Tuberous Sclerosis Association set new diagnostic criteria (see the box at right).

Clinical manifestations. The time course of tuberous sclerosis lesions is illustrated in the graph below.

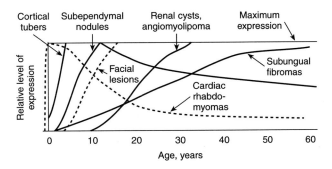

Time Course of TS Lesions

(Modified from Kwiatkowski DJ, Short P: Tuberous sclerosis, Arch Dermatol 130:349, 1994.)

DIAGNOSTIC CRITERIA FOR TUBEROUS SCLEROSIS COMPLEX

Primary features
  Facial angiofibromas*
  Multiple ungual fibromas*
  Cortical tuber (histologically confirmed)
  Subependymal nodule or giant cell astrocytoma (histologically confirmed)
  Multiple calcified subependymal nodules protruding into the ventricle (radiographic evidence)
  Multiple retinal astrocytomas
Secondary features
  Affected first-degree relative
  Cardiac rhabdomyoma (histologic or radiographic confirmation)
  Other retinal hamartoma or achromic patch*
  Cerebral tubers (radiographic confirmation)
  Noncalcified subependymal nodules (radiographic confirmation)
  Shagreen patch*
  Forehead plaque*
  Pulmonary lymphangiomyomatosis (histologic confirmation)
  Renal angiomyolipoma (radiographic or histologic confirmation)
  Renal cysts (histologic confirmation)
Tertiary features
  Hypomelanotic macules*
  "Confetti" skin lesions*
  Renal cysts (radiographic evidence)
  Randomly distributed enamel pits in deciduous and/or permanent teeth
  Hamartomatous rectal polyps (histologic confirmation)
  Bone cysts (radiographic evidence)
  Pulmonary lymphangiomyomatosis (radiographic evidence)
  Cerebral white-matter "migration tracts" or heterotopias (radiographic evidence)
  Gingival fibromas*
  Hamartoma of other organs (histologic confirmation)
  Infantile spasms

Definite TSC—Either one primary feature, two secondary features, or one secondary plus two tertiary features
Probable TSC—Either one secondary plus one tertiary feature, or three tertiary features
Suspect TSC—Either one secondary feature or two

From Roach ES et al: *J Child Neurol* 7:221, 1992.
*Histologic confirmation is not required if the lesion is clinically obvious.
TSC, tuberous sclerosis complex.

TUBEROUS SCLEROSIS

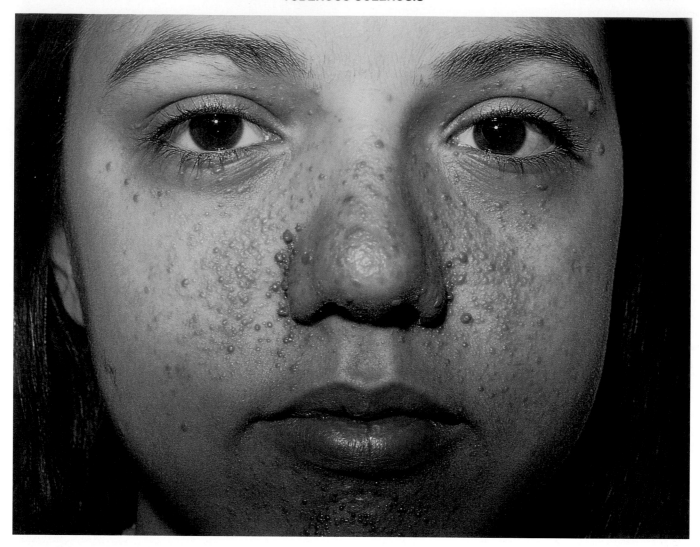

Figure 26-16 Adenoma sebaceum.

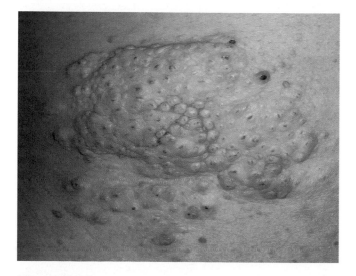

Figure 26-17
Shagreen patch is most commonly found in the lumbosacral region.

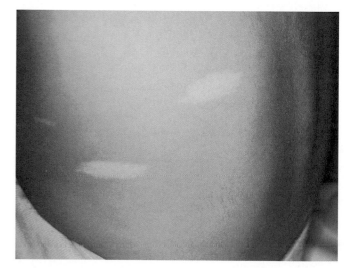

Figure 26-18
Hypopigmented macules.

Adenoma sebaceum. Adenoma sebaceum is the most common cutaneous manifestation of tuberous sclerosis.[75] The lesions consist of smooth, firm, 1- to 5-mm, yellow-pink papules with fine telangiectasia (Figure 26-16). Their color and location suggest an origin from sebaceous glands, but these growths are benign hamartomas composed of fibrous and vascular tissue (angiofibromas). The angiofibromas are located on the nasolabial folds, cheeks, chin, and, occasionally, on the forehead, scalp, and ears. The number varies from a few inconspicuous lesions to dense clusters of papules. They are rare at birth but may begin to appear by ages 2 to 3 and proliferate during puberty. They may be mistaken for multiple trichoepitheliomas, an autosomal dominant condition that appears on the central face. A secondary feature, the "forehead plaque," is a large angiofibroma.

Shagreen patch. The shagreen patch is highly characteristic of tuberous sclerosis and occurs in as many as 80% of patients; it occurs in early childhood and may be the first sign of disease. The lesion varies in size from 1 to 10 cm. There is usually one lesion, but several may be present. They are soft, flesh-colored-to-yellow plaques with an irregular surface that has been likened to pigskin (Figure 26-17). The lesion consists of dermal connective tissue and appears most commonly in the lumbosacral region.

Whitish macules and white tufts of hair. Hypomelanotic macules (oval, ash-leaf shaped, stippled, or "confetti shaped") are randomly distributed with a concentration on the arms, legs, and trunk. They are the earliest sign of tuberous sclerosis (Figure 26-18).[76] They are present in 40% to 90% of patients with the disease and number from 1 to 32 in affected individuals.[77-79] The white macules are present at birth and increase in number and size throughout life. They vary from 0.5 to 12 cm in diameter. The "confetti" macules are the rarest of the three types and consist of numerous 1- to 3-mm macules. The Wood's light can be used to accentuate the white macules and is particularly useful for examining patients with light skin. A biopsy shows melanocytes, thus excluding the diagnosis of vitiligo. Hypopigmented macules, present at birth, are not invariably associated with tuberous sclerosis, but their presence is an indication for further study. It is essential that the diagnosis be established as soon as possible so that parents can obtain genetic counseling. A tuft of white hair with no depigmentation of the scalp skin underlying the white tuft has been reported as an early sign of tuberous sclerosis.[80]

Periungual fibromas. Periungual fibromas appear at or after puberty in approximately 50% of cases. They are smooth, flesh-colored, conical projections that emerge from the nailfolds of the toenail and fingernail (Figure 26-19).

Systemic manifestations. Mental retardation occurs in less than 50% of cases. Subependymal nodules and cortical and white matter tubers are characteristic of tuberous sclerosis. Sclerotic patches (tubers) consisting of astrocytes and giant cells are scattered throughout the cortical gray matter. Calcium is deposited in tubers and may be detected shortly after birth by computed tomography (CT) scan, magnetic res-

onance imaging (MRI), or x-ray films and is found in 90% of affected children.[81,84] Brain lesions cause seizures in more than 90% of patients. Benign tumors consisting of vascular fibrous tissue and fat and smooth muscle are found in numerous organs, including the kidneys, liver, and gastrointestinal tract. Gray or yellow retinal plaques occur in 25% of cases. The incidence of enamel pitting in the adult is 100%. A dental disclosing solution swabbed on dry teeth exposes the pits.[82]

Genetic counseling. The patient's offspring, both male and female, have a 50% chance of inheriting this autosomal dominant disease. The penetrance is high, but expressivity is variable. Patients with normal parents acquire the disease from a new mutation. Linkage of tuberous sclerosis complex to markers on chromosome 9 is reported, but more than one locus may be responsible for the phenotype.[83] Currently no reliable method of prenatal diagnosis is available. For these reasons, subjects known to be at 50% risk should be assessed scrupulously to clarify their status. The National Tuberous Sclerosis Association provides information and support for physicians, patients, and families. The headquarters is at 8000 Corporate Drive, Suite 120, Landover, Maryland 20785; (800) 225-NTSA.

Diagnosis and management. The diagnosis of tuberous sclerosis must be sought in infants with white macules, white hair tufts, or other cutaneous signs. The diagnosis may be established by demonstrating brain calcifications that may occur in early infancy. MRI is the procedure of choice for the diagnosis of tuberous sclerosis. CT is more useful for detecting subependymal nodules, whereas MRI shows the number and location of cerebral cortical and subcortical lesions more accurately. When pre- and postcontrast MRI results are negative, CT is used to exclude small calcified subependymal nodules.[84] A positive scan result is often obtainable before the calcifications are present on skull x-ray films and even before the pathognomonic cutaneous findings appear. Facial angiofibromas may be surgically removed for cosmetic purposes by electrosurgery, cryosurgery, dermabrasion, or lasers.

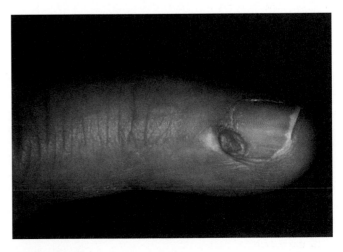

Figure 26-19
Tuberous sclerosis. Periungual fibromas.

Cancer-Associated Genodermatoses

An overview of the familial multiple cancer syndromes with cutaneous findings appears in the box below.

COWDEN'S DISEASE (MULTIPLE HAMARTOMA SYNDROME)

Cowden's disease (multiple hamartoma syndrome) is characterized by multiple hamartomas of ectodermal, endodermal, and mesodermal origin; a high incidence of malignant tumors of the breast and/or thyroid gland; and an autosomal dominant pattern of inheritance. The mucocutaneous manifestations are the most characteristic feature and are the key to diagnosis (see the box on p. 801).

Mucocutaneous lesions. Facial papules and oral mucosal papillomatosis are the most sensitive indicators of the disease. The asymptomatic cutaneous lesions are usually noticed at age 20, and no further progression of lesions is seen after the age of 30. The principal cutaneous lesion is a papule that may be smooth or keratotic. Cutaneous facial papules are of two types: Lichenoid, flesh-colored, flat-topped papules are found in the centrofacial and periorificial areas; and flesh-colored, elongated, verrucoid, papillomatous lesions are found clustered around the mouth, nose, eyes, and on the ears. The majority of these lesions are trichilemmomas.[85] The differential diagnosis of these facial papules includes Darier's disease and adenoma sebaceum

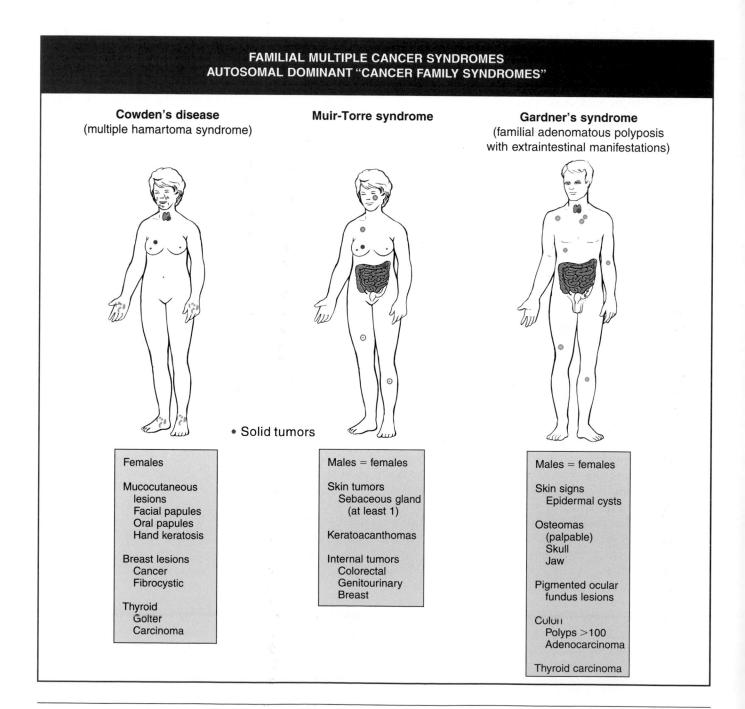

FAMILIAL MULTIPLE CANCER SYNDROMES
AUTOSOMAL DOMINANT "CANCER FAMILY SYNDROMES"

Cowden's disease
(multiple hamartoma syndrome)

Muir-Torre syndrome

Gardner's syndrome
(familial adenomatous polyposis with extraintestinal manifestations)

• Solid tumors

Females

Mucocutaneous
  lesions
  Facial papules
  Oral papules
  Hand keratosis

Breast lesions
  Cancer
  Fibrocystic

Thyroid
  Golter
  Carcinoma

Males = females

Skin tumors
  Sebaceous gland
    (at least 1)

Keratoacanthomas

Internal tumors
  Colorectal
  Genitourinary
  Breast

Males = females

Skin signs
  Epidermal cysts

Osteomas
  (palpable)
  Skull
  Jaw

Pigmented ocular
  fundus lesions

Colon
  Polyps >100
  Adenocarcinoma

Thyroid carcinoma

COWDEN'S SYNDROME

Mucocutaneous lesions—100%
(Constant and characteristic findings)
    Face—83%
        Lichenoid and verrucous papules
    Acral extremities—65%
        Hyperkeratotic and verrucous keratosis
    Palms and soles—48%
        Punctate keratoses
    Lips and oral mucosa—83%
        Papillomatosis
        Smooth and keratotic papular lesions
        Scrotal tongue
Thyroid tumors—67%
Fibrocystic breast disease—60%
Carcinoma of the breast >30%
Gastrointestinal polyps—40%
Genitourinary tract cysts and tumors—55%
Nervous system anomalies—19%
Eye lesions—13%
Skeletal abnormalities—37%
Lipomas

Modified from Starink TM: *J Am Acad Dermatol* 11:1127-1141, 1984.

found in tuberous sclerosis. Acral keratoses are located primarily on the dorsum of the hands and feet. They resemble flat warts (i.e., they are flesh-colored, flat-topped, papules 1 to 4 mm in diameter). Palmoplantar keratoses are isolated, pinpoint-to-pea-sized, translucent, hard papules that may show a central depression.[86]

The oral lesions are white, smooth-surfaced papules, 1 to 3 mm in diameter, that often coalesce, giving a cobblestone appearance. They are located primarily on the gingival, labial, and palatal surfaces.

Breast lesions. Breast lesions are the most important and potentially serious abnormality of Cowden's disease. Ductal adenocarcinoma occurs in more than 30% of patients, and fibrocystic disease occurs in 60% of patients. The median age of diagnosis of breast cancer is 41 years. All women with Cowden's disease should be considered for prophylactic bilateral total mastectomy by their third decade of life.[87,88]

Thyroid gland lesions. Palpable enlargement (goiter and adenoma) is the most frequently reported internal abnormality of Cowden's disease. Carcinoma is reported in several cases.

A wide variety of other abnormalities and malignancies have been reported, but the incidence is low.

MUIR-TORRE SYNDROME

Muir-Torre syndrome is an autosomal dominant genodermatosis characterized by at least one sebaceous gland tumor[89] and a minimum of one internal malignancy.

Skin tumors. The sebaceous gland tumors (adenoma, sebaceoma, epithelioma, or carcinoma) usually occur on the trunk, face, and scalp. They vary from small, asymptomatic papules or nodules that resemble cysts or benign tumors to waxy papules.[90] The syndrome may occur in individuals with a single sebaceous gland tumor.[89] Single or multiple keratoacanthomas occur in approximately 20% of patients. The median age for the appearance of the skin lesions is 53 years (range, 23 to 89 years).[91] Sebaceous gland tumors in the general population are rare. A tumor diagnosed as a sebaceous adenoma, sebaceous epithelioma, or sebaceous carcinoma should alert the clinician to the possibility of visceral cancer in both the patient and in family members. Sebaceous hyperplasia commonly seen on the face is not associated with malignancy.

Internal tumors. The most commonly associated neoplasms are colorectal (47%); 58% of these tumors occur proximal to or at the splenic flexure. Genitourinary tumors (21%), breast carcinomas (12%), and hematologic disorders (9%) are also common.[92] Fifty-three percent of patients develop one cancer, 37% develop two to three cancers, and 10% develop four to nine cancers. Cutaneous lesions occur before or concurrent with the diagnosis of the initial cancer in 63% of patients. The median age for the detection of the initial visceral neoplasm is 53 years (range, 23 to 89 years).[91] A few cases have been associated with polyps in the colon, but widespread gastrointestinal polyposis is rare. There is a relatively low potential for malignancy in both cutaneous and internal tumors, but metastasis from internal malignancies does occur, particularly from colon cancer.[93]

Epidemiology. Muir-Torre syndrome may appear de novo,[94] but there is often a variable family history of cutaneous and/or internal tumors. Males and females are equally affected. This may be one of the four subtypes of cancer family syndrome characterized by a genetically determined (autosomal dominant) predisposition to multiple visceral malignancies that arise at an early age and pursue a relatively benign course. As in cancer family syndrome, colon cancers in Muir-Torre syndrome are often more proximal to the splenic flexure than in the general populace.[95]

GARDNER'S SYNDROME

Gardner's syndrome (familial adenomatous polyposis with extraintestinal manifestations) is an autosomal dominantly transmitted disease with a similar penetrance in both sexes of nearly 100%. It consists of intestinal polyposis, epidermal cysts, multiple osteomas, mesenteric fibromas,[96] desmoid tumors,[97] pigmented ocular fundus lesions, unerupted teeth, and odontomas.[98] The incidence is approximately 1 of 8300 to 1 of 16,000 births.[99] The adenomatous polyposis coli (APC) gene on chromosome 5q21 is altered by point mutations in the germ line of Gardner's syndrome patients. The identification of these genes should aid in the counseling of patients with genetic predispositions to colorectal cancer.[100-102]

Cutaneous signs. Polyposis is a nearly constant feature, but epidermal cysts occur in approximately 35%. Epidermal cysts are frequently the presenting complaint and appear most often on the head and neck, but they frequently also occur in areas such as the legs, where epidermal cysts are rarely found. Gardner's syndrome should be considered in patients with epidermal cysts in unusual areas. The cysts can occur in childhood, but the average age at onset is 13 years.[103] They range from a few to many lesions and can be small or large enough to distort normal structures. Osteomas can be recognized clinically and radiographically in childhood. They most commonly appear on the head and neck and can be seen and felt.

Osteomas. Multiple osteomas, especially of the skull and jaws, are found in a number of affected and at-risk relatives. In some, these "markers" are found early in life, before the appearance of colonic polyps. Radiography of the jaws may serve as a valuable tool for the early detection of carriers of Gardner's syndrome.[104]

Pigmented ocular fundus lesions. Pigmented ocular fundus lesions are a reliable clinical marker for the disease and are found in 90% of patients and 47% of relatives who are at a 50% risk for Gardner's syndrome.[105,106] The presence of bilateral lesions, multiple lesions (more than four), or both is a specific and sensitive clinical marker for the syndrome. The lesions are discrete, darkly pigmented, and round, oval, or kidney shaped[107]; they range in size from 0.1 to 1 (or more) optic-disc diameters. One to 30 lesions may be present. Pigmented ocular lesions are found in infancy and are of value in the identification of persons at risk for Gardner's syndrome.[108]

Thyroid carcinoma. Carcinoma of the thyroid gland is frequently reported in these patients. It has the following characteristics: female predominance (89%), youth (average 23.6; range, 16 to 40 years), papillary form (88%), and multicentricity (70%).[109] Most (55.5%) thyroid carcinomas were discovered 1 to 17 years after familial adenomatous polyposis was identified, although some have been found before (29.6%) or at the same time (14.8%) it was diagnosed.[110] The high frequency of multicentric papillary thyroid carcinoma warrants aggressive diagnostic screening at regular intervals with neck palpation and ultrasonography.

Colonic polyps and cancer. Colonic polyps can be detected before the patient reaches puberty. They are usually asymptomatic, number greater than 100, and invariably progress to adenocarcinoma. Sulindac reduces the number and size of colorectal adenomas in patients with familial adenomatous polyposis, but its effect is incomplete, and it is unlikely to replace colectomy as primary therapy.[111] Gardner's syndrome patients who undergo aggressive bowel surgery when polyps are detected can have a normal life span. All family members should be examined. Genetic counseling is essential for this autosomal dominantly inherited disease.

Glucagonoma Syndrome

Glucagonoma syndrome (necrolytic migratory erythema) is characterized by elevated serum glucagon levels, a pancreatic alpha-cell tumor, abnormal glucose tolerance tests or diabetes, weight loss, hypoaminoacidemia, anemia, and a dermatitis referred to as *necrolytic migratory erythema*.[112-115] Most patients are women, ages 20 to 71. Reported glucagon levels of patients with glucagonoma syndrome range from 380 to 6750 pg/ml (normal, 100 to 200 pg/ml). A glucagon-secreting, islet-cell, pancreatic tumor is most frequently located in the tail of the pancreas, corresponding to the frequency of alpha cells in the normal pancreas. The tumors show evidence of hypervascularity, and selective, celiac axis arteriography is the most valuable preoperative technique for localizing these neoplasms and their common liver metastases.[116]

It is very difficult histologically to determine whether these tumors are benign or malignant. Most glucagonomas are malignant, and metastasis has occurred in 62%; the liver is the most common site. Patients with glucagonoma syndrome also have a number of other disorders, such as glossodynia (beefy, sore tongue), angular cheilitis, normochromic normocytic anemia, an elevated sedimentation

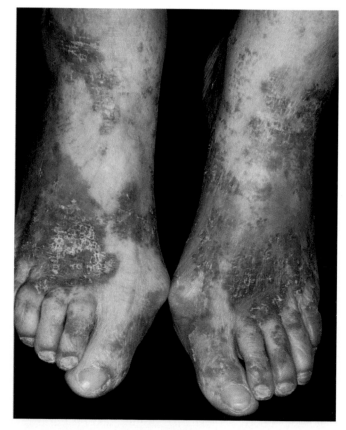

Figure 26-20
Glucagonoma syndrome. A gradually spreading irregular border. Central erythema, crusting, and hyperpigmentation are evident.

rate (30 to 100 mm/hour), and hypocholesterolemia. The tumors may secrete multiple hormones.[117]

Necrolytic migratory erythema. The dermatitis referred to as *necrolytic migratory erythema* begins as an erythematous area, progresses to superficial blisters, and gradually spreads ("migrates"), with central crusting and then healing, followed by hyperpigmentation 7 to 14 days after the initial erythema (Figure 26-20). The pattern is most evident on the perineum, lower legs, ankles, and feet. The process is more severe in areas of trauma and pressure. During its early evolution, necrolytic migratory erythema may elude recognition and be diagnosed as persistent subacute eczema. This early phase may last for months or years and precedes other clinical features of this syndrome.[118] The rash may be present with normal glucagon levels[119] and has been reported to improve with the depression of endocrine secretion by infusion of somatostatin,[120] somatostatin analogues,[121,122] and intravenous amino acids (Aminosyn).[123,124] The early histologic changes consist of cell death in the superficial epidermis; thus the designation *necrolytic*. The eruption clears shortly following resection of the tumor.[125,126] Dacarbazine cleared the eruption in one patient with an inoperative tumor.[127] The pathogenesis of necrolytic erythema is not understood. Hyperglucagonemia may not be a factor in its origin. Necrolytic migratory erythema has been reported in the absence of glucagonoma.[128] Hepatocellular dysfunction may be the key to the pathogenesis of the dermatitis.[129]

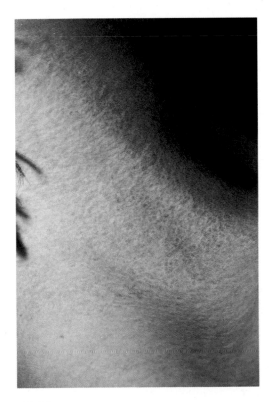

Figure 26-21
Pseudoxanthoma elasticum. Yellowish papules are found in flexural areas such as the neck and axillae.

Pseudoxanthoma Elasticum

Pseudoxanthoma elasticum (PXE) is an inherited defect of elastic tissue. There is both autosomal dominant and autosomal recessive inheritance. Ninety percent of patients appear to have an autosomal recessive inheritance pattern. The criteria for the diagnosis of PXE are listed in Table 26-4. All patients tend to merge into a single classic phenotype involving the skin, eyes, and cardiovascular system but with considerable variation in expression of the disorder. The name *pseudoxanthoma elasticum* refers only to the cutaneous aspect of the disease, although the skin is the least severely involved organ. The syndrome is characterized by flexurally distributed, yellowish papules; vascular complications, such as accelerated atherosclerosis; hypertension; intermittent claudication; gastrointestinal bleeding; angioid streaks in the ocular fundus; blindness; and many other disorders. Degenerative changes in the elastic fibers and connective tissue of the dermis, in the media and intima of the blood vessels, and in other organs cause the complications.

Skin lesions. The skin lesions consist of numerous tiny, yellowish papules arranged in lines in flexural areas. The most commonly affected sites are the neck and axillae (Figure 26-21). The appearance has been compared to the skin of a plucked chicken. The skin may be lax and hangs in folds. The lesions have a xanthomatous quality; thus the designation *pseudoxanthoma*. Degenerated and calcified elastic fibers are found internally and histologically in the skin.

Cardiovascular disease. In the absence of cardiac risk factors, patients with myocardial infarction or other signs of atherosclerotic vascular disease at an early age should be investigated for PXE. Calcification of the internal elastic laminae of the coronary arteries leads to narrowing of vessel lumina, resulting in symptoms similar to those of accelerated atherosclerosis.[130]

TABLE 26-4 Criteria for the Diagnosis of Pseudoxanthoma Elasticum

MAJOR CRITERIA

1. Characteristic skin involvement (yellow cobblestone lesions in flexural locations)
2. Characteristic histopathologic features of lesional skin (elastic tissue and calcium or von Kossa stains)
3. Characteristic ocular disease (angioid streaks, peau d'orange, or maculopathy) in adults older than 20 years of age

MINOR CRITERIA

1. Characteristic histopathologic features of nonlesional skin (elastic tissue and calcium or von Kossa stains)
2. Family history of PXE in first-degree relatives

From: Lebwohl M et al: *J Am Acad Dermatol* 30(1):103-107, 1994.

Ocular changes. Angioid streaks are present in the majority of patients with PXE. Angioid streaks look like irregular blood vessels. Degeneration of the elastic portion of Bruchs' membrane, a homogeneous layer that is located behind the retina, results in angioid streaks. Rents occur in Bruchs' membrane, followed by a proliferation of the pigment epithelium over the rents. Deep brown streaks simulating blood vessels radiate in a spokelike pattern directly beyond the optic disc. Retinal changes may first be observed after the age of 20. There may be a loss of central vision, and blindness may occur. Angioid streaks can also be found in Paget's disease and sickle cell anemia. Mottled hyperpigmentation is an early finding, consisting of a speckled, yellowish mottling of the posterior pole temporal to the macula. This appearance, called *peau d'orange*, is believed to be caused by changes in the retinal pigmented epithelium overlying a calcified and degenerating Bruchs' membrane. This finding is virtually pathognomonic of PXE and may be present in the first decade of the disease, prior to the appearance of the angioid streaks.[131]

Diagnosis. The absence of skin lesions should not be used to exclude the disorder. Histologic criteria are essential for the diagnosis of PXE. Fragmentation and clumping of elastic tissue occurs in the deep dermis of scars in randomly chosen sites and in normal-appearing flexural skin.[132,133] Verhoeff-van Gieson staining reveals the elastic tissue changes. Von Kossa stain shows calcified elastic tissue in the middle and deep dermis.

Eruptions of Pregnancy

Pregnant women experience a unique group of eruptions; some are well defined. Papular eruptions are the most common, but their status is confused by the variety of terms assigned to entities that appear to be closely related.

Three groups of diseases can be identified on the basis of primary lesions. The presence of no primary lesion but itching and excoriations indicates pruritus gravidarum. Pruritic papules, alone or concurrent with urticarial papules and plaques, indicates pruritic urticarial papules and plaques of pregnancy (PUPPP), prurigo gestationis, toxemic rash of pregnancy, or papular dermatitis of pregnancy. Vesicles and bullae arising from normal skin or from an urticarial base indicate herpes gestationis or impetigo herpetiformis.

The major concern with eruptions of pregnancy is the degree of discomfort produced and the potential for maternal and fetal morbidity and mortality. The majority of eruptions that occur during pregnancy are papular, are of a nonspecific nature, and clear after the mother delivers the child. The child is normal and unaffected by the disease. Itching is common during pregnancy; it causes discomfort, but it is benign and clears shortly after delivery.

The classification of the papular eruptions is confusing. The many diseases have been listed in preceding paragraphs. The only disease that has been carefully studied is PUPPP. It was thoroughly described in 1979, and most observers have discovered that the majority of papular eruptions of pregnancy conform to this well-defined category (see p. 140). Literature descriptions of other diseases varied slightly from those of PUPPP regarding the time of onset and distribution; therefore, unless further clarification is forthcoming, the papular eruptions of pregnancy are referred to as *PUPPP*. A papular eruption referred to as *papular dermatitis of pregnancy* associated with a 27% fetal mortality rate and elevated urinary chorionic gonadotropin has been reported, but there are only a few cases in the world literature. The vesicular and bullous diseases of pregnancy are very rare but very important. Rapid diagnosis and treatment may prevent potential serious complications.

PRURITUS GRAVIDARUM

Pruritus gravidarum is a condition of late pregnancy characterized by generalized itching without any primary lesion. It clears at delivery, may recur with successive pregnancies, and is benign. Pruritis occurs in approximately 3% to 14% of pregnant women and may be caused by the same diseases that affect nonpregnant women (e.g., urticaria, drug eruptions, scabies, atopic dermatitis, neurodermatitis, and pediculosis).

Prurigo gravidarum is characterized by generalized itching, with jaundice that results from bile salt accumulation in the skin. It usually appears in the last trimester of pregnancy and disappears at or shortly after delivery in 0.02% to 2.4% of pregnant women.[134] There are no lesions other than excoriations. Physiologic concentrations of estrogens and progestins are thought to interfere with hepatic excretion of bile salts and cause cholestasis in genetically predisposed women. A few patients, particularly those with itching early in pregnancy, become jaundiced and develop hepatomegaly, with laboratory evidence of hepatic cholestasis. The serum bilirubin levels may be normal or exceed 1.2 mg/100 ml, and serum transaminases may be elevated. Obstetric cholestasis has been associated with an increased incidence of premature labor, low fetal birth weight, and postpartum hemorrhage. Pruritus gravidarum clears spontaneously shortly after delivery but may recur with subsequent pregnancies or with use of estrogen-containing medications.

Mild itching is controlled with antipruritic lotions such as Sarna or Pramagel and oatmeal baths. Antihistamines do not control the pruritis caused by skin bile salt accumulation, but their sedative properties do offer some relief. Diphenhydramine and chlorpheniramine may be used safely during pregnancy. Severe cases are treated with the bile salt-sequestering ion-exchange resin cholestyramine, which binds bile acid in the intestine. It consistently relieves pruritis within 2 weeks, and the risks associated with cholestyramine use are minimal. Cholestyramine is distasteful and causes nausea, bloating, and constipation; but dosages of 12 to 16 gm daily cause infrequent side effects.[135]

HERPES GESTATIONIS

This rare, blistering disease of pregnancy is probably a variant of bullous pemphigoid and is described in Chapter Sixteen.

IMPETIGO HERPETIFORMIS

Impetigo herpetiformis is an extremely rare disease in which pustular lesions resemble pustular psoriasis; the disease may represent pustular psoriasis triggered by pregnancy. Superficial pustules appear at the advancing margin of mildly pruritic erythematous patches that originate in intertriginous areas. The lesions progress to involve wide areas of the skin. The fragile pustules rupture, leaving erosions that, after accumulating serum and crust, appear impetiginized. Hypocalcemia secondary to hypoparathyroidism is observed in some patients.[136] Without systemic steroids, the disease may be fatal for mother and fetus.

Guide to Information for Families with Inherited Skin Disorder

National Center for Education in Maternal and Child
  Health (NCEMCH)
38th and R Streets N.W.
Washington, DC 20057
(202) 625-8400

Alliance of Genetic Support Groups
1001 22nd Street, Suite 800
Washington, DC 20037
(202) 331-0942
(800) 336-GENE

National Organization for Rare Disorders (NORD)
P.O. Box 8923
New Fairfield, CT 06812
(203) 746-6518

National Neurofibromatosis Foundation, Inc.
141 Fifth Avenue, Suite 7-S
New York, NY 10010
(800) 323-7983 (outside New York)
(212) 460-8980

Tuberous Sclerosis Association of America, Inc.
  (TSAA)
P.O. Box 1305
Middleboro, MA 02370
(617) 947-8893

In addition to these organizations, most medical genetics centers are happy to provide information about such groups. The address and telephone number of the nearest center can be obtained by contacting the American Board of Medical Genetics, 9650 Rockville Pike, Bethesda, MD 20814; (301) 571-1825.

REFERENCES

1. McLean DI: Cutaneous paraneoplastic syndromes, *Arch Dermatol* 122:765-767, 1986.
2. Thiers BH: Dermatologic manifestations of internal cancer, CA-A CA, *J Clinicians* 36:130-148, 1986.
3. Callen JP: Skin signs of internal malignancy: fact, fancy, and fiction, *Semin Dermatol* 3:340-357, 1984.
4. Elewski BE, Gilgor RS: Eruptive lesions and malignancy, *Int J Dermatol* 24:617-629, 1985.
5. Ellis DL et al: Melanoma, growth factors, acanthosis nigricans, the sign of Leser-Trélat, and multiple acrochordons: a possible role for alpha-transforming growth factor in cutaneous paraneoplastic syndromes, *N Engl J Med* 317:1582-1587, 1987.
6. Abeloff MD: Paraneoplastic syndromes: a window on the biology of cancer, *N Engl J Med* 317:1598-1600, 1986.
7. Wilgenbus K, Lentner A, et al: Further evidence that acanthosis nigricans maligna is linked to enhanced secretion by the tumour of transforming growth factor alpha, *Arch Dermatol Res* 284:266-270, 1992.
8. Perez MI, Kohn SR: Cutaneous manifestations of diabetes mellitus, *J Am Acad Dermatol* 30:519-531, 1994.
9. Lowitt MH, Dover JS: Necrobiosis lipoidica, *J Am Acad Dermatol* 25:735-748, 1991.
10. Dwyer CM, Dick D: Ulceration in necrobiosis lipoidica—a case report and study, *Clin Exp Dermatol* 18:366-369, 1993.
11. Goette DK: Resolution of necrobiosis lipoidica with exclusive clobetasol propionate treatment, *J Am Acad Dermatol* 22:855-856, 1990.
12. Petzelbauer P, Wolff K, et al: Necrobiosis lipoidica: treatment with systemic corticosteroids, *Br J Dermatol* 126:542-545, 1992.
13. Noz KC, Korstanje MJ, et al: Ulcerating necrobiosis lipoidica effectively treated with pentoxifylline, *Clin Exp Dermatol* 18:78-79, 1993.
14. Statham B, Finlay AY, Marks R: A randomized double-blind comparison of an aspirin dipyridamole combination versus a placebo in the treatment of necrobiosis lipoidica, *Acta Derm Venereol* 61:270-271, 1981.
15. Eldor A, Diaz EG, Naparstek E: Treatment of diabetic necrobiosis with aspirin and dipyridamole, *N Engl J Med* 297:1033, 1977.
16. Beck H et al: Treatment of necrobiosis lipoidica with low-dose acetylsalicylic acid: a randomized double-blind trial, *Acta Derm Venereol* 65:230-234, 1985.
17. Karkavitsas K, Miller JA, Dowd PM, et al: Aspirin in the management of necrobiosis lipoidica, *Acta Derm Venereol* 62:183, 1982.
18. Unge G, Tornling G: Treatment of diabetic necrobiosis with aspirin or pipyridamole, *N Engl J Med* 299:1366, 1978.
19. Youshock E, Beninson J: Necrobiosis lipoidica: treatment with porcine dressings, split-thickness skin grafts and pressure garments: a case report and review of treatment modalities, *Angiology* 36:821-826, 1985.
20. Muhlbauer J: Granuloma annulare, *J Am Acad Dermatol* 3:217-230, 1980.
21. Huntley AC: The cutaneous manifestations of diabetes mellitus, *J Am Acad Dermatol* 7:427-455, 1982.
22. Muhlemann MF, Williams DRR: Localized granuloma annulare is associated with insulin-dependent diabetes mellitus, *Br J Dermatol* 111:325-329, 1984.
23. Haim S, Friedman-Birnbaum R, Shafrir A: Generalized granuloma annulare: relationship to diabetes mellitus as revealed in 8 cases, *Br J Dermatol* 83:302-305, 1970.
24. Friedman SJ, Winkelmann RK: Familial granuloma annulare: report of two cases and review of the literature, *J Am Acad Dermatol* 16:600-605, 1987.
25. Samlaska CP, Sandberg GD, et al: Generalized perforating granuloma annulare, *J Am Acad Dermatol* 27:319-322, 1992.
26. Davids JR, Kolman BH, et al: Subcutaneous granuloma annulare: recognition and treatment, *J Pediatr Orthop* 13:582-586, 1993.
27. Saied N, Schwartz RA, Estes SA: Treatment of generalized annulare with dapsone, *Arch Dermatol* 116:1345-1346, 1980.

28. Steiner A, Pehamberger H, Wolff K: Sulfone treatment of granuloma annulare, *J Am Acad Dermatol* 13:1004-1008, 1985.

29. Czarnecki DB, Gin D: The response of generalized granuloma annulare to dapsone, *Acta Derm Venereol* (Stockh) 66:82-84, 1986.

30. Schleicher SM, Milstein HJ: Resolution of disseminated granuloma annulare following isotretinoin therapy, *Cutis* Aug:147-148, 1985.

31. Botella-Estrada R, Guillen C, et al: Disseminated granuloma annulare: resolution with etretinate therapy, *J Am Acad Dermatol* 26:777, 1992.

32. Carlin MC, Ratz JL: A case of generalized granuloma annulare responding to hydroxychloroquine, *Cleve Clin J Med* 54:229-232, 1987.

33. Frankel DH, Medenica MM, Lorincz AL: Re: a case of generalized granuloma annulare responding to hydroxychloroquine, *Cleve Clin J Med* 55:117, 1988 (letter).

34. Stone OJ: Acanthosis nigricans—decreased extracellular matrix viscosity: cancer, obesity, diabetes, corticosteroids, somatotrophin, *Med Hypotheses* 40:154-157, 1993.

35. Hud J Jr, Cohen JB, et al: Prevalence and significance of acanthosis nigricans in an adult obese population, *Arch Dermatol* 128:941-944, 1992.

36. Cruz P Jr, Hud J Jr: Excess insulin binding to insulin-like growth factor receptors: proposed mechanism for acanthosis nigricans, *J Invest Dermatol* 98:82S-85S, 1992.

37. Tasjian D, Jarratt M: Familial acanthosis nigricans, *Arch Dermatol* 120:1351-1354, 1984.

38. Coates P, Shuttleworth D, et al: Resolution of nicotinic acid-induced acanthosis nigricans by substitution of an analogue (acipimox) in a patient with type V hyperlipidaemia, *Br J Dermatol* 126:412-414, 1992.

39. Pedro S: Drug-induced acanthosis nigricans, *N Engl J Med* 291:422, 1974.

40. Rigel DS, Jacobs MI: Malignant acanthosis nigricans: a review, *J Dermatol Surg Oncol* 6:923-927, 1980.

41. Curth HO et al: The site and histology of the cancer associated with acanthosis nigricans, *Cancer* 15:433-439, 1962.

42. Brown J, Winkelmann RK: Acanthosis nigricans: study of 90 cases, *Medicine* 47:33-56, 1968.

43. Moller DE, Flier JS: Insulin resistance—mechanisms, syndromes, and implications, *N Eng J Med* 325:938-948, 1991.

44. Stuart CA et al: Insulin resistance with acanthosis nigricans: the roles of obesity and androgen excess, *Metabolism* 35:197-205, 1986.

45. Stuart CA, Pate CJ, et al: Prevalence of acanthosis nigricans in an unselected population, *Am J Med* 87:269-272, 1989.

46. Plourde PV, Marks JG Jr, Hammond JM: Acanthosis nigricans and insulin resistance, *J Am Acad Dermatol* 10:887-891, 1984.

47. Cohen P, Harel C, et al: Insulin resistance and acanthosis nigricans: evidence for a postbinding defect in vivo, *Metabolism* 39:1006-1011, 1990.

48. Rendon MI, Cruz P Jr, et al: Acanthosis nigricans: a cutaneous marker of tissue resistance to insulin, *J Am Acad Dermatol* 21:461-469, 1989.

49. Grasinger CC, Wild RA, et al: Vulvar acanthosis nigricans: a marker for insulin resistance in hirsute women, *Fertil Steril* 59:583-586, 1993.

50. Darmstadt GL, Yokel BK, Horn TD: Treatment of acanthosis nigricans with tretinoin, *Arch Dermatol* 127:1139-1140, 1991.

51. Katz RA: Treatment of acanthosis nigricans with oral isotretinoin, *Arch Dermatol* 116:110-111, 1980.

52. Cruz PD Jr, East C, Bergstresser PR: Dermal, subcutaneous, and tendon xanthomas: diagnostic markers for specific lipoprotein disorders, *J Am Acad Dermatol* 19:95-111, 1988.

53. Fredrickson DS, Lees RS: A system for phenotyping hyperlipoproteinemia, *Circulation* 31:321-327, 1965.

54. Parker F: Xanthomas and hyperlipidemias, *J Am Acad Dermatol* 13:1-30, 1985.

55. Schaefer EJ, Levy RI: Pathogenesis and management of lipoprotein disorders, *N Engl J Med* 312:1300-1310, 1985.

56. Bergman R: The pathogenesis and clinical significance of xanthelasma palpebrarum, *J Am Acad Dermatol* 30:236-242, 1994.

57. Douste-Blazy P et al: Increased frequency of Apo E-ND phenotype and hyperapobeta-lipoproteinemia in normolipidemic subjects with xanthelasmas of the eyelids, *Ann Intern Med* 96:164-169, 1982.

58. Mulvihill JJ, Parry DM, et al: NIH conference. Neurofibromatosis 1 (Recklinghausen disease) and neurofibromatosis 2 (bilateral acoustic neurofibromatosis). An update, *Ann Intern Med* 113:39-52, 1990.

59. Crowe FW, Schull WJ, Neel JV: A clinical, pathologic, and genetic study of multiple neurofibromatosis, *Adv Neurol* 29:33-56, 1981.

60. Hope DG, Mulvihill JJ: Malignancy in neurofibromatosis, *Adv Neurol* 29:33-56, 1981.

61. Williamson TH, Garner A, et al: Structure of Lisch nodules in neurofibromatosis type 1, *Ophthalmic Paediatr Genet* 12:11-17, 1991.

62. Lewis RA, Riccardi VM: von Recklinghausen neurofibromatosis: incidence of iris hamartomata, *Ophthalmology* 88:348-354, 1981.

63. Lubs ML, Bauer MS, et al: Lisch nodules in neurofibromatosis type 1, *N Engl J Med* 324:1264-1266, 1991.

64. Toonstra J et al: Are Lisch nodules an ocular marker of the neurofibromatosis gene in otherwise unaffected family members? *Dermatologica* 174:232, 1987.

65. Sorensen SA, Mulvihill JJ, Nielsen A: Long-term follow-up of von Recklinghausen neurofibromatosis, *N Engl J Med* 314:1010-1015, 1986.

66. Neurofibromatosis Conference Statement: National Institutes of Health Consensus Development Conference, *Arch Neurol* 45:575-578, 1988.

67. Trattner A, David M, et al: Segmental neurofibromatosis, *J Am Acad Dermatol* 23:866-869, 1990.

68. Riccardi VM: Neurofibromatosis: the importance of localized or otherwise atypical forms, *Arch Dermatol* 123:882-883, 1987.

69. Roth RR, Martines R, James WD: Segmental neurofibromatosis, *Arch Dermatol* 123:917-920, 1987.

70. Miller M, Hall JG: Possible maternal effect on severity of neurofibromatosis, *Lancet* 11:1071, 1978.

71. Riccardi VM: Neurofibromatosis: past, present, and future, *N Engl J Med* 324:1283-1285, 1991.

72. Sloan JB, Fretzin DF, et al: Genetic counseling in segmental neurofibromatosis, *J Am Acad Dermatol* 22:461-467, 1990.

73. Truhan AP, Filipek PA: Magnetic resonance imaging. Its role in the neuroradiologic evaluation of neurofibromatosis, tuberous sclerosis, and Sturge-Weber syndrome, *Arch Dermatol* 129:219-226, 1993.

74. Shu HH, Mirowitz SA, et al: Neurofibromatosis: MR imaging findings involving the head and spine, *AJR* 160:159-164, 1993.

75. Nickel WR, Reed WB: Tuberous sclerosis, *Arch Dermatol* 85:209-226, 1962.

76. Hurwitz S, Braverman IM: White spots in tuberous sclerosis, *J Pediatr* 77:587-594, 1970.

77. Roth JC, Epstein CJ: Infantile spasms and hypopigmented macules: early manifestations of tuberous sclerosis, *Arch Neurol* 20:547-567, 1971.

78. Fois A et al: Early signs of tuberous sclerosis in infancy and childhood, *Helv Paediatr Acta* 28:313-321, 1973.

79. Jozwiak S: Diagnostic value of clinical features and supplementary investigations in tuberous sclerosis in children, *Acta Paediatr Hung* 32:71-88, 1992.

80. McWilliam RC, Stephenson JBP: Depigmented hair: the earliest sign of tuberous sclerosis, *Arch Dis Child* 53:961, 1978.

81. Burkhart CG, El-Shaar A: Computerized axial tomography in the early diagnosis of tuberous sclerosis, *J Am Acad Dermatol* 4:59-63, 1981.

82. Mlynarczyk G: Enamel pitting. A common sign of tuberous sclerosis, *Ann N Y Acad Sci* 615:367-369, 1991.

83. Northrup H, Kwiatkowski DJ, et al: Evidence for genetic heterogeneity in tuberous sclerosis: one locus on chromosome 9 and at least one locus elsewhere, *Am J Hum Genet* 51:709-720, 1992.

84. Menor F, Marti-Bonmati L, et al: Neuroimaging in tuberous sclerosis: a clinicoradiological evaluation in pediatric patients, *Pediatr Radiol* 22:485-489, 1992.

85. Brownstein MH et al: The dermatopathology of Cowden's syndrome, *Br J Dermatol* 100:667-673, 1979.
86. Salem OS, Steck WD: Cowden's disease (multiple hamartoma and neoplasia syndrome): a case report and review of the English literature, *J Am Acad Dermatol* 8:686-696, 1983.
87. Williard W, Borgen P, et al: Cowden's disease. A case report with analyses at the molecular level, *Cancer* 69:2969-2974, 1992.
88. Walton BJ et al: Cowden's disease: a further indication for prophylactic mastectomy, *Surgery* 90:82-86, 1986.
89. Rothenberg J, Lambert WC, et al: The Muir-Torre (Torre's) syndrome: the significance of a solitary sebaceous tumor, *J Am Acad Dermatol* 23:638-640, 1990.
90. Torre D: Multiple sebaceous tumors, *Arch Dermatol* 98:549-557, 1968.
91. Cohen PR, Kohn SR, et al: Association of sebaceous gland tumors and internal malignancy: the Muir-Torre syndrome, *Am J Med* 90:606-613, 1991.
92. Cohen PR: Muir-Torre syndrome in patients with hematologic malignancies, *Am J Hematol* 40:64-65, 1992.
93. Finan MC, Connolly SM: Sebaceous gland tumors and systemic disease: a clinicopathologic analysis, *Medicine* 63:232, 1984.
94. Bisceglia M, Zenarola P: Muir-Torre syndrome: a case report, *Tumori* 77:277-281, 1991.
95. Lynch HT, Lynch PM, Pester J, et al: The cancer family syndrome: rare cutaneous phenotypic linkage of Torre's syndrome, *Ann Intern Med* 141:607-611, 1981.
96. Burke AP, Sobin LH, et al: Mesenteric fibromatosis. A follow-up study, *Arch Pathol Lab Med* 114:832-835, 1990.
97. Zissiadis A, Harlaftis N, et al: Desmoid tumor in Gardner's syndrome, *Am Surg* 56:305-307, 1990.
98. Jones K, Korzcak P: The diagnostic significance and management of Gardner's syndrome, *Br J Oral Maxillofac Surg* 28:80-84, 1990.
99. Sanchez MA et al: Be aware of Gardner's syndrome: a review of the literature, *Am J Gastroenterol* 71:68-73, 1979.
100. Paraskeva C, Williams AC: Cell and molecular biology of gastrointestinal tract cancer, *Curr Opin Oncol* 4:707-713, 1992.
101. Pathak S, Hopwood VL, et al: Identification of colon cancer–predisposed individuals: a cytogenetic analysis, *Am J Gastroenterol* 86:679-684, 1991.
102. Powell SM, Petersen GM, et al: Molecular diagnosis of familial adenomatous polyposis, *N Engl J Med* 329:1982-1987, 1993.
103. Leppard B, Bussey HJR: Epidermoid cysts, polyposis coli and Gardner's syndrome, *Br J Surg* 62:387-393, 1975.
104. Halling F, Merten HA, et al: Clinical and radiological findings in Gardner's syndrome: a case report and follow-up study, *Dentomaxillofac Radiol* 21:93-98, 1992.
105. Traboulsi EI, Maumenee IH, et al: Congenital hypertrophy of the retinal pigment epithelium predicts colorectal polyposis in Gardner's syndrome, *Arch Ophthalmol* 108:525-526, 1990.
106. Iwama T, Mishima Y, et al: Association of congenital hypertrophy of the retinal pigment epithelium with familial adenomatous polyposis, *Br J Surg* 77:273-276, 1990.
107. Traboulsi EI, Murphy SF, et al: A clinicopathologic study of the eyes in familial adenomatous polyposis with extracolonic manifestations (Gardner's syndrome), *Am J Ophthalmol* 110:550-561, 1990.
108. Traboulsi EI et al: Prevalence and importance of pigmented ocular fundus lesions in Gardner's syndrome, *N Engl J Med* 316:661-667, 1987.
109. Kelly MD, Hugh TB, et al: Carcinoma of the thyroid gland and Gardner's syndrome, *Aust N Z J Surg* 63:505-509, 1993.
110. Bell B, Mazzaferri EL: Familial adenomatous polyposis (Gardner's syndrome) and thyroid carcinoma. A case report and review of the literature, *Dig Dis Sci* 38:185-190, 1993.
111. Giardiello FM, Hamilton SR, et al: Treatment of colonic and rectal adenomas with sulindac in familial adenomatous polyposis, *N Engl J Med* 328:1313-1316, 1993.
112. Binnick AN et al: Glucagonoma syndrome, *Arch Dermatol* 113:749-754, 1977.
113. Leichter S: Clinical and metabolic aspects of glucagonoma, *Medicine* 59:100-113, 1980.
114. Wynick D, Hammond PJ, et al: The glucagonoma syndrome, *Clin Dermatol* 11:93-97, 1993.
115. Kasper CS: Necrolytic migratory erythema: unresolved problems in diagnosis and pathogenesis. A case report and literature review, *Cutis* 49:120-122, 1992.
116. Wawrukiewicz AS et al: Glucagonoma and its angiographic diagnosis, *Cardiovasc Intervent Radiol* 5:318-324, 1982,
117. Dohlsten M, Hallberg T: Immunological studies in a patient with the glucagonoma syndrome, *Acta Med Scand* 218:251-255, 1985.
118. Hunt SJ, Narus VT, Abell E: Necrolytic migratory erythema: Dyskeratotic dermatitis, a clue to early diagnosis, *J Am Acad Dermatol* 24:473-477, 1991.
119. Hashizume T et al: Glucagonoma syndrome, *J Am Acad Dermatol* 19:377-383, 1988.
120. Elsborg L, Glenthoj A: Effect of somatostatin in necrolytic migratory erythema of glucagonoma, *Acta Med Scand* 218:245-249, 1985.
121. Wood SM, Kraenzlin ME, Adrian TE, et al: Treatment of patients with pancreatic endocrine tumours using a new long-acting somatostatin analogue: symptomatic and peptide responses, *Gut* 26:438-444, 1985.
122. Boden G et al: Treatment of inoperable glucagonoma with the long-acting somatostatin analogue SMS 201-995, *N Engl J Med* 314:1686-1688, 1986.
123. Norton JA et al: Amino acid deficiency and the skin rash associated with glucagonoma, *Ann Intern Med* 91:213-215, 1979.
124. Shepherd ME, Raimer SS, et al: Treatment of necrolytic migratory erythema in glucagonoma syndrome, *J Am Acad Dermatol* 25:925-928, 1991.
125. Reyes-Govea J, Holm A, et al: Response of glucagonomas to surgical excision and chemotherapy. Report of two cases and review of the literature, *Am Surg* 55:523-527, 1989.
126. Edney JA, Hofmann S, et al: Glucagonoma syndrome is an under-diagnosed clinical entity, *Am J Surg* 160:625-628, 1990.
127. van der Loos TLJM, Lambrecht ER, Lambers JCCA: Successful treatment of glucagonoma-related necrolytic migratory erythema with dacarbazine, *J Am Acad Dermatol* 16:468-472, 1987.
128. Marin-Kovich MP et al: Necrolytic migratory erythema without glucagonoma in patients with liver disease, *J Am Acad Dermatol* 32:604-609, 1995.
129. Kasper CS, McMurry K: Necrolytic migratory erythema without glucagonoma versus canine superficial necrolytic dermatitis: is hepatic impairment a clue to pathogenesis? *J Am Acad Dermatol* 25:534-541, 1991.
130. Lebwohl M et al: Brief report: occult pseudoxanthoma elasticum in patients with premature cardiovascular disease, *N Engl J Med* 329:1237-1239, 1993.
131. Pisani M, Rossi A, et al: Mottled hyperpigmentation of the fundus oculi associated with angioid streaks in pseudoxanthoma elasticum, *G Ital Dermatol Venereol* 125:569-574, 1990.
132. Lebwohl M et al: Diagnosis of pseudoxanthoma elasticum by scar biopsy in patients without characteristic skin lesions, *N Engl J Med* 317:347-350, 1987.
133. Hausser I, Anton-Lamprecht I: Early preclinical diagnosis of dominant pseudoxanthoma elasticum by specific ultrastructural changes of dermal elastic and collagen tissue in a family at risk, *Hum Genet* 87:693-700, 1991.
134. Winton GB, Lewis CW: Dermatosis of pregnancy, *J Am Acad Dermatol* 6:977-998, 1982.
135. Noguera X, Puig L, De Moragas JM: Prurigo gravidarum, *Cutis* 39:437-440, 1987.
136. Thio HB, Vermeer BJ: Hypocalcemia in impetigo herpetiformis: a secondary transient phenomenon? *Arch Dermatol* 127:1587-1588, 1991.

CHAPTER TWENTY-SEVEN

Dermatologic Surgical Procedures

Punch biopsy, shave biopsy, electrodesiccation and curettage, blunt dissection, and simple excision and suture closure are the basic techniques that physicians who treat skin disease should learn. One should be familiar with the more sophisticated techniques, such as dermabrasion and Mohs' micrographic surgery, so that referral to physicians who perform these techniques can be made at the proper time. The instruments used for most basic dermatologic surgical procedures are shown in Figure 27-1.

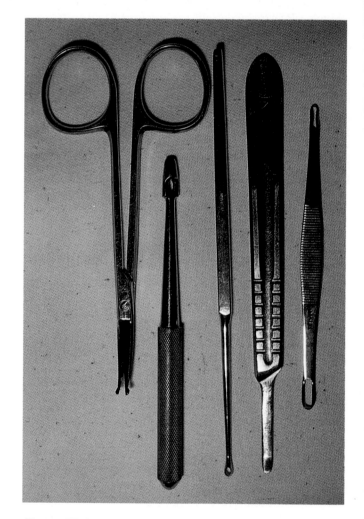

Figure 27-1
Instruments used for basic dermatologic surgical procedures. From left to right: curved probe-tipped scissors, 3-mm dermal punch, #1 curet, blunt dissector, Schamberg comedo expressor.

Local Anesthesia

Lidocaine (Xylocaine) 1% or 2%, with or without epinephrine, is used for most surgical procedures.[1] The onset of anesthesia is almost instantaneous, and the duration is adequate for most minor procedures. A 27- or, preferably, a 30-gauge needle is used.

Epinephrine. The vasoconstriction induced by epinephrine prevents absorption of lidocaine, prolongs anesthesia, and controls bleeding. Xylocaine with epinephrine is generally not used on fingertips. Very small quantities are usually tolerated on the nose and pinna.

Lidocaine allergy. Allergy to lidocaine is very rare.[2,3] Most patients who claim to be allergic have had a vasovagal response. Bacteriostatic saline is an alternative for patients who are allergic to lidocaine (see below).

Pain reduction. Anesthetics produce a sharp pain during skin infiltration. Pain is greater with rapid injections and can be minimized with slow injections through a 30-gauge needle. The needle should be inserted slowly but firmly into the dermis. Anesthesia is initiated by injecting a tiny amount of fluid; after a few seconds, infiltration is continued slowly until the skin surrounding the lesion blanches. Pinching the skin in the area to be injected either distracts the patient or blocks the transmission of pain impulses caused by the injections. A wheal can be raised by inserting the needle almost vertically. Penetration of the thick palm and sole skin is very painful. The area about the nostrils is very sensitive. Intrafollicular injection into the large follicles of the nose and cheeks minimizes pain. Superficial injections into the penis and vulva are well tolerated.

Painless anesthesia. Icing the lesion for 1 minute numbs the skin and minimizes needle-penetration pain. Adequate anesthesia with little or no infiltration pain can be induced with the following preparations. Bacteriostatic saline and lidocaine diluted with bacteriostatic saline solution are less painful than 1% lidocaine with sodium bicarbonate. It is unlikely that the pain of infiltration is a simple function of the pH of the anesthetic solution.[4]

Bacteriostatic saline. Commercially available bacteriostatic saline contains benzyl alcohol, which acts as a painless anesthetic. The anesthetic effect dissipates rapidly when injected subcutaneously. The volume of saline required to achieve anesthesia is at least 2 to 3 times that required when using 1% lidocaine and is of brief duration.

Saline and epinephrine. The addition of epinephrine 3 ml of 1 mg/ml (1:100,000 dil.) to 30 ml of bacteriostatic saline extends the duration of anesthesia from 4 minutes to 120 minutes. Bacteriostatic saline should not be used as an anesthetic for newborns.

Saline diluted with lidocaine. A mixture of saline (27 ml) and lidocaine 1% with or without epinephrine (3 ml) is also effective.

Buffered lidocaine. The addition of sodium bicarbonate reduces the pain produced by infiltration of lidocaine with or without epinephrine.[5] One milliliter of Neutra-Caine,* a 7.5% sodium bicarbonate buffer solution, is added to 5 ml of lidocaine or bupivacaine. Buffered lidocaine and epinephrine maintain greater than a 90% concentration 2 weeks after buffering when stored at 0° to 4° C. This permits batch buffering and storage for up to 2 weeks when properly refrigerated.[6] $NaHCO_3$ enhances the killing effect that has been described for lidocaine alone. The inability to recover common pathogenic bacteria from biopsy specimens could be the result of exposure to lidocaine buffered with $NaHCO_3$. Warming the local mixture to 40° C reduces the discomfort of injection even further.[7]

The ice-saline–lidocaine technique. This is a simple method of minimizing pain when obtaining local anesthesia. Cryogel packs are applied before the local anesthesic injection to minimize the pain of piercing the skin with the injection needle. The surgical field is then infiltrated with benzyl alcohol–containing normal saline. Subsequently, lidocaine with epinephrine can be infiltrated without discomfort.[8]

EMLA. EMLA is a mixture of 2.5% lidocaine and 2.5% prilocaine in an oil and water emulsion. EMLA should be applied to the desired area for approximately 1 hour under an occlusive dressing. It provides an effective analgesic making it useful for superficial surgery, split-thickness skin grafts, venipuncture, argon laser treatment, epilation, and debridement of infected ulcers. Other indications have included use in postherpetic neuralgia, hyperhidrosis, painful ulcers, and inhibition of itching and burning.[9]

Hemostasis

Monsel's solution (ferric subsulfate) is a valuable agent for providing rapid hemostasis. It is particularly effective in controlling bleeding after curettage of seborrheic keratosis and basal cell carcinoma. Immediate hemostasis is most efficiently achieved if the solution is applied when the wound is not bleeding. To exert tension and stop bleeding, the thumb and index finger are placed at the opposite edges of the wound and the skin is stretched. The blood is then wiped with gauze, the Monsel's solution is applied with a cotton-tipped applicator, and the tension is maintained for approximately 15 seconds. The lack of blood flow apparently allows more complete coagulation.

Monsel's artifact. When a biopsy is repeated, an area of skin that has been treated with Monsel's solution has a pigmented artifact that can interfere with histologic interpretation. The use of Monsel's solution should be avoided after biopsies of pigmented lesions or tumors that may prove to be diagnostic problems. The pathologist should be informed if Monsel's solution had been used.[10]

---

*Available from M.D., Inc., 6008/5748 Fort Henry Dr., Rt. 16, Kingsport, TN 37663; (615) 239-3410.

Wound Healing

Types of Cutaneous Wounds

Full-thickness wounds. The epidermis and the full thickness of the dermis are lost. The defect is deeper than the adnexa (hair follicles, eccrine sweat ducts). These wounds heal by contraction (associated with myofibroblast development), granulation tissue formation (with fibroplasia and neovascularization), and reepithelialization. Contraction causes a 40% decrease in the size of the wound. Epithelialization occurs from the wound edges.

Partial-thickness wounds. The epidermis and some portion of the dermis with parts of the adnexa remain in the wound bed. Such wounds are produced by shave excisions, curettage and electrodesiccation, dermabrasion, chemical peels, and carbon dioxide (CO_2) laser surgery. These wounds heal quickly through reepithelialization from the wound edges and adnexal structures in the base of the wound. Wound contraction is minimal when only the most superficial portion of the dermis has been lost.

Physiology of wound healing

Wound contraction and scar formation. Wound contraction begins at 1 week after the wound occurs. Light colonization with pathogenic bacteria may not interfere, but infection inhibits healing. Tensile strength in a wound increases progressively up to 1 year after the wound occurs. Tensile strength in a healed wound is always less than 80% of normal. Healing time is related to the logarithm of the area. The width of the wound is a better predictor of healing time than is the area in which the wound occurred. Wounds created by destructive techniques (e.g., cryosurgery, electrosurgery, laser surgery, and chemical cautery) heal more slowly than clean wounds created by scalpel or curet surgery.

Cellular changes. Neutrophils appear in a wound 6 hours after the event, reach their greatest number after 24 to 48 hours, and start to disappear after 72 hours. Neutrophils are not crucial to wound healing; neutropenia does not interfere with healing. Fibroblasts populate the wound after 48 to 72 hours. Their growth is enhanced by low oxygen and high lactate levels. Fibroblasts synthesize collagen and elastin.

Myofibroblasts are modified fibroblasts that resemble smooth muscle cells in morphology and function. They contain large amounts of contractile proteins and are responsible for wound contraction.[11]

Reepithelialization. Epidermal healing first depends on epidermal cell migration (first 24 hours) and later on epidermal cell mitosis, which peaks after 48 hours. Keratinocytes initially migrate over a matrix of fibronectin, fibrin, collagen, and elastin. This matrix acts as a structural support for cell migration. Epidermal migration and proliferation occur from the epithelial cells at the edge of the wound and from appendageal structures remaining in the wound bed. The rate of reepithelialization is directly related to the moistness of the wound. Open, dry wounds reepithelialize slower than occluded, moist wounds. The migration of keratinocytes beneath a dry crust is slower than migration over an occluded, moist wound, where the plane of epithelial cell migration lies near the wound surface (Figure 27-2).

Impairment of Wound Healing

Topical therapy. Topical steroids may interfere with healing because of their antiinflammatory action (Table 27-1).

Antiseptic solutions. One percent povidone-iodine, 3% hydrogen peroxide, and 0.5% chlorhexidine solutions are toxic for fibroblasts and keratinocytes and may delay the formation of granulation tissue.

Hemostatic solutions. Monsel's solution (ferric subsulfate), 30% aluminum chloride, and silver nitrate produce tissue necrosis and delay reepithelialization. The effect on small wounds is minimal.

Contact Dermatitis

Contact allergic reactions may occur with tapes and antibiotic ointments. Neomycin is a common sensitizer and should be avoided. Polysporin and Bacitracin are not common sensitizers.

Systemic factors. Malnutrition interferes with healing. Vitamin C and zinc deficiencies lead to poor healing. Systemic steroids in a dosage greater than 10 mg a day interfere with healing. Clinical experience suggests no impairment of wound healing for patients taking chemotherapeutic drugs.

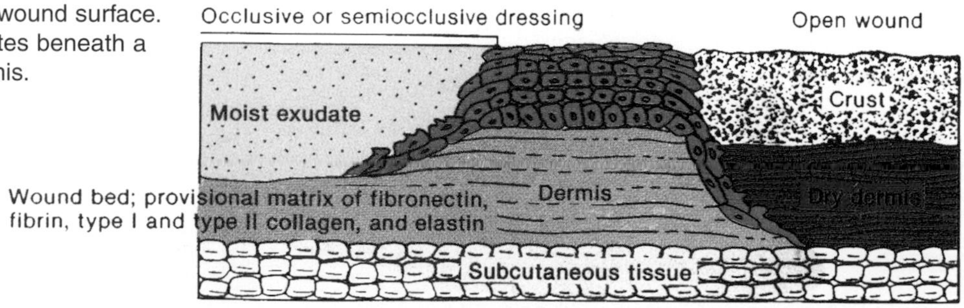

Figure 27-2
Occlusive dressing. The effects of tissue humidity on reepithelialization are shown. Occlusive dressings allow epithelialization to occur at the wound surface. In open wounds the epithelium migrates beneath a desiccated crust and devitalized dermis.

Occlusive or semiocclusive dressing   Open wound

Moist exudate   Crust

Wound bed; provisional matrix of fibronectin, fibrin, type I and type II collagen, and elastin   Dermis   Dry dermis

Subcutaneous tissue

TABLE 27-1 Topical Agents that Affect Epidermal Migration

Agents	Relative rate of healing (%)*
Triamcinolone acetonide ointment (0.1%)	−34
Furacin	−30
USP Petrolatum	−8
Eucerin	+5
Benoxyl lotion base (benzoyl peroxide preparation)	+14
Silvadene cream	+28
Neosporin ointment	+28
Telfa dressing	+14

*Compared with untreated

Wound dressings

Wound dressings—mechanism of action. Occlusion of wounds leads to faster healing.[12] The process of neovascularization within granulation tissue is stimulated by hypoxic conditions such as those that occur beneath occlusive, oxygen-impermeable dressings. Occlusive dressings prevent crust formation and drying of the wound bed. The rate of epithelialization is faster under occlusive dressings. Wound fluid under occlusive dressings is favorable to fibroblast proliferation. Adhesive occlusive dressings may remove newly formed epithelium. Hydrocolloid adhesive occlusive dressings prevent entry of bacteria into the wound. The use of occlusive dressings in chronic wounds leads to less pain, better granulation tissue, and painless wound debridement. In acute wounds, occlusive dressings promote bacterial growth but result in faster reepithelialization.

Function. Protection with dressings exerts pressure and maintains a moist wound environment. They reduce pain when applied to partial-thickness wounds. Topical antimicrobial agents that may enhance reepithelialization include neomycin, polymyxin B, Neosporin ointment, silver sulfadiazine, and 20% benzoyl peroxide lotion. Hexachlorophene, chlorhexidine, and alcohol may retard reepithelialization.[13]

Occlusive dressings. Crust formation is suppressed if the surface of the wound is kept moist by an occlusive film or by gauze applied over Polysporin. The level of adequate tissue humidity is then very close to the skin surface, and the epidermis migrates rapidly over the moist bed. Patients treated with occlusive dressings tend to have softer, smoother, smaller, and more superficial scars. There does not seem to be an increased incidence of infection with occlusive dressings. Occlusive dressings reduce wound pain. So-called oxygen-permeable membranes do not seem to transmit oxygen to the wound.[14] Many synthetic occlusive dressings are available for a variety of wounds (see the Formulary); examples of clinical uses include the following:

- Arterial and venous catheter sites
- Burns
- Decubitus ulcers
- Dermabrasion site after tattoo removal
- Leg ulcers following pinch grafts
- Mohs' micrographic wounds
- Skin graft donor sites
- Stasis ulcers
- Surgical incisions
- Traumatic wounds

Application techniques

OCCLUSIVE DRESSINGS. Occlusive dressings (Duoderm CGF, etc.) are best suited to chronic wounds, such as venous ulcers. Good preparation of surrounding skin by cleansing with hydrogen peroxide and drying with gauze ensures secure adhesion. Excess skin oil is removed with alcohol. At least 2.5 cm of margin around the wound should be allowed to prevent leakage. The length of time occlusive dressings should stay on a wound varies; dressings should be left in place until they start leaking fluid from their sides. Early removal of dressings can lead to stripping of delicate new epithelium. Initially, dressings usually need to be changed every other day. Thereafter they may be left in place for many days if excess fluid does not accumulate. Dressings applied over fresh wounds accumulate large amounts of fluid that can be removed by needle aspiration. Patients who disrupt new epithelium by careless removal of adherent dressings should use a nonadherent dressing such as Vigilon.[15] Dressings should not be applied to inflamed eczematous skin at the borders of stasis ulcers.

SEMIPERMEABLE DRESSINGS. Semipermeable dressings (Opsite, Tegaderm, Vigilon, and Biobrane) are an option for partial-thickness open wounds. These are changed when the amount of wound exudate becomes excessive. Vigilon is an oxygen-permeable dressing that consists of 4% polyethylene oxide and 96% water. It absorbs its own weight of exudate and, with the exterior polyethylene film removed, excess exudate can be absorbed by overlying absorbent dressings. Vigilon is nonadherent and maintains a moist wound environment. Vigilon is removed and a new dressing is applied every 24 to 48 hours.

Postoperative Wound Care (see the box below)

Partial and full-thickness open wounds

1. Avoid alcohol and aspirin in the immediate postoperative period.
2. Keep wounds covered and moist (e.g., with Polysporin or Bacitracin) to prevent crusts.
3. Bathing of granulating wounds is allowed. Avoid cleansing with hydrogen peroxide or povidone-iodine.
4. Undressed sutured wounds can be washed with soap and water twice a day starting the morning after surgery.

Sutured Wounds
Office

1. Semipermeable tape strips (e.g., Steristrips, Clearon skin closures) reduce tension across the suture line. Spaces left between the strips allow wound exudate to escape and to be absorbed by the overlying dressing.
2. A nonadherent primary dressing may then be applied, taped in place, and covered with a pressure dressing applied (bulky gauze) and secured by adhesive tape.
3. Tissue adhesives (tincture of benzoin, Mastisol) are applied to the skin to increase the adherence of tape to the skin.
4. Pressure dressings (applied for 24 to 36 hours) reduce the risk of hematoma formation following the excision of cysts.

Home. Small wounds do not require dressing for more than 24 to 48 hours.

1. Change dressing once or twice daily. The dressing may be left in place for uncomplicated dry wounds until the sutures are removed.
2. Cleanse with a mild liquid soap, sterile saline, or hydrogen peroxide solution.
3. An antibiotic ointment (e.g., Bacitracin) is applied and the wound is covered with a nonadherent dressing. The antibiotic ointment reduces the risk of the contact layer of the dressing adhering to the wound bed.
4. A pressure dressing is applied if required.

Excess granulation tissue. Granulation tissue is a loose collection of fibroblasts, inflammatory cells, and new vessels in an edematous matrix that forms at the base of open wounds. It provides a foundation for reepithelialization. Excessive granulation tissue rises above the wound surface, imposing a barrier to the inward-migrating epidermis. Certain areas, such as the scalp, temples, and lower legs, are prone to form exuberant granulation tissue in open surgical wounds or ulcers. Excess granulation tissue must be removed or suppressed. One technique is to curet the tissue and paint the open wound base daily with mercurochrome.

SCARLET RED GAUZE. Recurrent granulation tissue can be very effectively suppressed with scarlet red gauze, which is available in prepackaged wrappers. The deep purple-colored gauze is applied over the tissue, covered with white gauze, and secured with tape. The dressing is changed daily until reepithelialization is complete. The results can be amazing.

Scar formation. The evolution of a scar takes several months. New scars are thick and vascular, but gradually, over months, they become less vascular, nonbulky, and flat. Scars that remain thick (hypertrophic scars) or become inappropriately large (keloids) can be treated with intralesional steroids (see Chapter Twenty).

WOUND MANAGEMENT GUIDELINES

1. Use antiseptics for disinfection of intact skin only.
2. Select a method of wounding that minimizes tissue necrosis.
3. Use pinpoint electrocoagulation, pressure, topical thrombin, collagen, or gelatin rather than caustic agents to establish hemostasis.
4. Apply topical antibiotics to the wound instead of antiseptics to prevent wound infection and to accelerate healing.
5. Substitute tap water for hydrogen peroxide to cleanse wounds.
6. Use nonadherent occlusive dressing on wounds to accelerate healing.

From Brown CD, Zitelli JA: *J Dermatol Surg Oncol* 19:732-737, 1993.

Skin Biopsy

A skin biopsy can be performed simply in the office. Several techniques are practiced, and each has specific advantages (Table 27-2).

Choice of site. Generally, biopsies should not be taken from lesions below the knee if other sites are available. Specimens from this area are sometimes difficult for the pathologist to interpret, particularly specimens taken from older patients, in whom mild inflammation and pigmentation produced by stasis may be present. On the face, particularly in the elderly, the arteries are superficial at the following three locations: the temple lateral to the eyebrow (the temporal artery), the nasolabial fold as it intersects the alae (angular artery), and the supraorbital notch at the medial end of the brow (the supraorbital artery). Arteries may be injured by a deep punch biopsy at these sites.

Selection of lesion for biopsy. As a general rule, biopsies should be taken from lesions that are fresh but well developed. Very early lesions may not have developed diagnostic histologic features, and older lesions may be excoriated or crusted. However, it is important to perform biopsies of very early lesions for diagnosis of vesiculobullous diseases, such as pemphigus and dermatitis herpetiformis. Chronic diseases such as discoid lupus erythematosus may not develop diagnostic features for weeks; biopsies of older lesions should be performed in these cases.

PUNCH BIOPSY

A full thickness of skin can easily be obtained with a cylindric dermal punch biopsy tool. Disposable punches are very convenient (e.g., the Baker-Cummins punch). They are available in 2-mm, 3-mm, 3.5-mm, 4-mm, and 6-mm widths. The 3-mm punch is adequate for most lesions. Biopsies of the face may be peformed with a 2-mm punch to minimize scarring. The resulting wound has smooth, round edges and heals with a slightly depressed scar.

The procedure is adequate for the diagnosis of most tumors. If possible, lesions suspected of being malignant melanoma should be removed completely intact with an excisional biopsy. The quantity of tissue may be inadequate for diagnosis of inflammatory diseases and diseases of adipose tissue, such as erythema nodosum.

Suturing round or oval defects produced by the punch has been advocated by some authors, but suturing does not lead to satisfactory approximation of the margins. Healing by secondary intention is slow but cosmetically acceptable.

TABLE 27-2 Dermatologic Biopsy Techniques	
Type of biopsy	**Indications**
Punch	Most superficial inflammatory and bullous diseases; benign and malignant tumors except malignant melanoma
Shave	Superficial benign and malignant tumors (e.g., seborrheic keratosis, warts, dome-shaped nevi, and non-melanoma malignancies)
Excision	Deep inflammatory diseases (e.g., erythema nodosum); malignant melanoma

Punch biopsy technique. The site is prepared for biopsy with an alcohol pad; a sterile technique is not required. Local anesthesia is induced with 1% lidocaine with epinephrine. Epinephrine is avoided for biopsy near the fingertips. The injection is positioned around and under but not directly into the lesion.

The surrounding tissue is supported by stretching the skin with the thumb and index finger of the free hand. The punch is rotated back and forth between the thumb and forefinger while it is simultaneously pushed vertically into the tissue. Resistance is felt while the instrument penetrates through the dermis but ceases as the punch sinks quickly on entry into the subcutaneous tissue (Figure 27-3, *A* and *B*).

The punch is withdrawn and the cylindric piece of tissue is gently supported with smooth-tipped forceps; the specimen is cut deep with scissors to include subcutaneous tissue. Forceps with teeth may crush the specimen (Figure 27-3, *C*).

The tissue is immediately transferred to a preservative, and bleeding is controlled with Monsel's solution (Figure 27-3, *D*).

Figure 27-3 Punch biopsy.

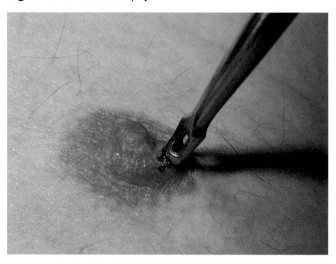

A, The dermal punch is rotated back and forth while gently advancing it through the dermis into the subcutaneous tissue.

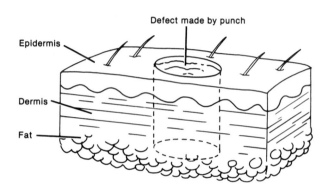

B, The punch should be introduced through the dermis and into the fat.

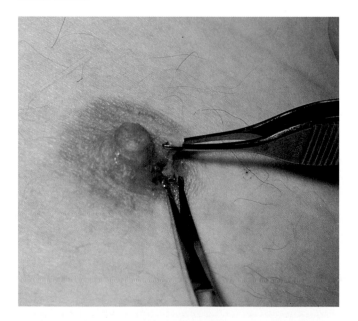

C, The cylindric piece of tissue is gently supported with forceps and cut deep to include subcutaneous tissue.

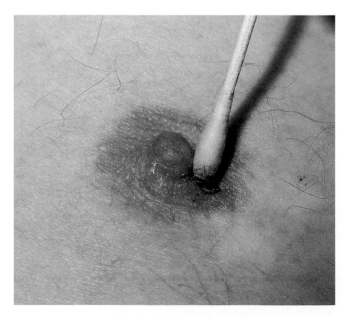

D, Bleeding is controlled with Monsel's solution.

SHAVE BIOPSY AND SHAVE EXCISION

Shave biopsy and shave excision are useful for elevated lesions and when a full thickness of tissue is unimportant. The technique, therefore, is not useful for most inflammatory skin diseases. Shave excision of nevi produces excellent cosmetic results. Any pigmented lesion suspected of being a melanoma should be totally removed by excisional biopsy.

Shave technique. The lesion is elevated from the surrounding skin by infiltration with lidocaine. The surrounding skin is supported with the thumb and forefinger of the free hand. The flat surface of a #15 surgical blade is laid against the skin next to the lesion. With long strokes, the blade is smoothly drawn through the lesion; back-and-forth sawing motions produce a jagged surface (Figure 27-4). Several strokes may be required around the periphery of larger lesions. The last attachment of skin may be severed more easily with scissors than with a scalpel blade. Rough edges and contours can be smoothed with electrocautery, and bleeding can be controlled with Monsel's solution.

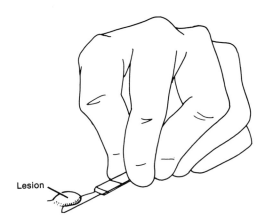

Figure 27-4
Shave excision. The curved surgical blade is laid flat on the skin surface and smoothly drawn through the base of the lesion.

Figure 27-6 Simple scissor excision.

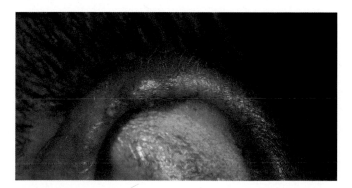

A, Chondrodermatitis nodularis chronica helicis before scissor excision.

SIMPLE SCISSOR EXCISION

Firm lesions that resist curettage may be removed by simple scissor excision. Polypoid and dome-shaped nevi, firm seborrheic keratoses, warts, and corns are removed by resting the curved section of curved, probe-pointed scissors on the skin surface and cutting about the border while slowly advancing the tip of the scissors toward the center of the lesion. The curet is used to remove any remaining tissue fragments. The resulting defect is usually smooth and remains on the same plane as the skin surface (Figures 27-5 and 27-6). Rough edges and contours can be smoothed with electrocautery.

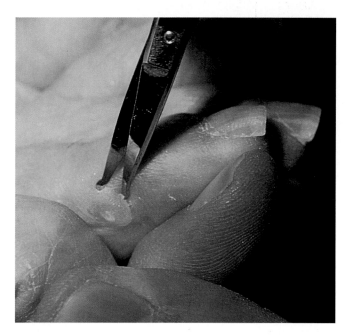

Figure 27-5
Scissor excision of a corn.

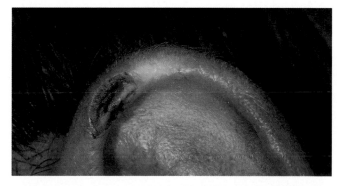

B, The lesion was excised, and the surface healed with a white smooth scar. Another lesion appeared anterior to the first and was excised by scissor excision. Note the exposed cartilage.

Electrodesiccation and Curettage

Indications. Electrodesiccation and curettage (D&C) is an invaluable technique for removing a variety of superficial skin lesions, such as seborrheic keratoses, basal cell epitheliomas, squamous cell carcinomas, pyogenic granulomas, granulation tissue, and genital warts. Electrodesiccation without curettage is sufficient for spider angiomas; small digitate, filiform, and genital warts; and small skin tags about the neck and axillae. The curet may be used without electrodesiccation to remove soft seborrheic and actinic keratoses and filiform warts.

Equipment. The required instruments are an electrodesiccation unit and a set of sharp dermal curets. Many inexpensive electrosurgical office units are capable of executing electrodesiccation, fulguration, and coagulation. Examples of commonly used electrosurgical office units are the Electricator, Hyfrecator, Bantam Bovie, and Ritter coagulator.

Pacemaker patients. Modern pacemakers are very resistant to electrical interference. Simple electrosurgery of small lesions on relatively healthy patients who have pacemakers poses negligible risks.[16]

TECHNIQUES—ELECTRODESICCATION

Electrodesiccation and fulguration are accomplished without the use of an indifferent electrode. The effects are superficial; electrodesiccation and fulguration are the techniques of choice for most dermatologic applications. Coagulation produces greater tissue destruction and requires the use of an indifferent electrode.[17]

Fulguration. The surface to be treated should be dry and relatively free of blood. The pointed electrode is held slightly away from the tissue surface; a "sparking" occurs, resulting in superficial dehydration (Figure 27-7, *A*). The tissues in the immediate surrounding area are charred. Hemostasis can be accomplished only if the field is dry.

Desiccation. The pointed electrode contacts the skin surface or is inserted slightly into the tissue (Figure 27-7, *B*). The resulting char of the tissue is essentially produced by fulguration. As with fulguration, hemostasis is possible only if the field is wiped dry.

Electrocoagulation. The bipolar setting is required. The active electrode (needle, small ball) is placed in contact with the tissue. Because of increased amperage, tissue necrosis tends to be more extensive than that produced by fulguration or desiccation. The greater production of heat and the conduction of current along vessels makes hemostasis possible in a bloody field.

Figure 27-7
A, Electrofulguration—the needle is held above the skin surface. **B**, Electrodesiccation—the needle touches the skin surface. *(From Boughton RS, Spencer SK:* J Am Acad Dermatol *862-867, 1987.)*

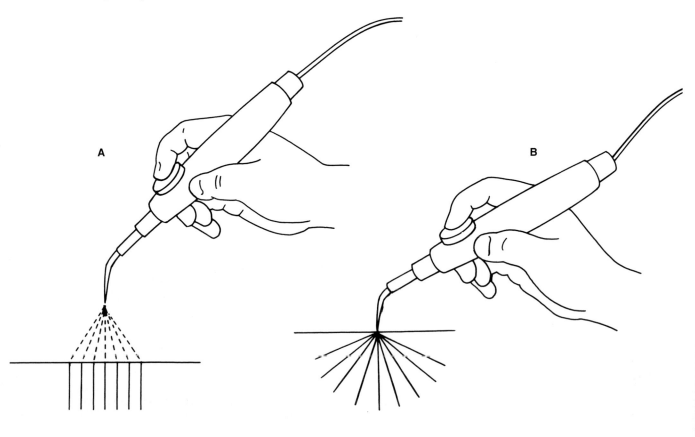

Curettage

Curettage is a scraping or scooping technique used to remove soft tumors, such as seborrheic keratoses, or tissues that have been softened by electrosurgery. Superficial growths are removed with minimal destruction of normal tissue. In many instances curettage is followed by electrodesiccation to control bleeding and destroy remaining fragments of tissue. Electrodesiccation, however, results in more hypopigmentation and scarring.

Indications. Seborrheic keratoses, warts, molluscum contagiosum, actinic keratoses, Bowen's disease, basal cell carcinoma, and squamous cell carcinoma may all be treated by curettage with or without electrosurgery.

Instruments. A dermal curet has a round or oval, sharp ring. Curets are available in diameters ranging from 1 to 7 mm. Instruments with smaller diameters are most useful for minor procedures.

TECHNIQUE—ELECTRODESICCATION AND CURETTAGE OF BASAL CELL CARCINOMA[18,19]

The technique for electrodesiccation and curettage of nodular basal cell carcinoma (BCC) is as follows: Local anesthesia is induced with lidocaine and epinephrine. The surrounding tissue is supported with the finger, and the soft, friable tumor is curretted until firm dermis is reached. The soft-textured tumor offers little resistance to the curet, and more than 90% of the tumor mass can be quickly removed. The entire surface and border is electrodesiccated or coagulated by slowly drawing the probe back and forth until a uniform char has been created at the base. The charred tissue is removed with the curet, and the desiccation and curettage is repeated two more times or until a normal tissue plane is observed and developed throughout. Desiccating and curetting is continued approximately 0.5 cm beyond the visible borders of the lesion to ensure that microscopic extensions of the tumor are destroyed. Active bleeding from the base may indicate residual tumor. Tumor-free dermis oozes blood in a uniform manner.

Bleeding is controlled with Monsel's solution. The wound may be left exposed to the air or may be covered with a bandage or light dressing. Daily washing with soap and water is encouraged. Hydrogen peroxide may be applied once or twice daily; antibiotic ointments are unnecessary. The patient returns in 7 to 10 days, and the adherent crust, if present, is removed.

Postoperative care. For large surgical defects that are allowed to heal by secondary intention, infection is prevented and crust formation is discouraged by the following method: The surgical site is painted daily with a thin film of 2% mercurochrome solution with a cotton swab and the skin surrounding the wound is cleaned with hydrogen peroxide and dried thoroughly. The area should be covered with a dry gauze. Bacitracin is used when the wound becomes dry.

TECHNIQUES—CURETTAGE

Local anesthesia is induced with lidocaine injected with a 27- or 30-gauge needle. Lidocaine can be delivered by jet injector into soft lesions such as warts and seborrheic keratoses. Jet injectors are not usually used on the face.

Pencil technique. The pencil technique is best for most soft lesions. Fine, precise movements are possible. The handle of the curet is grasped like a pencil between the thumb and the index and middle fingers. The base of the palm rests on the skin for stability. The skin around the lesion is stretched and held taut by the fingers of the surgeon's free hand. With several smooth, firm strokes (Figure 27-8, *A* and *B*), the curet is drawn through the tissue. The curet may be pulled toward the surgeon with the index finger[20,21] or pushed away with the thumb. The surgeon may actually feel the consistency of the tumor with the curet. This is very helpful when curetting nodular basal cell epithelioma, which has a firm, gelatin-like consistency. The dermis at the base of the tumor is very firm and resists curettage. The interface between the tumor and the dermis is not as distinct in elderly patients with actinically damaged dermal connective tissue. Bleeding is controlled with Monsel's solution.

Figure 27-8 Curettage technique.

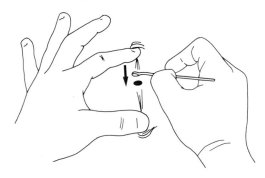

A, Pencil technique demonstrating method of holding curet and two-way tension planes for stabilizing the lesion.

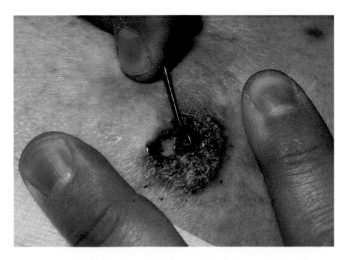

B, Curettage of an inflamed seborrheic keratosis with a #1 curet and the pencil technique.

Figure 27-9 Blunt dissection.

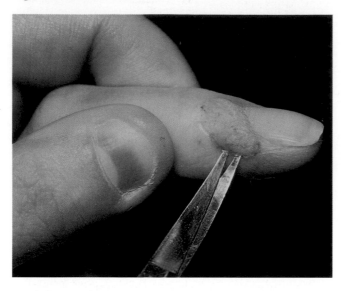

A, A plane of dissection is established by cutting circumferentially around the lesion with probe-tipped curved scissors.

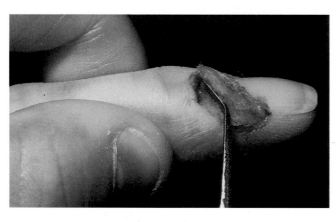

B, The blunt dissector is inserted in the plane of cleavage and firmly pressed against the lesion with several short firm strokes.

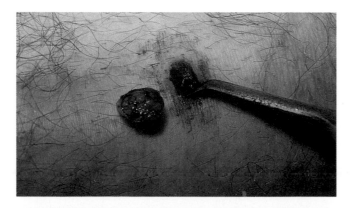

C, The blunt dissector is drawn firmly back and forth over the exposed surface to remove remaining fragments of tissue.

Blunt Dissection

Blunt dissection is a simple surgical procedure for removing epidermal tumors, such as warts[22,23] and keratoacanthoma[24]; the technique is fast, effective, and usually nonscarring. In many instances it is superior both to electrodesiccation and curettage and to excision because normal tissue is not disturbed.

Blunt dissectors are available commercially or may be homemade by altering the blade end of a Bard-Parker handle by flattening it with a grinding wheel and bending the tip approximately 30 degrees. A Schamberg acne expressor may also be used as a blunt dissecting instrument.

TECHNIQUE—BLUNT DISSECTION

The patient may be premedicated with analgesics for lesions in which postoperative pain is anticipated, such as with large plantar or periungual warts. The procedure is relatively painless when performed on areas other than the palms and soles.

Local anesthesia is induced with 2% lidocaine with epinephrine delivered.

A plane of dissection is established by inserting the tip of blunt-tipped scissors between the wart and normal skin and cutting the skin circumferentially (Figure 27-9, *A*).

The blunt dissector is inserted in the plane of cleavage; the intact lesion can be separated easily with short, firm strokes from the surrounding and underlying normal tissue (Figure 27-9, *B*). At the conclusion of this gross dissection, the blunt dissector is drawn firmly back and forth over the exposed surface of the bed to ensure that no tissue fragments remain (Figure 27-9, *C*).

Bleeding is controlled with Monsel's solution. A bandage is placed on the wound and the patient is advised to change it daily for 3 to 4 days. Thereafter, the wound is left exposed. The patient should be cautioned that moderate to intense pain may occur for 15 minutes to 2 hours after blunt dissection of periungual and plantar warts.

Cryosurgery

Small, superficial, nonmalignant lesions may be quickly and effectively treated by freezing with liquid nitrogen (boiling point −196° C). Cryosurgery for malignant lesions requires experience and sophisticated equipment with thermocouples that measure the depth of freeze.[25,26] Severe pain may result from freezing thick areas, such as the palms and soles, or areas that are anatomically confined, such as the area about the nails.[27] Lesions located on these areas are best treated with other methods. Epithelial cells, melanocytes, and nerve tissue are more susceptible to cold injury than is the connective tissue of the dermis and vessels.

Indications. Cryosurgery is very effective for common and genital warts, actinic keratoses, thin seborrheic keratoses, lentigines, and molluscum contagiosum.[28] The superficial portions of dermatofibromas and sebaceous hyperplasia can be destroyed by freezing. Thick seborrheic keratoses are best removed with the curet.

Equipment. Liquid nitrogen is available in most cities and may be stored in the office in 1- to 2-gallon tanks for approximately 10 days. Cotton swabs have been used to administer the nitrogen, but they are capable of transmitting virus particles. It is now recommended that nitrogen be administered with a direct spray or contact probe with an autoclavable tip.[29] A number of relatively inexpensive cryospray instruments are available, such as the Cry-Ac (Owen Instruments).

TECHNIQUE—CRYOSURGERY

Maximum tissue destruction occurs with rapid freezing and slow thawing. Repeated freeze-thaw cycles increase cell damage.[30] Pain is moderate to intense during freezing. The depth of freeze is approximately 1.5 × the lateral spread.[31] The end point of a 1- to 3-mm rim of freeze around the lesions corresponds to a thaw time of approximately 20 to 40 seconds and is adequate for epidermal lesions such as warts and actinic keratoses. Longer freeze-thaw times destroy portions of the dermis. The technique should be used conservatively; it is better to undertreat a lesion and re-treat it at a later date than to freeze it too vigorously, destroy excessive amounts of normal tissue, and create hypopigmentation.

THIN LESIONS. Seborrheic keratoses, flat warts, and actinic keratoses form a crust in 7 to 10 days and fall off. Broad, flat seborrheic keratoses may be frozen in sections (Figure 27-10, *A*); freezing from the center of a large lesion results in a freeze that is too deep.

THICK LESIONS. A hemorrhagic bulla must be created to treat warts effectively. Warts require more prolonged freezing than do thin seborrheic and actinic keratoses and heal in 2 to 3 weeks.

C&C (CRYOANESTHESIA AND CUTTING OR CURETTING). For raised lesions such as thick seborrheic keratoses and small dermal nevi (less than 5 mm), cryospray may be used to achieve quick cryoanesthesia. The raised portion is then removed with a curet or is cut flush to the skin surface with scissors or a scalpel. Treatment of nevi with the C&C method has an added advantage: any pigment that remains at the base of the lesion can be destroyed by short freezing the base.

"DIP-STICK" METHOD. A large cotton-tipped swab is prepared by winding the tip to a point. The applicator is dipped into the nitrogen tank, and the tip is immediately applied to the center of the lesion. A white, hard area of freeze rapidly propagates in all directions. The swab is removed after a 1- to 3-mm rim of freeze surrounding the lesion has been established. The swab is then discarded.

CRYOSPRAY. Benign, superficial lesions are usually treated for 5 to 15 seconds to establish a 1- to 3-mm rim of freeze extending beyond the lesion.

Postcryosurgery. Erythema and edema occur within minutes of thawing. Superficial freezing causes separation at the dermoepidermal junction and can produce a vesicle or bulla. Bullae are likely to occur on the arms and hands (Figure 27-10, *B*), and they can be large and hemorrhagic.

They resolve within a few days but sometimes require drainage if discomfort occurs. Cryosurgery wounds are slower to epithelialize than are laser or scalpel wounds.

Complications. Scarring is minimal with superficial freezing; the cosmetic results are equal to or better than those obtained with desiccation and curettage. If hypertrophic scarring; significant hypopigmentation or hyperpigmentation; or oozing, weeping wounds occur after treatment of warts or keratoses, freezing was too aggressive. Hyperpigmentation occurs in people with darker complexions. The trunk and legs are the areas most likely to form round, hyperpigmented macules after cryosurgery.

The nerves are superficial on the lateral aspects of the digits,[32] the angle of the jaw, and the ulnar fossa of the elbow. Cryosurgery should be avoided in these areas to prevent nerve damage.

Melanocytes are very sensitive to cold injury, and healing with hypopigmentation is common. Cryosurgery should be used with caution for dark-complected individuals.

Figure 27-10 Cryosurgery.

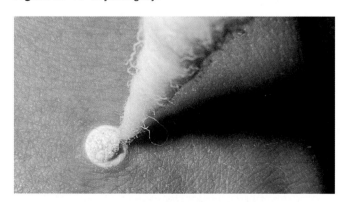

A, The nitrogen-soaked, cotton-tipped applicator is applied to the surface until a 1-mm rim of frozen tissue has been established.

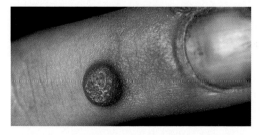

B, Hemorrhagic bullae can occur 24 to 48 hours after cryosurgery. This is most likely to occur on the arms and hands.

Figure 27-11 Extraction of cysts.

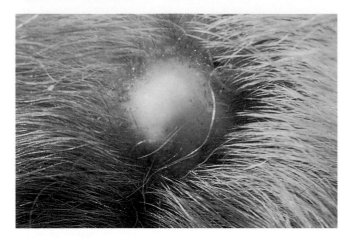

A, Make a linear incision (3 to 10 mm) through the skin and into the cyst with a pointed-tipped #11 surgical blade.

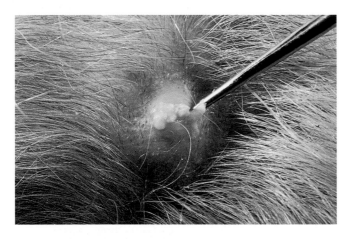

B, Insert a 1- to 3-mm curet through the incision and dislodge and remove as much of the cyst contents as possible. Compress the surrounding skin to force the cyst contents through the small incision.

Extraction of Cysts

A quick, simple technique is available for the removal of small epidermal (sebaceous) and pilar (scalp wens) cysts. Normal tissue is not removed, sutures are unnecessary, and there is little scarring.

TECHNIQUE—EXTRACTION OF CYSTS

After induction of local anesthesia, a linear incision (3 to 10 mm) is made through the skin and into the cyst with a pointed-tipped #11 surgical blade (Figure 27-11, *A*). The surrounding skin is compressed to force the cyst contents through the small incision. A 1- to 3-mm curet is inserted through the incision, and any remaining fragments of material are dislodged and removed (Figure 27-11, *B*). After total evacuation, firm pressure forces a part or all of the cyst wall through the incision, where it can be grasped with the forceps (Figure 27-11, *C*) and separated with scissors from connective tissue (Figure 27-11, *D*). To absorb blood and serum, the wound is compressed for several minutes, then covered with a small dressing. The area can be washed the next day.

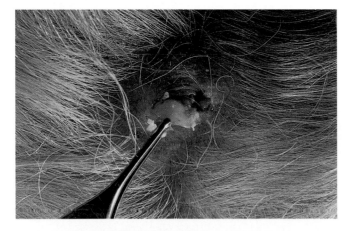

C, After total evacuation, firm pressure forces a part or all of the cyst wall through the incision. The cyst wall is grasped with forceps.

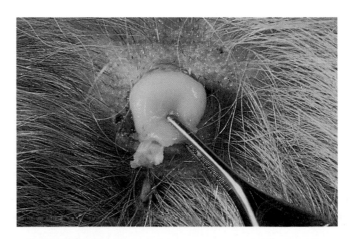

D, The cyst is separated with scissors from connective tissue and removed.

Figure 27-12 Dermabrasion.

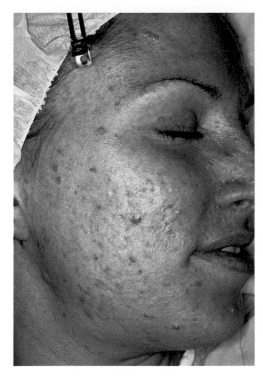

A, Pitted acne scars before dermabrasion.

Dermabrasion

Dermabrasion is a technique primarily used for removing pitted acne scars, but it is also useful for treating difficult photoaged skin problems and surgical scars.[33] Microscopic normalization of actinically damaged epidermis and papillary dermis follows dermabrasion for aged and photo-damaged skin.[34] Facial chemical peeling (phenol and trichloroacetic acid) is often used with dermabrasion.[35] The main advantage of dermabrasion over the chemical peel is the absence of severe depigmentation.[36]

Patients to be treated with dermabrasion must be carefully selected by physicians experienced in the technique. A diamond fraise is spun at high speeds and drawn over the skin surface so that the entire epidermis and upper dermis are removed. Residual portions of the skin adnexa (sweat ducts and hair follicles) proliferate and reepithelialize the smooth-planed surface. The use of dermabrasion is generally limited to the face, where adnexal structures are abundant (Figure 27-12; see also Figure 7-9). The patient experiences a deep warmth and throbbing sensation postoperatively. A crust forms and begins to peel. The length of time for complete reepithelialization varies with the depth of dermabrasion and the patient's age, but it generally requires 7 to 21 days. Direct sun exposure is avoided for several weeks after the procedure.

Complications include infection, change of color, scarring, loss of skin texture, and enlarged facial pores.[37] Hyperpigmentation occurs in most whites who have dark hair, dark eyes, or dark complexions, or those who tan easily. The pigmentation fades with time. Hypopigmentation occurs where dermabrasion has been deep. Hypertrophic scars can occur even after superficial dermabrasion.

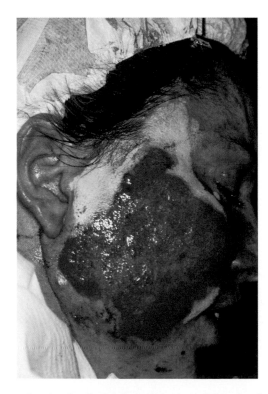

B, Immediately after facial dermabrasion of the cheeks. Trichloroacetic acid peeling (white color) was used on the edges to blend into the skin tone.

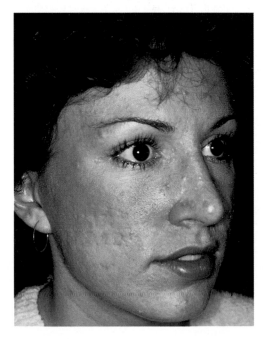

C, Same patient 6 months after dermabrasion. *(Courtesy June Robinson, M.D.)*

Mohs' Micrographic Surgery

Rather than increase in a sphere-shaped mass, certain skin tumors, such as basal cell epithelioma, transmit random, fingerlike projections into the surrounding connective tissue. These tumor strands may go undetected with standard desiccation and curettage or excision techniques, resulting in recurrence. In the past, multiple procedures were performed on unfortunate patients who, after a series of unsuccessful procedures, acquired a diffuse, poorly defined mass of substantial proportions.

In 1941, Frederick Mohs described a microscopically guided method of tracing and removing basal cell carcinomas.[38] Since then the technique has been used to treat many contiguously spreading skin cancers.[39] The procedure has been modified and is usually performed on fresh tissue in 1 day on an outpatient basis. Tissue is removed in thin layers, and all margins of the specimen are mapped to determine whether tumor remains. Cure rates are very high. The technique is tissue sparing: The tumor is precisely identified and maximum amounts of normal skin can be retained.[40]

TECHNIQUE—MOHS' MICROGRAPHIC SURGERY

The clinically apparent area is removed with a curet (Figure 27-13). In the past, a chemical fixative—zinc chloride paste—was applied and allowed to penetrate the tissue. Paste application resulted in the use of the now outdated term, *Mohs' chemosurgery*. Currently, the fixation step is omitted, thus the designation *fresh tissue technique*.[41,42]

A thin, horizontal layer of tissue is removed with a scalpel and divided into more convenient smaller specimens for frozen section. Two adjacent edges of tissue are dyed red and blue to provide spatial orientation. A diagram of the section is prepared, and the number and color coding is indicated on the map. Specimens are mounted in a cryostat and then sectioned. Cut sections are stained and microscopically examined.

The location of the tumor cells is indicated on a map and the above steps are repeated only in areas with tumor until a cancer-free plane is reached.

Figure 27-13
Microscopically guided excision of cutaneous tumors—Mohs' micrographic surgery.

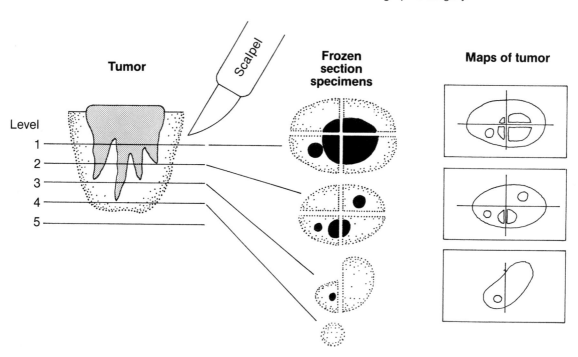

Tumor   Scalpel   **Frozen section specimens**   **Maps of tumor**

Level
1
2
3
4
5

Basal cell carcinoma with fingerlike projections of tumor in the dermis

Tumor sliced with scalpel and cut into quadrants before frozen section; dark areas represent tumor

Maps of tumor location drawn from frozen section specimens, indicating areas of remaining tumor that must be removed

The defect created by the fresh tissue technique can heal by secondary intention or can be closed primarily. Flaps were found to be preferable to skin grafts for facial repair, with forehead and nasolabial flaps particularly useful for the nose.[43] Cure rates of 94% to 99%[44] have been achieved (Figure 27-14).

The advantages of the microscopically controlled technique are that it preserves maximum amounts of normal tissue around the cancer, and it provides great reliability in determining adequate margins of excision. The disadvantage is that it is time-consuming, requiring hours or days to perform.

The indications for Mohs' micrographic surgery[45] are listed in the box below.

Figure 27-14 Mohs' micrographic surgery technique.

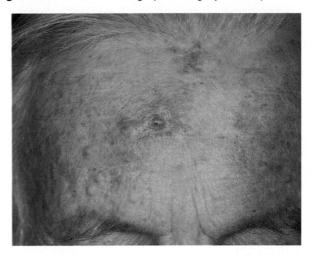

A, Sclerosing basal cell carcinoma. A small nodule is surrounded by an ill-defined erythematous area of induration.

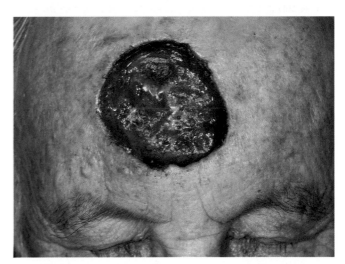

B, Mohs' micrographic surgery reveals the extent of the tumor shown, which clinically appeared to be rather small.

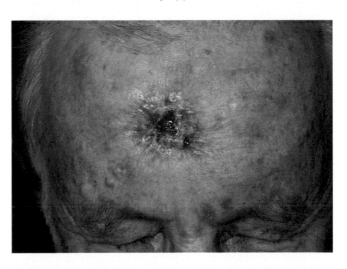

C, Six weeks after Mohs' micrographic surgery. The defect is healing by secondary intention.

INDICATIONS FOR MOHS' MICROGRAPHIC SURGERY

1. Extensive recurrent skin cancers that have not responded to aggressive conventional surgical techniques or radiation
2. Unusually large primary skin cancers of long duration
3. Poorly differentiated squamous cell carcinoma
4. Morpheaform or fibrotic basal cell carcinoma
5. Tumors with poorly demarcated clinical borders
6. Tumors on the face in locations where deeper invasion of the skin along natural skin planes is possible or the extent of the tumor is difficult to define, such as eyelids, nasal alae, nasolabial folds, and circumauricular areas
7. Areas where maximum conservation of tumor-free tissue is important for preservation of function, such as the penis or finger

Modified from Albright SD III: *J Am Acad Dermatol* 7:143, 1982.

Chemical Peels

Chemical peeling of facial skin is commonly performed by aesthetic surgeons. Peeling produces a controlled, partial-thickness chemical burn of the epidermis and the outer dermis. Several techniques are available to fine-tune the depth of the peel. Regeneration of peeled skin from follicular and eccrine duct epithelium results in a fresh, orderly, organized epidermis. In the dermis, a new 2- to 3-mm band of dense, compact, orderly collagen is formed between the epidermis and the underlying damaged dermis, which results in effective ablation of the fine wrinkles in the skin and a reduction of pigmentation. These clinical and histologic changes are long-lasting (15 to 20 years) and may be permanent for some patients. The local complications of peeling include pigmentation changes, scarring, milia, ectropion, infection, activation of herpes simplex, and toxic shock syndrome.[46] Chemical facial exfoliation can be deep, medium, or superficial, depending on the depth of penetration of the caustic agent used.

Deep peels to the deep reticular dermis. Phenol (carbolic acid), when used in the Baker's formula (3 ml phenol, 2 ml water, 8 drops 0.25% septisol [hexachlorophene soap], 3 drops croton oil), provides dramatic results but has the potential for systemic complications. Phenol is a protein precipitant that causes rapid denaturation of the surface keratin and other proteins in the epidermis and outer dermis. This burn injury extends to a depth of approximately 2 to 3 mm. Phenol is rapidly absorbed into the circulation and may cause cardiac arrhythmias. Full epithelialization occurs in 6 to 7 days. Phenol peels are best suited to fair-skinned women and can provide substantial improvement in rhytidosis and actinic damage.

Medium-depth peels to the outer papillary dermis. The results of medium-depth peels with trichloroacetic acid (TCA) are not as profound. TCA (35% to 50%) peels lighten pigmentary problems and improve rhytides with minimal potential for systemic toxicity, but local complications, including scarring and pigmentary changes, are still possible.

Superficial peels to the outer papillary dermis. Superficial peels with TCA (10% to 25%) and many other agents, when performed repeatedly, improve pigmentary irregularities and may improve some minor surface changes and impart a fresher appearance to facial skin.[47] Glycolic acid is an alpha hydroxy acid that is also used as a chemical peeling agent. Glycolic acid (50% to 70%) produces superficial peels that remove actinic keratoses, fine wrinkles, lentigines, melasma, and seborrheic keratoses. As with other peels, the depth of penetration can be titrated by the timed duration of the application of the acid. Peels are left on the skin for 3 to 7 minutes and can be repeated 3 to 4 times. Glycolic acid can be used to peel skin of all skin types with minimal risk.[48]

Dermal Implants

Soft tissue implants are now available for the treatment of facial wrinkles, acne scars, surgical defects, and plantar foot lesions. Bovine collagen (Zyderm I and II) is placed in the superficial dermis for correction of superficial wrinkle lines. Zyplast, a cross-linked bovine collagen product, is placed deeper and can raise depressed areas, such as those of acne scars, deep nasolabial folds, and surgical defects. Fibrel was approved in 1988 for the treatment of acne scars. The patient's plasma (autologous fibrin) is mixed with aminocaproic acid and exogenous porcine collagen. Fibrel may provide longer lasting corrections than Zyderm or Zyplast. Zyderm, Zyplast, and Fibrel have the consistency of a heavy cream. They are injected into the dermis with either a 27- or a 30-gauge needle.

Autologous fatty tissue injection is a surgical technique and does not require FDA approval. Adipocytes are harvested with a needle, washed, and reinjected. The poor viability of harvested cells has limited the effectiveness of this technique. Silicone has been used and misused for years and may never obtain FDA approval. It is the only product that gives a permanent correction. Several other products are under investigation or are available in other countries.

BOVINE DERMAL COLLAGEN IMPLANTS (ZYDERM AND ZYPLAST)

A processing technique using pepsin digestion removes the antigenic parts of the bovine collagen molecule. This refined collagen is available in two forms: type I collagen (Zyderm I and II) and cross-linked collagen (Zyplast) (Table 27-3). Zyplast is manufactured by adding glutaraldehyde during processing. This makes the collagen less immunogenic and enhances resistance to resorption. Saline-lidocaine–dispersed collagens are supplied in preloaded syringes and are injected through 30-gauge needles.

Duration of correction. Wrinkle and scar corrections last from 3 to 9 months. Optimum correction is retained longer with Zyplast, but deterioration at 3 to 9 months is rapid. Deterioration of correction with Zyderm begins earlier and is gradual.

Skin tests and adverse reactions. A 0.1-ml test injection is inserted into the volar forearm and observed for an untoward response after 72 hours and at the end of 4 weeks. Approximately 3% of patients have adverse test reactions and cannot receive Zyderm. It is claimed that double testing reduces the risk of treatment-associated reactions. The second test is administered during the 4-week follow-up visit. Approximately 1% to 2% of patients who do not react during the test period subsequently develop a localized hypersensitivity reaction at treatment sites after Zyderm implants.[49] Allergic reactions to Zyplast occur in less than 1% of patients. The allergic reaction results in erythema and induration and is the most common adverse reaction. These changes last for weeks but spontaneously resolve. A relatively common nonallergic reaction, erythema lasting weeks to months, occurs most frequently in the nasolabial folds after Zyplast implants. Abscesses as a manifestation of hypersensitivity to bovine collagen occur rarely (4 in 10,000 cases) and may persist for days to weeks. Periods of remission and exacerbation may occur from 1 month to more than 24 months. Localized tissue necrosis also occurs rarely (9 in 10,000 cases) after implantation and is probably the result of local vascular interruption and not hypersensitivity. More than half the reported cases involve the glabella. Evidence suggests that the increased vulnerability of the glabellar region is due to its unique vascular distribution.[50]

Safety issues. Patients treated with Zyderm who never displayed cutaneous reactions may develop significant levels of anti-Zyderm serum antibody. In one study, some of these patients progressively increased their antibody levels. Cross-reactivity between patient anti-bovine collagen sera and commercially prepared antibodies to human anti-collagen types I, II, and III was not observed. Given the frequency of current Zyderm use, it seems evident that for most patients, biologic exposure to collagen does not pose a health hazard.[51] Nevertheless, unanswered questions remain about the use of injectable collagen.[52]

Injection guidelines. For Zyderm I and Zyplast, the injection limit of a single patient over one year is 30 cc. Zyderm II carries a limit of 15 cc, and injecting a combination of any of these products is limited to a total of 30 cc per year.

Indications. Collagen implants are indicated for the dermal augmentation of acne scars, frown lines, nasolabial folds, periorbital fine lines,[53] the upper or lower lips,[54] depressed skin grafts, and many other soft tissue defects.[55,56] Soft, distensible lesions with smooth margins are the most amenable to correction, whereas "ice-pick" acne and tiny punched lesions do not respond as well (Figures 27-15 and 27-16).

Patient selection. Normal skin tension lines and lines of expression become deeper with age. These changes are most obvious in the nasolabial folds, glabella, forehead, lateral to the eyes, at the angles of the mouth, and radiating vertically from the lip margins (see Figures 27-15 through 27-17). The best results are obtained if the underlying skin is still elastic without much looseness or redundancy. The correction is not satisfactory for older patients with very lax underlying soft tissue.[57]

Techniques. Zyderm I is injected as superficially as possible in the upper dermis with the bevel of the needle down. Defects are overcorrected because saline is reabsorbed. Zyderm II is placed slightly deeper and does not flow as easily. Zyplast is placed in the mid-dermis serially in small volumes. The plane of the defect should rise only to the desired level of correction. The surgeon can mold the implant immediately after injection with firm index finger pressure. Zyplast is used most frequently for filling deep nasolabial folds, skin creases of the aging face, lip augmentation, scars, and facial atrophy.[58] Here the material is injected medially to the groove to avoid adding to the mass of the cheek.[59]

FIBREL

Fibrel was approved by the FDA in 1988 for the correction of depressed cutaneous scars. The components of Fibrel include gelatin powder (denatured porcine collagen types I and III) and E-aminocaproic acid. Just before use, Fibrel is mixed with the patient's plasma. It is hypothesized that the gelatin matrix implant induces a localized wound healing process that leads to regeneration of new soft tissue. A study showed that Fibril promotes new collagen synthesis and inflammatory response.[60] The antifibrinolytic action of E-aminocaproic acid has a fibrin-stabilizing effect. The

TABLE 27-3 Comparison of Injectable Collagen			
	Zyderm I	**Zyderm II**	**Zyplast**
Volume of augmentation achievable	+	++	+++
Duration of correction	3-8 months	3-8 months	3-8 months plus
Collagen (%)	35	65	98
Indications	Very shallow lines	Shallow lines	Deep lines and folds
Characteristics	Most versatile Most forgiving Flows easily	Flows, but beading possible	Full augmentation possible Persistent beading with overcorrection
Technique	Overcorrect by 150%-200% Blanch skin	Overcorrect by 50% Blanch skin	Just correct No blanch
Implantation site	Inject as superficially as possible in upper dermis Bevel of needle down	Upper dermis	Mid-dermis

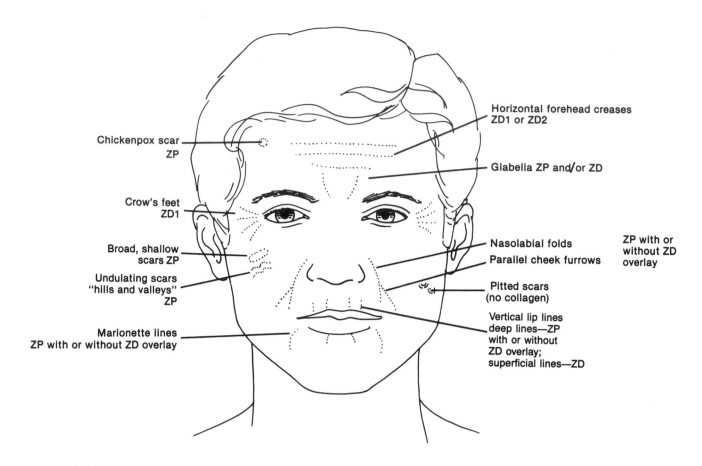

Chickenpox scar
ZP

Horizontal forehead creases
ZD1 or ZD2

Glabella ZP and/or ZD

Crow's feet
ZD1

Broad, shallow
scars ZP

Undulating scars
"hills and valleys"
ZP

Marionette lines
ZP with or without ZD overlay

Nasolabial folds

Parallel cheek furrows

Pitted scars
(no collagen)

Vertical lip lines
deep lines—ZP
with or without
ZD overlay;
superficial lines—ZD

ZP with or
without ZD
overlay

Figure 27-15
Zyderm collagen implants.

ZD1 = Zyderm I — for very shallow lines: superficial dermis
ZD2 = Zyderm II — for shallow lines: superficial dermis
ZP = Zyplast — for deep lines and folds: mid-dermis
ZD and ZP used in layered fashion for optimal effect

Figure 27-16 Dermal collagen implants.

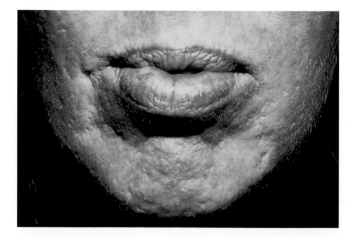

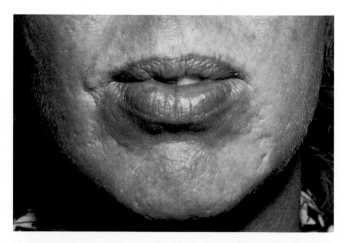

A, Multiple shallow scars are present on the cheeks.

B, Patient shown after bovine dermal collagen implants (Zyderm). *(Courtesy Collagen Corporation.)*

patients's plasma is used as a diluent to provide a source of supplemental fibrinogen.

The scar is first undermined with a special needle. When injected beneath a cutaneous depression, Fibrel elevates the depression and maintains the effect for up to a year or more. The incidence of adverse reactions is very low.[61] One study showed that one or two Fibrel treatments are effective in maintaining a greater than 50% correction of depressed cutaneous scars for up to 5 years, with negligible adverse sequelae and no untoward immunologic symptoms.[62]

Figure 27-17 Zyderm collagen implant; correction of marionette lines.

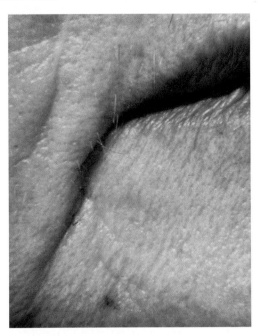

A, Deep fold at the angle of the mouth before implant.

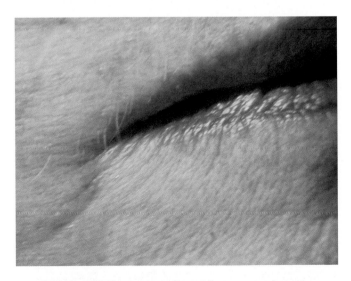

B, Correction after injection of 1 ml (one prepackaged syringe) of Zyplast. *(Courtesy Collagen Corporation.)*

Liposuction

Liposuction surgery is a safe technique when performed by a fully trained, experienced physician. Patients under 40 years of age with good skin elasticity are the best candidates, but patients ranging in age from 16 to over 70 can be successfully treated. Previously, body contouring by surgical excision of fat produced large scars. Fat is removed through half-inch incisions during liposuction.

Indications. With a variety of new instruments and techniques, virtually any area can be treated—the small pot belly, the spare tire, hips, lateral thighs, and "love handles" on men. Other appropriate areas include the male breasts (gynecomastia), the chin, the neck, anterior axillary fat folds, and the proximal arms. Lipomas are easily extracted. Liposuction is used by some surgeons during face-lift surgery.[63]

Technique. A radial tunneling procedure is used (Figure 27-18). A small cannula with a rounded aperture is inserted through a $1/2$-inch incision. The cannula is pushed into the fat to break it loose from the fibrous stroma. Multiple to-and-fro movements mechanically disrupt the fat and create tunnels. The loosened fat is removed with a very powerful suction.

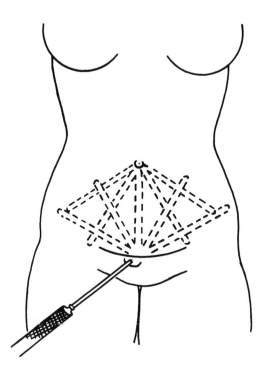

Figure 27-18
Liposuction. Site of incision and tunneling pattern for abdominal liposuction procedure.

Lasers

There are now several types of lasers used to treat cutaneous disease (Table 27-4).[64] CO_2 and argon lasers are generally available in many offices and hospitals. Neodymium yttrium aluminum garnet (Nd:YAG) and tunable dye lasers[65,66] are available at some medical centers. Lasers emit radiation of a specific wavelength. The choice of the laser depends on the absorption characteristics of the tissue. Each type of tissue absorbs radiation of only specific wavelengths and becomes heated. Parts of tissue that absorb light are called *chromophores*. A laser beam focused on the skin quickly heats and vaporizes the chromophores, destroying target tissue with minimal heat dissipation to adjacent tissues. Hemoglobin is the chromophore for the argon laser, and water the chromophore for the CO_2 laser. The amount of heat absorption and destruction depends on wavelength, power density, length of exposure, and tissue absorption. The output of most lasers is continuous; some are intermittent or pulsed.

The CO_2 laser. The CO_2 laser is the most versatile instrument for dermatologic purposes and is the most widely used form of laser therapy.[67] It is used as a cutting and vaporizing tool. The intense, invisible, infrared energy (10,600 nm) is absorbed by water. Soft tissues, which consist primarily of water, uniformly absorb the energy. The beam can be focused: A narrow beam concentrates tremendous energy, evaporates the tissue in a path only a fraction of a millimeter wide, and cuts with relative hemostasis, whereas a defocused beam delivers lower amounts of energy over a wider area and permits vaporization and ablation of larger lesions. Varying the power density controls the depth of vaporization. Numerous applications have been described for CO_2 laser treatment. The CO_2 laser may be the treatment of choice for only a limited number of diseases, such as extensive condyloma acuminatum, rhinophyma, and actinic cheilitis.[68] For other diseases, such as plantar and common warts, it remains an alternative tool that produces treatment results similar to those of standard surgical modalities that are much less expensive.

The argon laser. The light emitted by the argon laser is preferentially absorbed by hemoglobin. Its major role in dermatology is for the treatment of mature, nodular, port-wine stains; telangiectasias; small vascular lesions; and superficial pigmented lesions.[69]

Pulsed laser treatment of benign vascular lesions. Argon lasers were the first lasers used to treat port-wine stains in the mid 1970s. They produced scarring and pigmentary changes. The flashlamp-pumped pulsed dye laser has revolutionized the treatment of port-wine stains in infants and in adults, where resolution of the port-wine stain is excellent, with a scarring rate of approximately 1% and only occasional temporary hyperpigmentation.[70,71] It is based on the fact that hemoglobin absorbs yellow light (577 to 585 nm), and the 360- to 450-microsecond pulse duration is shorter than the thermal relaxation time (time required for the target tissue to lose 50% of its heat) of blood vessels, thus limiting nonspecific thermal damage to the surrounding collagen. Multiple treatment sessions are required. Infants are more compliant than young children.[72] There is a postoperative purpuric appearance in which the skin becomes grey to black for 7 to 10 days following treatment. Some therapists treat hemangiomas in the evolution or involution stages. Superficial lesions respond best.[73] The candela flash lamp–pumped dye laser is safe and effective for the treatment of facial telangiectasia.[74]

Pulsed laser therapy of pigmented lesions and tattoos. Melanosomes are 1-μ organelles of melanocytes that are destroyed when submicrosecond pulse durations are used. Melanin absorbs energy from the ultraviolet regions to the near infrared regions and, therefore, allows many different wavelengths to be used. Selective destruction of melanosomes can be accomplished using a variety of instruments, all of which have been FDA approved for treating benign pigmented epidermal and dermal lesions. These

---

TABLE 27-4 Lasers in Dermatologic Surgery

Type	Wavelength (nm)	Application
Argon	488-514	Vascular and other pigmented lesions
Carbon dioxide	10,600	Cutting, vaporization, coagulation of all tissues (bone more difficult)
Copper vapor	578	Vascular lesions
Dye laser—flashlamp pumped	577-585	Vascular lesions
Dye laser— argon laser–pumped	630	Photodynamic therapy
	577	Vascular lesions
Gold vapor	628	Photodynamic therapy
Neodymium:YAG	1,064	Deep coagulation, vascular lesions, tattoos
Ruby laser—*Q*-switched	694	Tattoos, nonvascular pigmented lesions

From Garden JM, Geronemus RG: *J Dermatol Surg Oncol* 16:156, 1990.

include the candela pigmented lesion dye laser (510 nm), the frequency-doubled Q-switched Nd:YAG laser (532 nm), the Q-switched ruby laser (694 nm), and the Q-switched Nd:YAG laser (1064 nm).

Tattoos. Q-switched lasers can remove tattoos without residual scarring. The Q-switched ruby laser (694 nm) effectively removes blue-black and green ink, but may treat other colors less efficiently. It is frequently associated with transient pigmentary changes, including rare depigmentation. The Q-switched Nd:YAG laser at 1064 nm quickly removes black ink and, less efficiently, other colors; pigmentary changes are much less frequent.[75] The 532-nm wavelength treats red ink effectively, but leads to temporary hypopigmentation. Transient textural changes may be noted, but scarring is rare. Efficacy of ink removal depends on the wavelength used for the targeted pigment.[76]

Pigmented lesions. The candela pigmented lesion dye laser treats café-au-lait macules, lentigines, seborrheic keratoses, postinflammatory hyperpigmentation,[77] and red tattoos.[78] Epidermal melasma responds more reliably than melasma with a strong dermal component. Transient hypopigmentation and hyperpigmentation resolve in 4 to 6 months. The Q-switched ruby laser is effective for treating epidermal pigmented[79] lesions and some dermal pigmented lesions (nevus of Ota).[80]

REFERENCES

1. Grekin RC, Auletta MJ: Local anesthesia in dermatologic surgery, *J Am Acad Dermatol* 19:599-614, 1988.
2. Ruzicka T, Gerstmeier M, Przybilla B, et al: Allergy to local anesthetics: comparison of patch test with prick and intradermal test results, *J Am Acad Dermatol* 16:1202-1208, 1987.
3. Glinert RJ, Zachary CB: Local anesthetic allergy. Its recognition and avoidance, *J Dermatol Surg Oncol* 17:491-496, 1991.
4. Lugo-Janer G, Padial M, et al: Less painful alternatives for local anesthesia, *J Dermatol Surg Oncol* 19:237-240, 1993.
5. McKay W, Morris R, Mushlin P: Sodium bicarbonate attenuates pain on skin infiltration with lidocaine, with or without epinephrine, *Anesth Analg* 66:572-574, 1987.
6. Larson PO, Ragi G, et al: Stability of buffered lidocaine and epinephrine used for local anesthesia, *J Dermatol Surg Oncol* 17:411-414, 1991.
7. Mader TJ et al: Reducing pain of local anesthetic infiltration: Warming and buffering have a synergistic effect, *Ann Emerg Med* 23:550-554, 1994.
8. Swinehart JM: The ice-saline-Xylocaine technique. A simple method for minimizing pain in obtaining local anesthesia, *J Dermatol Surg Oncol* 18:28-30, 1992.
9. Lycka BA: EMLA. A new and effective topical anesthetic, *J Dermatol Surg Oncol* 18:859-862, 1992.
10. Olmstead PM, Lund HZ, Leonard DD: Monsel's solution: a histologic nuisance, *J Am Acad Dermatol* 3:492-498, 1980.
11. Telfer NR, Moy RL: Wound care after office procedures, *J Dermatol Surg Oncol* 19:722-731, 1993.
12. Eaglstein WH: Occlusive dressings, *J Dermatol Surg Oncol* 19:716-720, 1993.
13. Brown CD, Zitelli JA: A review of topical agents for wounds and methods of wounding. Guidelines for wound management, *J Dermatol Surg Oncol* 19:732-737, 1993.
14. Varghese MC, Balin AK, Carter DM, et al: Local environment of chronic wounds under synthetic dressings, *Arch Dermatol* 122:52-57, 1986.
15. Falanga V: Occlusive wound dressings: why, when, which? *Arch Dermatol* 124:872-877, 1988.
16. Sebben JE: Electrosurgery and cardiac pacemakers, *J Am Acad Dermatol* 9:457-463, 1983.
17. Boughton RS, Spencer SK: Electrosurgical fundamentals, *J Am Acad Dermatol* 16:862-867, 1987.
18. Whelan CS, Deckers PJ: Electrocoagulation for skin cancer: An old oncologic tool revisited, *Cancer* 47:2280-2287, 1981.
19. Salasche SJ: Curettage and electrodesiccation in the treatment of midfacial basal cell epithelioma, *J Am Acad Dermatol* 8:496-503, 1983.
20. Adam JE: The technic of curettage surgery, *J Am Acad Dermatol* 15:697-702, 1986.
21. Mohs FE: The technic of curettage surgery, *J Am Acad Dermatol* 16:886, 1987 (letter).
22. Pringle WM, Helms BC: Treatment of plantar warts by blunt dissection, *Arch Dermatol* 108:79-82, 1973.
23. Habif TP, Graf FA: Extirpation of subungual and periungual warts by blunt dissection, *J Dermatol Surg Oncol* 7:553-555, 1981.
24. Habif TP: Extirpation of keratoacanthomas by blunt dissection, *J Dermatol Surg Oncol* 6:652-654, 1980.
25. Kuflik EG, Gage AA: The five-year cure rate achieved by cryosurgery for skin cancer, *J Am Acad Dermatol* 24:1002-1004, 1991.
26. Torre D: Cryosurgery of basal cell carcinoma, *J Am Acad Dermatol* 15:917-929, 1986.
27. Kuflik EG: Specific indications for cryosurgery of the nail unit Myxoid cysts and periungual verrucae, *J Dermatol Surg Oncol* 18: 702-706, 1992.
28. Kuflik EG: Cryosurgery updated, *J Am Acad Dermatol* 31:925-944, 1994.
29. Boulier IC, Myskowski PL, et al: Disposable attachments in cryosurgery: a useful adjunct in the treatment of HIV-associated neoplasms, *J Dermatol Surg Oncol* 17:277-278, 1991.

30. Farrant J, Walter CA: The cryobiological basis for cryosurgery, *J Dermatol Surg Oncol* 3:403-407, 1977.

31. Torre D: Understanding the relationship between lateral spread of freeze and depth of freeze, *J Dermatol Surg Oncol* 5:51-53, 1979.

32. Elton RF: Complications of cutaneous cryosurgery, *J Am Acad Dermatol* 8:513-519, 1983.

33. Katz BE, Oca AG: A controlled study of the effectiveness of spot dermabrasion ('scarabrasion') on the appearance of surgical scars, *J Am Acad Dermatol* 24:462-466, 1991.

34. Benedetto AV, Griffin TD, et al: Dermabrasion: therapy and prophylaxis of the photoaged face, *J Am Acad Dermatol* 27:439-447, 1992.

35. Stuzin JM, Baker TJ, et al: Treatment of photoaging. Facial chemical peeling (phenol and trichloroacetic acid) and dermabrasion, *Clin Plast Surg* 20:9-25, 1993.

36. Niechajev I, Ljungqvist A: Perioral dermabrasion: clinical and experimental studies, *Aesthetic Plast Surg* 16:11-20, 1992.

37. Fulton J Jr.: The prevention and management of postdermabrasion complications, *J Dermatol Surg Oncol* 17:431-437, 1991.

38. Mohs FE: Chemosurgery, a microscopically controlled method of cancer excision, *Arch Surg* 42:279, 1941.

39. Bennett RG: Current concepts in Mohs micrographic surgery, *Dermatol Clin* 9:777-788, 1991.

40. Roenigk RK: Mohs' micrographic surgery, *Mayo Clin Proc* 63:175-183, 1988.

41. Tromovitch TA, Stegman SJ: Microscopic-controlled excision of cutaneous tumors: chemosurgery, fresh tissue technique, *Cancer* 41:653-658, 1978.

42. Amonette RA: Mohs' technique: chemosurgery and fresh tissue surgery, In Epstein E, Epstein E Jr, editors: *Techniques in skin surgery*, Philadelphia, 1979, Lea & Febiger.

43. Rudolph R, Miller SH: Reconstruction after Mohs cancer excision, *Clin Plast Surg* 20:157-165, 1993.

44. Mohs FE: *Chemosurgery, microscopically controlled surgery for skin cancer*, Springfield, Ill, 1978, Charles C Thomas.

45. Albright SD: Treatment of skin cancer using multiple modalities, *J Am Acad Dermatol* 7:143-171, 1982.

46. Peters W: The chemical peel, *Ann Plast Surg* 26:564-571, 1991.

47. Matarasso SL, Glogau RG: Chemical face peels, *Dermatol Clin* 9:131-150, 1991.

48. Moy LS, Murad H, et al: Glycolic acid peels for the treatment of wrinkles and photoaging, *J Dermatol Surg Oncol* 19:243-246, 1993.

49. Stegman SJ, Chu S, Armstrong RC: Adverse reactions to bovine collagen implants: clinical and histologic features, *J Dermatol Surg Oncol* 14 (suppl 1):39-48, 1988.

50. Hanke CW, Higley HR, et al: Abscess formation and local necrosis after treatment with Zyderm or Zyplast collagen implant, *J Am Acad Dermatol* 25:319-326, 1991.

51. Hanke CW et al: Risk assessment of polymyositis/dermatomyositis after treatment with injectable bovine collagen implants, *J Am Acad Dermatol* (in press).

52. Frank DH, Vakassian L, et al: Human antibody response following multiple injections of bovine collagen, *Plast Reconstr Surg* 87:1080-1088, 1991.

53. Elson ML: Soft tissue augmentation of periorbital fine lines and the orbital groove with Zyderm-I and fine-gauge needles, *J Dermatol Surg Oncol* 18:779-782, 1992.

54. Gonzalez Ulloa M: The sensuous lip, *Aesthetic Plast Surg* 16:231-236, 1992.

55. Elson ML: Clinical assessment of Zyplast implant: a year of experience for soft tissue contour correction, *J Am Acad Dermatol* 18:707-713, 1988.

56. Pollack SV: Silicone, fibrel, and collagen implantation for facial lines and wrinkles, *J Dermatol Surg Oncol* 16:957-961, 1990.

57. Bailin PL, Bailin MD: Collagen implantation: clinical applications and lesion selection, *J Dermatol Surg Oncol* 14(suppl 1):21-26, 1988.

58. Matti BA, Nicolle FV: Clinical use of Zyplast in correction of age- and disease-related contour deficiencies of the face, *Aesthetic Plast Surg* 14:227-234, 1990.

59. Klein AW: Indications and implantation techniques for the various formulations of injectable collagen, *J Dermatol Surg Oncol* 14(suppl 1):27-30, 1988.

60. Gold MH: The fibrel mechanism of action study, *J Dermatol Surg Oncol* 20:586-590, 1994.

61. Millikan L et al: Treatment of depressed cutaneous scars with gelatin matrix implant: a multicenter study, *J Am Acad Dermatol* 16:1155-1162, 1987.

62. Millikan L, Banks K, et al: A 5-year safety and efficacy evaluation with fibrel in the correction of cutaneous scars following one or two treatments, *J Dermatol Surg Oncol* 17:223-229, 1991.

63. Field LM: Lipo-suction surgery: a review, *J Dermatol Surg Oncol* 10:530-538, 1984.

64. Dover JS, Kilmer SL, et al: What's new in cutaneous laser surgery, *J Dermatol Surg Oncol* 19:295-298, 1993.

65. Tan OT et al: Histologic responses of port-wine stains treated by argon, carbon dioxide, and tunable dye lasers, *Arch Dermatol* 122:1016-1022, 1986.

66. Garden JM, Polla LL, Tan OT: The treatment of port-wine stains by the pulsed dye laser, *Arch Dermatol* 124:889-896, 1988.

67. Olbricht SM: Use of the carbon dioxide laser in dermatologic surgery. A clinically relevant update for 1993, *J Dermatol Surg Oncol* 19:364-369, 1993.

68. Olbricht SM, Arndt KA: Carbon dioxide laser treatment of cutaneous disorders, *Mayo Clin Proc* 63:297-300, 1988.

69. McBurney EI: Clinical usefulness of the argon laser for the 1990s, *J Dermatol Surg Oncol* 19:358-362, 1993.

70. Garden JM, Bakus AD: Clinical efficacy of the pulsed dye laser in the treatment of vascular lesions, *J Dermatol Surg Oncol* 19:321-326, 1993.

71. Wheeland RG: Treatment of port-wine stains for the 1990s, *J Dermatol Surg Oncol* 19:348-356, 1993.

72. Goldman MP, Fitzpatrick RE, et al: Treatment of port-wine stains (capillary malformation) with the flashlamp-pumped pulsed dye laser, *J Pediatr* 122:71-77, 1993.

73. Geronemus RG: Pulsed dye laser treatment of vascular lesions in children, *J Dermatol Surg Oncol* 19:303-310, 1993.

74. Ruiz-Esparza J, Goldman MP, et al: Flash lamp-pumped dye laser treatment of telangiectasia, *J Dermatol Surg Oncol* 19:1000-1003, 1993.

75. Kilmer SL, Lee MS, et al: The Q-switched Nd:YAG laser effectively treats tattoos. A controlled, dose-response study, *Arch Dermatol* 129:971-978, 1993.

76. Kilmer SL, Anderson RR: Clinical use of the Q-switched ruby and the Q-switched Nd:YAG (1064 nm and 532 nm) lasers for treatment of tattoos, *J Dermatol Surg Oncol* 19:330-338, 1993.

77. Fitzpatrick RE, Goldman MP, et al: Laser treatment of benign pigmented epidermal lesions using a 300 n-second pulse and 510 nm wavelength, *J Dermatol Surg Oncol* 19:341-347, 1993.

78. Grekin RC, Shelton RM, et al: 510-nm pigmented lesion dye laser. Its characteristics and clinical uses, *J Dermatol Surg Oncol* 19:380-387, 1993.

79. Goldberg DJ: Benign pigmented lesions of the skin. Treatment with the Q-switched ruby laser, *J Dermatol Surg Oncol* 19:376-379, 1993.

80. Goldberg DJ, Nychay SG: Q-switched ruby laser treatment of nevus of Ota, *J Dermatol Surg Oncol* 18:817-821, 1992.

Appendix

1. Nystatin tablet 1,000,000 units three times a day for 2 weeks, followed by nystatin tablet 500,000 units three times a day for 2 weeks
2. Nystatin tablet 1,000,000 units, dissolve in mouth twice daily for 1 week
3. Miconazole vaginal cream, insert in vaginal tract before bedtime for 2 weeks

THE SALICYLATE, AZO DYE, AND BENZOIC ACID–FREE DIET: THE FOLLOWING FOODS MAY BE EATEN

Bread	Asparagus	Tangerines	Olives	Pears	Artichokes
Sugar	Wax beans	Cereals (not flavored)	Bean sprouts	Rice	Green beans
Eggs	Broccoli	Salad oils (not flavored)	Beets	Butter	Beet greens
Beef	Carrots	Milk	Brussels sprouts	Cream	Cabbage
Fish	Swiss chard	Chicken	Cauliflower	Turkey	Celery
Mushrooms	Lettuce	Lettuce	Chives	Parsley	Eggplant
Crackers	Pumpkin	Potatoes	Onions	Plain rolls	Pineapples
Pork	Squash	Veal	Radishes	Lamb	Spinach
Beans	Dates	Peanuts	Turnip greens	Cottage cheese	Turnips
Corn	Mango	Lima beans	Figs	Parsnips	Loganberries

SOURCES OF SALICYLATES, AZO DYES, AND BENZOIC ACID

Foods containing natural salicylate

Almonds	Currants	Nectarines
Apples	Dewberries	Oranges
Apricots	Gooseberries	Peaches
Bananas	Grapefruit	Pickles
Blackberries	Grapes or raisins	Plums or prunes
Blueberries	Green peas	Raspberries
Boysenberries	Green peppers	Strawberries
Cherries	Lemons	Tabasco peppers
Cucumbers	Melons	Tomatoes

Foods containing salicylates, azo dyes, or benzoic acid

Most foods containing color or flavors, such as breakfast cereals (Cheerios, Sugar Jets, Bran Flakes, Product 19, Raisin Bran, Sugar Pops), bakery goods (dinner rolls, cinnamon rolls, cake mixes, frosting mixes, cookie mixes, tarts, turnovers, brownie mixes), puddings, mints, flavored candies, flavored chips (Whistles, taco chips), ice cream, jellies, jams; macaroni and spaghetti (certain brands), some packaged and canned soups, mayonnaise, salad dressings, luncheon meats (salami, bologna), frankfurters, oleomargarine, ketchup (certain brands), mustard, cider and wine vinegars, canned fish (anchovies, herring, sardines, caviar, cleaned shellfish), fruit gelatins, some cheeses, flavored sauces, surface-treated fish (can be washed away)

Beverages containing salicylates, azo dyes, or benzoic acid

Root beer	Gin	Fruit juices
Cider	Distilled liquor (except vodka)	Kool-aids
Wine	Flavored colas	Beer

Drugs and other products

Aspirin and aspirin-containing compounds (hundreds of preparations), toothpaste and toothpowder, mint flavors, mouthwashes, lozenges, gum, some antihistamines

Dermatologic Formulary

■ ACNE MEDICATIONS

Retin-A

Base concentration		Packaging
Cream	0.025%	20 gm
		45 gm
	0.05%	20 gm
		45 gm
	0.1%	20 gm
		45 gm
Gel	0.01%	15 gm
		45 gm
	0.025%	15 gm
		45 gm
Liquid	0.05%	28 ml

Benzoyl Peroxide Cleansers

Product	Formulation	Packaging
Benzac AC wash 2.5%	Liquid 2.5%	8 oz.
Benzac AC wash 5%	Liquid 5%	8 oz.
Benzac AC wash 10%	Liquid 10%	8 oz.
Benzac W wash (Rx)	Liquid 5%	4 oz, 8 oz.
Benzac W wash (Rx)	Liquid 10%	8 oz.
Brevoxyl Cleansing Lotion (Rx)	Liquid 4%	10.5 oz.
Desquam-X 5% wash (Rx)	Liquid 5%	150 ml
Desquam-X 10% wash (Rx)	Liquid 10%	150 ml
Desquam-X 10% bar (Rx)	Bar 10%	4 oz bar
Panoxyl 5 bar (otc)	Bar 5%	4 oz bar
Panoxyl 10 bar (otc)	Bar 10%	4 oz bar

Benzoyl Peroxide Gels (2.5%)

Product	Base	Packaging
Benzac W 2.5	Water	60, 90 gm
Benzac AC 2.5%	Water	60, 90 gm
Clear By Design (otc)	Water	45, 90 gm
Desquam-X 2.5%	Water	1.5 oz
Desquam-E 2.5	Water	1.5 oz
Panoxyl AQ 2.5	Water	60, 120 gm

Benzoyl Peroxide Gels (4%)

Product	Base	Packaging
Brevoxyl (Rx)	Water	42.5, 90 gm

Benzoyl Peroxide Gels (5%)

Product	Base	Packaging
Benoxyl 5 (otc)	Water	1 oz, 2 oz
Benzac 5	12% alcohol	60 gm
Benzac AC 5%	Water	60, 90 gm
Benzac W 5	Water	60, 90 gm
5-Benzagel	14% alcohol	42.5, 85 gm
Desquam-X 5	Water	45, 90 gm
Desquam-E 5	Water	1.5 oz
Neutragena Acne Mask 5%		2 oz tube
Panoxyl 5	20% alcohol	60, 120 gm
Panoxyl AQ 5	Water	60, 120 gm
Sulfoxyl Regular 5 (contains 2.5% sulfur)	Water	30 ml

Benzoyl Peroxide Gels (10%)

Product	Base	Packaging
Acne-Aid (otc)	Flesh tinted	1.8 oz
Benoxyl 10 (otc)	Water	1 oz, 2 oz
Benzac 10	12% alcohol	60 gm
Benzac AC 10%	Water	60, 90 gm
Benzac W 10	Water	60, 90 gm
10-Benzagel	14% alcohol	42.5, 85 gm
Desquam-X 10	Water	42.5, 85 gm
Desquam-E 10	Water	1.5 oz
Panoxyl 10	20% alcohol	60, 120 gm
Panoxyl AQ 10	Water	60, 120 gm
Sulfoxyl Strong 10 (contains 5% sulfur)	Water	2 oz

Topical Antibiotics for Acne

Product	Antibiotics	Base*	Packaging
Akne-mycin	2% erythromycin	Petrolatum	25 gm ointment
A/T/S	2% erythromycin	66% alcohol, pg	60 ml liquid
A/T/S gel	2% erythromycin	92% alcohol	60 ml liquid
Benzamycin	3% erythromycin 5% benzoyl peroxide	16% alcohol	23.3 gm gel
Cleocin T	1% clindamycin	50% alcohol, pg	30, 60 ml liquid
			30, 60 ml gel
		Water based	60 ml lotion
		50% alcohol	#60 pledgets
Emgel	2% erythromycin	77% alcohol, pg	27, 50 gm gel
Erycette	2% erythromycin	66% alcohol, pg	#60 swabs
EryDerm	2% erythromycin	77% alcohol, peg	60 ml liquid
Erygel	2% erythromycin	92% alcohol	30, 60 gm gel
Erymax	2% erythromycin	66% alcohol, pg	2 oz, 4 oz liquid
Metrogel†	0.75% metronidazole	pg	30, 45 gm gel
Staticin	1.5% erythromycin	55% alcohol, pg	60 ml liquid
Theramycin Z	2% erythromycin	Zinc acetate	60 ml liquid
Topicycline	2% tetracycline	40% alcohol	70 ml liquid
T-Stat	2% erythromycin	71.2% alcohol, pg	60 ml liquid
T-Stat	2% erythromycin	71.2% alcohol, pg	#60 swabs

*pg, Propylene glycol; peg, polyethylene glycol.
† For treatment of rosacea.

Drying-Keratolytic Preparations

Product	Sulfur	Salicylic acid	Resorcinol	Other	Packaging
Acne drying gel (otc)	—	—	—	Witch hazel and alcohol	0.75 oz
Acnomel cream (otc)	8%	—	2%	11% alcohol	28 gm tinted
Allercreme oil regulating lotion (absorbs sebum) (otc)	—	—	—	Acrylates copolymer	4 oz jar
Fostril lotion (otc)	2%	—	—	6% laureth 4	30 ml
Komed lotion (otc)	—	2%	—	8% sodium thiosulfate 25% isopropyl alcohol	52.5 ml
Komed HC (Rx)	—	2%	—	0.5% hydrocortisone acetate 8% sodium thiosulfate 25% isopropyl alcohol	52.5 ml
Novacet lotion (Rx)	5%	—	—	10% sodium sulfacetomide	30 gm tube
Rezamid lotion (otc)	5%	—	2%	28.5% alcohol, 0.5% parachlorometraxylenol	60 ml tinted
Saligel acne gel (otc)	—	5%	—	14% alcohol	60 gm
Sulfacet-R lotion (Rx)	5%	—	—	10% sodium sulfacetamide	25 gm
Sulforcin lotion (otc)	5%	—	2%	11.65% alcohol	60 ml tinted
Sulfoxyl lotion regular (Rx)	2%	—	—	5% Benzoyl peroxide	59 ml
Sulfoxyl lotion strong (Rx)	5%	—	—	10% Benzoyl peroxide	59 ml
Xerac alcohol gel 4% (otc)	4%	—	—	44% isopropyl alcohol	1.5 oz

Medicated Bar Cleansers for Acne

Product	Active ingredient	Packaging
Acne-Aid Cleansing Bar	6.3% surfactant	4, 5.8 oz bars
Fostex bar	2% sulfur	Bar
Salicylic acid soap	2% salicylic acid	4 oz bar
Salicylic acid and sulfur soap	3% salicylic acid, 5% sulfur	4.1 oz bar
SAStid soap	10% sulfur; 3% salicylic acid	4.1 oz bar
Sulpho-Lac soap	5% sulfur	Bar
Sulfur soap	10% sulfur	116 gm bar

Medicated Cleansers for Acne

Product	Active ingredient	Packaging
Brasivol	Aluminum oxide scrub particles	Base, fine, medium, rough
Fomac foam	2% salicylic acid	3 oz bottle
Ionax Foam	0.2% benzalkonium CL	75, 150 gm can
Ionax Astringent	Five cleansing ingredients	8 oz bottle
Neutrogena Oil-Free Acne Wash	2% salicylic acid	6 oz pump
Seba-Nil	Oil-removing base	8, 16 oz bottles
SalAc	2% salicylic acid	6 oz bottle

Isotretinoin (Accutane)

Accutane capsules	10 mg
	20 mg
	40 mg

Dosing Isotretinoin by Body Weight

Body weight		Total mg/day		
Kilograms	Pounds	0.5 mg/kg	1 mg/kg	2 mg/kg
40	88	20	40	80
50	110	25	50	100
60	132	30	60	120
70	154	35	70	140
80	176	40	80	160
90	198	45	90	180
100	220	50	100	200

■ ANTIBIOTICS (ORAL)

Generic	Brand name	Preparation*	Adult dosage (mg; unless noted)
Cephalosporins			
First-generation			
Cephradine	Velosef	250, 500 mg	1-2 gm/24h (bid, qid)
Cephalexin	Keflex	250, 500 mg	250-1000 qid
Cefadroxil	Duricef	500, 1000 mg	1 gm-24h (qd-bid)
Second-generation			
Cefaclor	Ceclor	250, 500 mg	250-500 tid
Cefuroxime	Ceftin	125, 250, 500 mg	250-500 bid
Cefprozil	Cefzil	250, 500 mg 125 mg/5 ml 250 mg/5 ml	250 bid-500 qd
Third-generation			
Cefixime	Suprax	200, 400 mg	200 bid, 400 qd
Fluoroquinolones			
Ofloxacin	Floxin	200, 300, 400 mg	200-400 mg q12h
Ciprofloxacin	Cipro	500, 750 mg	500-750 bid
Macrolides			
Erythromycin (ethylstearate)	E.E.S., E-Mycin, Pediamycin	250, 400 mg	250-800 qid*
Erythromycin (enteric coated)	ERYC, Ery-Tab, E-Mycin	125, 250, 330, 500 mg	250-500 q6h*
Clarithromycin	Biaxin	250, 500 mg	250-500 mg bid
Azithromycin	Zithromax	250 mg	500 mg first day 250 qd × 4 days
Penicillins			
Ampicillin	Amcill	250, 500 mg	250-500 qid
Penicillin V	Pen-Vee K, etc.	250, 500 mg	250-500 qid
Dicloxacillin	Dynapen	125, 250, 500 mg	125-500 q6h
Cloxacillin	Generic	250, 500 mg	500 mg qid
Amoxicillin	Generic	250, 500 mg	250-500 tid
Amoxicillin clavulanate	Augmentin	250, 500 mg	250-500 q8h
Sulfonamides, sulfones			
Sulfamethoxazole-trimethoprim	Bactrim DS, Septra DS	800 mg/160 mg	1 tablet bid
Dapsone	Generic	25, 100 mg	50-300 mg qid
Tetracyclines			
Clindamycin	Cleocin	75, 150, 300 mg	150-300 q6h
Demeclocycline	Declomycin	150 mg	150 mg qid, or 300 mg bid
Doxycycline	Monodox, Vibramycin	50, 100 mg	100-200/24h (qd-bid)
Minocycline	Minocin, Dynacin	50, 100 mg	100-200/24h (qd-bid)

*Many preparations available in liquid form.

■ ANTIBIOTICS (TOPICAL)*

Generic name	Brand name	Preparation*
Bacitracin	Baciguent ointment	15, 30, 120 gm
Chloramphenicol	Chloromycetin cream	30 gm
Clioquinol (iodochlorhydroxyquin)	Vioform lotion	15, 30 gm
Clioquinol and 1% HC	Vioform lotion	15 ml
Clioquinol and 0.5% HC	Vioform HC mild cream, ointment	15, 30 gm
Gentamycin	Garamycin cream, ointment	15 gm
Gramicidin and hydrocortisone (HC) acetate	Cortisporin ointment	15 gm
Iodoquinol and 0.5% or 1% HC	Vytone	1 oz tube
Mafenide acetate	Sulfamylon cream	60, 120, 480 gm
Metronidazole	MetroGel	1 oz, 45 gm
Mupirocin 2%	Bactroban ointment	15, 30 gm
Neomycin		7.5-60 gm
Nitrofurazone	Furacin cream	30 gm
Polymyxin and bacitracin	Polysporin ointment (many brands)	15, 30 gm (ointment)
	Neosporin powder	10 gm (powder)
Polymyxin, neomycin, and bacitracin	Neosporin (many brands)	15, 30 gm
Povidone-iodine	Betadine ointment	30 gm
Silver sulfadiazine	Silvadene creme	20, 50, 400, 1000 gm
Sulfacetamide sodium	Sebizon lotion	85 gm
Tetracycline HCl	Achromycin ointment	14.2, 30 gm

*Topical antibiotics for acne are listed in the acne medication section.

■ ANTIFUNGAL AGENTS (ORAL)

Brand name	Generic name	Packaging
Diflucan	Fluconazole	50, 100, 200 mg
Fulvicin-U/F	Griseofulvin microsize	250, 500 mg
Grifulvin V	Griseofulvin microsize	250, 500 mg; 125 mg/5 ml in 4 oz bottle
Grisactin	Griseofulvin microsize	250, 500 mg
Fulvicin-P/G	Griseofulvin ultramicrosize	125, 165, 250, 330 mg
Gris-PEG	Griseofulvin ultramicrosize	125, 250 mg
Grisactin Ultra	Griseofulvin ultramicrosize	125, 250 mg
Nizoral	Ketoconazole	200 mg
Lamisil	Terbinafine	250 mg
Sporanox	Itraconazole	100 mg
Mycelex troches for oral *Candida*		10 mg troche; bottle of 70 or 140
		Dissolve 5/day in mouth for 14 days

■ ANTIFUNGAL AGENTS (TOPICAL)

Topical Agents Active Against Dermatophytes and Candida

Brand name	Generic name	Packaging
Exelderm	Sulconazole	15, 30, 60 gm cream
		30 ml solution
Fungoid Creme	Miconazole	2 oz cream
Fungoid&HC	Miconazole	30-1 gm packets cream
Halotex	Haloprogin	15, 30 gm cream
Lamisil	Terbinafine hydrochloride cream	15, 30 gm cream
Loprox	Ciclopirox olamine	15, 30, 90 gm cream
		30, 60 ml lotion
Lotrimin	Clotrimazole	15, 30, 45, 90 gm cream
		10, 30 ml lotion
Lotrisone*	Clotrimazole and betamethasone dipropionate	15, 45 gm cream
Monistat-Derm	Miconazole	15, 30, 85 gm cream
		30, 60 ml lotion
Mycelex	Clotrimazole	15, 30, 45, 90 gm cream
		10, 30, ml lotion
Naftin	Naftifine	15, 30, 60 gm cream
		20, 40, 60 gm gel
Nizoral	Ketoconazole	15, 30, 60 gm
Oxistat	Oxiconazole	15, 30, 60 gm cream
		30 ml lotion
Spectazole	Econazole	15, 30, 85 gm cream

*A preparation containing an antifungal agent and potent topical steroid; it is useful for inflamed fungal infections. Potent topical steroids should be used only for short durations in intertriginous areas such as the groin. Change to an antifungal agent once inflammation is controlled.

Topical Agents Active Against Candida

Brand name	Generic name	Packaging
Fungizone	Amphotericin B	20 gm cream
		30 ml lotion
		20 gm ointment
Fungoid Tincture	Miconazole	2 oz bottle liquid
Mycostatin	Nystatin	15, 30 gm cream
		15, 30 gm ointment
		60 ml suspension (oral)
Mycolog II*	Nystatin and triamcinolone	15, 30, 60, 120 gm cream or ointment
Mycelex troches†	Clotrimazole	10 mg troche
		Bottle of 70 or 140

*A preparation containing an anti-*Candida* agent and topical steroid; it is useful for inflamed yeast infections. Topical steroids should be used only for short durations in intertriginous areas such as the groin. Change to an anti-*Candida* agent once inflammation is controlled.

†Dissolve in mouth 5/day for 14 days.

Over-the-Counter Topical Agents Active Against Dermatophytes

Brand name	Generic name	Packaging
Antinea	6% benzoic acid 3% salicylic acid	1 oz
Desenex	Undecylenic acid	45 ml spray bottle
		42.5 gm foam
		30 gm ointment
Micatin	Miconazole*	15 gm cream
Tinactin	Tolnaftate	15 gm cream
		10 ml solution
Zeasorb-AF	Miconazole 2%	70 g bottle

* Also active against *Candida*.

Agents Effective for Treating Tinea Versicolor

Brand name	Generic name	Packaging*	Directions
DHS Zinc (or any other zinc shampoo)	2% pyrithione zinc	6 oz, 12 oz	Apply to trunk, arms, and thighs for 10 min; shower off; reapply to affected area; shower on rising Repeat for 14 days
Exsel	2.5% selenium sulfide	120 ml lotion	Apply daily for 10 min for 7 consecutive days
Exelderm	Sulconazole	60 gm	qd for 14 days
Halotex	Haloprogin	30 gm cream	qd for 14 days
Loprox	Ciclopirox olamine	90 gm cream	qd for 14 days
Lotrimin	Clotrimazole	90 gm cream	qd for 14 days
Monistat-Derm	Miconazole	85 gm cream	bid 3 weeks
Mycelex	Clotrimazole	90 gm cream	qd for 14 days
Sebulex	2% sulfur, 2% salicylic acid	240 ml lotion	Apply qhs, wash off in morning, for 7 days
Selsun	2.5% selenium sulfide	120 ml lotion	Apply daily for 10 min for 7 consecutive days
Spectazole	Econazole	85 gm cream	qd for 14 days
Tinactin	Tolnaftate	15 gm	qd for 14 days
Tinver	25% sodium thiosulfate, 1% salicylic acid	180 ml	bid 21 days
Nizoral	Ketaconazole	200 mg tablet	Single 400 mg dose each month or 200 mg qd 5 days
		15, 30, 60 gm tubes	
		60 gm cream	qd for 14 days
Diflucan	Fluconazole	50, 100, 200 mg	Single 300-mg dose each month
Sporanox	Itraconazole	100 mg	200 mg for 7 days

*Many sizes of these preparations are available. Generally it is most economical to prescribe the largest-size container because a large area must be treated.

■ ANTIHISTAMINES

Generic name	Brand name	Preparation	Adult dose	Sedative effect
Alkylamines				
Brompheniramine	Dimetane	4 mg 8 mg timed release (TR) 12 mg, TR 2 mg/5 ml 10 mg/ml injection	4 mg q4-6h q8-12h q12h Up to 24 mg/24h	+
Chlorpheniramine	Chlor-Trimeton	4 mg 8 mg, TR 12 mg, TR 2 mg/5 ml 10 mg/ml injection for IV, IM, or SC 100 mg/ml injection for IM or SC	4-8 mg q4-12h Up to 24 mg/d	+
Dexchlorpheniramine	Polaramine	4 mg 4 mg, TR 6 mg, TR 2 mg/5 ml	2 mg q4-6h 4 mg q8-12h 6 mg q8-12h	+
Triprolidine	Actidil	2.5 mg 1.25 mg/5 ml	2.5 mg q4-6h	+
Ethanolamines				
Clemastine	Tavist-1 Tavist	1.34 mg 2.68 mg 0.67 mg/5 ml	1.34-2.68 mg q8-12h	++
Diphenhydramine	Benadryl	25 mg 50 mg 12.5 mg/tsp 10 mg/ml injection 50 mg/ml injection	25-50 mg q6-8h	+++
Ethylenediamines				
Tripelennamine	PBZ	25 mg 50 mg 37.5 mg/5 ml	25-50 mg q4-6h up to 600 mg/d	++
Phenothiazines				
Promethazine	Phenergan	12.5 mg 25 mg	12.5 mg q8h 25 mg qhs	+++
Piperazines				
Hydroxyzine HCl	Atarax	10, 25, 50, 100 mg	10-100 mg q4-8h	+
Hydroxyzine pamoate	Vistaril Pamoate	10, 25, 50, 100 mg	10-100 mg q4-8h	+
Piperidines				
Azatadine	Optimine	1 mg	1-2 mg q12h	++
Cyproheptadine	Periactin	4 mg 2 mg/5 ml	4-8 mg q8h up to 32 mg/d	+
_H_2 Blockers_				
Cimetidine	Tagamet	200, 300, 400 mg	400 mg bid	0
Famotidine	Pepcid	20-40 mg	20-40 mg qhs	0
Nizatidine	Axid	150, 300 mg	300 qhs	0
Ranitidine	Zantac	150, 300 mg	150 mg bid	0
_H_1 and H_2 Blockers_				
Doxipen	Adapin	10 mg 25 mg	10-25 mg q6-8h	+++
Doxipen	Zonalon	30 gm tubes—cream	qid	+
Nonsedating				
Astemizole	Hismanal	10 mg	30 mg day 1 20 mg day 2 10 mg qd thereafter	0
Loratadine	Claritin	10 mg	10 mg qd	0
Terfenadine	Seldane	60 mg	60 mg q12h	0

▪ ANTINEOPLASTIC AGENTS (TOPICAL)

Product	Fluorouracil	Packaging
Efudex	2% fluorouracil	10 ml liquid
	5% fluorouracil	10 ml liquid
	5% fluorouracil	25 gm cream
Fluoroplex	1% fluorouracil	30 ml solution
	1% fluorouracil	30 gm cream
Actinex	10% masoprocol	30 gm cream

▪ ANTIPERSPIRANTS

Brand name	Active ingredient	Packaging
Certan-dri (otc)	Aluminum chloride (hexahydrate)	1, 2 oz roll-on
		Pump spray nonaerosol
Drysol (Rx)	20% aluminum chloride (hexahydrate) in 93% anhydrous ethyl alcohol	37.5 ml bottle
		35 ml bottle with Dab-O-Matic applicator
Lazerformalyde Solution (Rx)	10% formaldehyde	3 oz roll-on
Formaldehyde-10 spray	10% formaldehyde	2 oz spray bottle
Xerac AC (Rx)	6.25% aluminum chloride (hexahydrate) in 96% anhydrous ethyl alcohol	35, 60 ml bottles with Dab-O-Matic applicator

Drionic Therapy for Hyperhidrosis (Iontophoresis)

Iontophoresis (the application of low-level electric current to the surface of the skin) results in reduced production of sweat at that site. A battery-operated device conforming to the shape of the treated area, using tap water–wetted pads in contact with the skin of the palms, soles, or axillae, is available for patient self-use. Four to 15 treatments 20 minutes long inhibits sweat for up to 6 weeks; 95% of patients showed improvement in 2 weeks, and 86% remained improved at 6 weeks. Minor retreatment every 6 weeks is needed to sustain inhibition. Biopsies reveal hyperkeratotic plugs within sweat ducts following treatment.

Three devices (Drionic Hands, Drionic Axillae, Drionic Feet) are available at $125.00 per pair. They may be ordered by the patient from General Medical Co, Dept DM-8, 1935 Armacost Ave, Los Angeles, CA 90025.

More complicated devices are available from other manufacturers.

▪ ANTIPRURITIC LOTIONS

Brand name	Active ingredient	Packaging
PrameGel	1% pramoxine, 0.5% menthol	
Sarna	0.5% each of camphor, menthol	7.5 oz bottle

▪ ANTIVIRAL AGENTS

Famvir (famciclovir), 500 mg tablets
Valtrex (valacyclovir), 500 mg capsules
Zovirax (acyclovir), 200, 400, 800 mg capsules
Zovirax ointment 5%, 3 and 15 gm tubes

Topical Therapy for Postherpetic Neuralgia

Zostrix (capsaicin, 0.025% cream), 1.5 oz, 3 oz tubes (otc)
Zostrix-HP (capsaicin, 0.075% cream), 1 oz, 2 oz tubes (otc)

■ CONTRACEPTIVES (ORAL)

Drug	Progestin (mg)	Estrogen (ethinyl estradiol μg)
Desogen	Desogestrel 0.15	30
Ortho-Cept	Desogestrel 0.15	30
Ortho-Cyclen	Norgestimate 0.25	35
Ortho Tri-Cyclen	Norgestimate 0.25	35
Ovcon-35	Norethindrone 0.4	
Brevicon 21, 28	Norethindrone 0.5	35
Modicon 21, 28	Norethindrone 0.5	35
Ortho-Novum 7/7/7*	Norethindrone 0.5, 0.75, 1.0	35
Ortho-Novum 10-11*	Norethindrone 0.5, 1.0	35
N.E.E. 10/11 21, 28	Norethindrone 0.5, 1.0	35
Tri-Norinyl*	Norethindrone 0.5, 1.0, 0.5	35
Norinyl 1 + 35 21, 28	Norethindrone 1.0	35
Ortho 1/35 21	Norethindrone 1.0	35
Demulen 1/50 21, 28	Ethynodiol diacetate 1.0	50
Demulen 1/35 21, 28	Ethynodiol diacetate 1.0	35
Triphasil 21, 28	Levonorgestrel 0.05, 0.075, 0.125	30, 40, 30
Tri-Levlen 21, 28	Levonorgestrel 0.05, 0.075, 0.125	30, 40, 30
Levlen 21, 28	Levonorgestrol 0.15	30
Nordette 21, 28	Levonorgestrol 0.15	30
Lo/Ovral 21, 28	Norgestrel 0.3	30
Ovral	Norgestrel 0.5	50
Loestrin 1/20	Norethindrone 1.0	20
Loestrin 1.5/30	Norethindrone 1.5	30

Less

ANDROGENICITY

More

Modified from The Medical Letter 34 (885), Dec. 11, 1992; and Dickey RP: *Managing contraceptive pill patients*, ed 4, Durant, OK, 1986, Creative Informatics.

*Many oral contraceptives are available in both 21- and 28-day regimens.

Total androgenic effect of a pill depends on the balance between the estrogen and progestin agent. Pills with low androgenicity are better for acne, alopecia, and hirsutism. Individual response to pills varies. Some women with acne improve with pills with high androgenicity.

■ CORTICOSTEROIDS (TOPICAL)

Listed by potency group: group I is the most potent.

Group	Brand name	%	Generic name	Tube size (gm; unless noted)
I	Condran Tape		Flurandrenolide	24″ × 3″, 80″ × 3″ roll
	Temovate cream	0.05	Clobetasol propionate	15, 30, 45, 60
	Temovate ointment	0.05		15, 30, 45, 60
	Temovate gel	0.05		15, 30, 60
	Temovate emollient	0.05		15, 30, 60
	Temovate solution	0.05		25, 50 ml
	Ultravate cream	0.05	Halobetasol propionate	15, 50
	Ultravate ointment	0.05		15, 50
	Diprolene lotion	0.05	Augmented betamethasone dipropionate	30 ml, 60 ml
	Diprolene ointment	0.05		15, 45
	Diprolene gel	0.05		15, 45
	Psorcon ointment	0.05	Diflorasone diacetate	15, 30, 60
II	Alphatrex ointment	0.05	Betamethasone dipropionate	15, 45
	Cyclocort ointment	0.1	Amcinonide	15, 30, 60
	Diprolene AF cream	0.05	Augmented betamethasone dipropionate	15, 45
	Diprosone ointment	0.05	Betamethasone dipropionate	15, 45
	Florone ointment	0.05	Diflorisone diacetate	15, 30 60
	Halog cream	0.1	Halcinonide	15, 30, 60, 240
	Halog ointment	0.1		15, 30, 60, 240
	Halog solution	0.1		20, 60 ml
	Halog-E cream	0.1		15, 30, 60
	Lidex cream	0.05	Fluocinonide	15, 30, 60, 120
	Lidex gel	0.05		15, 30, 60, 120
	Lidex ointment	0.05		15, 30, 60, 120
	Lidex solution	0.05		20, 60 ml
	Lidex-E cream	0.05		15, 30, 60, 120
	Maxiflor ointment	0.05	Diflorasone diacetate	15, 30, 60
	Maxivate cream	0.05	Betamethasone dipropionate	15, 45
	Maxivate ointment	0.05		15, 45
	Topicort cream	0.25	Desoximetasone	15, 60, 120
	Topicort gel	0.05		15, 60
	Topicort ointment	0.25		15, 60
III	Alphatrex cream	0.05	Betamethasone dipropionate	15, 45
	Alphatrex lotion	0.05		60 ml
	Aristocort cream	0.5	Triamcinolone acetonide	15, 240
	Aristocort ointment	0.5		15, 240
	Aristocort A cream	0.5		15, 240
	Aristocort A ointment	0.5		15
	Benisone gel	0.025	Betamethasone benzoate	15, 60
	Betatrex ointment	0.1	Betamethasone valerate	15, 45
	Cutivate ointment	0.005	Fluticasone propionate	15, 30, 60
	Cyclocort lotion	0.1	Amcinonide	20, 60 ml
	Diprosone cream	0.05	Betamethasone dipropionate	15, 45
	Elocon ointment	0.1	Mometasone furoate	15, 45
	Florone cream	0.05	Diflorasone diacetate	15, 30, 60
	Florone E emollient	0.05		15, 30, 60
	Kenalog cream	0.5	Triamcinolone acetonide	20
	Kenalog ointment	0.5		20
	Maxiflor cream	0.05	Diflorasone diacetate	15, 30, 60
	Maxivate lotion	0.05	Betamethasone dipropionate	60 ml
	Trymex cream	0.5	Triamcinolone acetonide	15
	Topicort LP cream	0.05	Desoximetasone	15, 60
	Uticort gel	0.025	Betamethasone benzoate	15, 60
	Uticort ointment	0.025		15, 60
	Valisone ointment	0.1	Betamethasone valerate	15, 45
IV	Aristocort ointment	0.1	Triamcinolone acetonide	15, 60, 240, 2400
	Benisone ointment	0.025	Betamethasone benzoate	15, 60
	Cordran ointment	0.05	Flurandrenolide	15, 30, 60
	Cyclocort cream	0.1	Amcinonide	15, 30, 60
	Elocon cream	0.1	Mometasone furoate	15, 45
	Elocon lotion	0.1		30, 60 ml
	Fluonide ointment	0.025	Fluocinolone acetonide	60

Group	Brand name	%	Generic name	Tube size (gm; unless noted)
IV	Halog cream	0.025	Halcinonide	15, 60, 240
	Halog ointment	0.025		15, 60, 240
	Kenalog ointment	0.1	Triamcinolone acetonide	15, 60, 80, 240, 2520
	Synalar ointment	0.025	Fluocinolone acetonide	15, 30, 60, 120, 425
	Synalar HP cream	0.2		12
	Trymex ointment	0.1	Triamcinolone acetonide	15, 80
	Westcort ointment	0.2	Hydrocortisone	15, 45, 60
V	Aristocort cream	0.1	Triamcinolone acetonide	15, 60, 240, 2520
	Benisone cream	0.025	Betamethasone benzoate	15, 60
	Beta-Val cream	0.1	Betamethasone valerate	15, 45
	Betatrex cream	0.1	Betamethasone valerate	15, 45
	Betatrex lotion	0.1		15, 60 ml
	Cloderm cream	0.1	Clocortolone pivalate	15, 45
	Cordran cream	0.05	Flurandrenolide	15, 30, 60
	Cordran lotion	0.5		15, 60 ml
	Cordran ointment	0.025		30, 60
	Cutivate cream	0.05	Fluticasone propionate	15, 30, 60
	Dermatop cream	0.1	Prednicarbate	15, 60
	DesOwen ointment	0.05	Desonide	15, 60
	Fluonide cream	0.025	Fluocinolone acetonide	15, 60
	Kenalog cream	0.1	Triamcinolone acetonide	15, 60, 80, 240, 2520
	Kenalog lotion	0.1		15, 60 ml
	Kenalog ointment	0.025		15, 60, 80, 240
	Locoid cream	0.1	Hydrocortisone butyrate	15, 45
	Locoid ointment	0.1		15, 45
	Locoid solution			20, 60 cc
	Synalar cream	0.025	Fluocinolone acetonide	15, 30, 60, 425
	Synemol cream	0.025	Fluocinolone acetonide	15, 30, 60
	Tridesilon ointment	0.05	Desonide	15, 60
	Trymex cream	0.1	Triamcinolone acetonide	15, 80, 480
	Trymex ointment	0.025		15, 80
	Uticort cream	0.025	Betamethasone benzoate	15, 60
	Uticort lotion	0.025		15, 60 ml
	Valisone cream	0.1	Betamethasone valerate	15, 45, 110, 430
	Valisone lotion	0.1		20, 60 ml
	Westcort cream	0.2	Hydrocortisone	15, 45, 60
VI	Aclovate cream	0.05	Prednicarbate	15, 60
	Aclovate ointment	0.05	Prednicarbate	15, 60
	Aristocort cream	0.025	Triamcinolone acetonide	15, 60, 240, 2520
	DesOwen cream	0.05	Desonide	15, 60, 90
	DesOwen ointment			15, 60
	DesOwen lotion			2, 4 oz
	Fluonid cream	0.01	Fluocinolone acetonide	15, 60
	Fluonid solution	0.01		20, 60 ml
	Kenalog cream	0.025	Triamcinolone acetonide	15, 60, 80, 240, 2520
	Kenalog lotion	0.025		60 ml
	Locorten cream	0.03	Flumethasone pivalate	15, 60
	Synalar cream	0.01	Fluocinolone acetonide	15, 45, 60, 425
	Synalar solution	0.01		20, 60 ml
	Tridesilon cream	0.05	Desonide	15, 60
	Trymex cream	0.025	Triamcinolone acetonide	15, 80, 480
	Valisone cream	0.01	Betamethasone valerate	15, 60
VII	Celestone cream	0.2	Betamethasone valerate	15
	Decaderm gel	0.1	Dexamethasone	15, 30
	Epifoam	1.0	Hydrocortisone acetate	10
	Hytone cream	1.0	Hydrocortisone	1
		2.5		1, 2 oz
	Hytone lotion	1.0		4 oz
		2.5		2 oz
	Hytone ointment	1.0		1
		2.5		1 oz
	Lacticare HC lotion	1.0	Hydrocortisone	4 oz
		2.5		2 oz
	Medrol cream	0.25	Methylprednisolone	7.5, 30, 45
	Oxylone cream	0.025	Fluoromethalone	15, 60, 120
	Synacort cream	1.0	Hydrocortisone	15, 30, 60
		2.5		30

■ CORTICOSTEROIDS (TOPICAL)

Alphabetical list by brand name.
Group I is the most potent.

Group	Brand name	%	Generic name	Tube size (gm; unless noted)
VI	Aclovate cream	0.05	Alclomatasone dipropionate	15, 45, 60
VI	Aclovate ointment	0.05		15, 45, 60
III	Alphatrex cream	0.05	Betamethasone dipropionate	15, 45
III	Alphatrex lotion	0.05		60 ml
II	Alphatrex ointment	0.05		15, 45
III	Aristocort cream	0.5	Triamcinolone acetonide	15, 240
V	Aristocort cream	0.1		15, 60, 240, 5.25 lb jar
VI	Aristocort cream	0.025		15, 60, 240, 5.25 lb jar
III	Aristocort ointment	0.5		15
IV	Aristocort cream	0.1		15, 60, 240, 2400
III	Aristocort A cream	0.5		15
V	Aristocort A cream	0.1		15, 60, 240
VI	Aristocort A cream	0.025		15, 60
III	Aristocort A ointment	0.5		15
IV	Aristocort A cream	0.1		15, 60
V	Benisone cream	0.025	Betamethasone benzoate	15, 60
III	Benisone gel	0.025		15, 60
IV	Benisone ointment	0.025		15, 60
V	Beta-Val cream	0.1	Betamethasone valerate	15, 45
V	Betatrex cream	0.1		15, 45
V	Betratrex lotion	0.1		15, 60 ml
III	Betratrex ointment	0.1		15, 45
VII	Celestone cream	0.2	Betamethasone	15
V	Cloderm cream	0.1	Clocortolone privalate	15, 45
V	Cordran cream	0.05	Flurandrenolide	15, 30, 60, 225
V	Cordran lotion	0.05		15, 60 ml
IV	Cordran ointment	0.05		15, 30, 60, 225
V	Cordran ointment	0.025		30, 60, 225
III	Cutivate ointment	0.005	Fluticasone propionate	
V	Cutivate cream	0.05		
IV	Cyclocort cream	0.1	Amcinonide	15, 30, 60
III	Cyclocort lotion			20, 60 ml
II	Cyclocort ointment	0.1		15, 30, 60
VII	Decaderm gel	0.1	Dexamethasone	15, 30
V	Dermatop cream		Prednicarbate	15, 60
VI	DesOwen cream	0.05	Desonide	15, 60, 90
V	DesOwen ointment			15, 60
VI	DesOwen lotion			2, 4 oz
I	Diprolene creme	0.05	Betamethasone dipropionate	15, 45
II	Diprolene lotion	0.05		30, 60 ml
I	Diprolene ointment	0.05		15, 45
III	Diprosone cream	0.05	Betamethasone dipropionate	15, 45
III	Diprosone lotion	0.05		20, 60 ml
II	Diprosone ointment	0.05		15, 45
IV	Elcon creme	0.1	Mometasone furoate	15, 45
IV	Elcon lotion	0.1		30, 60 ml
III	Elcon ointment	0.1		15, 45
III	Florone cream	0.05	Diflorasone diacetate	15, 30, 60
II	Florone ointment	0.05		15, 30, 60
III	Florone E emollient	0.05		15, 30, 60
V	Fluonid cream	0.025	Fluocinolone acetonide	15, 60
VI	Fluonid cream	0.01		15, 60
IV	Fluonide ointment	0.025		60
VI	Fluonid solution	0.01		20, 60 ml
II	Halog cream	0.1	Halcinonide	15, 30, 60, 240
IV	Halog cream	0.025		15, 60, 240
II	Halog ointment	0.1		15, 30, 60, 240
IV	Halog ointment	0.025		15, 60, 240
II	Halog solution	0.1		20, 60 ml
II	Halog-E cream	0.1	Halcinonide	15, 30, 60

Group	Brand name	%	Generic name	Tube size (gm; unless noted)
VII	Hytone cream	1.0	Hydrocortisone	1
VII	Hytone cream	2.5		1, 2 oz
VII	Hytone lotion	1.0		4 oz
VII	Hytone lotion	2.5		2 oz
VII	Hytone ointment	1.0		1 oz
VII	Hytone ointment	2.5		1 oz
III	Kenalog cream	0.5	Triamcinolone acetonide	20
V	Kenalog cream	0.1		15, 60, 80, 240, 2520
VI	Kenalog cream	0.025		15, 60, 80, 240, 2520
V	Kenalog lotion	0.1		15, 60 ml
VI	Kenalog lotion	0.025		60 ml
III	Kenalog ointment	0.5		20
IV	Kenalog ointment	0.1		15, 60, 80, 240, 2520
V	Kenalog ointment	0.025		15, 60, 80, 240
VII	Lacticare lotion	1.0	Hydrocortisone	4 oz
VII	Lacticare lotion	2.5	Hydrocortisone	2 oz
II	Lidex cream	0.05	Fluocinonide	15, 30, 60, 120
II	Lidex gel	0.05		15, 30, 60, 120
II	Lidex ointment	0.05		15, 30, 60, 120
II	Lidex solution	0.05		20, 60 ml
II	Lidex-E cream	0.05		15, 30, 60, 120
V	Locoid cream	0.1	Hydrocortisone butyrate	15, 45
V	Locoid ointment	0.1		15, 45
VI	Locorten cream	0.03	Flumethasone pivalate	15, 60
III	Maxiflor cream	0.05	Diflorasone diacetate	15, 30, 60
II	Maxiflor ointment	0.05		15, 30, 60
II	Maxivate cream	0.05	Betamethasone dipropionate	15, 45
III	Maxivate lotion	0.05		60 ml
II	Maxivate ointment	0.05		15, 45
VII	Medrol cream	0.25	Methylprednisolone	7.5, 30, 45
VII	Oxylone cream	0.025	Fluoromethalone	15, 60, 120
I	Psorcon ointment	0.05	Diflorasone diacetate	15, 30, 60
VII	Synacort cream	1.0	Hydrocortisone	15, 30, 60
VII	Synacort cream	2.5		30
V	Synalar cream	0.025	Fluocinolone acetonide	15, 30, 60, 425
VI	Synalar cream	0.01		15, 30, 60, 425
IV	Synalar ointment	0.025		15, 30, 60, 425
VI	Synalar solution	0.01		20, 60 ml
IV	Synalar-HP cream	0.2		12
V	Synemol cream	0.025	Fluocinolone acetonide	15, 30, 60
I	Temovate cream	0.05	Clobetasol propionate	15, 30, 45, 60
I	Temovate ointment	0.05		15, 30, 45, 60
I	Temovate gel			15, 30, 60
I	Temovate-E			15, 30, 60
I	Temovate solution			25, 50 ml
II	Topicort cream	0.25	Desoximetasone	15, 60, 120
II	Topicort gel	0.05		15, 60
II	Topicort ointment	0.25		15, 60
III	Topicort LP cream	0.05		15, 60
VI	Tridesilon cream	0.05	Desonide	15, 60
V	Tridesilon ointment	0.05		15, 60
III	Trymex cream	0.5	Triamcinolone acetonide	15
V	Trymex cream	0.1		15, 80, 480
VI	Trymex cream	0.025		15, 80, 480
IV	Trymex ointment	0.1		15, 80
V	Trymex ointment	0.025		15, 80
I	Ultravate cream	.05	Halobetasol propionate	15, 50
I	Ultravate ointment	.05		15, 50
III	Uticort gel	0.025		15, 60
V	Uticort lotion	0.025		15, 60 ml
III	Uticort ointment	0.025		15, 60
V	Valisone cream	0.1	Betamethasone valerate	15, 45, 110, 430
VI		0.01		15, 60
V	Valisone lotion	0.1	Betamethasone valerate	20, 60 ml
III	Valisone ointment	0.1		15, 45
V	Westcort cream	0.2	Hydrocortisone valerate	15, 45, 60, 120
V	Westcort ointment	0.2		15, 45, 60

■ CORTICOSTEROID SPRAYS, TAPE, AND OTIC SOLUTION

Brand name	%	Generic name	Packaging
Aeroseb-Dex spray		Dexamethasone (0.02 mg/sec)	58 ml
Cordran tape		Flurandrenolide (4 µg/cm²)	24″ × 3″ and 80″ × 3″
Decaspray		Dexamethasone (0.075 mg/sec)	25 ml
Diprosone spray	0.1	Betamethasone dipropionate	85 ml
Kenalog in Orabase	0.1	Triamcinolone acetonide	5 gm
Kenalog spray	0.2	Triamcinolone acetonide	23, 63 ml
Tridesilon otic solution	0.05	Desonide (plus 2% acetic acid)	10 ml

■ CORTICOSTEROIDS (ORAL)

Generic name	Brand name	Preparation	Equivalent dose (mg)
Betamethasone	Celestone	0.6 mg, 0.6 mg/5 ml	0.6
Cortisol (hydrocortisone)	Cortef	5, 10, 20 mg	20
	Hydrocortone	10, 20 mg	20
Cortisone	Cortone	25 mg	25
Dexamethasone	Decadron	0.25, 0.5, 0.75, 1.5, 4, 6 mg	0.75
Dexamethasone	Hexadrol	0.5, 0.75, 1.5, 4 mg, 5 mg/5ml	0.75
Methylprednisolone	Medrol	2, 4, 8, 16, 24, 32 mg	4
Paramethasone	Haldrone	1, 2 mg	2
Prednisolone	Delta-Cortef	5 mg	5
	Prelone	15 mg/5 ml	5
Prednisone	Deltasone	1, 2.5, 5, 10, 20, 50 mg	5
	Liquid Pred	5 mg/5 ml	5
	Metricorten	1, 5 mg	5
	Orasone	1, 5, 10, 20, 50 mg	5
Triamcinolone	Aristocort	1, 2, 4, 8, 16 mg, 2 mg/5 ml	4
	Kenacort	1, 2, 4, 8 mg, 4 mg/5ml	4

■ DEPIGMENTING AND COSMETIC COVERING AGENTS

Skin Bleaches and Depigmenting Agents

Brand name	Active ingredient	Sun protectant	Packaging
Benoquin cream (Rx)*	20% monobenzone	None	1¼ oz tube
Eldopaque Forte 4% cream (Rx)†	4% hydroquinone	Sunblock	1 oz tube
Eldoquin Forte 4% cream (Rx)	4% hydroquinone	None	1 oz tube
Melanex topical solution‡	3% hydroquinone	None	1 oz bottle
Solaquin Forte 4% cream (Rx)	4% hydroquinone	Sunscreen	1 oz tube
Solaquin Forte 4% gel (Rx)	4% hydroquinone	Sunscreen	1 oz tube
Ultraquin	Hydroquinone crystals for compounding		

*Indicated for extensive vitiligo to depigment entire body.
†Flesh-tinted cream base.
‡Packaged with a narrow plastic and broad tip sponge applicator.

Masking Agents (Cosmetic Covering Agents)

Brand name	Base	Packaging	Shades
Covermark*	Cream	1, 3 oz	10 different shades
	Stick	0.18 oz	7 different shades
	Crayon	—	3 different shades
Dermablend cover cream*	Cream	⅜ oz/1½ oz	8 different shades
Erace	Stick	—	
Faye-Mendelsohn	Cream	0.58 oz	2 shades for blending
Dy-O-Derm†	Liquid	4 oz	
Vitady†	Liquid	½, 2 oz	

*Waterproof concealing makeup.
†A solution to mask vitiligo; transmits most UVA radiation, so it can be used concurrently with psoralens in vitiligo therapy.

■ HAIR RESTORATION PRODUCT

Rogaine   Minoxidil solution   60 ml bottle

■ LUBRICATING AGENTS

Emollients

Emollients are complex mixtures containing many ingredients. They are listed under their primary ingredient.

Emollients Containing Urea

Urea promotes hydration and removal of excess keratin.

Product	Active Ingredients	Packaging
Aqua Care cream	2% urea	75 gm
Aqua Care/HP		
Cream	10% urea	75 gm
Lotion		8 oz
Atrac-Tain		
Cream	10% urea, 5% lactic acid	2 oz
Lotion	5% urea, 2.5% lactic acid	4, 8 oz
Carmol 10 lotion	10% urea	6 oz
Carmol 20 cream	20% urea	3 oz
Medco 40	40% urea	2, 4 oz
Nutraplus	10% urea	
Cream		90 gm, 1 lb
Lotion		8, 16 oz
Rea-lo cream	30% urea	60 gm, 1 lb
U-Lactin	10% urea, lactic acid	2, 4 oz
Ultra Mide lotion	25% urea	8 oz
Ureacin-10 lotion	10% urea, 3% lactic acid	8 oz
Ureacin-20 cream	20% urea, 3% lactic acid	2.5 oz

Emollients Containing Lactic Acid

Lactic acid promotes hydration and removal of excess keratin.

Product	Active Ingredients	Packaging
Epilyt lotion	5%	4 oz
Lac-Hydrin cream (Rx)	12%	225, 400 gm bottles
Lacticare lotion	5%	8, 12 oz bottles
Lactinol lotion	10%	8 oz
Lactinol-E cream	10%	4 oz
Penecare cream	7.5%	4 oz
Penecare lotion	5%	8 oz
Purpose dry skin cream	—	90 gm
U-Lactin lotion	—	8 oz

Emollients Containing Glycolic Acid

Product	Active Ingredients	Packaging
Aqua Glycolic face cream	10%	2 oz
Aqua Glycolic facial cleanser		8, 12 oz
Aqua Glycolic hand/body lotion	14%	4, 8 oz bottles
Aqua Glycolic shampoo	14%	8 oz
Aqua Glyde astringent	11%	8 oz
Aqua Glyde shave and aftershave		4 oz

Gel That Removes Excess Keratin

Keralyt gel, 6% salicylic acid and propylene glycol, 1 oz

Emollients Containing Mineral Oil

Lotions

Allercreme Ultra emollient
Cetaphil
Complex-15
Dermassage
Formula 405
Hydrisinol
Jeri-Lotion
Keri
Lacticare
Lubriderm
Neutrogena moisture (SPF-5 PABA)
Nivea moisturizing
Nivea skin oil
Nutraderm, Nutraderm 30
Theraplex Clear
Ultra-Derm

Creams

Candermyl
Cetaphil
DML Forté
Eucerin
Formula 405
Hydrisinol
Keri
Lubriderm
Nivea moisturizing
Nutraderm
Purpose dry skin

Spray

Alpha Keri

Emollients Containing Glycerin

Corn Huskers Lotion
Curel Skin Lotion
Keri Light
Nutraderm 30 lotion
Neutrogena Norwegian Formula emulsion
  (scented and unscented)
Neutrogena Norwegian Formula emulsion hand cream
  (scented and unscented)
Shepard's Dry Skin Care
Wibi Lotion

Ointments

Ointments containing petrolatum

Aquaphor
Dermasil lotion, cream
DML Forté
Eucerin
Hydrophilic petrolatum
Moisturel
Theraplex emollient
Wondra

Greaseless ointments

Acid Mantle
Unibase

Bath Oils

Alpha-Keri therapeutic
Aveeno Bath
Jeri-Bath
Lubath
NutraDerm
Ultra-Derm

■ POWDERS, PROTECTING LOTIONS, AND PROTECTING BARRIER CREAMS

Powders

Brand name	Generic name	Size	Use
Breezee Mist Antifungal Foot Powder	10% undecyclenic acid	4 oz	Drying
	Cornstarch		Drying
Pedi-Pro Foot Powder		2 oz	
	Talcum		Drying, mildly absorptive
Zeasorb	Talcum, cellulose, acrylic	75, 240 gm	Drying, absorptive
Zeasorb-AF	Talcum, cellulose, acrylic Miconazole Nitrate 2%		

Protecting Lotions

Brand name	Generic name	Size	Use
Calamine	Zinc oxide, ferric oxide		Cooling, drying shake
	Zinc oxide, 12.5% lotion	30, 60 ml	Protecting, lubricating

Protecting Barrier Creams

Brand/generic name	Size	Use
Dermaguard	2, 12 oz	Industrial (protects against acids)
Desitin ointment	30, 60, 120, 240, 480 gm	Protective ointment
Ivy Shield	1.25, 4, 16 oz	Helps prevent poison ivy and oak dermatitis
Kerodex 51	120, 480 gm	Protective cream for dry, oily work
Kerodex 71	120, 480 gm	Protective cream (water repellent)
pH-Stabil	60, 240 gm	Protective cream
Zinc oxide		
20% ointment	60 gm	Protective ointment
25% paste	30, 60, 480 gm	Protective paste

■ PSORIASIS AND SEBORRHEIC DERMATITIS (SHAMPOOS)

Antimicrobial Antiseborrheic Shampoos (Pyrithione Zinc and Others)

Brand name	Active ingredient	Packaging
Betadine	7.5% povidone-iodine	118 ml
Capitrol (Rx)	2% chloroxine	85 gm
Danex	1% pyrithione zinc	120 ml
DHS Zinc	2% pyrithione zinc	6, 12 oz
FS Shampoo (Rx)	0.01% fluocinolone acetonide	120 ml
Head & Shoulders	2% pyrithione zinc	51, 75, 120, 210 gm cream 120, 210, 330, 450 ml lotion
Metasep	2% parachlorometraxylenol	120 ml
Nizoral	2% ketoconazole	4 oz
Sebulon	2% pyrithione zinc	120, 240 ml
Theraplex Z Shampoo	2% zinc pyrithione	8 oz
Zincon Dandruff Shampoo	1% pyrithione zinc	120, 240 ml
ZNP Bar	2% pyrithione zinc	4.2 oz bar

Antiseborrheic Preparations

Brand name	Active ingredient	Packaging
Nizoral cream	Ketoconazole	15, 30, 60 gm
Sebizon	10% Sulfacetamide sodium	85 gm

Corticosteroid, Tar, and Other Medicated Scalp Preparations

Brand name	Active ingredient	Base	Packaging
Barseb HC	1% hydrocortisone, 0.5% salicylic acid	45% isopropyl alcohol	52.5 ml
Barseb Thera-spray	0.6% hydrocortisone, 0.48% salicylic acid	Aerosol	120 gm
Derma-smoothe/FS (Rx)	Fluocinolone acetonide 0.01%	Peanut oil	120 ml
P & S	Less than 1% phenol, NaCl	Paraffin oil	120, 240 ml
10% liquor carbonis detergens in nivea oil*	Liquor carbonis detergens, 8, 16 oz	Nivea oil	Prescribe
Neutrogena tar gel solution	2% coal tar, 2% salicylic acid	Alcohol free	2 oz
Texacort solution	1% hydrocortisone solution	Solution	30 ml

*Pharmacist compounded.

Selenium Sulfide Shampoos

Brand name	Concentration	Packaging
Exsel	2.5%	120 ml
Selsun	2.5%	120 ml
Selsun Blue	1%	120, 210, 330 ml

Sulfur and Salicylic Acid Shampoos

Product	Sulfur	Salicylic acid	Packaging
Ionil Plus		2%	240 ml
Meted	5%	3%	120 ml
Sebulex	2%	2%	120 ml 120, 240 ml
Sulfoam	2%		4, 8, 16 oz
Tiseb	—	2%	8 oz
Vanseb	2%	1%	90 gm cream 120 ml lotion
Xseb	—	4%	4, 8 oz
P & S	—	2%	4, 8 oz

Tar and Tar-Combination Shampoos

Brand name	Concentration	Packaging
Denorex	2% coal tar gel	60, 120 ml
	2% coal tar lotion	120, 240 ml
DHS Tar	0.5% coal tar USP	4, 8, 16 oz
DHS Tar gel	0.5% coal tar USP	8 oz
Ionil-T	5% coal tar, 2% salicylic acid	120 ml, 240 ml, pt, qt
Ionil-T Plus	2% crude coal tar	240 ml
Liquor carbonis detergens	10-15% coal tar	Any amount in Green soap*
Neutrogena T/gel	2% Newtar	4.4, 8.5, 16 oz
Neutrogena T/gel extra strength	4% Newtar (1% coal tar)	6 oz
Neutrogena T/sal	3% salicylic acid	4.5 oz
Packer's pine tar	0.82% pine tar	180 ml
Pentrax tar	4.3% crude coal tar	120, 240 ml
Polytar	1% mixture of tars	180, 360 ml
Sebutone	0.5% coal tar, 2% salicylic acid, 2% sulfur	120, 240 gm lotion
Tegrin Medicated	5% coal tar extract	60, 132 ml cream 112.5, 198 ml lotion
Theraplex T shampoo	1% coal tar	8 oz
Tiseb-T	0.5% coal tar product	
Vanseb-T	5% coal tar	120 ml lotion
Xseb-T	2% crude coal tar	4, 8 oz
Zetar	1% whole coal tar	180 ml

*Pharmacist compounded.

■ PSORIASIS MEDICATIONS (ORAL)

Psoralens

Brand name	Active Ingredient	Packaging
Oxsoralen lotion	Methoxsalen 1% lotion	1 oz bottle
Oxsoralen-Ultra	Methoxsalen (liquid form)	10 mg capsules, bottle of 50 (green capsules)
8-MOP	Methoxsalen (crystalline form)	10 mg capsules, bottle of 30 (pink capsules)
Trisoralen tablets	Trioxsalen	5 mg tablets, bottles of 28, 100

Recommended Oxsoralen-Ultra Dosage According to Weight

Patients weight		Dose	
(kg)	(lbs)	Low	High
<30	<65	10	10
30-50	65-100	10	20
51-65	101-145	20	30
66-80	146-175	20	40
81-90	176-200	30	50
91-115	200-250	30	60
>115	>250	40	70

Etretinate (Tegison)

Capsules   10, 25 mg

Methotrexate

Tablets	2.5 mg	
Injection	2.5 mg/ml	2 ml vials
Preservative-free injection	25 mg/ml	2,4,8 ml vials
Powder for injection	20, 50, 100, 250 mg	20 ml vials or single-use vials

■ PSORIASIS MEDICATIONS (TOPICAL)

Anthralin (Dithranol)

Brand name	Concentration (%)	Base	Packaging
Anthra-Derm	0.1, 0.25, 0.5, 1	Ointment	1.5 oz, 42.5 gm tubes
Drithocreme	0.1, 0.25, 0.5	Cream	50 gm tube
Drithocreme HP 1%	1	Cream	50 gm tube
Dritho-Scalp	0.25, 0.5	Cream	50 gm tube*
Lasan	0.4	Ointment	60 gm tube

*With special applicator.

Anthralin stain-prevention treatment

Brand name	Active ingredient	Packaging	Use
CuraStain	Triethanolamine	4 oz cream or spray	Dermatologic stain remover; apply to surrounding skin and lesions before wash-off. Apply to lesions after wash-off.

Anthralin paste (instructions for the pharmacist)

Anthralin	%*
Salicylic acid	4%
Paraffin	5%
Zinc oxide paste (qs)	100%

1. Heat the zinc oxide in the mixing bowl of a variable-speed mixer and the paraffin in a water bath.
2. Levigate the powders in a small amount of mineral oil.
3. When the zinc oxide is soft and the paraffin melted, shake all ingredients and mix until the product is somewhat congealed.
4. Package into 2 oz ointment jars.

*Concentrations of 2% or 4% are compounded.

Topical Vitamin D₃ Analog

Brand name	Active ingredient	Packaging
Dovonex Ointment	Calcipotriene .05	30, 60, 100 gm tubes
Dovonex Cream	Calcipotriene .05	30, 60, 100 gm tubes

Occlusive Dressing (Self-Adhesive) for Psoriasis

Brand name	Size	Packaging
Actiderm*	3½″ × 5″	Box of 5
Restore for Psoriasis	4″ × 4″	Box of 5
	8″ × 8″	Box of 3

*Approved for use with or without topical corticosteroids.

Tar-Containing Bath Oil

Brand name	Size	Packaging
Balnetar	2.5% coal tar	240 ml
Doak Oil	2% tar distillate	240 ml
Doak Oil Forte	5% tar distillate	120 ml
Lavatar	33.3% tar distillate	120, 480 ml
Polytar Bath	25% polytar	240 ml
Zetar emulsion (Rx)	30% whole coal tar	177 ml (6 oz)

Tar Creams and Solution

Brand name	Concentration	Other ingredient	Base	Packaging
Aqua Tar	2.5% coal tar extract	—	Gel (water base)	90 gm
Doak Tar Lotion	5% tar distillate	—	Lotion	4 oz
Estar	5% coal tar	13.8% alcohol	Gel	90 gm
Fototar	2% coal tar, USP	—	Cream	85 gm, 1 lb jar
Fototar Stik	5% coal tar, USP	—	Wax	15 gm
Ichthyol	10% ichthammol	—	Ointment	30 gm
Liquor carbonis detergens*	20% coal tar solution	—	Solution	4 oz, pt, gal
Mazon cream	0.18% coal tar	1% salicylic acid, 1% resorcinol, 0.5% benzoic acid	Cream	
Oxipor VHC	48.5% coal tar solution	1% salicylic acid	Lotion	2 oz, 4 oz
P & S Plus	8% coal tar solution	2% salicylic acid	Gel	105 gm
Packer's	5.87% pine tar		Soap	
PolyTar Soap	Blend of tars		Soap	Bar
Pragmatar	4% coal tar distillate	3% salicylic acid, 3% sulfur	Ointment	
PsoriGel	7.5% coal tar solution	1% alcohol	Gel	4 oz
T/Derm	5% coal tar extract	Alcohol free	Oil	4 oz
Tegrin Medicated	5% crude coal tar extract		Lotion	6 oz
			Cream	60, 132 gm
Unguentum Bossi	5% Tar distillate	5% ammoniated Hg	Ointment	60, 480 gm

*Used by the pharmacist for compounding in Unibase and other ointment bases.

Gel That Removes Excess Keratin

Keralyt Gel, 6% salicylic acid and propylene glycol, 1 oz

■ SCABICIDES AND PEDICULOCIDES

Scabicides

Brand name	Generic name	Packaging
Elimite	Permethrin	5% cream: 60 gm
Eurax*	Crotamiton	10% cream: 60 gm
		10% lotion: 2 oz, 1 pt
Kwell	Lindane	1% cream: 2 oz, 16 oz
		1% lotion: 2 oz, 16 oz
Kwell shampoo	Lindane	1% lotion: 2 oz, 16 oz
—	Sulfur	5%-10% precipitated
		sulfur in petrolatum†
	Ivermectin‡	6 mg tablets‡

*Eurax has been reported to be less effective than lindane.
†Pharmacist compounded.
‡See p. 453.

Pediculocides

Brand name	Generic name	Packaging
A-200 (otc)	0.33% pyrethrins	30 gm gel
A-200 Pyrinate Gel shampoo (otc)	0.17% pyrethrins	2, 4 oz shampoo
NIX cream rinse	Permethrin	2 oz
Ovide	0.5% malathion	Lotion 2 oz
R & C shampoo (otc)	0.3% pyrethrins	2, 4 oz shampoo
RID (otc)	0.3% pyrethrins	2 oz, 4 oz, 1 gal liquid
Step 2*	8% formic acid	Cream rinse
	Lindane	Bulk

*For removal of lice eggs (nits); does not kill lice.

■ SHAMPOO—FRAGRANCE FREE, DYE FREE

DHS Clear, 8, 16 oz

■ SOAP-FREE CLEANSERS

Often used in the management of atopic dermatitis.

Aquanil lotion	8, 16 oz
Cetaphil lotion	4, 8, 16 oz
Moisturel sensitive skin cleanser	8.75 oz
Neutragena—nondrying	5.5 oz
SFC lotion	8, 16 oz

■ SOAPS—BAR (MILD, NONIRRITATING)

Alpha-Keri	Dove	Oilatum
Basis glycerin	Neutrogena dry skin	Purpose
Basis superfatted	Nivea Creme	Shepard's moisturizing
Cetaphil		

■ SUNSCREENS*

Ultraviolet light
UVA (320-400 nm)—Photoaging, suntan, carcinogenic, penetrates to fat.
UVB (290-320 nm)—Sunburn, suntan, carcinogenic, penetrates epidermis.

UVB absorbers
PABA esters
  Amyl dimethyl PABA (Padimate A or Escolol 506)
  Octyl dimethyl PABA (Padimate O or Escolol 507)
Salicylates
  Homomenthyl salicylate (homosalate)
Cinnamates
  2-ethyl-hexyl p-methoxycinnamate (Parsol MCX)

UVA absorbers
Benzophenones
  Oxybenzone
  Dioxybenzone
  Avobenzone or Parsol 1789
  Benzophenone-3

UVA + UVB absorbers
Physical sunscreens
  Titanium dioxide
  Zinc oxide
  Red ferric oxide

Brand name	Active ingredient	SPF†
Bain de Soleil	7% octyldimethyl PABA, 2.5% oxybenzone, 0.5% dioxybenzone	15
Cancer Garde-33	8% octyl-p-dimethylaminobenzoate, 7.5% octyl-p-methoxycinnamate, 5% titanium dioxide, 3% oxybenzone	33
Durascreen 15	Methoxycinnamate, salicylate, oxybenzone	15
Durascreen 30	Methoxycinnamate, salicylate, oxybenzone, titanium dioxide	30
PreSun-15	Octylmethoxycinnamate, oxybenzone, octylsalicylate	15
PreSun-29	Octylmethoxycinnamate, oxybenzone, octylsalicylate	29
Shade UVAGUARD	3% parsol 1789 (avobenzone), 7.5% octylmethoxycinnamate, 3% oxybenzone	15
Solbar PF 15 cream	Oxybenzone USP, octylmethoxycinnamate	15
Solbar PF 15 liquid	Oxybenzone USP, octylmethoxycinnamate, alcohol 40	15
Solbar PF 50	Oxybenzone USP, octylmethoxycinnamate, octrocrylene	50
Sundown-15	7% octyldimethyl PABA, 5% octylsalicylate, 4% oxybenzone	15
Sundown-24	Octyldimethyl PABA, oxybenzone	24
Sundown-30	Octylmethoxycinnamate, octylsalicylate, oxybenzone, titanium dioxide	30
Tis screen-15	3% 2-hydroxy-4-methoxybenzophenone	15
Total Eclipse-15	2.5% glyceryl PABA, 2.5% octyldimethyl PABA, 2.5% oxybenzone	15
Physical Sunscreens		
Absorbs all wavelengths of light.		
A-Fil	Titanium dioxide, zinc oxide, talcum, kaolin, iron oxide, or red veterinary petrolatum	6
Clinique		6
Covermark		6
Reflecta		6
RV Paque		6

*Many other products are available.
†SPF, Sun protection factor.
NOTE: PABA and its esters and preservatives in sunscreens may occasionally cause allergic contact photodermatitis and allergic contact dermatitis. Allergic patients should be given a product containing a different active ingredient.

■ ULCER MEDICATIONS

Topical Enzyme Preparations

Dissolve and facilitate removal of necrotic tissue in healing wounds.

Brand name	Generic name	Packaging
Elase	Fibrinolysin, desoxyribonuclease	30 ml powder
Elase-Chloromycetin	Fibrinolysin, desoxyribonuclease, chloamphenicol	10, 30 gm ointment
Granulex	Trypsin, balsam Peru	60, 120 gm aerosol castor oil
Panafil	Papain, urea, chlorophyll derivatives	30 gm, 1 pound
Panafil White	Papain, urea	30 gm
Santyl	Collagenase	15 gm, 30 gm ointment
Travase	Sutilains	14.2 gm ointment

Synthetic Dressings

Type/brand name	Properties	Use
Hydrocolloid membranes Comfeel Ulcus DuoDerm (regular and extra thin)	Conforms to body surface, opaque (flesh colored)	Debridement of necrotic wounds, ulcers
Hydrophilized polyurethane Omiderm	Transparent, semipermeable, transmits topical medication	Ulcers, dermabrasions, skin disease (pemphigus, etc.)
Monifilament nylon membrane N-terface	Nonadherent, transmits fluids	Skin grafts, dermabrasion
Polyethylene oxide/water membranes Spenco Second Skin Vigilon	Semitransparent, nonadherent	Ulcers, dermabrasion
Polyurethane membranes OpsSite Ensure Tegaderm Accuderm Bioclusive	Translucent, self-adherent, gas permeable, fluid impermeable	Ulcers, sutured wounds, IV lines
Silicone/nylon membrane Biobrane	Semipermeable, coated with collagen peptides, decreases water vapor loss, adherent	Burns

Absorbing Granules

Debrisan Wound Cleansing Beads DuoDerm granules Bard Absorption dressing	25, 60, and 4 gm packets in boxes of 7 or 14
Iodosorb Wound Cleansing Gel	2 oz

■ VAGINAL ANTI-*CANDIDA* AGENTS

Topical Therapy for Acute Candida Vaginitis

Drug	Formulation	Dosage
Butoconazole	Cream	5 gm at bedtime for 3 days
Clotrimazole	Cream, 1% Cream, 10% Vaginal tablet, 100 mg Vaginal tablet, 500 mg	5 gm at bedtime for 7 to 14 days 5 gm single application 1 tablet at bedtime for 7 days or 2 tablets at bedtime for 7 days 1 tablet once
Miconazole	Cream, 2% Vaginal suppository, 100 mg Vaginal suppository, 200 mg Vaginal suppository, 1200 mg	5 gm at bedtime for 7 days 1 suppository at bedtime for 7 days 1 suppository at bedtime for 3 days 1 suppository once
Econazole	Vaginal tablet, 150 mg	1 tablet at bedtime for 3 days
Fenticonazole	Cream, 2%	5 gm at bedtime for 7 days
Tioconazole	Cream, 2% Cream, 6.5%	5 gm at bedtime for 3 days 5 gm at bedtime in a single dose
Terconazole	Cream, 0.4% Cream, 0.8% Vaginal suppository	5 gm at bedtime for 7 days 5 gm at bedtime for 3 days 80 mg at bedtime for 3 days
Nystatin	Vaginal tablet, 100,000 U	1 tablet at bedtime for 14 days

Preparation for Restoration and Maintenance of Vaginal Acidity

Aci-Jel therapeutic vaginal jelly, 0.921% acetic acid, 85 gm tube, 1 full applicator morning and evening

■ WART MEDICATIONS

Keratolytic Combinations for Treating Warts and Molluscum Contagiosum

Brand name	Salicylic acid	Lactic acid	Podophyllin	Cantharidin	Packaging
Cantharone Plus	30%	—	5%	1%	7.5 ml
Duofilm	16.7%	16.7%	—	—	15 ml
Verrex	30%	—	10%	—	7.5 ml
Verrusol	30%	—	5%	1%	7.5 ml
Viranol solution	16.7%	16.7%	—	—	10 ml

Silver Nitrate

Product	Silver nitrate	Packaging
Silver nitrate	10%	30 ml solution
Silver nitrate	10%	30 gm ointment
Silver nitrate sticks		Packages of 12

Cantharidin

Brand name	Cantharidin	Packaging
Cantharone	0.7% in film-forming vehicle	7.5 ml
Verr-Canth	0.7% in film-forming vehicle	7.5 ml

Salicylic Acid Preparations for Treating Warts, Calluses, and Hyperkeratotic Skin (all otc)

Brand name	Salicylic acid(%)	Packaging
Compound W		
Liquid	17	9.3 ml liquid
Gel	17	7.5 gm gel
Duoplant	17	14 gm gel
Keralyt	6	30 gm gel
Mediplast	40	Plaster
Occlusal-HP	17	10 ml liquid
Salacid	25	
Salactic	17	1.5 ml film
Salonil	40	
Sal-Acid Plaster	40	14 pkg
Sal-Plant	17	14 gm gel
Trans-Plantar	21	Cartons of 20 mm 25 patches, securing tapes, and cleaning file
Trans-Ver-Sal	15	Cartons of 6, 12, or 20 mm (15 or 40 pads), securing tapes, and emery file

Podophyllin/Podofilox

Brand name	Podophyllin	Packaging
Condylox	0.5% podofilox (podophyllotoxin)	3.5 ml
Pod-Ben-25	25% in tincture benzoin	30 ml
Podoben	25%, 10% benzoin, 72% isopropyl alcohol	5 ml
Podofin	25% in tincture benzoin	7.5 ml
—	Podophyllin in tincture of benzoin or alcohol	Compounded

Interferon

Intron-A (interferon alfa-2b), recombinant injection

Chloroacetic Acids—Keratolytic and Cauterizing

Brand name	Active ingredient	Packaging
Bichloracetic acid	Dichloroacetic acid	Treatment kit, 15 ml
Monocete solution	80% monochloroacetic acid*	15 ml
Mono-Chlor	80% monochloroacetic acid	15 ml
Tri-Chlor	80% trichloroacetic acid	15 ml

*Monochloroacetic acid is the most deeply destructive.

■ WET DRESSINGS

Generic/brand name	Active ingredient
Acetic acid	Vinegar is 5% acetic acid
AluWets crystals	Aluminum chloride hexahydrate
Buro-Sol powder	Aluminum acetate
Burow's Solution (Domeboro, Bluboro, Pedi-Boro, Buro-Sol)	Aluminum acetate
Domeboro otic solution	2% acetic acid (60 ml)
Domeboro powder, Bluboro, Pedi-Boro	Aluminum sulfate, calcium acetate (boxes of 12, 100 packets)
Domeboro tablets, Bluboro, Pedi-Boro	Aluminum sulfate, calcium acetate (boxes of 2, 100 tablets)
Potassium permanganate	0.025%-0.1%, stains skin purple
Silver nitrate	0.1%-0.5%, stains skin black (prepared by pharmacist)

Index

---

*Page numbers in italics indicate illustrations;
t indicates tables.

QUANTITY OF CREAM TO APPLY AND DISPENSE

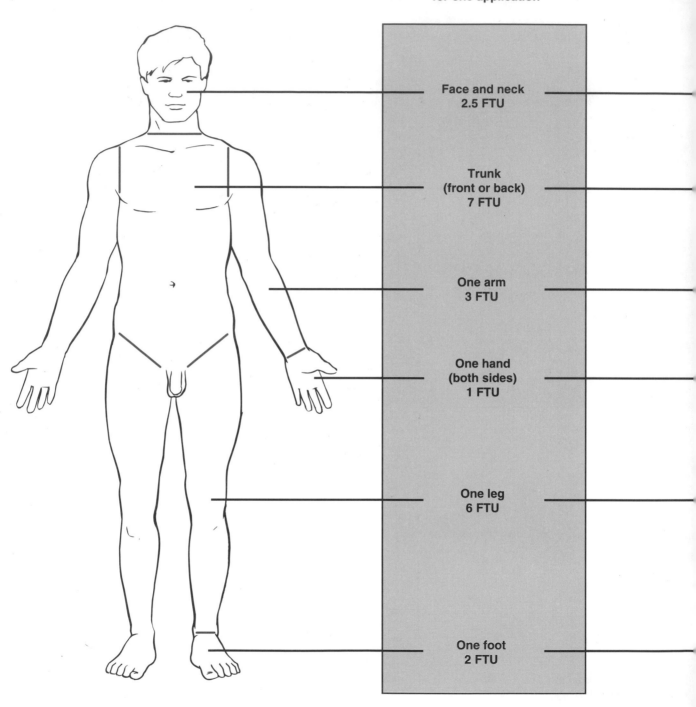

Fingertip units required for one application

Face and neck
2.5 FTU

Trunk
(front or back)
7 FTU

One arm
3 FTU

One hand
(both sides)
1 FTU

One leg
6 FTU

One foot
2 FTU

Modified from Long CC, Finlay AY: The fingertip unit: a new practical measure, *Clin Exp Dermatol* 16:444-447, 1991.